Strategies For Health

A COMPREHENSIVE GUIDE TO HEALING YOURSELF NATURALLY

Steven Horne, RH (AHG)

Fulton Books, Inc.
Meadville, PA

Published by Fulton Books 2021

ISBN 978-1-63710-253-4 (paperback)
ISBN 978-1-63710-254-1 (digital)

Printed in the United States of America

Table of Contents

Important Notice

This material is for educational purposes only. It is not intended to replace the services of licensed health care providers. Always obtain competent medical advice for all serious or persistent illness. If you use any of the procedures in this material to treat any disease in yourself or others without the assistance of licensed health care providers, you are doing so at your own risk.

Acknowledgments

This book is the result of a database my company created to store information on herbal remedies, nutritional supplements, and other natural remedies. We've been collecting this information for over twenty years. Besides my own research and clinical experience, I have relied on many of my associates in natural healing for advice and contributions to this information. I would especially like to acknowledge Kimberly Balas, ND, Thomas Easley, RH(AHG), and Matthew Wood, RH(AHG), who have helped develop the body system's approach and energetic system on which this book is based. David Horne has spent many hours working on the programming and organization of the database as well as editing the information. Other employees who have put significant effort into the database in previous years include Kenneth Hepworth, Leslie Lechner, Diana Horne, and Amanda Steiner.

Section One

Finding Your Healing Strategy

Congratulations! You're about to learn incredibly powerful truths about healing.

If you have a desire to be healthier, start by setting a goal to be healthy. Once you set a goal, you need a strategy to help you achieve it and that's what this book, and specifically this introduction, will help you do.

In part one, I'll explain why you need a strategy for healing. You'll learn why treating disease is not the same as building health and why trying to relieve symptoms doesn't produce long-term health. You'll also learn the difference between disease care and real health care as well as how you can take responsibility for your health. Modern medicine tends to disempower people by making them feel dependent on drugs, surgeries, or other treatments for health. I prefer to empower people with knowledge so they can confidently take responsibility for their own health rather than make them dependent on me for help and advice.

In part two, I'll take you step-by-step through the process of developing a strategy for healing that will ensure you are able to achieve your goal of lasting health. The first step I'll talk about in building health is to adopt a proper attitude about your life and health. You won't get well if you don't believe you can get well.

Next, I'll explain why you should concentrate on working on your overall health and not just look for a remedy for your disease. So in my second strategy for healing, I'll suggest some healthy habits you should cultivate.

Next, I'll talk about using some basic supplements to enhance your healthy lifestyle habits and diet. These supplements are ones that can improve the overall health of most Americans. So your third step will be to see if any of these supplements are important for you.

In step four, I'll get down to the basics of how to select specific health remedies for your individual needs. I'll help you learn how to think in terms of body systems and biological terrain when selecting remedies (particularly herbs) rather than disease symptoms. This is a major paradigm shift for most people, but if you can make the shift you'll get far more dependable and long-lasting results.

In my forty years of writing and teaching about herbalism and natural healing I've trained hundreds of natural health practitioners in the principles you're about to learn. They, in turn, have successfully used these principles to help tens of thousands of people regain their health.

The strategies I'm sharing with you work. So whether you're just looking to help yourself and your family or whether you're using this book as a guide to help you help others, please take the time to read this introduction carefully and apply the strategy it explains. You'll get better results if you do.

Part I
Why We Need Healing Strategies

When I first started using natural remedies, I thought that the main difference between modern medicine and natural medicine was the remedies that were used. A popular slogan in those days was "I use herbs instead." We were choosing to use herbs in place of drugs to treat diseases.

During this early period, I would look up a disease in an herb book and see what herbs people had used for it. I was relying on something one of my early herb teachers, Edward Milo Millet, called the historical uses approach. Sometimes I got great results using this approach, but other times I was disappointed as remedies failed to work as I expected.

These inconsistent results continued to frustrate me until I finally realized that natural healing was about more than substituting herbs for drugs. It was an entirely different way of approaching health and disease.

Even though I had switched to using herbs, I was still using allopathy. Allopathy means "against the symptom," and refers to a system of medicine where the goal is to counteract symptoms. So I was using herbs the same way I had used medications: to counteract disease symptoms. When I had a cough, I took herbs to try to suppress the cough. If I was constipated, I used an herbal laxative instead of a drug laxative. If I had a headache, I wanted an herb to relieve the pain, just like a painkiller would.

My disappointments were never because herbs weren't effective. They were because I was using them ineffectively. I was thinking of herbs as symptom relievers, substitutes for drugs, when I needed to see them as remedies to support the normal healing process. Switching from drugs to herbs, while an improvement, wasn't enough. I needed to change my approach as well.

Once I started to understand this new approach to natural healing, I stopped being frustrated by inconsistent results.

A New Understanding of Disease

The understanding that I came to and that has helped me use herbs and other natural remedies so much more effectively was this:

The symptoms of a disease are not the problem—they are the results or effects of the problem, not the cause.

While simple to state, this idea can be hard to understand. To illustrate what I mean, try imagining that you're driving and a warning light starts blinking on the dashboard. It is the "low oil pressure" indicator. The flashing red light is a constant irritation and reminder that something is wrong. You want the problem to go away. Disconnecting or covering up the light would make the light stop blinking, but the oil pressure would still be low.

The reason I was getting disappointing results was that I was only trying to make the warning indicator (disease symptoms) go away without understanding what the actual problem was. I never asked what my body was telling me when I had a cough or was constipated or had a headache.

Headaches are a great example of what I'm talking about. Headaches are not really a disease; they are a warning indicator. They can be a sign of dehydration. They are frequently a sign of stress or poor posture. If you push yourself too hard or don't support your body's alignment, this can make your neck and shoulder muscles tense, which irritate nerves and inhibit blood flow to the head. Headaches can also be signs of food allergies, magnesium deficiency, indigestion, and liver congestion.

A painkiller would stop the pain of the headache and an herbal analgesic could do the same, but neither of them would do anything to address the underlying reason your head is hurting. They are both just covering up or disconnecting the warning light.

Once I realized that the symptoms were not the disease and I started to look deeper, I got much better results. For each of the different underlying problems of headaches, there are corresponding solutions. Hydration, improved posture and relaxation, removing allergens, taking enzymes or magnesium, decongesting the liver, or making dietary changes. Using the historical uses approach was hit-or-miss. If I happened to pick the right remedy for the cause of the headache, the remedy worked great. If not, I was disappointed. It was my lack of understanding of root causes that was the problem, not the herbs themselves.

What is true for headaches is true for other ailments. Naming a disease isn't enough information to know what's causing the problem. The name of a disease is just a shorthand for describing a list of symptoms. Without digging deeper, all you'll ever get is symptomatic relief.

Drugs Offer Symptomatic Relief

Drug companies know they are relieving symptoms. If you listen carefully to drug commercials, they don't say that the drug cures the disease. They say that it relieves symptoms. The drug isn't fixing the underlying problem; it's just temporarily di‍

> *The radical shift in my thinking came because I realized that symptoms weren't the problem. They were the results or effects of the problem, not the cause of the problem.*

connecting the symptomatic warning lights. The underlying cause usually remains unresolved. With this in mind, it should be no surprise that you won't find anyone who has cured their allergies, asthma, high blood pressure, autoimmune disease, arthritis, diabetes, COPD, Alzheimer's disease, or other chronic health issues with pharmaceutical drugs.

The very fact that modern medicine typically asserts that many diseases are incurable is an admission that the remedies they are providing do not actually cure. If you think about it, it's good for business. If you actually cure someone, they don't need your product anymore. On the other hand, if you offer them symptomatic relief, you have a regular, sometimes lifetime, customer.

Unfortunately, using remedies, even herbal ones, to relieve symptoms means you're never fixing the cause of your problems, which means you'll gradually get weaker and sicker for the rest of your life. You'll also need stronger medicines and/or larger doses to control these symptoms as time goes on.

I'm writing this because I'm tired of seeing people struggle with this disease-treatment, symptom-relieving approach to health. I want to help you understand how to shift your thought processes away from treating diseases (relieving symptoms) like I did and to discover how to actually remove the causes of ill health.

The Danger in a Name

There is a problem inherent in trying to name a disease. Imagine that the joints in your hands are becoming more swollen and painful. You might also notice they are a little red and perhaps slightly warmer than surrounding tissues. So you go to the doctor and tell him this. He examines your joints and says, "You have arthritis." You now have a name for your problem, but you really know nothing that you didn't already know. Here's why.

Arthritis is a Latin word. *Arthro* means "joint" and *itis* means "inflammation." So *arthritis* means "inflammation of the joint." The classic symptoms of inflammation are heat, swelling, redness, and/or pain. Thus, arthritis means you have heat, swelling, redness, and/or pain in your joints. Thus, you told your doctor about your symptoms in English, and he told you about your symptoms in Latin. In the end, you've learned nothing new about what's wrong with you.

In a practical example of this problem, I once had a client who had pain and swelling in the area of her pancreas. She spent $800 to receive a diagnosis of idiosyncratic pancreatitis. Again, translating the Latin, *idiosyncratic* means "of unknown origin." *Pancreatitis* is inflammation of the pancreas. Essentially, she went to the doctor asking, "Why am I hurting here?" and the diagnosis basically says, "You're hurting there and we don't know why."

It's vital you understand the implications of this. Plant this idea firmly in your mind—a disease name doesn't tell you what's really wrong. You have to dig deeper than that or you're not going to get well. To further help you understand this, let me refer you to a wonderful book on real diagnosis written in 1874 book by the eclectic physician John M. Scudder. It's called *Specific Diagnosis*. In it, Dr. Scudder states.

> Diagnosis has reference to the classification of disease according to received nosology [a fancy word for the classification of diseases]; that it means naming the affliction…[the doctors] travail in diagnosis until a suitable name is delivered. And then they consult their memory and books for recipes to throw at this name, which to them seems almost an entity. It looks absurd when thus plainly stated, yet it is true to a far greater extent than the majority suppose…

> The student would certainly think, from this teaching, that getting a name for a disease, was the first and principal object in medical practice…men pride themselves on their skill in naming diseases—calling it diagnosis. What can be more natural than that medicines should be prescribed at names, when so much trouble is taken to affix them?

This idea of prescribing treatments based on disease names is firmly entrenched in modern medicine, so it's no wonder that most sick people expect an herbalist and natural healer to do the same thing. Dr. Scudder claimed this practice was not just ineffective; it was actually worthless.

> "Do you mean to say," asks the reader, "that the present system of nosology [disease classification] is useless?" Yes, so far as curing the sick is concerned… Not only useless, but worthless—a curse to physician and patient—preventing the one from learning the healing art, and the other from getting well.

To put this problem in a different way, I refer to the pioneer herbalist Samuel Thomson in his book *New Guide to Health*:

> …it is evidently immaterial what is the name, or color of the disease, whether bilious, yellow, scarlet or spotted; whether it is simple or complicated, or whether nature has one enemy or more. Names are arbitrary things, the knowledge of a name is the cumin and anise, but in the knowledge of the origin of a malady, and its antidote, lies the weightier matters of this science. This knowledge makes the genuine physician; all without it is real quackery.

As Thomson says, having a name doesn't help you understand the underlying root of the problem, nor does it tell you the antidote or cure. Without understanding the "origin of the malady," there isn't an effective way to correct the condition.

The Curse of Modern Medicine

The obsession with naming diseases is worse today than it was in Scudder's or Thomson's time. Today, medical doctors have to deal with an incredibly intricate classification system, IDC (International Classification of Diseases) codes. These are alphanumeric designations given to every diagnosis, description of symptoms, and cause of death attributed to human beings. The codes are developed, monitored, and copyrighted by the World Health Organization (WHO).

As a result, medical diagnosis has largely become assigning the proper IDC code to a person's symptoms. This is absolutely essential for insurance or Medicare billing purposes, which is how most doctors get paid.

Treatment is then rendered using CPT (Current Procedural Terminology) codes published by the American Medical Association, designed to provide a uniform data set that could be used to describe medical, surgical, and diagnostic services rendered to patients with that computer code.

This is problematic because it leads to cookbook medicine where there is little to no room for doctors to use their own observation, analysis, and approach. These fixed codes and treatments prevent doctors from straying too far from the highly reductionist, symptom-oriented standard procedures. If doctors do so they risk censorship, or worse, the loss of their licenses.

We need to break free of this trap of naming diseases and prescribing treatments based on these names if we want real health. If you are a natural health practitioner, such as a traditional naturopath or herbalist, it's also important to break away from these disease names if you want to help people without running into legal trouble. Instead, we need to learn to focus on identifying and removing the causes of ill health, which is not only legally safe, but actually more effective.

Redefining Diseases and Symptoms

In learning how to rethink the way we approach health, we'll return to Dr. Scudder's *Specific Diagnosis*.

> Man has but one life, and it is the same in all parts. The normal manifestations of this life we call health; the abnormal manifestations of it disease. If we can always think of disease as a method of life, in a living body, we will have gotten rid of an old error… Disease, then, is not an entity—something to be forcibly expelled from a living body—but is actually a method of life.

The thought that helped me grasp what Scudder is saying here came when I realized that dead bodies don't produce disease symptoms; they just decompose (fall apart). All disease symptoms are produced only in living bodies. Therefore, they are manifestations of the life force within the body trying to correct whatever is causing the body distress.

So when you experience any disease, you're experiencing an imbalance in the manifestation of the life within you. There is a lack of ease (dis-ease) in the way your life is going. Whether the body is fighting against an external irritation such as a toxin, injury, or microbe or whether it's dealing with some kind of nutritional deficiency or imbalanced lifestyle (i.e., lack of sleep or exercise), the internal balance of the body has been disrupted.

You can't separate this imbalance from yourself by giving it a name and attacking it. But this is exactly what most people try to do.

A Practical Approach to Symptoms

Let me share with you the most important thing I ever discovered about health. It was part of this big paradigm shift I experienced. I realized that the symptoms of acute infectious diseases (e.g., colds, flu, measles, chicken pox) did not arise directly from the infection; they are actually caused by the body's immune defenses fighting the infection. In other words, they are the body's attempts at a cure.

This is exactly what Scudder is telling us. Acute disease symptoms are a manifestation of the power of life within the body, not the power of disease.

Realizing this, I recognized that trying to suppress or eliminate these symptoms was actually working against the immune system. A practical example of this is fever. A low fever (103 and below) is created by the body to inhibit viral replication. The fever slows the spread of the virus, allowing time for the immune system to fight the infection. Lowering the fever with aspirin or Tylenol actually aids the virus and interferes with the natural immune responses.

Here's another practical example. Inflammation is often seen as a bad thing, but inflammation, like fever, is part of the body's innate immune responses. Acute inflammation sequesters a damaged area and draws in white blood cells to clean up microbes and debris. It also slows the spread of toxins in venomous bites. So inflammation is actually a good thing.

Inflammation only becomes a problem when the irritation or damage that caused the inflammation isn't fixed. For example, if you have a splinter and don't remove it, the presence of the splinter creates an ongoing irritation and a chronic inflammatory response.

Even when the source of the irritation is gone, the body needs certain nutrients to reverse the inflammatory response and create a healing response in its place. If it is lacking in certain nutrients, such as omega-3 essential fatty acids, zinc, or vitamin C, it may have trouble reversing the inflammation, even after the irritation is removed.

In either case, using an anti-inflammatory to interfere with the inflammatory response isn't going to fix anything if the source of the damage is still present. To fix the problem, the source of the damage must be removed. At that point, an anti-inflammatory herb, or nutrients that aid healing, may become helpful in returning the tissues to their normal state of health.

Processes of Elimination

Continuing with the idea that symptoms are not the problem, consider that many acute disease symptoms actually involve the body trying to eliminate the irritants, which are the real cause of the problem. For example, coughing or sneezing is an attempt to flush irritants (i.e., dust, pollen, chemicals, microbes) from the respiratory passages. Interfering with that process is actually interfering with the body's attempts to heal itself, which prolongs the irritation and makes the problem last longer.

Nausea, vomiting, and diarrhea serve a similar function in the digestive tract. Vomiting is a defense mechanism that eliminates irritating material from the stomach. If you eat spoiled food, the faster you throw up, the sooner you'll feel better. Trying to inhibit vomiting would actually make you sicker.

Diarrhea flushes irritants from the intestines. If it's a short run of diarrhea, it's actually a healing process. Of course, if the diarrhea doesn't stop, it's like chronic inflammation. It will dehydrate you rapidly and can even kill you, but this doesn't change the fact that it's a protective mechanism. It's an effect, not a cause, of disease.

As I previously mentioned, this is the most important thing I ever learned about healing, because once I recognized these symptoms as healing processes, a manifestation of the process of life, not of disease and death, I quit trying to suppress them. Instead, I started thinking in a different direction. I started asking, "What is my body trying to do, and how can I help it?" That made all the difference. By working with the symptoms instead of against them, I found I could throw off most acute illnesses in less than twenty-four hours instead of being sick for days.

Years ago, I read an article in the *Wall Street Journal* that reported on a study that had discovered that taking antihistamines to dry up a runny nose doubled the time it took to recover from a cold. I lost the article, but it reinforced the idea that the symptoms of the cold are the immune system's way of curing it.

I summarized this understanding in one phrase: "the cold is the cure." People say there is no cure for the common cold, but it's obvious that the body knows how to cure a cold because people get colds and recover all the time. The

> *I quit trying to suppress symptoms. Instead, I started thinking in a different direction. I started asking, "What is my body trying to do, and how can I help it?" That made all the difference.*

problem is that they want to get rid of the symptoms (the immune responses that are aiding in recovery) and not have to experience the discomfort associated with the body's cure.

Messages from the Body

To further deepen your understanding of symptoms, you need to understand how the body communicates its needs. It sends its messages through bodily sensations such as hunger, thirst, fatigue, restlessness, shivering, sweating, and gasping. These sensations are related to the basic things the body needs to survive—oxygen, water, food, rest, activity (exercise). and protection from the elements. If you feel thirsty, then you need water; tired, you need rest; and so forth. You can also gasp for air, shiver with cold, or sweat to cool down.

These messages can be thought of as symptoms and each symptom requires an appropriate response, which is to give the body what it needs. Only the appropriate response will work. Eating doesn't satisfy the need for water, and exercise doesn't correct the need for sleep. Drinking ice water won't help when we're shivering, and sleep won't satisfy the hunger for food.

It's human nature, however, to search for shortcuts, to get rid of the messenger without responding appropriately to the message. For example, a woman once brought her elderly mother to me for a consult. When I talked to her and reviewed her symptoms and lifestyle, it was clear to me that she was severely dehydrated. She only drank two cups of tea each day (and tea is a diuretic). I said that the best thing she could do to restore her health and relieve her symptoms would be to drink six to eight cups of plain water each day.

The woman didn't want to do this. She didn't like the taste of water. The daughter asked if there was some herb or nutrient I could give her that would help her. I told her that this was impossible. You can't heal a plant dying from a lack of water by adding nutrients to the soil. So our conversation turned to trying to figure out a way to flavor the water so she would drink more of it.

You Can't Fix Lack of Sleep with Supplements

Here's another example—fatigue. People usually need around eight hours of sleep per day, but a large percentage of the population get much less than they need. As a result, they are chronically tired. To cope with this, they use caffeinated beverages, including so-called energy drinks. It's an allopathic self-medication for their fatigue and a perfect example of the difference between symptom relief and cure. Plants that contain caffeine, such as coffee, cola nuts, guarana, and yerba santa are all natural, herbal remedies, but this does not make them appropriate remedies for fatigue.

Understanding what caffeine does when you feel tired is a practical example of the difference between treating a symptom and fixing the cause, as well as a lesson in why you need to pay attention to the body's messages and respond appropriately. Here's how caffeine works.

There's a neurotransmitter in the brain called adenosine. This chemical is released when the body needs rest. It causes tiredness when it attaches to certain receptors in the brain, which prompts you to rest or sleep. Caffeine attaches to these receptors and blocks them. In other words, it works by blocking the message that you are tired. Metaphorically, it's like trying to turn off the fuel gauge in your car that tells you you're low on gas so you can keep driving without having to stop and refuel. If you did this with a car, you'd just run out of gas.

Unlike a car, however, the body has redundant, backup systems. When you're tired and you keep pushing yourself, the stress response, also known as the fight-or-flight response, kicks in to help keep you going. The sympathetic nervous system and adrenal glands respond to this situation the same way it responds when you're tired and about to go to sleep and something frightens you. You get a temporary energy boost, but when it's over you're even more tired than you were before because you've drained some of your body's reserve energy. The caffeine didn't create more energy, it just forced you to tap into a backup energy system.

Fortunately, the body is clever in working around this attempt to cheat nature and gain energy without rest. It adapts to the caffeine by building more receptors for adenosine. Now the message can get through in spite of the presence of the caffeine. However, with the increase in adenosine receptors, caffeine becomes required to feel normal. Because of these additional adenosine receptors, skipping that daily dose of coffee or soda will leave you feeling tired even when your body really isn't.

Once your body adapts, to get the same stimulation you first did from caffeine, a higher dose is required. Eventually this will stop working because it will lead to nervous exhaustion. All your energy reserves will become drained and the caffeine won't work anymore. Your energy levels will crash in spite of it. This is accompanied by anxiety, insomnia, and other side effects of the caffeine.

At this point the only thing that will cure the fatigue is rest, but the high dose of caffeine required just to stay alert interferes with the ability to rest. The solution is to stop caffeine entirely, which will allow the body to start downregulating the number of adenosine receptors. There will be a period of withdrawal when you do this, during which you'll temporarily feel worse while the body readjusts, but you won't be able to rebuild your energy reserves if you don't do this.

I've come to recognize that symptom-relieving drugs and even herbs generally bypass with the body's internal messaging systems in similar ways. The chemicals in these substances inhibit or stimulate various messaging systems, which interferes with the body's ability to communicate its needs. The body will attempt to override this interference, which will in turn require a different drug or herb or a stronger dose.

It also means that there will be side effects, since the real problem has never been addressed or corrected. This is why it is vitally important to learn to read the body's messages clearly and make an appropriate response that provides exactly what the body actually needs.

Warning Messages from the Body

The examples I listed above, thirst and fatigue, concern what the body needs. However, the body also has ways of telling you what it doesn't need, that is, what isn't good for it. The primary way it does this is through some form of discomfort or pain.

For example, if you touch a hot pan or cut yourself with a knife, the pain tells you that what you did caused injury. Applying something to help the burn or cut heal makes sense, but it would be foolish to continue to touch hot pans without a hot pad or to be careless with knives just because you can apply a remedy that helps the burn or cut to heal. Fortunately, pain is a pretty effective teacher, and most of us learn how to be more careful to avoid future injury.

Unfortunately, most people are often less willing to let pain be a teacher when it comes to chronic illness. Pleasure, the sense that the body is getting what it needs, cannot be experienced through overindulgence. Yet people often do things to excess that are pleasurable only in moderation. They may also continue to do things that the body initially reacted to with discomfort, such as smoking, until the body adapts to them and they become habitual.

Indigestion, headaches, stiffness, and other symptoms of pain or distress are always a message that there are unhealthy things that need to be changed. The problem is that we often fail to make the connection between our behaviors and these minor sufferings. We are taught that these things just happen. Thus, we take antacids, analgesics, anti-inflammatories, or other symptom-relieving medications to ease the discomfort, but never really try to figure out what is going on that is causing the discomfort.

So again, if you want to be healthy, you should start paying attention to minor pains and discomfort for what they are—messages about how well you are or aren't taking care of your body. Pain teaches you to be careful and avoid injury. Discomfort teaches you how to avoid excesses in food, drink, and behavior. When these initial gentle messages are ignored, the body eventually starts sending stronger messages in the form of greater pain and discomfort until you start paying attention again.

Taking Responsibility

People involved in natural healing are often critical of orthodox medicine and its symptom-treating orientation. However, in fairness, orthodox medicine is just trying to provide what most people want. Consider this idea in light of this famous statement by Henry David Thoreau: "For every thousand hacking at the leaves of evil, there is one striking at the root." Applying this idea to health care, we could say that for every thousand patients seeking relief from the symptoms of disease, there is only one seeking to remove the root cause.

Generally speaking, it's human nature to want symptomatic relief, because it means that you can continue to eat, drink, and live the way you always have without examining any your behavior. Instead of seeking to change behavior, you can put off the consequences of your behavior by taking medications or submitting to some medical procedure.

Modern medical care has its place. It has excellent diagnostic systems and amazingly effective, symptom-relieving treatments for most diseases. Symptomatic treatment is not evil, because it's important to help ease people's suffering. Giving a soldier wounded on the battlefield a shot of morphine doesn't help his wounds to heal, but it certainly eases his suffering. A person in a highly unstable condition, such as extremely high blood pressure or heart rate, can be stabilized through the use of drugs.

It's human nature to want symptomatic relief, because it means that you can continue to eat, drink, and live the way you always have without examining any your behavior. Instead of seeking to change behavior, you can put off the consequences of your behavior by taking medications or submitting to some medical procedure.

So don't misunderstand: allopathic care is useful, but it is misleading to call it health care. It should be called *disease care* because it's focused on easing disease. And if that's what you're after—symptomatic relief—modern medicine is exactly what you should rely on. In fact, we currently have the best disease care system in the history of the world.

But *health care* is not the same as disease care. Health care should be focused on building good health, rather than treating diseases. Doctors don't have very much training in health care; they aren't taught very much about nutrition or cultivating a person's belief in their ability to heal. They do make some general lifestyle recommendations, but they aren't fitness coaches, stress-management experts, or nutritionists, and they are definitely not herbalists.

Occasionally you'll find holistically minded medical doctors, but they are the exception rather than the rule. So medical doctors are generally not good sources for information on either herbal medicine or nutritional supplements unless they have taken the time to independently study these subjects on their own. Thus, if you want to build good health instead of just treating diseases, you need to seek out other sources of information, like this book.

Health Care

Modern medical research is primarily focused on finding ways to treat disease. In his book, *Specific Diagnosis*, Dr. Scudder suggests that doctors should study health instead of disease. They should first learn what a healthy, living body is like. What a person can learn from dissecting a dead body is limited since the life process is no longer operational. Dr. Scudder advocates diagnosis that involves keen observation of living human beings.

I've discovered that this is the beginning point of genuine health care and the real basis of natural healing. Natural healing starts with the questions, "What is natural to the human body?" and "What is a healthy way to think, eat, and live?" As one who believes in a divine Creator, I assume that there is an orderly cause and effect at work in all aspects of life. I want to know, "How did the Creator intend for us to live?" I want to know what acts in harmony with the principle of life, so I can recognize what is not acting in harmony with life.

As a person seeks to understand this, they can start to see how they are deviating from the ideal of good health. If they are working with others, they can see how their clients' bodies and lives are out of balance. Aiding the healing process now has the goal of guiding a person toward a healthier life. One does not have to understand the various diseases that afflict a person to do this; they just need to help the person gain greater health, knowing that the power to heal lies within the body itself.

I call this approach to health care treatment by prevention. As the pioneer herbalist Samuel Thomson put it, "that same thing that will prevent disease will cure it." In other words, natural healing starts treating a person by encouraging them to do the same things they should have done to stay healthy in the first place.

Disease Treatment versus Health Building

Even though this book lists ailments and remedies that may help them, the book was not written to be an allopathic, cookbook approach to healing. I've taught the treatment-by-prevention idea for years, taking various approaches in an attempt to help people shift their health paradigm. In my doing so, it has never ceased to amaze me what will happen after I've taught these concepts and the question-and-answer period starts. People will always ask, "What do you do for…?" and give me the name of a disease. They do this without providing me any information about the person who has the disease, their health history, lifestyle. or diet.

It's clear to me that it takes a major paradigm shift to grasp the idea of getting rid of disease by building health. So this book was created to build a bridge between people's desire to treat their diseases. By listing ailments and then trying to point them in the direction of things they can do to rebuild their health I am attempting to switch their thought processes from disease care to health care.

In order to get the most from this book, it's important that you grasp the essential differences between the disease-treatment approach to health most people are familiar with and the health-building approach I've introducing. Here are the fundamental differences between them.

The Disease-Treatment Approach

First, in the disease-treatment approach each disease is treated as if it were a separate and distinct entity. The body is not viewed as a whole, and the disease is seen, not as an abnormal life process, but something that is a separate and distinct entity to be fought against or expelled. As a result, the language is one of war: "I'm going to fight this disease," "I'm going to win this battle against cancer," or "We need to kill those parasites."

In contrast, the health-building approach assumes that all of a person's health problems are seen as a part of an inter-connected whole. Symptoms are seen as signals that the body is out of balance. The symptoms are indications of one or more of the four following real issues:

The body lacks something it needs to be healthy.

The body is being exposed to something that is irritating or damaging it.

The body is trying to expel what is irritating it.

The body is trying to cope with the imbalances in a person's diet, lifestyle, emotions, or attitudes.

Thus, the diseases one is experiencing provide clues as to what these underlying problems might be, but they do not provide sufficient information to determine what needs to be done. They need to share more than just the name of a disease; they need to share health history, diet, and lifestyle as well as how their body isn't healthy (symptoms). It also helps to understand what problems and stresses they are struggling with in life and what their current attitudes and emotions are.

Second, in the disease-treatment approach, the therapy is based on the nature of the disease and the goal of the therapy is to relieve the disease symptoms. Remedies that relieve symptoms quickly are seen as better than remedies that act more slowly, even if the slower acting remedies produce better health in the long run.

The Health-Building Approach

In contrast, the health-building approach builds the therapy around the person. In this approach, we evaluate the person's lifestyle, diet, mindset, emotions, and history to try to discover what is causing their health problems.

Symptoms are indications of one or more of the four following real issues:

The body lacks something it needs to be healthy.

The body is being exposed to something that is irritating or damaging it.

The body is trying to expel what is irritating it.

The body is trying to cope with the imbalances in a person's diet, lifestyle, emotions, or attitudes.

Having all this information allows us to start forming a theory of "What did it?" It's like solving a detective mystery. We collect the clues and then decide who the most likely suspects are. Does the person need to change their diet? Do they need more exercise? Are they suffering from sleep deprivation? Is their body toxic and in need of fasting and detoxification?

In essence, we line up the suspects and pick the ones that are probably causing the most injury to the body. We then create a strategy for eliminating these suspects (causes). As Samuel Thomson put it, "If we remove the cause, the effect [disease] will cease."

The strategy is unique to the person because we understand that the body can only be as healthy as its weakest link. If the weakest link is diet and nutritional deficiencies, we work on that first. If the weakest link is excessive exposure to some kind of toxin or irritant, we eliminate that first and help the body clean itself out.

Once we form the strategy, we test it by implementing it. We observe if the body (as a whole) begins to move toward a greater state of health. If it does, we're on the right track. We may tweak the strategy and make it better, but our overall approach is valid. If following the strategy doesn't move the body toward health (the person stays the same or gets worse), we reevaluate the situation and change the strategy.

Which Approach Will You Take?

To summarize, the disease-treatment approach bases its recommendations on the individual diseases a person has, while the health-building approach bases its recommendations on an evaluation of what is causing all the imbalances (diseases and symptoms) in the person's life and is based on helping the body return to an overall state of better health.

Again, because it's so important to grasp the difference, let me restate this in another way. To build health, we need more information than a disease name. First, we need to know all the ailments a person has because we have to look at them all as manifestations of the same underlying imbalances in a person's body. Then, we need to get information about their diet, lifestyle, and mental/emotional state. From this we can formulate a strategy for improving their overall health so the body can repair and rebalance itself.

In part two of this introduction, we'll go through the process of developing a health-building strategy for yourself or others. If you follow the four steps laid out in this process you're more likely to get the results you desire.

Part II
Developing a Healing Strategy Step-by-Step

To get the most out of this book, I've laid out a four-step process to developing a health-building strategy. You can use this process on yourself, or if you are a practitioner, you can use it with your clients. For best results, use all four steps. Don't skip any of them. Each step helps you accomplish the next one.

Many people are tempted to skip to the last step. If you're helping others, you may need to adjust the steps to accommodate people as you help them to shift their paradigm, but again, all four steps are essential to real health.

Healing Strategy Step 1:
Believe You Can Get Well

The power of thought in health is demonstrated by the existence of placebo effect, which most people know about but have been taught to see as a negative rather than a positive thing. *Placebo* means "I will please" and refers to the fact that a certain percentage of people will get well on any treatment, as long as they believe it will help them. The percentage varies, but it is around 25 to 33 percent (about one-fourth to one-third of all patients). The very fact that believing a sugar pill will help you feel better causes some people to feel better demonstrates the incredible power of the mind in healing.

The reason double-blind, placebo-controlled studies are the gold standard for medical research is that they are the only way to rule out placebo effect. *Double-blind* means that neither the doctor nor the patient knows if they are getting the real remedy or the placebo. When they did single-blind studies, where the doctor knew if the patient was getting the drug or the placebo, they found the success rate for the drug was much higher. Why? Because the doctor had more confidence in the new drug than in the placebo, and even though he did not tell the patient, his confidence, or lack of it, was somehow picked up by the people in the study.

The implications of this are incredible. It suggests that you have about a 30 percent chance of getting well if you believe that what you are doing will make you well, even if what you are doing has no physical effect. It also suggests that you can get well just because you believe in the doctor or healer who is helping you.

I've studied positive thinking from the secular perspective and faith from the spiritual perspective, and both perspectives teach me the same thing. The thoughts you choose to hold in your mind have real power in what you experience in your life, as do the words you speak. So why not start by believing you can be well?

I talk about how to do this under the *Affirmation and Visualization* strategy in the "Specific Strategies" section. Study this strategy and put it firmly into your mind that you are healthy. Take your focus away from disease and put it onto health. If you are helping others, use it to boost your confidence that you can help them experience greater health.

The Nocebo Effect and Voodoo Hexes

The power of the mind in health is also demonstrated by nocebo effect, something which most people haven't heard about. *Nocebo* means "not pleasing." The research into the nocebo effect shows that not only can your mind help you heal; it can also make you sick.

This research involves giving a person a placebo and telling them that it's a drug with potential for side effects. When this is done, some people will experience side effects on the placebo. For instance, people taking sugar pills believing they are chemotherapy drugs will experience nausea and lose their hair. The percentage is roughly the same for the placebo effect, about 25 to 30 percent.

Furthermore, just as having faith in your doctor or practitioner can help you heal, statements made by a doctor or practitioner you trust can also interfere with your healing, that is, if you choose to believe them. A negative statement that programs your mind that you have an "incurable disease" or that you have only "a short time left to live" can become a voodoo hex. A voodoo hex is when someone you trust tells you something bad is going to happen and you believe them so that your mind goes about creating the negative thing.

Doctors and others are often well-meaning when they make these statements. In their minds, they are just being realistic. But the nocebo effect shows that this is an ill-advised practice. Doctors are not gods. They do not know how long a person has to live or what God has in mind for a person's life. People are often miraculously cured from "incurable" diseases.

It is wrong to take away hope. I personally do not believe that any disease is incurable. I do believe that some people are incurable, often because they are unable, or more likely unwilling, to do what they need to do to get well. I also do not believe in the idea of false hope. Hope and its accompanying principle of faith are needed in people's lives to motivate them to do something about their condition.

A person who loses hope may become filled with despair. A person who believes a voodoo hex about their health will stop seeking solutions to their problems. Instead, they will mentally and emotionally prepare to die, often fulfilling the doctor's prophecy about how long they have left to live.

Exercising Faith to Be Healed

I've read many stories and have personally seen examples of people who temporarily override a voodoo hex given on how long they have to live. If a person has a significant event, such as the birth of a grandchild or the graduation or marriage of a son or daughter, that is scheduled to take place after the six or twelve months they've been told they have left, they often determine to live to see that event. So they extend their live another two or three months simply via their mental determination to do so. Then, shortly after the event, they pass away.

The research into the nocebo effect shows that not only can your mind help you heal; it can also make you sick.

This also shows the power of the mind. If you believe your life still has purpose, you will find a way to survive to fulfill that purpose. This is why I encourage people who have been given a death hex to continue to plan for life and to make the most of whatever time they have left. I have always counseled these people to *not* believe what they have been told. I assure them that no one knows when they are going to die except God. I point out that a perfectly healthy person can be killed tomorrow in a tragic accident and that people who think they are going to die often live miraculously for many more years.

So I encourage them to treat each day as a gift and focus on enjoying and utilizing whatever time they have left in life to the fullest. This helps turn their mindset around. It helps them shift their thoughts away from thoughts of dying toward thoughts of living.

I also tell people with a death hex, "Suppose God miraculously grants you another five years of life. What are you going to do with it? What changes will you make? What will you do differently?" I ask them to think, "Why should God give you more time if you're just going to continue to live your life as you do now? Could your sickness be a wake-up call that's trying to get you to rethink your life and make appropriate changes, to perhaps repent in some way?"

Perhaps the best way to illustrate what I'm talking about is to tell you two stories with very different endings. Although I could tell you many others, these two should be sufficient to illustrate the difference attitude makes in healing.

A Miraculous Change of Attitude

The first deals with a young man I worked with in the late 1980s who had been diagnosed with AIDS. I had read several books written by doctors who had successfully treated AIDS holistically, but I had never personally worked with someone with this condition.

As I talked with him, I was trying to instill hope in him by sharing what I had read, but I could tell that he wasn't hearing me. He looked defeated and hopeless. As I prayed for guidance about how to help him, a thought came to me. I asked him, "Is it your time to die? Is God telling you it's time for you to come home?"

When I said this, he looked me in the eye for the first time and said, "It's funny you should ask me that, because last night I was praying and I had a strong feeling that God has a purpose for me and wants me to live."

I slapped my knee and said boldly, "Well there you have it. If God wants you to live, how can you die? Think about that."

When I saw him a week later, his entire attitude had changed. He knew that he had a purpose for living and was confident he could recover. Over the next few months, we both researched his condition and tried different things to build his health. The last time I saw him he was the longest-sur-viving AIDS patient in Utah, having outlived everyone else who had contracted the disease. He was still healthy and told me that doctors were studying what he did to see if they could help others.

Focusing on Death Instead of Life

The second story does not have such a happy ending. The wife of one of my best friends was diagnosed with gall bladder cancer. The doctor told her that 98 percent of people who get this type of cancer die within a year. In spite of how rare this form of cancer is, I actually met two people within one week who had cured themselves naturally of cancer of the liver and gallbladder and offered to share what they had learned.

She declined. She said that her family would oppose her taking an alternative route and to please them she was going to take the medical route.

Six months into her treatment, she related a dream to me and asked me for an interpretation. In the dream she saw a forest after a forest fire. It was a scene of death and desolation. Behind her, she could hear birds chirping and leaves rustling, and she knew that behind her was a green forest that had not been touched by the fire. However, she could not take her eyes off the burned out forest to turn around and look at the green one.

I said a quick prayer to myself, asking for inspiration to interpret her dream, and this is what I was given. I knew that she had a tendency to hang onto all the bad things that had happened in the past and had difficulty letting go of them. I told her that she was focused on the negative side of life, including her disease and the possibility she might die. I told her she needed to shift her mental focus and start focusing on the good things in life and think about life instead of death.

She said that she felt I had interpreted her dream correctly, but over the months that followed, she still seemed unable to shift her focus. When the chemotherapy was causing problems with her digestive tract I could not persuade her to take even a little slippery elm or aloe vera juice to soothe her digestive system, because her doctor had forbidden her to take any herbs. She continued to dwell on the negative things of life and died exactly twelve months from the time she was diagnosed.

Developing Faith and a Positive Mental Attitude

If you've come to understand the importance of mental attitude in your life and in your health, you understand a basic truth. You have to focus the mind on what you want, not on what you don't want. When you're focused on what you don't want, you are actually thinking about what you don't want. In fact, when you are against something, you tend to actually strengthen it.

I've observed this in trying to change people's minds. If you attack the other person's position, they get defensive, dig in mentally and emotionally, and resist the attack. Attacking a person's position, therefore, tends to entrench them more deeply into that position. This is just one example of this general principle.

Here's another. Try searching for "Not <something>" on the internet. The "something" can be replaced by anything you want. Take the word *cancer* for instance. Search for "not cancer" on the web. What will you get? Information about cancer, of course.

> *Fighting against a disease, which is the entire allopathic mindset, actually reinforces the disease. I know that's a strange concept for most people, but allow me to elaborate. By assuming the position that you must attack the disease or defend against it, you are mentally giving power to the disease.*

Your brain works in the same way. If you're telling yourself, "I'm going to fight this cancer," "I'm going to beat this cancer," or "I'm going to win the battle against cancer," what is your brain thinking about? It's thinking about cancer. It's not thinking about health.

In other words, fighting against a disease, which is the entire allopathic mindset, actually reinforces the disease. I know that's a strange concept for most people, but allow me to elaborate. By assuming the position that you must attack the disease or defend against it, you are mentally giving power to the disease. You are seeing it as something that is strong and powerful, which must be overcome.

There's a scripture that says, "Faith is the substance of things hoped for, the evidence of things not seen." (Heb. 11:1). What this means is that faith is exercised by focusing on what you hope for (not what is) and holding the evidence in your mind of what has not yet come to pass. In other words, faith is exercised by seeing the end result and picturing it as if it were already yours.

This is why it's essential that you change the nature of the very questions you are asking in your mind. Stop thinking, "How can I get rid of this disease?" That's a disease focus, not a health focus, and it leads you to seek symptomatic relief instead of real healing. Instead, ask yourself, "What do I need to do to be healthy?" That's a health focus and will shift your mind from thinking about disease to thinking about health.

Negative Mental Attitude versus Positive Mental Attitude

If you want a high level of wellness in your life, I encourage you to shift your thinking about everything in life (not just health and disease). This is important, because health is not just physical. Your entire mental and emotional world affects your physical body. So do your finances and personal relationships. So try to let go of as many negative mental attitudes (NMA) as you can and replace them with positive mental attitudes (PMA). The table at the bottom of this page lists some areas of your life you should examine and work to shift your mind from NMA to PMA.

The more you can make this switch from NMA to PMA the better off you will be in every area of your life. It's part of doing the "check up from the neck up" and healing from the head down.

Healing Unresolved Trauma and Abuse

Much of the NMAs people have and the emotional burdens that accompany them are due to unresolved problems from the past, especially from childhood. When someone has been unable to heal mentally and emotionally from difficult events, they tend to go into a state of constant fear (stress and anxiety), grief (sadness and depression), or anger (irritability

Negative Thinking (NMA)	**Positive Thinking (PMA)**
Thinking about what you don't have	Being grateful for what you do have
Worrying about your problems	Praying and believing that God can help you find solutions to your problems
Worrying about bad things that might happen in the future	Setting goals to get what you want and focusing your mind on achieving them
Thinking about all the things you don't like about your life	Thinking about all the good things in your life
Focusing on the weaknesses and shortcoming of yourself and others	Seeing the good in yourself and those around you
Trying to avoid stress and problems	Making time for pleasure and finding ways to enjoy life
Dwelling on the bad things that have happened to you in the past	Forgiving those who have hurt or offended you and letting go of the past
Feeding your mind with negative and discouraging information, news, and entertainment	Feeding your mind with positive and inspiring information, news, and entertainment

and loss of temper). It's hard to have a PMA and feel happy, loving, and peaceful when you are carrying around a burden of unresolved traumatic and abusive experiences.

If you have been abused or mistreated in the past and are still troubled by it, it means you've never recovered from it and it may be playing a role in your ill health. I've particularly found this to be the case with people who have suffered from multiple health problems and severe illness for most of their life. A big part of my own healing work has been addressing these issues with people.

This is why there are many specific strategies for dealing with mental and emotional health listed under various diseases in this book. Please do not ignore these in developing your healing strategy. For instance, *Counseling or Therapy* or *Emotional Healing Work* are often essential to a person's recovery. Please read these therapies if you suffer from the effects of trauma and abuse and desire to be well.

Other Mental and Emotional Aids

If you are currently under a lot of stress, that's a big factor in your health problems too. The stress response creates contribute to the nervous and glandular system which listed in the "Conditions" section, but it's really one of the major underlying causes of many diseases. Stress is if you experience a lot of stress, study this condition and the various ways to help it.

Also read about the specific strategies *Stress Management* and *Pleasure Prescription*. These strategies help a person build resistance to the stresses of life.

The *Flower Essences* and *Aromatherapy* strategies may also help you make adjustments to your mental attitude and emotions. For this reason, there are flower essences and essential oils listed under various health conditions.

The reason I've stressed this first step in developing a health-building strategy is that it's very hard to motivate yourself to change your diet and lifestyle if you don't believe you can get well and discipline your mind to form a positive mental attitude. If you're working with others, their negative attitudes and emotions will interfere with everything else you try to do.

My experience is that people who shift their attitude and work on their thoughts and emotions get far better results with natural remedies than people who don't. In fact, resolving people's mental attitude and emotional stress is often the only thing some people need to get well. Even when you're drugs or medical treatments, you'll get better results your thinking and learn how

Healing Strategy Step 2:
Form Healthy Habits

The second step in creating health in your life is to cultivate healthy habits. Your life is controlled by habits, which are simply ways of interacting with the world that have been repeated often enough that they become automatic. Habits operate without conscious effort. For example, when you were learning to walk or drive a car, you had to think about what you were doing and focus attention on it. Once you learned these skills, you can do them without focusing your mental attention on them. They become automatic.

Most of your habits of living, including the way you eat, how much exercise you get, and how well you sleep were acquired without conscious thought or effort. You absorbed these habits from your family, friends, and society. As a result, many of these habits are not healthy, and your body tries to tell you so through messages of discomfort and disease.

It is difficult to change your habits if you don't have a sense of purpose and a positive mental attitude. Without these, people tend to "live to eat" rather than "eat to live." When you have a love for yourself and others and you have positive goals and plans for life, it is easier to take care of your body by adopting healthy habits of eating and living.

Changing from unhealthy habits to healthy ones is where you apply the concept of treatment by prevention. In other words, you treat diseases by building good health habits. If you want real health, this is an essential step, because contrary to the general attitude of society, there are *no shortcuts* that produce genuine health. All remedies and practitioners that promise health without cultivating healthy habits are just going to temporarily relieve symptoms.

It takes about two to three weeks of concentrated effort to form a new habit. So if you can motivate yourself to change some aspect of your diet or lifestyle for just a few weeks, you'll start to do it automatically. It will become part of your lifestyle.

Let me share a firsthand experience with this. When first I decided to stop eating refined sugar and white flour, I experienced incredible cravings. I literally went through withdrawal for about two weeks. However, after about three weeks, these foods actually lost their appeal. I started to feel so good that it was easy to avoid them because I started to recognize how bad I felt when I ate them. In fact, my taste buds changed so that I started craving healthier food and actually didn't like the taste of the empty-calorie, junk food I'd been attracted to before. That's an example of how habit force takes over for will-power if you can just stick with something for a few weeks.

Tactics for Improving Health Habits

Realizing that it's difficult to change habits, I often employ the following tactics when trying to help others implement this part of the healing strategy. If you are using this book to help others, these are great ways to go about helping people change their habits. If you are using it for yourself, it's easier to motivate yourself following these principles.

First, I don't try to change everything about a client's diet and lifestyle at once. If a person feels overwhelmed with too many things to do, they don't do anything. So I usually start with only one or two recommendations. These could be something as simple as avoiding one problematic food or ingredient, taking a walk every day, or drinking more water each day.

Second, I ask them to commit to this change for only a short period. I usually start by asking them to do something for two weeks. If they say this is too hard, I ask if they can do it for a week. Whatever time we agree on, I ask them to verbally promise me they will do this for that period of time. This way, they don't feel like they're committing to something forever.

Third, I schedule a follow-up appointment to check up on their progress after the agreed-upon period. The follow-up is important as one of the best ways to increase a person's will-power is to hold them accountable by making them have to report on their progress.

If you aren't working with a practitioner, I suggest you find a good friend and verbally commit to the change you want to make. Promise them you will report on your progress at a set date. This works, because most of us don't like to admit failure to another person. It's a major reason that support groups like Alcoholics Anonymous are successful in helping people make important life changes.

Fourth, in the case of giving up an unhealthy food, I tell clients that after avoiding it for the agreed-upon period, they can indulge themselves by treating themselves with it as a reward. What typically happens is this; they give up the unhealthy food or substance for a week or two and start to feel better. As soon as they treat themselves to it, they feel worse, which reinforces in their mind the connection between the unhealthy substance and their ill health. This gives them greater will-power in the future, because everyone is naturally motivated to feel good.

For example, I remember asking a teenager who clearly had a milk allergy causing his sinus problems to give up dairy products. He didn't want to, as he loved milk and ice cream. I finally got him to commit to avoiding dairy for one week with the promise that he could reward himself by eating as much ice cream as he

wanted after the week was over. I also gave him some herbs to help decongest his sinuses.

When I saw him again, he reported that his sinus problems got better while he was taking the herbs and avoiding the dairy. As soon as he rewarded himself with the ice cream, however, he went right back to where he started, as his sinuses plugged back up again. He told me that the dairy products lost their temptation when he realized they were contributing to his sinus problems.

Creating Habits of Health

To help you create better health habits, I'm going to give you a list of seven questions to ask yourself. You can also ask these questions to people you are trying to help. As you ask each question, think about your answers and decide the areas in which you need to improve your health habits. Then, write them down.

Once you have written down the ways in which you can improve your health habits, pick one from the list and set a goal to work on it for two to three weeks. Find someone you trust whom you can report to. After working on it, pick a second one and repeat the process.

Each healthy habit you make will increase your energy and your overall sense of well-being. This provides you with more motivation and willpower to work on the next one. You will soon find that following a healthy lifestyle is easier than living an unhealthy life. Your sense of well-being, high energy level and clarity of thought will make it easy not to slip back into your old unhealthy habits. With that understanding, here are the seven basic questions to consider when seeking to form healthier habits.

1. Are you eating a healthy diet?

Many people know their diet isn't healthy, but they make no effort to change. Others think they are following a healthy diet because they've adopted a particular dietary plan or philosophy. While I've seen healthy people who have adopted a variety of diets (vegan, vegetarian, or paleo, for example), I believe that the best diet plan to follow is the one that makes you feel great. If you're not feeling great, then consider what you might do differently. I recommend people pay less attention to dietary philosophy and more attention to their own body.

> *Don't try to change everything about a client's diet and lifestyle at once. If a person feels overwhelmed with too many things to do, they don't do anything.*

How do you feel an hour or two after you feel bloated or stuffy fog or some for foods, you probably shouldn't be eating them, even if they appear to be perfectly healthy for other people.

There are many suggestions for helping you adopt a healthier diet in the "Specific Strategies" section of this book. If you're new to natural health start with the *Eat Healthy* strategy. Beyond these basic ideas, there are special diets that may be helpful with certain health problems. These special diets include *Alkalize the Body, Blood Type Diet, Gluten Free Diet, Gut Healing Diet, Ketogenic Diet,* and *Low Glycemic Diet.* When one of these special diets is listed under a health condition pay close attention to it for more specific dietary suggestions.

There are also specific nutrients and foods that aid specific health conditions. Again, these are listed under the ailments in the "Conditions" section. When you look up ailments, pay close attention to these special nutrients or foods (especially if they show up under more than one problem you have). These include the strategies *Bone Broth, Eat Enzyme-Rich Foods, Friendly Flora, Healthy Fats, Increase Dietary Fiber*, and *Mineralization*.

Don't be overwhelmed by the many options. Start by picking one or two things you can do and do them for a couple of weeks. Then try something else. Everyone is genetically different and has their own unique circumstances, so the diet that works for one person may not necessarily work for someone else. Just pay attention to the messages your body is giving and try to find the foods that help you feel good and have better energy and mood when you eat them.

2. Are you getting enough sleep?

Sleep is absolutely critical to health, and generally speaking, most people need between eight and nine hours per night. Unfortunately, many people get only six hours or less. That's very detrimental to health, for many reasons. Here are a few.

First, healing takes place in the deepest part of sleep at night. If you are being shortchanged on sleep by even one hour each night, it interferes with your body's ability to heal.

Second, sleep is essential to mental and emotional health. Again, being shortchanged on sleep by just one or two hours per night can make you irritable, depressed, and/or inefficient in your work. Many accidents occur because people weren't getting enough sleep.

Third, sleep aids detoxification in your body. Your body does internal housekeeping during the hours of sleep. It's hard for your cells to detoxify if you aren't getting enough sleep.

Sleep patterns are also habit patterns. If you cultivate the habit of going to bed at a specific time and waking up at a specific time each day, your body will fall into a natural rhythm around this schedule and it will become easier to get adequate sleep.

So if you're not getting eight to nine hours of sleep per night, follow the *Sleep* strategy. If you're having trouble sleeping, look up *Insomnia* in the "Conditions" section for suggestions on how to improve your sleep.

3. Are you getting enough exercise?

Many people in modern society are too sedentary. There are also those for whom exercise is an obsession and they look forward to it. This is again an illustration of habit force. If you develop a habit of exercise, it becomes easy and automatic, but it takes a couple of weeks of effort to get the habit going.

At minimum almost everyone should be getting an hour of light exercise three times a week. Even better would be thirty to sixty minutes of exercise daily. Exercise doesn't necessarily mean working out at the gym, although that's an option; it can be as simple as walking or swimming. The important thing is to try to find an activity that will be enjoyable, as this helps to motivate you to do it.

If you aren't getting exercise, follow the *Exercise* strategy. If you have trouble exercising, you can also look up *Exercise (Performance)* and *Exercise (Recovery)* in the "Conditions" section for supplements that may help you exercise better or recover faster from sore muscles or other problems associated with exercise.

4. Do you have good posture?

Closely related to exercise is good posture. Poor posture, and the structural imbalances it creates, can cause stress and pain in the body. Headaches, neck pain, back pain, leg pain and more can be related to poor posture.

Posture is also habitual. Habits like slouching in a chair, leaning forward as you walk, and hanging your head are all absorbed from childhood and other environmental factors. Correcting these poor habits of posture will not only ease physical pain but also improve emotional mood.

For example, standing up straight and throwing your shoulders back actually aid self-esteem and reduces depression. Walk upright with good posture will aids self-confidence and positivity. So the benefits aren't just physical, they're also emotional.

If you do heavy lifting, work at a computer, or perform other tasks regularly that stress the body's structural alignment read the *Good Posture* strategy. This strategy will be found under many specific conditions, as it is often a contributing factor in various physical and emotional health problems.

5. Are you drinking enough water?

It's a good practice to drink about half an ounce of water for each pound of body weight every day. Most people don't get enough water, and dehydration contributes to pain and chronic illness. Fruit juice, sugary drinks, coffee, and alcohol don't count, but herbal teas can, as long as they aren't strongly diuretic. Get in the habit of drinking water regularly.

For more information on the importance of water, read the *Hydration* strategy. Many ailments in the "Conditions" section can be aided by better hydration, so pay attention to this therapy when it comes up. You can also read about *Dehydration* in the "Conditions" section.

6. Are you avoiding harmful substances?

There are many things many people consume regularly that aren't good for health. If you have a strong constitution and an otherwise-healthy lifestyle, you can probably tolerate some of these things in moderation. But they are never good in excess, and if you are sick, especially with certain health problems, it's wise to avoid them completely. These substances include illegal drugs, alcohol, tobacco, caffeinated beverages, and refined sugar. It's also wise to minimize exposure to chemicals in general. If any of the following strategies are listed in the health problem you are looking up in the "Conditions" section, please pay attention to them: *Avoid Caffeine, Avoid Sugar, Avoid Xenoestrogens, Eliminate Allergy-Causing Foods, Eliminate FODMAPs, Eliminate Salycilates, Reduce Chemical Exposure*, and *Reduce Electromagnetic Exposure*.

Again, the use of many substances harmful to health is a habit. And you correct a bad habit by substituting it with a new, good habit. When trying to eliminate a harmful substance from your diet or lifestyle, pick a positive, more healthy substance or influence you can use as a substitute reward to help you generate a new, good habit to take its place. For instance, you can drink water instead of soda pop, chew a sugar-free gum instead of smoking, and eat a healthy snack instead of something with sugar.

7. Do you need to fast or detoxify?

If you are exposed to chemicals in your workplace or live in an area of the country where there is a lot of environmental pollution, it's wise to do some detoxification therapy on a regular basis. The most basic of all detoxification therapies, and one of the oldest of all healing practices, is fasting. Fasting helps you gain discipline over your body and your appetites. It clears your body of disease processes caused by food allergies. It helps rebalance the friendly flora in your gut. Fasting is an important therapy when you are acutely ill, as it's not wise to eat any heavy food when you're fighting an infection. It is also a spiritual practice that helps you attune yourself to the divine.

Just about everyone can benefit from some form of periodic fasting. So I would encourage you to develop a habit of periodic fasting, by following the *Fasting* strategy.

Detoxification is also important when detoxification strategies are listed under one or more of the conditions you are experiencing. Detoxification strategies include: *Caster Oil Pack, Colon Cleanse, Colon Hydrotherapy, Epsom Salt Bath, Gall Bladder Flush, Heavy Metal Cleanse, Liver Detoxification, Oral Chelation*, and *Sweat Bath*.

Most of your success in healing the body will come from these seven things. You will get far better, faster and more lasting results from adopting these basic health practices than from just taking herbs and supplements. So again, don't skip this vital step in developing your personal strategy for healing. And if you're working with clients, don't let them skip this step either. This short anonymous poem I found in the *Health Poetry Prescription* by Earnest Endeavor sums up the basic idea quite nicely.

The Six Best Doctors

The six best doctors anywhere—
And no one can deny it—
Are Doctors Sunshine, Water, Air,
Rest, Exercise and Diet.
These six will gladly you attend,
If only you are willing.
The mind they'll clear, your ills they'll mend,
And charge you not a shilling.

Healing Strategy Step 3:

Take Some Basic Supplements

Before selecting specific supplements for health problems, there are several basic supplements that are vital to your overall health that you should consider first. The body doesn't heal selectively, which means that anything you do to improve your overall health will aid your recovery from any specific health challenges you may have.

What follows is a list of seven basic supplements that most people find helpful. The list grew out of a conversation I had with two colleagues over lunch. The first was a holistic medical doctor, Dr. Hugo Rodier, and the second was a naturopath who has been a longtime friend and business associate, Dr. Kimberly Balas. In our discussion, we agreed that most people could recover from at least 50 percent of their ailments if they just ate a healthier diet and used four basic supplements. Over the next couple of years, Dr. Balas and I expanded the list to the seven you'll find here.

I personally use many of these supplements, not necessarily every day, but fairly regularly. I consider them a form of nutritional health insurance, something that can make up for some of the deficiencies in modern diets and the stresses associated with modern living.

Basic Supplement No. 1: Digestive Enzymes

In the 1930s, Francis Pottenger did a series of experiments feeding cats cooked and raw food. Cats fed exclusively on raw meat and milk thrived for generation after generation, while cats fed cooked milk or meat developed allergies, arthritis, and numerous other diseases common in modern civilization.

Part of the reason for this difference is that raw foods contain enzymes, which are deactivated or destroyed during cooking. Since most people in modern society eat primarily cooked foods, most people can benefit from taking enzymes to make it easier to digest their food and get the nutrition they need from it.

From ...ds also contain enzyme inhibitors, so foods that come to be...s can also be hard to digest, unless they are soaked ...rouuing process or eaten with enzymes. These foods include grains, nuts, and legumes. The need for enzymes becomes even more important when you recognize that many processed foods contain preservatives, which often act as enzyme inhibitors.

You can get these enzymes naturally by following the strategy *Eat Enzyme Rich Foods*. Many people, including myself, find that they need supplementary enzymes and other digestive secretions like betaine hydrochloric acid (HCl) and bile salts. For example, people with blood type A tend to be naturally low in HCl production.

Most people also need enzyme supplements as they get older. It has been estimated that about half of the population over fifty has low stomach acid. Elderly people usually need enzyme supplements, as do people recovering from chronic health problems.

There are two basic types of digestive enzyme supplements to consider. The first are plant enzymes, which are the same type of enzymes found in raw foods. The second are digestive enzymes, which are the same digestive secretions produced by the body. Plant enzymes include proteases (which aid in protein digestion), amylases (which aid starch and sugar digestion), and lipases (which help break down fats). There are also enzymes that help break down plant fibers, such as cellulase.

Anyone whose diet is over 30 percent cooked food and is suffering from any health problems, but especially diges- ...blems, should take a good plant enzyme ... off the digestive tract, ...utrients, and

improves overall health. I've even mixed plant enzymes into the food of children who have been diagnosed with failure to thrive and had them start to develop normally again.

Digestive enzymes include pepsin and pancreatic enzymes. Although they aren't enzymes, two other similar supplements that aid digestion are betaine hydrochloric acid and bile salts. For people over fifty or people who are recovering from long term illness I recommend a *Digestive Support Formula* that contains all of these digestive secretions. People over fifty, especially those who have the A blood type, often benefit from taking a *Betaine HCl* supplement as well.

Basic Supplement No. 2 Minerals

Unless someone is growing their own food using organic methods in mineral-rich soil, they are going to need to supplement their minerals regularly. Agricultural practices over the past one hundred years have severely depleted the soil, which in turn has severely depleted the mineral content of foods. Just like your guts need probiotics to maintain health, plants need microbes in the soil to maintain their health. Soil fungii and bacteria help make minerals bioavailable to plants. Chemical farming sterilizes the soil, kills these microbes, and interferes with the mineral absorption of the plants.

It is difficult to find documentation of this fact because the knowledge seems to be suppressed, but I have seen studies that document this. In one, four-thousand grain samples were taken from four Midwestern states over a four-year period. These samples were then analyzed for their mineral content. During this period, the following mineral reductions were measured: copper levels dropped 68 percent, sodium levels 55 percent, calcium levels 41 percent, iron levels 26 percent, magnesium 22 percent. Even levels of phosphorus and potassium, both of which are found in the commercial fertilizers, dropped—phosphorus by 8 percent and potassium by 28 percent. This shows that the plants were not able to utilize these elements even though they were present in the soil. (De Wayne Ashmead "Without Chelation You're Dead" *World Health and Ecology*, 8 no. 2 (1976): 3)

Another study I found was conducted by Firman E. Baer of Rutger's University. He compared the mineral content of organically grown foods with non-organically grown foods. The study showed significant differences in the mineral content. For example, organically grown snap beans had twice the phosphorus content, three times the calcium content, four times the magnesium content, over three times the potassium content, and 22 times more iron than their chemically grown counterparts.

In another example, spinach grown in organic soil had twice the phosphorus content, twice the calcium content, four times the magnesium content, three times the potassium content, and nearly 80 times the iron content of commercially grown spinach. (https://www.organicphuket.com/minerals-organic-versus-conventional/)

When Weston Price, author of the classic book *Nutrition and Physical Degeneration*, toured the world in the 1930s, he found the indigenous people, living on traditional diets, had far more macro minerals in their diet than people living on modern, refined foods. They obtained about four times the amount of calcium and magnesium, for example. He didn't test for trace mineral content, where I suspect the difference would be even greater.

It is clearly important to supplement with minerals, particularly trace minerals. For this reason, I think a *Colloidal Minerals Formula* or *Joan Patton's Herbal Minerals* will benefit most people, but it will be especially helpful for people who have a lot of structural problems such as tooth decay, problems with bones and joints, and muscle aches and pains. When *Mineralization* is a recommended strategy for a condition, seriously consider a supplements like these.

You will also find specific minerals mentioned for various ailments. Pay attention to these recommendations, especially if the same mineral shows up as helpful for more than one health problem you have. For general health, you might also consider the following minerals as supplements.

People often supplement with calcium, but I have personally found that more people are deficient in magnesium than calcium. It's been estimated that about 70 percent of the population is magnesium deficient, and I find it very helpful for people with muscle tension, anxiety, insomnia, hypersensitivity, low energy, and migraine headaches.

Zinc is another common mineral deficiency. It's important for immunity, male reproductive function, a calm nervous system, and would healing. Many women also need iron, but I recommend getting it primarily from food sources or herbs.

Basic Supplement No. 3
Vitamins

A *Multiple Vitamin and Mineral* supplement is helpful for anyone who consumes a diet that contains a lot of refined or processed foods, but it can even be helpful for people who are trying to eat healthy. Reduced mineral uptake in the soil also reduces vitamin content in food. Plus, vitamins deteriorate as food is stored and shipped. Most "fresh" produce in the supermarket is already two weeks old when it reaches the consumer, which means it has already lost some of its vitamin content.

Fat-soluble vitamins are a particular problem as most people aren't getting enough of them. Weston Price, mentioned earlier, found that indigenous people had ten times more fat-soluble

vitamins in their diets as people living on modern foods. Of particular importance is vitamin D_3. It has been estimated that 90 percent of the population is deficient in it. Many people are also deficient in vitamins A, E, and K. These fat-soluble vitamins boost the immune system, help prevent cardiovascular disease, and are critical to the health of bones, teeth, and joints.

Weston Price also found that native people had about four times more water-soluble vitamins in their diets. Unless you eat a lot of fresh, raw fruits and vegetables, you can probably use extra vitamin C. If you eat refined sugar of any kind, white flour, and white rice, you likely need more B-complex as well. Vegetarians, and especially vegans, are often deficient in vitamin B12.

While supplementing with specific vitamins may be helpful for some conditions, I recommend you start with a good *Multiple Vitamin and Mineral*, along with a trace mineral supplement, for basic nutrition. Then, if you still have indications of specific deficiencies, add in the individual vitamins or minerals. Don't overdo supplementation with vitamins and minerals, as more is not necessarily better. Try to get most of your nutrition from eating healthy food.

Basic Supplement No. 4
Essential Fatty Acids

Contrary to all the propaganda that suggests otherwise, you need fats in your diet. Fats are critical for the cell membranes, brain and nerve function, and immunity. Extremely low-fat diets can actually be harmful. The problem is that most Americans are eating the wrong kinds of fat in the form of refined vegetable oils, margarine, and shortening. As a result, most people are getting too many harmful transfats, too many omega-6 essential fatty acids (EFAs), and not getting enough omega-3 EFAs.

Omega-3 EFAs are important for immune functions, regulating inflammatory processes, cardiovascular and brain health, and the formation of cell membranes. The best sources of omega-3 fatty acids are wild game, milk, meat and eggs from grass-fed, pastured animals, and deep-ocean or wild-caught fish. Farm-raised fish and animals raised in confinement on animal feed tend to be lower in omega-3 EFAs. If you aren't eating these types of foods, you eat a lot of fried foods (like chips and French fries), and/or you use a lot of vegetable oils, I recommend taking an omega-3 fatty acid supplement. You can learn more about good fats by reading the *Healthy Fats* strategy. For even more information, read the article "Fat Facts" at stevenhorne.com.

Basic Supplement No. 5
Probiotics

Most people associate bacteria with disease, but not all bacteria are bad. In fact, there is utilization of living disinfectan...

confusion in the immune system. This is because the friendly bacteria in your digestive tract, known as friendly flora, or the microbiome, are part of your natural immunity.

Friendly flora create a biofilm, a sort of living blanket that coats the intestinal tract and inhibits other species of microorganisms from gaining a foothold. They also improve the body's ability to digest fats and proteins. And synthesize vitamins, such as B_1, B_2, B_6, B_{12}, folic acid, and biotin. They also help eliminate certain substances in the digestive tract, such as ammonia, cholesterol, and excess hormones.

The microbiome is disrupted by the excessive use of antibiotics and other medications, as well as by excessive consumption of refined carbohydrates and processed foods. The microbiome is developed in infancy through nursing. If you weren't nursed as an infant for at least six months, have taken numerous courses of antibiotics, or have issues with the immune or intestinal system, a probiotic supplement might be in order. You can also eat fermented foods to naturally supplement both enzymes and probiotics. Read the *Friendly Flora* strategy for more information.

Basic Supplement No. 6
Fiber

Fiber is very important in daily cleansing of the body. If you are eating fiber rich fruits and vegetables every day, including edible skins and seeds, you'll get plenty of fiber from your diet. However, if you're like most people, you peel the few fruits and vegetables you do eat and have a diet consisting primarily of low-fiber foods like refined carbohydrates and animal proteins. If this describes you, you should definitely take a fiber supplement.

Fiber has numerous benefits. It absorbs bile from the gallbladder to help keep cholesterol levels balanced, slows the release of sugar into the blood to stabilize blood sugar, absorbs toxins in the intestinal tract, reduces irritation in the gut, and provides food for friendly bacteria. And of course, it helps with maintaining regular elimination.

Just taking one teaspoonful of a *Fiber Blend* first thing in the morning, along with a large glass of water, can make a dramatic difference in your general health. The water is important because without it fiber can actually constipate you.

You may need to start with a smaller amount and work up so your body gets used to the extra fiber. If your colon transit time is slow, then you should probably take a *Stimulant Laxative Formula* with the fiber for a week or two. If you experience a lot of gas and bloating when you take fiber, you probably have small intestinal bacterial overgrowth (SIBO) or dysbiosis. Look these conditions up and get this under control first.

Basic Supplement No. 7
Antioxidants

Experts suggest that the majority of chronic and degenerative diseases are caused by oxidative stress, also known as free radical damage, which is also associated with chronic inflammation. Free radical damage also causes the cosmetic problems associated with aging—dry skin, wrinkles, age spots, and the like. This is why many nutritionists recommend eating five to seven half-cup servings of brightly colored fruits and vegetables and green leafy vegetables every day. These foods contain large quantities of antioxidant nutrients, which protect the body from oxidative damage.

This isn't that difficult to do if you eat the fruits or vegetables before you eat anything else. So for example, try eating an apple, orange, banana, or a cup of berries for breakfast. That's your first two servings. Then eat some carrot or celery sticks or a salad at the start of lunch. That's one or two more servings. Then put a cup of vegetables like broccoli, cauliflower, green beans, zucchini, or squash on your dinner plate and eat them first. Right there you'd have five or six servings.

If you're not doing this, you might consider supplementing your antioxidants. Many vitamins, such as vitamins C and D are antioxidant, so your multiple vitamin and mineral helps in this area, but you can also take an *Antioxidant Formula*. There are also individual herbs with powerful antioxidant properties too.

That's it—seven basic supplements that can benefit most people's general health. Consider which of these supplements are appropriate for you as step 3 in developing your personal strategy for healing. Use them for about one month, along with developing healthier habits and many of your health problems will disappear. You can then use step 4 to find ways of correcting your remaining health issues.

Healing Strategy Step 4

Selecting Specific Remedies

Most of your ability to heal comes from following the general principles covered in the first three steps. So you may be able to skip step 4 completely.

This follows the 80/20 rule—that is to say you'll achieve 80 percent of your ability to heal with steps 1 through 3. These are the general principles of healing. Only the remaining 20 percent of your results will come from using specific remedies.

The most important thing to remember when selecting specific remedies is avoid thinking of them as treatments for specific diseases. Instead, look at them as ways of correcting two factors: (1) balancing biological terrain and (2) strengthening weak body systems. You should do this because you'll get better, more consistent results when you do.

In addition, if you are selling or recommending herbs and supplements, you can't legally recommend them based on disease names unless you're a licensed medical professional. According to FDA regulations, any product that is labeled as being able to "cure, prevent, treat, or mitigate" a disease is considered a drug. While I think this stance is ridiculous, since it even makes water become a drug if you suggest it will prevent or treat a disease, it's important to understand what you can and cannot say about herbs and supplements if you happen to be selling them.

The claims that are legal are called structure/function claims. These are claims that suggest that a product can help to maintain, regulate, or promote normal, healthy bodily functions. When you select and/or recommend supplements based on how they affect biological terrain and body systems, you're doing so based on what's going on in the structure and function of the body and staying within the appropriate legal guidelines.

To use a simple, practical example, if I say that cascara sagrada will relieve your constipation, I'm making a drug claim, since constipation is a disease. On the other hand, if I explain that cascara sagrada contains anthraquinone glycosides which support normal peristalsis of the colon, I'm making a structure/function claim. Learning how to talk about herbs and supplements as supports for rebalancing biological terrain and supporting weak body systems not only helps you stay on the right side of the law, it's also the more accurate way to talk about these remedies.

Going back to the example, here's why. Constipation has many causes. A person may be constipated because they are dehydrated, don't get enough fiber in their diet, have an imbalance in their gut flora, or are experiencing a drug side effect. So while cascara sagrada may stimulate bowel movements, it isn't necessarily correcting the underlying reason a person is constipated. Saying it stimulates the peristaltic movements of the colon is accurate and based on biological terrain and body systems. Stimulation is the effect cascara has on the biological terrain, while the colon is the body system where it exhibits this action.

In many of the conditions listed in this book I go to great lengths to discuss the common underlying causes of those ailments. This is important because many conditions have multiple potential causes. Figuring out which causes apply in a given situation is critical when it comes to selecting specific remedies. The bottom line is this: you have to select remedies based on the person and what their body needs and not the name of the disease with which they've been diagnosed.

To accomplish this, I base my selection of specific remedies on three primary factors. The first is remedies that are needed for one of the therapies discussed in the various strat-

egies mentioned in this book. Second, I might select remedies to help the condition of the tissues, which I'm calling the biological terrain. I will explain biological terrain later.

Finally, I also select remedies based on which body systems are weak and need to be strengthened or supported. The "Systems" section in this book is designed to help you select remedies based on body systems. It is placed directly after this section for a purpose, which is to stress the vital importance of learning to work with systems rather than symptoms.

Understanding the Body

To explain the concept of biological terrain and body systems and why this is an effective approach to health care, I need to provide a little background about how the body works. The body is really a community of over one hundred trillion individual cells. If these cells are healthy, the body is healthy.

Cells have five basic needs for health and when these basic needs are met, they will be healthy. First, each requires a constant supply of oxygen. Second, cells require a constant supply of nutrients. The trick, of course, is that these nutrients must be balanced. Too much of one nutrient or a deficiency of another and the cells aren't going to be happy. That's why a basic, healthy diet is essential.

Third, oxygen and nutrients must be dissolved in the water in which cells live. Since the body is mostly water, that's why hydration is so important.

The fourth need cells have is a regulated temperature. If the body gets too cold, cells freeze and die. If they get too hot, they also die. The body temperature is maintained at about 98.6 for optimal health; it can't shift more than ten degrees in either direction without endangering health and life. This heat is generated by metabolizing nutrients using oxygen.

The fifth and final thing cells require is a constant removal of waste material. As cells utilize oxygen and nutrients, they put off waste, much like a burning fire puts off smoke and ash. Hence, the fluid cells live in must be constantly moving in order to carry away the cellular waste products. If the fluid stagnates and waste materials aren't removed, the cells will suffocate in their own waste. This is why aiding detoxification is a basic therapy in natural healing.

Homeostasis and Body Systems

The balanced state, in which all these cellular needs are being met, is called homeostasis. Research suggests that cells will be healthy as long as homeostasis is maintained. This was proved in the 1930s, when Dr. Alexis Carrel, a two-time Nobel Prize winning scientist who performed the first kidney transplant and the head of the Rockefeller Research Institute, conducted an experiment using a small piece of tissue from an embryonic chicken.

His team cultivated this tissue in a flask. They provided it with nutrients, oxygen, and water. They filtered the water to remove the toxic wastes and kept the temperature regulated. By doing this they were able to keep that piece of chicken heart growing for more than thirty years, far past the life span of a normal chicken.

Dr. Carrel said that when the fluid bathing the cells was maintained with sufficient oxygen and nutrients, "the cell colonies remain indefinitely in the same state of activity. They never grow old. Colonies obtained from a heart fragment removed in January 1912, from a chick embryo, are growing as actively today as 23 years ago." [Alexis Carrel, *Man the Unknown*, (New York: Halcyon House, 1938), 173.]

What this means is that maintaining homeostasis, or internal balance, is the key to health. When the body gets out of balance, we get sick because cells don't function properly. If the body gets too far out of balance, we die. When we talk about balancing biological terrain, we're talking about doing things to help keep this homeostatic balance.

Specialization and Cooperation

In order to maintain homeostasis, the cells of the body have become specialized to perform specific functions. These cells are organized into systems that work together to maintain the balance of homeostasis.

It helps to think of this like a community. Each individual needs food, clothing, shelter, transportation, communication, and so forth. However, individuals don't provide all these things for themselves. They specialize in certain services that they provide for the rest of the community.

In the same way, each group of tissues that forms an organ or system that does something for the whole body and, in turn, receives what it needs from the whole body. The cells are joined together for the common good, and they depend on one another. This means that the body can never be stronger than its weakest system. Dr. Arthur C. Guyton in his *Textbook of Medical Physiology*, put it this way.

Each cell benefits from homeostasis, and in turn each cell contributes its share toward the maintenance of homeostasis. This reciprocal interplay provides continuous automaticity

of the body [that is, the sharing of the work load makes the body able to function on its own without outside help] until one or more functional systems lose their ability to contribute their share of function. When this happens, all of the cells of the body suffer. Extreme dysfunction leads to death, while moderate dysfunction leads to sickness. [Arthur C. Guyton, *Textbook of Medical Physiology*, 6th ed., (Philadelphia: W.B. Saunders Company, 1981), 7]

What this means is that you can't just be sick in one part of the body. If any organ isn't working properly, the whole body is sick. That's why I stress that the body can be no healthier than its weakest system. It also means that when you can identify the body systems that are the weakest links and the strengthen them, the health of the entire body improves. The illnesses provide clues to which systems are weak, but you need to learn to look deeper than observing the organs and tissues where the symptoms are manifesting.

For example, Hashimoto's thyroiditis is an autoimmune disease of the thyroid gland. The immune system is producing antibodies to target thyroid tissue for destruction.

In many of the conditions listed in this book I go to great lengths to discuss the common underlying causes of those ailments. This is important because many conditions have multiple potential causes. Figuring out which causes apply in a given situation is critical when it comes to selecting specific remedies.

This means is that the root problem isn't with the thyroid gland, even though it is where symptoms are manifesting. The problem is with the immune system, which is improperly tagging thyroid tissue, and this, in turn, often leads back to the health of the intestinal tract. Wherever possible, these types of relationships are explained under various health conditions.

What you need to do is figure out which systems are not working properly and then restore balance to their structure and function. Often it's just one or two body systems that are causing all the problems in the other systems. Based on my experience, the most common systems where root causes are found are (1) the digestive and intestinal system, (2) the liver, (3) the glands, usually the thyroid and/or adrenals, (4) the nervous system, usually due to stress, and 5) the kidneys and/or lymphatics. When these systems are restored to health, other systems automatically return to normal function.

Chemical Messaging

The body helps to maintain homeostasis through various communications systems that send chemical messages to adjust cellular function to maintain homeostasis. I previously referred to one of these chemical messengers, adenosine, when we talked about caffeine. Like caffeine, many drugs work by targeting various chemical messaging systems in the body, either stimulating or inhibiting them.

Herbs also talk to the body's chemical messaging systems, but they do so in much more subtle and complex ways. While a drug generally works on only one chemical messaging system, herbs influence multiple chemical messaging systems, nudging body functions in one direction or another. So in my experience, herbs are better at restoring a healthy balance to body's functions.

How an herb moves the body towards balance is called an herb's energetics. I'll explain more about energetics shortly, but I want to point out that the energetics for different herbal remedies are prominently featured in that herbs listing in the "Remedies" section.

Comments on Evidence-Based Medicine

Before explaining herbal energetics, I want to comment on the current trend in herbal and natural medicine. It is called evidence-based medicine. This means one is looking for scientific research to back up the use of an herb or nutrient in a particular disease.

While I think looking at research about herbs and nutrients is helpful, I find that this approach is too strongly linked to allopathic concepts of disease care. In other words, the studies are typically done to test a remedy's effect on a particular disease or symptom. As is true of all such research, a percentage of people will do well and others not so well. This is because the treatment is aimed at the disease, not at the person.

To help you understand this better, let me refer to a concept from traditional Chinese medicine (TCM) which states, "Different diseases, one treatment; one disease, different treatments." What this means is that a Chinese physician will treat all the diseases a person has as if they were one disease. He is not treating the individual manifestations of disease but rather the overall picture of how a person is out of balance. It also means that five patients complaining of the same disease may get five different treatments because each person has a unique constitution and the overall pattern of their illnesses is different.

This approach stands in stark contrast to the approach of Western medicine, which focuses its treatment programs on the disease. Western medicine calls a treatment effective if 60 to 70 percent of their test subjects improve on the treatment, but what about the other 30 to 40 percent that the treatment didn't help and in some cases made the person worse? No attempt is made to understand why some people respond to the treatment and some don't. As long as statistical averages are in their favor, the treatment will be employed. (That's not good if you're one of the people the treatment makes worse!)

That's why you need to learn to look at the overall person and see the big picture when it comes to health. That's what holistic health care is all about. Returning to the first part of this introduction, the question "What should I do for my arthritis (or asthma, backache, or other specific problem)?" is really the wrong question. In natural healing you should be asking, "What imbalance in the person's biological terrain and body systems has given rise to this condition?"

When the overall pattern of imbalance is corrected, the body starts to rebuild health and the diseased condition will improve naturally. It's not that herbs and nutrients are incapable of offering symptomatic relief. You can use them to ease symptoms; it's just that you shouldn't stop at symptomatic treatments. TCM practitioners regard offering symptomatic relief as inferior medicine. Superior medicine addresses the underlying imbalances that result in a person's overall health improving.

Understanding Biological Terrain

With that understanding, let's explain the model of biological terrain used in this book. Traditional systems of herbal medicine around the world used energetic models based on elements (such as the Western system of air, water, fire, and earth) to explain patterns of imbalance in the body and classify how remedies corrected them.

Although the metaphorical models of traditional systems of medicine have much to teach us about how herbs work, they can be puzzling to people trained in Western analytical thinking. Fortunately, my friend and fellow herbalist Matthew Wood has created a Western model of biological terrain, that is easier for most people to understand. I have adopted this system and find it very useful in teaching how the terrain gets imbalanced and what herbs can be used to restore balance.

This system looks at two opposing imbalances in three different biological areas. These three factors are the metabolic rate or energy level (how active or inactive the tissues are), tissue density (the balance between the solids and liquids in the body), and muscle tension (whether muscles are overly relaxed or overly tense).

Metabolic rate can become imbalanced by becoming hyperactive (hot) or underactive (cold). Wood labeled the hyperactive state *irritation*, and the underactive state *depression*.

The second factor, tissue density, relates to the balance of minerals to fluids (water and fats). Tissues can become too damp, resulting in congestion and swelling, or too dry, resulting in rigidity and brittleness. Wood calls the damp state *stagnation*, and the dry state *atrophy*.

The final pair of imbalances relate to muscle tone. Too much tension in the muscles causes cramping or spasticity, which also reduces flow, movement, and secretion. Too little tension in the muscles, an atonic or lax condition, causes a loss of structural integrity and excessive drainage or flow. Wood calls the tense state *constriction*, and the atonic state *relaxation*.

I'll provide a more in-depth description of each state in a moment, but first I want to talk about biological terrain as a progression of unhealed tissue damage. I want to explain how nearly all illnesses are simply unhealed damage in body tissues.

The Disease Process, pH and Energy

I see the first four tissue states as a progression of the disease process, which begins in the acute (irritation) stage and then moves through the other three stages—subacute (stagnation), chronic (depression), and degenerative (atrophy). These four stages of disease are associated with the pH of the biological terrain and the energy potential in the tissues.

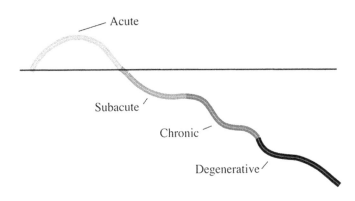

Normal Tissues

The normal pH of the blood and lymph, which form the internal environment or biological terrain of the body, is 7.4. This pH represents an energy potential of about -0.25 millivolts, which means it has electrons it can donate to chemical reactions. This state is represented by the horizontal line labeled normal in the graph above.

Acute Inflammation and Hyperactivity

The body responds to all tissue damage (injury, infection, poisoning) with inflammation, which makes inflammation the starting point for all diseases. It is a hyperactive tissue state in which energy levels are elevated as represented in the peak labeled "acute" above. In the biological terrain model this is called it irritation.

According to Dr. Jerry Tennat in his book *Healing is Voltage*, the pH in inflamed tissues rises to about 7.88, which raises the voltage potential to about -0.50 millivolts of electrical potential, as shown in the table on the next page, which was adapted from his work. At this point tissue color

changes from a normal pink to red and becomes physically warmer. This state is also associated with acute, throbbing pain, which discourages using the damaged body part so it can rest and heal.

This elevated pH and voltage is necessary for healing, something demonstrated by the fact that animals who are able to regenerate lost tails or legs (such as lizards) start the regenerative process with increased electrical activity at the site of injury. Research also shows that low-voltage electrical current can be used to stimulate healing in tissues that were not previously healing. In addition, this is likely the basis for healing by touch, as electrical energy can pass from one person to another through touch, providing the added energy needed for healing. Using energy for healing is discussed in detail in my *Fundamentals of Natural Healing* course.

Subacute Tissue Stagnation

If the damage is not healed and the inflammation is not reversed, the area that was damaged becomes congested and stagnant. This is the subacute stage of the disease process, where the energy level drops below the normal level as shown in the graph. Voltage drops below the normal level at this point. The voltages on the table below aren't precise but give a general indication of what happens.

As the energy potential lowers, fluid movement slows down. Inflammation always involves swelling, which sequesters the damaged area until white blood cells can come in and clean up the damage. This process prevents the spread of toxins and infection, but if the area isn't cleared of fluid, the swelling becomes continuous.

The tissues in the congested area don't get enough oxygen and nutrients, and toxins also start to accumulate at the site of injury, creating a swampy condition in the tissues. This subacute disease state is associated with the tissue state of stagnation.

Chronic Tissue Depression and Hypoactivity

If healing does not occur during the subacute phase, the disease progresses into a chronic state. Here the pH and potential energy for healing diminishes further, causing tissues to become seriously underactive. Tissue function becomes greatly diminished, which corresponds to the tissue state of depression.

Tissues at this point often become pale and cool to the touch. If infection is present, however, they may be dark red or purplish in color. This is where chronic inflammation sets in along with chronic disease symptoms, as other areas of the body seek to make up for the deficient function.

Cell pH	Voltage	Tissue Condition
7.88	-50 mV	Acute Inflammation
7.61	-35 mV	Normal for kids
7.53	-30 mV	
7.44	-25 mV	Normal for adults
7.35	-20 mV	Subacute
7.26	-15 mV	Tired
7.18	-10 mV	Sick
7.09	-5 mV	Chronic
7.00	0 mV	Polarity Shift
6.83	+20 mV	Degenerative
6.48	+30 mV	Cancer occurs

Degeneration and Tissue Atrophy

When the pH of the biological terrain drops below neutral (7.0), the biological terrain moves from being alkaline to becoming acid. An acid environment doesn't have electrons to donate for healing; instead, it is hungry for electrons and draws them from surrounding tissues.

This is the same thing that free radicals do. Free radicals steal electrons from other molecules, destabilizing them. A continuous acidic environment causes the tissues to begin structurally breaking down, which is what happens in the degenerative state of disease. This is the state of tissue state of atrophy.

The Six Tissue States

The other two tissue states involve nerve function and muscle tone and are not part of the disease progression. Nevertheless, recognizing them is important as they involve flow and movement in the body.

Having explained the progression of disease, here's a summary of all six tissue states. If you can recognize these imbalances in your own or other people's bodies, you will be able to more intelligently select herbal remedies that will restore them to health.

Irritation (Hot)

Irritation is the overactive state. It is associated with fever and inflammation. When tissues are irritated, they are warm, red, and painful to the touch. They are also typically swollen. Since the body responds initially to all damage by using inflammation to sequester the injured area and call in white blood cells to clean up infection or toxins, any tissue that was recently injured will be inflamed. Inflammation and fever also accompany acute infection. In addition, all diseases that end in "itis" are inflammatory diseases, and this means they involve irritated tissues.

Remedies that help to reduce this inflammation, heat, or fever are said to be *cooling*, which means they are typically anti-inflammatory, antioxidant, and febrifuge (fever-reducing). These are typically sour, mucilaginous, or bitter herbs.

Depression (Cold)

The underactive state is called depression. Here the tissues lack functional activity. They don't respond to stimulus because they aren't strong enough to respond. All hypoactive organs and tissues would be depressed organs and tissues. These tissues will typically be pale and cool to the touch. When the energy of the whole body is depressed, the pulse will be slow and often weak. The person will be tired and chill easily.

If infection is present (and bacterial and fungal infection usually doesn't settle into tissues unless they first become depressed), the area may be a dark red or purplish color and there may be heat, but the heat is due to the microbial activity, not the activity of the tissues.

This is the tissue state of chronic inflammation, which is now thought to be at the root of all chronic and degenerative disease. Remedies that correct this tissue state are said to be *warming* and include pungent and aromatic herbs, some acrid herbs (known as diffusives), and some sweet tonic herbs. Essential oils primarily work on depressed tissues as well. These remedies help awaken these weakened tissues back into activity.

Stagnation (Damp)

The damp state is called stagnation. It is characterized by swollen tissues, which can take the form of swelling after injury, edema, or congested lymph nodes. Swelling often accompanies inflammation and will persist if the injured tissue doesn't heal properly. With just a little practice, it's easy to feel when tissues are swollen. They feel spongy or water logged.

The lack of fluid movement in the tissues creates a type of swampy environment. It's a toxic environment, which has also been called torpor. Remedies that reduce stagnation or torpor have traditionally been called alteratives or blood purifiers. They are diuretic and/or lymph moving in nature and tend to be *drying*. They can also be thought of as cleansing or detoxifying. Bitter or salty herbs are the primary drying remedies, but astringents, aromatics, and pungent herbs are also drying.

Atrophy (Dry)

Atrophy is the final result of unhealed tissue damage. In this stage of disease, tissues begin to dry out, become with-

"Remedies" section of this book are classified based on their type and their energetics. Here's how this system works.

Based on the six tissue states, Thomas Easley and I developed a system of classifying herbal remedies according to their basic actions. These nine basic energetic classifications are used to balance the six tissue states and are defined in three categories, as follows.

Remedies Affecting Function

Herbs can affect how the body functions metabolically, either speeding up or slowing down metabolism. A higher metabolism causes tissues to become not only more active but also physically warmer, while a lower metabolism causes tissues to become less active and physically cooler.

Cooling

Herbs that are classified as cooling are herbs that reduce tissue irritation. They are typically anti-inflammatory, fever-reducing (febrifuge), and/or antioxidant. Most herbs in this are sour, bitter and/or mucilant. Cooling can also be used to describe herbs that are calming to body functions—that is they reduce hyperactivity (overactivity) of organs and tissues.

Warming

Remedies that are classified as warming have the opposite energy of herbs that are cooling and are used to counteract tissue depression. Warming herbs stimulate tissue activity and help to overcome tissues that have become hypoactive (underactive). Remedies in this category are typically aromatic or pungent, but some sweet herbs also have a warming quality.

Neutral

Some herbs are neither warming nor cooling but rather promote a balanced metabolism. These remedies are said to be neutral and can be used with both tissue irritation and depression.

Remedies Affecting Structure

Herbs also affect the structure of the body that maintains a balance between rigidity (tone) and fluidity. High rigidity is associated with dryness, a loss of water and fats in the tissues. High fluidity is associated with dampness, where the tissues are swollen and water-logged.

Drying

Remedies that are drying are used to clear lymphatic congestion and promote the excretion of excess water through the kidneys. They counteract the tissue state of stagnation or dampness, reducing edema, relieving swelling, and shrinking swollen lymph nodes. Bitter herbs are the primary drying agents, although astringents, aromatic, and pungent herbs also tend to be drying.

Moistening

Remedies that are moistening help to restore normal flexibility and softness to tissues that have become too hard, brittle, or dry. They counteract the tissue state of atrophy and help to rebuild tissue that has started to degenerate. Herbs that are oily, mucilaginous, and sweet tend to counteract atrophy and dryness.

Balancing

Some remedies help to balance both dry and damp tissue. Primarily salty herbs, these remedies will help both stagnation and atrophy. Salty herbs supply mineral electrolytes, which help rebuild weakened tissue and also move stagnant fluid.

Remedies Affecting Tone

Remedies that affect tone help muscles and tissues to either tighten up when they are too loose or relax when they are too tense. This helps control the flow of fluids and movement in the body.

Relaxing

Remedies that are relaxing help muscles to relax, relieving tension, spasticity, and cramping. This allows fluids to flow more freely through the body. Relaxing herbs can dilate arteries to lower blood pressure, dilate bronchi to ease breathing, or open sweat glands to induce perspiration. They also assist muscle movement by reducing tension in the muscles. This can also relieve spastic, shooting pains caused by constriction and cramping of tissues. Antispasmodics and some aromatics and bitters that act as relaxing nervines exhibit this action.

Constricting

The primary constricting remedies are astringents. These tighten tissues that have become too loose and are allowing fluids to leak. Constricting remedies can act as styptics to control bleeding, can reduce mucus secretion, stop excess sweating, relieve urinary incontinence, and counteract diarrhea. They can also reduce swelling.

Nourishing

Remedies that work primarily by supplying nutrients tissues need to repair themselves and maintain normal cellular functions are nourishing. Like balancing or neutral herbs, they are remedies that help to nutritionally restore balance to the biological terrain.

Twelve Basic Categories of Herbs

To further aid a person's understanding of herbs and how they work, I've created a system of twelve basic categories of herbs. Here's an overview of these categories, which are based primarily on an herb's taste, smell and texture.

It's actually quite amazing how much you can learn about the actions of an herb just by using your senses. This is because the herbs primary constituents, which are the second factor in each category, are the chemicals your senses are detecting.

These chemicals give the herb its third basis of classification, which is its primary actions or medicinal properties. Each herb has its own unique properties, but it also has general properties that work to balance the body's tissue states and organs.

It's easiest to think of this in relationship to food. Different foods have their unique characteristics, but they also fall into broad categories, like leafy green vegetables, starchy foods, proteins, and so forth. If you're looking for a starchy food you can choose between a variety of them, such as grains, potatoes, and yams, and still get the starch your body needs. Likewise, if you want a green salad, you can use lettuce, spinach, baby beet greens, or kale. If it's protein you can have fish, poultry, red meat, dairy, eggs, or legumes.

Here are the twelve basic categories of herbs with a description of their sensory characteristics (taste, smell and texture). This is followed by their energetics (how they affect the biological terrain of the body) and the primary constituents that give them these characteristics and basic actions.

Acrid Herbs

Acrid herbs have a bitter, nasty, burning taste and are one of the least pleasant remedies to take in liquid form. Their primary action is relaxing, which means they relieve the tissue state of constriction. Their action is opposite that of astringents, which tighten tissue. In addition to being relaxing, acrid herbs may also be cooling, drying, and diffusive (meaning they help open up and move things). Their principal active constituents are resins and alkaloids.

Terrain	Action	Effect
Remedies for Tissue Function	Cooling	Reduces irritation
	Neutral	No effect
	Warming	Relieves depression
Remedies for Tissue Density	Drying	Relieves stagnation
	Balancing	Balances fluids and solids
	Moistening	Relieves atrophy
Remedies for Tissue Tone	Relaxing	Relieves constriction
	Nourishing	Supports tissue health
	Constricting	Relieves relaxation

Aromatic Herbs

These are herbs with a large amount of volatile or essential oil, giving them a strong fragrance. Aromatics are stimulating (warming) and drying. They help to remove moisture and stagnation from tissues acting as carminatives, diaphoretics, and digestive stimulants. They can also have nervine properties. Aromatics help overcome tissue depression.

Astringent Herbs

Astringent herbs have a slightly bitter flavor accompanied by a drying, puckering sensation in the mouth. This is due to the presence of tannins. There are also some saponins and alkaloids that have constricting or toning effects that, like tannins, help to arrest discharge and bleeding and shrink swollen tissues.

Bitter Stimulant Herbs (Alkaloidal Bitters)

These are herbs with a bitter taste that have stimulating or metabolic-boosting properties. They are stimulating, which means they are initially warming or energizing, but lead to energy discharge and a cooling effect. They are also drying. Their primary constituents are alkaloids (like caffeine) with stimulating effects.

Fragrant Bitter Herbs

The presence of a bitter taste coupled with a strong aroma is what characterizes these herbs, which often contain sesquiterpene lactones or triterpenes. They are warming and drying and act as strong digestive stimulants. Many are antiparasitic, and a few act as relaxing nervines.

Mucilant Herbs

These herbs are recognized primarily by texture, rather than taste or smell. They have a slippery, slimy texture when moist, coupled with a bland or slightly sweet flavor. This is due to mucopolysaccharides (mucilage and gums) and glycosaminoglycans, which give these plants cooling, moistening, and soothing effects. They help with tissue irritation and atrophy (hot and dry conditions).

Oily Herbs

These herbs have a slightly oily nature and texture due to the presence of vegetable oils. They typically contain essential fatty acids (omega-3 or omega-6) and/or medium chain saturated fatty acids. They are cooling, moistening, and nourishing in nature. They can also be lubricating. They counteract dryness and heat, relieving the tissue states of atrophy and irritation.

Pungent Herbs

These are spicy herbs with a biting aroma and a spicy, burning taste. They are closely related to aromatics but owe their actions to oleoresins, allylsulfides, alkamides, and essential oils with monoterpenes. They are very warming (stimulating) and drying, counteracting tissue depression.

Relaxing Bitter Herbs

These are bitter-tasting herbs that have relaxing or loosening qualities. They often stimulate elimination via laxative or diuretic actions. They may contain compounds like diterpenes, glycosides, anthraquinone glycosides, and some alkaloids. They are cooling and drying in nature and help overcome stagnation.

Salty Herbs

The taste of salty in herbs is a mild, grassy flavor with a weak salty flavor that takes practice for one to learn to detect. These herbs contain minerals, specifically salts of magnesium, potassium, sodium, and calcium. This makes them balancing to moisture in the body. They may relieve either stagnation or atrophy or both. They also support kidney and lymphatic function and help build structures like bones and teeth.

Sour Herbs

Herbs with a puckering, sour flavor, like lemons, signal the presence of fruit acids, like vitamin C (ascorbic acid), malic acid, and citric acid, as well as flavonoids. They typically have antioxidant properties that cool and soothe irritated tissues. They are also nourishing and can be fluid balancing.

Sweet (Tonic) Herbs

Sweet or tonic herbs typically have a mildly sweet flavor, sometimes having a slightly bitter quality as well. There sweetness could be compared to that of dark chocolate. They contain polysaccharides, saponins, and glycosides and are typically used to build up weakened conditions and overcome atrophy. They may also be adaptogenic or slightly nutritive.

Tips for Using Remedies

Selecting appropriate specific remedies skillfully takes practice and experience, but understanding biological terrain and the actions of herbs will help you develop this skill more rapidly. Don't be afraid to experiment, however. Unless otherwise indicated, the remedies in this guide are extremely safe, but here are some additional guidelines that will help you.

Don't try to do too many things at once. It can be overwhelming to make too many dietary changes or to take too many supplements. If your plan feels burdensome or overwhelming, pare it down to something you can comfortably handle. Otherwise, you are unlikely to follow through with the program.

This includes limiting the herbs and supplements you pick. There seems to be an almost-universal belief that "if a little is good, more is better." This is rarely the case. I've found that people who take too many herbs and nutritional supplements generally don't get good results. It's a good idea to start with no more than two to four formulas or supplements. If you take too many supplements it's difficult to tell what is working and what is not.

When putting a program together to resolve a health problem, you need to monitor progress. Try keeping a journal or log where you can make notes about changes you observe. For serious health problems, I recommend working with a competent health practitioner. (You can search for one at findanherbalist.com or on the website for the American Herbalist's Guild (americanherbalistsguild.com/member-profiles).

How Quickly Should You See Results?

People have been told that herbs and supplements are slow acting, so they will often take an herbal formula or supplement for a month or more without seeing any results. Herbs and supplements work faster than that!

The perception that herbs and supplements work slowly is due to the difference between healing and symptomatic relief. Drugs generally offer rapid symptomatic relief, but rarely do they actually restore a person's health. Herbs and supplements may not offer rapid symptomatic relief, but they can actually restore a person's health.

Healing takes time. There is no instant relief when it comes to healing a wound or a broken bone. The process takes time. The same is true for healing from chronic or degenerative conditions. It can take months to experience substantial recovery; however, it doesn't take months to start seeing results.

Generally speaking, herbs actually work quite rapidly in terms of speeding the healing process. So here's a general guide to when you should start seeing results.

With acute conditions, such as colds, flu, and minor injuries, you'll generally see improvement in anywhere from two to eight hours. If you see no improvement after twenty-four hours, what you're using probably isn't working. In this case, try something else. If the herb or supplement is helpful, you can take it until symptoms are gone, and then generally for one to two more days to make sure everything has completely returned to normal.

With chronic conditions, you will usually notice some improvement in two to five days if the herb or supplement is helpful. If you see no improvement after ten days, then the herb or supplement you are taking probably isn't going to work, and you can re-evaluate your strategy and try something different. If the herb or supplement is helpful, then you can resume taking it and continue until the problem resolves itself. Once the problem is resolved, it is often helpful to continue taking it at a slightly lower dose for an additional two to four weeks. You will probably need to take the supplements for at least three to six months (and occasionally a year or two) for a complete recovery.

If symptoms recur after discontinuing the product, you can start using the supplement again until symptoms subside. Then you may need to stay on a lower dose for several months to a year.

With serious degenerative diseases, such as cancer, heart disease, and diabetes, it may be hard to detect any subjectively noticeable improvement for a couple of weeks. This is why some type of objective monitoring is necessary to help determine if the program is working. This could be monitoring a person's bloodwork, their appearance and energy level, or other observable signs. If you see no improvement after four weeks, the program probably isn't working and the strategy needs to be reevaluated.

With these serious diseases it is generally insufficient to expect herbs or supplements alone to restore a person to health. Attitude changes, lifestyle changes and a proper diet are essential to restoring health.

Don't give up if you don't get it right the first time you try. Even well-trained, experienced practitioners don't always get a program right on the first try. In traditional Chinese medicine (TCM) it has been said that the first prescription is part of the diagnosis. The reason doctors *practice* medicine, is that they do the same thing. If their first prescription doesn't work, they reevaluate and try something different. There's no harm in doing the same thing yourself, or others, as long as you're using nontoxic herbs and supplements.

Adjusting Dosages

Herbal formulas and nutritional supplements are accompanied by a manufacturer's suggested dose. Assume that this dose is meant for an average-size adult (about 150 pounds). If you are larger, you may need a slightly higher dose; smaller, you may need a lower dose. If you are sensitive to substances, you may need to start with a lower dose too.

If the herb or supplement is safe for children (and there is no suggested dose for children), adjust the dose by weight. So for a 50 pound child, take one-third of the suggested adult dose. For smaller children take one-fourth to one-fifth of the recommended adult dose. For larger children, adjust the dose upward.

Dosages with herbs are not as critical as they are with drugs because the potential for adverse reactions is much smaller. In addition, most manufacturers recommend conservative, safe doses for the general public. In many cases, you can safely double (or even triple) the recommended dosage. Still, when trying a new supplement it is a good idea to start with a smaller dose, make sure you tolerate the product well, and then adjust the dose upward if the supplement is having a positive effect but the dose isn't quite strong enough.

Dealing with Negative Reactions

Everyone is biochemically different and even with relatively safe herbs and supplements, people will sometimes react negatively to a product. The most common adverse effects of herbs are digestive upset, nausea, diarrhea, and headaches. Skin rashes can also occur. These reactions are not life-threatening, so don't be alarmed; however, don't ignore them either.

These signs are often symptoms of rapid detoxification—meaning you're detoxifying too quickly. If these reactions occur, stop taking the herbs or supplements, drink lots of water, and wait a few days. When symptoms have subsided, you can try taking the supplement in a lower dose. If symptoms reappear, stop taking the herb, formula, or supplement and don't take it again as you may have an allergy or intolerance to it. Otherwise, you can gradually increase the dose.

Unskilled herbalists sometimes blame all adverse reactions on a detoxification process; however, both herbs and nutritional supplements can have adverse reactions in some people. Examples of adverse reactions include (but are not limited to) increased anxiety, bloating, increased heart rate, increased blood pressure, and dizziness. Again, these reactions are not life-threatening, but they are signs that the supplement or herb should be immediately discontinued.

If you go off the herb or supplement for a couple of days, the symptoms generally will stop (unless they are being caused by something other than the herb or supplement). To double-check if the herb or supplement was actually at fault (sometimes these apparent reactions are just coincidences), you can again try the herb or supplement at a lower dose, as described above.

If you have questions about adverse reactions, you may wish to consult with a competent herbalist. (If you don't know a competent herbalist, you can search for one at findanherbalist.com or americanherbalistsguild.com.) Medical doctors generally know very little about herbs, and have limited training in nutrition, so they are usually not reliable sources of information on herbs or nutritional supplements.

Index of Systems

Section Two

Systems

Using the Body Systems, Organs & Tissues and the Chinese Energetic System for Healing

In the introduction I discussed the importance of working with biological terrain and body systems instead of trying to treat diseases. In this section, we cover indications for the six basic biological terrain imbalances and remedies that help each of them. We also introduce the eleven major body systems and discuss the indications for basic imbalances in each of them. We also include remedies for specific organs and tissues within that system.

Most body systems have a section that helps you identify the six tissue terrains from the biological terrain model for that system. Remedies to rebalance these biological terrain issues for that system are listed under each terrain. Some systems also contain information on enhancing or inhibiting specific chemical messengers (such as hormones or neurotransmitters) within that system.

The exceptions are the nervous, glandular, reproductive, immune, and endocannabinoid system (found under other systems and organs), which do not fit the biological terrain model. These systems are generally broken down into various parts that may be over active or under active.

There is also a section on health patterns in traditional Chinese medicine, which I have also found helpful in balancing a person's constitution and improving their overall health. Again there are indications for each imbalance and a list of remedies to correct them.

Remedies for Biological Terrain

The human body can be divided into eleven major systems. Each of these systems contributes something to the body as a whole, and each system is dependent on all the other systems of the body to work properly. If one system becomes damaged, all systems are adversely affected and overall health suffers. Thus, improving the health of one weak system improves the health of the body as a whole.

Most body systems have a section that helps you identify the six tissue terrains from the biological terrain model for that system. Remedies to rebalance these biological terrain issues for that system are listed under each terrain.

The exceptions are the nervous, glandular, reproductive, immune, and endocannabinoid system (found under other systems and organs), which do not fit the biological terrain model. These systems are generally broken down into various parts that may be over-active or under-active.

Many systems also contain listings for remedies for specific organs or tissues within that system. Some systems also contain information on enhancing or inhibiting specific chemical messengers (such as hormones or neurotransmitters) within that system.

We have a set of ABC+D Body Systems charts that show this material in simplified form which you can purchase if you wish to learn this system. There is also a course, the ABC+D Approach to Natural Healing which can train you further in understanding how to do this.

On the next the pages you will find a copy of the Body System's Questionnaire, which is a simple tool you can use to see which body systems need the most support. Pads of these questionnaires are available at stevenhorne.com if you wish to use them in consulting. For personal use, you can simply copy these pages and fill them out for yourself or your family members.

Once you determine which system(s) are the weakest, look up that system and see if you can identify the correct biological terrain imbalance(s) so you can select effective remedies. The systems are listed in the order they are found on the questionnaire, and not in alphabetical order.

The Body Systems Questionnaire

Instructions: Read through the items listed on the left hand side of the table, if it applies to you circle all the numbers on the row to the right of it. If it doesn't or you don't know don't mark anything. Some questions only apply to men ( ) or women ( ). When you have finished reviewing the list, total all the numbers you have circled in each column.

	1	2	3	4	5	6	7	8	9	10	11	12	13
Absent-mindedness or memory loss						1	2				1		
Acid indigestion, heartburn or acid reflux	2						1						
Anger, irritability, easily upset		2				1	1					1	
Anxiety, nervousness or excessive fear	1				1		2				2		
Arthritis, joint pains, joint stiffness			1		1		2						
Asthma	1		1	3			1		1				
Bad breath or body odor			1		1								
Brittle nails or other nail problems	1						2						
Burning or painful urination					2							1	2
Cholesterol over 275 mg/dL		1				1		1	4	2			
Cholesterol under 175 mg/dL		1					2	1			2	1	2
Chronic fatigue or lack of stamina	1			1		1	1	1	2		1		1
Chronic muscle tension or muscle cramps						1	2						
Chronic or frequent dry cough		1	2				1						
Chronic post nasal drip	1		1	2			1						
Cold hands and feet, low body temperature						1			5				
Cold sores or mouth ulcers (canker sores)	1						1						
COPD, emphysema, chronic lung disease	1		1	3			1	2					
Coughing yellow or green mucus			2				1						
Cravings for fats or fatty foods		1				1				2			
Cravings for sweets or sugary foods	1									4	2		
Dark circles under eyes				1			1		1				
Depression, feeling down or discouraged		1	1				1		3		1		2
Diabetes, blood sugar over 90 mg/dL	1	1				1	2			5	1	1	
Difficulty breathing, shortness of breath			1	3			1						
Difficulty getting to sleep		1				2							
Difficulty starting urination					1								3
Dizzy or light headed						1	1				1	1	
Dry skin		1					1		3				
Eczema, psoriasis or severe acne		2			1		2	1	1	1	1	1	1
Erectile dysfunction					1								3
Excess mucous production			1	2									
Excessive intestinal gas, flatulence	2	1	2				1						
Family history of diabetes		1				1				2			
Family history of heart disease						2							
Page 1 Totals													

	1	2	3	4	5	6	7	8	9	10	11	12
Feeling burned out or exhausted							1		1		2		1
Food allergies	2	1						2				
Food sits heavy on stomach after meals	2		1									
Frequent belching or bloating	1	1	2					1				
Frequent mental and emotional stress	1						2				2	1
Frequent mood swings, moody		1	1				1			2	2	1
Frequent neck and shoulder pain							1	1				
Frequent nighttime urination				2							2	3
Frequent thirst, dry mouth	1		1		1					3	1	
Frequent urge to urinate, frequent urination				3				1				2
General feeling of weakness, lingering chronic illness	2	1	1					2	2	1	1	1
Grief, sadness, self-pity				2		1	1		1			
Gingivitis, gum disease, bleeding gums						2		1				
Groggy or tired feelings in the morning	1	2					1				1	
Hair loss or thinning	1					1		1		3		
Hard dry stool or straining to eliminate		2										
Hay fever, respiratory allergies, allergic rhinitis	1		1	3				1				
Headache, feeling of pressure or tension	1						1	1				
Headaches, migraines with pounding or throbbing pain		2				1	1					
Heavy menstrual bleeding		1						1			2	
Hemorrhoid or anal fistula		1	2			1		1				
High blood pressure, hypertension					1	2	1			2		
Hot flashes and night sweats										1	1	3
Infertility							1		1		2	3
Inflammatory bowel disorders, colitis, Crohn's disease			2					1		1		
Irregular heart rate (arrhythmia)						2	1					
Irregular menstrual cycle							1		1		1	1
Itchy nose, ears or skin		1	1	1				1				
Kidney stones, calcium deposits				2								
Leg cramps, restless leg syndrome				1		1	2					
Less than 1 bowel elimination per day	1		2					1				
Loose stool or diarrhea			2									
Loss of appetite or poor appetite	2		1				1					
Loss of self confidence and motivation		1					1				1	2
Loss of sexual desire							1		3		1	3	3
Lower back pain					1			2				
Menstrual cramps							1	1			2	
Muddled thinking or mental confusion			1				1		3	1	2	1	1
Muscle pain and stiffness					1			2				
Page 2 Totals												

	Digestive	Hepatic	Intestinal	Respiratory	Urinary	Circulatory	Nervous	Structural	Immune	Thyroid	Pancreas	Adrenal	Female Reproductive	Male Reproductive
Muscle weakness or weak legs, knees					1	1		2						
Night sweats					1							1	3	
Osteoporosis, weakening of the bones					1			2					1	
Overweight, difficulty losing weight	2	1					1			3	3			2
Pain in mid to upper back				1		1		2						
Pain or tension in the chest		1		1		1								
Pale complexion or anemia	1					1			1					
Premenstrual syndrome, PMS		1											3	
Prostate problems		1												3
Puffiness under the eyes					2							1		
Rapid heart rate (tachycardia)						1	1			1				
Respiratory infections (frequent)	1		1	2					2					
Restless disturbed sleep, frequent waking		1			1		1					2		1
Restless dreams or nightmares		1										1		
Scanty urination or dark colored urine					2									
Sinus headaches			1	2										
Sinusitis or chronic sinus congestion			1	2					1					
Skin ulcerations or wounds not healing						1		2	1		2			
Swollen lymph nodes		1	1	2					2					
Triglycerides over 200 mg/dL		1				1				3	1			
Underweight or unable to gain weight	2						1	1		1	1			
Urinary tract infections (frequent)					3				1				1	
Vaginal discharge, infection									2				2	
Vaginal dryness													2	
Varicose veins or spider veins		2				2			1					
Water retention or edema				1	3	1							1	
Totals from Page 3														
Totals from Page 1														
Totals from Page 2														
Grand Totals														
Body System	Digestive	Hepatic	Intestinal	Respiratory	Urinary	Circulatory	Nervous	Structural	Immune	Thyroid	Pancreas	Adrenal	Female Reproductive	Male Reproductive

0-5 points	This system **probably doesn't need** any specific herbal and/or nutritional support
5-15 points	This system **may need** some general herbal and/or nutritional support
15-25 points	This system **could probably** benefit from some specific herbal and/or nutritional support
25-35 points	This system is in **critical need** of specific herbal and/or nutritional support

This quiz is from *Strategies for Health* – ©2021 Tree of Light – stevenhorne.com

General Irritation   *Overactive/Hot*

Irritation is the easiest of all tissue imbalances to recognize because it is the body's initial response to all damage. Anytime the body suffers injury, tissues respond through a process called inflammation. In the case of infection, the body may also respond to the irritation with fever. So fever and inflammation are the imbalances in biological terrain we are calling tissue irritation.

As the term in-*flame*-ation suggests, damaged tissues become hyper or overheated, because whatever is damaging the tissues is irritating them. It doesn't matter what the nature of the irritation is (pathogen, toxin, or mechanical stress); the tissues go into a hyper-state of function to discharge the irritant and affect repairs.

These irritated tissues feel hot to the touch and will also appear red. Redness is a major sign of irritation, whether it is a bright-red tongue or a flushed, red face. Swelling and pain are also associated with inflammation and the irritated tissue state. The pain associated with irritation is acute and typically feels sharp or stabbing.

The suffix *itis* is Latin for *inflammation*. So many disease names are simply Latin terms telling us where the inflammation or irritation is located. For example, tonsillitis (inflamed tonsils) appendicitis (inflamed appendix), or arthritis (inflamed joint).

Irritated tissues need to be cooled and soothed. Traditional herbal remedies for irritated tissues are often sour in taste, which is a possible sign of plants with high antioxidant properties. Burning is an oxidative process, so when tissues are burning (en-flamed) antioxidants, which are also typically anti-inflammatory, are indicated.

A scarlet or magenta colored tongue, an elevated temperature and a rapid pulse are major signs of systemic irritation. In addition, the pH tends to become overalkaline.

Indications for General Irritation

Tissues: Red, warm, usually swollen

Tongue: Red, often pointed or elongated

Pulse: Rapid, often floating

Pain: Acute, often sharp

Emotional State: Restless, agitated, irritated, angry, aggressive, frustrated

Iridology: White fibers

The following cooling and soothing remedies can help.

Formulas: Anti-Inflammatory Pain, Antioxidant, and Chinese Yang-Reducing

Herbs: Açaí, **aloe vera**, andrographis, bilberry, chrysanthemum, cranberry, devil's claw, **elderberry**, elderflower, forsythia, grape seed extract, hawthorn, honeysuckle, **lemon**, **lycium**, **mangosteen**, noni, rose hips, **turmeric**, willow bark, and yarrow

Supplements: Alpha-lipoic acid, Co-Q10, curcumin, MSM, vitamin A, **vitamin C**, and vitamin E

Essential Oils: Chamomile (Roman), helichrysum, and rose

General Depression   *Underactive/Cold*

When we speak of tissue depression, we're not talking about feeling emotionally down; we're referring to a state where tissues are sluggish and not responding appropriately to irritation. The overall symptoms of tissue depression include a general feeling of tissue coolness and fatigue. Any part of the body that appears pale or excessively white and feels cool to the touch is depressed. So a tired person, with a pale complexion and cool skin, has a depressed biological terrain.

Low-grade irritation is sometimes present with tissue depression, but the tissue color is purplish or blackish (such as the color of a bruise) and there is still coolness and fatigue. This is a state of chronic, low-grade inflammation, not the acute inflammation that follows immediately after injury. In addition, all organs that are underactive, as in hypothyroidism (low or depressed thyroid activity), are depressed organs.

To restore balance to the biological terrain depressed tissues must be stimulated or warmed. This is typically done with pungent or aromatic herbs, such as capsicum and ginger. All essential oils are also warming in the sense that they stimulate sluggish tissues back into activity.

Slow pulse, pale tongue, and chronic weakness are all signs of systemic depression. The pH tends to be overly acid in tissue depression.

Indications for General Depression

Tissues: Pale, cool to the touch, but may also be slightly warm and purplish-red (like a bruise)

Tongue: Pale, whitish or dark reddish purple

Pulse: Slow, often deep

Pain: Chronic, usually dull

Emotional State: Lethargic, tired, discouraged, overwhelmed, depressed

Iridology: Dark fibers

The following warming and stimulating remedies can help.

Formulas: Circulatory, **Mitochondria Energy,** and Topical Analgesic

Herbs: Capsicum, cinnamon, clove, **garlic, ginger,** guarana, guggul, horseradish, juniper berries, **oregano,**

peppermint, **rosemary**, sweet annie, tea, green or black, **thyme**, and yerba maté

Supplements: **Vitamin B-complex**, vitamin B_1, **vitamin B_{12}**, vitamin B_2, and vitamin B_3

Essential Oils: Atlas cedarwood, **cinnamon**, clove, juniper, lemon, peppermint, rosemary, spearmint, and wintergreen

General Stagnation   *Torpid/Damp*

Just think of a swamp and you'll immediately have the intuitive understanding of this tissue condition. The tissues are bogged down with stagnant fluid, creating a toxic environment around the cells. Fluid retention, swollen lymph nodes, congested lungs and sinuses, and a sluggish digestive tract are all examples of stagnant conditions in the tissues.

A stagnant biological terrain was traditionally considered to be the underlying cause of many health problems, such as skin-eruptive diseases like acne, rashes, and eczema. It has also been traditionally linked with the development of growths like boils, uterine fibroids, cystic breasts, and even tumors.

The eclectic doctors in the Western herbal tradition called this tissue state torpor. They called the herbs that removed this stagnation alteratives. Alteratives have also been called blood purifiers. They are indicated whenever the body is damp, swollen, congested, and toxic.

You can identify stagnation by any kind of swelling or congestion. This includes edema, swollen lymph nodes, and cysts. Oily skin and hair and excess mucus production are also signs of stagnation.

In stagnation, there are insufficient mineral salts to keep fluids moving. Salty herbs, rich in mineral electrolytes, and simple bitters are generally indicated in tissue stagnation.

Indications for General Stagnation

Tissues: Swollen, spongy, water-logged, whitish when depressed

Tongue: Swollen and damp, often with scalloped edges, may have a heavy mucus coating

Pulse: Rolling or slippery

Pain: Dull, congestive

Emotional State: Sad, grieving, fearful, hurt, sluggish

Iridology: Uric acid diathesis, straw yellow color, hydrogenoid subtype

The following drying and cleansing remedies can help.

Formulas: Ayurvedic Skin Healing, **Detoxifying**, Hepatoprotective, **Lymph Cleansing**, and Lymphatic Infection

Herbs: Alfalfa, black walnut, **burdock**, chickweed, **dandelion**, **echinacea**, gentian, goldenseal, **milk thistle**,

myrrh, neem, Oregon grape, **red clover**, **turmeric**, **yellow dock**, and yucca

Supplements: Bacillus coagulans, **berberine**, and N-acetyl cysteine

Essential Oils: Cajeput, eucalyptus, **frankincense**, juniper, **myrrh**, pine, and tea tree

General Atrophy   *Rigid/Dry*

The opposite condition to stagnation, atrophy involves an accumulation of minerals with a loss of fluid in the form of water or fat (oil). This occurs with increasing frequency as people age. The bodies of young children tend to be moist, supple, and very flexible, but as people age, they come increasingly dry, withered, and stiff. The skin becomes increasingly dry and wrinkled, joints become painful and inflexible due to a lack of lubrication, and mobility and all parts of the body begin to lose fluidity and function.

This state, which we call atrophy, isn't due to just a lack of water, although dehydration can be a factor that contributes to atrophy. It's also due to a lack of lubricating healthy fats and fat-soluble vitamins, as well as increasing imbalances in metabolism due to the disrupted glandular functions that are part of what is now called metabolic syndrome.

Mineral deposits such as stones and bone spurs and the loss of movement and flexibility are major signs of systemic atrophy. Hardening of any tissue and general degeneration of tissues are also part of tissue atrophy.

Tissue atrophy is primarily corrected using oily, mucilant, or sweet herbs. Some salty alteratives may also be helpful.

Indications for General Atrophy

Tissues: Dry, shrunken, cracked, brittle, hard

Tongue: Dry, often cracked or fissured, may appear shriveled, often dark purple or reddish-black in color

Pulse: Thin, weak and/or deep

Pain: None or chronic, stiff, achy, constant

Emotional State: Rigid, inflexible, hardened, insensitive

Iridology: Dark-brown or black pigments, crypts, stairstep or honeycomb lacuna

The following moistening and building remedies can help.

Formulas: Chinese Earth-Increasing, **Chinese Qi and Blood Tonic**, GLA Oil, Herbal Calcium, Intestinal Soothing, and **Vulnerary**

Herbs: Aloe vera, astragalus, black currant oil, borage oil, **cordyceps**, dulse, evening primrose oil, **ginseng (American)**, **ginseng (Asian/Korean)**, he shou wu, horsetail, Irish moss, **licorice**, **marshmallow**, mullein, oat straw, plantain, psyllium, rehmannia, reishi, **slippery elm**, wild yam, and yam (Chinese)

Supplements: Omega-3 DHA, omega-3 EPA, omega-6 GLA, **vitamin A**, vitamin B₁₂, **vitamin D**, and **vitamin E**

Essential Oils: Anise, fennel, grapefruit (pink), orange (sweet), patchouli, and red mandarin

General Constriction *Spastic/Tense*

Constriction refers to an excess of tension or tone of muscles. The obvious example of this is muscle cramps or spasms, but there are many other conditions caused by the tissue state of constriction.

Constriction inhibits flow, so high blood pressure is a sign of constriction in the arteries. Sharp, shooting pains are also signs of constriction. Chronic stiffness and high anxiety are also associated with constriction.

By blocking flow and movement, constriction can create conditions that are jerky, sudden, unpredictable, irregular, and alternating, something the Chinese call "wind" disorders. These include problems like alternating diarrhea and constipation or alternating chills and fever. Anytime you have a condition that moves around or shifts from one extreme to another, tissue constriction may be involved.

Constriction is corrected by acrid herbs with an antispasmodic action or aromatic or bitter nervines that help tissues relax. Magnesium is typically deficient in systemic tissue constriction.

Indications for General Constriction

Tissues: Spastic, tense, cramped

Tongue: Quivering

Pulse: Wiry or tense

Pain: Sharp, stabbing, or shooting, often migrating from one location to another

Emotional State: Stressed, tired, overwhelmed, anxious, nervous, high-strung, reckless

Iridology: Contraction furrows, tight collarette

The following relaxing remedies can help.

Formulas: Antispasmodic Ear, Antispasmodic, Chinese Fire-Decreasing, Fibromyalgia, and Jeannie Burgess' Stress

Herbs: Agrimony, black cohosh, black haw, chamomile, cramp bark, hops, **kava kava, lobelia,** mimosa, motherwort, passion flower, valerian, vervain (blue), and **wild yam**

Supplements: Magnesium and vitamin B-complex

Essential Oils: Chamomile (Roman), clary sage, **jasmine, lavender, marjoram, rose,** and ylang ylang

General Relaxation *Atonic/Loose*

Relaxation is a loose or atonic state of the tissues that is characterized by an excess flow of fluids. Copious discharges of urine, mucus, or sweat, as well as bleeding and watery diarrhea are all signs of an overly relaxed biological terrain. Leaky gut syndrome, varicose veins, and hemorrhoids are also examples of tissue relaxation.

Anytime you see excessive discharge, secretion, drainage, or flow or tissues that are bleeding, oozing, seeping or leaking there is a state of tissue relaxation. Severe localized swelling may also be a sign of relaxation.

Relaxation is corrected with astringent herbs or herbs rich in trace minerals and nutrients that help restore tone to tissues. There may be deficiencies of vitamin C and its accompanying bioflavonoids as well as calcium, silica, and other minerals.

Indications for General Relaxation

Tissues: Weak, easily damaged, excessively porous, draining or discharging fluids

Tongue: Swollen, flabby

Pulse: Non-resistant, relaxed, languid

Emotional State: Changeable, fearful, compliant, yielding, withdrawing, enabling

Iridology: Radial furrows, expanded, discolored or broken collarette, connective tissue or polyglandular type

The following toning remedies can help.

Formulas: Colloidal Mineral, Herbal Calcium, Vein Tonic, **Watkin's Hair, Skin, and and Nails**

Herbs: Bayberry, black walnut, blackberry root, **calendula, cinnamon,** eyebright, horse chestnut, **horsetail,** kudzu, lady's mantle, plantain, red raspberry, rose hips, rosemary, sage, shepherd's purse, tea, uva ursi, **white oak bark,** and **yarrow**

Supplements: Bioflavonoids, calcium, **charcoal,** clay (bentonite), collagen, silicon, and **vitamin C**

Essential Oils: Cypress, geranium, **lemon,** myrrh, and rosemary

Digestive System

Because problems with digestion are the root cause of many people's health problems, the digestive system is a great place to start. It is a common root cause of about 30-50% of most people's health problems.

The digestive system works to provide the nutrients your body needs from food in order to function. Each cell must be bathed in fluid containing amino acids, sugars, fatty acids, vitamins and minerals to carry out its work. The foods we consume contain these nutrients in more complex forms, such as proteins, starches and fats. Since the body can't utilize these nutrients in their whole form, they must be processed and digested before the bloodstream can transport them to each cell.

In the process of digestion, proteins are broken down into amino acids. Carbohydrates (starches and complex sugars) are broken down into simple sugars. Fats are broken down into fatty acids and glycerin. Fat-soluble vitamins must be made water-soluble. Minerals enter a colloidal suspension (a highly-dissolved state) and become chelated (bonded) to amino acids or fatty acids for absorption. Breaking these nutrients down into their simplest form is the responsibility of the digestive system.

The old saying, "You are what you eat" doesn't reflect the complete truth. A person could be eating the most nutrient-rich food in the world, but if his or her digestive system is too weak to break the food down and absorb it, that person would still starve. It would be more accurate to say that, "you are what you are able to digest, assimilate, and utilize from what you eat." This is why a healthy digestive system is the beginning of a healthy body, and why we focus on this system first. What good does it do to eat well or take supplements to feed and support other body systems if the digestive system can't deliver them to the bloodstream for distribution and utilization?

Common symptoms that the digestive system is a primary system to work on include the following:

Indications for Digestive System

- Abdominal pain or discomfort
- Acid indigestion, heartburn or acid reflux (GERD)
- Bloating, belching or intestinal gas
- Cravings for sugary foods
- Food allergies
- Frequent problems with bad breath
- Frequent indigestion or stomachache
- Groggy feeling in the morning
- Heavy feeling in stomach after meals
- Loss of appetite or poor appetite
- Loss of smell or taste
- Under weight or unable to gain weight

Digestive Irritation   *Overactive/Hot*

Digestive irritation is where the stomach, duodenum, or esophagus is inflamed and/or the stomach is hyperactive in its acidic secretions. This generally occurs in younger people and is often caused by stress, eating on the run, overeating, dehydration, or over-consumption of spicy foods. Although ulceration is part of digestive irritation, it is also a condition of atrophy in this case and many of the remedies for digestive atrophy are more helpful.

Staying hydrated, eating smaller meals in a relaxed environment, and avoiding spicy foods will help. It also helps to be careful with the combinations of foods you eat.

Indications for Digestive Irritation

Iridology: Bright white stomach zone

Tongue: Red (especially in the center), often pointed or elongated

Pulse: Generally rapid, possibly floating

Emotional State: Difficulty relaxing, getting absorbed in study or work

- Acute acid reflux, heartburn
- Digestive upset with good appetite
- Food digests quickly
- Rapid colon transit time
- Digestive upset immediately after eating
- Person generally young, under the age of thirty
- Discomfort or pain from stimulants, spicy or pungent foods

The following cooling and soothing remedies can help.

Formulas: Children's Colic, Christopher's Gallbladder, and H. Pylori-Fighting

Herbs: Catnip, **chamomile**, cherry, **fennel**, licorice, marshmallow, **meadowsweet**, sage, slippery elm, turkey rhubarb, and yarrow

Supplements: Calcium, **potassium**, sodium alginate, and sodium bicarbonate

Digestive Depression   *Underactive/Cold*

Many people who suffer from acid indigestion don't have an overactive stomach; instead, the stomach is actually underactive and there is a lack of hydrochloric acid production. This results in bacterial fermentation in the digestive tract that causes acid production.

If your indigestion occurs about an hour after eating, you may have digestive depression. Another sign is belching and bloating after meals.

A basic correction is to drink aromatic herb teas with meals or take *Digestive Bitters Formulas* twenty to thirty minutes prior to meals. Supplementation with betaine hydrochloric acid or digestive enzymes can be helpful as well as eating smaller meals and chewing food slowly and thoroughly.

Indications for Digestive Depression

Iridology: Dark stomach zone

Tongue: Dark, often with heavy yellow or brown coating

Pulse: Slow and/or weak

- Digestive upset with poor appetite
- Tendency to nausea, belching, burping
- Food sits heavy on stomach with dull, drowsy feeling after eating
- Indigestion starts about one hour after eating
- Frequent belching and/or bad taste in mouth

- Person generally older, usually over age 50
- Discomfort from eating sugary and starchy foods

The following warming and stimulating remedies can help.

Formulas: Antifungal EO, Children's Colic, **Chinese Earth-Decreasing**, **Christopher's Carminative**, Digestive Settling EO, Digestive Support, Ed Millet's Herbal Crisis, Herbal Composition, Jeannie Burgess' Allergy-Lung, **Papaya Enzyme**, and Stabilized Allicin

Herbs: Black pepper, **cardamom**, chamomile, **cinnamon**, clove, fennel, **ginger**, and **peppermint**

Supplements: Amylase and protease

Essential Oils: Peppermint

Digestive Stagnation   *Torpid/Damp*

Digestive depression and digestive stagnation often go hand in hand. In digestive stagnation there is a lack of motility in the stomach and small intestines so that food does not move rapidly enough through the digestive system. This is state also leads to imbalanced in intestinal microbes and parasites.

Aromatics and bitters stimulate both digestive secretion and digestive motility. Digestive enzymes may be helpful as well as taking Digestive Bitters Formulas twenty to thirty minutes prior to meals.

Indications for Digestive Stagnation

Iridology: Discolored stomach zone

Tongue: Swollen and damp with heavy white or yellow mucus coat, often pale

Pulse: Rolling or slippery

Emotional State: Mental obsession and worry

- Heavy feeling in stomach after eating that may last for hours
- Bad taste in the mouth
- Heavy mucus production
- Gas, bloating, belching, burping after eating
- Severe gas with sensation of abdominal pressure
- Sugar cravings
- Difficulty digesting proteins
- Heavy mucus production

The following drying and cleansing remedies can help.

Formulas: Anti-Fungal, Antifungal EO, Antiparasitic, Chinese Balanced Cleansing, **Chinese Earth-Decreasing**, Detoxifying, Digestive Settling EO, Flu and Vomiting, **Herbal Bitters**, Liver Cleanse, **Papaya Enzyme**, Plant Enzyme, Steven Horne's Children's Composition, and Yeast Cleansing

Herbs: Angelica, artichoke, chamomile, **dandelion**, **gentian**, **goldenseal**, myrrh, **orange (bitter)**, turkey rhubarb, turmeric, and yellow dock

Supplements: **Berberine**, bromelain, curcumin, and protease

Digestive Atrophy   *Rigid/Dry*

Digestive atrophy involves a weakness of the upper digestive system that results in poor digestion of food and weakness in the body as a whole. There is usually a deficiency in the production of hydrochloric acid (HCl) and enzymes as well as a lack of mucus secretions in the stomach to protect it from stomach acid. This may result in ulceration.

Don't use HCl or protease enzymes if there is ulceration. Stick to soothing mucilaginous herbs. If the problem is just digestive weakness take HCl or enzymes and make sure to drink adequate amounts of water in between meals. Try taking a pinch of natural salt with a glass of water twenty to thirty minutes prior to meals.

Indications for Digestive Atrophy

Iridology: Comb teeth, dark stomach zone

Tongue: Dry, red or pale, withered in severe cases, often with a large crack down the center

Pulse: Thin and slow, or thin and weak

Emotional State: Nervous, weak

- Poor protein and fat digestion, cravings for sugar and carbohydrates
- Thin, unable to gain weight, rapid weight loss
- Very poor appetite
- Pale, anemic-looking
- Cold limbs
- Person generally sickly or elderly

The following moistening and building remedies can help.

Formulas: **Chinese Earth-Increasing**, Chinese Wood-Decreasing, Fat-Absorbing Fiber, and Plant Enzyme

Herbs: **Aloe vera**, astragalus, **atractylodes**, **ginseng (American)**, **ginseng (Asian/Korean)**, **licorice**, marshmallow, Saint John's wort, saw palmetto, slippery elm, and wild yam

Supplements: Amylase, lipase, protease, and zinc

Digestive Constriction   *Spastic/Tense*

In digestive constriction the stomach is tense and tends to move upward into the opening in the diaphragm for the esophogus. (See the strategy *Hiatal Hernia Correction*.) This creates the symptoms listed below. This is common in people with chronic illness and poor digestion.

Indications for Digestive Constriction

Iridology: Tight collarette, contraction furrows

Pulse: Tense or wiry

Emotional State: Weak gut instincts or lack of gut instincts, chronic suppression of anger

- Difficulty swallowing
- Sensation of a lump in the throat
- Can't take an abdominal breath
- Sensations of pressure in the chest
- Tension in the solar plexus
- Bloating pains that release with belching or flatulence
- General weakness and low resistance to disease

The following relaxing remedies can help.

Formulas: Chinese Earth-Increasing and Jeannie Burgess' Stress

Herbs: Catnip, chamomile, cramp bark, **lobelia**, Saint John's wort, and wild yam

Digestive Relaxation　　　*Atonic/Loose*

Digestive relaxation is mostly found in children who spit up easily after eating. In adults there is a dull, heavy feeling in the stomach after eating, accompanied by a feeling of nausea.

Indications for Digestive Relaxation

Iridology: Loose fiber structure in stomach zone

Tongue: Thick, moist, flabby and scalloped

- Tendency for nausea and vomiting
- Heavy, full feeling even after small meals
- Thin, copious mucus secretion causing indigestion
- Indigestion in children

The following toning remedies can help.

Herbs: Bayberry, pau d'arco, plantain, and **red raspberry**

Supplements: Calcium, **charcoal**, and clay (bentonite)

Specific Digestive Tissues

The following are remedies that may help with specific digestive organs.

Esophagus　　　*Body Part*

The esophagus is the tube that goes from the mouth to the stomach, through which food is swallowed. It may be irritated by acid reflux or by substances being swallowed. It can also become constricted, inhibiting swallowing. Sipping or sucking on soothing mucilaginous herbs can soothe an irritated esophagus.

Herbs: Aloe vera, licorice, lobelia, and slippery elm

Pancreas Head　　　*Gland*

The pancreatic head secretes digestive enzymes to help digest food in the small intestines. These pancreatic enzymes

include trypsin, which breaks the protein fragments from the stomach into free amino acids; amylase, which finishes the process of breaking starches and complex sugars into simple sugars; and lipase, which breaks fats down into fatty acids and glycerin. Fats also need bile to break them down. Bile is formed in the liver and stored in the gallbladder, which squeezes it out when it is needed in digestion.

Formulas: Chinese Earth-Decreasing, Christopher's Carminative, **Digestive Support**, Flu and Vomiting, and **Herbal Bitters**

Herbs: Dandelion and gentian

Supplements: Amylase, lipase, **pancreatin**, protease, and **sodium bicarbonate**

Parotids (Salivary Glands)

The parotids or salivary glands produce a watery secretion composed of water, electrolytes, mucus and enzymes necessary for digestion. As food is chewed, it mixes with oral saliva where enzymes and other constituents begin the process of predigestion.

Formulas: Herbal Potassium

Herbs: Horsetail, sage, white oak, and yucca

Supplements: Chlorophyll and zinc

Stomach　　　*Organ*

The stomach has been considered the seat of disease and death by some traditional healers. Hippocrates thought that all disease starts in the stomach. Samuel Thomson thought that the stomach is the place where the flow of life-energy begins and that clearing the stomach automatically helps alleviate disease. It is likely that every person with any kind of serious chronic disease, including candida, chronic sinus problems, PMS, hypoglycemia, migraine headaches, chronic fatigue, arthritis, and even cancer and autoimmune disorders, has a problem with their digestive system in general and their stomach in particular.

When we ingest food, it is held initially in the upper portion of the stomach. This gives digestive enzymes from saliva and any enzymes naturally present in the food a chance to do some predigestion. This is one of the major reasons that many raw foods digest better than cooked foods. The enzymes present in raw food can do as much as 30 to 40 percent of the digestion before the stomach even begins to work on it.

In the lower portion of the stomach, food is mixed with hydrochloric acid and pepsin. Rennin is also produced by the stomach to break down the proteins in milk. Acid and enzyme secretion is controlled by nerves that are triggered by the smell or taste of food. Hydrochloric acid causes the cells of the food you eat to swell and burst. Together with pepsin, this acid breaks down long chains of protein into smaller fragments called proteases, peptones, and polypeptides. The acid also causes minerals like calcium and iron to break down into fine particles and form a colloidal suspension. This is the first essential step for the assimilation of these minerals. The hydrochloric acid also kills harmful microorganisms that may have been ingested with the food. Thus, this acid is part of the body's complex and thorough immune system.

Because the stomach requires strong acid to break down food, this acid must be carefully controlled. To protect the lining of the stomach from being digested as well, the stomach wall is lined with a thick coat of mucus. A valve at the top of the stomach prevents acid from moving up into the esophagus. When this valve fails to function properly, usually due to hiatal hernia, heartburn or acid reflux occurs.

A valve at the bottom of the stomach keeps food in the stomach until it is ready to be released into the duodenum (the first turn of the small intestines). If the body knows there is not enough bicarbonate solution in the pancreas to neutralize the acid, the valve at the bottom of the stomach won't open because the duodenum and the rest of the small intestines do not have this thick mucus coating. When the valve doesn't open, pressure builds up, contributing to the development of a hiatal hernia and acid reflux or a wearing down of the stomach lining, resulting in ulcers.

The substance that leaves the stomach in small spurts is called chyme. As the chyme passes through the first turn of the small intestine, enzymes from the pancreas, and bile from the gallbladder are secreted onto the food along with an alkaline solution containing bicarbonate. Baking soda is a combination of this bicarbonate and sodium (sodium bicarbonate) and has been used as a traditional remedy for occasional acid indigestion. If the bile and pancreatic secretions fail to neutralize stomach acid, then the duodenum can get burned, causing duodenal ulcers.

Formulas: Betaine HCl, **Children's Colic**, **Chinese Earth-Decreasing**, Chinese Earth-Increasing, **Christopher's Carminative**, Digestive Settling EO, **Digestive Support**, Flu and Vomiting, H. Pylori-Fighting, **Natural Antacid**, Papaya Enzyme, **Plant Enzyme**, and Pregnancy Tea

Herbs: Aloe vera, bayberry, blessed thistle, **catnip**, chamomile, chickweed, dandelion, fennel, **goldenseal**, hops, **licorice**, lobelia, passion flower, **safflower**, saw palmetto, slippery elm, turmeric, white oak, and yarrow

Supplements: Sodium bicarbonate and zinc

Essential Oils: Peppermint

Hepatic System

The hepatic system consists of the liver and the gallbladder and imbalances in it are a frequent underlying cause of many health problems.

It is closely tied to the digestive system because it produces the bile salts that emulsify fats for digestion. However, it does much more than aid in the digestion and assimilation of nutrients.

The liver itself has over five hundred functions. In traditional Chinese medicine it is associated with the wood element and the ability of all the organs and systems to harmonize their functions.

All blood from the digestive system is filtered through the liver before being distributed throughout the body. The liver stores nutrients and processes them for use by the body. It stores sugar in the form of glycogen, to be released when the blood sugar is low. It forms proteins and makes cholesterol to transport fatty acids through the blood-stream.

The liver also is the major organ of internal detoxification. In a two-stage process, it removes toxins and spent metabolic processes (like hormones and neurotransmitters that are no longer needed) for removal from the body. People who suffer from allergies or sensitivity to chemicals often have liver issues.

An important clue that you need to work on your liver is when you have a hard time figuring out what is wrong with you. Another important clue that your liver needs support is if you tend to be angry and irritable or unassertive and overly compliant.

In my experience, the hepatic system is also a frequent underlying cause of many health problems. Symptoms you may need to work with this system include the following.

Indications for Hepatic System

- Anemia
- Cravings for fat or difficulty digesting fats
- Difficulty falling asleep
- Environmental sensitivity
- Excessive anger or irritability
- Feeling groggy in the morning
- Food or respiratory allergies
- Frequent feelings of fatigue
- Generally not feeling well, with no specific symptoms
- High cholesterol
- Hypochondriac feelings
- Migraine headaches
- PMS problems (women)
- Skin problems (e.g. acne, rashes, eczema)
- Varicose veins
- Working around chemicals

Hepatic Irritation *Overactive/Hot*

Inflammation of the liver is known as hepatitis, a severe condition for which medical attention should be sought. However, one can have a mildly irritated liver that is not severe enough to be diagnosed as hepatitis. When the liver is irritated avoid all processed foods, spicy foods, food additives, and other irritating substances. Fasting with plain water or water with lemon or black cherry juice can be helpful.

Indications for Hepatic Irritation

Iridology: Biliary constitution, white fibers in liver/gallbladder area

Tongue: Bright red, especially on the sides

Pulse: Full, rapid, forceful

Emotional State: Tendency to anger and irritably

- Pain or tenderness under right rib cage
- Irritation and redness around the eyes
- Reddish, ruddy complexion, with tendency for flushing of the face
- Tendency to high blood pressure
- In severe cases: yellowish cast to the skin, severe flu-like symptoms (seek medical assistance)

The following cooling and soothing remedies can help.

Formulas: Antioxidant, **Chinese Wood-Decreasing**, and Hepatoprotective

Herbs: Dandelion, **lemon juice**, **lycium**, **mangosteen**, **milk thistle**, and schisandra

Supplements: Bioflavonoids, MSM, **SAM-e**, and **vitamin C**

Essential Oils: Helichrysum

Hepatic Depression *Underactive/Cold*

An underactive or weak liver can create a host of vague and shifting symptoms that make a person feel like they are a hypochondriac because they can't figure out what's wrong with them. They just don't feel good, but can't pinpoint the reason.

In addition to supplements, one can strengthen the liver by avoiding overeating and snacking between meals and by reducing one's exposure to chemicals. Fasting once or twice each month for twenty-four hours with plain water or water with lemon or black cherry juice can also be helpful.

Indications for Hepatic Depression

Iridology: Biliary constitution; brown or dark-brown pigments

Tongue: Dirty yellow coating on tongue, sometimes brownish

Pulse: Thin, weak

Emotional State: Difficulty expressing anger, with tendency toward lethargy and depression

- Pale, anemic
- Dull, glazed eyes
- Lack of appetite
- General malaise
- Frequent dull headaches
- Severe body or foot odor
- Chronic skin conditions
- Puffiness and pressure under right rib cage
- Vague symptoms, feeling like a hypochondriac

The following warming and stimulating remedies can help.

Formulas: Chinese Wood-Increasing and Hepatoprotective

Herbs: Angelica, **bupleurum**, chamomile, cinnamon, dandelion, **dong quai**, fennel, feverfew, fringe tree, ginger, horseradish, milk thistle, rosemary, and **turmeric**

Supplements: Curcumin, indole-3-carbinol, MSM, **N-acetyl cysteine, SAM-e**, and **vitamin B-complex**

Hepatic Stagnation *Torpid/Damp*

The liver gets a significant portion of its blood through the portal vein, which comes from the digestive tract. If the digestive system is congested, the blood supply to the liver can easily be congested. This can result in a stuffy feeling in the abdomen and under the right rib cage along with other symptoms below.

In severe cases (gallbladder obstruction), seek medical attention. The strategy *Gall Bladder Flush* may be helpful for gallbladder congestion. Coffee enemas or enemas with bitter herbs like those listed above stimulate liver detoxification. See the strategy *Colon Hydrotherapy*.

Indications for Hepatic Stagnation

Iridology: Biliary constitution, dark fibers or lacuna in liver area

Tongue: Heavy coating

Pulse: Slippery or rolling

Emotional State: Frustration, difficulty relaxing

- Puffy around eyes
- Bloated, stuffy feeling
- Acute pain under right rib cage
- Difficulty digesting fats, greasy stools or light colored stools
- Difficulty getting to sleep (night hawk)
- Morning grogginess
- Frequent headaches or migraines
- Tendency to bloating and constipation
- Chronic skin conditions

The following drying and cleansing remedies can help.

Formulas: Ayurvedic Skin Healing, Blood Purifier, Chinese Balanced Cleansing, Chinese Fire-Increasing, Chinese Wood-Decreasing, Christopher's Gallbladder, **Detoxifying**, Heavy Metal Cleansing, **Hepatoprotective**, Herbal Bitters, and Liver Cleanse

Herbs: Artichoke, **barberry**, blessed thistle, blue flag, burdock, celandine, **dandelion root**, **fringe tree**, **milk thistle**, Oregon grape, **turmeric**, and **yellow dock**

Supplements: Berberine, curcumin, and N-acetyl cysteine

Hepatic Atrophy   *Rigid/Dry*

With continued exposure to toxins and poor nutrition over time the liver can start to atrophy and fail to function adequately. A severe form of this is cirrhosis of the liver. The liver can eventually start to fail, requiring a liver transplant. To help rebuild a liver that is atrophying, it is essential to avoid all chemicals, food additives, processed foods, and even spicy foods. Fresh vegetable juices (especially beet roots and greens, celery, chard) can be helpful along with some of the listed supplements.

Indications for Hepatic Atrophy

Iridology: Biliary constitution, dark fibers or pigments in liver area

Tongue: Dry tongue, withered on the sides

Pulse: Weak or slightly tense

Emotional State: Lack of will-power, depression

- Dark, sunken eyes
- Dry skin
- Thin and pale, poor digestion
- Lack of appetite for fats and proteins, but cravings for sugar after or between meals
- Fatigue and weakness
- Chronic liver damage, history of drinking or drug use or exposure to chemicals

The following moistening and building remedies can help.

Formulas: Chinese Wood-Increasing and Hepatoprotective

Herbs: Baical skullcap, **beet**, **burdock**, chickweed, licorice, olive, peony, **reishi**, **schisandra**, shitake, and wild yam

Supplements: CBD, **N-acetyl cysteine**, **omega-3 EFAs**, and **vitamin A**

Hepatic Constriction   *Spastic/Tense*

Circulation to the liver can be constricted, or the bile ducts can become constricted which results in pain under the right rib cage and other symptoms. In severe cases (gallbladder obstruction), seek medical attention. Otherwise, avoid caffeine (e.g. coffee, tea, guarana, energy drinks) and pungent herbs like capsicum and garlic. A gallbladder flush may be helpful, along with herbs, to relax the liver and gallbladder.

Indications for Hepatic Constriction

Iridology: Biliary constitution, contraction furrows

Pulse: Wiry, tense, obstructed

Emotional State: Suppression of anger, followed by sudden outbursts of anger

- Alternating diarrhea and constipation
- Light colored stools
- Difficulty digesting fats, indigestion from eating fats
- Acute shooting or spastic pain under right rib cage, sometimes in chest

The following relaxing remedies can help.

Formulas: Christopher's Gallbladder

Herbs: Agrimony, bupleurum, cramp bark, lobelia, vervain (blue), and **wild yam**

Supplements: **Magnesium** and SAM-e

Hepatic Relaxation   *Atonic/Loose*

This condition of the liver often accompanies liver stagnation. When venous circulation through the liver is poor, it contributes to venous congestion in general, which can cause hemorrhoids, varicose veins, and other problems. Eating fresh berries every day can be helpful, along with herbs, to tone the venous circulation and aid liver function.

Indications for Hepatic Relaxation

Iridology: Lacuna in liver area

Tongue: Swollen on the sides

Pulse: Non-resistant

- Tendency to hemorrhoids
- Tendency to varicose veins
- Weeping eczema
- Puffy, sagging eyes
- Heavy menstrual bleeding and menstrual pain
- Prostate problems in men, uterine fibroids in women

The following toning remedies can help.

Formulas: Vein Tonic

Herbs: Bayberry, bilberry, **butcher's broom**, green tea extract, **horse chestnut**, **pau d'arco**, sage, schisandra, **white oak**, and yarrow

Supplements: Bioflavonoids

Specific Hepatic Tissues

Here is some information and remedy lists for the specific organs in the hepatic system.

Gallbladder   *Organ*

The gallbladder is a small pear-shaped muscular sack that acts as a storage tank for bile. Bile is made in the liver by liver cells and sent through tiny ducts or canals to the duodenum (small intestine). The gallbladder stores the bile to have it available in larger quantities for secretion when a meal is eaten. Bile is a mixture of bile salts, lipids, cholesterol, pigments, proteins and sodium.

The ingestion of food and especially fats causes the release of the hormone cholecystokinin, which in turn signals the relaxation of the valve at the end of the common bile duct, which lets the bile enter the small intestine. It also signals the contraction of the gallbladder to squirt the concentrated liquid bile into the small intestine where it helps with the emulsification or breakdown of fats in the meal.

Healthy bile appears yellow from the breakdown of dead red blood cells and causes the golden-brown color of healthy stools. Jaundice, a yellow coloring of the skin, results when bile is not excreted. The bile salts act like a detergent, allowing the fats to mix with water so they can be carried safely through the bloodstream. They are reabsorbed along with the nutrients and sent back to the liver.

Formulas: Chinese Wood-Decreasing, **Christopher's Gallbladder**, Detoxifying, Digestive Support, Fat-Absorbing Fiber, Fiber, **Herbal Bitters**, **Lipase Enzyme**, and Liver Cleanse

Herbs: Blessed thistle, blue flag, burdock, cascara sagrada, chickweed, **dandelion**, devil's claw, **fringe tree**, goldenseal, hydrangea, kelp, **milk thistle**, mullein, **Oregon grape**, **turmeric**, **wild yam**, and **yellow dock**

Supplements: Berberine, lecithin, lipase, and magnesium

Essential Oils: Orange (sweet) and thyme

Liver   *Organ*

The liver is the largest internal organ, weighing more than three pounds. It is located on the right side of the body just underneath the dome of the diaphragm, and its triangular shape appears reddish-brown in color. Much of what the liver does is not fully known, but its main functions include receiving and delivering nutrients to other parts of the body, producing many different substances for different systems, storing blood and fat, and filtering out and destroying wastes, and harmful substances.

The liver functions on a cellular level, greatly increasing the efficiency of the organ. Each lobule is surrounded by veins and arteries that allow this organ to receive nutrient-rich blood from the digestive system, take what it needs, and send the rest to other parts of the body.

Each lobule also produces bile and bile salts, which are then collected, stored, and concentrated in the gallbladder until they are needed to aid digestion. The liver also produces glycogen, a product of fat, carbohydrate, and protein metabolism, which maintains blood glucose levels. Other liver products include substances to aid in the production of red blood cells, blood clotting, vitamin A, and urea.

Many of these products are stored in the liver until they are needed. The liver also stores vitamins A, D, and K, iron, and copper along with fats that the body cannot immediately use. At any given time, the liver contains approximately 20 percent of the body's blood, which is released into the circulatory system as needed.

As blood flows through the liver, harmful substances are filtered or neutralized. For example, dead red blood cells are collected, and the iron from each is removed and then used for new blood cells. Other poisonous substances, such as alcohol and drugs, heavily tax the liver and lead to organ malfunction. The gallbladder serves as the elimination organ for the liver. Some of the neutralized waste products are dumped into the intestines through the bile for elimination from the body. The bile is nature's natural laxative, as it helps to stimulate bowel elimination.

Because of the vital importance of this organ and the many body systems it serves, a liver that malfunctions can lead to serious consequences. In fact, the health of the liver in many ways determines the health of the individual. In Cherokee medicine, it is considered the seat of healing. In Chinese medicine, it is the home of the wood element, the element of life. Maybe that's why we intuitively named it the *live*-r. The Chinese also consider the liver to be the ruler of the blood. In Western medicine, most of the herbs that are used to aid liver function have been called blood purifiers, showing this relationship between the liver and the blood.

When the liver is moderately dysfunctional, a host of vague symptoms can occur. These symptoms are due to toxins being able to bypass the liver and get into the general circulation. They are also due to nutritional imbalances in the biochemistry of the blood.

Formulas: Antioxidant, Chinese Balanced Cleansing, Chinese Qi-Regulating, **Chinese Wood-Decreasing**, **Chinese Wood-Increasing**, Christopher's Herbal Iron, **Detoxifying**, Essiac Immune Tea, Heavy Metal Cleansing, Hepatoprotective, Ivy Bridge's Cleansing, **Liver Cleanse**, Methylated B Vitamin, Proanthocyanidins, and **Skinny**

Herbs: Bee pollen, **blessed thistle**, **bupleurum**, **burdock**, chamomile, **chickweed**, **dandelion**, echinacea, ginger, hops, licorice, **milk thistle**, olive, Oregon grape, psyllium, **red clover**, rose, Saint John's wort, **schisandra**, spirulina, **turmeric**, vervain (blue), wood betony, and yellow dock

Supplements: 7-keto, alpha-lipoic acid, chlorophyll, chromium, Co-Q10, colostrum, indole-3-carbinol, iron, lecithin, **N-acetyl cysteine**, omega-6 CLA, protease, **SAM-e**, vitamin B-complex, vitamin B_3, vitamin B_6, **vitamin C**, and vitamin E

Essential Oils: Bergamot, grapefruit (pink), helichrysum, jasmine, lemon, red mandarin, and rose

Intestinal System

Many people have found their overall health improves when they do a better job of regulating their elimination. Keeping the intestinal system is important for both assimilating nutrients and removing waste materials and for supporting a healthy immune system.

The intestinal system extends from the duodenum to the anus and includes both the small and large intestines. The small intestine is involved with the digestion and assimilation of food. The large intestine is primarily involved with the storage and disposal of waste material.

When the intestinal system is functioning normally, two to three bowel movements per day are common, although variations in diet will affect the frequency of bowel movements. A general rule of thumb is that the longer waste material stays in the body, the more toxic it becomes and the more it affects how you feel. It is important, therefore, to give your body sufficient healthy fluids, foods, and fiber to ensure the proper functioning of your intestinal system.

The microbiome in the intestinal system is a critical part of the immune system. Imbalances in the microbiome contribute to a wide variety of health problems, including leaky gut and small intestinal bacterial overgrowth (SIBO). These, in turn, are contributing factors in autoimmune disorders, allergies, respiratory congestion and sinus problems and general feelings of sluggishness and poor health.

Indications for Intestinal System

- Abdominal pain or discomfort
- Asthma and other chronic lung problems
- Autoimmune disorders
- Bloating, belching or intestinal gas
- Cancer
- Chronic sinus problems
- Constipation (bowel movements fewer than once per day)
- Depression or anxiety
- Diarrhea or loose stools
- Food or respiratory allergies
- General poor health
- Hard, dry stools
- Hemorrhoids or anal fistula

- History of heavy antibiotic use
- Inflammatory bowel disorders
- Leaky gut syndrome
- Low-fiber diet
- Straining to eliminate
- Weak immune system

Intestinal Irritation   *Overactive/Hot*

The intestines can become irritated and inflamed when we ingest harmful substances, overeat, mix incompatible foods or have issues digesting certain foods. In it's severe form, this involves inflammatory bowel disorders. Sour or mucilaginous remedies are generally helpful in cooling and soothing the intestinal system.

Indications for Intestinal Irritation

Iridology: Jagged collarette

Tongue: Red, often pointy, with yellow coating at the back, occasionally with sores or bumps at the back or geographic tongue

Pulse: Rapid and superficial

Emotional State: Anxious, stressed, nervous

- Acute pain and discomfort in lower abdominal area
- Stool tends to be loose, occasional diarrhea
- Rapid colon transit time
- Inflammatory bowel diseases (seek medical attention)

The following cooling and soothing remedies can help.

Formulas: Chinese Yang-Reducing, **Intestinal Soothing**, and Pepsin Intestinal

Herbs: Aloe vera, black walnut, boswellia, **cat's claw**, **chamomile**, cherry, **licorice**, **marshmallow**, **plantain**, rose hips, **slippery elm**, wild yam, and yellow dock

Supplements: Bromelain, **omega-3 EFAs**, and vitamin C

Essential Oils: Chamomile (Roman)

Intestinal Depression   *Underactive/Cold*

Intestinal depression is a condition where there is reduced function of the intestinal tract, typically resulting in reduced motility of the intestines (colon transit time) and a lack of normal secretion to digest food. It is typically associated with intestinal stagnation, creating a cooler, damper intestinal tract. Aromatic herbs can be used to stimulate digestive secretions and motility. Enzymes can be taken to aid digestion or taken between meals to help clear out congestion. Avoid sugars and simple starches with intestinal depression.

Indications for Intestinal Depression

Iridology: Dark color inside of collarette, central heterochromia

Tongue: Dark red or purplish, often with heavy white coating at the back

Pulse: Slow, weak, and deep

Emotional State: Can't let go

- Sluggish bowel eliminations (fewer than one movement per day) with sluggish transit time
- Stool dark with strong odor
- Tendency to gas, bloating and flatulence
- Chronic bad breath and/or body odor
- Tendency toward chronic sinus problems and respiratory congestion

The following warming and stimulating remedies can help.

Formulas: Chinese Earth-Decreasing, Gentle Bowel Cleansing, **Ivy Bridge's Cleansing**, **Parasite Cleansing**, and **Stimulant Laxative**

Herbs: Capsicum, **cinnamon**, **clove**, **garlic**, **ginger**, horseradish, mugwort, oregano, **peppermint**, sweet annie, and wormwood

Supplements: Bromelain and **protease**

Essential Oils: Cinnamon, **clove**, lime, and oregano

Intestinal Stagnation   *Torpid/Damp*

Intestinal stagnation is associated with excessive fermentation and toxicity in the digestive tract. There is typically an imbalance in the intestinal microbiome. It is usually associated with intestinal depression.

Herbal laxatives can be used short-term to increase motility and move things more quickly through the system. Bitters can be used to rebalance the microbiome. An *Herbal Bitters Formula* can help to restore digestive function.

To keep the intestines moving, stay well hydrated and make sure you are consuming adequate fiber. Magnesium, vitamin C and triphala may also be helpful for maintenance of intestinal health.

Indications for Intestinal Stagnation

Iridology: Lacuna inside collarette, loose collarette

Tongue: Thick yellow mucus coating at the back of the tongue

Emotional State: Holding onto the past, "full of it"

- Regular but sluggish bowel movements (every two to three days or more)
- Stool like thick logs
- Stuffy, bloated feeling in abdomen
- Chronic skin conditions
- Tendency for chronic sinus problems and respiratory congestion
- Tendency toward weight gain in abdominal area

The following drying and cleansing remedies can help.

Formulas: Anti-Fungal, Antiparasitic, **Chinese Balanced Cleansing**, **Detoxifying**, Ed Millet's Herbal Crisis, **Herbal Bitters**, Herbal Composition, Intestinal Detoxification, **Ivy Bridge's Cleansing**, Parasite Cleansing, Pepsin Intestinal, **Stimulant Laxative**, and Yeast Cleansing

Herbs: Barberry, black walnut, **buckthorn**, **butternut bark**, **cascara sagrada**, senna, **turkey rhubarb**, and yellow dock

Supplements: Berberine, clay (bentonite), magnesium, and vitamin C

Intestinal Atrophy   *Rigid/Dry*

Intestinal atrophy involves dryness and weakness of the intestinal membranes. Soothing, mucilaginous fibers help to moisten and soothe intestinal tissues. Rebalancing friendly flora with probiotics is also helpful.

Indications for Intestinal Atrophy

Iridology: Central heterochromia

Tongue: Dry, sometimes withered or cracked

Pulse: Weak or thin and slow or rapid and weak

Emotional State: Nervous, stuck in the past

- Infrequent bowel movements
- Dry, hard round ball-like stool, difficult to pass
- Dry mouth, with frequent thirst and urination
- Constipation from dehydration
- Anal fissure (fistula)

The following moistening and building remedies can help.

Formulas: **Chinese Earth-Increasing**, **Chinese Yin-Increasing**, Fiber, **Gentle Bowel Cleansing**, GLA Oil, **Gut-Healing Fiber**, Irritable Bowel Fiber, Lung Moistening, and Vulnerary

Herbs: **Aloe vera**, **flax**, guar gum, licorice, **marshmallow**, plantain, **psyllium**, and **slippery elm**

Supplements: Omega-3 EFAs

Intestinal Constriction   *Spastic/Tense*

People who get constipated from stress and have irregular bowel movements, or bowel movements that alternate between diarrhea and constipation, suffer from intestinal constriction. Antispasmodics and nervines that help the colon relax are helpful.

Indications for Intestinal Constriction

Iridology: Jagged or irregular collarette, tight collarette

Pulse: Wiry, tense, or obstructed pulse

Emotional State: Tendency for mood swings, difficulty letting go of things

- Constipation from stress, bowel moves easier when relaxed
- Erratic bowel movement schedule
- Chronic need for stimulant laxatives
- Cramping, explosive bowel movements
- Cramping pains in the colon, intestinal griping
- Sharp pains in abdomen, coming and going at irregular intervals

The following relaxing remedies can help.

Formulas: Antispasmodic
Herbs: Catnip, chamomile, cramp bark, **lobelia**, and **wild yam**
Supplements: Magnesium

Intestinal Relaxation *Atonic/Loose*

Intestinal relaxation involves frequent bowel elimination or watery, unformed stools. It also takes the form of the condition, leaky gut. Astringents can be used to tone the bowel to reduce discharge and tone the gut wall. Charcoal is also helpful as are the soothing mucilaginous fibers listed under *Intestinal Atrophy*.

Indications for Intestinal Relaxation

Iridology: Loose or broken collarette
Tongue: Damp with heavy white coating
Pulse: Passive, non-resistant

- Diarrhea or watery, loose stool
- Leaky gut syndrome
- Mucus in stool
- Hemorrhoids or anal fistula, weak rectal muscles
- Blood in stool (seek medical attention)

The following toning remedies can help.

Formulas: Ed Millet's Herbal Crisis, Gut-Healing Fiber, and Internal Bleeding
Herbs: Bayberry, **black walnut**, **blackberry root**, cat's claw, cinnamon, collinsonia, **goldenseal**, red raspberry, and white oak
Supplements: Bacillus coagulans, **charcoal**, and **L-glutamine**

Specific Intestinal Tissues

Here are some specific digestive organs and remedies that may be helpful for them.

Appendix *Organ*

The appendix sits at the junction of the small intestine and large intestine in the lower right abdomen. It is a thin tubular protrusion about four inches long. The function of the appendix is not fully known, although new theories are emerging.

One is that the appendix acts as a storehouse for good bacteria, rebooting the digestive system after diarrhea-related illnesses. Other experts believe the appendix is just a useless remnant from our evolutionary past. Surgical removal of the appendix causes no observable health problems.

In recent years, scientists have learned that the appendix serves an important role in the human fetus and in young adults. Endocrine cells have been found in the appendix of the human fetus during the eleventh week of development. Endocrine cells in the fetal appendix have been shown to produce biogenic amines and peptide hormones, which are compounds that assist with various biological control mechanisms.

In adult humans, the appendix is now believed to contribute to certain immune functions. Lymphoid tissue begins to accumulate in the appendix shortly after birth and reaches a peak between the second and third decades of life, decreasing rapidly thereafter and practically disappearing after the age of sixty.

In light of these findings, the appendix appears to expose white blood cells to the wide variety of antigens (foreign substances) present in the gastrointestinal tract. We can logically assume, then, that the appendix helps to suppress potentially destructive antibody responses while promoting local immunity. The appendix draws antigens from the intestines and reacts to these contents.

Formulas: Intestinal Soothing, Liquid Lymph, and Lymph Cleansing
Herbs: Goldenseal and Oregon grape
Supplements: Berberine

Large Intestines (Colon) *Organ*

The large intestine, or colon, is a key part of the digestive system. A typical adult colon is approximately five feet long. It is not as long as the small intestine, but the colon is roughly two and a half inches in diameter—three times the girth of the small intestine.

By the time the liquified food (chyme) reaches the colon, a large part of the nutrients has been absorbed. The chyme passes from the small intestine to the colon via the ileocecal valve. This valve opens and closes by the action of a sphincter muscle, which allows the chyme to pass from the small intestine to the colon while keeping the contents of the colon from backing up into the small intestine.

As the final link in the digestive chain, it is the colon's job to (1) absorb any remaining water and electrolytes from the chyme, (2) continue moving the waste material along its way, and (3) store the waste material until it is time for it to be expelled. The colon moves material through by involuntary wavelike contractions, made possible by smooth muscles within the colon wall, a process that is known as peristalsis.

The colon is also colonized by several pounds of microorganisms, known collectively as the friendly flora. A healthy colon should contain about 70 percent or more of beneficial bacteria, primarily various species of *Lactobacillus* bacteria and about 30 percent or less of other organisms such as *E. coli* and yeast. Unfortunately, some health experts estimate that most Westerners have 70 percent or more of the harmful bacteria and 30 percent or less of the beneficial bacteria—just the opposite of what is required for optimal health. The chief reasons for this are improper diet and prescription drug use—primarily antibiotics.

Formulas: Anti-Fungal, Fiber, **Gentle Bowel Cleansing**, Gut Immune, Intestinal Detoxification, **Intestinal Soothing**, Irritable Bowel Fiber, **Ivy Bridge's Cleansing**, Parasite Cleansing, **Probiotic**, **Stimulant Laxative**, Weight Loss Cleansing, and Yeast Cleansing

Herbs: Aloe vera, bayberry, black walnut, buckthorn, **cascara sagrada**, psyllium, and turkey rhubarb

Supplements: **Charcoal**, **chlorophyll**, **magnesium**, and vitamin C

Essential Oils: Peppermint

Rectum   *Body Part*

The rectum is a muscular ring at the end of the large intestine. Its primary function is to keep the intestine sealed shut until the need to pass feces arises. When that occurs, it assists in moving the feces out of the body.

The rectum also functions as a temporary storage site for fecal matter before it is eliminated from the body through the anal canal. As the food you eat passes through the digestive system, it is broken down and nutrients are absorbed in the stomach and, small and large intestines. Fecal matter, which includes digestive juices, bacteria and fiber, continues to move into the lower portion of the large intestine or the rectum. The rectum holds the feces until one pushes it out of the body by having a bowel movement.

The rectum is made up of muscular walls that are able to expand to hold fecal matter. As the rectum expand, it sends a signal to the brain that you need to have a bowel movement. Muscles in and around the anal canal control this action. Older children and adults are able to control these muscles, relaxing them to release the feces from the rectum or contracting them to avoid having a bowel movement.

Straining to pass stool through the rectum can result in varicose veins in the rectum (commonly known as hemorrhoids) or tiny tears called anal fistula. Adequate fiber and proper hydration keep the stool soft and help to prevent these problems, while astringents like white oak bark and collinsonia can aid healing.

Formulas: Fiber, Healing Salve, **Irritable Bowel Fiber**, and Vein Tonic

Herbs: Collinsonia, marshmallow, slippery elm, and **white oak**

Supplements: Nanoparticle silver

Essential Oils: Geranium

Small Intestines   *Organ*

Despite its name, the small intestine is the lengthiest part of the digestive system and plays an important role in the digestion and absorption of the food you eat. The small intestine has three parts: the duodenum, the jejunum and the ileum.

The duodenum is the first portion of the small intestine. It is tolerant to low pH levels because it receives the still very acidic contents of the stomach. The pancreatic duct releases pancreatic enzymes that reduce the acidity of the digesting food before it reaches parts of the small intestine that aren't tolerant. The bile duct, which carries bile from the liver, also empties into the duodenum and is responsible for breaking down fats within the food. The duodenum is the shortest part of the small intestine, measuring less than ten inches long, and continues the digestive process that began in the stomach.

The jejunum is the next section of the small intestine. Digestion continues in this section under the action of bile and pancreatic secretions.

To maximize the surface area for absorption, the inner surface of the small intestine is lined with tiny finger-like protuberances, called microvilli. This increases the ability of the body to absorb nutrients into the blood.

The ileum is the final part of the small intestine and is responsible for the absorption of vitamin B-12 and the final processing of carbohydrates and proteins. The end of the ileum is where the small and large intestines meet, and it's also where the appendix is located.

Formulas: Blood Sugar Control, Digestive Support, Fat-Absorbing Fiber, Fiber, **Gentle Bowel Cleansing**, **Gut Immune**, **Herbal Bitters**, **Intestinal Soothing**, Lipase Enzyme, Papaya Enzyme, **Pepsin Intestinal**, and Plant Enzyme

Herbs: Aloe vera, bayberry, **ginger**, **marshmallow**, **peppermint**, and **slippery elm**

Supplements: Sodium alginate

Essential Oils: Peppermint

Respiratory System

The respiratory system is seldom a primary source of health problems. Although once there are problems in the respiratory system, they contribute to an overall decline in health due to a lack of oxygenation of the tissues.

The primary job of the respiratory system is to provide oxygen to the bloodstream and remove carbon dioxide as a waste material. Oxygen is essential to every cell because it allows nutrients to be burned, providing the necessary energy for the cell to function. Deprived of oxygen, body tissues begin to die in minutes.

When the cells burn their fuel, they give off carbon dioxide, a waste material that is picked up by the bloodstream and transported back to the lungs for elimination. Thus, the lungs are an organ of both assimilation (absorbing oxygen) and elimination (removing carbon dioxide). This process is known as respiration.

Respiration, or breathing, requires a great deal of space in the body and uses more energy than you may realize. We take in air through the nose and mouth, then it travels through the larynx, the voice box, down the trachea and into the two bronchial passages in the lungs. These tubes have unique qualities that make breathing easier. Rings of cartilage surround each passageway to keep it open at all times.

The airways are also lined with a mucous membrane to catch dust, germs, and other foreign particles that otherwise would enter the body every time you open your mouth or take a breath. These particles are trapped in the mucus and then moved upward by tiny hairlike projections called cilia. Cilia also line the sinuses. The sinuses normally push mucus to the back of the throat, while the lungs push the mucus to the top of the air passageway. The mucus is then swallowed and expelled by the digestive tract.

Indications for Respiratory System

- Asthma
- Chronic or frequent cough
- COPD
- Excess mucus production
- Frequent respiratory infections
- Hay fever and respiratory allergies
- Itchy nose or ears
- Post nasal drip
- Sinus headaches
- Sinusitis or chronic sinus congestion
- Wheezing or shortness of breath

Respiratory Irritation   *Overactive/Hot*

When respiratory membranes are irritated, they typically produce excess mucus to try to flush the irritant. The irritation can be an allergic reaction to dust or pollen or a reaction to an airborne chemical irritant. You also have this condition in the early stages of a cold, where mucus drainage is thin and watery. When respiratory passages are irritated, drink lots of water to aid the flushing process and take remedies that soothe and cool the irritated membranes.

Indications for Respiratory Irritation

Iridology: Lymphatic constitution, hydrogenoid subtype, white in lung area

Tongue: Red (especially in the front middle area) and pointy

Pulse: Rapid and floating

Emotional State: Acute grief, shock and sadness

- Thin, watery mucus drainage, often burning to tissues
- Irritation, redness, and itchiness to eyes and nose
- Rhinitis and hay fever
- Productive cough with clear or white mucus
- Acute respiratory infection, early stages of a cold

The following cooling and soothing remedies can help.

Formulas: Antioxidant, Jeannie Burgess' Allergy-Lung, Seasonal Cold and Flu, and **Steven Horne's Anti-Allergy**

Herbs: Butterbur, **elderberry**, **eyebright**, goldenrod, **lemon juice**, mangosteen, mullein, **nettle, stinging**, **osha**, plantain, **pleurisy**, rose hips, thyme, turmeric, and **wild cherry bark**

Supplements: Bromelain, Co-Q10, MSM, **quercetin**, and **vitamin C**

Essential Oils: Anise, cypress, **eucalyptus**, and peppermint

Respiratory Depression *Underactive/Cold*

In respiratory depression, the respiratory tissues have been weakened by damage, irritation, or infection. Mucus is not moving efficiently, which contributes to respiratory stagnation (discussed next). The body needs aromatics or essential oils that will stimulate productive cough or sinus drainage to flush irritants, infection, or mucus from the system. Drink lots of water, take aromatic herbs for the lungs, and/or inhale essential oils in steam.

Indications for Respiratory Depression

Iridology: Lymphatic constitution, darkness in lung area

Tongue: Pale, with heavy mucus coating

Pulse: Weak and deep

Emotional State: Chronic, repressed grief; cold, insensitive, lacking compassion for others, unable to cry or show vulnerability

- Chronic lung or sinus infections
- Poor resistance to infection
- Pale complexion
- Wheezing, shortness of breath
- Conditions aggravated by cold weather
- Pale cheeks

The following warming and stimulating remedies can help.

Formulas: Chinese Metal-Increasing, **Ed Millet's Herbal Crisis, Fire Cider, Lung-Supporting EO, Stabilized Allicin,** Steven Horne's Horehound Cough, and Topical Analgesic

Herbs: Fenugreek, **garlic,** grindelia, horehound, **horseradish, pine bark,** rosemary, **thyme,** typhonium, and **yerba santa**

Supplements: Vitamin C and **zinc**

Essential Oils: Atlas cedarwood, **camphor, eucalyptus, menthol, pine,** rosemary, sandalwood, and thyme

Respiratory Stagnation *Torpid/Damp*

In respiratory stagnation, there is excessive productive of thick mucus that is difficult to move. Air passages are constricted due tot he presence of this mucus which is typically slightly discolored (yellow or greenish). Remedies are used that loosen the mucus and help move it from the system. Drink lots of water when taking these remedies.

Indications for Respiratory Stagnation

Iridology: Lymphatic constitution, hydrogenoid subtype

Tongue: Swollen or damp with heavy white or yellowish coating

Pulse: Slippery or rolling

Emotional State: Internalized sadness, feeling stifled or smothered

- Thick mucus, often discolored yellow
- Subacute infection, Later stages of a cold
- Chronic sinus problems
- Bronchitis, asthma and other respiratory conditions with heavy mucus production
- History of frequent ear infections
- Symptoms aggravated by dampness

The following drying and cleansing remedies can help.

Formulas: Anti-Snoring, **Chinese Metal-Decreasing,** Christopher's Sinus, **Ed Millet's Herbal Crisis, Fire Cider, Herbal Composition,** Jeannie Burgess' Allergy-Lung, Lung Moistening, Lung-Supporting EO, Seasonal Cold and Flu, **Sinus,** Steven Horne's Anti-Allergy, and Steven Horne's Horehound Cough

Herbs: Cherry, coltsfoot, elecampane, **goldenseal,** grindelia, **horehound,** myrrh, orange (bitter), Oregon grape, osha, thyme, and **yerba santa**

Supplements: Berberine

Essential Oils: Atlas cedarwood, camphor, **eucalyptus,** frankincense, myrrh, and **pine**

Respiratory Atrophy *Rigid/Dry*

In respiratory atrophy, the respiratory passages become dehydrated and weakened. They are also dry, which can result in dry, hacking coughs or chronically congested sinus passages. Drink water with a pinch of natural salt to help hydrate the respiratory tissues and use these cooling and building remedies.

Indications for Respiratory Atrophy

Iridology: Lymphatic constitution

Tongue: Dry, possibly thin, and cracked

Pulse: Thin, weak, deep

Emotional State: Deeply repressed grief and sadness, hardness of heart, stoic

- Dry, irritated, unproductive cough
- Wheezing and difficulty breathing
- Mucus difficult to expel
- Symptoms aggravated by dry weather and wind
- Sunken cheeks, sallow face
- History of smoking
- Diagnosis of COPD, emphysema, or chronic asthma

The following moistening and building remedies can help.

Formulas: Ayurvedic Bronchial Decongestant, **Chinese Metal-Increasing,** Lung Moistening, and Vulnerary

Herbs: Astragalus, balloon flower, bamboo, **codonopsis, cordyceps,** elecampane, **fritillary bulb, licorice,** loquat, **marshmallow, mullein,** plantain, **pleurisy root,** and slippery elm

Supplements: Vitamin A and vitamin D

Essential Oils: Patchouli and rose

Respiratory Constriction *Spastic/Tense*

There are muscles in the bronchial passages that open airways to allow more air into the lungs or constrict to allow less. When there is constriction of the airways, breathing becomes difficult. Stress and a weakness of the adrenal glands can contribute to respiratory constriction. Use antispasmodic remedies that relax the tissues to help open the airways.

Indications for Respiratory Constriction

Iridology: Contraction furrows

Pulse: Wiry, hard, tense, or bounding

Emotional State: Feeling stifled, smothered, overly controlled, unable to be free

- Spastic or cough
- Acute asthma attacks and asthma associated with anxiety
- Bronchial constriction due to tension, stress, or weak adrenals
- Spastic pains in chest associated with breathing

- Difficult or painful breathing, gasping for air
- Respiratory symptoms with sudden, rapid onset
- Symptoms worse from movement

The following relaxing remedies can help.

Formulas: Antispasmodic, Ayurvedic Bronchial Decongestant, Chinese Metal-Decreasing, and Steven Horne's Horehound Cough

Herbs: Balloon flower, black cohosh, khella, **lobelia, pleurisy, skunk cabbage,** and yerba santa

Essential Oils: Anise, **cajeput, clary sage,** cypress, eucalyptus, fennel, and **thyme**

Respiratory Relaxation   *Atonic/Loose*

When respiratory membranes are overly relaxed there is an excessive discharge of mucus that usually tends to be thin and watery. There may also be bleeding from the sinuses or lungs, which calls for remedies that tone mucous membranes.

Indications for Respiratory Relaxation

Iridology: Hydrogenoid subtype

Tongue: Swollen; thick, damp coating

Pulse: Relaxed, possibly rolling or slippery

Emotional State: Chronic sadness, internalized crying

- Excessive production of thin, watery mucus with drippy secretions
- Swollen lymph glands or tonsils
- Swollen Eustachian tubes, resulting in frequent earaches
- Nosebleeds
- Coughing blood (reddish mucus)

The following toning remedies can help.

Formulas: Steven Horne's Sinus Snuff

Herbs: Bayberry, eyebright, horsetail, sage, and **yerba santa**

Supplements: Silicon

Essential Oils: Frankincense and myrrh

Specific Respiratory Tissues

Here is a description of some of the major parts of the respiratory system and remedies that may be helpful for them.

Bronchi   *Body Part*

The bronchial tubes descend from the trachea through bronchial passageways into the lungs. They contain muscles that expand to allow greater airflow or contract to restrict airflow. When the bronchial passages become inflamed you get bronchitis. Chronic constriction of the bronchial passages from inflammation, mucus or contraction (or any combination of these factors) contributes to asthma. Specific direct aids for the bronchi include the following.

Formulas: Antihistamine, Antispasmodic, **Ayurvedic Bronchial Decongestant,** Chinese Metal-Decreasing, Chinese Metal-Increasing, **Jeannie Burgess' Allergy-Lung,** and Lymphatic Infection

Herbs: Black cohosh, catnip, chamomile, **cordyceps, elecampane,** fenugreek, garlic, **horehound, lobelia,** mullein, and Oregon grape

Essential Oils: Atlas cedarwood, **eucalyptus, frankincense, ravensara,** rosemary, and thyme

Lungs   *Organ*

The lungs are cone-shaped pink organs that are fairly passive. They have a spongy texture that allows them to expand and contract as the diaphragm and rib muscles change the size of the entire chest cavity. Inside the lungs, the bronchial tubes, with a structure some have compared to an upside-down tree, subdivide into smaller and smaller tubes called bronchioles. These tubes end in bunches of tiny round air sacs called alveoli, which are small, balloon-like sacs at the end of the small air passages in the lungs.

Oxygen is inhaled and absorbed into the bloodstream through the thin walls of each alveolus by way of the pulmonary veins. Carbon dioxide from the pulmonary artery is exhaled as a waste product of the lungs. The greater the surface area the lungs have for gas exchange, the greater their efficiency to absorb oxygen. The seven hundred million or more alveoli found in both lungs—if flattened out—would cover an area of fifty to one hundred square yards. This is approximately the size of a tennis court, and it is all neatly folded and bundled into the chest cavity.

Muscles near the lungs help expand and contract (tighten) the lungs to allow breathing. These muscles include the diaphragm, the intercostal muscles, the abdominal muscles, and the muscles in the neck and collarbone area.

Formulas: Broken and Hardened Hearts FE, Chinese Metal-Decreasing, **Chinese Metal-Increasing,** Disinfectant EO, Fire Cider, Grief and Sadness FE, Immune-Boosting, **Jeannie Burgess' Allergy-Lung, Lung Moistening,** Seasonal Cold and Flu, Topical Analgesic, and Vulnerary

Herbs: Astragalus, black cohosh, **cordyceps,** devil's claw, **garlic,** goldenseal, horsetail, licorice, lobelia, marshmallow, mullein, and Saint John's wort

Essential Oils: Eucalyptus, frankincense, **pine,** rosemary, and thyme

Sinuses   *Body Part*

The function of the sinuses is not clear, but theories include humidification and warming of incoming air, lightening of the skull, improvement of vocal resonance, absorption of shock to the face or skull, and secretion of mucus to assist with air filtration. The sinuses are lined with the mucoperiosteum, which is thinner and has fewer blood vessels and glands than the mucosa of the nasal cavity. Cilia sweep mucus out of the sinuses and into the nasal passages for elimination. This makes healthy sinuses self-cleaning, but certain airborne pollutants and pathogens can overcome its defenses and cause infection from time to time, which can congest and plug up the sinuses.

Formulas: Antihistamine, **Christopher's Sinus**, Disinfectant EO, Ed Millet's Herbal Crisis, Fire Cider, Jeannie Burgess' Allergy-Lung, **Sinus**, **Steven Horne's Sinus Snuff**, and Topical Analgesic

Herbs: Bayberry, burdock, **eyebright**, **fenugreek**, goldenseal, and **thyme**

Supplements: Nanoparticle silver, vitamin A, vitamin C, and xylitol

Essential Oils: Cajeput, eucalyptus, pine, ravensara, tea tree, and thyme

Circulatory System

Poor circulation affects every part of the body because good circulation is essential to the delivery of oxygen and nutrients to every cell and the removal of carbon dioxide and other wastes.

The main function of the circulatory system is to provide all living cells in our bodies with oxygen and essential nutrients, then to take away each cell's waste. It is an amazing highway that travels through the entire body, connecting all the cells together. This complex system is made up of the heart, arteries, and veins.

The heart pumps the blood through the arteries, the largest blood vessels in the body. The arteries branch out to all parts of the body, getting smaller and smaller as they reach the extremities of the body. The smallest blood vessels are called capillaries. Here, the nutrient-waste exchange is made and then the nutrient-deficient blood, carrying waste, returns to the heart by way of the veins.

The circulatory system strongly affects the health of every other system in the body. Every part of the body needs a supply of oxygen and nutrients from the blood and the removal of carbon dioxide and wastes. When circulation becomes impaired, degeneration sets in wherever the blood can't reach.

The circulatory system is also a vital part of the immune system as it carries white blood cells and other immune factors like antibodies. It is also the avenue for delivery of endocrine hormones to tissues.

Indications for Circulatory System

- Anemia
- Chest pain
- Cold hands and feet
- Diabetes or metabolic syndrome
- Family history of heart disease
- Gingivitis or gum disease
- Heart palpitations
- High or low blood pressure
- High cholesterol or triglycerides
- Irregular heart beat, arrhythmia
- Rapid heart beat, tachycardia
- Swelling in lower extremities
- Varicose veins or spider veins
- Wounds that won't heal in the extremities

Circulatory Irritation   *Overactive/Hot*

Circulatory irritation is the beginning of most circulatory health problems, including the hardening of the arteries which leads to heart attacks and strokes. Remedies that help to reduce circulatory irritation, including eating lots of brightly colored fresh fruits and vegetables will help prevent circulatory problems.

Indications for Circulatory Irritation

Pulse: Strong, rapid and full, or rapid and irregular

Tongue: Elongated with red tip or red dots on tip

Emotional State: Restless, overstimulated, heartbroken, workaholic

- Gum disease (gingivitis)
- Reddish complexion, red ears, reddish nose
- Spider veins on nose or cheeks
- Metabolic syndrome or diabetes with high blood pressure
- Tachycardia or heart palpitations
- Cardiac hypertrophy
- Heart feels weak, pain in the region of the heart and shoulder

The following cooling and soothing remedies can help.

Formulas: Antioxidant, Cardiovascular Nutritional, and Irritable Bowel Fiber

Herbs: Bilberry, ginkgo, grape skin and seeds, **hawthorn**, lemon balm, **linden**, lycium, **mangosteen (fruit and pericarp)**, rose hips, tea (green), **turmeric**, willow, and yarrow

Supplements: Bioflavonoids, **Co-Q10**, curcumin, resveratrol, **vitamin A**, **vitamin C**, **vitamin D**, and **vitamin E**

Circulatory Depression   *Underactive/Cold*

Circulatory depression is the lack of good circulation throughout the body. Without a good blood supply, no tissue of the body can be healthy. Many aromatic herbs can stimulate circulation to help keep blood flow going to all parts of the body. Regular exercise is also important for good blood flow.

Indications for Circulatory Depression

Pulse: Slow, deep, feeble or rapid and weak; may also be irregular

Tongue: Bluish cast or pale, possibly swollen or dark red

Emotional State: Chronically heartbroken, emotionally depressed, lacking courage or motivation

- Poor circulation, cold hands and feet
- Vertical crease in left earlobe
- Pale or anemic OR may have a bluish or dark cast
- Poor wound healing
- Fatigue and lethargy
- Tendency to edema
- Sensation of heaviness in the chest or angina
- Shortness of breath

The following warming and stimulating remedies can help.

Formulas: Circulatory, **Fire Cider**, and Heart Health

Herbs: Arjuna, black pepper, **capsicum**, cinnamon, dong quai, **garlic**, ginger, nettle leaf and seed, **prickly ash**, rosemary, and turmeric

Supplements: Co-Q10, curcumin, **L-carnitine**, magnesium, and **vitamin B$_3$**

Essential Oils: Cinnamon, clove, **rosemary**, and thyme

Circulatory Stagnation *Torpid/Damp*

If blood becomes too thick and doesn't flow well through the arteries and veins, blood clots can develop. These can cause thrombosis, heart attacks and strokes. Regular exercise and staying properly hydrated help prevent circulatory stagnation as do remedies that naturally thin the blood and improve blood flow.

Indications for Circulatory Stagnation

Iridology: Lipemic diathesis, pinguicula, hematogenic constitution

Tongue: Swollen, damp

Pulse: Full

Emotional State: Awake at night, excessive thinking

- Thick blood, dehydration
- Tendency for blood clot formation (thrombosis)
- Congestive heart failure, fluid around the heart
- Heart disease with rheumatism, arthritis or skin eruptions
- Tendency to edema and constipation
- Dull hangover sensations with difficulty rising in the morning
- Lack of physical activity, sedentary lifestyle

The following drying and cleansing remedies can help.

Formulas: Cardiovascular Antioxidant, Oral Chelation, and **Vein Tonic**

Herbs: Alfalfa, **artichoke**, **butcher's broom**, dandelion, goldenseal, **guggul**, **horse chestnut**, nettle leaf, **orange (bergamot)**, Oregon grape, red yeast rice, rehmannia, reishi, and **turmeric**

Supplements: Chlorophyll and **vitamin E**

Circulatory Atrophy *Rigid/Dry*

Plaque forming in the arteries is the major symptom of cardiovascular atrophy. As blood vessels lose flexibility, blood flow is impeded and the risk of clots forming increases. High blood pressure and irregularities of the heart can also be part of the picture. Congestive heart failure is also a severe form of circulatory atrophy.

Indications for Circulatory Atrophy

Iridology: Lipemic diathesis, bordered meander (sclera)

Pulse: Feels hard, inflexible; may be irregular

Emotional State: Emotionally rigid, hardness of heart

- Arteriosclerosis, hardening of the arteries
- Heavy dental plaque formation
- High blood pressure
- Wounds don't heal
- Ringing in the ears
- Hands and feet chronically cold
- Memory loss, absent mindedness, difficulty concentrating, tendency to fall asleep when sitting
- Problems with heart valves

The following moistening and building remedies can help.

Formulas: Broken and Hardened Hearts FE, Cardiovascular Antioxidant, Heart Health, **Nitric Oxide Boosting**, and **Oral Chelation**

Herbs: Arjuna, coleus, ginseng (Asian/Korean), **hawthorn**, **night-blooming cereus**, and **reishi**

Supplements: Co-Q10, krill oil, **magnesium**, omega-3 DHA, **omega-3 EFAs**, **vitamin A**, **vitamin C**, **vitamin D**, and **vitamin E**

Essential Oils: Cypress, geranium, juniper, and lemon

Circulatory Constriction *Spastic/Tense*

Arteries contain small muscles that contract to decrease blood flow and relax to increase blood flow. This is regulated by a chemical messenger called nitric oxide (NO). As arteries become increasingly narrow, blood pressure increases. Helping blood vessels relax through lifestyle changes such as stress management and supplements is important to circulatory health.

Indications for Circulatory Constriction

Iridology: Contraction furrows, pulsing pupils

Tongue: Possibly quivering

Pulse: Wiry, tense or bounding

Emotional State: Emotionally tense, nervous, difficulty relaxing; obsessive thought patterns; person feels regret as if they had lost the chance for a happy life

- High blood pressure
- Cardiac arrhythmia (irregular heart rate), often associated with stress
- Angina (chest pain) associated with stress and nervous tension

The following relaxing remedies can help.

Formulas: Blood Pressure Reducing, Broken and Hardened Hearts FE, Cardiovascular Nutritional, Male Performance, and **Nitric Oxide Boosting**

Herbs: Arjuna, **beet**, black cohosh, capsicum, coleus, cramp bark, garlic, hawthorn, **khella**, **linden**, **lobelia**, motherwort, and **olive leaf**

Supplements: L-arginine and **magnesium**

Essential Oils: Bergamot, chamomile (Roman), **lavender**, **marjoram**, neroli, and **ylang ylang**

Circulatory Relaxation   *Atonic/Loose*

When blood vessels lose tone, as in varicose veins or aneurysm, they need toning agents to restore their structural integrity. You can apply various astringents topically (where possible) or use toning remedies internally. Bleeding of any kind would also be considered a problem of circulatory relaxation.

Indications for Circulatory Relaxation

Iridology: Vessel pools or meandering vessels (sclera)

Tongue: Possible bluish cast

Pulse: Relaxed, non-resistant

- Aneurysm
- Bleeding or discharge of blood
- Varicose veins, spider veins or easy bruising
- Thick prominent, visible veins
- Tendency for hemorrhoids or anal fistula
- Tendency for nose bleeds or easy bleeding
- Tired, sore legs
- Bluish or dark cast to the complexion
- Uterine fibroids and endometriosis in women
- prostate swelling and prostatitis in men

The following toning remedies can help.

Formulas: Internal Bleeding and **Vein Tonic**

Herbs: Bayberry, bilberry, **butcher's broom**, **calendula**, collinsonia, **horse chestnut**, lady's mantle, rose hips, **shepherd's purse**, tienchi ginseng, **white oak bark**, and **yarrow**

Supplements: Bioflavonoids, silicon, **vitamin C**, and vitamin E

Essential Oils: Cypress, geranium, juniper, **lemon**, and rosemary

Specific Circulatory Tissues

Here are some specific remedies for various parts of the circulatory system.

Arteries   *Tissue*

Arteries are blood vessels, the strong and elastic tubes that carry oxygen-rich blood away from the heart. As the arteries move away from the heart, they divide into smaller vessels. The largest arteries are about as thick as a thumb. The smallest arteries are thinner than hair. These thinner arteries are called arterioles. Arteries carry bright-red blood, which comes from the oxygen that they carry. The arteries have a one-cell-thick lining that produces a chemical messenger called nitric oxide. Nitric oxide dilates blood vessels to maintain normal blood pressure. Arteries can also develop arterial plaque, which causes heart disease. Here are some of the direct aids that promote healthy arteries and arterial blood flow.

Formulas: Antioxidant, **Blood Pressure Reducing**, **Cardiovascular Antioxidant**, Cardiovascular Nutritional, Cholesterol-Regulating, **Circulatory**, **Nitric Oxide Boosting**, Oral Chelation, and Stabilized Allicin

Herbs: Bilberry, **capsicum**, coleus, ginkgo, hawthorn, and linden

Supplements: Vitamin A, **vitamin C**, vitamin D, and **vitamin E**

Blood   *Tissue*

Blood carries nutrients, water, oxygen, and waste products to and from the body's cells. It is pumped by the heart through thousands of miles of blood vessels. A young person has about four quarts of blood in his or her body, whereas an adult has about five quarts. Much more than a red liquid, blood is made up of liquids, solids, and small amounts of oxygen and carbon dioxide.

Red blood cells are responsible for carrying oxygen and carbon dioxide. Red blood cells pick up oxygen in the lungs and transport it to all the cells in the body. After delivering the oxygen to the cells, it gathers up the carbon dioxide (a waste gas produced as our cells work) and transports it back to the lungs where it is removed from the body through exhaling (breathing out). There are about five million red blood cells in one drop of blood.

White blood cells help the body fight off germs. As germs enter the body, white blood cells attack and destroy them. When you develop an infection, your body will produce more white blood cells to help fight it.

Platelets are blood cells that help stop bleeding. When we cut ourselves and blood leaks out, platelets in our blood come to the site and plug the opening. As the platelets stick to the opening, they attract more platelets, fibers and other blood cells to help seal the broken blood vessel. When the platelets have finished their job, the wound stops bleeding.

Plasma makes up about half of the body's blood. There are billions of living blood cells floating in plasma. Plasma carries the blood cells and other components throughout the body. Plasma is 95 percent water and the other 5 percent is made up of dissolved substances, including salts.

Red blood cells, white blood cells and platelets are all made by the bone marrow, whereas plasma is made in the liver. Blood-building remedies can be helpful for anemia, monthly blood loss through menstruation, or just a lack of good-quality blood or blood volume.

Formulas: Chinese Qi and Blood Tonic, Chinese Wood-Decreasing, **Chinese Wood-Increasing**, **Christopher's Herbal Iron**, Internal Bleeding, Methyl B12 Vitamin, Nattokinase Enzyme, Pet Supplement, and Pregnancy Tea

Herbs: Alfalfa, beet, blessed thistle, burdock, chickweed, **dong quai**, **nettle, stinging, peony**, and **yellow dock**

Supplements: Chlorophyll, **iron**, **vitamin B-complex**, vitamin B$_9$, **vitamin C**, vitamin E, and zinc

Capillaries   *Tissue*

Capillaries are tiny blood vessels as thin or thinner than the hairs on your head. Capillaries connect arteries to veins. Through a process known as microcirculation, food nutrients, oxygen, and wastes pass in and out of your blood through the capillary walls. Capillaries are only one cell thick. Capillary health is essential to delivering oxygen and nutrients to the tissues and removing waste.

Formulas: Antioxidant, Liquid Lymph, Oral Chelation, and **Vein Tonic**

Herbs: Butcher's broom, echinacea, **ginkgo**, hawthorn, **prickly ash**, **rose**, and yarrow

Supplements: Vitamin C and vitamin E

Essential Oils: Neroli

Heart   *Organ*

Throughout history, the heart has been viewed as the center of human emotions and the most vital organ to life. The heart is approximately the size of a man's fist and is located slightly off-center in the lower chest. Each of the two sides of the heart is a separate pump made up of two chambers, the atrium and the ventricle, which, along with one-way valves, keep blood flowing in the right direction. The right side of the heart pumps blood to the lungs, where it receives a healthy supply of oxygen. The blood then returns to the left side of the heart, which pumps the oxygenated blood to the body. The oxygen-depleted blood returns from the body to the right side of the heart, and the cycle continues.

This cycle operates every minute of our lives. The heart beats an average of seventy times per minute, pumping over ten pints of blood through the body even when it is at rest. It is estimated that the heart beats a total of 2.5 billion times over the course of one's life, although this is a conservative estimate.

To perform at this level, the heart requires its own blood vessels. These are called coronary arteries and cardiac veins. Their only job is to supply the cardiac muscle with the nutrients and oxygen it needs. This muscle is thick and strong and is surrounded on the outside by the pericardium and on the inside by the endocardium. These layers serve as protection for the heart and also prevent blood from leaking out of the heart into the chest cavity.

Formulas: Brain-Heart, Broken and Hardened Hearts FE, Cardiovascular Antioxidant, Chinese Fire-Increasing, Cholesterol-Regulating, Circulatory, Garcinia Fat-Burning, Grief and Sadness FE, **Heart Health**, **Nitric Oxide Boosting**, and **Oral Chelation**

Herbs: Arjuna, astragalus, black cohosh, blessed thistle, cordyceps, eleuthero, gotu kola, **hawthorn**, olive, passion flower, red raspberry, red yeast rice, safflower, and valerian

Supplements: Calcium, **Co-Q10**, iron, krill oil, **L-carnitine**, lecithin, **magnesium**, **vitamin C**, **vitamin D**, and **vitamin E**

Essential Oils: Clove and rose

Spleen   *Organ*

The spleen is a fist-shaped purple organ about four inches long that resides in the upper far left part of the abdomen and to the left of the stomach. It is protected by the rib cage, so you can't easily feel it unless it becomes abnormally enlarged.

The spleen has a variety of functions in the body. It assists the immune system by acting as a filter for blood. It does this by recycling old red blood cells and storing platelets and white blood cells. The spleen also helps fight certain kinds of bacteria that cause pneumonia and meningitis.

An enlarged spleen is generally caused by viral mononucleosis ("mono"), liver disease, blood cancers (lymphoma and leukemia), or other conditions. The spleen is also vulnerable to injury. A ruptured spleen can cause serious internal bleeding and is a life-threatening emergency.

Formulas: Chinese Earth-Increasing, Essiac Immune Tea, and Immune-Boosting

Herbs: Chamomile, chickweed, dandelion, devil's claw, licorice, milk thistle, red clover, Saint John's wort, **white oak**, and yellow dock

Supplements: Chlorophyll, lecithin, vitamin B-complex, and vitamin B$_9$

Essential Oils: Patchouli

Veins   *Tissue*

Veins carry oxygen-depleted blood back to the heart. Veins differ from arteries in structure and function. For example, arteries are more muscular than veins, whereas veins are often closer to the skin and contain valves to help keep blood flowing toward the heart. Poor venous circulation can result in fluid retention, varicose veins, hemorrhoids, spider veins and increased risk of blood clots. A list of specific direct aids that tone and strengthen the veins follows.

Formulas: Antioxidant, Nattokinase Enzyme, **Oral Chelation**, and **Vein Tonic**

Herbs: Bilberry, **butcher's broom**, feverfew, **horse chestnut**, and rose

Supplements: Bioflavonoids, vitamin C, and **vitamin C**

Essential Oils: Geranium

Structural System

The health of the structural system is dependent on the health of other systems such as digestion and circulation. If you want to work on the structural system, you should also consider working with these other systems.

The structural system consists of the bones, muscles, skin, hair, and connective tissue. It forms the framework of the body and allows us to move, as well as the body's protective coverings and the connective tissue that hold the body together.

The skeletal system serves as the body's framework. And, the bones double as a storehouse for minerals. The bone marrow is where both red and white blood cells are made. The bones also serve to protect vital organs like the brain, spinal column, heart and lungs.

The muscular system moves the body and holds the skeletal system in place. Muscles power the heartbeat, breathing, digestion, and other automatic processes.

The skin and membranes form the protective barriers of the body and are the body's first line of immune defense. The skin is also an important sensory organ and helps to regulate body temperature.

Indications for Structural System

- Arthritis or joint pain
- Back or neck pain
- Brittle fingernails
- Broken bones
- Cramps or spasms
- Crooked teeth
- Dental problems, many cavities and root canals
- Gout
- Injuries (sprains, bruises, cuts, etc.)
- Muscle tension
- Osteoporosis
- Skin problems, like eczema and psoriasis
- Stiff, aching, or painful muscles
- Teeth grinding
- Weak legs, knees, or ankles

Structural Irritation   *Overactive/Hot*

The inflammatory response to damage or irritation is what we are labeling structural irritation. It involves swollen, red and painful tissues in any part of the structural system. Remedies that ease pain and inflammation are helpful for structural irritation.

Indications for Structural Irritation

Iridology: Whitish fibers, uric acid diathesis, overacid or febrile subtype

Tongue: Bright red, often pointed

Pulse: Rapid, floating, superficial

Emotional State: Irritable, short temper, emotionally reactive, but quick to let go

- Acute inflammation (heat, swelling, redness and pain)
- Tissues appear red, often swollen
- Tissues feel warm and tender to the touch
- Acute, sharp pain in tissues
- Aftermath of acute injury or trauma (e.g. bumps, abrasions, sprains, burns)
- Aftermath of surgery

The following cooling and soothing remedies can help.

Formulas: Analgesic Nerve, **Anti-Inflammatory Pain**, Ayurvedic Skin Healing, **CBD Anti-inflammatory**, **CBD Topical Analgesic**, Healing Salve, Joint Healing Nutrients, Proanthocyanidins, Shock and Injury FE, Stan Malstrom's Herbal Aspirin, and Topical Analgesic

Herbs: Aloe vera juice or gel, **arnica**, black cohosh, **boswellia**, chickweed, **comfrey**, **devil's claw**, **mangosteen pericarp**, marshmallow, **plantain**, rehmannia, slippery elm, **turmeric**, willow bark, and yarrow

Supplements: Curcumin, MSM, vitamin C, and vitamin E

Essential Oils: Lavender, **menthol**, rose, and **wintergreen**

Structural Depression *Underactive/Cold*

Structural depression involves a loss of function and warmth in structural tissues. It is a weakened state of the tissues, which generally require aromatics, essential oils, and other warming remedies to restore circulation and energy. Tissue that has weakened and become infected can also benefit from remedies for structural depression. In this case, there is a dark reddish or purplish color to the tissues, such as you find in a bruise, rather than the bright-red color of structural irritation.

Indications for Structural Depression

Iridology: Dark fibers, grayish colored iris

Tongue: Pale or dark reddish/purplish

Pulse: Slow, thin and weak, may be rapid and non-resistant

Emotional State: Slow to react, sometimes stubborn; doesn't anger easily, but once angry finds it difficult to let go

- Tissues appear whitish or pale; or dark red with a bluish, purple-black color (bruising)
- Tissues cool to the touch
- Dull, chronic aching pain
- Wounds and injuries not healing properly
- Infected wounds and injuries with pus formation

The following warming and stimulating remedies can help.

Formulas: Analgesic EO, Enzyme Spray, and Topical Analgesic

Herbs: Capsicum, cinnamon, clove, **garlic**, ginger, **myrrh**, **prickly ash**, and thyme

Supplements: Zinc

Essential Oils: Camphor, cinnamon, clove, eucalyptus, **myrrh**, oregano, **tea tree**, and **thyme**

Structural Stagnation *Torpid/Damp*

Whenever structural tissues are swollen, there is structural stagnation. Structural stagnation is a sign of poor blood and lymph flow through the area. Skin-eruptive diseases are also considered a form of structural stagnation. Alteratives are used to promote the flow of lymph and help the body remove irritants. Some aromatics and essential oils may also be helpful.

Indications for Structural Stagnation

Iridology: Lacuna, connective tissue weakness

Tongue: Swollen, damp with heavy mucus coating

Pulse: Rolling, slippery, sluggish

Emotional State: Spontaneous, changeable, emotionally driven

- Tissues swollen, spongy to the touch
- Swollen joints, with dull persistent pain
- Swollen lymph nodes
- Tissues irritated from exposure to chemicals or irritants
- Skin-eruptive conditions such as acne, oozing rashes, pox
- Boils, abscesses

The following drying and cleansing remedies can help.

Formulas: Ayurvedic Skin Healing, **Blood Purifier**, Detoxifying, **Herbal Arthritis**, and Topical Analgesic

Herbs: Alfalfa, **black walnut**, **burdock**, chaparral, dandelion root, devil's claw, goldenseal, myrrh, Oregon grape, **pau d'arco**, **red clover**, **turmeric**, yarrow, yellow dock, and **yucca**

Supplements: Chlorophyll and **curcumin**

Essential Oils: Cinnamon, frankincense, grapefruit (pink), and lemon

Structural Atrophy *Rigid/Dry*

When tissues become weak, brittle, dried out, and/or inflexible, they have atrophied. Structural atrophy involves this kind of degenerative condition in tissues. Remedies that supply nutrients to moisten and rebuild tissues, including various mucilaginous and nutritive herbs, are helpful. Many of these remedies can also help injuries to heal and/or keep structural tissues healthy.

Indications for Structural Atrophy

Iridology: Pigments, heterochromia

Tongue: Red (especially in the center), often pointed or elongated

Pulse: Generally rapid, possibly floating

Emotional State: Analytical, mental, thoughtful, slow to change mind

- Tissues are dry, rough or leathery, thin and brittle
- Brittle nails, hair, skin and bones
- Diagnosis of osteoarthritis or osteoporosis
- Loss of many teeth to decay
- Broken bones, sprains and other injuries slow to heal
- General structural weakness and degeneration

The following moistening and building remedies can help.

Formulas: Colloidal Mineral, Healing Salve, Herbal Calcium, **Joan Patton's Herbal Minerals**, Joint Healing Nutrients, and **Skeletal Support**

Herbs: Alfalfa, **aloe vera**, ashwagandha, chickweed, **comfrey**, dulse, eucommia, flax seed, **horsetail**, kelp, licorice, marshmallow, mullein, **plantain**, rehmannia, **slippery elm**, and **teasel**

Supplements: Calcium, **chondroitin**, **collagen**, **glucosamine**, and omega-3 EPA

Essential Oils: Jasmine, rose, sandalwood, and ylang ylang

Structural Constriction   *Spastic/Tense*

Muscle spasms and cramps are the major signs of structural constriction, which can also involve muscle tension and shooting pains. Remedies that relax muscles are indicated in structural constriction.

Indications for Structural Constriction

Iridology: Contraction furrows, tight collarette

Tongue: Possibly quivering

Pulse: Tense, wiry

Emotional State: Tense, nervous, and high-strung; lacks flexibility and grace in movements

- Muscle cramping and spasm
- Chronic muscle tension
- Sharp stabbing or shooting pain
- Pains that migrate from one location to another
- Intermittent sharp, pain in muscles or joints
- Tension headaches
- General stiffness and inflexibility

The following relaxing remedies can help.

Formulas: Analgesic Nerve, **Antispasmodic**, **Fibromyalgia**, Herbal Potassium, and Jeannie Burgess' Stress

Herbs: Agrimony, black cohosh, cramp bark, **kava kava**, khella, **lobelia**, skullcap, skunk cabbage, valerian, and wild yam

Supplements: Magnesium

Essential Oils: Chamomile (Roman), clary sage, **jasmine**, **lavender**, marjoram, sandalwood, and **ylang ylang**

Structural Relaxation   *Atonic/Loose*

When structural tissues lack tone or suffer from excessive discharge (e.g. oozing, bleeding) remedies that tone the structure are indicated.

Indications for Structural Relaxation

Iridology: Connective tissue type, polyglandular type

Emotional State: Spontaneous, changeable, emotionally driven, burns out rapidly

- Internal hemorrhage or external bleeding
- Oozing wounds, injuries or damaged tissues
- Wounds with pus
- Insect bites and stings
- Poison ivy or poison oak
- Severe swelling
- Swelling associated with sprains and other minor injuries
- Ulcerations

The following toning remedies can help.

Formulas: Colloidal Mineral, Herbal Tooth Powder, Joan Patton's Herbal Minerals, Skeletal Support, Watkin's Hair, Skin, and and Nails

Herbs: Bayberry, **calendula**, **goldenseal**, **horsetail**, red raspberry, rose hips, **white oak bark**, and **yarrow**

Supplements: Calcium and silicon

Essential Oils: Geranium, juniper, and lemon

Specific Structural Tissues

What follows are remedies for specific structural organs and tissues.

Bones   *Tissue*

The skeletal system is comprised of all the different bones in the body and the joints that connect them. The system's basic function is to provide support and structure for the body. The skeletal system also protects vital organs, assists in body movement and helps to produce blood cells. Bones also serve as a storehouse for minerals. Old bone is continually being reabsorbed, and new bone laid down.

Bone tissue has characteristics that are unique from any other tissue. It is one of the hardest tissues in the body, but it is not completely solid. Internal cavities are the site of bone cell production, and blood vessels reach these cavities through a central canal. These cavities do not detract from the strength of the bone, the resistance of which equals that of iron—four times the strength of concrete.

Along with their strength, our bones are also remarkable because of their flexibility and lightness. The skeleton accounts for only 14 percent of the total body weight. The flexibility of our bones comes from collagen, which makes up part of the bone composition. The other components are calcium and phosphorus, which form rigid crystals for strength. Bone also has the unique ability to heal a break in itself without scarring.

Formulas: Chinese Water-Increasing, **Colloidal Mineral**, Herbal Arthritis, Herbal Calcium, **Joan Patton's Herbal Minerals**, **Joint Healing Nutrients**, Pet

Supplement, **Skeletal Support**, Vulnerary, **Watkin's Hair, Skin, and and Nails**

Herbs: Alfalfa, bee pollen, **comfrey**, dulse, **horsetail**, hydrangea, mullein, **rehmannia**, slippery elm, and white oak

Supplements: Boron, **calcium**, copper, krill oil, L-lysine, magnesium, manganese, vitamin C, **vitamin D**, and zinc

Gums   *Tissue*

When gums become inflamed they can recede, causing teeth to become loose. Although flossing and cleaning the teeth help to prevent gum inflammation, it is really a systemic problem showing that there is inflammation throughout the body, particularly in the cardiovascular system. Along with keeping teeth clean, increasing intake of antioxidants will help keep gums healthy. Here are some specific direct aids for the gums.

Formulas: Anti-Inflammatory Pain, Antioxidant, **Chinese Yang-Reducing**, and **Herbal Tooth Powder**

Herbs: Bayberry, **black walnut**, goldenseal, juniper, and **white oak**

Supplements: Co-Q10, **nanoparticle silver**, and xylitol

Essential Oils: Clove, geranium, and myrrh

Hair   *Tissue*

Unhealthy hair is a sign of other problems in the body such as poor nutrition, poor circulation, or thyroid problems, which must be addressed to keep the hair healthy. Hair color depends on trace minerals. Essential oils can be added to shampoo to aid hair health.

Formulas: Chinese Water-Increasing and **Watkin's Hair, Skin, and Nails**

Herbs: Dulse, **horsetail**, kelp, rosemary, sage, and yarrow

Supplements: MSM, vitamin B_5, vitamin E, and **zinc**

Essential Oils: Clary sage, lemongrass, and **rosemary**

Joints   *Tissue*

Joints are the places where bones join together. Joints allow movement in the body. Joints contain ligaments that connect bones together. There is also a cushion of cartilage and fluid that allows the bones to glide over one another without wear and tear. When joints are damaged, arthritis, pain, and stiffness can set in.

Formulas: Analgesic EO, Analgesic Nerve, Anti-Inflammatory Pain, General Analgesic, **Herbal Arthritis**, **Joint Healing Nutrients**, Watkin's Hair, Skin, and and Nails

Herbs: Alfalfa, boswellia, **horsetail**, **turmeric**, willow, and **yucca**

Supplements: Chondroitin, collagen, **curcumin**, and glucosamine

Essential Oils: Wintergreen

Muscles   *Tissue*

The muscular system, another aspect of the body's structure, is responsible for the muscular workings of each organ (such as the heart), as well as body movement. The bones of the skeleton make the body a system of levers, and muscles move these levers.

Muscles are not as solid as they appear. They are really made up of bundles of muscle fiber. Nerves attach to these fibers, and with an electrical impulse from the brain, several muscles work together to perform a fairly simple function, such as moving a finger, or a complex movement, such as slam-dunking a basketball.

The nerve signals from the brain cause the muscle fibers they are communicating with to slide over one another. This causes the whole muscle to contract and provide the desired movement. Contraction is the only way muscles work. In other words, muscles pull on the bones rather than push.

Skeletal muscle is the most abundant tissue in our bodies. A healthy, trained muscular system makes everyday tasks easier, and feats of athletic prowess possible.

Formulas: Analgesic EO, **Antispasmodic**, Colloidal Mineral, Electrolyte Drink, **Fibromyalgia**, General Analgesic, Topical Analgesic, **Vulnerary**, Whole Food Green Drink, and **Whole Food Protein**

Herbs: Alfalfa, bee pollen, chamomile, comfrey, dong quai, hops, kava kava, lobelia, **safflower**, valerian, and **yucca**

Supplements: Calcium, Co-Q10, lecithin, **magnesium**, MSM, vitamin B-complex, vitamin B_5, vitamin B_6, vitamin C, and vitamin E

Essential Oils: Marjoram and neroli

Nails   *Tissue*

Like hair, the health of fingernails depends on the overall health of the body. Problems with fingernails can signal specific health issues. Brittle nails can be a sign of a lack of minerals like calcium and silica. Nail fungus can be a sign of reduced immunity or systemic yeast infection. Problems with fingernails can also indicate circulatory problems, a lack of protein or other nutrients, and thyroid problems.

Formulas: Algae, Enzyme Spray, GLA Oil, **Watkin's Hair, Skin, and Nails**, **Whole Food Green Drink**, and Whole Food Protein

Herbs: Black walnut, calendula, **dulse**, **horsetail**, and kelp

Supplements: MSM, omega-3 EFAs, **silicon**, vitamin B-complex, and **zinc**

Essential Oils: Tea tree

Skin   *Tissue*

The skin is the external covering of the body. It is a protective layer of the body that protects it from harmful external influences.

There are millions of living organisms in a person's skin, including some bacteria that help the skin defend itself against infection. Skin also secrets a fluid to lubricate as well as defend against toxic substances. As a selective barrier, skin keeps out infection but allows water and heat to pass through.

If the skin covering your body was laid out flat, it would measure between twelve and twenty square feet. Skin makes up 12 percent of your body weight and is composed of three layers—the epidermis, the dermis, and the subcutis. The epidermis is the outer layer, which is also the thinnest, but just how thin it is depends on where it is on the body. For example, on the feet the epidermis is very thick, while it is very thin on the eyelids. The epidermis is the location of nerve endings, which allows us to respond to the gentlest touch.

The middle layer, or dermis, is where injured tissue is repaired, and it is also the location of the skin's blood vessels and sweat glands. Both the blood vessels and the sweat glands contribute to temperature control—an important function of the skin. For example, in cold weather, blood flow slows down and hairs are pulled erect to trap a layer of air next to the skin to provide extra insulation. In hot weather, sweat is secreted from the sweat glands. The moisture evaporates off the surface of the skin, drawing heat out of the body.

The subcutis, or subcutaneous layer, is the bottom layer of skin. Its tissue is made mostly of lipids, providing a cushion for bones, organs and muscles against bumps. It also acts as insulation.

Skin also protects the body with its pigments. Melanocytes carry the pigment and absorb harmful ultraviolet radiation, turning it into infrared rays. Melanocytes also account for the difference in people's skin color.

Formulas: **Ayurvedic Skin Healing**, Blood Purifier, CBD Topical Analgesic, Chinese Wood-Increasing, Detoxifying, **Enzyme Spray**, **Healing Salve**, Shock and Injury FE, Topical Analgesic, **Vulnerary**, **Watkin's Hair, Skin, and and Nails**

Herbs: Aloe vera, bayberry, black walnut, **burdock**, chamomile, chickweed, **dulse**, echinacea, feverfew, goldenseal, gotu kola, **horsetail**, juniper, **kelp**, marshmallow, Oregon grape, passion flower, psyllium, **red clover**, safflower, sage, saw palmetto, slippery elm, white oak, yarrow, and yellow dock

Supplements: Charcoal, iron, MSM, omega-3 DHA, **omega-3 EFAs**, vitamin B$_3$, **vitamin C**, **vitamin E**, and **zinc**

Essential Oils: Bergamot, clary sage, grapefruit (pink), helichrysum, jasmine, lavender, lemongrass, marjoram, myrrh, neroli, red mandarin, rose, rosemary, sandalwood, and wintergreen

Sweat Glands

The sweat glands help the body with thermoregulation. They open to allow sweat to cool the body and close to conserve heat. Remedies that help the sweat glands can be very valuable in fighting colds and fevers. Herbs that open the sweat glands are called diaphoretics or sudorifics.

Formulas: Ed Millet's Herbal Crisis, Fire Cider, Paavo Airola's Cold, and **Steven Horne's Children's Composition**

Herbs: Boneset, capsicum, catnip, chamomile, elder, ginger, lobelia, peppermint, **sage**, and **yarrow**

Essential Oils: Cinnamon

Spinal Discs   *Tissue*

In between the vertebrae are the spinal discs, doughnut-shaped cushions, whose soft centers are encased in a tougher exterior. The spinal discs carry the weight of the upper body from one vertebrae to the next, while allowing the vertebra to move so the spine can flex.

When the spine is chronically curved, it places excessive stress on one part of the disc. Instead of being distributed evenly across the disc, the weight is pushed to one side. As the discs are chronically distressed, especially in someone with a nutrient-deficient diet, they start to wear out. They may bulge out and eventually rupture. They may also thin out so they no longer provide adequate cushioning between the vertebrae. As discs weaken, osteoarthritis may occur, causing further deterioration of the spine.

The spinal column is also the protective housing for the spinal cord, which carries nerve impulses from the brain to the body and from the body back to the brain. Peripheral nerves exit the spinal column in between the vertebrae. These nerves are what allow you to feel and move, and they also help to regulate the function of all the organs and glands.

Poor alignment of the spinal column can put pressure on the nerves, which is why chiropractic care or other body work that helps to better align the spinal vertebrae often appears to help the function of internal organs like digestion, breathing, and circulation. People who do exercises that help to stretch and align the back, such as yoga, also notice overall improvement of body function.

When the misalignment becomes severe enough to cause discs to slip or rupture, more noticeable problems occur.

Slipped or ruptured discs put pressure on nerves, which can cause neck, arm, or leg pain. There may even be sensations of numbness or tingling in parts of the body supplied by those nerves. Muscles may even weaken, impairing movement.

Formulas: Anti-Inflammatory Pain, **CBD Topical Analgesic**, Chinese Water-Decreasing, **Chinese Water-Increasing**, **Enzyme Spray**, Topical Analgesic, and Vulnerary

Herbs: Capsicum, **goldenseal**, lobelia, and mullein

Supplements: CBD

Teeth   *Tissue*

Although the teeth appear to be solid and permanent, they (like bones) are constantly needing to be remineralized. Adequate levels of minerals and fat-soluble vitamins like D_3 actually help prevent tooth decay. Natural remedies can fight the bacteria in plaque and help mineralize the teeth.

Formulas: **Colloidal Mineral**, Herbal Calcium, **Herbal Tooth Powder**, **Joan Patton's Herbal Minerals**, and Pet Supplement

Herbs: Alfalfa, **black walnut**, and **white oak**

Supplements: Calcium, krill oil, **vitamin D**, and xylitol

Essential Oils: Clove

Urinary System

Problems with the urinary system affect every part of the body because of the role this system plays in detoxification, in fluid and mineral balance, and in regulating blood pressure.

The urinary system consists of the kidneys and bladder. It is responsible for filtering wastes from the bloodstream and eliminating them from the body. The urinary system also participates in the regulation of fluids and minerals in the body and helps to regulate blood pressure.

Poor urinary function can cause lymphatic congestion and edema (water retention). In traditional Chinese medicine, weakness of the kidneys is also linked with structural problems, such as back pain, bone loss, and joint problems, due to its role in regulating pH and mineral balance. There is also a link between urinary problems and reproductive problems in both men and women.

Indications for Urinary System

- Bladder infections
- Blood in the urine
- Burning or painful urination
- Copious, pale urine
- Difficulty starting urination
- Excessive perspiration or night sweats
- Frequent pale urine

- Frequent urination
- Gout
- Kidney stones
- Pain in the mid to low back
- Puffiness under eyes
- Scant, dark urine
- Swollen lymph nodes
- Urinary incontinence (dribbling)
- Urinary tract infections (UTIs)
- Water retention or edema
- Weak knees or legs

Urinary Irritation   *Overactive/Hot*

Urinary irritation involves any acute inflammatory reactions in the urinary organs or passages. This is typically due to infection, but may also be caused by irritants being eliminated via the urinary passages.

Indications for Urinary Irritation

Iridology: Lymphatic constitution, white fibers in kidney area

Tongue: Bright red

Pulse: Rapid, often floating

Emotional State: Irritable, angry, "pissed"

pH: Acid urine, alkaline saliva

- Dark or cloudy urine with strong odor
- Burning, scalding, or painful urination
- Frequent urge to urinate, with scant production of urine
- Heat and heavy sensations in the lumbar region of the back
- Diagnosis of acute urinary tract infections

The following cooling and soothing remedies can help.

Formulas: Liquid Kidney, Urinary Support, and **UTI Prevention**

Herbs: **Corn silk**, **cranberry**, lemon juice, **marshmallow**, mulberry (white) root bark, noni, **pipsissewa**, pygeum, quince (Asian), and yarrow

Supplements: Vitamin C

Urinary Depression   *Underactive/Cold*

In urinary depression, fluid accumulates in the body because of decreased function of the urinary organs. Stimulating diuretics are used to increase the output of the urinary system. Ample amounts of water need to be consumed when taking these remedies.

Indications for Urinary Depression

Iridology: Lymphatic constitution, uric acid diathesis, overacid or febrile subtype, hydrogenoid subtype

Tongue: Pale, damp, and swollen; usually with a heavy coating

Pulse: Weak, deep

Emotional State: Chronic fear, uncertainty, indecisive

pH: Alkaline urine, alkaline saliva

- Scant urine with fluid retention
- Chronic or pitting edema
- Swollen ankles, toes, fingers
- Paleness and puffiness under eyes
- Cold, stiff, heavy feeling in back

The following warming and stimulating remedies can help.

Formulas: Diuretic and Liquid Kidney

Herbs: Buchu, celery seed, **juniper berry**, kava kava, parsley, siler, and **uva ursi**

Essential Oils: Juniper

Urinary Stagnation   *Torpid/Damp*

Urinary stagnation typically involves edema, coupled with sluggish lymphatic function. It may also involve urinary tract infections, creating chronic irritation of the urinary passages.

Indications for Urinary Stagnation

Iridology: Lymphatic constitution, hydrogenoid subtype, straw-yellow color in iris

Tongue: Pale with moist coating; swollen with scalloped edges

Pulse: Rolling or slippery, lacks sharpness

Emotional State: Fearful, timid, wishy-washy

pH: Alkaline urine, acid saliva

- Scanty and clear urine
- Water retention, edema
- Eyes puffy, dull and listless
- Skin stays white for two or more seconds when pressed
- Frequent backache
- Chronic urinary tract infections

The following drying and cleansing remedies can help.

Formulas: Chinese Water-Decreasing, Diuretic, Prostate, **Urinary Immune**, and UTI Prevention

Herbs: Achyranthes, burdock, celery seed, **cleavers, dandelion leaf, goldenseal**, gravel root, hoelen, hydrangea, **lemon juice**, pipsissewa, pygeum, and red clover

Supplements: Berberine

Essential Oils: Grapefruit (pink) and lemon

Urinary Atrophy   *Rigid/Dry*

In urinary atrophy, the kidneys lose some of their filtering ability—that is, they become inefficient at removing irritants, such as acid waste from the system. This tends to show up not only as chronic urinary tract issues but also as a weakening of the structural system. It may also involve the formation of kidney stones.

Indications for Urinary Atrophy

Iridology: Uric acid diathesis, overacid or febrile subtype

Tongue: Dry, may be cracked or withered

Pulse: Weak, slightly tense

Emotional State: Rigid, inflexible, dogmatic, fanatical

pH: Acid urine, acid saliva

- Low back pain or frequent back pain
- Hips will not stay in alignment
- Weak knees and ankles
- Tendency to arthritis and osteoporosis
- Erectile dysfunction, infertility
- Formation of stones or calcifications

The following moistening and building remedies can help.

Formulas: Chinese Water-Increasing, Herbal Potassium, and Urinary Support

Herbs: Astragalus, cleavers, **eucommia, goldenrod, gravel root, horsetail, hydrangea, lemon juice**, marshmallow, mulberry (white) root bark, **nettle leaf and seed**, and noni

Supplements: Magnesium and potassium

Urinary Constriction   *Spastic/Tense*

Sharp pains in the urinary passages or difficulty with urination may be signs of constricted urinary passages or the passage of stones. Antispasmodic remedies that help open the urinary passages may be helpful.

Indications for Urinary Constriction

Iridology: Contraction furrows

Tongue: Quivering

Pulse: Wiry, resistant

Emotional State: Holding on, unable to let go

- Sharp, spastic pains in kidneys or bladder or when urinating
- Edema that comes and goes
- Dark, scant urine alternating with pale, clear urine
- Urinary pain from passing stones

The following relaxing remedies can help.

Formulas: Prostate

Herbs: Agrimony, gravel root, hydrangea, **kava kava**, lemon, and lobelia

Supplements: Magnesium

Urinary Relaxation *Atonic/Loose*

Incontinence and blood in the urine are common signs of urinary relaxation. Remedies that tone urinary passages are indicated.

Indications for Urinary Relaxation

Iridology: Lacuna in urinary area

Tongue: Pale, moist

Pulse: Passive, non-resistant

- Copious, pale urine
- Frequent urination
- Incontinence, dribbling
- Pus or blood in urine
- Nighttime urination
- Weakness and soreness in lower back
- Nocturnal emission in men
- Vaginal discharge in women

The following toning remedies can help.

Formulas: Watkin's Hair, Skin, and Nails

Herbs: Horsetail, pau d'arco, red raspberry, sage, and **uva ursi**

Supplements: Silicon

Specific Urinary Tissues

The following are remedies for specific urinary organs and tissues.

Bladder *Organ*

The bladder holds the urine created by the kidneys until it can be eliminated.

Formulas: Chinese Water-Decreasing, Chinese Water-Increasing, Diuretic, **Liquid Kidney**, Urinary Immune, Urinary Support, and **UTI Prevention**

Herbs: Corn silk, **goldenseal**, horsetail, hydrangea, juniper, licorice, **marshmallow**, Oregon grape, red clover, Saint John's wort, **uva ursi**, and yarrow

Kidneys *Organ*

The main functions of the kidneys are controlling body fluid concentrations and filtering wastes out of the blood. The kidneys also play a role in regulating fluid-mineral balance for structural health and blood pressure.

The kidneys are paired and located in the upper abdomen, where they are protected by the spine and surrounding organs. An average kidney is four inches long, three inches wide, and two inches deep, weighing about five ounces.

Inside each kidney, there are approximately one million nephrons, each of which helps filter the blood. The blood that flows through the kidneys is carrying the byproducts of dead cells from throughout the body. These byproducts include carbon and oxygen (which can be exhaled), hydrogen (which combines with oxygen to form water), and nitrogen. Concentrated amounts of nitrogen in the body can be toxic. This nitrogen is converted to urea in the liver. Urea, along with other foreign substances, is filtered out of the body through the kidneys.

The nephrons pull water, salts, and glucose out of the blood stream, although red blood cells and proteins are too large to pass through the filter. Along the same tubes of the nephron, some water, salt, and glucose are periodically reabsorbed into the bloodstream. But the selective filter doesn't allow urea and other poisonous substances back into the bloodstream.

Urea combines with water to form urine. As more water is reabsorbed in the kidneys, the urine becomes more and more concentrated. The exact concentration levels depend on the body's needs at any given time. The kidneys control body fluid concentration by regulating how much water and salt is reabsorbed. Therefore, if the body needs more salt, the salt concentration in the urine will be less. Also, if you drink more water than your body can use at one time, more water is expelled, also bringing the urine concentration down.

Drinking adequate amounts of water is essential for healthy kidneys along with getting adequate mineral electrolytes, particularly potassium.

Formulas: Chinese Water-Decreasing, **Chinese Water-Increasing**, **Diuretic**, **Herbal Potassium**, Liquid Kidney, Liquid Lymph, and **Urinary Support**

Herbs: Cleavers, dandelion, eucommia, **goldenrod**, horsetail, juniper, kava kava, **nettle, stinging**, noni, and **parsley**

Supplements: Potassium

Glandular System

The glandular system regulates numerous body functions and imbalances in hormones that contribute to many varied health issues. There are three main glands that can be root causes of numerous health problems.

First, problems with the pancreas and blood sugar regulation lead to metabolic syndrome and diabetes, which are linked with increased risk of cancer and other degenerative diseases. Second, the thyroid affects the entire metabolism and energy level, as well as circulation, intestinal function, and immunity. Finally, the adrenal glands help us cope with stress, regulate blood sugar and inflammatory responses, and create the building blocks for reproductive hormones.

The glandular system is a communication network that controls and regulates a vast range of things within our bodies, including sleep, growth, sexual development, metabolism, body temperature, tissue repair and the generation of energy.

The human body has two types of glands—endocrine glands, which secrete hormones into the bloodstream, where they are carried to specific tissues or organs to stimulate a particular reaction, and exocrine glands, which secrete fluids through a duct or a tube. The endocrine glands include the pituitary, pineal, thyroid, parathyroid, thymus, hypothalamus, pancreas, adrenal, and sex glands. The exocrine glands include the tear, salivary, and sweat glands.

Glands can become weakened by stress, poor diet, or the presence of dangerous chemicals. As we age hormonal communication tends to become more confused, which results in a loss of health and stamina.

Indications for Glandular System

- Burning sensations in hands and feet (adrenal, pancreas)
- Cold hands and feet (thyroid)
- Dark circles under eyes (adrenal)
- Dry skin (thyroid)
- Excess weight (pancreas, adrenal, thyroid)
- Fatigue in the afternoons (pancreas, adrenal)
- Fatigue, chronic or excessive (adrenal, thyroid)
- High levels of stress (adrenal)
- Feeling exhausted, burned-out (adrenal, thyroid)
- Frequent thirst and urination (pancreas, adrenal)
- Hair loss or thinning (thyroid)
- Low body temperature, easily chilled (thyroid)
- Mental confusion, brain fog (adrenal, pancreas, thyroid)
- Mood swings (adrenal)
- Restless, disturbed sleep (adrenal)
- Restless dreams or nightmares (adrenal)
- Waking up unable to go back to sleep (adrenal, pancreas)

Adrenal   *Gland*

There are two adrenal glands, one on the upper part of each kidney. They work with the kidneys to control fluid and mineral concentrations in the body. The adrenal glands also control the metabolism of glucose and the adrenaline rush you may feel in response to stressful or dangerous situations. The adrenal glands are small—each about the size of a grape. When weakened, however, they can cause big problems, including occasional sleeplessness and low libido. Adrenal problems are widespread due to stress and the excessive use of sugar and caffeine.

Adrenal Irritation   *Overactive/Hot*

Adrenal irritation is essentially stress initiating the fight-flight-freeze response. Remedies that help calm the adrenal function and reduce stress aid adrenal irritation.

Indications for Adrenal Irritation

Iridology: Dilated pupils

Pulse: Rapid, tense

- Aftermath of traumatic or stressful situations
- Excessive consumption of caffeine and sugar
- Rapid heart rate, increased blood pressure
- Muscle tension
- Poor digestion
- Constipation
- Metal obsession, situational anxiety

The following adrenal calming remedies can help.

Formulas: Anti-Anxiety, **Anti-Stress B-Complex**, Ashwagandha Complex, and Shock and Injury FE

Herbs: **Ashwagandha**, astragalus, chamomile, cordyceps, **eleuthero**, ginseng (American), ginseng (Asian/Korean), gynostemma, **holy basil**, **kava kava**, magnolia bark, passion flower, reishi, rhodiola, **schisandra**, and **vervain (blue)**

Supplements: Vitamin B-complex

Essential Oils: **Chamomile (Roman)**, **lavender**, rose, and ylang ylang

Adrenal Depression   *Underactive/Cold*

Chronic stress leads to a feeling of hypervigilance and exhaustion. We often call this state adrenal fatigue or burnout. Remedies that build and support the adrenal glands are helpful for adrenal depression.

Indications for Adrenal Depression

Iridology: Pulsing pupils

Tongue: Quivering

Pulse: Rapid, but feeble

- Feeling overwhelmed and exhausted
- Feeling unable to cope with life
- Fatigue and lack of stamina with insomnia
- Dark circles under eyes
- Tendency for low blood pressure or sudden drop in blood pressure when moving from sitting to standing position
- Tachycardia and heart palpitations
- Sensation of pressure in chest (angina)
- Cravings for sweets
- Emotionally sensitive, easily moved to anger or tears

The following adrenal building remedies can help.

Formulas: Adaptogen-Immune, **Adrenal Glandular**, and **Chinese Fire-Increasing**

Herbs: Ashwagandha, astragalus, biota seed, **borage**, **cordyceps**, eleuthero, **ginseng (Asian/Korean)**, gynostemma, he shou wu, holy basil, **licorice**, reishi, **schisandra**, and suma

Supplements: Pantothenic acid, **vitamin B-complex**, **vitamin C**, and zinc

Adrenal Cortex   *Tissue*

Situated along the perimeter of the adrenal gland, the adrenal cortex mediates the stress response through the production of mineralocorticoids and glucocorticoids, including aldosterone and cortisol respectively. It is also a secondary site for synthesizing sex hormones, like progesterone, estrogen and testosterone.

Formulas: Adrenal Glandular and **DHEA with Herbs**

Herbs: Ginseng (American), **ginseng (Asian/Korean)**, **licorice**, and maca

Supplements: DHEA

Essential Oils: Pine

Adrenal Medulla   *Tissue*

The adrenal medulla is part of the adrenal gland and is located at the center of the gland. It secretes epinephrine (adrenaline), norepinephrine (noradrenaline), and a small amount of dopamine in response to stimulation by the sympathetic nervous system. Notable effects of adrenaline and noradrenaline include increased heart rate and blood pressure, blood vessel constriction in the skin, and gastrointestinal tract, bronchiole dilation, and decreased metabolism—all of which are characteristic of the fight-or-flight response.

Formulas: Anti-Stress B-Complex, Chinese Yin-Increasing, Jeannie Burgess' Stress, and **Shock and Injury FE**

Herbs: Chamomile, eleuthero, kava kava, **passion flower**, reishi, and valerian

Supplements: Vitamin B_5

Essential Oils: Lavender, pine, and ylang ylang

Pancreas   *Gland*

The tail of the pancreas is located anatomically left near the spleen. It secretes insulin and glucagon to regulate blood sugar levels. Damage to the insulin-producing cells in this part of the pancreas results in type 1 diabetes. Problems with the pancreatic tail contribute to blood sugar imbalances like hypoglycemia, syndrome X, and type 2 diabetes.

Pancreatic Irritation   *Overactive/Hot*

This is the prediabetic stage of pancreatic problems. The pancreas is hypersecreting insulin because of too many simple carbohydrates in the diet. This results in metabolic syndrome, a precursor to many chronic and degenerative diseases, but it also causes hypoglycemic drops in blood sugar in many people. Remedies that stabilize blood sugar and reduce sugar cravings are helpful.

Indications for Pancreatic Irritation

Medical Indications

- Medical diagnosis of metabolic syndrome or early stages of type 2 diabetes
- Fasting blood glucose > 90
- A1c > 5.7

Iridology: Orange discoloration in iris, marking in pancreatic areas

Other Indications

- Sugar cravings, high carbohydrate diets
- Weakness or dizziness when fasting
- Weight gain, especially around waist
- Waist hip ratio greater than 1:1 in males and 0.8:1 in women
- Triglycerides over 200, HDL below 35

The following pancreatic tail calming remedies can help.

Formulas: Algae, Chinese Yin-Increasing, Hypoglycemic, Whole Food Green Drink, and **Whole Food Protein**

Herbs: Bee pollen, beet root, blue-green algae, chlorella, **coconut oil**, **garcina fruit rind extract**, **licorice**, **spirulina**, and **stevia**

Supplements: Berberine, **chromium**, L-glutamine, and xylitol

Pancreatic Depression   *Underactive/Cold*

Pancreatic depression is associated with diabetes. Either the insulin isn't working anymore due to insulin resistance in type 2 diabetes or due to a lack of insulin in type 1 diabetes.

Indications for Pancreatic Depression

Medical Indications

- Medical diagnosis of type 1 or type 2 diabetes
- Low insulin levels (type 1)
- High insulin levels (type 2)

Iridology: Orange discoloration in iris, marking in pancreatic areas

Other Indications

- Constant thirst with frequent urination
- Dizziness or light-headedness after eating carbohydrates

• Symptoms develop after vaccination or exposure to toxins

The following pancreatic tail building remedies can help.

Formulas: Blood Sugar Control

Herbs: Bitter melon, **cinnamon**, fenugreek, ginseng (American), goldenseal, **gymnema**, jambul, **nopal**, and stevia

Supplements: Alpha-lipoic acid, chromium GTF, omega-3 EFAs, vanadium, xylitol, and zinc

Hypothalamus   *Gland*

The hypothalamus is a portion of the brain that contains a number of small nuclei with a variety of functions. One of the most important functions of the hypothalamus is to link the nervous system to the endocrine system via the pituitary gland. The hypothalamus is located below the thalamus, just above the brain stem. In humans, the hypothalamus is roughly the size of an almond.

The hypothalamus is responsible for certain metabolic processes and other activities of the autonomic nervous system. It synthesizes and secretes certain neurohormones that either stimulate or inhibit the secretion of pituitary hormones. The hypothalamus controls body temperature, hunger, thirst, fatigue, sleep, and circadian cycles.

Formulas: 5-HTP Adaptogen and Herbal Potassium

Herbs: Bee pollen, red raspberry, sage, and yarrow

Supplements: Chlorophyll and MSM

Essential Oils: Clary sage, jasmine, patchouli, thyme, and ylang ylang

Parathyroid   *Gland*

The parathyroid glands are small endocrine glands attached to the thyroid that produce parathyroid hormone. They control the levels of calcium and phosphorus in the body, which allows the nervous and muscular systems to function properly. When blood calcium levels drop below a certain point, calcium-sensing receptors in the parathyroid gland are activated to release hormone into the blood.

Formulas: Hypothyroid, Skeletal Support, **Watkin's Hair, Skin, and and Nails**

Herbs: Damiana, **horsetail**, **kelp**, valerian, and white oak

Supplements: 7-keto and **vitamin D**

Pineal   *Gland*

The pineal gland is a pine cone shaped-gland of the endocrine system located in the center of the brain. The pineal gland produces several important hormones, including melatonin. Melatonin influences sexual development and sleep-wake cycles. The pineal gland is composed of cells called pine-alocytes and cells of the nervous system called glial cells. The pineal gland connects the endocrine system with the nervous system in that it converts nerve signals from the sympathetic system of the peripheral nervous system into hormone signals.

Formulas: 5-HTP Adaptogen, Anti-Stress B-Complex, Suma Adaptogen, **Watkin's Hair, Skin, and and Nails**

Herbs: Alfalfa, black cohosh, dong quai, ginger, goldenseal, gotu kola, horsetail, kelp, spirulina, and wood betony

Supplements: Lecithin, **melatonin**, vitamin B-complex, and zinc

Essential Oils: Clary sage, **frankincense**, **jasmine**, lavender, **patchouli**, **sandalwood**, and ylang ylang

Pituitary   *Gland*

The pituitary gland is considered the master gland. It is located at the base of the skull, between the optic nerves, and is attached to the brain. It receives messages from the brain and then secretes various hormones to regulate hormone production in other glands. The pituitary is referred to as the master gland because it controls hormone functions such as our temperature, thyroid activity, growth during childhood, urine production, testosterone production in males, and ovulation and estrogen production in females. In effect, the gland functions as a thermostat that controls all other glands that are responsible for hormone secretion. It is a critical part of the body's ability to respond to the environment. The pituitary gland actually functions as two separate compartments with an anterior portion and a posterior portion.

Pituitary (Anterior)   *Gland*

The anterior gland is actually made of a separate collection of individual cells that act as functional units that are dedicated to produce a specific regulatory hormone messenger or factor. These factors are secreted in response to the outside environment and the internal bodily responses to that environment. These pituitary factors then travel through a rich blood network into the bloodstream and eventually reach their specific target gland. They then stimulate the target gland to produce the appropriate type and amount of hormone so the body can respond to the environment correctly.

The anterior pituitary produces growth hormones, the thyroid stimulating hormone (TSH), the adrenocorticotrophic hormone (ACTH), the follicle-stimulating hormone (FSH), the luteinizing hormone (LH), and prolactin. These hormones regulate the thyroid, adrenal and reproductive glands.

Formulas: Algae, Female Cycle, **General Glandular, Target Mineral Thyroid**, and Whole Food Green Drink

Herbs: Alfalfa, **bee pollen**, **chaste tree**, devil's claw, sage, and **spirulina**

Supplements: Co-Q10 and vitamin B-complex

Pituitary (Posterior)   *Gland*

The posterior pituitary secretes the hormone oxytocin, which causes the contraction of the uterine muscles during the final stage of pregnancy to stimulate the birthing process. The posterior pituitary also stimulates the ejection, or letdown, of milk from the mammary glands following pregnancy. In addition, it produces the antidiuretic hormone vasopressin, which helps the kidneys to reabsorb water and maintain proper fluid balance.

Formulas: Herbal Potassium

Herbs: Alfalfa, blessed thistle, catnip, gotu kola, hops, parsley, and rose

Thyroid   *Gland*

The thyroid gland is located in the neck just below the larynx. The thyroid's main function is to control metabolism. More specifically, the thyroid gland controls how quickly the body uses energy, makes proteins, and controls how sensitive the body should be to other hormones.

The thyroid regulates these processes by producing the hormones triiodothyronine and thyroxine. The most common problems of the thyroid gland consist of an overactive thyroid gland, hyperthyroidism, and an underactive thyroid gland, hypothyroidism.

Thyroid Irritation   *Overactive/Hot*

Overactivity of the thyroid gland is typically due to autoimmune reactions. Remedies that reduce thyroid irritation, balance the glandular system or calm immune reactions are helpful.

Indications for Thyroid Irritation

Medical Indications

- Elevated T3 and/or T4 levels, with low TSH
- Medical diagnosis of Graves' disease or other hyperactive thyroid condition

Other Indications

- Fine brittle hair, hair loss
- Goiter with red skin over thyroid area
- Hyperactive, nervous, irritable, restless
- Thin, difficulty gaining weight
- Bulging eyes
- Rapid heart rate and/or heart palpitations
- Tendency to nausea, vomiting, diarrhea
- Increased appetite, weight loss
- Intolerance to heat
- Low cholesterol

The following thyroid calming remedies can help.

Formulas: Adrenal Glandular, Chinese Fire-Decreasing, **Chinese Fire-Increasing**, and **Thyroid Calming**

Herbs: Bugleweed, eleuthero, hops, **lemon balm**, licorice, and **motherwort**

Supplements: Magnesium, selenium, and vitamin B$_5$

Thyroid Depression   *Overactive/Hot*

Low thyroid may be caused by iodine deficiency or by an autoimmune reaction. These are remedies that can support thyroid function or balance immune reactions.

Indications for Thyroid Depression

Medical Indications

- Medical diagnosis of hypothyroidism or Hashitmoto's thyroiditis
- Low T3 and/or T4 levels, with high TSH

Other Indications

- Thinning hair, hair loss
- Puffy face
- Enlarged thyroid
- Dry, coarse, dull skin
- Poor appetite and constipation
- Low body temperature, easily chilled
- Weight gain, difficulty losing weight
- Infertility, loss of libido, heavy menstruation
- Slow heartbeat
- High cholesterol
- Depression with fatigue

The following thyroid building remedies can help.

Formulas: Ashwagandha Complex, **Hypothyroid**, Target Mineral Thyroid, and **Thyroid Glandular**

Herbs: Ashwagandha, **black walnut**, bladderwrack, coconut oil, coleus, **dulse**, he shou wu, Irish moss, **kelp**, **nettle, and stinging**

Supplements: Iodine, MSM, SAM-e, and **selenium**

Specific Hormones

Here are the hormones related to the glandular system.

Adrenocorticotropic Hormone

Adrenocorticotropic hormone (ACTH) stimulates production of adrenal hormones. The remedies listed here are believed to reduce the secretion of this hormone to lower stress levels.

Herbs: Eleuthero, **holy basil**, rhodiola, and schisandra

Aldosterone   *Hormone*

Aldosterone is an adrenal hormone that regulates sodium and potassium balance. It reduces urine output and helps tissues hold onto fluid. It reduces the formation of urine by reducing amount of water excreted by kidneys and constricts blood vessels to increase blood pressure.

Formulas: Herbal Potassium

Herbs: Licorice

Essential Oils: Pine, rosemary, and thyme

Cortisol   *Hormone*

Cortisol is an adrenal hormone that influences metabolism. It is a stress hormone, but it is also anti-inflammatory.

Excessive cortisol leads to rapid aging, but deficient cortisol can be a factor in excessive immune activity (autoimmune disorders) and inflammation.

Low Cortisol

Low levels of cortisol can occur when the adrenal glands become weakened, often from chronic stress. Since cortisol suppresses inflammation, low cortisol levels may be involved in chronic inflammation. The corticosteroid drugs used to control inflammation mimic cortisol in the body.

Indications for Low Cortisol

- Chronic inflammation
- Autoimmune disorders
- Long term stress
- PTSD

The following cortisol supporting remedies can help.

Formulas: Adrenal Glandular, Chinese Qi and Blood Tonic, and DHEA with Herbs

Herbs: Licorice, wild yam, and yucca

High Cortisol

Cortisol is released when the fight-or-flight response is initiated, so high levels of cortisol will occur when a person is under a lot of stress. High cortisol causes premature aging, suppression of the immune system and may contribute to weight gain. Adaptogens can help to decrease or modulate stress and reduce cortisol levels.

Indications for High Cortisol

- Severe stress or trauma
- Weight gain associated with stress
- Premature aging (e.g. gray hair, wrinkles)
- Use of corticosteroid drugs

The following cortisol calming remedies can help.

Formulas: Ashwagandha Complex and Cortisol-Reducing

Follicle Stimulating Hormone

Follicle stimulating hormone (FSH) stimulates testes to produce sperm in males. In women, it stimulates follicle to develop an egg, and ovaries to produce estrogen. Most of these remedies calm the production of FSH or help to balance its production.

Herbs: Chaste tree, maca, mugwort, and willow

Growth Hormone

Growth hormone (somatotropin) is secreted during deep sleep. It regulates growth and tissue repair.

Supplements: L-arginine

Luteinizing Hormone

In females, luteinizing hormone (LH) stimulates ovaries to produce progesterone during the latter half of the menstrual cycle. In males, it stimulates testes to produce testosterone.

Herbs: Chaste tree, hops, mugwort, oat, and willow

Oxytocin   *Hormone*

Oxytocin is released by the posterior pituitary. It causes uterine contractions during childbirth. (The drug Pitocin is a synthetic version of oxytocin.) It also causes lactiferous duct contraction to release breast milk. It also causes menstrual cramping. It creates feelings of emotional bonding, improving empathy and compassion. It has been called the love hormone because it promotes feelings of contentment, reductions in anxiety, and feelings of calmness and security.

Herbs: Blue cohosh, cannabis, **cocoa**, lady's mantle, and shepherd's purse

Prolactin   *Hormone*

After childbirth, prolactin assists other hormones in initiating and sustaining milk production. It is also released after orgasm reducing sexual drive.

Herbs: Fennel, sage, and vervain (blue)

Thyroid-Stimulating Hormone

Thyroid-stimulating hormone (TSH) or thyrotropin, stimulates production of thyroxin in the thyroid.

Formulas: Target Mineral Thyroid

Thyroxin   *Hormone*

Thyroxin (T4) is the storage form of the thyroid formula. It is converted to the more active form T3 as it is needed. This conversion primarily takes place the liver.

Formulas: Hypothyroid and **Thyroid Glandular**

Herbs: Ashwagandha, bladderwrack, **dulse**, Irish moss, and **kelp**

Supplements: Iodine

Tri-iodothyronine   *Hormone*

Tri-iodothyronine (T3) is the more active form of the thyroid hormone. It regulates metabolism and body weight. It also plays a role in fertility and menstruation. It helps regulate cholesterol and aids the health of skin and hair. It also aids memory, concentration, and sleep. It is also important for energy levels and for keeping bones healthy.

Formulas: Hypothyroid and **Thyroid Glandular**

Herbs: Ashwagandha, **black walnut**, coleus, **dulse**, guggul, Irish moss, **kelp**, saw palmetto, and schisandra

Supplements: Iodine

Reproductive System

Problems with the reproductive system are always dependent on other systems and overall health. Nevertheless, there are situations where you need to directly support the reproductive system.

The reproductive system is part of the glandular system but goes beyond the function of hormonal regulation of the body into the perpetuation of the species. It involves the reproductive glands (testicles in males and ovaries in females) and also the reproductive organs: uterus, vagina, and penis. Hence, it is generally considered its own system. Reproductive health is important not only for individual health but also for the health of relationships between husband and wife. It helps form and strengthen the bonds of love that unite a family.

The reproductive glands use cholesterol to produce sex hormones. These hormones form the sex organs in a developing fetus and also stimulate changes in the body during puberty. Malfunction in the reproductive system is a serious, personal matter that can deeply affect self-esteem and happiness.

Reproductive Hormones

This section lists direct aids for balancing reproductive hormones.

Estrogen   *Hormone*

There are three different estrogens produced in the body. They are estriol, estrone, and estradiol. In the female body, estrogen is balanced with progesterone, with estrogen being dominant during the first half of the menstrual cycle. The balance of estrogen can be either too high or too low in the body; however, the more common problem is high estrogen.

High Estrogen

When estrogen levels are too high remedies that help to breakdown estrogen or enhance progesterone are needed.

Indications for High Estrogen

- PMS with irritability, anxiety, mood swings
- Low sex drive
- Uterine fibroids
- Heavy menstrual bleeding (menorrhagia)
- Headaches, migraines
- Nervous tension, panic attacks
- Tendency to miscarriage
- Fibrocystic breasts

The following estrogen calming remedies can help.

Formulas: Female Cycle

Herbs: Chaste tree, **false unicorn**, flax seed hull (lignans), red clover, and wild yam

Supplements: Indole-3-carbinol, SAM-e, **vitamin B$_6$**, and vitamin B$_9$

Low Estrogen

A few women experience low estrogen during childbearing years, but it is a more common problem after menopause. Remedies that enhance estrogen or contain phytoestrogens may be helpful.

Indications for Low Estrogen

- Vaginal dryness, painful intercourse
- Hot flashes, night sweats
- Decreased breast size
- Low sex drive
- Thinning skin
- Forgetfulness, mental confusion, brain fog
- Wrinkles, acne, oily skin

The following estrogen supporting remedies can help.

Formulas: DHEA with Herbs and Menopause Support EO

Herbs: Black cohosh, **dong quai**, hops, kudzu, licorice, and **maca**

Supplements: DHEA

Essential Oils: Clary sage, geranium, and grapefruit (pink)

Progesterone   *Hormone*

Progesterone is important for regulating ovulation, menstruation, and maintaining pregnancy. Progesterone is sometimes used to cause menstrual periods in women who have not yet reached menopause but are not having periods due to a lack of progesterone in the body. Like estrogen, it can be too high or too low.

High Progesterone

High progesterone is not a common problem, but it can be an issue for some women.

Indications for High Progesterone

- PMS with depression, sadness, and mental confusion
- Fatigue, drowsiness
- Forgetfulness
- Increased appetite
- Painful swollen breasts
- Cystitis, bladder infections
- Yeast infections
- Taking birth control pills

The following progesterone calming remedies can help.

Formulas: DHEA with Herbs and Female Tonic
Herbs: Black cohosh and blue cohosh
Supplements: L-tyrosine, **magnesium**, and vitamin B_6
Essential Oils: Bergamot, clary sage, geranium, and rose

Low Progesterone

Low progesterone is often coupled with high estrogen. It can also be a problem after menopause.

Indications for Low Progesterone

- Miscarriage
- Irregular menstrual cycle
- Infertility
- Nervous tension
- Low bone density
- Vaginal dryness and painful intercourse
- Low sex drive

The following progesterone supporting remedies can help.

Formulas: Female Cycle
Herbs: Chaste tree, **false unicorn**, lady's mantle, parsley, wild yam, and yarrow
Supplements: Magnesium and vitamin B_6

Testosterone   *Hormone*

Testosterone is the principal male reproductive hormone and is largely responsible for male growth and development, although it is present in the female body as well. Testosterone is a steroid hormone from the androgen group that is primarily secreted in the testes.

High Testosterone

Although, high testosterone isn't often a problem for men, it can be problem for some women.

Indications for High Testosterone

- Highly assertive
- Logical, detached, unemotional
- Excess facial hair and baldness in women

The following testosterone calming remedies can help.

Herbs: Black cohosh, **hops**, and licorice
Essential Oils: Grapefruit (pink)

Low Testosterone

Low testosterone in men can lead to problems like muscle weakness and sexual disorders such as erectile dysfunction. It is a common problem for many men as they grow older.

Indications for Low Testosterone

- Loss of energy and stamina
- Depression
- Loss of muscle mass and weight gain
- Erectile dysfunction or lack of firm erections
- Loss of libido (sex drive)
- Loss of emotional drive
- Increased risk of heart disease
- Low self esteem
- Reduced athletic performance

The following testosterone supporting remedies can help.

Formulas: DHEA with Herbs and Male Performance
Herbs: Cordyceps, **eleuthero**, **epimedium**, **ginseng (Asian/ Korean)**, **maca**, **muira puama**, and nettle root
Supplements: DHEA, vitamin B_5, and zinc
Essential Oils: Cinnamon, lemon, and sandalwood

DHEA   *Hormone*

DHEA is made in the adrenal glands from pregnenolone, which is made from cholesterol. It is the precursor to the reproductive hormones estrogen and testosterone.

High DHEA

DHEA levels are seldom too high, except during the "raging hormone" period of puberty. If DHEA is too high it is usually because people are taking too much DHEA as a supplement. With high DHEA, avoid DHEA supplements and adrenal glandulars.

Indications for High DHEA

- Acne
- Excessive libido

- Irritability
- Insomnia
- Breast swelling and tenderness in women
- Facial hair in women

The following dhea calming remedies can help.

Herbs: Cordyceps, **eleuthero**, and suma

Low DHEA

Excessive stress over a long periods can cause the body to produce more cortisol and less DHEA. DHEA also declines with age. Supporting the adrenals with glandulars or adaptogens, as well as supplementing with DHEA, may be helpful.

Indications for Low DHEA

- Flabby muscles
- Auto-immune disorders
- High cholesterol
- Decreased libido
- Fatigue
- Allergies
- Chronic inflammation
- Low testosterone in men

The following dhea supporting remedies can help.

Formulas: Adrenal Glandular and **DHEA with Herbs**

Herbs: Ginseng (Asian/Korean), licorice, **maca**, schisandra, and suma

Supplements: DHEA

Female Reproductive System

The primary role of the female reproductive system is to produce eggs, facilitate fertilization and regulate pregnancy. The female reproductive cycle is governed by several processes involving hormones from the pituitary and the ovaries. The cycle begins with the first day of menstruation. The pituitary secretes the follicle-stimulating hormone (FSH) shortly thereafter. This causes a maturation of a follicle in the ovary and the development of an egg. It also stimulates the follicle to secrete estrogen. Estrogen is the dominant hormone during the first half of the cycle (about day 3 to day 14). Estrogen has a catabolic effect. Under the influence of estrogen, the body fluids thin out and fats and proteins are broken down.

A short time later, during the first half of the cycle, the pituitary starts secreting luteinizing hormone. That further stimulates the secretion of estrogen and causes the follicle to release the mature egg—a process called ovulation. Ovulation takes place about halfway through the cycle.

The follicle where the egg was produced now develops into the corpus luteum or yellow body. The corpus luteum begins to secrete progesterone, the hormone that dominates the second half of the cycle. Under the influence of progesterone, the body begins to synthesize fats and proteins and thickens the body fluids. Thus, progesterone has more of an anabolic effect. It is during this second half of the cycle that many women experience PMS symptoms because their body becomes congested.

If fertilization occurs and pregnancy results, the corpus luteum develops further and secretes progesterone throughout the pregnancy to halt the monthly cycles. Birth control pills are a synthetic form of progesterone and work in the same manner.

The hormone prolactin is secreted by the pituitary during the latter half of the cycle to maintain the corpus luteum and stimulate progesterone and estrogen production. If pregnancy does not occur, there is a small spike of estrogen during the second half of the cycle and the period starts over again.

Indications for Female Reproductive System

- Cravings for chocolate with periods
- Depression with periods
- Edema or bloating associated with periods
- Heavy menstrual bleeding
- Hot flashes and/or night sweats
- Infertility
- Irritability with periods
- Lack of sexual desire
- Menstrual cramps
- Painful menstruation
- PMS symptoms
- Post-menopausal symptoms
- Pregnancy and nursing
- Vaginal discharge or dryness

Breasts   *Body Part*

The mammary glands or breasts secrete milk used to feed infants. Both men and women develop breasts from the same embryological tissues, but at puberty female sex hormones, mainly estrogen, promote the more prominent breast development that does not occur in men.

Formulas: Enzyme Spray, Liquid Lymph, Mushroom Immune, **Phytoestrogen Breast**, and Standardized Acetogenin

Herbs: Aloe vera, blessed thistle, mullein, **saw palmetto**, and slippery elm

Supplements: Indole-3-carbinol, lutein, and nanoparticle silver

Essential Oils: Clary sage, clove, **frankincense**, helichrysum, and ylang ylang

Ovaries   *Gland*

The ovaries are small paired organs located near the pelvic cavity of females. Ovaries produce the female egg cells. The eggs are fertilized by sperm from the male and a zygote is formed. The development of the zygote to a complete human baby takes place in the female reproductive system over a gestational period of about nine months. The ovaries also produce estrogen and progesterone during a woman's childbearing years.

Formulas: Chinese Wood-Decreasing, **Chrisopher's Menopause**, and **Female Tonic**

Herbs: Aloe vera, **black cohosh**, blessed thistle, chaste tree, **damiana**, dong quai, and **wild yam**

Supplements: Magnesium and **vitamin B$_6$**

Essential Oils: Frankincense

Uterus   *Body Part*

The uterus (or womb) is the major reproductive organ in females. It is home to the developing fetus, produces secretions of the female reproductive system, and allows the passage of sperm to the fallopian tubes, where the sperm fertilize the egg.

Formulas: Female Tonic

Herbs: Astragalus, black cohosh, blessed thistle, chamomile, chickweed, dong quai, horsetail, **lady's mantle**, parsley, **red raspberry**, uva ursi, white oak, wild yam, and **yarrow**

Essential Oils: Clove and frankincense

Vagina   *Body Part*

The vagina is the tract leading to the uterus. It receives the penis during sexual intercourse. Like the intestines, it contains friendly microbes that help protect it from infection. Imbalances in these microbes can lead to infections or inflammation.

Formulas: **Anti-Fungal** and Probiotic

Herbs: Aloe vera, bayberry, **pau d'arco**, and slippery elm

Supplements: **Nanoparticle silver**

Essential Oils: Geranium, lavender, myrrh, and sandalwood

Male Reproductive System

The primary role of the male reproductive system is to produce sperm to fertilize the egg produced by the female reproductive system. It consists of the testicles, testes, prostate gland and penis.

Indications for Male Reproductive System

• Difficult urination

• Erectile dysfunction

• Infertility

• Lack of sex drive

• Loss of self-confidence and drive

• Nighttime urination

• Prostate problems

Prostate   *Gland*

The prostate gland is located just underneath the bladder and produces a fluid that delivers sperm upon ejaculation. The prostate stores and secretes a slightly alkaline fluid that helps neutralize the acidity of the vaginal tract, prolonging the life span of the sperm. To work properly, the prostate needs the male hormones androgen, which is responsible for male sex characteristics, and testosterone, which is produced mainly by the testicles. However, it is the hormone dihydro-testosterone that regulates the prostate.

One of the common health problems in older men is a swelling of the prostate, which makes urination difficult. Fortunately, there are a number of good herbal remedies that can help this problem. Other common problems related to this include impotency and infertility.

Formulas: Antiparasitic, Chinese Water-Increasing, **Prostate**, and UTI Prevention

Herbs: Buchu, echinacea, **nettle root**, pumpkin seed, **pygeum**, red raspberry, **saw palmetto**, and white sage

Supplements: **Equol**, indole-3-carbinol, **lycopene, omega-3 EFAs**, and **zinc**

Testes   *Gland*

The testes are components of both the reproductive and endocrine systems. For the reproductive system, they produce sperm, and for the endocrine system, they produce the male reproductive hormones responsible for masculine characteristics.

Formulas: **DHEA with Herbs** and **Male Performance**

Herbs: Black walnut, **ginseng (Asian/Korean)**, and **maca**

Supplements: Lecithin and **zinc**

Essential Oils: Pine

Immune System

The immune system is not a single system but a complex set of processes that involve multiple body systems. These include the digestive system, lymphatic system, circulatory system, skin and more. It is roughly divided into three parts. There are the protective surfaces of the body, the skin and mucous membranes, which create mechanical barriers. Then there are the cell-mediated immune responses, the innate immune system, and the adaptive immune system.

The innate immune system consists of inflammatory responses (that sequester damaged tissues) and three kinds of white blood cells: macrophages, neutrophils and natural killer cells. The innate immune system functions as a first line of defense when the skin or mucous membranes are damaged to allow infection to enter the body. This system is nonspecific—meaning, it doesn't look for any particular kind of invader. It works on viruses, bacteria, and even cancer cells.

The adaptive immune system consists of two kinds of white blood cells, B-cells and T-cells, along with antibodies, which are used to tag specific cells for destruction. The adaptive immune system resides primarily in the blood and lymph and protects you against specific microbes. It is the part of the immune system a vaccine is supposed to stimulate to cause you to develop immunity. The thymus helps to program these immune cells.

At its most fundamental level, the immune system is the ability of the body to distinguish between what belongs in the body from what does not belong in the body, then to remove what does not belong. In this sense, immunity and good eliminative function are intimately connected.

Indications for Immune System

- Any disease that ends in "itis" (e.g. tonsilitis, laryngitis)
- Allergic reactions
- Autoimmune disease of any kind
- Cancer
- Infections of any kind (viral, bacterial, fungal)
- Lymphatic congestion
- Swollen lymph nodes

Formulas: Gut Immune, H. Pylori-Fighting, Heavy Metal Cleansing, Hemp Oil with Terpenes, Hepatoprotective, Herbal Composition, Immune-Boosting, Jeannie Burgess' Thymus, Liquid Lymph, Lung-Supporting EO, Lymph Cleansing, Lymphatic Infection, Methyl B12 Vitamin, Mushroom Immune, Nitric Oxide Boosting, Paavo Airola's Cold, Personal Boundaries FE, Phytoestrogen Breast, **Plant Enzyme**, Proanthocyanidins, Probiotic, Refreshing and Cleansing EO, Seasonal Cold and Flu, Standardized Acetogenin, Steven Horne's Children's Composition, Urinary Immune, Whole Food Green Drink, and Yeast Cleansing

Herbs: **Astragalus**, black walnut, **cordyceps**, devil's claw, echinacea, eleuthero, goldenseal, olive, Oregon grape, red clover, turmeric, vervain (blue), and yarrow

Supplements: Alpha-lipoic acid, colostrum, krill oil, L-lysine, MSM, **nanoparticle silver**, omega-3 EFAs, protease, sodium alginate, vitamin C, vitamin D, and zinc

Essential Oils: Clove, eucalyptus, frankincense, lemon, myrrh, rosemary, tea tree, and thyme

Four Stages of Disease

Natural remedies generally work by altering the biological terrain to make it inhospitable to disease agents and/or by strengthening the immune responses. Therefore, it's less important to know whether you are dealing with a virus, bacteria, or fungus than it is to know what stage the disease is in. The following are the four stages of the disease process with remedies to aid the body's ability to remove infection in each stage.

Acute Stage   *Irritation*

The acute stage is the initial stage of infectious disease where an organism gains a foothold in the body, usually through damage to the skin or mucous membranes. This invokes an inflammatory response where the body seeks to flush the irritant. It may also trigger a fever, which slows viral replication and increases the immune reactions. These remedies are helpful during this stage.

Indications for Acute Stage

Tongue: Bright red, often elongated

Pulse: Rapid, superficial

- Initial stages of acute contagious diseases (first twenty-four to forty-eight hours)
- Fever
- Thin, watery or white mucus
- Coughing, sneezing, sinus drainage
- Nausea, vomiting, or diarrhea
- Pox, rashes, skin eruptions

The following acute immune support remedies can help.

Formulas: **Children's Elderberry Cold and Flu**, **Chinese Fire-Decreasing**, Cold Lozenges, **Elderberry Cold and Flu**, Jeannie Burgess' Allergy-Lung, and Paavo Airola's Cold

Herbs: Astragalus, **boneset**, chamomile, **chrysanthemum**, **elderberry/flower**, forsythia fruit, **garlic**, **ginger**, **honeysuckle**, isatis, **lemon balm**, lemon juice, **peppermint**, rose hips, thyme, and **yarrow flower**

Supplements: **Nanoparticle silver**, vitamin A, **vitamin C**, vitamin D, and **zinc**

Essential Oils: Cajeput, cinnamon, clove, **eucalyptus**, lemon, **pine**, **tea tree**, and **thyme**

Subacute Stage   *Stagnation*

If the body is unable to flush out the agent of infection with 24-48 hours the system starts to become sluggish and stagnation settles in, signaling the subacute stage of disease. Remedies that boost immune responses are helpful, but even better are remedies that clear lymphatic passages and aid thin mucus secretions. Bitters are usually more helpful at this point.

Indications for Subacute Stage

Tongue: Damp, swollen, heavily coated

Pulse: Slippery, rolling

- Later stages of acute contagious diseases (after twenty-four to forty-eight hours)
- Low grade fever
- Swelling
- Feeling sluggish and worn out
- Lymphatic congestion, swollen lymph nodes
- Sore throats and earaches
- Congestion in lungs and sinuses, mucus difficult to expel
- Loss of appetite
- Frequent digestive upset, gas, belching, bloating

The following subacute immune support remedies can help.

Formulas: Antibacterial, Liquid Lymph, Lymph Cleansing, and **Lymphatic Infection**

Herbs: Amur cork, andrographis, boneset, coptis, **echinacea**, **goldenseal**, myrrh, **olive leaf**, Oregon grape, pau d'arco, red root, usnea, **vervain (blue)**, and yarrow

Supplements: Berberine, **nanoparticle silver**, **protease**, vitamin C, vitamin D, and zinc

Essential Oils: Frankincense and **myrrh**

Chronic Stage   *Depression*

When infection becomes more deep-seated, chronic remedies that stimulate the immune response and boost the body's defensive abilities are helpful.

Indications for Chronic Stage

Tongue: Dark reddish/purple or pale with small red spots, may have heavy yellow coating

Pulse: Rapid, but feeble

- Lingering, low-grade, chronic infections
- Long term sickness, slow convalescence
- Chronic, low grade fever or alternating fever with chills
- Weight loss, fatigue, general weakness
- Chronic cough or sinus congestion
- Chronic skin conditions

The following chronic immune support remedies can help.

Formulas: Chinese Qi and Blood Tonic, Chinese Qi-Increasing, **Chinese Wind-Heat Evil**, **Immune-Boosting**, Mushroom Immune, and **Yeast Cleansing**

Herbs: Astragalus, cat's claw, **cordyceps**, **echinacea**, **garlic**, lemon balm, lomatium, maitake, **olive leaf**, **oregano**, Oregon grape, **pau d'arco**, reishi, Saint John's wort, shitake, **spilanthes**, and thlaspi

Supplements: Berberine, beta-glucans, caprylic acid, colostrum, **nanoparticle silver**, **propolis**, selenium, **vitamin D**, and zinc

Essential Oils: Frankincense and **oregano**

Degenerative Stage   *Atrophy*

When infections are severe or long-lasting, medical attention should be sought. However, there are some strong infection-fighting remedies that may be helpful in recovery.

Indications for Degenerative Stage

Tongue: Dry, may be shriveled or cracked; may be blackish in severe cases

Pulse: Weak, thin, deep

- Chronic immune weakness with frequent infections and fatigue
- Chronic respiratory problems
- Pus filled wounds, oozing sores
- Bad body odor, may smell like rotten meat or ammonia
- Antibiotic resistant infections
- Person may be near death in severe cases
- Medical diagnosis of AIDS

The following degenerative immune support remedies can help.

Formulas: Chinese Qi and Blood Tonic and Immune-Boosting

Herbs: Astragalus, **baptisia**, **cordyceps**, **echinacea**, **garlic**, lobelia, maitake, mugwort, **pawpaw**, **red root**, reishi, sweet annie, **thuja**, and wormwood

Supplements: Beta-glucans, colostrum, **nanoparticle silver**, propolis, **vitamin A**, **vitamin C**, and **vitamin D**

Essential Oils: Cinnamon, eucalyptus, oregano, tea tree, and thyme

Immune Activity

The immune system may be overreacting or under reacting. This determines whether you need to boost or modulate immune reactions.

Hyperactive Immune Activity   *Overactive*

When the immune system overreacts, people get allergies, some cases of asthma, and autoimmune disorders. They also tend to have chronic, low-grade inflammation. Avoid immune stimulants and obtain medical assistance, especially in severe allergies or autoimmune reactions.

Indications for Hyperactive Immune Activity

Medical Indications

- Autoimmune conditions
- Multiple sclerosis (MS)

Immune System - 81

- Rheumatoid arthritis
- Fibromyalgia
- Myasthenia gravis
- Chronic fatigue syndrome
- Amyotrophic lateral sclerosis (ALS)/Lou Gerhig's disease
- Lupus (systemic lupus eyrthematosus)
- Scleroderma
- Hashimoto's thyroiditis
- Graves' disease
- Autoimmune hepatitis
- Type 1 diabetes

Other Indications

- Vaccine reactions
- Conditions worsen with immune stimulants
- Chronic inflammation

The following immune calming or modulating remedies can help.

Formulas: Fibromyalgia, **Steven Horne's Anti-Allergy**, and Whole Food Green Drink

Herbs: Aloe vera, **ashwagandha**, astragalus, **black walnut**, boswellia, chamomile, **cordyceps**, devil's claw, eleuthero, **licorice**, maitake, reishi, **schisandra**, turmeric, and **yucca**

Supplements: Colostrum, curcumin, magnesium, **omega-3 EFAs**, vitamin D, and zinc

Hypoactive Immune Activity   *Underactive*

When the immune system is weak, people are prone to catch infections easily and are susceptible to disease like cancer where the immune system is underactive.

Indications for Hypoactive Immune Activity

Medical Indications

- Psoriasis
- Cancer
- Reduced white blood cell count

Other Indications

- Chronic infections
- Poor resistance to disease
- Poor immunity
- Cysts
- Abscesses
- Growths and lumps
- Chronic swollen lymph nodes or severe lymphatic swelling
- Changes in moles
- Warts

The following immune boosting or stimulating remedies can help.

Formulas: Essiac Immune Tea, **Immune-Boosting**, and **Mushroom Immune**

Herbs: Astragalus, burdock, cat's claw, **chaga**, **chaparral**, cordyceps, **echinacea**, goldenseal, **maitake**, pau d'arco, **paw paw standardized extract**, red clover, red root, reishi, shitake, and venus fly trap

Supplements: Beta-glucans and **protease (between meals)**

Essential Oils: Frankincense and myrrh

Specific Immune Tissues

The following organs and tissues relate to the immune system.

Lymphatics

The lymphatic system is a complementary system to the circulatory system. It removes fluid from the spaces around the cells (known as lymph) and transports it back to the circulatory system through a series of one-way ducts. The lymphatic system is also an important part of the immune system. On its way back to the circulatory system, the lymph passes through the lymph nodes (or lymph glands). These are present in large numbers in the neck, breast, armpits, and groin and house many white blood cells, which can identify and fight invading organisms. The lymph nodes may become congested, inflamed, and swollen. Lymphatic congestion also contributes to fluid retention, sore throats, earaches, tender breasts, and other problems.

Lymphatic direct aids help lymph flow more freely, creating better lymphatic drainage. This helps the body detoxify and the immune system work better.

Formulas: Chinese Water-Decreasing, Essiac Immune Tea, Liquid Kidney, **Liquid Lymph**, **Lymph Cleansing**, and **Lymphatic Infection**

Herbs: Burdock, calendula, **cleavers**, echinacea, kelp, lobelia, marshmallow, **mullein**, **Oregon grape**, plantain, **red clover**, **red root**, sage, stillingia, vervain (blue), yarrow, and yellow dock

Supplements: Nanoparticle silver

Essential Oils: Bergamot, geranium, grapefruit (pink), helichrysum, and orange (sweet)

Peyer's Patches   *Tissue*

Peyer's patches (also known as aggregated lymphoid nodules) are elongated thickenings of the intestinal lining. They have similarities to lymph nodes and are part of the immune system in the intestines.

Formulas: Gut Immune

Herbs: Bupleurum

Prostaglandins   *Hormone*

Prostaglandins are hormone-like substances released by all the cells in the body. They influence surrounding cells and influence things like pain and inflammation and tissue healing. The remedies listed here reduce inflammation and pain and promote healing of tissues by influencing prostaglandins.

Formulas: Analgesic Nerve, Anti-Inflammatory Pain, CBD Anti-inflammatory, **CBD Topical Analgesic,** GLA Oil, and Stan Malstrom's Herbal Aspirin

Herbs: Amur cork, black cohosh, meadowsweet, and **willow**

Supplements: CBD and omega-6 CLA

Essential Oils: Wintergreen

Mucous Membranes   *Tissue*

The mucous membranes line the digestive, respiratory, and urinary passages. These membranes act as a primary line of immune defense.

Formulas: Christopher's Sinus, **Ed Millet's Herbal Crisis, H. Pylori-Fighting,** Herbal Composition, Intestinal Soothing, Jeannie Burgess' Allergy-Lung, Pepsin Intestinal, Sinus, and Vulnerary

Herbs: Aloe vera, bayberry, black walnut, goldenseal, licorice, marshmallow, red raspberry, rose, sage, slippery elm, uva ursi, and **yarrow**

Supplements: Vitamin C

Essential Oils: Bergamot and myrrh

Thymus   *Gland*

The thymus gland is a specialized, butterfly-shaped organ of the human immune system. Located in the center of the chest under the breastbone, it is also one of the most important glands in the body because it helps to regulate the immune system.

The primary function of the thymus gland is to produce and process lymphocytes or T-cells. Lymphocytes are white blood cells that protect the body by producing antibodies that stop the invasion of foreign agents, bacteria, and viruses. They also prevent the growth of abnormal cells like cancer cells.

The thymus gland produces a hormone called thymosin, which stimulates the T-cells in the other lymphatic organs to mature. It also produces a hormone called thymopoietin, which is protein present in the messenger RNA.

The thymus gland is very active in children, as it helps develop the immune system. In some cases, the thymus gland may become underactive, leaving the person more prone to infections.

Formulas: Chinese Qi and Blood Tonic, Essiac Immune Tea, and **Jeannie Burgess' Thymus**

Herbs: Echinacea, rose, **thyme,** and yarrow

Supplements: Zinc

Essential Oils: Bergamot

Tonsils   *Tissue*

The tonsils are oval-shaped tissues located at each side of the throat. The fundamental immunological roles of tonsils have yet to be understood. Like other organs of the lymphatic system, the tonsils may be involved in helping fight off infections, especially upper respiratory infections, but there is no conclusive evidence to that effect.

Tonsils tend to reach their largest size near puberty, and they gradually shrink thereafter. However, they are largest relative to the diameter of the throat in young children. Tonsillitis is a disorder in which the tonsils are inflamed (sore and swollen). Tonsil enlargement can affect speech, making the voice sound hypernasal. Tonsillitis becomes a serious problem if the tonsils obstruct the airway or interfere with swallowing, or if the person suffers from frequent recurring tonsillitis. In older people, swollen tonsils may indicate a viral infection or a tumor.

Formulas: Liquid Lymph, **Lymph Cleansing, Lymphatic Infection,** and Stabilized Allicin

Herbs: Echinacea, lobelia, mullein, red clover, **red root,** and sage

Supplements: Berberine and **nanoparticle silver**

Nervous System

Since the nervous system controls all body processes, problems with the nerves can affect every other system. However, problems with the nerves may also involve imbalances in other body systems too.

The nervous system controls and regulates all voluntary and involuntary activities of the body. It consists of the brain, spinal cord, and peripheral nerves. The nerves are divided into two major branches, the central nervous system and the autonomic nervous system.

The central nervous system manages sensory input and directs voluntary muscle movement.

The autonomic nervous system controls all the automatic processes of the body such as regulating breathing, heartbeat and digestion.

Because the nervous system is complex, we have broken it down into multiple components, including sections for each of the senses and all the major neurotransmitters.

Indications for Nervous System

- Absent-mindedness
- Alcoholism
- Anxiety, nervousness
- Chronic muscle tension
- Difficulty getting to sleep

- Dizziness or light-headedness
- Excitability, difficulty relaxing
- Feeling depressed or discouraged
- Headaches of all kinds
- Loss of memory
- Neurodegenerative disorders
- Neuropathy
- Panic attacks
- Poor concentration
- Poor memory
- Shaky hands

Autonomic Nervous System (ANS)

The autonomic nervous system includes the parasympathetic, sympathetic, and enteric nervous systems.

The parasympathetic nervous system is responsible for regulating internal organs and glands, which occurs unconsciously. The parasympathetic system specifically is responsible for stimulation of rest-and-digest activities that occur when the body is at rest, including sexual arousal, salivation, tear production, urination, digestion, and defecation. Its action is described as being complementary to the sympathetic nervous system, which is responsible for stimulating activities associated with the fight-or-flight response.

The sympathetic nervous system's general action is to mobilize the body's resources under stress, by inducing the fight-or-flight response. It is, however, constantly active at a basal level to maintain homeostasis. Alongside the other two components of the autonomic nervous system, the sympathetic nervous system aids in the control of most of the body's internal organs.

Parasympathetic-Dominant ANS

In general, the parasympathetic nervous system is responsible for helping you relax, digest, and wind down. Excessive parasympathetic function is associated with difficulty concentrating and excessive nervous system stimulation. Remedies to reduce parasympathetic activity and increase sympathetic activity to create better balance are helpful.

Indications for Parasympathetic-Dominant ANS

Iridology: Small pupils (miosis)

Tongue: Light red or with red tip, quivering

Pulse: Thin and wiry

Emotional State: Likes to take risks, live on the edge; hyperactive; has poor attention span; has difficulty focusing

- Tendency for low blood pressure
- Rapid digestion and metabolism

- Dislikes gentle touch, prefers firm touch
- Agitated by small noises
- Relaxing nervines act like stimulants

The following nerve stimulating remedies can help.

Formulas: Stimulating Energy and **Vandergriff's Energy Booster**

Herbs: Bee pollen, cinnamon, cocoa, **coffee green bean**, eleuthero, **guarana**, licorice, orange (bitter), **rosemary**, **schisandra**, tea, yarrow, and yerba maté

Supplements: Copper, iodine, and L-tyrosine

Essential Oils: Cinnamon, lemon, and rosemary

Sympathetic-Dominant ANS

Sympathetic nerves are activated by stress and help us be alert and focused. Too much sympathetic activity creates a tendency for restlessness and anxiety, as well as poor digestion and high blood pressure. Remedies that activate the parasympathetic nervous system and calm the sympathetic help to restore balance.

Indications for Sympathetic-Dominant ANS

Iridology: Enlarged pupils (mydriasis)

Pulse: Rapid, full, wiry, or hard; tendency to palpitations

Emotional State: Restless, nervous, constantly busy, high strung, overexcited, stressed, anxious, irritable

- Tendency for high blood pressure
- Poor digestion, frequent digestive upset
- Insomnia with difficulty relaxing and getting to sleep
- Chronic muscle tension
- Tension headaches

The following nerve calming remedies can help.

Formulas: Anti-Anxiety, CBD Relaxing, **Chinese Fire-Decreasing**, **Herbal Sleep Aid**, and **Jeannie Burgess' Stress**

Herbs: California poppy, catnip, chamomile, hops, **kanna**, kava kava, mimosa, **passion flower**, **skullcap**, valerian, and **vervain (blue)**

Supplements: **L-threonine**, **magnesium**, vitamin B-complex, and **zinc**

Essential Oils: Chamomile (Roman), **jasmine**, **lavender**, and **ylang ylang**

Solar Plexus   *Tissue*

The solar plexus is an area of the body just under the sternum (breastbone). There is an important nerve center here that connects with the digestive organs and provides us with a sixth sense, often referred to as gut instinct. The solar plexus is actually a complex network of nerves (plexus) located in the upper abdomen, where the celiac trunk, superior mesenteric artery, and renal arteries branch from the abdominal aorta.

Herbs: Chamomile, dandelion, and **Saint John's wort**

Central Nervous System

The central nervous system (CNS) nerves are involved in muscle movement and sensory input. They also regulate pain. The peripheral nerves integrate information they receive and transmit it to the brain.

Formulas: Anti-Stress B-Complex, Antispasmodic Ear, **Antispasmodic**, Balancing EO, Brain and Memory Protection, Brain Calming, Calming and Relaxing EO, **CBD Relaxing**, Chinese Fire-Decreasing, **Chinese Fire-Increasing**, Chinese Qi and Blood Tonic, Christopher's Nervine, GLA Oil, **Jeannie Burgess' Stress**, Mood Lifting EO, Refreshing and Cleansing EO, Renewing and Releasing EO, Suma Adaptogen, **Watkin's Hair, Skin, and and Nails**

Herbs: Black cohosh, chamomile, damiana, feverfew, gotu kola, hops, **kava kava**, lobelia, olive, passion flower, **Saint John's wort**, valerian, vervain (blue), wild yam, **wood betony**, and yellow dock

Supplements: Alpha-lipoic acid, calcium, krill oil, L-glutamine, lecithin, magnesium, omega-3 DHA, **omega-3 EFAs**, **vitamin B-complex**, vitamin B_3, vitamin B_5, and vitamin B_6

Essential Oils: Bergamot, chamomile (Roman), clary sage, frankincense, geranium, **helichrysum**, **lavender**, lemongrass, neroli, orange (sweet), and red mandarin

Nerve Irritation (Pain)

The central nervous system sends pain signals to alert you that something is wrong in the body. Reducing pain signaling while healing can be helpful in promoting rest and sleep. Calming pain signals is also helpful for people experiencing chronic pain or nerve irritation. However, ultimately, the cause of the pain must be discovered and corrected.

Indications for Nerve Irritation (Pain)

- General aches and pains
- Headaches, arthritis, muscle aches
- Pain due to surgery, injury or trauma
- Neuralgia

The following nerve soothers remedies can help.

Formulas: **Analgesic EO**, Analgesic Nerve, **Anti-Inflammatory Pain**, **CBD Anti-inflammatory**, **CBD Topical Analgesic**, General Analgesic, and Stan Malstrom's Herbal Aspirin

Herbs: Black cohosh, boswellia, butterbur, **California poppy**, **corydalis**, **dogwood (Jamaican)**, feverfew, hops, Indian pipe, **kava kava**, **lobelia**, meadowsweet, periwinkle, Saint John's wort, **turmeric**, valerian, willow, and wood betony

Supplements: CBD, curcumin, MSM, and omega-3 EFAs

Essential Oils: Camphor, helichrysum, lavender, **menthol**, and **wintergreen**

Nerve Depression (Exhaustion)

After long periods of stress, the nerves can become depleted causing a person to feel chronically tired and anxious. Nourishing nervines and adaptogens can help restore nerve function and calm shaking feelings.

Indications for Nerve Depression (Exhaustion)

Iridology: Pulsing pupils

Tongue: Quivering

Pulse: Weakly tense

- Feeling overwhelmed or burned out
- Trembling hands, shaky feelings
- Restless sleep, disturbed dreams, frequent waking

The following nourishing adaptogens remedies can help.

Formulas: Adrenal Glandular, Ashwagandha Complex, Chinese Fire-Increasing, and Chinese Qi-Increasing

Herbs: Ashwagandha, astragalus, biota, codonopsis, **cordyceps**, **ginseng (American)**, ginseng (Asian/Korean), gynostemma, **holy basil**, jujube, **oat**, **reishi**, schisandra, **skullcap**, and suma

Supplements: Magnesium, omega-3 EFAs, **vitamin B-complex**, vitamin B_{12}, **vitamin B_5**, and **vitamin C**

Essential Oils: Clary sage and **lavender**

Nerve Atrophy (Damage)

Nerves can become damaged and in need of regenerative tonics to help them heal.

Indications for Nerve Atrophy (Damage)

- Numbness, tingling or loss of sensation
- Nerve damage from injury or surgery
- Peripheral neuropathy, neuralgia
- Vaccine damage
- Learning and behavioral problems in children

Herbs: Chamomile, **horsetail**, jujube, **oat**, rosemary, rosemary, **Saint John's wort**, and wood betony

Supplements: Omega-3 DHA, **omega-3 EFAs**, and vitamin B-complex

Essential Oils: Helichrysum and lavender

Nerve Constriction (Tension)

Spasms, cramping, and tight muscles signal the need for remedies that help relax the muscles and nerves.

Indications for Nerve Constriction (Tension)

- Spasms and cramps
- Neck or back pain with tight muscles
- Tendency for high blood pressure
- Stomach cramps
- Tension headaches
- Tics, twitching
- Tremors, palsy

The following nerve tonics remedies can help.

Formulas: Antispasmodic Ear, **Antispasmodic**, and Fibromyalgia

Herbs: Black cohosh, black haw, cramp bark, **kava kava**, khella, **lobelia**, passion flower, **skunk cabbage**, valerian, and wild yam

Supplements: Magnesium and potassium

Essential Oils: Clary sage, **jasmine**, **lavender**, neroli, orange (sweet), and **ylang ylang**

Brain   *Organ*

The brain is the center of the nervous system. Enclosed in the cranium, the brain makes up about two percent of the body's weight (about three pounds) and contains approximately ten billion nerve cells. The brain is protected by the skull and a cushion of fluid surrounding it, while a constant supply of oxygen-rich blood comes directly from the heart to keep the fragile cells of the brain alive. Collectively, the brain not only controls the body's organs and muscles but also manages an individual's emotions, memories, thoughts, reasoning, imagination, creativity, knowledge and everything that makes us who we are. The brain stem controls breathing, heart rate, and other autonomic processes that are independent of conscious brain functions.

The neocortex is the center of higher-order thinking, learning, and memory. The cerebellum is responsible for the body's balance, posture, and coordination of movement. The frontal lobes are associated with executive functions such as self-control, planning, reasoning, and abstract thought. The occipital lobe is that portion of the brain that is devoted to vision.

Remedies listed here help the brain and to a lesser degree the spinal nerves.

Formulas: Algae, Attention-Focus, **Brain and Memory Protection**, Brain Calming, **Brain-Heart**, Chinese Fire-Increasing, Chinese Qi-Regulating, Herbal Sleep Aid,

Memory Enhancing, Mood Lifting EO, Renewing and Releasing EO, Suma Adaptogen, Watkin's Hair, Skin, and Nails, and Whole Food Protein

Herbs: Feverfew, **ginkgo**, **gotu kola**, and turmeric

Supplements: Alpha-lipoic acid, krill oil, L-glutamine, lecithin, magnesium, omega-3 DHA, **omega-3 EFAs**, vitamin B-complex, vitamin B_3, vitamin B_6, vitamin B_9, vitamin C, and zinc

Essential Oils: Peppermint

Brain Irritation

Brain irritation is indicated when the brain is overstimulated and overreacting and there are feelings of agitation or anxiety. The following remedies can help calm brain function and help a person stay relaxed and focused.

Indications for Brain Irritation

- Medical diagnosis of anxiety disorders (e.g. OCD, PTSD)
- Phobias, panic attacks
- Rapid heartbeat or palpitations
- Tightness in the chest
- Excessive sweating
- Tendency toward addictive and antisocial behavior
- Excessive anger or aggression

The following brain calming aids remedies can help.

Formulas: Algae, **Anti-Anxiety**, Attention-Focus, and **Brain Calming**

Herbs: Bacopa, **blue-green algae**, chamomile, ginkgo, hawthorn, **jujube**, **lemon balm**, licorice, oat, **passion flower**, and **spirulina**

Supplements: GABA, L-glutamine, magnesium, omega-3 DHA, **omega-3 EFAs**, vitamin B-complex, and **zinc**

Brain Depression

When the brain is not adequately stimulated, people feels tired and unmotivated. The following remedies may help by stimulating the parts of the brain responsible for focus, drive, and ambition.

Indications for Brain Depression

- Medical diagnosis of depression
- Excessive fatigue, excessive sleep
- Lack of motivation or drive
- Loss of interest in life, withdrawal

The following mood lifting aids remedies can help.

Formulas: 5-HTP Adaptogen, **Ashwagandha Complex**, Chinese Qi and Blood Tonic, **Chinese Qi-Regulating**, and Chinese Wood-Increasing

Herbs: Ashwagandha, **black cohosh**, **bupleurum**, cyperus, **damiana**, ginkgo, **kava kava**, **lemon balm**, **mimosa**, perilla, rosemary, and **Saint John's wort**

Supplements: **Lithium**, magnesium, **SAM-e**, **vitamin B$_{12}$**, vitamin B$_6$, **vitamin B$_9$**, and vitamin D

Essential Oils: **Bergamot**, geranium, grapefruit (pink), jasmine, **lemongrass**, **neroli**, orange (sweet), rose, **rosemary**, and ylang ylang

Brain Atrophy

Brain atrophy is indicated when memory and cognition begin to decline. This is most commonly due to age. The following remedies may help aid memory, concentration, and the ability of the brain to process and learn information.

Indications for Brain Atrophy

- Medical diagnosis of Alzheimer's or severe dementia
- Increasing loss of memory, forgetfulness, absent-mindedness
- Difficulty with concentration or focus

Formulas: **Brain and Memory Protection**, **Memory Enhancing**, Watkin's Hair, Skin, and and Nails

Herbs: Ashwagandha, **bacopa**, **ginkgo**, **gotu kola**, periwinkle, **rosemary**, and sage

Supplements: Alpha-lipoic acid, **huperzine A**, **magnesium**, N-acetyl cysteine, omega-3 DHA, and vitamin B-complex

Essential Oils: **Peppermint** and **rosemary**

Senses

The sensory system is part of the nervous system and supplies information to the brain about the outside world.

Hearing　　　　　　　　　　　*Body Part*

The following are direct aids that are used to help solve problems with hearing, such as ringing in the ears and ear infections.

Formulas: **Antispasmodic Ear**, Brain-Heart, and Lymphatic Infection

Herbs: Aloe vera, echinacea, ginkgo, **lobelia**, and mullein

Supplements: Vitamin B-complex and xylitol

Essential Oils: Helichrysum, **lavender**, and tea tree

Sight　　　　　　　　　　　　　*Organ*

The following are direct aids that are used to help solve problems with the sight, such as eye infections, macular degeneration, and retinopathy.

Formulas: **Antioxidant Eye**, Chinese Wood-Increasing, Chinese Yang-Reducing, **Herbal Eyewash**, Nitric Oxide Boosting, and Oral Chelation

Herbs: **Bilberry**, **chamomile**, chickweed, **eyebright**, goldenseal, gotu kola, horsetail, lobelia, passion flower, red raspberry, tea, white oak, and yarrow

Supplements: **Lutein**, N-acetyl cysteine, and omega-3 DHA

Smell　　　　　　　　　　　　*Sense*

The following are direct aids that are used to help solve problems with the sense of smell, especially when caused by congestion.

Formulas: Jeannie Burgess' Allergy-Lung and Sinus

Supplements: **Zinc**

Taste　　　　　　　　　　　　*Sense*

The following are direct aids that are used to help solve problems with the sense of taste.

Supplements: Vitamin B-complex and **zinc**

Neurotransmitters

The direct aids in this next section enhance the function of specific neurotransmitters within the nervous system.

Acetylcholine　　　　　*Neurotransmitter*

The following may help increase levels of acetylcholine, or contain substances that bind to receptor sites for acetylcholine. This neurotransmitter helps with memory and muscle tone. It is deficient in Alzheimer's disease.

Formulas: Attention-Focus, **Brain and Memory Protection**, Memory Enhancing, Watkin's Hair, Skin, and and Nails

Herbs: Sage

Supplements: Lecithin

Essential Oils: Rosemary

Dopamine　　　　　　　　*Neurotransmitter*

The following remedies may help increase dopamine levels. Dopamine is a neurotransmitter involved in mood, muscle coordination, and sexual drive.

Formulas: Chinese Qi-Regulating, Mood Lifting EO, and Self-Responsibility FE

Herbs: Velvet bean

Supplements: **L-phenylalaine**, **L-tyrosine**, magnesium, SAM-e, vitamin B$_3$, vitamin B$_6$, and **vitamin C**

Epinephrine   *Neurotransmitter*

The following remedies either enhance epinephrine or stimulate receptor sites for epinephrine.

Formulas: Stimulating Energy and Vandergriff's Energy Booster

Herbs: Cocoa, **coffee**, **guarana**, **orange (bitter)**, sage, and yerba maté

Supplements: **Copper**, iron, **L-tyrosine**, vitamin B_3, vitamin B_6, and vitamin C

Essential Oils: Pine, rosemary, and thyme

GABA   *Neurotransmitter*

GABA is a neurotransmitter that calms down excessive nervous firing in the brain. It may be deficient in ADHD, epilepsy and schizophrenia. The following either enhance GABA or stimulate GABA receptors.

Formulas: Attention-Focus and **Brain Calming**

Herbs: **Ashwagandha**, hops, **kava kava**, lemon balm, **passion flower**, **skullcap**, and valerian

Supplements: **GABA**, L-glutamine, and L-threonine

Serotonin   *Neurotransmitter*

The following remedies may help increase serotonin levels in the body. Serotonin is a mood-elevating neurotransmitter.

Formulas: **5-HTP Adaptogen** and Mood Lifting EO

Herbs: Eleuthero, ginkgo, kava kava, passion flower, rhodiola, **Saint John's wort**, tea, and yerba maté

Supplements: **L-tryptophan**, vitamin B_3, and vitamin B_6

Substance P   *Neurotransmitter*

Substance P is the neurotransmitter that transmits pain signals. These remedies decrease the action of substance P, helping to relieve pain.

Formulas: Anti-Inflammatory Pain, **CBD Topical Analgesic**, and **Topical Analgesic**

Herbs: **Capsicum** and clove

Supplements: CBD

Essential Oils: **Camphor**, **clove**, and **menthol**

Other Organs and Systems

There are some parts of the body that don't fit neatly into a body system, they are listed here.

Endocannabinoid System

The endocannabinoid system (ECS) is a recent discovery. Researchers found the ECS while researching the effects of cannabis. The system, and the compounds used in it, were named after the cannabis plant in the same way opioid receptors were named for the opiates from the poppy plant.

The ECS appears to help maintain homeostasis, the normal balance of healthy conditions in the body. This balance is maintained through chemical messengers that respond to injuries, stress, or other problems to help the body cope, adapt, and eventually heal.

For example, when the body is injured, chemical messengers like prostaglandins and substance P evoke an inflammatory response and pain signals. Pain lets us know the body has been damaged, and the inflammation alerts the immune system. The ECS activates to gradually reverse these signals and return the system to normal equilibrium.

The same thing happens when something causes us to feel stressed. The fight-or-flight response kicks in to prime our body to react with the difficult or dangerous situation. Once the challenge is over, the ECS helps the body return to its normal relaxed state.

This means that the ECS plays a critical role in our ability to heal, both from physical injury and from emotional distress. Researchers are suggesting that many chronic illnesses may involve a malfunctioning of the ECS, which prevents the body from returning to homeostasis.

The ECS consists of two types of receptors on cell membranes throughout the body, known as CB_1 and CB_2 receptors.

CB1 Receptors

CB_1 receptors are primarily found in the brain and nervous system, although they are also located in the heart and circulatory system, the male and female reproductive system, the digestive organs, the gastrointestinal tract, and other organs. Primarily CB_1 receptors help balance the neurotransmitter system, including stress responses, pain and mood.

Formulas: **CBD Relaxing** and Hemp Oil with Terpenes

Herbs: Cannabis, **cocoa**, and **kava kava**

Supplements: CBD

CB2 Receptors

CB_2 receptors are found primarily in the immune system and organs with immune functions, such as the spleen, tonsils, skin, lungs, liver and gastrointestinal tract. CB_2 receptors can also be found in the brain, heart, kidneys, pancreas, bones and gallbladder. Primarily, CB_2 receptors help modulate immune processes and inflammation.

Formulas: CBD Anti-inflammatory and **CBD Topical Analgesic**

Herbs: Black pepper and cannabis

Supplements: CBD

Essential Oils: Copaiba

Eustachian Tubes   *Tissue*

The Eustachian tubes run from the throat to the inner ear and help to equalize air pressure on both sides of the eardrum. When your ears pop changing altitude, the pressure is being adjusted via the eustachian tubes. These tubes can swell, often due to an allergic reaction. This does allow the pressure to equalize, or the inner ear to drain, which can cause pressure and pain. Children who get frequent ear infections often have problems with their eustachian tubes.

Formulas: Antihistamine and Liquid Lymph

Herbs: Eyebright and nettle, stinging

Mitochondria   *Other*

Inside of the cells of every plant, animal and human being you will find small structures called mitochondria. These rod-shaped organelles (cellular organs) are the power plants for cells. Their job is to convert the calories from carbohydrates, fats, and proteins into energy the cells can use. They provide every cellular process with the energy it needs to function using a cyclic process known as the Krebs cycle.

Researchers are now discovering that mitochondria do more than produce energy. They also play a role in the synthesis of fatty acids, the regulation of cellular levels of amino acids and enzyme cofactors, balancing levels of heme (the iron compound that forms the basis of hemoglobin), calcium balance, neurotransmitter synthesis, and insulin secretion.

Mitochondria also produce reactive oxygen species (free radicals) that can damage their own structures as well as other structures in the cell if there aren't enough antioxidants present to regulate them. They also play a role in apoptosis, which is the mechanism that triggers cells to die. Apoptosis is the process by which the body gets rid of virally infected cells and cancer cells. Without apoptosis, multicellular organisms can't protect themselves from cells that have started to malfunction.

As all this research is coming forth, science is discovering that mitochondrial dysfunction is involved in numerous degenerative diseases. First, since mitochondria produce energy, anyone who has serious, long-lasting fatigue probably has mitochondrial dysfunction. Mitochondrial problems are also involved in diabetes, deafness, and neuropathy. It's also being proposed that health conditions such as cancer, diabetes, fibromyalgia, and serious mental illnesses (such as schizophrenia and bipolar disease) may result from mitochondrial dysfunction, although the research on the role mitochondria play in all these diseases isn't clear yet.

Formulas: Detoxifying, Methyl B12 Vitamin, Methylated B Vitamin, and **Mitochondria Energy**

Supplements: Alpha-lipoic acid, Co-Q10, L-carnitine, **magnesium, manganese,** N-acetyl cysteine, **vitamin B-complex, vitamin B_1,** vitamin B_{12}, **vitamin B_2,** vitamin C, vitamin D, vitamin E, and zinc

Vocal Cords   *Body Part*

The vocal cords vibrate, allowing you to sing and speak. They can become irritated and inflamed, creating problems with the voice.

Herbs: Collinsonia, lobelia, and **sage**

Chinese Energetic System

Traditional Chinese medicine has a useful system for understanding imbalance in the body. This section presents some of the basic elements of the Chinese system and some formulas and single herbs that are used with it.

Chi

People with the Western mindset tend to think of health merely in mechanical or physical terms. This is not true in Chinese medicine. The entire Chinese system, which includes herbalism, massage therapy, and acupuncture, is based on the theory that all things have an energy field. This energy, which flows in, through, and around our bodies is called chi. Acupuncture charts show lines of energy flow through the body called meridians. The meridians carry the life-energy, the chi, through the various organs and parts of the body.

If the flow of life energy through the organ is either excessive or blocked, then that organ will become diseased in some way. The energy field is like a matrix that controls the physical structure of the body and the way the cells line up within that structure. Thus, all illness is a manifestation of imbalanced energies in the body.

If there is too much energy flowing through a part of the body, we could say that that part of the body is stressed. To stress something is to place too much pressure or emphasis on it. Hence, a body part with too much energy flowing through it is overemphasized or stressed. On the other hand, if there is too little energy flowing through a body part, then that body part would be said to be weakened.

Formulas and herbs increase chi (like those listed below), improve energy and stamina. Unblocking stuck chi can also relieve pain. Enhancing chi also promotes healing, especially when one is experiencing weakness.

Formulas: Chinese Qi and Blood Tonic, Chinese Qi-Increasing, Chinese Qi-Regulating, and Chinese Wind-Heat Evil

Herbs: Astragalus, atractylodes, codonopsis, cordyceps, **ginseng (Asian/Korean)**, and licorice

Yin and Yang

The notion of chi is connected to the concept of yin and yang. The concept of yin and yang pervades all of traditional Chinese thought, not just in medicine, but in other forms of science and art as well. The concept of yin and yang is the idea that everything has its opposite.

You can think of yin and yang as two basic forces operating in nature. One is an inward force that is hidden and unmanifest. It is contractive, downward, and negative. The other is is an outward force that changes things. It is expansive, linear, and positive.

The outward force is the yang force and is associated with heaven, light, up, daytime, male traits, and function. The inward force is the yin force and is associated with darkness, winter, nighttime, female traits, and structure.

According to Chinese medicine, there are two types of energy in the body, the yin energy and the yang energy. The yang energy is the outward energy that is used to perform the daily tasks of work and play. The yin energy is the energy that is held in reserve for emergencies.

Excess Yang

When disease first strikes, it is on an acute level; that is to say, the symptoms are all superficial or on the surface. Acute symptoms include such things as vomiting, runny noses, diarrhea, rashes, hives, and coughing.

In Western herbalism, these acute symptoms are recognized as the body's efforts to heal itself, to get rid of the toxins that are accumulating in the system. In Chinese herbalism, these are yang symptoms. They can be overcome by bringing some of our yin energy reserves to the surface to fight off the illness. Yang energy is associated with fever, heat, and inflammation.

Formulas: Chinese Wind-Heat Evil and Chinese Yang-Reducing

Herbs: Amur cork, baical skullcap, burdock, and chrysanthemum

Deficient Yin

However, disease may progress to a more chronic level. That is the level of more deep-seated troubles, such as lung weakness, glandular fatigue, poor circulation, and poor digestion. Western herbalism recognizes that these are symptoms that the organs have lost their vitality and become weak. There are no acute symptoms associated with these problems because the body organs have become too weak to expel the toxins.

In Chinese herbalism, these would be yin symptoms. The disease has overcome the yin energy or the hidden energy reserves of the body, so there are no reserves for emergencies. These disorders must be overcome by building up the yin energy reserves.

Deficient yin can also be associated with heat, but this heat is accompanied by weakness. The heat is caused by the lack of the moist, cooling yin energy. Yin deficiency also leads to dryness in the tissues.

Formulas: Chinese Yin-Increasing

Herbs: Asparagus (Chinese), **ginseng (American)**, ophiopogon, and **solomon's seal**

The Five Elements

All ancient cultures had elemental theories. The American Indians, the East Indians, and many other cultures have utilized elemental theories. The idea behind elemental theories is similar to the notion of yin and yang. It bears the idea that there are certain basic forces, or elements, of which everything is made.

It is easiest to think of this in terms of color. All the visible colors are composed of the three primary colors: red, yellow, and blue. So although there are thousands of subtle shades of color, each is simply a different combination of the three primary colors. A true elemental theory would be something like the three primary colors; that is, it would identify the primary elements of which everything we see (and don't see) is made.

The Chinese utilized a system of five elements. These five elements are wood, fire, earth, metal and water. According to the theory of the five elements, the essence of these five things is found in everything, including people.

The formulas for balancing the five elements are divided into two categories, formulas for stressed (excess) conditions and formulas for weakened (deficient) conditions. These may be generally considered as formulas for acute health problems related to certain organs and formulas for chronic health problems related to certain organs.

The formulas in the stressed category relieve yang conditions. They correct conditions of excess or overactive energy. This is typically brought on as the body is trying to rid itself of something that is irritating it. Thus, the stressed formulas help the body get rid of excesses or cleanse itself.

The formulas in the weakened category relieve yin conditions. They help rebuild energy reserves when they are depleted and the body is in a chronic and/or degenerative condition. They build up or nourish the yin energy reserves.

Wood Element

Wood represents the principle of life and the renewal of life. The wood element represents your ability to spread out into our environment in an aggressive manner and then stop, contemplate and plan a new strategy for action. It is that part of nature that is cyclic, flowing with the changing seasons and environmental conditions.

An inability to exhibit the characteristics of the wood element may be a sign of imbalance. This can manifest as either a deficiency (weakened wood) or an excess (stressed wood). For example, people with excessive wood might feel continually irritable and always on edge.

They would tend to be angry and pushy and always planning ways to get ahead. People who are deficient in wood, on the other hand, might have the inability to express anger or feelings of frustration and inner conflict. They might find it difficult to move forward in a constructive manner.

In physical terms, the Chinese associate the liver/gallbladder with the wood element. The Chinese associate decision making and the abilities of planning and judgment with the liver. The emotions of anger and resentment are said to damage the liver and gallbladder. Western culture also associates anger with the liver and gallbladder with sayings like, "This really galls me." Resentment is also spoken of as bitterness. The gallbladder is the home of the bitter bile and of bitterness in the personality.

Physical symptoms of wood imbalances also center on the liver and gallbladder. However the liver and gallbladder affect numerous other body systems, so there are many other physical symptoms of wood imbalance.

Stressed Wood

Symptoms of liver problems are usually associated with a "touch of the flu." These same symptoms in France have been called a liver crisis. When the liver energy is overactive (i.e., stressed), here are some of the symptoms that typically occur: nausea, diarrhea, fatigue, stiff and aching muscles, cold hands and feet, anger and defensiveness, migraine headaches, other headaches, gallbladder attack, flu-like symptoms, discomfort, swelling and/or tenderness underneath right rib cage, dizziness and puffy eyelids, difficulty getting to sleep followed by difficulty awakening in the morning (a sort of hangover feeling), and skin eruptions (acne, pimples, rashes).

Physically a person with excess wood is prone to a congested liver and gallbladder and emotionally they are prone to anger, irritability and frustration, aggression and depression. Indications of excess wood energy include hypoglycemia, migraine headaches, allergies, poor fat metabolism, abdominal pain and distention and skin problems.

Formulas: Chinese Wood-Decreasing and Detoxifying
Herbs: Bupleurum

Weakened Wood

When the liver is in a weakened (or underactive) condition, it will probably manifest symptoms of liver stress periodically, along with the following: hypoglycemia, PMS, food allergies, chronic fatigue, depression, despondency, despair ("What's the use, why fight it anymore?"), hypochondriac feelings, changeable health, doctors not finding what's wrong, immune system weakness, candida, poor bowel elimination, gas and indigestion, poor fat digestion, liver spots on the skin.

A person lacking in wood energy will have a tendency to feel frustrated, depressed, discouraged, and indecisive, with occasional bouts of sudden anger.

Formulas: Chinese Qi-Regulating and **Chinese Wood-Increasing**

Herbs: Dong quai, lycium, **peony**, **rehmannia**, and reishi

Fire Element

Fire is associated with warmth and light. Fire is very active, dynamic, colorful, energetic, and lively and contains the spark of vitality. We speak of a person as being "all fired up" or "on fire". Fire also represents the ability to transform things, and we use fire or energy in manufacturing.

A person with a balanced fire element is warm and friendly, loving and kind. Their hands and feet tend to be warm. They have a normal sexual appetite and response. They have imagination and joy in their lives.

But, if the fire element becomes too abundant, there will be excessive energy in the top half of the body, since fire tends to rise. A person with an excess of fire is often insecure on the inside so they seek constant attention from others, excitement, and diversions. This pursuit of joy and happiness puts excessive stress on the body, especially the heart. They also tend to have vivid dreams, high ideals, and a strong imagination.

Too little fire might result in not being able to finish what is started. Lack of fire could also be called burnout or the loss of energy and drive. Lack of fire energy manifests as fatigue coupled with anxiety that makes relaxing difficult.

The organs associated with the fire element are broken into two groups. The first is composed of the heart (yin) and small intestines (yang). The second is composed of the triple warmer (yang) and circulation/sex (yin). The triple warmer is thought to control the metabolic rate and keep the body warm. It is probably connected with the glandular system (thyroid and adrenals). The circulation/sex meridian is associated with the reproductive glands and the circulation of blood. It is related to physical warmth (good circulation) and sexual drive.

The circulatory system and the heating system of the body are associated with the fire element. The heart is seen by the Chinese as the home of insight and understanding. Courage is also associated with the heart, as in faint-hearted or lion-hearted.

The intestines are sorters, and like the refiner's fire, they separate the good from the bad. The Chinese have the philosophy that the body heat (life energy) is created by three burners (centers) in the main trunk of the body. They call this the triple warmer and associate it with the fire element as well. The sexual drive is associated with the fire element in both Chinese herbalism and in Western expression. We speak of love as burning with passion, and lack of desire as frigidity.

Stressed Fire

Stress and excessive tension, irritability, restlessness, insomnia, and other nervous disorders are the most prominent physical symptoms of too much fire. Symptoms of being fire-stressed also include feeling high-strung, overactive, tense, and nervous; difficulty relaxing; restlessness; convulsions; dizziness; tossing and turning at night; mental diseases; incoherent speech; unreasonable weeping and laughing; anxiety; fright; excitability; heart palpitations; overactive thyroid; and overtaxed adrenals.

A person with too much fire is prone to excessive excitement, restlessness, anxiety, and insomnia, conditions associated with excessive stress.

Formulas: Anti-Stress B-Complex, **Chinese Fire-Decreasing**, and Jeannie Burgess' Stress

Herbs: Biota, jujube, **mimosa**, polygala, and **reishi**

Supplements: Amber (succinum), **magnesium**, and vitamin B-complex

Weakened Fire

Lack of fire is known as burnout. It is what happens after being under stress for long period of time and no longer being able to cope. Symptoms of fire deficiency include feeling tired, nervous exhaustion, adrenal exhaustion, enervation, muddled thinking, forgetfulness, low thyroid function, waking up frequently, lack of sexual drive (frigidity), mental confusion, poor memory, restless dreaming, dry skin, low body temperature, cold hands and feet, poor circulation, fatigue, and the inability to speak clearly.

One of the surest indicators I have found for a weakened fire element is fatigue coupled with the inability to sleep soundly. These people don't have trouble getting to sleep (that is a wood element problem) but they have trouble staying asleep. They either wake up frequently needing to urinate, or they simply wake up after four or five hours of sleep and lie awake thinking about their problems.

Sometimes the stress of life just gets to be too much and a person starts to feel burned-out. This shows the subconscious association of fire with passion, excitement and motivation. This same association exists in Chinese medicine. When a person becomes deficient in fire energy, they become tired and nervous, feel overwhelmed, vulnerable, and broken hearted, and lose sexual desire.

Formulas: Ashwagandha Complex and **Chinese Fire-Increasing**

Herbs: Broomrape, **eleuthero**, ginseng (Asian/Korean), and **schisandra**

Earth Element

The earth is the grounding element. It holds things down and keeps them in place. Being stable, basic, deep-rooted, centered, grounded, and fertile are all characteristics associated with the earth element within us.

The emotions of sympathy and compassion are associated with the earth. They are the mothering emotions. The earth element is associated with mothering. We often speak of Mother Earth because the earth nourishes us and provides us with food, clothing, and shelter. Hence, the desire to nourish, care for, and protect others is an earthy feeling.

People who are too earthy or motherly might have a tendency to worry a lot about others. Sympathy has an effect on the stomach. We commonly warn people not to worry too much or they'll get ulcers. The epitome of an earth-stressed personality would be the stereotypical overprotective mother who dotes and fusses over everyone.

People with a deficiency of the earth element would be nervous, flighty, unstable, imbalanced, or otherwise unearthed. They also might be egocentric—that is, they are deficient in the emotion of compassion and have no feelings of nurturing others. Another sign of deficiency would be the inability to digest or process things, including information.

The stomach is associated with the earth element in Chinese herbalism. The stomach is the home of nourishment.

The Chinese also associate the spleen with the earth element, but this is not the organ we think of as the spleen in the West; instead, it is the ability to turn the food we eat into flesh, or, in other words, the ability we have to metabolize and utilize nutrition. Hence, it probably has more to do with the pancreas than the spleen.

Stressed Earth

Physiologically, an earth-excess condition would be characterized by acute indigestion with pain in the stomach area and loss of appetite. The belching of a rotten egg taste and smell shows that proteins are not being digested properly in the stomach. Here is a complete list of earth-stressed symptoms: belching, gas, foul breath, sour stomach, nausea, bloating, loose stool, sugar cravings, and cravings for junk food. Worry, general emotional upset and projection of fears into the future are emotional symptoms of an overactive earth element.

Sometimes, however, this energy is excessive and needs to be calmed down, as when we have an upset stomach and acid indigestion. This often comes because we have overloaded our digestive organs and they become congested. The result is stomach pain, bloating, gas, indigestion, sore stomach, foul belching, a heavy feeling in our stomach, and loss of appetite.

The nurturing, mothering energy can also become excessive on the emotional side too. Excess mothering quickly becomes smothering, plagued by constant fears, worries, and a general sense of being off-balance.

Formulas: Chinese Earth-Decreasing and Christopher's Carminative

Herbs: Hawthorn, hyssop, and **peppermint**

Weakened Earth

Physically, earth-weakened people have underactive stomachs and digestive systems. Because of their difficulty digesting food they may become sallow, pale, weak, cold, fatigued, and even anorexic. Here is a more complete list: general weakness, poor muscle tone, poor physical development, loss of energy, cold limbs, cramping, tension in the solar plexus, difficulty swallowing capsules, sensation of lump in throat, overstimulated thyroid, inability to gain or lose weight, long-term physical weakness. Emotionally, being unable to cope with new situations, clinging to the past, deep-seated worries and fears and repressed anger may indicate an earth-weakness.

When a person has an inability to properly digest and metabolize food, they tend to lose muscle mass. They may become very thin and pale, or simply overweight with a lack of muscle tone. The Chinese associate these symptoms with a deficiency of spleen chi (or energy). The traditional Chinese name for this formula, *wen zhong*, means warm the center, referring to the power of this formula to warm up or enhance digestive energy.

Formulas: Chinese Earth-Increasing and Digestive Support

Herbs: Astragalus, **ginseng (American)**, ginseng (Asian/Korean), and **saw palmetto**

Metal Element

The metal element is important for defense. It is used to make swords and shields for our defense. Metal invokes ideas of substance, structure, and strength. The metal element is associated with autumn because this is the time of year when all things begin to consolidate within themselves. They begin to pull in their reserves and store up for the coming winter. Although life appears to fade on the surface, it is still present, deep within things.

The metal element is associated with mucus or phlegm and the emotions of sorrow and grief. Prolonged sorrow and grief might weaken a person's ability to stand up for themselves.

Excessive metal behavior could be characterized by the age of the knights. In addition to wearing metal armor, they were hyper-defensive. They fought crusades or wars in the name of religion. Excess metal leads to defensiveness, rebelliousness, militancy, and an excessive need to assert one's opinion. We can all think of the person who jumps to the defensive under the slightest provocation. Marches bring out the metal in people because the brass (metal) instruments stir the adrenal glands to action.

The Chinese associate the metal element with the colon and the lungs. However, it is more practical to think of the metal element as associated with the immune system. The skin and the mucous membranes (which line the lungs and digestive tract) are like a shield to protect our bodies from harmful substances and allow only life-giving nutrients to pass. The inner and outer skins can be thought of as our first line of defense. The lungs are the major center of this defense for the respiratory tract and are thought to receive the life force, Chi. The bowel is the center for the digestive tract, and the intestines drain away the dregs.

There is a strong connection between respiratory problems and grief. Sinus problems, for example, may be a symptom of inner tears or crying. A chronic cough may be difficulty in getting something off your chest. Note that older people often die of pneumonia after the death of their spouses. Inability to express and release grief will cause deep-seated lung problems, such as asthma, chronic bronchitis, pneumonia and dry coughing. It may also cause a person to become hardened and unable to get close to others. Many times in clinical practice we have traced the origin of a chronic lung problem back to unresolved grief. As the person is able to sob and weep, thereby releasing the grief, the respiratory problems improve.

Stressed Metal

Metal-stressed symptoms are associated with respiratory congestion. Symptoms center on acute congestion of the respiratory system, probably caused by poor lymphatic circulation due to digestive problems and bowel obstructions. Specifically, shallow breathing, wheezing, cough, sinus congestion, lymphatic swelling, asthma attack, and excessive grieving or sadness are all metal-stressed symptoms.

Formulas: Chinese Metal-Decreasing and Jeannie Burgess' Allergy-Lung

Herbs: Coltsfoot, loquat, mulberry, and perilla

Weakened Metal

A deficiency or breakdown in the metal element would be associated with chronic weakness of the respiratory system, such as emphysema, chronic lung infections, frequent colds, and flu. In metal weakness, the lungs become dry and inflexible. Specific symptoms include pallor, fatigue, shortness of breath, excessive perspiration, poor appetite, feeble speaking, shortness of breath, tension in chest, repressed or

deep-seated grief, hardness of heart, inability to feel close to others, weakened immune response, inability to stand up and defend oneself, disintegration, or an inability to express sorrow and grief.

Formulas: Chinese Metal-Increasing

Herbs: Astragalus and cordyceps

Water Element

Water is fluid and changing, taking whatever shape it is given. Its form is determined by its container, or the lack of one. The nature of water is to be serene and submissive, but in excess it can be violent and as inundating as a flood. Water is essential to life, and the Chinese consider the water element to be the most basic of all the elements.

The energy of water is also expressed in the flow of blood and lymph and our own ability to be fluid and flexible. The emotion associated with water is fear, and excessive fear is thought to damage the kidneys. This is expressed in the expression, "He was so scared he wet his pants." Also, the adrenals, situated on top of the kidneys, are the glands that respond most violently to fear.

According to Chinese philosophy, the kidneys are the gate of self-expression. People whose kidneys are weak were often subjected to undue fears by their parents. Because they were constantly warned about the dangers of doing big things, such as climbing trees, swimming, and running, they tend to channel their energy into doing small things such as painting, and mechanical tinkering. The connections with these problems and fear are very clear. We speak of someone as being spineless, unstable, having a yellow streak down the spine, and weak-kneed.

A lack of the water element would lead to a lack of fluidity (brittleness) or the ability to change, submit, and compromise. Water flows down, so the water problems would show up in the lower half of the body. With too much of the element of water, one might become too fluid and unable to stand up for oneself and would become weak-kneed. People who are excessive in water tend to start many projects (water is nourishing to the roots of things), but they are too wishy-washy to see them through to completion.

Stressed Water

The major symptom of a water-stressed constitution is water retention. The excess water (edema) needs to be removed from the system. Other symptoms that may indicate stress on the water element include late-afternoon sluggishness, heavy feelings, backache, leg pains, headaches, neck and shoulder pain, prostate problems, PMS, burning urination, and bladder infections. Emotionally, being wishy-washy, indecisive, uncertain, fearful, and timid are symptoms of stressed water.

Water-stressed herbs are diuretics, which enhance kidney function.

Formulas: Chinese Water-Decreasing and Diuretic

Herbs: Buchu, corn silk, hoelen, and juniper

Weakened Water

A water-weakened condition is associated with chronic kidney weakness. This kidney weakness also leads to a deterioration in the structural system. A sort of brittleness settles into the body that creates arthritis, stiffness, weakness of knees and ankles, chronic back and leg pain, brittle bones (osteoporosis), one hip higher than the other, one shoulder drooping lower than the other, curvature of the spine, and more easily fractured bones. Other possible symptoms include impotence and fatigue. Hardened in attitudes, inflexible, unable to adapt or change due to fear of change, rigid, and inflexible in thinking patterns may also signal a water-weakened condition.

The connection between the kidneys and the structural system can be explained largely as follows. When people eat a heavy protein diet, it creates acid waste in their blood. If the kidneys are weak, they cannot filter the waste out of the blood, so to keep the body pH balanced, the body robs the bones, muscles, and connective tissue of calcium to neutralize the acid in the blood. This weakens the structural system of the body.

Specifically, weakness of the structural system creates an unstable condition of the pelvis, where one hip is higher than the other. This makes one leg appear to be longer than the other. This syndrome puts pressure on the muscles of the lower back, causing low back pain, sciatic nerve pain, weakness of the knees, stress on the ankles, contortions of the spine, and headaches. Millions of people suffer from these problems, so it is clear that a water-weakened constitution is quite common.

Water-weakened conditions are resolved through herbs that soothe and build the kidneys and remove the acid waste from the blood. Reducing protein consumption and drinking plenty of pure water are absolutely essential to rebuilding weakened kidneys.

Formulas: Chinese Water-Increasing

Herbs: Eucommia, goldenrod, horsetail, nettle, stinging, and **noni**

What Is Your Chinese Constitutional Type?

To find out, look at the list of symptoms in each category. If you currently have a problem with that symptom, put a check in the column marked **present problem** across from the symptom. If the problem has also been a problem in the past, put a check in the column marked **past problem**. If you used to have a problem with that symptom, but it is no longer a problem, you should still put a check mark in the past problem column. If the problem has been a particularly serious one, put two check marks in the box.

Total the number of check marks in each column, then place the combined total of both columns in the last box. See the example below:

Symptom	Present Problem	Past Problem
Puffy eyelids	✓	✓
Gall bladder problems	✓	✓✓
Skin conditions (acne or rashes)		✓
Present and Past Subtotals	2	4
Combined Total for Excess Wood	6	

After completing the entire questionnaire and totaling your scores, record them here. Adding each row and column gives you your total scores for each element and for excess and deficient symptoms.

Take this quiz online at http://treelite.com/quizzes/

Element	Combined Total Excess	Combined Total Deficient	Total Excess + Deficient
Wood			
Fire			
Earth			
Metal			
Water			
Yang/Yin			
Sagging Chi			
Deficient Chi			
Total Excess and Deficient Columns Here			

Symptoms for Excess Wood

Symptom	Present Problem	Past Problem
Hypoglycemia (low blood sugar)		
Migraine headaches		
Allergies (food or respiratory)		
PMS (premenstrual syndrome)		
Problems with fat digestion or metabolism		
Discomfort under right side of rib cage		
Fatigue in the mornings		
Hypochondriac feelings		
Lower abdominal pain and distention		
Sensation of foreign body (lump) in the throat		
Angry, irritable feelings		
Puffy eyelids		
Gallbladder problems		
Skin conditions (acne or rashes)		
Present and Past Subtotals		
Combined Total for Excess Wood		

Symptoms for Deficient Wood

Symptom	Present Problem	Past Problem
General fatigue		
Lower back pain or weak legs		
Scant menstruation with prolonged cycle (women only) or anemia (women or men)		
Severe abdominal pain		
Blurring of vision		
Dryness of the eyes		
Pale complexion		
Hypochondriac feelings		
Hypoglycemia (low blood sugar)		
Depression or bipolar mood disorder		
Feeling discouragement or despair		
Dry skin around eyes		
Chronic liver problems (e.g., hepatitis, cirrhosis)		
Inflammatory bowel disease (e.g., colitis, Crohn's)		
Present and Past Subtotals		
Combined Total for Deficient Wood		

This quiz is from *Strategies for Health* – ©2021 Tree of Light – stevenhorne.com

Symptoms for Excess Fire

Symptom	Present Problem	Past Problem
Nervous or high-strung personality		
Mania or excessive enthusiasm		
Dizzy or light-headed feelings		
Restless or "always on the go"		
Tension headaches		
Irritable or fidgety		
Anxiety or panic attacks		
Muscle tension		
Heart palpitations		
Easily moved to tears or laughter		
Difficulty getting to sleep		
Absentmindedness and forgetfulness		
Fast or loud talker		
Red tip on tongue		
Present and Past Subtotals		
Combined Total for Excess Fire		

Symptoms for Excess Earth

Symptom	Present Problem	Past Problem
Frequent bad breath		
Belching after meals		
Bad taste in mouth		
Abdominal pain or discomfort		
Intestinal gas and bloating		
Cravings for sugar		
Sour or acid stomach		
Temporary loss of appetite		
Frequent nausea		
Chronic worry		
Thick coating on tongue		
Acid reflux		
Fear for the future		
Feeling off-balance		
Present and Past Subtotals		
Combined Total for Excess Earth		

Symptoms for Deficient Fire

Symptom	Present Problem	Past Problem
Extreme fatigue with restless sleep patterns		
Sensation of pressure or pain on the right side of the chest		
Lack of sexual desire, or impotency		
Muddled or confused thinking		
Waking up frequently at night		
Restless or disturbing dreams		
Night sweats or excessive perspiration		
Feeling overwhelmed		
Feeling burned out		
Nervous exhaustion or trembling		
Feeling vulnerable or brokenhearted		
Quivering tongue		
Dark circles under eyes		
Burning sensations in the hands, feet or heart		
Present and Past Subtotals		
Combined Total for Deficient Fire		

Symptoms for Deficient Earth

Symptom	Present Problem	Past Problem
Poor protein digestion		
General weakness		
Poor muscle tone		
Inability to gain or lose weight		
Intestinal cramping		
Food sits heavy on stomach after eating		
Stomach pain aggravated by cold		
Chronically poor appetite		
Difficulty swallowing capsules		
Hiatal hernia or tension in the solar plexus		
Pale tongue with moist white coating		
Chronic worries and fears		
Clinging to the past		
Unable to cope with new situations		
Present and Past Subtotals		
Combined Total for Deficient Earth		

This quiz is from Strategies for Health *– ©2021 Tree of Light – stevenhorne.com*

Symptoms for Excess Metal

Symptom	Present Problem	Past Problem
Congested lungs and sinuses		
Coughing		
Wheezing		
Asthma		
Bronchitis		
Allergies or hay fever		
Sinus headaches		
Swollen lymph nodes		
Sensation of fullness in chest		
Fluid in lungs or chest		
White or pale mucus		
Thick, white coating on tongue		
Excessive grieving		
Sadness		
Present and Past Subtotals		
Combined Total for Excess Metal		

Symptoms for Excess Water

Symptom	Present Problem	Past Problem
Scanty or clear urine		
Edema or water retention		
Heavy, sluggish feelings		
Sluggish feeling in late afternoon		
Backache		
Leg, neck or shoulder pain		
Prostate problems (men); PMS with fluid retention (women)		
Burning Urination		
Bladder infections		
Damp tongue with white moist coating		
Teeth marks on edges of tongue		
Wishy-washy		
Timid and fearful		
Uncertain and indecisive		
Present and Past Subtotals		
Combined Total for Excess Water		

Symptoms for Deficient Metal

Symptom	Present Problem	Past Problem
Chronic lung infections		
Frequent colds and flu		
Pallor (pale and sickly looking)		
Fatigue		
Tightness in chest		
Feeble speaking (soft or low voice)		
Dry cough		
Excessive perspiration or night sweats		
Shortness of breath		
Dry cough		
Pale tongue		
Repressed or deep-seated grief		
Aloof and emotionally distant		
Unable to cry or express sadness		
Present and Past Subtotals		
Combined Total for Deficient Metal		

Symptoms for Deficient Water

Symptom	Present Problem	Past Problem
Spinal misalignment, chiropractic adjustments don't hold		
Frequent and urgent urination		
Weak and brittle bones, osteoporosis		
Impotence (men) Loss of sexual desire (women)		
Dribbling following urination		
Low back pain (lumbar region)		
Prostate problems (men); PMS with fluid retention (women)		
Ringing in the ears		
Graying of the hair		
Weak knees or ankles		
Pale tongue, tendency to be dry		
Hardened, inflexible attitudes		
Fear of change, difficulty adapting		
Rigid and inflexible thinking patterns		
Present and Past Subtotals		
Combined Total for Deficient Water		

Symptoms for Excess Yang

Symptom	Present Problem	Past Problem
Fever or fever with chills		
Headache		
Sore throat		
Eye irritation (red or bloodshot eyes)		
Gum irritation (e.g., gingivitis, bleeding gums)		
Skin infections or acute rashes		
Earaches		
Nosebleeds		
Chronic inflammation		
Sensations of heat or burning		
Irritability or excitement		
Flushing of the face		
Bright-red tongue		
Rapid heartbeat		
Present and Past Subtotals		
Combined Total for Excess Yang		

Symptoms for Sagging Chi

Symptom	Present Problem	Past Problem
Depression		
Feelings of heaviness		
Worry and nervousness		
Hysteria or neurosis		
Insomnia		
Tightness in the chest		
Prolapse of colon or uterus		
Sensation of lump in the throat		
Heavy feeling in the back of the head		
Nightmares or restless dreams		
Migrating pains		
Chest pains		
Hypersensitivity		
Headaches or dizziness		
Present and Past Subtotals		
Combined Total for Sagging Chi		

Symptoms for Deficient Yin

Symptom	Present Problem	Past Problem
Constant thirst		
Frequent urination		
Dry mouth		
Dry eyes		
Night sweats		
Ringing in the ears		
Dry cough		
Burning sensations in hands and feet		
Constipation with dry, hard stool		
Confusion and poor memory		
Burning skin		
Dry sore throat		
Dry red tongue		
Hypoglycemia or diabetes		
Present and Past Subtotals		
Combined Total for Deficient Yin		

Symptoms for Deficient Chi

Symptom	Present Problem	Past Problem
Extreme or chronic fatigue		
General weakness		
Shortness of breath		
Cold and pale skin		
Hair loss		
Slow recovery from illness		
Frequent chills		
Anorexia or muscle wasting		
Poor appetite		
Discouragement, sadness or fear		
Impotency (males) or loss of sexual desire (males or females)		
Frequent illness (low immune system)		
Weakness of the legs		
Pale tongue		
Present and Past Subtotals		
Combined Total for Deficient Chi		

This questionnaire may be used in conjuction with *Strategies for Health*.
An interactive version is available for free at http://treelite.com/quizzes/ – ©2021 Tree of Light – stevenhorne.com

Section Three

Strategies

Techniques, Diets, Cleanses, and Therapies for Healing

This section is the heart of this book. These strategies are basic things a person can do to improve their health. These therapies include basic diet and lifestyle changes, techniques for using certain types of remedies and instructions on basic holistic healing techniques.

Studying this section will give you an overview of many things you can do to improve your overall health and overcome disease in general. When looking up any condition pay close attention to the therapies listed for that condition and check them out before considering specific herbs, supplements, and essential oils as these therapies work on the underlying or root causes of health problems.

Affirmation and Visualization

The discovery that what you think influences your immune system via the nervous system has given rise to the science of psychoneuroimmunology. Basically, positive thoughts enhance our health and well-being, while negative thoughts detract from it.

What is the difference between a positive thought and a negative one? It's very simple. Positive thinking is focusing our mind on what we want, while negative thinking is focusing our mind on what we don't want. So when we're focused on thinking about a disease we have and how we want to get rid of it, we're actually thinking negatively. "I'm going to fight this cancer," in other words, is *not* a positive thought because the focus is on the disease.

Positive thinking would entail thinking something like, "I'm getting stronger and healthier every day." This is focused on the goal of what you want, not the elimination of what you don't want.

Affirmation and visualization are two tools that you can employ to help you create positive thoughts that will enhance your health and your ability to heal. Affirmation is auditory and verbal, while visualization is visual and nonverbal. Of the two, visualization is the more powerful, but both can be helpful, so try combining them for the best effect. Here's how to use these mental tools for healing.

Using Affirmations

An *affirmation* is a present-tense statement that affirms what I want as if I actually have it. Thus, if I had a broken bone and I wanted to speed the healing of that bone I would affirm, "My bone is whole and strong." Notice the present-tense in the statement, "My bone *is*." This is a vital key to making affirmations work because it is laying hold of what you desire in the present tense. If you say, "My bone *will be* whole and strong," this places the fulfillment in the future, not the present, and does not convey the same power. If a direct statement like that is difficult to use, a less-direct but equally effective statement would be, "My bone is healing as it should."

Examples of healing affirmations for yourself or others would include statements such as these:

My body is healthy and strong.

My body is healing as it should.

You will feel better starting now.

Your body is recovering nicely.

To get the most benefit out of an affirmation, you should write it down and post it somewhere you will see it every day. A good place is your bathroom mirror. That way, when you brush your teeth in the morning and again in the evening, you can read the affirmations out loud. It is very important to repeat the affirmation aloud, as hearing yourself say it makes it stronger.

During the day, when negative thoughts arise, simply replace them with your affirmation. So, as you start to worry about the disease or problem, simply start saying your affirmation. Since your mind cannot hold two thoughts at the same time, the positive thought crowds out the negative thought.

If you are a person of faith, affirmation can be helpful when combined with prayer. Pray for the outcome you desire and then affirm that the matter is now in God's hands. Faith is holding in your mind the outcome you desire as if you already have it. "Now faith is the substance of things hoped for, the evidence of things not seen" (Heb. 11:1). Another way of saying this is that faith gives us confidence or assurance in what we hope for. I think of faith as the exercise of a positive mental attitude that includes God's will.

So always ask in your prayer that God's will be done and that whatever happens will be for the good of all concerned. God may have a better plan for you than you have for yourself. Also, be open to guidance, as one way God answers prayers is by helping us to understand the changes we need to make in our lives to achieve the outcome we desire. Therefore, it doesn't hurt to be prayerful about your choice of herbs, supplements, lifestyle changes, and so forth.

Using Visualization

The second method for helping to create positive thoughts is visualization. *Visualization* involves getting into a relaxed state and breathing deeply while you picture the final result you desire in your mind. Again, it is important to see what you want, not what you don't want, and to picture yourself having it in the present, not in the future.

For instance, cancer patients have practiced visualizing their white blood cells gobbling up the cancer cells and destroying them. If you have an injury, visualize your body healed and whole again. It has been proved in studies that such visualization actually enhances immunity and tissue repair.

Both of these techniques are enhanced by practicing deep breathing and relaxation, as is done in meditation. As one breathes deeply, tissues are oxygenated, which fans the spark of life and increases the flame of life throughout the body. Breath is called the "breath of life" because it is intimately connected with the vital force. To breathe is to connect with feelings, to be alive. Shallow breathing causes a person to stifle his or her feelings by deadening the body.

So start the healing process by breathing deeply and allowing the body to relax. Then you can pick one of the foregoing methods for "laying hold" on the health you want before you actually have it. Although we've linked these techniques to specific conditions in which they may be particularly helpful, affirmation and visualization can be helpful with any health or non-health-related problems.

Alkalize the Body

While nutrients are important, life is not simply chemistry. It's a little understood fact that health is highly dependent on energy.

Think about it. Living tissue is not static like the parts in your cell phone or car. Living tissue is constantly growing, changing, adapting and moving. If you zoom in on the activity of the cell in any living creature, you will see that hundreds of chemical and mechanical processes are taking place thousands of times per second.

These life reactions take energy, and that energy is primarily electrical. The vitality of your physical body, therefore, is dependent upon a steady flow of electrons to operate your muscles, circulation, nerves, and every other tissue.

A loss of energy and vitality is the first sign you are losing health. Another early sign is that your brain gets foggy—you can't think clearly. It's only after you continue to lose energy that you start to feel sick. When you lose even more energy, you experience chronic pain in your body.

So if you're sick or experience any type of chronic pain (headaches, backache, etc.) or are simply tired and not thinking as clearly as you'd like, you need to increase the energy stores in your body. In fact, if you're experiencing any chronic or degenerative disease, you need to boost your body's energy reserves, as nothing in the body can heal if energy stores are too low.

Your Body's Battery Pack

The body generates electrical energy and it also stores this energy, much like a battery does. The more your internal battery packs are charged up, the more vitality you experience and the faster you heal when injured. A high-energy charge creates a relaxed, but energized state of being, a clear mind, and an overall sense of well-being.

In contrast, the more rundown your internal batteries, the more tired and sick you feel. It appears that all chronic disease may involve a loss of electrical potential. It's chronic, simply because the body doesn't have enough energy reserves to initiate healing.

pH and Energy

To understand the bioelectric nature of the body, we need to understand pH as a measure of the electrical potential of a solution because the body uses an alkaline pH to store and supply energy.

Pure water (H_2O) has a neutral pH of 7, as shown on the scale above. It's neutral because the electrical charges in water are in perfect balance. When water ionizes, it splits into two components, H+ (hydrogen atom missing an electron, or in other words a single proton, and OH- (an oxygen and hydrogen pair with an extra electron). The H+ is acid; the OH- is alkaline. As shown, the lower the pH, the more acid a solution is; the higher numbers reflect more alkalinity.

So pH is essentially a measurement of electrical charge. If a solution needs electrons, it is acid. If it is alkaline, it has extra electrons to donate.

It's these differences in electrical charges that allow for the creation of the batteries. A battery contains an acid substance with a positive charge (deficient electrons) and an alkaline substance with a negative charge (extra electrons), separated by a third substance.

When you make a connection between the negative (alkaline) terminal and the positive (acid) terminal, the electrons in the alkaline substance begin to flow to the acid substance. This creates an electrical current.

The body also maintains pH differentials that store energy. The normal pH of blood and lymph is about 7.4, a slightly alkaline state. A pH of 7.44 provides an electrical potential of about twenty-five millivolts (-25 mV), according to the book *Healing is Voltage* by the holistic doctor Jerry Tennat.

It Takes Energy to Heal

When the body is damaged, it needs raw materials (nutrients) to make repairs, but it also needs energy—specifically electrical energy. When tissues are damaged, there is an increase in pH at the site of injury. At a pH of 7.88, the electrical energy increases to -50 mV, double the normal of -25 mV. Tissues change from pink to red, and we experience acute throbbing pain. This encourages us not to use the damaged body part, so we allow it to rest and heal. When the repairs are completed, pH returns to normal and the pain and redness subside.

The fact that it takes increased electrical energy for tissues to repair is also demonstrated by the fact that animals who are able to regenerate lost tails or legs (such as lizards) start the regenerative process with increased electrical activity at the site of injury. It is also demonstrated by the fact that low-voltage electrical current can be used to stimulate tissues to heal that were not previously healing. It's also the basis for healing by touch, as electrical energy can pass from one person to another, aiding healing.

Acid pH = Low Energy = Chronic Disease

When the pH is too low, there is not enough electrical energy for healing. The result is chronic inflammation and dull, aching pains. Less energy potential also means fatigue, brain fog, and increased aches and pains. Muscles become tense as they lose energy and become more acidic. If the tissues become too acidic, cells mutate in order to survive and become cancerous.

In order to keep the blood pH balanced, the body has numerous buffering systems. The digestive, respiratory, and urinary systems, play critical roles in pH balance as do the mineral reserves held in bones and muscle. These buffering systems are critical to life because only a slight deviation in blood pH would end your life.

Testing the Charge on Your Cellular Batteries

A simple way to get a readout on your cellular energy level is to check the pH of your urine and saliva. This is easily done with pH test strips, which are available both online and in many pharmacies.

Saliva is made primarily from lymph and provides a good window into the pH of your lymphatic fluid. This is the best indicator of your current cellular voltage.

Urinary pH tells what the body is trying to eliminate. In obtaining electrical charges from food, the body generates acid waste, which is removed via the kidneys. If your urinary pH is too low, you are generating too much acid in your system that isn't being properly buffered.

Additionally, pH levels vary throughout the day so to get a good reading you should check your pH twice daily for at least three or four days. The first test should be when you wake up, and the second test should be later in the day, either before dinner or before bedtime.

Urinary pH should be lowest (more acid) in the morning, when the body is dumping acid generated while you were sleeping. Urinary pH should be higher (more alkaline) later in the day.

To check urine pH, urinate for a couple of seconds and then catch a urine sample in a cup midway through urination. Dip the strip into the urine sample. Compare the color of the strip with the key that comes with the test paper and record your reading.

To check saliva pH, do so before eating or brushing your teeth. Spit a couple of times to clear the saliva in your mouth and then spit onto a spoon and dip the test strip in the saliva. Don't put the strip in your mouth. As before, compare the color to the provided key and record your reading.

After checking your pH for several days, average your readings. According to Dr. Tennat, your cellular pH tends to be about 0.8 units higher than your saliva pH. So if your cellular batteries are properly charged, your salivary pH should average about 6.5 to 6.7, which puts your cellular pH around the desired 7.4 (7.3 to 7.5).

Your urinary pH will typically be lower (more acid), but should average higher than 6.0. If your readings are lower than this, you are generating too much acid and your buffering systems are overwhelmed.

Remember that an overacid pH means your body doesn't have enough electrical energy to keep you healthy. So you need to recharge your cellular batteries by alkalizing your pH.

Recharging Your Cellular Batteries

If your body is overacid, the first thing you need to do is build up your reserves of alkalizing minerals. Seven elements act as electrolytes to create energy flow. The four alkalizing mineral electrolytes are calcium, magnesium, potassium and sodium. They combine with three acid-forming elements (phosphorus, sulfur, and chlorine) in various ways to form twelve different mineral salts. These salts include calcium chloride, calcium phosphate, magnesium sulfate, potassium chloride, and so forth.

When the body is acidic, it is a good indication that you aren't getting enough calcium, magnesium, and/or potassium. Most people get plenty of sodium through table salt, sodium chloride. However, if you need to alkalize the system quickly, a teaspoon of baking soda (sodium bicarbonate) dissolved in a little water will rapidly alkalize the system.

Alkalizing Minerals

If you feel tense, nervous and tired, you're probably depleted in magnesium, a common mineral deficiency. An over-acid system borrows magnesium from the muscles and nerves, which results in tense muscles, muscle spasms, nervousness, and poor sleep. Most people can take between 200 and 800 mg daily.

An over-acid system also causes the body to draw calcium from tissues to buffer the acids. Calcium is a less-common deficiency than magnesium but should be supplemented with magnesium when the body is overacid. Calcium carbonate, in particular, is a powerful acid buffer, which is why it is used in over-the-counter antacids, but it is not the best form of calcium to get calcium into your bones and tissues.

Kidney Function, Hydration and pH

As previously mentioned, a primary job of the kidneys is to remove acid waste. The kidneys need water to dilute the acid and eliminate it. If you aren't drinking enough water, your urine becomes overly acidic and is very irritating to the urinary passages, which makes you need to urinate frequently and can cause discomfort during urination. Unfortunately, this can make people drink less water, not more, compounding the problem.

To balance your pH, you need to drink about half ounce of clean water per pound of body weight per day. That's over two quarts for a 150-pound person (see the *Hydration* strategy). Milk, juice, coffee, and soda pop don't count, but herbal teas do.

The Chinese recognized a connection between the health of the kidneys, bones, and muscles thousands of years ago. In traditional Chinese medicine, kidney qi (chi) deficiency— that is, a weakness of kidney energy—is characterized by low back pain, weak knees and ankles, muscle pain, weak joints, and other structural problems.

Remember that when the kidneys can't filter the acid, the body has to use its reserves of potassium, magnesium, and calcium to buffer the acids. This weakens the muscles, bones, joints, and other tissues that need these minerals. The excess calcium passing through the kidneys also makes a person prone to kidney stones.

Drinking more water and taking a *Chinese Water-Increasing Formula* will help to rectify this situation. This Chinese tonic helps the kidneys flush the acid more efficiently and improves structure strength and muscle tone.

Stress and pH

Your body has a natural daily pH cycle that follows the activity of the autonomic nervous system. During the day, your batteries are discharging under the influence of the sympathetic nervous system and the pH of your urine and saliva will be slightly more acid. At night, when your body is rebuilding energy under the influence of the parasympathetic nervous system, your pH readings will be more alkaline.

Stress activates the sympathetic nervous system and causes your pH to be more acidic. So so the caffeinated beverages people think are giving them more energy, such as coffee, cola drinks, and energy drinks, are draining their energy reserves and driving the system to be more acid. The carbon dioxide and phosphates in soda pop make it one of the most acid-forming drinks you can consume. If you want more energy, alkalize and drink more water.

If you're under a lot of stress and feeling depleted, try taking a *Chinese Mineral Qi Adaptagen Formula* (one of the *Colloidal Mineral Formulas*). It contains potassium, trace minerals, and various Chinese herbal tonics. This will add more of the alkalizing mineral potassium to your system (which also aids kidney function) and will help reduce your stress level. It will alkalize your pH and increase your energy reserves.

The Alkalizing Effects of Antioxidants

Food isn't just a source of calories and nutrients; it's also a source of electrical energy. Raw food has more electrical energy than cooked or processed food. Fresh food has more energy than food that has been in storage for a long time, even if it's still raw.

Living foods spoil through a process called oxidation, which involves a loss of their electrical energy. We've all seen this when we cut into an apple and shortly after it starts to turn brown. The browning is the result of free radicals stealing electrons from the apple tissues, a process called oxidation.

But if we dip the cut apple into some water with fresh lemon juice added to it, it will take longer for the apple to turn brown. The lemon juice helps preserve the apple from spoiling because it contains antioxidants like vitamin C and citric acid.

An antioxidant donates an electron to the free radical. This stabilizes the free radical and prevents tissue damage. This is like the electron moving from the alkaline side of a battery to the acid side. So antioxidants help to preserve the electrical energy and alkaline pH.

It also helps us understand why it isn't the pH of the food that determines whether it helps to acidify or alkalize the body. Lemon juice is sour and acidic, but it is ultimately alkalizing in the body because of its antioxidants. Many sour fruits are high in antioxidants and have an alkalizing effect. Traditionally, sour fruits are considered cooling because they help inflamed tissues to heal.

ORAC (oxygen radical absorbance capacity) is a term used to describe antioxidant potential. Many people find that an *Antioxidant Formula* not only protects them against free radicals but it also alkalizes their system, gives them an energy pick-up, reduces chronic inflammation and pain, and improves their overall health.

Respiration and pH

The lungs are one of the major systems that buffer pH. Oxygenated blood helps alkalize the body, while a high level of CO2 in the blood makes it more acidic. The Deep Breathing strategy helps one stay more alkalized as it oxygenates the blood.

Many people have also found that drinking liquid chlorophyll helps to oxygenate the blood and create a more alkaline pH. Combining chlorophyll with a liquid *Antioxidant Formula* (like the *Antioxidant Mangosteen Formula*) provides quick, caffeine-free, alkalizing energy pick up.

If you have respiratory problems, try taking cordyceps or a *Chinese Metal-Increasing Formula*. This will strengthen the ability of your lungs to buffer pH.

Diet and pH

In the long run, adopting a more alkaline diet is essential to maintaining a properly energized body. To keep things simple, eat more fresh and, where possible, raw fruits and vegetables. These foods are alkalizing due to their live, high-energy state, the antioxidants nutrients they contain, and the alkalizing mineral electrolytes in them, like calcium, magnesium, and potassium.

On the other hand, meat and seeds (grains and legumes) tend to be more acid-forming. This is because the metabolism of protein for fuel creates more acid waste and the predominant minerals in these foods tend to be the more acid-forming phosphorus and sulfur. Refined and processed foods also tend to be acid-forming because they have been denatured and contain less electrical energy.

Raw milk and fermented dairy tend to be pH balancing, but pasteurized milk, cheese, and ice cream are more acid-forming. Fats and oils like coconut oil and olive oil, are pH neutral.

Ideally, about 60 to 80 percent of your diet should be alkaline foods and the remainder acid-forming foods. For more detailed information on what foods are acid-forming and which are alkalizing, consult Tree of Light's *Blood Type, pH and Nutrition* charts.

Additional Tips to Increase Electrical Energy

The earth itself is a source of electrical energy. When you walk barefoot in the grass or the sand, hug a tree, or lie on the ground you absorb electrons from the earth. That's why we sense that connecting with the earth grounds us.

Running water is also highly charged and donates electrons, which is why taking a shower helps us feel refreshed. The same thing can be said for swimming or wading in the ocean.

Touch can also transfer electrical energy. When a parent hugs or massages a sick child, it transfers electrical energy that aids healing. When a healthy person touches a sick person it helps them heal.

The important thing to remember is that your health doesn't just depend on nutrients; it also depends on energy. Following some of the above tips will help provide more electrical energy so you can charge your body for greater health and vitality.

Aromatherapy

Aromatherapy is a term coined by the French cosmetic chemist Rene-Maurice Gattefosse in 1937. After an explosion in his laboratory, Gattefosse inserted his painfully burned arm into a nearby vat of lavender oil. He was amazed at the miraculous way the lavender oil instantly relieved the pain and began an immediate process of healing. The arm subsequently healed quickly and without scarring.

Today, aromatherapy is the use of essential oils for mental, emotional, and physical healing. Essential oils are volatile compounds found in plants. They are responsible for the aroma or smell of the plant. These nonfatty oils are distilled or expressed from herbs, flowers, and trees.

Although individual essential oils have their own qualities, in general essential oils are antibacterial, antiviral, and antifungal. They tend to stimulate circulation, boost immune responses, increase blood oxygen levels, and stimulate cellular growth and repair. They also have strong effects on the nerves and endocrine glands because the sense of smell directly affects the hypothalamus, which regulates the pituitary and acts as the switching station for the brain. This means that essential oils can also help enhance a person's mood, soothe stress, calm negative emotions, and enhance glandular functions.

Essential oils are potent and highly concentrated remedies. Generally speaking, it is unwise to take most essential oils internally. Those that are safe for internal use should only be used in drop doses that are highly diluted and then only for short periods (less than two weeks). The best use of aromatherapy oils is topical.

Even then, essential oils should not be used undiluted on the skin for open wounds or burns, exceptions being oils like lavender or tea tree. If in doubt, always conduct a patch test to be certain. To do a patch test, double the concentration you plan to use, apply it inside the forearm, and monitor for redness, itching, or swelling. If there are any signs of irritation, don't use the oil topically, at least not without properly diluting it.

Essential oils should never be used on or around the eyes. If eye contact occurs, the most effective method of flushing is to use a fatty substance that will absorb the oil. Using water will just spread the oil onto the mucous membrane lining of the eye, causing additional irritation. Some examples of substances to use include butter, cold milk, or vegetable oil. After applying the fatty substance, wash thoroughly with water for five minutes. This also works for spills on the skin.

Overuse and excess dosages can lead to skin irritations, headaches, nausea, and a feeling of unease. Always use a more diluted amount with children. And as with any concentrated substance, keep essential oils out of the reach of children and do not leave a bottle of oil that has no orifice reducer where a child could take off the cap and consume its contents.

Specific Ways to Use Essential Oils

Here are a few of the major ways essential oils can be used.

Topical application (neat). The term *neat* is used to describe the application of an essential oil to the skin without any dilution. You simply apply one or two drops of oil directly to the afflicted area and rub it in. Only do this with oils that are nontoxic and non-irritating to the skin.

Topical application (diluted). Many oils are safe to use if you dilute them in a fixed oil (such as olive oil) before applying topically to afflicted areas. You can usually dilute oils ten to one (10:1) or twenty to one (20:1), but some oils need to be diluted even more.

Massage. Create your own massage oil by adding twelve to eighteen drops of an essential oil per one ounce of a massage oil or a pure vegetable oil like olive. For children, reduce the amount of essential oil by half. Use for a full massage or spot massage at pressure points for a quick effect.

Inhalation. A simple and easy way to introduce oils to your senses is to take the lid off the bottle and breath deeply. It is very effective, and you can use it anytime and anywhere.

Steam inhalation. This is a technique for helping relieve congestion in the lungs and sinuses. It can also help with respiratory infection. Heat a pan of water until it starts to boil. Remove the pan from the heat and add ten to twenty drops of essential oils to the water. Cover your head with a towel and lean over the pan of water to inhale the steam.

Diffuser. This is the best way to disperse oils into the air. This device consists of a glass nebulizer attached to a pump that forces air though, creating a fine mist that lingers for a long time. This is an extremely therapeutic use and can kill germs in the air to prevent the spread of infection.

Hydrosol. Create a natural air freshener by adding forty to fifty drops of your favorite oil or oil blend to a two ounce glass bottle of pure water with a spray mister. This is great for home, work, or car. Shake well before each use. Always use glass, not plastic, bottles.

Baths. Add eight to fifteen drops of an essential oil to the tub with a small amount of a natural, odorless soap, such as Dr. Bronner's Supermild Baby Soap. Mix the oil in with a capful of soap and hold under the faucet while drawing the bath. The soap emulsifies the oil so it will mix into the water. Baths are very effective for absorbing the oils through the skin as well as for their emotional effects.

Compress. Add six drops of an essential oil to a bowl of hot or cold water. Submerse a cloth in the water, wring it out, and place it on the area needing healing. Hot compresses are useful for muscular pain and cramp relief, and cold compresses are useful for swelling or headache.

Internal use. Although I rarely using essential oils internally, there are some applications where it is appropriate to do so. Where oils are safe for internal use, the best way to take them is to dilute them ten to one (10:1) or twenty to one (20:1) in olive oil or coconut oil. This means you use ten to twenty drops of the fixed oil to one drop of the essential oil. Take one or two drops of the diluted oils, once or twice daily for three to four days. With the exception of peppermint oil, I never recommend using essential oils internally for more than two weeks.

Avoid Caffeine

If you're one of those people who just can't get moving in the morning without your cup of coffee or tea (or perhaps a cola of some kind), you have lots of company. Nearly 80 percent of the world's population uses caffeine in some form. Many of us laughingly state there is no life before coffee, feeling our bodies and minds work sluggishly and far from peak ability until adequate quantities of the stimulant are ingested. Yet while we read with dismay the inroads drugs have made into our society as a whole, rarely do we stop to consider that caffeine is a drug (yes, legal, but nonetheless a drug).

How Caffeine Works

Because of its long history of use, caffeine has been more extensively studied than nearly any other ingredient in the food supply. Caffeine is a naturally occurring substance found in numerous plant species throughout the world. It belongs to a group of compounds known as xanthines (or methylxanthines), along with theophylline (used in medicine to dilate bronchi and ease breathing in asthma and emphysema) and theobromine. These chemicals are all stimulants to the central nervous system, producing different effects on various parts of the body.

Caffeine primarily works by attaching to receptors for a neurotransmitter called adenosine in the brain, which blocks the signal that you are tired. This causes you to keep going even though your body is low in energy. The body responds to this in the same way it does to stress, by activating stress hormones (cortisol and epinephrine) to keep you active.

However, the body learns to adapt to the caffeine by producing more adenosine receptors to get the message through that you are tired, which is why more caffeine is needed to get the same affect. If you drink a single cup of coffee per day, the body simply adapts to it so that you need to have the coffee so you don't feel tired because of the extra adenosine receptors in your brain.

Effects of Caffeine

Caffeine has a number of effects on the body. It acts on the cardiovascular system, raising blood pressure and heart rate. Respiratory effects include increased breathing rate and dilation of the bronchi, which enables easier breathing. By revving our metabolism to higher rates, caffeine can help burn more calories; conversely, by initially lowering blood sugar, it can cause us to eat more, especially sweets. Both digestive and urinary systems are stimulated, producing increased urine output and mild laxative effects.

Consumption of about two cups of coffee has been proved to improve clarity and speed of thinking, and decrease drowsiness and fatigue. Typically, effects vary with individuals; however, most of caffeine's effects are dose-related and time-related, as anyone who's ever had insomnia after drinking an after-dinner cup of coffee can attest. Unlike many other drugs, caffeine does not accumulate in the body, therefore it requires repeated "hits" to maintain the effects.

When to Avoid Caffeine

Caffeine-bearing herbs are also fairly strong medicine. Regular, daily use of caffeine-bearing plants can and does cause adrenal fatigue or "burnout" in many people. According to Paul Berger, ND, the eclectic physicians of the last century described a condition they called caffeinism—an illness created by the regular consumption of caffeine. Symptoms of excess caffeine consumption include chronic fatigue, jittery nerves, anxiety, insomnia, overly aggressive behavior, and hyperactivity. So while caffeine-bearing plants can be used safely for medicine, I discourage their daily use for most people.

In my experience regular, use of caffeine can contribute to high blood pressure and insomnia. Even though the research suggests it's not involved, I also recommend not using it if

you have breast cysts. Definitely avoid it if you have hyperthyroidism, irritability, sleep difficulties, nervousness, and adrenal fatigue. Also, caffeinated sodas tend to be acidifying (see *Alkalize the Body* therapy) due to the caffeine.

Eliminating caffeinated beverages can have withdrawal symptoms such as feel tired or getting a headache. You may even feel a bit depressed.

Adaptogens may be helpful in transitioning off caffeine. These include American or Asian ginseng, eleuthero, or schizandra. B-complex vitamins and vitamin C can help boost energy naturally by supporting the adrenal function. Vitamin B-5 (pantothenic acid) is very helpful if the adrenal glands have become exhausted from excess consumption of caffeine.

It may help to substitute a caffeine-free beverage such as an herbal tea for black tea, an herbal coffee substitute for coffee, or sparkling water with a little fruit juice added for sodas. By focusing on healthy substitutes instead of just eliminating the caffeinated beverages, you will ease the transition.

Avoid Sugar

Sugar is a highly addictive substance and the average American consumes between 125 and 175 pounds of refined sugar per year. That's about one-third to one-half pound per day! Most of this is in the form of table sugar (sucrose) or high-fructose corn syrup. Both products are a mixture of glucose and fructose, and both have the same health-destroying effects.

Grains also contain a lot of starch, which is broken down into sugar by the digestive tract. Refined grains convert rapidly into simple sugars and have the same problems as refined sugars. Alcohol also rapidly converts to simple sugars and contributes to blood sugar imbalances.

These simple sugars are addictive for several reasons. First, sugar stimulates the reward centers in the brain, causing a release of dopamine, in an almost identical manner as nicotine, cocaine, and amphetamines. When we consume sugar regularly, this dopamine response that feels so pleasurable becomes blunted, causing cravings for more sugar.

Another reason sugar is addictive is that niacin is required for the conversion of glucose into energy. Niacin is also required for the production of the mood-enhancing neurotransmitter serotonin, which is also involved with sleep, pain reduction, and blood sugar regulation. Sugar causes a release of serotonin, which initially makes us feel good, but it also depletes niacin, the precursor for replenishing serotonin. This causes a reduction in serotonin and mood, which causes the person to crave more sugar, creating a vicious cycle.

The body needs other nutrients, including B-vitamins, vitamin C, and many minerals such as chromium, vanadium, zinc, and magnesium, to convert sugar into energy. In whole foods, the nutrients required to metabolize sugar are present along with the sugar, so the body is more able to properly control and regulate energy production and mood, causing less cravings.

Sugar and Hormonal Balance

Sugar also upsets the body's hormonal balance. The pancreas keeps blood sugar levels stable by secreting two hormones, insulin and glucagon. When there is too much sugar in the blood (hyperglycemia), the pancreas secretes insulin to drive this sugar into storage. When the blood sugar level drops too low (hypoglycemia), the pancreas secretes glucagon to bring sugar out of storage.

Insulin depresses glucagon production, and glucagon depresses insulin production. This relationship, which is much like a hormonal teeter-totter, is called a hormonal axis.

When large quantities of glucose enter the bloodstream, the pancreas secretes insulin, suppressing glucagon production. The more insulin we secrete, the more we become resistant to insulin, requiring more and more insulin to accomplish the same job. When the sugar in the blood has been used up, the body has a hard time mobilizing sugar from storage. The result is reactive hypoglycemia, a sudden drop in blood sugar.

As our blood sugar drops below normal levels from reactive hypoglycemia, our body releases cortisol and epinephrine, causing cravings for sugar, which jacks the sugar level up again. This is like a blood sugar roller coaster ride, and your mood goes up and down with it. Blood sugar levels have a powerful impact on the brain, so sugar can contribute to hyperactivity, irritability, depression, and nervousness.

These high insulin levels cause fat stores to increase as the body tries to find ways to store the sugar. So avoiding sugar is essential for long-term weight loss.

High insulin levels also depress the production of prostaglandins that control inflammation. Chronic inflammation sets in, which sets the stage for heart disease, cancer, and inflammation in the brain, which contributes to the destruction of brain cells.

Breaking Sugar Addiction

The body is programmed to crave sugars because sugars are rare in the natural world. Thus, when people relied on hunting and gathering, finding a good plant source of sugar or starch allowed them to store energy as fat to fuel the body until the next source of food could be found. In modern society, where sugars and starches are so readily available, this mechanism works against instinct, which makes it really difficult to kick the sugar and carbohydrate habit.

So instead of just trying to avoid refined sugar and simple carbohydrates, we need to start by consciously consuming complex carbohydrates, like fresh fruits, vegetables, and whole grains in place of products containing refined sugar and refined carbohydrates like white flour and white rice. Some people get benefit from switching to more natural sugars in place of refined sugar, such as raw honey, real maple syrup, freeze-dried sugar cane juice, and other natural sugars. Because these sugars contain more nutrients than refined sugar, the body's need for nutrients is better met, increasing satiety and causing less cravings.

Eating a breakfast high in protein will also help with overcoming sugar addiction! If you break your fast in the morning by eating simple carbohydrates, such as a pastry, doughnut, toast, or breakfast cereal (even the whole grain varieties), you trigger an insulin reaction that starts you on the blood sugar roller-coaster ride all day. Conversely, when you break your fast with high-protein foods, you stimulate the release of glucagon, which mobilizes stored reserves of sugar and lowers insulin production.

Consider eggs, whole milk yogurt, and meats (preferably organic) for breakfast. At the very least, make a smoothie with whole fruits and protein powder. If you crave carbohydrates and sugar, avoid eating fruit, fruit juice, and even whole-grain cereal at breakfast until your metabolism stabilizes. Once you don't crave these simple sugars anymore, you can probably have some of these foods for breakfast too.

See instructions for the *low-glycemic Diet* strategy, as this is the ultimate answer to sugar cravings. If you feel bad when eating proteins, you might have issues breaking down the proteins due to low stomach acid. See Low Stomach Acid in the conditions section for more information.

You can also try using adaptogens as they also tend to balance blood sugar levels. B-complex vitamins and magnesium help the body utilize sugar properly and can be very helpful in overcoming sugar addiction. If your fasting blood sugar is over 100, consider using a *Blood Sugar Control Formula* to help control blood sugar levels.

Excessive cravings for sweets or food in general can also come from a lack of sweetness (joy) in one's life, which causes one to excessively seek pleasure through food. Learning to find other ways to have joy and pleasure in one's life can be helpful.

Avoid Xenoestrogens

Over fifty years ago it was discovered that chemicals in our environment were having a negative impact on the reproductive capability of wild animals. In spite of this, our society has continued to accept and use these chemicals because they offer "quick fixes" in modern agriculture. Some of these chemicals have now been dubbed as xenoestrogens.

To understand the nature of xenoestrogens, we need to start by recognizing that the term *estrogen* does not refer to a specific hormone. An estrogen is any natural or artificial substance that induces estrus (female fertility and desire to mate). The human body makes three different estrogens—estriol, estrone, and estradiol. Xenoestrogens are chemical compounds from environmental pollutants that bond to estrogen receptor sites. *Xeno* is a Greek word meaning "foreigner, stranger, or alien." So *xenoestrogens* are foreign or alien estrogens.

Xenoestrogens can disrupt the function of the endocrine system in two ways. First, they can mimic natural hormones and turn on cellular processes at the wrong time or simply overstimulate them. A second way they can disrupt the body's hormonal processes is to bond to receptor sites without stimulating them, blocking normal hormonal processes. The results of this bonding can be cellular damage, the inappropriate activation of genes, or the disruption of normal hormonal processes.

Although these chemicals have been "tested" for safety, they have all been tested individually, not collectively. One experiment showed that, when ten commonly encountered chemicals were mixed at a tenth of their individually active dose, the potency (measured as cell proliferation) was ten times higher than expected. So the synergistic effect of these chemicals is dangerous.

Furthermore, they do not readily degrade or break down in the environment. In fact, they tend to accumulate in the fatty tissues of animals and concentrate the higher up the food chain you go.

Xenoestrogens have been documented as causes in reproductive dysfunction and mutations in wild birds, frogs, reptiles, and even mammals. However, the first species of animals to be affected were birds of prey, because they sit at the top of the food chain. The problems these chemicals have caused in wild animals should have clued us into the harm they are causing human beings, but commercial interests have continued to push for their use.

Harmful Effects of Xenoestrogens

Some of the possible effects these xenoestrogens are having on human beings include thus:

Early onset of puberty in young girls (precocious puberty).

Increases in breast and prostate cancer. These tissues contain estrogen receptor sites and are extremely prone to genetic damage and the stimulation of excess growth by xenoestrogens. Other cancers of the reproductive organs may also be caused by xenoestrogens.

Uterine fibroids and other reproductive disorders in women. By over stimulating uterine tissue, excessive tissue growth is encouraged.

Decrease in male fertility and an increase in prostate problems, including prostate cancer.

Sources of Xenostrogens

Some of the chemicals that appear to have serious reproductive and endocrine disruptive effects include the following:

Pesticides (such as 2,4-D, DDT)

Organochlorides (such as dioxin, PPBs, PCBs)

Heavy metals (cadmium, lead and mercury)

Plastic ingredients (particularly soft plastics)

Hormones fed to chickens and cows to increase egg and milk production

Cosmetics

Both men and women need to become keenly aware of xenoestrogens, avoiding them as much as they possibly can. Organic fruits and vegetables should be purchased whenever available, and commercial produce should be washed in a natural soap, like Dr. Bronners, to remove pesticide residues. Use only organic meat, dairy, and eggs. Use glass or paper cartons instead of plastic containers where possible. Do not microwave food in plastic containers or put hot food in plastic containers. Avoid chemicals in general wherever possible.

Another strategy to minimize exposure to xenoestrogens is to use natural, plant-based estrogens to tie up estrogen receptor sites. Phytoestrogens are chemicals in plants that also bond to estrogen receptor sites. However, phytoestrogens have a much weaker estrogenic effect than natural estrogens or xenoestrogens. The theory is that by consuming foods rich in phytoestrogens, receptor sites will be tied up, resulting in less estrogen stimulation.

Soy products and other legumes (beans and peas) are rich in phytoestrogens. We do not, however, recommend large quantities of soy, especially for men, because soy has a very strong estrogenic effect of its own. So we recommend using a variety of legumes, if you can tolerate them. Other good sources include dark-green vegetables and whole grains. Herbal sources include red clover, flax seeds, licorice, and hops.

Because our exposure to chemicals is so high in modern society, it is also wise to support the liver's ability to detoxify estrogens. Indole-3-carbinol, SAM-e, cruciferous vegetables, onions, and garlic all support the detoxification pathways that rid the body of excess estrogens.

Blood Type Diet

Research done by Dr. Peter D'Adamo and Dr. James D'Adamo has demonstrated that there is a strong correlation between your blood type and the foods and supplements you need to consume for optimal health. Dr. D'Adamo has widely promoted this concept in several popular books, including *Eat Right for Your Type* and *Live Right for Your Type*.

The blood has to identify structures that are part of the body versus those that are not, so it knows what to keep and what to eliminate. Foods contain lectins, chemicals that are involved in this identification process. The theory of the blood type diet is that lectins that are incompatible with one's blood type create negative immune reactions, such as agglutination of the blood, inhibited digestion and absorption of nutrients, and hyper immune reactions. In practice, it is a good place to start in screening for foods that may not be compatible with your metabolism.

In the blood type diet a food is classified as an "avoid" because it produces negative lectin reactions in that blood type, which means the food can act as an irritant to the body. On the other hand, foods that are labeled "beneficial" are highly compatible with that type. These foods actually serve as a type of medicine, strengthening health and preventing disease. Foods that are "neutral" merely supply nourishment. They do not have negative lectin reactions, but they also do not have positive, healing properties.

In addition, different blood types are prone to certain basic health risks, which means that there are basic supplements that are often helpful for people with that blood type. There are also some general lifestyle recommendations for each blood type.

Here's a brief description of each of the four blood types. For more information, including a list of foods that are considered beneficial, neutral, or avoid, check out our *Blood Type, pH and Nutrition* charts at treelite.com.

Blood Type O

Blood type O is the predominant blood type in the world. People with this blood type tend to be strong and self-reliant. They tend to have good digestion and a strong immune system. They can eat more meat, but they need to balance protein intake with vegetables (especially green-leafy ones). If they eat too many high-glycemic starches like bread and potatoes, they can become over acidic (see the *Alkalize the Body* strategy), putting stress on the kidneys. They are prone to *H. pylori* infections, ulcers, and intestinal inflammation. Deglycyrrhizinated licorice (DGL), slippery elm, marshmallow, ginger, and turmeric can help control intestinal inflammation.

Higher levels of catecholamines, dopamine and epinephrine, can make them aggressive when stressed, moody, and more prone to problems like bipolar disorder, depression, and schizophrenia. They are also more prone to hyperactivity as children.

Consumption of red meat, especially for breakfast, helps stabilize their mood. If they crave wheat, they should eat pro-tein instead. They may benefit from supplementation with L-tyrosine and glutamine to stabilize their neurotransmitters but should avoid kava kava and Saint John's wort because Saint John's wort inhibits the breakdown of catecholamines.

The *Antistress B-Complex Formula*, methylated B_{12}, and folate may be beneficial. Taking 5-HTP may help ease depression.

They also tend to have hyperactive immune responses, such as allergies, inflammatory diseases, and auto-immune reactions, especially autoimmune thyroid disease or Hashimoto's thyroiditis. They are also more prone to heart disease, stroke, and blood-clotting disorders. Supplements that can help include omega-3 EFAs, adaptogens (especially rhodiola, astragalus, ashwagandha), and colostrum.

Strengths: Strong digestive and immune system, natural defenses against infections, efficient metabolism and preservation of nutrients.

Weaknesses: Immune system can become overactive, intolerant to new dietary and environmental conditions.

Beneficial Activities: Intense, competitive workouts like running, aerobics, martial arts and contact sports.

Major Avoids: Grains (wheat, corn), dairy, beans (kidney, navy, pinto, lentils), nuts (cashews, peanuts, pistachios), vegetables (cauliflower, potatoes), fruits (oranges, tangerines).

Major Beneficials: red meat (beef, buffalo, lamb, venison), fish (sea bass, cod, halibut, snapper, yellowtail), beans (adzuki, black-eyed peas), nuts and seeds (flax, pumpkin, walnut), vegetables (beet greens, Swiss chard, broccoli, kale), fruits (cherries, plums).

Blood Type A

Blood type A is the second most predominant blood type in the world. People with this blood type tend to be settled, cooperative and orderly. They adapt well to dietary and environmental changes. They tend to have less efficient digestive systems and less reactive immune systems.

Eating large quantities of animal proteins, especially red meat, can create problems, partly because of a tendency toward low production of hydrochloric acid (HCl), which is needed to digest protein and absorb minerals. Therefore, they often benefit from taking digestive bitters prior to meals to stimulate HCl production or by taking betaine HCl supplements. Adopting a primarily vegetarian diet may also help. Certain fermented foods, especially fermented vegetables, can also be beneficial.

People with blood type A are more likely to overproduce cortisol under stress and have a hard time breaking it down. This can make it more difficult for them to recover from stress and lead to insomnia, anxiety, obsessive-compulsive behavior, and brain fog. They often benefit from B-complex vitamins with vitamin C, relaxing nervine herbs (especially chamomile, lavender, passionflower, and skullcap), adaptogens (ashwagandha, eleuthero, schizandra, holy basil, and ginseng) and other stress-reducing remedies. Melatonin can be helpful for problems with sleep. Zinc can help reduce excess cortisol and reduce anxiety.

Beneficial Activities: More calming, relaxing, and centering exercises like yoga, tai chi, walking, and swimming tend to be the most beneficial. Breathing exercises and singing can also be helpful.

Activities to Avoid: Activities that create stress, including violent movies, arguments, large crowds, caffeine, and lack of sleep should be avoided.

Strengths: Adapts well to dietary and environmental changes; immune system preserves and metabolizes nutrients more easily; cooperative, creative.

Weaknesses: Prone to anxiety, sensitive digestive tract, vulnerable immune system open to microbial invasion.

Major Avoids: Meat (beef, pork), seafood (bass, catfish, grouper, haddock, halibut, oyster, scallop), dairy, wheat, lima beans, nuts (Brazil, pistachio), vegetables ((tomatoes, potatoes, peppers), fruits (oranges, mangoes, papaya).

Major Beneficials: fish (cod, perch, snapper, salmon, sardine, trout), grains (amaranth, rye, oat), beans (black, pinto, soy, lentils), nuts/seeds (peanut, pumpkin, walnut), vegetables (beet greens, broccoli, carrot, onions, Swiss chard), fruits (berries, grapefruit, lemon, lime).

Blood Type B

Blood type B's are a rarer blood type. They tend to be balanced, flexible, and creative. They have strong immune systems and adapt well to dietary and environmental changes.

They are omnivores and do well on both plant and animal foods. They do well with meat, with the exception of chicken, and they are the only type that readily tolerates dairy products.

People with Blood Type B have naturally high cortisol levels, which causes them to overreact to stress, can disrupt sleep, and suppress immune activity. This can also lead them to react in an overly emotional manner to stress and suffer from lethargy and a lack of motivation. Melatonin and methylated B_{12} can help them have a better sleep cycle, reducing stress. Adaptogens such as ginseng, eleuthero, ashwagandha and holy basil can help, along with vitamin C, B-complex vitamins, and zinc.

They are susceptible to bacterial infections and low-grade viral infections. They can be prone to chronic fatigue, lupus, MS, severe influenza, urinary tract infections, sinus infections, overgrowth of E. coli in the intestines, and staph infections.

Elderberry, medicinal mushrooms like maitake and reshi, astragalus, and licorice root can help to improve immune response. Cranberry can help prevent urinary tract infections.

They are also prone to blood sugar problems, depression, low thyroid hormones, and high blood pressure. Supplements that can help to balance out their blood sugar and improve circulatory function include magnesium, Co-Q10, L-carnitine, chromium, zinc, and alpha lipoic acid. Berberine, cinnamon, and other herbs that help to regulate blood sugar levels may also help.

Beneficial Activities: Moderate physical activities like hiking, cycling, tennis and swimming.

Strengths: Strong immune system, versatile with dietary changes, balanced nervous system.

Weaknesses: Vulnerable to viruses, autoimmune disorders, strong reaction to foods, memory loss.

Major Avoids: Meat (chicken, duck, quail, pork), seafood (clam, crab, lobster, mussels, shrimp, yellowtail), grains (corn, wheat, rye), beans (black, garbanzo, lentils, mung, soy), nuts (peanuts, cashews, pistachio), tomatoes, olives.

Major Beneficials: meat (goat, lamb, venison), seafood (caviar, cod, halibut, salmon, sardine, dairy (cow milk, goat milk, cottage cheese, yogurt, feta), grains (oat, rice), beans (kidney, lima), walnuts, vegetables (beet, cabbage, carrot, peppers, yams), fruits (papaya, pineapple).

Blood Type AB

Blood type AB is the rarest of the blood types. It is a cross between blood type A and blood type B, having a blend of the characteristics of both. People with blood type AB tend to be very adaptable to modern civilization and tend to be both charismatic and mysterious.

They tend to have a sensitive digestive tract and an overly tolerant immune system, which makes them more prone to infections. They may experience chronic, low-grade viral infections, as well as respiratory and ear infections. They are also more prone to parasites and abnormal cell proliferation.

They tend to have higher levels of the catecholamines (epinephrine and norepinephrine) and lower levels of dopamine, which can cause them to feel angry and alienated from others. They can also overreact to stressful situations and exhibit extreme introversion. Boosting levels of L-tyrosine can help to balance their neurotransmitters. Cordyceps, gynostemma, sangre de grado, and danshen root can also be helpful. Glutamine can help produce more of the calming neurotransmitters. Glutathione can be used to help aid in recovery from stress.

They tend to have low levels of hydrochloric acid (HCl), making it difficult for them to digest proteins. Taking digestive bitters prior to meals to stimulate acid production or taking betaine HCl supplements helps.

They have high levels of clotting factors, which make them more prone to forming blood clots. Nattozimes may be helpful in reducing clotting tendencies. L-arginine is also useful in enhancing nitric oxide to dilate blood vessels and reduce pressure.

Strengths: Some benefits of both A and B types; designed to deal with modern conditions; mixed diet.

Weaknesses: Sensitive digestive tract, over-tolerant immune system that allows for microbial invasion, introversion, tendency to feel alienated from others

Beneficial Activities: Calming, centering exercises like yoga or tai chi, combined with moderate activities like hiking, cycling, tennis.

Major Avoids: Meat (red meat, pork chicken), seafood (clam, crab, lobster, shrimp, oyster, yellowtail) corn, lima and kidney beans, wheat, seeds (sunflower, pumpkin), peppers, fruits (banana, orange)

Blood type is only a starting point in helping you determine what foods and lifestyles are healthy or unhealthy for you. Always pay attention to how you feel and determine what is the best diet and lifestyle for you individually.

Bodywork

The structural alignment of the body is important in health. Good posture and structural alignment prevent excessive strain on joints and muscles. It also helps nerve function. Injuries and various emotional stresses can throw the body out of balance structurally, causing muscle tension, pain, stress on the joints, and even pressure on nerves.

There are a number of body work techniques that may be helpful in restoring alignment, easing pain and improving structural function. These include massage therapy, chiropractic care, Rolfing, shiatsu, and the Bowen technique. There are also techniques for training the body to move in a more-aware and less-stiff pattern, such as the Alexander technique and the Feldenkrais method.

Massage Therapy: Massage is one of the most widely recognized bodywork techniques. It can be helpful for back pain, tense muscles, lymphatic congestion and the relief of stress. I've found regular massage is very helpful for maintaining good overall health. I've personally used massage to relieve backache, neck pain, headaches, and muscle cramps with family and friends as described in the *Lymph-Moving Pain Relief* strategy.

Chiropractic Care: I've used a chiropractor like a primary-care physician for most of my life. Chiropractic care does more than help the spine, it promotes healing of the body in general by aiding nerve flow and function. A good chiropractor can often do body work besides adjusting the spine. Chiropractic may be helpful for backache, arthritis, headaches and migraines, pains, sciatica, scoliosis whiplash, and injury recovery.

Rolfing: This is a deep-tissue therapy that realigns the entire body. I went through a series of Rolfing sessions many years ago and it helped my entire body, including improving my ability to breath deeply from my diaphragm. Rolfing can be helpful for releasing trauma held in the tissues, thus aiding emotional healing. It's much more intense than massage or chiropractic.

Shiatsu: This is a traditional Japanese form of bodywork that involves stretching and the use of trigger points. I've had some massage where shiatsu was employed. I think it's effective but don't have as much experience with it.

Bowen Technique: I've been worked on by some Bowen practitioners. The technique is very subtle, but effective. It involves very gentle rolling motions across the muscles, tendons, and fascia.

I've read about the Alexander technique and the Feldenkrais method and think both of them can be very useful for relieving muscle tension and stress throughout the body to restore a more balanced and graceful structural system. I think they are particularly helpful for releasing trauma and injury in the tissues.

I recommend you employ some type of bodywork for most types of joint and muscle pain as well as recovery from both physical and emotional trauma. At the very least, work on your posture with the *Good Posture* therapy.

Bone Broth

Bone broth is a nourishing food that supplies nutrients and minerals needed for the health of bones, teeth, joints and the gastrointestinal tract. It is used to help heal the GI tract in intestinal inflammation and leaky gut syndrome. It is also helpful for improving structural health in conditions like arthritis, broken bones, and osteoporosis.

Here are the directions for making bone broth.

Ingredients

2 lbs. beef or chicken bones (from organic, grass-fed animals if possible; chicken necks and oxtails also make good stock; you can also use the bones and scraps of meat left over from roasting a chicken or turkey)

3 gallons of cold filtered water

1/2 cup good quality apple cider vinegar (optional, but it draws more minerals from the bones)

1 tablespoon of a natural salt

(You can optionally add vegetables, and it's okay if these vegetables are slightly wilted. This is a good way to use up vegetables that are still good but a little past their prime.)

3 onions, coarsely chopped

3 carrots, coarsely chopped

3 celery sticks, coarsely chopped

(You can also optionally add seasonings)

several sprigs of fresh thyme, tied together

1 tsp. dried green peppercorns, crushed

1 bunch parsley

Instructions

When using beef bones with meat still on them, it works best to roast the bones in the oven until the meat is slightly cooked. This is an optional, not an essential step, but I think it makes the broth taste better.

Place the bones in a very large stockpot with the vinegar and cover with the water. Let stand for one hour, then add the vegetables to the stockpot. Bring the water to a boil and allow to boil for about twenty to thirty minutes. A large amount of scum (looks like bubbles/oil slick) will often come to the top. This needs to be skimmed off with a spoon and discarded. After you have skimmed off the scum, reduce the heat and add the seasonings. A Crock Pot or slow-cooker can also be used to simmer the stock if you are leaving the house for an extended period.

Simmer for at least twelve hours and up to seventy-two hours. I usually simmer mine for twenty-four hours. Add fresh parsley in the final ten minutes.

Finally, remove bones with tongs and discard. Strain the rest of the stock into a large bowl. Place the pot in the sink and surround with cold water and/or ice to partially cool, then place in the refrigerator until cold. Fat will congeal at the top and can be skimmed off. Stock may thicken with the natural gelatin in it. This is not only normal, it's a sign you've made good stock. Stock can be kept in the refrigerator for seven to ten days or placed into containers and frozen for later use. (Be sure to allow room for expansion during freezing.) Stock can be warmed and consumed as is or can be used as a base for soups.

Castor Oil Pack

Castor oil packs are used topically to break up congestion and help to soften hardened tissue. To make a castor oil pack, you will need the following:

1/4 cup castor oil

8 drops essential oil, such as lavender (optional)

A soft cloth

Combine the castor oil and the essential oils. Soak the cloth in the oil so the cloth is saturated but not dripping.

Fold the cloth and place it in a baking dish and put the dish in the oven at 350 degrees for about 20 minutes. It should be warm, but not hot. As an alternative, you can heat the oil and the cloth in a crock pot. This is slower, but produces a more steady heat.

Place folded cloth directly over painful area. Cover with a towel to keep it warm. You can also put a hot water bottle over the pack. Use the pack once a day for 30 to 60 minutes. Rinse off the oil after each use.

Colon Hydrotherapy

The fastest way to cleanse the bowel is with an enema or colonic. Clearing the colon in this manner can be helpful in a wide range of conditions. The procedures are simple, safe, and effective.

You can use just plain water as an enema solution; however, I recommend that you use purified water, not tap water. An enema is more effective, though, when you use an herbal solution. What you use in the enema will depend on what you're trying to achieve. Here are some options:

Garlic (for infections, fever, parasites)

Catnip, chamomile, peppermint (for colds, fevers)

Lobelia or blue vervain (for spasms, tension)

Oregon grape (for infection)

Herbal Composition Formula (for fevers, acute illness)

Herbal Crisis Formula (colds, flu, fevers)

Probiotics (to improve intestinal microbiome)

Coffee (traditionally used for liver detoxification and cancer therapy)

These are not the only things you can use, just some basic examples.

Always test the enema solution to make sure it is warm, not hot or cold. If you place a couple of drops on your wrist, it should feel neutral in temperature (like testing a baby bottle).

Directions for Adults

Fill the enema bag with lukewarm purified water or an enema solution. Lie on your left side. Lubricate the end of the enema tip and the rectal area and gently insert the tip into the rectum. Allow the solution to flow into the colon. If there is any sense of pressure or pain, stop the flow immediately and gently massage the area where you feel the discomfort. If it does not go away after a minute or two, get up and expel. If it does go away, release a little more fluid into the colon.

Once the fluid flows freely into the colon while you're lying on your side, you can move to your back and continue the procedure. Finish the procedure by lying on your right side. Remember, any-time you feel pain or discomfort, massage that area and then expel the liquid and start again. You may need to fill the bag and repeat the process three or four times before you will really begin to get the colon clean. In fact, the first few times you try this, you may not be able to cleanse the entire colon. You may encounter spasms or other obstructions that won't want to move. Don't be discouraged; it took me several months of doing an enema once per week before I was able to get fluid past the halfway point in my colon due to a muscle spasm in my transverse colon. I finally learned to use lobelia or lavender oil to relax that spasm and clean out the entire length of the colon.

An even more effective method of cleansing the colon is to get a colonic from a colon therapist. A colonic is much more effective than an enema for cleansing the colon. You can also obtain a colonic board that you can use in your own home.

Directions for Children

To give an enema to a baby or a young child you will need a bulb syringe, some petroleum jelly or similar lubricant, and an enema solution. For children, a weaker solution of garlic or herbs like catnip, fennel, chamomile, and blue vervain work well.

For an older child you can use an enema bag in place of the bulb syringe. Before giving any child an enema, however, I urge you to try the procedure on yourself.

Place a towel on the floor and lay the child on his or her back or left side on the towel. When doing this with a baby, place a diaper on top of the towel. Explain to the child that this procedure will be uncomfortable, but it will help him or her feel better. Be gentle, but firm. If you were taking the child to the doctor, the child might have to get a shot or have blood drawn which would hurt far more, but you'd probably make them hold still for that anyway. An enema is nowhere near as uncomfortable as a shot, and I've often told children that. I have always talked to my children in a loving but firm manner when doing this procedure.

Lubricate the anal opening and the tip of the syringe. Fill the syringe with the enema solution by squeezing the syringe and then sucking up the solution. Turn the syringe upright and squeeze any remaining air out of it. Refill the rest of the way so that the syringe is completely full. Gently insert the tip of the syringe into the anus. Then give a gentle squeeze. If you encounter strong resistance or the child seems to be in pain stop squeezing and withdraw the syringe. Make sure you don't "suck" with the syringe as you withdraw.

If nothing comes out, repeat the process again. It may take several tries before anything passes, but don't be concerned, just patient. Putting in a small amount of fluid every five minutes will not hurt the bowel. In fact, small children often get dehydrated when they are feverish from not drinking enough fluids, so the body could be absorbing all the liquid that you have put into the bowel.

With an older child, tell them they can go "potty" if they feel that they need to. If they don't, then repeat the process. Then wait a minute or two and put a little more fluid in.

With a baby, on the other hand, put a diaper on the baby's bottom after putting one syringeful into the rectum and then wrap the diaper in a towel. (Enemas can make the stool "runny," and you don't want it to leak onto you.) Then cuddle and hold the baby for a few minutes. Again, if nothing comes out after about ten to twenty minutes, repeat the procedure.

The stool should be soft. If only a small amount of hard stool is passed, you may still need to repeat the process again, until a soft stool passes. The trick is to get the bowel to move freely.

Compress or Fomentation

A compress is simply a cotton ball or gauze pad soaked in a tea or decoction and applied to an area of the body. You can also use liquid herbal extracts, diluted with water. A fomentation is like a compress, but covers a larger area of the body. Here one soaks a piece of cloth (like a clean washcloth or towel) in a tea, decoction, or water with an added tincture or extract.

Compresses and fomentations can be applied either warm or cold, depending on the need. Cold is better for soothing heat and inflammation, warm for easing pain and reducing swelling. They can used to accelerate healing of wounds or muscle injuries. They can be applied over itchy skin or dermatitis. A cold compress is sometimes used for headaches. To make a compress:

1. submerge cloth or cotton in the herbal liquid, or apply a tincture directly to a cotton ball or gauze pad,

2. squeeze out the excess liquid, if any,

3. hold the cotton ball, gauze pad, or cloth against the affected area,

4. when it cools or dries, repeat the process using a fresh mixture.

The following are examples of herbs that can be used in compresses and fomentations:

Calendula: astringent, stops bleeding, dries tissue

Chamomile: soothing, relaxing, anti-inflammatory

Comfrey: speeds tissue healing, reduces swelling

Elderflower: cooling and anti-inflammatory

Plantain: draws poisons, speeds healing, helpful for bites and stings

Yarrow: anti-inflammatory, shrinks swelling, stops bleeding

White Oak: astringent, reduces swelling, dries tissue

Counseling or Therapy

Mental and emotional problems are real, but they are not necessary biochemical in nature. Unresolved trauma and life events that haven't been processed can leave a person stuck in negative ways of thinking and feeling.

One of the oldest and most helpful ways to overcome mental and emotional problems is through counseling or some type of therapy. While a professional counselor will be necessary for many situations, there are other options as well. A trusted friend who is willing to listen without passing judgment or giving too much advice can work wonders. A person can also talk to a religious leader, pastor, or minister who can listen and offer comfort and support.

The point is that the person who has been abused or suffered serious trauma needs to process what has happened to them and make sense of it. This is why people often talk spontaneously about their problems and suffering as soon as they have a sympathetic, listening ear.

It's important to find someone who will gently guide the person's thought processes without labeling the suffering person, which unfortunately, is often done in modern psychology. Labeling mental and emotional problems isn't really helpful for fixing them. In fact, they often perpetuate the problem rather than help solve it by stigmatizing it, that is making the person feel like the problem is part of who they are.

For example, if a child is rebellious, they may be labeled with "oppositional defiant disorder." Once they have been labeled this way, rebellious behaviors may come to be expected, and normalized. Other stigmatizing labels include ADD/ADHD, social anxiety disorder, depression, bipolar disorder, and mental illness.

So in seeking someone to work with, find someone whose approach is based on empathy, love and gentle guidance to help the person work through their problems, rather than a "diagnose and fix" model. The following are some resources you can look to for more information on this approach.

Doctor Peter R. Breggin has spoken out strongly against the use of drugs and biomedical therapies in favor of therapy based on empathy and love. I highly recommend his books *Toxic Psychiatry* and *The Heart of Being Helpful*. To learn more, visit his website breggin.com.

Harvey Jackins teaches people how to help each other heal emotionally by using empathetic listening skills in a program called re-evaluation counseling. His book The Human Side of Human Beings helps you understand the problems created by trauma and what needs to happen for healing. His website is rc.org.

Peter A. Levine has written a series of books on the effects of trauma and trauma recovery. A good book to start

with is In *An Unspoken Voice: How the Body Releases Trauma and Restores Goodness*. His website is somatic-experiencing.com.

I've also developed my own approach to counseling people. It's discussed under the *Emotional Healing Work* strategy.

Deep Breathing

Oxygen is the most important "nutrient" the body needs for healing, and yet we seldom think about oxygen when we think about health. However, chronically ill people are almost always shallow breathers.

Healthy cells require a highly oxygenated environment. A low-oxygen environment in the body favors infections and can ultimately lead to the development of cancer. Oxygen helps the body stay more alkaline and makes metabolism more efficient so we get more energy out of the food we eat. Deep breathing also pumps the lymphatic system which removes waste material from around the cells.

Ideally, a person should be able to take a deep breath from their diaphragm, which means their stomach will rise up as they breathe in and fall as they breathe out.

To practice deep breathing, start by lying on your back on the floor. Inhale slowly and deeply for the count of four. If you are breathing correctly, your belly should rise as you inhale. Hold your breath for the count of four and then exhale for the count of four. Your belly should fall as you exhale. Then pause for a count of four before taking another breath.

If your belly does not rise as you inhale and fall as you exhale and you have to move your chest to breathe deeply you probably have a hiatal hernia. Do the exercises for correcting this so you can open up your diaphragm and breathe more freely.

After practicing inhaling and exhaling for the count of four, see if you can gradually increase the count on your inhalation and exhalation. You do not need to hold for longer than the count of four after the inhalation and exhalation. A trick to strengthening your diaphragm and deepening your capacity to breathe is to force as much air out of your lungs as possible when you exhale. This allows you to take an even deeper breath on the next inhalation.

If you practice deep breathing at least once per day for fifteen to twenty minutes you will find that your breathing naturally becomes slower and deeper. You will feel emotionally calmer and more centered, too. You may also notice an increase in mental clarity and energy.

Detoxification

Although medical science tends to discredit the idea of detoxification (also referred to as cleansing or colon cleansing), natural healers have long stressed the importance of maintaining good elimination for better health. After all, every day our body manufactures waste in the process of metabolism, which has to be eliminated. If you think about it, just about any system or machine needs some kind of regular cleaning to run properly.

For example, plumbers know that pipes can get clogged and drains need to be cleaned. Auto mechanics realize that oil and other fluids need to be regularly changed. Even electronic equipment needs to be cleaned periodically to keep dust from damaging circuits. It makes sense that this is also true for our bodies.

Most of us strive to keep the outside of the body clean, but few pay much attention to keeping clean on the inside. Most people who have done some internal cleansing, however, have noted numerous improvements in their general health.

Detoxification is about two things. One is minimizing your exposure to toxins in the first place, and the other is using herbs, supplements, hydrotherapy, fasting, or other natural means to improve the function of eliminative organs.

Since, detoxification is the process of getting rid of what is either harmful or no longer useful, doing a cleanse simply involves supporting the body's natural detoxification systems to eliminate metabolic waste and environmental toxins more efficiently. Generally, this means using herbs that have been found to improve liver and kidney function, bind toxins, increase lymphatic flow, open the sweat glands, and encourage elimination from the bowels. It may also involve destroying harmful organisms (yeast, bacteria, or parasites).

Here are the basic elements of a good detoxification program.

Water

The most important tool for cleansing is water, because all eliminative processes require water. Most people do not drink enough water. Experts suggest we should have about half an ounce of water per pound of body weight each day. On a cleanse, one might need a little more. Since the quality of water is also important, drink the purest water you can find. See the *Hydration* strategy for more information on the importance of water.

Fiber

The second most important tool for cleansing is fiber. Dietary fiber binds toxins in the intestinal tract and bulks the stool to promote normal and healthy elimination. Most Americans do not get enough fiber in their diet, so a good *Fiber Blend Formula* should be part of any good cleanse. See the *Increase Dietary Fiber* strategy for additional information on the importance of fiber.

Detoxifying Herbs

The third tool needed for a good cleanse is a blend of herbs that support the liver, kidneys, colon, and lymphatics. The liver utilizes enzyme systems that neutralize toxins and prepare them to be flushed through the kidneys or colon (via the gallbladder). Water and fiber then carry these toxins away. See the *Liver Detoxification* strategy for more information on how the liver aids detoxification.

Many good herbal formulas for supporting this process are available. These formulas are listed in the book as *Detoxifying Formulas* and *Blood Purifier Formulas*.

For people with extremely sluggish elimination, a *Stimulant Laxative Formula* may also be helpful. However, herbal laxatives should not be used long-term because people tend to become dependent on them. For long-term problems with sluggish elimination, consider using a *Gentle Laxative Formula*, which will help to tone and rebuild the intestinal system. Magnesium and vitamin C are also helpful for restoring normal bowel tone and function.

Diet

Traditionally, a detoxification program or cleanse has involved fasting or at least partial fasting. In fact, fasting for twenty-four hours, consuming only water, one day per month is a good detoxification practice for general health. A modified form of fasting is called the juice fast. You can read more about fasting and juice fasting under the *Fasting* strategy.

Since most detoxification programs last two weeks or more, it is better to adopt a semi fasting state during the cleanse. Simply avoid all refined and processed foods during the cleanse and eat lots of fresh fruits and vegetables. This aids the cleansing process by not burdening the body with more cooked, processed foods, and chemical additives.

The nice thing about making this a time to clean up your diet is that cleaning out the body tends to reduce your craving for junk food, anyway. So by the time you have finished the cleansing program, it will be easier to maintain a healthy eating program. It can also help you identify foods that cause allergic reactions.

Other Suggestions

Cleansing can also be aided by various forms of hydrotherapy. For instance, enemas and colonics can be helpful as long as they aren't overdone (see the *Colon Hydrotherapy* strategy). Generally speaking, enemas and colonics shouldn't be done more than once or twice per week and never for a period longer than a few months without taking a break.

Sweat baths, steam baths, or saunas are also useful as they encourage detoxification through the skin. These may be done more frequently. See the *Sweat Bath* strategy.

Foot soaks or foot spa baths are also helpful in the detoxification process. Again, once or twice a week for a limited period is more than enough.

Remember that cleansing takes the good out with the bad, so you should alternate cleansing with a program of rebuilding and good nutrition. When it comes to cleansing, more is not better.

Sample Cleansing Programs

There are prepackaged detoxification programs you can use. My favorites are *Ivy Bridge's Cleansing Program* and the *Chinese Balanced Cleansing Program*. It's also fairly easy to put together your own. Here are two basic cleansing programs to choose from:

Basic Cleanse

Here's a great basic two to four week cleansing program. For two weeks take the following.

Two capsules of a *Detoxifying Formula* two or three times daily.

One or two capsules of a *Plant Enzyme Formula* or a *Digestive Support Formula* with each meal

Once per day about thirty minutes before breakfast, take a *Fiber Blend Formula* in a large glass of water or juice. Start with half a teaspoon and gradually increase to the one to two heaping teaspoons to help the body get used to taking the fiber.

Drink half an ounce of purified water per pound of body weight each day. If you do not drink enough water, the fiber will actually constipate you.

The above supplies the three main items needed in a cleanse. Optionally, you can add the following:

If the bowels move less than twice daily add two to four capsules of a *Gentle Laxative Formula* or one or two capsules of a *Stimulant Laxative Formula* before bedtime

You can also take 500 to 1,000 mg of magnesium and 1,000 to 5,000 mg of vitamin C to encourage bowel movements

These are only basic suggestions; both the amounts and the products may be varied to account for individual circumstances.

This cleanse should be done for a maximum of two to four weeks. It is rarely necessary or wise to continue a cleanse longer than this. Over cleansing can be a problem as cleansing depletes the body of nutrients as well as eliminating toxins.

Daily Internal Housekeeping

Doing a complete cleansing program is like doing a major cleanup job in your home, washing walls and carpets while throwing away things you no longer need. However, we also do little housekeeping chores every day to keep our homes clean, such as washing dishes, vacuuming. or putting away clothes.

Our body also needs to do its daily cleaning for us to stay in good health. We can help our body do its "housekeeping" by taking some supplements that keep the colon and eliminative organs working properly. This prevents the buildup of toxins in the first place. Drinking plenty of water and making sure we get enough fiber are the most important aspects of daily cleansing.

Ivy Bridge, an herbalist in Tustin, California has long recommended a once-a-day cleansing program called Ivy's Recipe, which is also the basis for the prepackaged *Ivy Bridge's Cleansing Program*. Her basic program is thus:

2 tbsp. aloe vera juice

2 tbsp. liquid chlorophyll

1 heaping tsp. *Fiber Blend Formula*.

These ingredients are blended in a glass of apple juice and taken first thing in the morning. Ivy also recommended taking two capsules of cascara sagrada, but using stimulant laxatives daily isn't a wise idea. If you are having problems with constipation try a *Gentle Laxative Formula* with the cleanse.

Other prepackaged detoxification programs you can find in this book include the *Parasite Cleansing Program*, the *Weight Loss Cleansing Program* and the *Yeast Cleansing Program*. There are also find suggestions for detoxification under the *Heavy Metal Cleanse* and *Liver Detoxification* strategies.

Douche

Douching is the practice of flushing the vagina with water or other fluids in a similar manner to the use of an enema for the colon. There are prepackaged douches one can buy at the local pharmacy, or one can make one's own. Modern medicine generally discourages the process of douching, and it is definitely not something that should be done regularly. However, many women have found that an herbal douche can be used to help fight a vaginal infection and rebalance the friendly flora of the vaginal area.

It is important to properly clean the douche bag or syringe you are using so as not to introduce bacteria into the vaginal area. After cleaning it with warm soapy water and rinsing thoroughly with hot water, fill the douche bag or syringe with the liquid you are using. Then insert the end into the vagina.

Squeeze to release the fluid up your vagina until all the douche mixture has been used. Then take a shower, remembering to wash the outside of the vagina with mild soap.

Several possible remedies for douching include:

Pau d'arco tea for vaginal yeast infections.

Chamomile tea for vaginal irritation.

Water with colloidal silver for bacterial or yeast infections.

Two teaspoons of apple cider vinegar in two cups of lukewarm water for vaginal odor and vaginal infections.

Probiotics mixed in water to repopulate the friendly flora of the vaginal walls.

Don't douche when pregnant. Also, don't douche regularly as it upsets the balance of friendly flora in the vaginal tract.

A safer way to help clear up infections, odor or irritation in the vaginal area is to take a sitz bath.

Drawing Bath

A drawing bath is used to draw or pull toxins from the body, primarily through the oil glands on the skin. Sweat baths help eliminate water-soluble toxins, while drawing baths help eliminate fat-soluble toxins. Drawing baths are useful for skin eruptive diseases and heavy metal detoxification.

There are a couple of ways to make a drawing bath. For instance, decoctions of blood-purifying herbs can be used in baths. Simmer a handful of the herb or herbs you want to use in a large pot with a couple of gallons of water in it for about twenty to thirty minutes. Strain and add to the bath.

You can also use commercially prepared liquid herbal extracts in a bath. You need a full two-ounce bottle in a bath, however, so while convenient, it can be rather expensive. Both blood-purifying herbs and some mucilaginous herbs can be used. Oatmeal also makes a good drawing bath but needs to be kept in a cheesecloth bag to prevent clogging your drain.

The best agent for a drawing bath, however, especially when detoxifying heavy metals, is clay. A fine clay like Redmond clay can be added to the bathwater. Use about one cup for a standard bath. Soak for twenty to thirty minutes and then rinse off. The clay is fine enough that it won't clog drains if you flush a lot of water down the drain after the bath. Hydrated bentonite can also be used in drawing baths.

Eat Enzyme-Rich Foods

Enzymes regulate numerous body functions and minerals act as catalysts for enzymes, so the two work hand in hand to promote health. Enzymes are natural components of living things, so they are found in raw foods. However, heat deactivates or destroys enzymes.

Cultured foods like live-culture yogurt and sauerkraut are also rich in enzymes. These foods are regularly consumed in many cultures and appear to contribute greatly to gastrointestinal health, but few Americans consume them regularly. And if these foods have been heated past 120 degrees, the enzymes are deactivated. To compound the problem, most processed foods contain enzyme inhibitors, which are added to processed foods to prevent spoilage and increase shelf life.

Ideally, a large percentage of a person's food should be raw, but few people are able to do this in modern society. This fact, compounded with the other problems I've discussed, means many people need to take an enzyme supplement to make up for the enzymes they don't get in their diets. A *Plant Enzyme Formula* is a good way to do this.

It is also possible to stimulate the body's own digestive secretions. Generally speaking, bitter-tasting herbs and pungent or aromatic herbs will stimulate digestive secretions. This includes bitter greens eaten raw in a salad, as long as they are not coated with sweet or creamy salad dressings, just an oil and vinegar dressing. *Digestive Bitter Tonics* can be helpful in stimulating enzyme production too.

Eat Healthy

Eating healthy is about choosing to eat foods that will improve your health and avoiding ones that will harm it. Dietary needs differ with your genetics (constitution), where you live, the stresses you're exposed to, and the health problems you have. So there isn't one diet that is perfect for everybody, but there are fundamentals that you can follow to improve your basic nutrition and in turn improve your health. The following are some basic principles to help you:

Focus on eating fresh whole, unprocessed foods.

Avoid added sugars and refined/simple starches.

Read labels so you know what is in the food you eat.

Pay attention to what your tasting and how you feel after you eat.

Your body cannot function properly or heal itself without adequate amounts of amino acids from proteins, fatty acids from fats, vitamins, minerals, and other phytochemicals found in whole natural foods.

Many modern diseases stem from a lack of good nutrition. This was demonstrated back in the 1930s by the work of Dr. Weston Price. Dr. Price spent ten years traveling around the world, studying the dental and general health of many groups of indigenous people and people living in modern society and published the results of his life's work in a book called *Nutrition and Physical Degeneration*.

Dr. Price discovered that everywhere he went, indigenous peoples were healthy and robust when they ate the natural foods found in their environment. On the other hand, when these people were introduced to white flour, refined sugar, processed oils and modern commercial foods, they began to experience the health problems common to Western man. Here we focus on the fundamentals of a healthy diet based on what Dr. Price learned.

Fuel Your Body with Nutritionally Dense Food

Glucose, the sugar found in blood, is one of the primary fuel sources for muscle and brain activity. When your blood sugar level gets low, you can feel tired, nervous, irritable, or stressed. You may also have a hard time concentrating or thinking straight. However, if blood sugar levels get too high, you can feel restless and agitated, gain weight, and experience increased inflammation throughout the body. Keeping blood sugar balanced is important for both physical and emotional health.

The complex carbohydrates found in fruits and vegetables provide sugars that are released gradually into the blood stream, helping to maintain stable blood sugar levels. Fruits and vegetables contain sugars, but they are always accompanied by the vitamins and minerals (such as B complex, chromium, zinc, and magnesium) that are necessary to process these carbohydrates into energy.

In contrast, simple carbohydrates like white flour, refined sugar, and high-fructose corn syrup have been stripped of these nutrients. This means that the sugars in these foods cannot be processed into energy without robbing the body's nutritional reserves. This is why simple carbohydrates are also called empty-calorie foods, while fresh vegetables and fruits are considered nutritionally dense foods.

The ratio of caloric value (potential fuel) to the content of noncaloric essential nutrients like vitamins and minerals determines the nutritional density. Nutritionally dense foods have a high ratio of nutrients to calories. Empty-calorie foods supply low amounts of nutrients and high amounts of calories.

Consuming these empty-calorie foods has been linked with heart disease, cancer, chronic intestinal dysbiosis (imbalances in yeast and bacteria in the gut), obesity, inflammatory diseases of all kinds, and even mood disorders, like hyperactivity, anxiety, and depression.

In contrast, nearly all experts in nutrition now acknowledge that a diet that contains five to nine servings of vegetables and fruits have a positive impact on health. Eating a nutrient-dense diet reduces the risk of heart disease, cancer, and other chronic and degenerative diseases by reducing inflammation and oxidative damage in the body.

Many people do not like fresh vegetables or fruits because their taste buds have been jaded by junk food. While changing your diet, focus on the positive rather than the negative. Focus on eating the healthy food first, rather than focusing on having to avoid the junk food. When you eat your fruits and vegetables first, you'll feel more nutritionally satisfied and have less room for high-glycemic, simple carbohydrates. In fact, over time, you may find yourself naturally craving vegetables instead of pastries and a piece of organic fruit instead of a candy bar, because your body will start to prefer the nutrient-dense food.

Avoid Junk Foods

The growing sales of processed foods that are devoid of minerals, vitamins, and other vital nutrition has correlated with the dramatic increase in obesity, diabetes, digestive disorders, and inflammatory diseases, along with the continuing high rates of heart disease and cancer.

It is important to understand that there is no shame in whatever you're eating in your current diet. There are many reasons you currently eat the way you do and understanding this can help you make informed choices in the future to improve your health.

Our brains are hardwired to value calorie-dense foods, because for much of human history starvation was a real possibility. Junk foods satisfy a place deep inside of us, a remnant of survival programming that food manufacturers take advantage of. However, with practice we can learn to acknowledge the desire to consume junk food and minimize or eliminate junk foods.

Some of the biggest reasons are cost, convenience, and access. Because of their popularity and various political factors, like farm subsidies, processed foods tend to be cheap and available everywhere. High-quality, nutritionally dense foods tend to be more expensive and, in some places, just aren't available at all. These areas have been called food deserts. Many people have also grown up eating this way for their whole lives; if you were raised eating certain foods it can be challenging to change. But you can change if you want; you may need to spend a bit more, plan ahead, or go out of your way, but you can change the way you eat.

Fatigue, anxiety, depression, and addiction are all reasons people eat junk foods. They can give you a burst of energy by spiking your blood sugar, which spikes a neurotransmitter called dopamine in the brain. Dopamine is associated with addiction, and refined sugar and carbohydrates are very addictive. Also, when you're tired, junk foods offer a temporary boost of energy. They don't provide sustained energy, however. The energy boost is usually followed by an energy letdown an hour or two later.

When people are unhappy in their lives, they tend to self-medicate by eating junk food. This can help mask feelings of anxiety and depression by boosting dopamine, endorphins, and serotonin. This is also part of our survival programing, which is designed to make us feel emotionally good when consuming calorie-dense foods.

All of this leads to addiction, a.k.a. ritualistic compulsive self comforting. Once someone is used to energizing and self-medicating with junk food, it can be hard to change, especially when other forms of comfort and connection are lacking. It may be important to focus on improving other areas and finding connection and support to help with this.

No matter what reasons a person may have for eating junk food, there is one big reason to change—their health. Getting junk food out of one's life will help a person lose weight, feel happier emotionally, increase their energy, and improve their mental clarity, and start the healing process from whatever diseases are afflicting them.

Balance Protein, Fats, and Carbohydrates

Everyone will need slightly different proportions of protein, fat, and carbohydrates. Most people will have a good diet if they imagine their plate is divided into three parts. One-third of your plate should be some high quality protein source, and the other two-thirds should be composed primarily of fruits and vegetables. There should also be some quality fat in the diet. Since fats are very high-calorie sources, we only need a small amount of fat (about one tablespoonful) to make up one-third of our caloric intake.

It's best to focus on low-glycemic carbohydrates, not high-glycemic carbohydrates. low-glycemic carbohydrates are foods which do not rapidly release sugar into the blood stream, which means they do not trigger the release of large amounts of insulin. This is particularly important if you are trying to lose weight.

low-glycemic foods to focus on include all non-starchy vegetables, including zucchini, green beans, lettuce, chard, beets, broccoli, cabbage, cauliflower, peas, celery, onions, bell peppers, and turnips. Some fruits are also low-glycemic, such as most berries (raspberries, strawberries, blackberries, etc.). Others, which are very sugary, such as dates and pineapple are high-glycemic.

Vegetables that are sources of complex carbohydrates, but are not low-glycemic include potatoes and grains, like wheat, corn and rice. Complex carbohydrates that are not low-glycemic are wholesome foods, but because they trigger more insulin production (and therefore more fat storage), they need to be consumed in smaller portions than low-glycemic carbohydrates. See the *low-glycemic Diet* strategy for more information.

In transitioning into this diet, you will tend to have cravings for higher carbohydrate foods while your body makes the adjustment. The next tip deals with this issue.

Focus on the Positive

When you try to make a positive change by denying yourself something, you'll find it very difficult to change. This is why dieting usually doesn't work. People restrict their caloric intake, deny themselves foods they love, and at some point their psyche rebels and they binge.

Don't think in terms of self-denial, but rather in terms of self-nurturing. Instead of focusing on trying to eliminate junk foods, simply start crowding them out of your diet by focusing on eating nutritionally dense natural foods. For instance, when you feel hungry, try eating an apple and some almonds or walnuts first. Then eat those chips. Have some baby carrots or celery sticks first, then eat the pastry.

When making this change, you won't crave the nutritious food at first, but as you learn to prepare whole, natural foods in place of refined and processed foods, you'll not only start feeling better and thinking more clearly but you might also realize that junk food doesn't taste as good. Soon you'll find them easy to avoid.

Healthy Substitutions

The most difficult addiction to overcome is the addiction to refined sugars. The best way to break this addiction is to start eating more protein and vegetables while treating yourself to more nutritionally-dense treats. Use raw honey, real maple syrup, freeze-dried sugar cane juice, coconut sugar, date sugar, or other natural sugars instead of refined sugar. These foods will give you vitamins and minerals with the sugar, which will satisfy your cravings with fewer calories.

If you have a serious sugar addiction, eat protein (eggs and meat) for breakfast with no carbohydrates (cereal, toast, juice, etc.). Do this until your metabolism starts to adapt to the lower carbohydrate intake. If you have problems digesting protein for breakfast, your liver is probably congested. Avoid eating late at night and take hydrochloric acid and/or enzyme supplements with breakfast.

You can also substitute whole grains for refined flours. Whole-grain products are more nourishing and filling than white bread and white rice, so you won't eat as much. You don't want to eat a lot of grain products because they are also high-glycemic carbohydrates. Also consider the fact that grains (particularly wheat and corn) are major food allergens for many people. So try some alternative grains, like millet, amaranth, quinoa, and buckwheat, as they tend not to trigger allergic reactions.

You can take a similar approach to fats. Don't think of fats as bad. Your body needs fats; it just needs the right kinds of fats. Start using real butter (preferably from grass-fed cows), ghee (clarified butter), and coconut oil in cooking. You can also use extra-virgin olive oil and flaxseed oil for salads. Also satisfy your cravings for fats by eating naturally fatty whole foods like eggs, whole-milk dairy products (as long as you're not allergic or sensitive to dairy or eggs), fatty fish like wild-caught salmon, fat from grass-fed meat, nuts and seeds (walnuts, pecans, flax, and chia seeds for example), and avocados.

It may also help to take fish-liver oil or an omega-3 fatty acid supplement. You may also benefit by taking some fat-soluble vitamins like A, D_3, and K_2. These will supply you with the fat-soluble vitamins your body is missing and craving.

Enjoy the Color, Taste and Smell of Food

Get reacquainted with the wonderful color, flavor, and aroma of natural foods, especially fruits and vegetables. Go to a local farmer's market to reacquaint your senses with the delight of natural foods. Get a few cookbooks that teach you how to cook with fresh vegetables and other natural foods, so you know how to prepare flavorful meals. As your taste buds learn to appreciate natural foods, the artificially sweetened, flavored, and preserved foods will lose their appeal.

Eliminate Allergy-Causing Foods

An underlying cause of many people's health problems is food allergies. Food allergies can cause migraine headaches, irritability, hyperactivity, inflammatory diseases of all kinds and can contribute to respiratory congestion.

The most common foods that cause allergic reactions are grains containing gluten (wheat, rye and barley) and dairy products. Corn, eggs, oranges and other citrus fruits, nuts, peanuts, sulfites, food additives, dyes, chocolate, strawberries, shellfish, and soy products are others. Interestingly, many of these foods have been highly "tampered with" through genetic modification, modern agricultural methods, and/or excessive processing.

If you suspect that some of your health problems may be related to food allergies, you can start by trying a simple experiment. Stop eating foods that you suspect allergies to and see if your symptoms subside. The foods listed above are a good place to start.

If symptoms improve, wait at least seven days, then reintroduce suspected foods one at a time to see if symptoms reappear. Wait twenty-four hours and watch for reactions. Look for these signs, as they indicate a probable reaction to a food: dark circles under the eyes; redness of the ears, face or eyes; a glassy look; an increased pulse rate; or mood changes. If no changes or symptoms occur, try introducing another suspect food.

You can also fast for a few days, consuming only water or juice. If symptoms improve, then food allergies may be involved. Again, reintroduce the suspect foods one at a time and watch for reactions.

Still another method for isolating suspected food allergies is muscle-response testing. Simply name each of the suspected allergy-causing foods and muscle-test for it. A weak response indicates the body is not handling that food very well. In one case, muscle testing revealed that a person with a wheat allergy wasn't allergic to wheat at all; he was allergic to the pesticide residues on the grain. By switching to organically grown wheat, the problem disappeared.

If you don't know how to muscle-test, another method is to take the pulse, eat a small amount of a food, and test the pulse again. Any food that raises the pulse more than six beats per minute after ingestion is probably an allergen.

Another thing to watch for in identifying food allergens is by paying attention to food cravings. Food allergy is generally linked with food addiction. It is much like any other addiction, cigarettes, alcohol, or even refined sugar. Although the substance isn't good for the body, it adapts to its presence. When the substance is withdrawn and the body starts to "cleanse" itself of the irritant, the person feels "dis-ease."

Once you've identified allergy-causing foods you simply have to eliminate them from your diet. It is possible that after they have been eliminated for a sufficient period of time (often a year or more) that they can slowly be reintroduced into the diet. Homeopathic remedies are also available to help desensitize a person to an allergy-causing food.

Many nutritionists say that the best way to combat food allergies is to adopt a "rotation diet." This means that a person's diet should be increased to include a wide variety of nonallergenic fruits and vegetables, seeds and nuts, and grains such brown rice, millet, amaranth, and barley. Eat one food one day, then you should wait three or four days to eat that particular food again. Increasing the types of foods eaten, as well as rotating them through the diet, will help to greatly reduce food allergy responses.

Eliminate FODMAPs

If you have frequent acid indigestion, burping, belching, bloating, gas, or irritable bowel syndrome try eliminating foods containing FODMAPs (fermentable oligosaccharides, disaccharides, monosaccharide and polyols) for a period. Foods high in FODMAPs contribute to small intestinal bacterial overgrowth and leaky gut syndrome because they serve as food for intestinal bacteria. You can find a list of foods high in FODMAPs online (such as ibsdiets.org/fodmap-diet/fodmap-food-list/ or https://www.dietvsdisease.org/low-fod-maps-food-list/). High FODMAP foods are also marked on the food lists on our *Blood Type, pH, and Nutrition* charts.

Eliminate Salicylates

While salicylates (natural aspirin compounds) are common in many foods and herbs, modern diets are much higher in salicylates than traditional diets and when combined with modern food additives may contribute to irritability, restlessness, difficulty focusing, oppositional defiance and other behavioral problems, especially in children. People who suffer from migraines, rashes, irritable bowel, asthma, chronic sinus problems, tinnitus, arthritis and mood disorders like anxiety and depression, may also be sensitive to salicylates. Herbs that contain salicylates include willow bark, meadowsweat, black cohosh, and wintergreen. You can find a list of foods high in salicylates online (such as diet-vsdisease.org/salicylate-intolerance/ or https://www.drugs.com/article/low-salicylate-diet.html). High salycilate foods are also marked on the food lists on our *Blood Type, pH, and Nutrition* charts.

Emotional Healing Work

Research shows that positive thoughts and emotions enhance healing. The tools of affirmation and visualization are helpful for creating positive thoughts, but our emotional state is not based solely on our thoughts as many believe. While it is true that our thoughts influence our emotions, it is also true that our emotions influence our thoughts.

I call the process of helping people work through their negative emotions *emotional healing work*. Emotional healing work is *not* about making negative emotions go away, something many people try to do. This is because both our positive and our negative emotions play an important role in our lives. The goal is not to eliminate negative emotions but to turn them into positive opportunities for growth and healing.

Negative emotions are like pain. We may not like pain, but if we didn't feel pain, we wouldn't know what was harmful to the body. Without pain to warn us, we would injure ourselves and never know it. Without the discomfort associated with disease symptoms, we would not know that we were sick and would not be motivated to seek healing. So whether we like it or not, pain and discomfort are necessary aspects of life.

What pain does for the body, negative emotions do for the soul. Negative emotions tell us when something is wrong in our lives, which needs to be identified and healed. Feeling excessively afraid, angry, sad, or even depressed is a sign that a particular behavior or attitude is harmful to us. So just like pain can teach us to avoid injuring our body or cause us to seek help, negative emotions can teach us how to stop harming our soul and cause us to make positive changes in our lives.

Unfortunately, few people learn the lessons that pain and negative emotions are trying to teach. When it comes to pain, most people seek symptomatic treatment. Without identifying the cause of the pain and discomfort (disease symptoms), people typically take drugs that merely mask the symptoms. This provides temporary relief, but the real problems are never resolved and overall health deteriorates over time. This form of medicine is known as allopathy, which literally means "against the symptom."

As explained in the beginning of this book, one of the hardest tasks a natural healer faces is to help people under-stand that natural healing is not designed to provide symptomatic relief. Natural healing is about identifying the root causes of health problems and fixing them. The true natural healer doesn't treat diseases, per se, but rather looks at the habits and lifestyle of the person to determine what they are doing that is harming their body. The "cure" is to fix the cause, and in the case of emotions, the cause involves how we relate to other people and situations.

When the physical cause is addressed in disease, the physical effect (the disease symptoms) disappears. When the cause of a negative emotion is identified and the person takes steps to change their attitudes and behaviors (rather than seeking to change the attitudes and behaviors of others), emotional healing can take place.

Just as allopathic medicine is targeted at suppressing symptoms, our culture practices "emotional allopathy"—meaning people are taught to just try to make the negative feelings go away without understanding what is causing them. People do this in a variety of ways. For example, they may take drugs to suppress their depression or anxiety, but they may also seek to numb their emotional pain through alcohol, eating, sex, or other addictions.

There are also more subtle ways people practice emotional allopathy on themselves or others. For instance, most of us have been taught to suppress one or more emotional responses by denying what we are feeling. We may also learn to project the responsibility for what we feel outward through blame. That is, we seek to restore our sense of well-being through attacking others, playing the victim, or otherwise trying to make others responsible for our emotional well-being and happiness.

Our Hearts Hold the Key

All this is unfortunate, because the feelings we experience in our heart are the key to discovering our ultimate happiness. Just as pain can help us realize something is wrong and cause us to seek healing, our negative emotions can motivate us to make the changes in our life that will ultimately bring us joy, love, peace, and happiness. We just have to be willing to listen to our heart and understand what these feelings are trying to tell us.

Unfortunately, most of us have been told over and over that we can't trust our heart and our emotions. Instead of learning to listen to our negative feelings and understand them, we're encouraged to deny, ignore, or suppress them, in which case we often react to them unconsciously. Rarely are we helped to understand and use them in constructive ways.

Running away from our emotions is like running away from the monster in a childhood nightmare. As long as we deny, suppress, or otherwise try to "get rid of" a feeling, it will continue to chase us. As the title of a book by Carol Truman so eloquently states, *Feelings Buried Alive, Never Die*.

Denying one's feelings isn't the only way one may try to deal with them. One may also try to blame what they feel on others. Now, it is true that we can have a negative emotional reaction to the behavior of others. For instance, I'm sure that all of us would be scared if someone were pointing a gun to our head and threatening our life, but these reactions to the behavior of others are only temporary. Our overall mood and our typical emotional reactions (or personality) are based on what is inside of us, not what is happening in the world around us.

To demonstrate the truth of this idea, think about someone you dislike. It is quite likely that there are other people who love that person. It is also likely that others may dislike people you love. What is true for people is also true for life events. A situation that might evoke feelings of hurt or anger in you might not provoke the same reaction in someone else. You might be scared to death in a situation that another person might view as an interesting challenge.

As you contemplate this, you will see that your emotional reactions are not primarily caused by the world around you; they are primarily the result of what is inside of you. More specifically, your emotional reactions are caused by how you choose to respond to a given situation, which is often based on your beliefs and thought processes.

Emotional healing work involves learning to get in touch with our emotions and acknowledging rather than denying them. It involves learning to feel what our heart is telling us, rather than just blaming what we feel on everyone else and insisting that they change so we can feel good.

If you are lucky enough to find someone who can help you through the process of understanding your emotions, it is certainly worth seeking out their help. For example, you may wish to utilize a counselor or a minister to help you work through your unresolved emotional wounds (as suggested in the *Counseling or Therapy* strategy). If you do not have someone you can work with, here are some self-help techniques extracted from my book *The Heart's Key to Health, Happiness, and Success*.

Step 1: Practice making your mind shut up so you can listen to your heart.

If you already practice some form of meditation, this step won't be hard for you. If you've never tried meditating, it takes some practice to learn how to quiet the mind. Most of the time our minds are constantly "chattering with words." These words express our worries, cares, desires, plans, schemes, and an endless stream of social conditioning.

There are many techniques for reaching this meditative state of mind and you are free to use any technique that works for you. However, if you do not currently have a technique, here is a very simple one that I use.

First, find a quiet environment. Ideally, this is done in the wilds of nature, but most modern people don't have easy access to wilderness environments, so a private room or place of worship is fine.

Second, you need to get into a comfortable position and allow your body to relax. When first getting started, it can be helpful to lie down and allow every part of your body to sink deeply into the floor or the earth. However, it is also easy to fall asleep when doing this, so you may find that it is easier to quiet the mind and stay awake while sitting up. The way I do this is to sit or lie down and allow my body to sink into the earth. I imagine gravity as the arms of Mother Earth and relax into the embrace of it.

Third, you will need a focal point for your mind. Some people gaze at a candle or repeat a phrase, verse, scriptural passage, mantra, or prayer over and over, such as the Jesus prayer from orthodox Christianity, "Lord Jesus Christ, Son of God, have mercy on me a sinner." Dr. Herbert Bensen, M.D. and author of *The Relaxation Response*, suggested repeating the word *one* over and over in your mind.

I have found that breathing alone can be an effective focus point. Simply start by breathing slowly and deeply making the inhalation, exhalation and the pauses in between them equal. Directions for doing this can be found under the strategy for *Deep Breathing*. The breathing and counting become the point of focus for the mind that stills the monkey chatter in the brain.

Fourth, you will need to adopt a passive attitude. This means that whatever comes to your mind, you observe it passively without judging or analyzing it. You just notice it and then return to your single point of focus. It is especially important to not judge or analyze how well you're doing in the process. Just relax and "let go."

The goal is to reach the state where there are no words in your mind, where you are "thinking" without language. Yes, this is possible. This is the state of mind where you can observe your own thoughts, feelings, and actions as if you were an objective, outside party.

Step 2: Tune into your feelings and bodily sensations.

Once you learn to quiet your mind, this exercise is the next step. Even if you haven't been able to completely quiet your mental chatter, as long as you have reached a relaxed state of body, you can try this. In fact, tuning into your body and your feelings can be used as a point of focus to reach this quiet state of mind.

Simply ask yourself, "What am I feeling?" or "How do I feel?" while you continue to breathe deeply. Stay focused on your body. Your head will often want to provide an immediate answer in words, but this is not the real answer to the question you are asking. What you want are not words, but sensations in your body. You want to actually feel something in your body.

Don't be surprised if you have a hard time feeling your bodily sensations and answering the question, "How do I feel?" We are so used to the idea that their feelings don't matter (and that nobody cares how we feel) that it can be difficult for us to connect with our feelings. This shows how disconnected from our hearts we can be and is a sign of deeply buried emotions.

To help you tune into your feelings, it may help to get more specific. Think about a problem, worry or concern that you have and then ask, "How does this make me feel?" Breathe deeply, and again, notice any sensations that arise in your body.

When you actually do get in touch with a bodily sensation, feeling, or emotion, you should turn your attention to it. Allow yourself to just experience the sensation or emotion without trying to make it go away or change it.

It helps to breathe into the area of your body where you are feeling it. You do this by imagining your breath moving into that part of your body as you inhale. This works because it sends energy to that part of the body, enlivening it and intensifying the feeling. Your awareness will also follow your breath.

If the feeling is an actual emotion, then notice where you feel that emotion. Is it in your heart, your stomach, or your gut? What does the feeling feel like? All feelings are experienced through bodily sensations. Is the feeling warm or cool, tense or relaxed, pleasant or painful? Whatever it is, turn your attention on it and just experience it.

What you feel may not be an emotion. It may be a physical sensation such as pain or tension. If this is the case, treat it the same way you would an emotion. Don't resist it or fight it; just allow it to be. Breathe deeply into the area where you feel the tension or pain. Then, as you exhale, imagine that pain or tension flowing back out of your body with your breath.

You may even try asking the pain or tension, "What do you want?" or "What are you trying to tell me?" If your brain tries to answer, ignore it, keep breathing and keep asking the part of your body that's in discomfort the question. You may need to do this for several minutes, but don't be surprised when your body actually answers you. Oh, and you will know that it was your body (not your head) that answered the question, because often the pain and tension will dissipate once it has delivered its message.

Step 3: Use questions and question-affirmations to deepen your understanding of your emotions and find healing.

The most powerful tool for emotional healing is something I call the question-affirmation. To understand this tool,

you first have to know what an affirmation is. An *affirmation* is a present tense statement that affirms what one wants as if one actually has it. See the *Affirmation and Visualization* strategy for more information on how to create affirmations.

A question-affirmation is an affirmation that is used to explore your feelings about that affirmation. It turns the affirmation into a question by asking, "How would I feel if…?". This allows you to explore and uncover negative belief systems surrounding the affirmation.

Here's an example of how this technique works. The story is a composite of several real case histories.

A woman went to a nutritionist for help with a weight problem. She wanted to be attractive so she could get married. She was put on a weight loss program that worked beautifully for a few weeks. Then, suddenly, the weight came back on and she wound up even heavier than before. This had happened every time she tried to lose weight.

The nutritionist was also familiar with emotional healing techniques. He did some investigation and probed into the woman's past to see when she had first started to gain weight. It was discovered that when she was five, an uncle had attempted to sexually molest her. Fortunately, he had been caught before he could actually perpetrate the deed.

However, it was a very emotionally upsetting time. In the midst of this pain and trauma, her mother had blurted out, "It's a shame she's not fat! Fat girls never get molested." Within the year, the girl had started to gain weight.

Since our subconscious mind is wired to avoid pain and suffering, the girl's mind laid hold on the mother's words. To protect her from being molested in the future, it caused her to gain weight. She couldn't lose weight because her subconscious mind was programmed with a belief that the weight was necessary to protect her from pain and suffering. Of course, it didn't protect her from pain and suffering, so the belief was an illusion or a lie.

The problem with regular affirmations is that in situations like these, they will actually backfire. If the woman starts to affirm, "I am thin and beautiful," the subconscious fear that says, "Being thin and beautiful means you will get sexually molested," kicks in gear, which can sabotage her efforts to lose weight.

The question-affirmation would allow her to uncover the buried feelings surrounding the weight issue by asking, "What would it feel like if I were thin and beautiful?" By examining this question, the feelings of fear and pain will surface and the illusions, which underlie these buried emotions, are forced to reveal themselves. By bringing them to the light of awareness, they can be changed and healed.

When the subconscious mind sees that a particular belief is a lie, it instantly reprograms itself, because we are hardwired to want happiness. As soon as we perceive that a changed course of action will result in positive emotions, the desire for these positive emotions kicks in gear and behavior patterns start to change naturally.

Examples of question-affirmations would include thus:

> What would it feel like if it was all right for me to cry?
>
> What would it feel like if it was okay for me to feel my fears?
>
> What would it feel like if I was free to laugh?

The possible uses of this tool are endless, so be creative with it and remember that whatever comes up, just try to feel it and accept it. Don't try to make it go away.

Questions in general are useful for healing, even when they aren't linked to a positive affirmation. For example, one time I had an earache that lasted for over a month. Nothing I tried seemed to help, including going to a medical doctor. So I went into a quiet, meditative state and asked myself the question, "What would I hear if I could hear clearly?" I only had to ask myself this question twice when I suddenly knew why y emotions were shutting down my hearing. As soon as he resolved to do something to change the situation, my ears started to heal.

For help in identifying emotional issues that may be linked with your health problems, consider getting the book, *You Can Heal Your Life* by Louise L. Hay. There is an entire free training program on how I do my emotional healing work on my YouTube channel. You can access all the recordings and handouts at stevenhorne.com/program/Free-Emotional-Healing-Training-Program. There is also a set of *Emotional Healing Charts* we created to assist people in doing emotional healing work using flower essences and aromatherapy.

Enhance Nitric Oxide

Nitric oxide (NO) is a simple molecule composed of one atom of nitrogen and one atom of oxygen. It is highly reactive and only lasts a few seconds in the body after it is created, but it plays a critical role in overall health because of its ability to enhance blood flow.

In 1998, the Nobel Peace Prize for Physiology or Medicine was awarded to three researchers for their discoveries concerning nitric oxide as a signaling molecule in the cardiovascular system. These researchers found that the lining of the blood vessels produce NO in order to relax the muscles in the blood vessels, thereby reducing blood pressure and allowing greater blood flow.

The research into NO explains why nitroglycerine works as a treatment for angina (chest pain from narrowed arteries). Nitroglycerine is transformed into nitrite, which is then converted to NO, causing an immediate relaxing of blood vessels.

Since that time, researchers have found numerous health benefits from enhancing NO production in the body, starting with its ability to greatly enhance cardiovascular health. In fact, NO may be a critical factor in helping to reduce cardiovascular disease in general.

Nitric Oxide and Cardiovascular Health

To start, declining levels of NO may be the cause of essential hypertension (high blood pressure from unknown causes), something that plagues millions of people. High blood pressure is a major risk factor for strokes and heart attacks. It also causes kidney damage and increasing NO levels appears to be a major way of getting blood pressure back into normal ranges.

The research suggests that increasing NO levels can help prevent, slow or even reverse arterial plaque, thereby helping to keep arteries healthy and flexible. It can also help prevent thrombosis, the formation of blood clots in the circulatory system that cause heart attacks, strokes, and other problems.

Reduced blood flow from a lack of NO is also one of the causes of erectile dysfunction (ED) in men. In fact, many drugs for ED work by increasing NO levels.

Another benefit of NO is that increased levels can improve athletic performance by helping more blood (and oxygen) get to the muscles. Adequate levels of NO will help reduce muscle soreness after exercise.

The Many Health Benefits of Nitric Oxide

The benefits of NO don't stop with aiding circulation. Increased NO levels have also been shown to increase cellular sensitivity to insulin, making it helpful for people with diabetes. It also reduces diabetic complications, such as blindness, foot and leg ulcers, and kidney disease.

There is also a link between NO and chronic inflammation. While the mechanisms involved in this link are still being explored, it appears that chronic inflammation reduces NO production, whereas enhancing NO production is linked with reduced inflammation. What the research shows is that enhancing NO production may help relieve the chronic inflammation involved in asthma and arthritis.

Finally, it appears that NO plays a critical role in the brain. Low levels are associated with memory loss and depression. There is also evidence that higher levels of NO can improve bone density and aid the immune system in fighting infections.

All this may be linked to the simple fact that nothing in the body can be healthy or heal without an adequate supply of blood. Anything that interferes with how well the blood can supply oxygen and nutrients to the tissues is ultimately going to lead to health problems.

Endothelial Dysfunction and Low NO

The endothelium or endothelial lining is a layer of cells, just one cell thick, lining the arteries. Because these cells produce nitric oxide to signal the artery muscles to relax and increase blood flow, they play a vital role in managing oxygen and nutrient distribution to every other cell of the body.

Endothelial dysfunction occurs when the endothelial lining is damaged. This means that less nitric oxide will be released, resulting in less blood flow to the tissues. This is an underlying factor in chronic and degenerative disease because tissue health cannot be maintained without adequate blood flow.

Chronic inflammation, one of the major underlying factors in chronic and degenerative disease, contributes to low levels of NO and endothelial dysfunction. The more inflammation that is present in the body, the lower the levels of NO produced by the endothelium. Thus, all the factors that contribute to chronic inflammation are also involved.

Another major factor is mitochondrial dysfunction. Mitochondria are tiny cellular structures involved in energy production and many other body processes. They produce electrical energy or heat depending on the needs of the body. They also produce heme to produce hemoglobin and nitric oxide, both of which help deliver oxygen to the tissues. Mitochondria can also produce free radicals, which can be involved in tissue damage and chronic inflammation. See the condition *Mitochondrial Dysfunction* for additional information.

Understanding all the different ways NO production is linked with inflammation, energy production, and overall health is still being explored by researchers. However, we do know a lot about how you can improve your NO production and overall health. What follows are a few simple ways to do so.

Exercise and NO

Exercising is one of the best ways to enhance NO production. Thirty to sixty minutes a day of walking, swimming, riding a bike, lifting some weights, or engaging in any other form of moderate exercise greatly increases NO levels, which helps reverse endothelial dysfunction and improve blood flow throughout the body.

Exercise helps prevent cardiovascular disease, reduces your risk of stroke, helps lower blood pressure, balances blood fats and triglycerides, reduces inflammation, eases leg pain, and helps you lose weight. It doesn't matter how old you are, as soon as you start a program of regular physical activity you start to see the benefits within a few weeks (see *Exercise* strategy).

If you struggle to exercise, you're in luck. The relationship between exercise and NO levels is reciprocal. That is to say, not only does exercise enhance NO, NO also enhances the ability to exercise. Several studies have shown that increasing blood levels of nitrates, a precursor to NO production, results in greater efficiency in energy production and oxygen utilization in the muscles during exercise. The research was done using beet juice to supply the nitrates.

This means that enhancing NO can help you exercise longer and with less fatigue and get even more dramatic results than those seen with exercise alone. This is particularly important to know if you are overweight, asthmatic, diabetic, already have heart disease, or any other condition that makes exercise difficult. By enhancing NO, you can jump start your exercise program.

NO Production with Nutrition

While exercising is critical to healthy NO production, supplementation can spark the energy to get started while both enhancing the production of NO and the health of the endothelial lining. We'll start by looking at the two pathways in the body for creating NO and the nutrients that support them.

L-Arginine

The first NO pathway involves nitric oxide synthase (NOS) enzymes, which produce NO from the amino acid L-arginine. There are three forms of these NOS enzymes in the body.

The first is neuronal nitric oxide synthase (nNOS or NOS I). which is found in the brain. It aids blood flow in the brain and helps brain and nerve development. Thus, NO is essential to maintaining brain and nerve function.

The second NOS is immune nitric oxide synthase (iNOS or NOS II). It signals immune defenses to help the body fight infection. Thus, NO is also important for immunity and the regulation of chronic inflammation.

The final NOS enzyme is the one I've referred to previously. It's endothelial nitric oxide synthase (eNOS or NOS III) which produces nitric oxide to dilate arteries and enhance blood flow.

Supplementation with L-arginine helps increase nitric oxide production by all three of these enzymes. L-arginine supplements have been used to help cardiovascular disease, angina, intermittent claudication, dementia, erectile dysfunction, improve immune function, and increase athletic performance. Another amino acid, L-citrulline can help to recycle L-arginine and make it more effective. The body also requires oxygen to convert arginine to NO.

Nitrates

Another way the body makes NO is from nitrate (NO_3) and nitrite (NO_2). Nitrates are naturally found in many common vegetables, including lettuce, arugula, spinach, parsley, cabbage, and turnips. Beets, however, are one of the best sources.

Dietary nitrates are absorbed in the stomach and intestines. They are carried through the bloodstream to the salivary glands, which extract the nitrates and concentrate them in the salvia. Bacteria in the mouth convert the nitrates to nitrite, which is swallowed and converted into NO under the influence of hydrochloric acid.

Nitrites produce NO without oxygen, which means they can help enhance NO when oxygen levels are low. This is important because as we age, oxygen levels in tissues tend to fall. Oxygen levels are also low in many chronic diseases.

At one time people were concerned about the safety of nitrates because of their use as preservatives in processed meats. It turns out that natural nitrates and nitrites in vegetables aren't harmful to human health; instead, they are important phytonutrients.

Other Nutrients

Vitamin D_3 is an antioxidant that helps protect the endothelial lining from damage and is also a cofactor in the activation of nitric oxide synthetase, the enzyme that produces nitric oxide. Low levels of vitamin D_3 contribute to reduced levels of nitric oxide, and experts suggest that upward of 90 percent of the population may be deficient in vitamin D_3.

Magnesium is essential in mitochondrial energy production and therefore in the synthesis of nitric oxide in endothelial cells. Vitamin C has a protective effect on the endothelial cells, preventing endothelial dysfunction. B vitamins, such as B_1 (thiamine), B-3 (niacin), B_6 (pyridoxine) and B_9 (folic acid) are absolutely critical to energy production within all mitochondria, including the nitric-oxide producing mitochondria in the endothelial cells. Niacin, taken as a single is helpful for opening up blood flow.

Finally, vitamin K_2, a vitamin involved in blood clotting, has been discovered to assist vitamin D_3 in maintaining the health of the endothelium. It helps to mobilize calcium and keep it from depositing in the artery walls, thus preventing hardening of the arteries.

In addition to exercise and supplements, it should be obvious that a diet rich in vegetables (like beets, chard, lettuce, and other sources of nitrate) is highly beneficial for circulation. It's also helpful to avoid refined sugar and to not smoke. You can also use a *Nitric Oxide Boosting Formula* to increase your production of NO.

Epsom Salt Bath

Epsom salt is magnesium sulfate. Soaking in a warm to hot bath containing this salt of magnesium is a great way to reduce stress, ease muscle tension, eliminate toxins, and relax. To take an Epsom salt bath simply add two cups of Epsom salt to the bathwater. You can also add five to ten drops of one of your favorite essential oils. Good choices for relaxing include lavender and rose. Be sure to mix the essential oils with a small amount of a natural, unscented soap like Dr. Bronner's Supermind Baby Soap so they will disperse in the water. Soak in the bath for fifteen to twenty minutes. Feel free to light candles and listen to relaxing music too. An Epsom salt bath is a good activity to include in the *Pleasure Prescription* strategy for countering stress.

Exercise

Over the past few decades, Americans have become increasingly sedentary. Many of us work forty hours a week (or more) at a desk job and then come home to watch TV, play video games, or surf the web.

Statistics suggest that children spend twenty to forty hours a week at these sedentary activities. Participation in outdoor activities has diminished. Because of safety concerns, many parents don't let their children play outside and explore anymore. Even state and federal parks are seeing fewer visitors each year as people find all their entertainment inside their homes.

This trend is dangerous to our health. No matter how well we eat or what supplements we take, nutrition alone is not enough to ensure good health. Physical activity is essential to maintain optimum weight, regulate blood sugar, maintain emotional health, and reduce the risk of degenerative diseases, like heart disease.

So to be healthy, we need to get out of our chairs and get involved in more physical activities. Yes, we're talking about exercise. We all know we should get regular exercise, but how many of us actually do it? Judging by the number of Americans who are out of shape, overweight, and depressed, a large percentage of us are not getting the physical activity we need to stay healthy.

For many of us, the thought of exercise is hard to bear. There are many reasons to loathe exercising. It might remind you of sweaty high school gym classes. You may feel too busy or too stressed to exercise. Some of us are just too embarrassed by how out of shape we are. You may believe that exercise is all "no pain, no gain" and has to be difficult and grueling. And some of us have injuries or illnesses that make exercise very difficult. Well, if you shudder at the thought of exercise for any of these (or other) reasons, then here is some good news; you don't have to do anything that difficult. You just have to get moving.

One of the best forms of exercise is simply walking. If you walk for just thirty minutes a day, you activate enzymes that help the body burn fat. If you can walk sixty minutes a day that's even better. You can also try swimming or playing any kind of sport several times a week. If that's too difficult, you can just start lymphasizing.

Lymphasizing

What is lymphasizing? It's a term coined in the early 1980s by lymphologist Dr. C. Samuel West to describe gently bouncing up and down on a mini trampoline without having your feet leave the mat. This gentle up and down movement is similar to the motion we make when we bounce a crying baby up and down. This gentle movement does wonders for health because it doesn't take strenuous physical activity and provides most of the health benefits of exercise.

It's called *lymphasizing* because this type of movement stimulates lymphatic flow. This is important because unlike the circulatory system, the lymphatic system lacks a pump, so lymph flow is largely passive. Gently bouncing up and down on a mini-trampoline greatly increases lymphatic flow, hence "lymphasizing."

Of course, you don't really need a mini trampoline to get the benefits of lymphasizing. Any kind of activity that gets you moving and breathing deeply is a form of lymphasizing, including just taking a walk. Yoga and tai chi can also be thought of as lymphasizing because they involve non-strenuous movement performed with deep breathing. Any activity that just gets you moving without stress and pain while breathing deeply can be considered lymphasizing. Doing this non-stressful activity for just twenty to thirty minutes a day will make a big difference in your health.

Exercise and Inflammation?

When cells are damaged due to trauma, toxins or nutritional deficiencies, a process called inflammation is started. We now know that inflammation is the "mother of all diseases," meaning that heart disease, cancer, diabetes, arthritis, asthma, dementia, and a host of other chronic and degenerative diseases are all linked to chronic inflammation.

Part of the inflammatory process is the movement of fluid and protein out of the blood stream and into the tissue spaces. This is the cause of one of the four classic symptoms of inflammation—swelling. The other three are heat, redness, and pain. Once you realize that the only way for the fluid and protein causing this swelling to be removed is through the lymphatic system, you understand why lymphasizing—i.e., physical movement and deep breathing—is essential to staying healthy. You cannot reduce inflammation and properly detoxify your cells without it.

When you remove the excess fluid from around your cells, they are able to get more oxygen and nutrients. Your cells' energy production increases, which gives you more energy. The more sedentary you are, the less energy you will have, which will contribute to fatigue and depression.

For someone who is chronically ill or "burned out" from stress, rigorous exercise can actually be counterproductive because it increases the output of stress hormones and may further damage already weakened tissues. Lymphasizing, on the other hand, will rebuild health, even if you are seriously ill. The key is to start slowly and build up gradually, but be consistent about it.

If you can only walk or bounce on a mini trampoline for five minutes the first day without feeling tired or stressed, then do it for five minutes. Then try it for six minutes the next day and seven minutes the day after that. This regular physical movement will gradually detoxify your cells and renew your health and energy. It will also elevate your mood and mental abilities. Have you ever noticed how your head "clears" when you take a walk?

Resistance Exercise

Lymphasizing is something everyone can do, but if you're well enough to do so, a little resistance training is also beneficial. Resistance exercise, such as lifting weights, is very beneficial for health. Muscle burns more energy than fat, so the more muscle you have the less likely you are to gain weight. Exercise that makes muscles "burn" also helps muscles take up sugar without the need for insulin, which helps with metabolic syndrome and type 2 diabetes. Stronger muscles also take stress off joints to aid arthritis and joint disorders.

Resistance exercise is also helpful for bone strength as we get older. The stress put on the bones by this exercise stimulates the body to increase bone mass, reducing the risk of osteoporosis and fractures.

If you need help motivating yourself to do exercise, here are a few tips. First, find someone to exercise with can provide accountability and extra motivation. This could even be a dog you need to take for a walk every day.

Second, pick a form of exercise that's pleasant for you. You want to make your exercise time pleasant and fun. If you're doing something enjoyable it will make it easier to motivate yourself to stick with it until it becomes a habit.

Finally, if you feel tired and sore after exercise, you can aid recovery by taking a *Nitric Oxide Boosting Formula* prior to exercise and/or an *Electrolyte Drink Powder* afterwards. These can help you feel better, making it easier to keep going until you develop the habit. You can find additional suggestions under the condition *Exercise (Recovery)*.

Fasting

Have you ever noticed that little children and animals tend to shun food when they are sick? There is a reason for this. In most acute illness, the body is congested, and when the body is congested, it does little good to put more food into it. It just clogs the system more.

Think of it this way: Suppose the drain in your kitchen sink got plugged up and you were unable to wash dishes. You wouldn't continue to make more meals and dirty more dishes until you'd gotten the drain unplugged, right? Well, when you are sick, it's often a sign that one or more of the "drains" in your body are clogged. If you take time to unclog the drain before you resume eating, your food will digest better and the body will metabolize it more efficiently.

Okay, maybe you're not into the kitchen stuff, so here's another analogy for those of you who are more mechanically inclined. Think of what happens to a car when the air filter is dirty, the oil needs to be changed, and the carburetor and spark plugs are getting fouled. The car no longer burns fuel efficiently, which reduces performance. It also increases the amount of "gunk" being generated by the engine, which causes the engine to get even more clogged up. If one takes the time to clean the carburetor, change the oil, and replace the spark plugs and filters, the engine will burn cleaner and more efficiently.

Just like an automotive engine or our household plumbing, the body gets "clogged" periodically. When this happens, the body needs a nutritional "lube, oil, and filter service" or an herbal "drain opener" to clean it out so that it can run efficiently again.

Of course, I'm not suggesting that cleansing is the only thing we need to keep the body healthy. Obviously, the body also needs exercise, rest, and good nutrition. But, the body isn't going to be able to utilize good nutrition properly if it's congested, and you won't feel like exercising when your metabolic "engine" isn't running efficiently. You probably won't sleep very well when the body's drains are plugged either. So in many cases, if you want to improve your health, a good place to start is by doing a cleanse.

The most basic of all cleanses is a fast. In fact, fasting is one of the oldest and most effective natural healing techniques. As mentioned earlier, it's also instinctive, since small children and animals don't eat when they don't feel well.

"Starving" Illness

Some of us have been taught to "eat to keep up strength" when we're sick, but this is bad advice. Even though everyone has heard the sage wisdom of the famous Greek physician Hippocrates, "Feed a cold and starve a fever," practically nobody understands what it means. His advice becomes clearer if you render it as "if you feed a cold, you will have to starve a fever." In other words, it's not wise to feed a cold or a fever. Both need to be "starved" out with fasting because these illnesses are signs the body is congested with metabolic waste.

Many modern Western herbalists and naturopaths have discovered the incredible value of "starving" colds, flu, fevers, and other acute ailments. So next time you feel a cold or flu coming on, stop eating and do some cleansing! Putting

food into the body when you're ill is like running more water into a sink with a plugged drain—it's just going to make the problem worse.

Of course, while water is not likely to help a plugged kitchen drain, water is exactly what the body needs when its "drains" are clogged. The old adage "Go to bed, rest, and drink plenty of fluids," is probably the best advice ever written as basic therapy for acute illness. Every eliminative channel of the body needs water to function properly. Simply resting and flushing the system with liquids will help you get over most colds, flu, and other minor ailments faster than an OTC (over-the-counter) medication.

A twenty-four hour fast one day per month is a good basic health-building practice. Periodically, longer fasts can be utilized. For most people, a three-day fast is sufficient, but people have fasted for as long as forty days. I don't recommend long fasts for health purposes, however.

Juice Fasting

People who are hypoglycemic—that is, they suffer from low blood sugar—have a hard time fasting. If you're one of these people, it's probably better to do a juice fast. It's also better to do a juice fast if you're going to fast for more than twenty-four hours. A juice fast involves abstaining from solid food and drinking some kind of fresh fruit or vegetable juice whenever you feel hungry. Plenty of water should also be consumed while on a juice fast. The famous herbalist, Dr. John Christopher, described this type of juice fast cleansing in his booklet *Dr. Christopher's Three-Day Cleansing Program*.

When juice fasting, it's important to have a supply of fresh, raw juice. This means one will either need to own a juicer or have a source to buy fresh, unpasteurized juice. It is best to stick with one type of juice for the duration of the fast. Raw unfiltered apple juice is a good choice because it has a mild laxative action. However, if one has blood sugar issues, it should be diluted half and half with water, or the person should opt to use vegetable juices (such as carrot, celery and beet juice), as they don't raise blood sugar levels as much.

One of the easiest (and most effective) juice fasts is to drink lemon water sweetened with real maple syrup. Grade-B maple syrup is preferred because it has a higher mineral content than grade-A maple syrup, which is more sugary. However, you can use either. You can make the lemon drink anyway you want, but a good recipe is the juice of four lemons in a half gallon of water with about an equal amount of maple syrup as lemon juice.

Lemon is great because it helps both the liver and the kidneys flush toxins. If you're interested in learning more about this cleanse, read *The Master Cleanser*, by Stanley Burroughs, which explains how to do this type of juice fasting.

The twenty-four-hour fast or a two- or three-day juice fast once a month can have many health benefits. First, it eliminates allergy-causing foods from the diet, which results in the elimination of allergy-induced health symptoms. Juice fasting can help reduce chronic pain, relieve digestive upset, clear thought processes, create stronger resistance to disease, and increase energy.

A fast should always be broken by eating a meal of fresh fruits or vegetables. Never "pig out" when breaking a fast! Eat light at first and gradually reintroduce heavier foods.

People with serious gut health issues should probably not juice fast or do long total fasts. Instead, they can do a "fast" using bone broth for twenty-four to forty-eight hours. See *Gut Healing Diet* for more information on this type of diet.

Intermittent Fasting

One final way to incorporate fasting into your health program is to use intermittent fasting. This is a program of daily fasting where you do not eat for a period of sixteen hours. So for example, you can eat from either 7 a.m. until 3 p.m. (skipping dinner) or eat from 12 p.m. to 8 p.m. (skipping breakfast). When you're not eating, drink plenty of water. You can also drink unsweetened tea or coffee. This gives your body sixteen hours each day to detoxify and is very beneficial for overcoming SIBO, leaky gut, and other digestive system problems.

Flower Essence

Flower essences are vibrational (homeopathic-like) remedies made from the flowers of plants. They are used to help a person find healing on an emotional rather than a physical or mental level.

Dr. Edward Bach, an English medical doctor and homeopath, discovered how to use flowers for emotional healing and created the first thirty-eight flower essence remedies, known collectively as Bach Flower Essences. He also created an "emotional first aid" blend of five flower essences, called Rescue Remedy, which is the most widely used flower essence product.

Dr. Bach was frustrated by the symptomatic approach of modern medicine. He felt that medical doctors focused too much on the pathology (the disease symptoms) and not enough on the patient. Bach was a pioneer in understanding gut microflora. He developed homeopathic "vaccines" called Bach nosodes to adjust the friendly flora of the gut to improve health. He was also an advocate of healthy diet and detoxification of the GI tract as a route to good health.

As he observed patients, he began to notice that certain illnesses tended to go with certain personality traits. He also noticed that a patient's emotional state had a lot to do with

healing. He came to believe that unresolved emotional conflicts created disharmony between the soul and the mind. In Bach's mind, health was created by restoring internal harmony, with health being "the true realization of what we are… We are children of God."

Bach wanted to create a system of healing that wouldn't destroy living things and that would be gentle and effective in nature. It is believed that he created flower essences after sampling the morning dew on flowers and feeling the energy of the flower in the dew. He matched the vibration or energy of the plant with the emotional vibration of the person.

Since the time of Edward Bach, many people have followed in his footsteps developing additional flower remedies for emotional healing. Two major pioneers in flower essence therapy are Patricia Kaminski and Richard Katz, founders of the Flower Essence Society (FES) in Nevada City, California. They have created hundreds of North American flower remedies.

Another modern flower essence practitioner is Ian White, who created a line of remedies from Australian wildflowers. There is also a line of tree flower essences. Today, there are dozens of people who are continuing to discover plants that can help us heal emotionally. When working with the emotional issues that are underneath many of our physical health problems, flower essences can be a great ally.

At the very least, keep a bottle of the *Shock and Injury FE Blend* on hand. It can be very helpful for centering one's emotions during times of trauma or stress and can even be applied topically to help minor injuries to heal faster.

A good guide to using flower essences is the *Flower Essence Repertory* by Patricia Kaminski and Richard Katz. It references the thirty-eight English flower remedies created by Edward Bach, plus about one hundred North American flower remedies. You can also consult my book *The Heart's Key to Health Happiness and Success* and our *Essential Tools for Emotional Healing Chart*.

You can use flower remedies by taking four to ten drops under the tongue two or three times per day or as needed. Wait five minutes before eating or drinking. You can also add four to ten drops to a glass of water and drink it. Add fifteen to twenty drops to a spray bottle filled with four to eight ounces of purified water and shake vertically ten to twenty times to create a spray form of the product which can be sprayed into a room. You can also apply flower essences to the pulse points on the wrist or use them in baths or soaks.

Additional training on using flower essences can be found in the free emotional healing training class at stevenhorne.com/program/Free-Emotional-Healing-Training-Program. I also recommend checking out the website for Flower Essence Services (fesflowers.com/) and FlorAlive (floralive.com/).

Forgiveness

During the course of our lives, people will do things that harm us physically or hurt us emotionally. The words or actions that inflict these wounds may have intended harm or they may have been done without a full understanding of their consequences. While there is a time and place for seeking justice, many times the hurt from these things lingers with a person for years like a festering emotional wound. The inability to let go of past hurts and wrongs through the process of forgiveness can leave a person feeling bitter, angry, resentful, and otherwise emotionally scarred.

The inability to forgive can manifest in a variety of mental and emotional problems such as addiction, which can be a way of trying to escape the pain in one's past. It can also be involved in anxiety, depression, and excessive anger.

In my observation, these emotional wounds can contribute to physical health problems too. Resentment can literally "eat you alive" through a disease called cancer. Unhealed trauma from sexual abuse can cause reproductive problems in women. The inability to forgive oneself can also contribute to the attack against oneself going on in autoimmune disorders.

So how does one forgive? To start with forgiveness is not about forgetting or burying the pain in one's past. It is not about ignoring the injury you received either. A person who says, "I may forgive but I will never forget," doesn't understand what forgiveness is, because forgiveness releases the pain so that the memory of the trauma no longer brings up pain.

The word forgive is composed of the parts "fore" and "give." When you give something to someone in love there can be no pain or trauma associated with the act. When someone takes something from you, however, we feel a sense of pain and betrayal. Forgiveness is the act of giving afore. That is, it is the act of turning a trespass by another into an act of giving on your part. What you give away is released, and there is no more emotional pain involved with it.

It isn't always easy to forgive; it often takes calling upon the Higher Power through prayer to help us do it. But it's well worth it. But laying aside the spiritual aspect of forgiveness, I'm going to provide you with two practical tools I've used to help people forgive others and release the pain of the past.

Before I explain these two techniques, first let me talk about the process of figuring out who you need to forgive. At the very least, you should consider doing these techniques on yourself and your parents. Do this even if you don't consciously recognize any need to do so. Just about everyone has things from their past they need to forgive themselves for, and no one has perfect parents. There is often at least one situation, if not several situations, in which we feel our parents weren't fair with us.

Next, think of anyone you feel has abused or hurt you in your life. This could be siblings, friends, ex-lovers or ex-spouses, current spouses or lovers, business partners or associates, and so forth. Make a list of all these people, then pick one of the following techniques to help you forgive them.

When I'm doing forgiveness work with others, I use the second technique combined with muscle testing to help them identify who they need to forgive. I have the person say, "I have forgiven [name of the person] completely." Then, I test them. If they test strong on the statement, they don't need to forgive that person. If they test weak, they have forgiveness work to do.

Forgiveness Journal

The first tool involves getting a notebook that you will write in. Starting with the first person on your list, you write the following: "[Your first name] forgives [name of the person] completely." Since my name is Steven I would write the following if I were doing this: "Steven forgives himself completely" or "Steven forgives his mother (or father) completely."

As you write, memories may surface where you felt wronged by the person you are forgiving. Let's say you remember a time when one of your parents punished you unjustly for something you didn't do. You add this issue to the end of the statement. So if I were doing this for myself, I might write something like, "Steven forgives his [parent] completely for punishing him for something his brother did."

You write this extended statement until the feeling of peace comes over you, then you go back to the general statement that you forgive the person completely. The person who taught me this technique suggested we should write this 490 times for each person (that's 7 times 70). You don't actually have to count the number of times; you just have to do it until a complete feeling of peace comes over you as you write it.

That's your signal that you've successfully "let go" of your past hurts with that individual and you can move onto the next person on your list. When you can write, "[your name] has forgiven *everyone* who has *ever* wronged [him or her]," with perfect peace, you are done.

Forgiveness Affirmation

If you don't use muscle testing, you can still do this technique. You should have a complete feeling of peace when you make the statement that you have forgiven someone completely. If you don't have a feeling of peace, there is something you need to forgive them for. Here's the process you go through to do this.

Sit or lay down in a comfortable position. Breathe deeply. Then ask the following question out loud, "What would it feel like if I forgave [name of the person] completely?" Take another deep breath, notice how you are feeling, and then repeat the question. If negative feelings come up such as anger, fear, or sadness, pay attention to these feelings.

If painful memories surface, add them to the statement, "What would it feel like if I forgave [name of the person] completely for [whatever they did to hurt you]?" Again, allow yourself to feel and acknowledge any negative emotions that surface.

At some point these negative feelings will shift and good feelings will start to take their place. You may feel lighter, more peaceful, more relaxed, or happier. Recognize that this is what you will feel if you let go of the past and forgive this person, then say out loud, three times, "I forgive [name of the person] completely." If you feel a sense of peace after saying this, you are done. Move onto the next person until you have forgiven everyone on your list.

For more information, please see my YouTube video on forgiveness. (https://youtube.com/watch?v=yC69ekYzJME)

Friendly Flora

Bacteria tend to be associated with disease and thought of as something to be eliminated and destroyed. This has created an almost-obsessive use of disinfectants. But, not all bacteria are bad. It is the action of bacteria, for example, that allows milk to be fermented to create cheese, yoghurt and kefir. Bacteria also create other fermented foods such as sauerkraut and tofu. Another benefit of bacteria is that they breakdown minerals in the soil and make them available to the roots of plants.

Our body's roots—i.e., the place where we absorb water and nutrients—are the intestinal tract, and bacteria play an important role there. In fact, there are about three to four pounds of friendly microorganisms living in the intestinal tract, most of them bacteria. A proper balance of these microbes is essential to good health, because they are part of a symbiotic relationship. Many strains of bacteria are actually part of your body's natural ecosystem. They serve to help protect our bodies against unfriendly microbes.

There are many different species of beneficial bacteria inhabiting the intestines. Many belong to the genus *Lactobacillus*. These include *L. acidophilus*, one of the first strains sold as a supplement. Another genus containing species of friendly bacteria is *Bifidobacterium*, sometimes referred to as Bifidophilus. A third major group belong to the *Streptococcus* genus. There are many others.

The good bacteria inhabiting the intestines are called *friendly flora* or *probiotics*. *Biotic* is from a Greek word that refers to life. So *pro*-biotic means favorable to life. This is in contrast to the word *anti*-biotic, which literally means against life. They are collectively known as the *microflora* or *microbiome*. An imbalance in the microbiome is called *dysbiosis*.

Antibiotics weaken the immune system because they destroy the friendly flora. These friendly flora are actually part of the immune system. Friendly bacteria enhance the immune system in several ways. First of all, they form a sort of living blanket that coats the intestinal tract and inhibits other species of microorganisms from gaining a foothold on the intestinal mucosa. They compete with other microbes for food, which also holds down the growth of infectious organisms.

Friendly bacteria even produce chemicals that are deadly to harmful forms of bacteria, so they act as natural antibiotic agents against harmful bacteria. Another benefit of friendly bacteria is that they have a stimulating effect on the body's immune system. For instance, animal studies showed that *S. thermophilus* and *L. bulgaricus* increased proliferation of lymphocytes, stimulated B lymphocytes, and activated macrophages.

A well-known benefit of friendly flora is their ability to keep yeast such as *Candida albicans* in check. When antibiotics, chemotherapy, chlorine, or other chemicals or drugs destroy some of the friendly flora, yeast multiply out of control. They secrete a toxin that weakens the intestinal membranes and reduces the immune response. Probiotics are the antidote to this problem, helping to restore a healthy intestinal microflora.

Probiotics also help overall colon health. They reduce the risk of inflammatory bowel disorders such as colitis, Crohn's disease, and irritable bowel syndrome. They also reduce the risk of colon cancer. They should be used as part of a natural treatment plan for these diseases.

A healthy intestinal microflora improves the body's ability to digest fats and proteins. Probiotics synthesize certain vitamins the body needs, including B_1, B_2, B_6, B_{12}, folic acid, and biotin. The synthesis of B_{12} by probiotics is particularly important for vegetarians, who are not getting this vitamin in their diets.

The friendly flora also help detoxify certain poisons in the digestive tract. For instance, they help break down ammonia, cholesterol, and excess hormones.

Finally, about 70 percent of the energy requirements of the intestinal mucosa come from fatty acids produced as a by-product of bacterial fermentation. This means that the intestinal microflora actually helps feed the intestinal lining, demonstrating how vital this synergistic relationship is to health.

In fact, a healthy intestinal microbiome is such an important part of total health that some researchers feel it should be considered as an independent body system. The intestinal microbiome is a highly adaptable system, as it changes constantly, adapting itself to both diet and environment. It is easy to see why a balanced intestinal microbiome is such an important factor in a healthy body.

Probiotics can be obtained from yoghurt, kefir, and other fermented dairy foods containing live bacterial cultures. They can also be found in naturally fermented pickles, kim-chi, and sauerkraut in the refrigerated section of the health food store. Fermented soy products like miso can also help. There are many good recipes for making your own fermented foods in *Nourishing Traditions* by Sally Fallon, one of my favorite books on nutrition.

When looking for a probiotic supplement, look for one that contains several strains of bacteria such as acidophilus, bifidophilus, and others. Make certain that the product is stored in the refrigerator, as the bacteria are living organisms and will die quickly when stored at room temperature.

Gallbladder Flush

The gallbladder flush is a natural procedure that has been used to ease gallbladder attacks and potentially pass gall stones. It has been around for years and many people have had good success in using it. How it works isn't totally clear, but one explanation is that the large amount of olive oil ingested on the gallbladder flush sends the gallbladder into spasms which eject small stones and may also clear bile ducts.

The procedure is controversial and there is a slight risk, which is that a large stone may get stuck in the bile ducts resulting in the need for surgery. However, in over thirty years of experience, I have only had one report of this happening. Besides, surgery is the standard treatment for this condition and surgery carries a much higher risk than this procedure, which makes me think that it is worth trying first. If it fails, then go for the surgery.

Here's the standard way to do a gallbladder flush. Start by fasting for twenty-four to forty-eight hours on fresh, raw apple juice or fresh-squeezed grapefruit juice. Malic acid, an ingredient in the apple juice, is reported to soften the stones, but persons with hypoglycemia or yeast infections will do better on grapefruit juice. If using grapefruit juice, supplement with magnesium and malic acid (as in the *Fibromyalgia Formula*) for a similar effect.

Just before going to bed at the close of the fast, drink half a cup of olive oil and half a cup of lemon (or grapefruit) juice. Mix these together thoroughly like you would shake up a salad dressing. The lemon juice cuts the olive oil and makes it more palatable. It sounds and smells worse than

it tastes. Next, lie on your right side for a half-hour before going to sleep. In the morning, if you don't have a bowel movement, take an enema. This procedure may need to be repeated two days in a row.

Generally, you will pass some dark-black or green objects that look like shriveled peas the day after drinking the olive oil and lemon juice. These objects are not gallstones. Gallstones that can be passed are much smaller than this, generally less than two millimeters in diameter. Chemical analysis of these objects shows they are composed of soap, and are created by the bile interacting with the oil.

The controversy of this procedure is whether the stones actually pass or it just eases the pain and discomfort of the gallbladder attack and allows the problem to become asymptomatic again. You see, most people with gallstones don't know they have them, because they cause no symptoms. Whether stones are passing or not, this procedure typically eases gallbladder pain and allows the person to resume a normal life without surgery.

I have seen a number of versions of this procedure, but they all rely on olive oil. This may be because olive oil acts as a solvent of cholesterol, the chief constituent of most gallstones. Some gallstones, however, are calcium based.

One variation that seems to work particularly well is to take a dose of Epsom salt about two or three hours prior to taking the olive oil and lemon juice. Follow the directions on the box of Epsom salts as per the dosage.

Certain herbs may also enhance the procedure. Herbs called cholagogues increase the flow of bile and help to dissolve stones slowly over a period of weeks and months. Herbs that have this property include dandelion root, artichoke, barberry bark, yellow dock root, fringe tree bark, turmeric, and celandine. A *Chologogue Formula* containing any of these can be taken before attempting the gallbladder flush to increase its effectiveness, or afterwards to continue improving gallbladder function.

In fact, taking these herbs regularly for a year or more may even help to dissolve larger stones. I would recommend a combination of artichoke, barberry, fringetree, and turmeric, as these seem to be especially good at helping the gallbladder to heal and potentially to remove stones. You can also take six teaspoons of olive oil mixed with six teaspoons of lemon juice each evening while taking the herbs. This is a slower and gentler way to do the gallbladder flush

If gall stones are calcium-based, then hydrangea and magnesium will be helpful in dissolving them. Take these herbs during the fast and for several months after the gallbladder flush.

If the procedure does not bring relief, medical help should be sought.

Gluten-Free Diet

Gluten is a protein structure found in wheat and other grains. The inability to handle gluten causes celiac disease but is also involved in other inflammatory bowel disorders. Gluten intolerance can cause inflammation in the joints, skin, respiratory tract, and brain without any obvious gut symptoms. Gluten may also trigger autoimmune reactions in Hashimoto's disease, rheumatoid arthritis, and other auto-immune problems.

Since there are no nutrients in gluten-containing foods that you can't get more easily and efficiently from foods that don't contain gluten there are no nutritional deficiencies one could develop by avoiding gluten. There are, however, many potential health benefits to avoiding or eliminating it.

Foods containing gluten include wheat (includes bulgur, durum flour, farina, graham flour, semolina), barley (malt, malt flavoring, and malt vinegar are usually made from barley), rye, triticale (a cross between wheat and rye), spelt, and kamut.

Gluten-free grains and grain alternatives you can use instead include amaranth, buckwheat, coconut flour, corn (hominy and cornmeal), flax, millet, potato flour, quinoa, rice, sorghum, soy flour, and teff.

Many foods contain wheat or other gluten grains, so you need to be vigilant in looking at ingredients. Look for foods that say "gluten-free" on the package. Ask about gluten in foods when eating out at restaurants.

Good Posture

Your spinal column is a marvel of structural engineering. It is designed to hold the body upright, but unlike a rigid column or pole, it also has to be able to bend and move.

To allow this to happen, the backbone is composed of many smaller bones called vertebrae, which are held in place by ligaments, tendons, and muscles. These muscles exist in pairs, which help to balance the spine and hold it erect. When the spine moves, muscles on one side contract, while the muscles on the other side relax and stretch.

When you are standing up straight, the weight of the upper body is distributed down the spine and the muscle tension is balanced on each side of the body. When you're not standing erect, or holding your head up straight, the muscles in the spine are forced to hold up the weight of your body and/or head against gravity. Muscles on one side of the body are tensing against the force of gravity, while muscles on the other side are permanently contracted and unable to stretch.

Poor posture causes muscle fatigue and pain. It can produce backache or back pain, as well as pain in the knees, legs, shoulders, neck, and head. Headaches are often caused by problems with posture related to the head. Sciatic nerve pain can also be caused by bad posture. Here are some ways to avoid these problems and help to reverse them when they occur.

Straighten Up Your Act

Since poor posture is a major contributor to back problems, do things to improve your posture. For example, practice standing straight by standing with your back against a wall. Stretch out your back and try to align your back against the wall.

Also practice sitting up straight when working at a computer or desk. Move the computer monitor so it is at eye level to keep your head straight. Don't bend your head downward to work on a cell phone or tablet. Try bringing the device up to eye level so you can keep your neck straight. If you can't, stretching backward periodically will relax the muscles in your back and neck.

Make Sure Your Hips Are Aligned

Check the alignment of your hips by standing in front of a mirror and placing your fingers on the hip bones on both sides of your body. Notice if they are level. If they are not (that is, if one hip is higher than the other), this could be causing your back pain. It can also cause neck and shoulder pain because the pelvis is the foundation for the spine. If the pelvis is out of alignment, then the whole spine will be stressed all the way to the neck.

If your pelvis is out of alignment, body work along with exercise and improving your posture will often correct the alignment. Seek out a chiropractor who works with muscles and connective tissue, a well-trained massage therapist who can do deep-tissue work or other body-worker who can assist you in getting your pelvis and spine in alignment.

A simple self-help technique is to walk and stand putting most of your weight on the longer leg. This helps to compress the longer leg and stretch the shorter leg, which brings your pelvis back into alignment. You can also massage the muscles in your lower abdomen and buttocks.

Stretch and Move Your Spine

Practice bending and stretching your spine in different directions to keep it flexible. If you work at a desk or sit a lot, try stretching backward several times a day. This helps to balance the muscles on both sides of the spine, which alleviates tension and fatigue.

If you're really stiff, try the *Herbal Back Adjustment* strategy. Also try he therapies under the *Bodywork* strategy or an exercise program that focuses on stretching muscles, like yoga.

Gut-Healing Diet

In people with healthy GI tracts, food is completely digested, the nutrients absorbed, and the non-nutritive components eliminated. In people with impaired digestion and intestinal irritation, however, undigested food proteins are absorbed into the bloodstream, causing an inflammatory immune response that can manifest as a host of other disorders including migraines, autoimmune diseases, allergies, Hashimoto's thyroiditis, GERD, inflammatory bowel disease (IBD), and irritable bowel syndrome (IBS).

In these situations, diet is absolutely essential to healing the gastrointestinal tract. There are four possible diets one can follow, which are briefly described below.

Here are the basics of four gut-healing diets. Resources for learning more can be included with each description.

Specific Carbohydrate Diet (SCD)

The Specific Carbohydrate Diet works well for people who need a black-and-white list of foods they can and cannot eat. It has allowed (legal) foods and not allowed (illegal) foods. The diet allows meat, fats, non-starchy vegetables, ripe fruit, nuts and seeds, some beans, and lactose-free dairy. It also allows glucose and honey. The inclusion of dairy foods and honey make this diet easier for some people to follow. Improvement should be seen in a month if the diet is going to work. If it doesn't, switch to another diet. (Resources: breakingtheviciouscycle.info, https://healthygut.com/about-the-scd-diet/, and https://www.dietvsdisease.org/specific-carbohydrate-diet/.)

GAPS Diet

The GAPS diet differs from the SCD diet because it doesn't allow dairy products, honey, gelatin, or store bought fruit juice. GAPS also allows vegetables in soups. The GAPS diet has stages, an introductory diet that should be followed before moving into the full GAPS diet. It depends on the severity of the problem how fast or slow a person can move through the stages. This diet was originally designed to help with severe mental and emotional issues and can be very helpful for problems like autism. (Resources: https://www.thegoodgut.org/the-complete-guide-to-the-gaps-diet/, and gaps.me, and gapsdiet.com.)

FODMAP Diet

FODMAP is an acronym that stands for fermentable oligosaccharides, disaccharides, monosaccharide and polyols. These are carbohydrates that are difficult to digest and become fermented by bacteria, causing bloating and discomfort. Foods that are high in FODMAPs include wheat, rye, onions, legumes, dairy products, fructose, and sweeteners like sorbitol and xylitol. By removing potential triggers to digestive distress and then slowly reintroducing them, you'll be able to pinpoint your food intolerances and adjust your diet accordingly. See *Eliminate FODMAPs* strategy.

Paleo Diet

Unlike the others, Paleo isn't a set diet. Instead, it's a philosophy about eating, with several variations. The idea is to eat foods that were traditionally eaten by hunter-gatherer people for thousands of years before modern agriculture and processed foods. Strict Paleo is grain-free, legume-free, and dairy-free, but as people get healthier there are several variations of Paleo that allow and encourage certain dairy products. Resources: https://thepaleodiet.com/, https://paleodiet.org/food-list/, and https://ultimatepaleoguide.com/paleo101/.) There are also numerous books about the Paleo diet.

Here are some basic things you can follow, even if you don't pick one of these diets.

For starters, all simple sugars and refined carbohydrates should be eliminated from the diet. This includes refined sugars of all kinds, white flour, and white rice. All gluten-bearing grains should also be eliminated, which include wheat, spelt, kamut, rye, and barley. In fact, it is a good idea to eliminate all grains from the diet, at least in the beginning until the gut has healed.

Dairy may also be problematic because the bacteria love to feast on the sugar in dairy, lactose. Many people also have problems with a milk protein called A1 beta-casein. Modern dairy cows (Holstein) have this protein, which releases a peptide called BCM 7. This protein can cause neurological impairment, autoimmune reactions (including type 1 diabetes), inflammation of the blood vessels, reduced intestinal motility, and excess mucus secretion.

Goat milk products and some traditional breeds of cattle do not have A1 beta-casein. So goat milk products and cultured dairy foods can be beneficial for some people; other people may have to eliminate all dairy foods.

Eat a diet comprised exclusively of fresh, nutrient-dense vegetables, whole fruits, and proteins (fish, eggs, and meat). Cultured foods, especially cultured vegetables, are especially beneficial.

Healthy Fats

You need fats in your diet to stay healthy. Fats play critical roles in good health. Brain and nerve tissue, for instance, requires the proper kind of fats, and low-fat diets can harm the intelligence of children. The heart burns fat as its primary source of fuel. Fats are burned to keep the body warm in cold weather and are necessary for the production of many hormones.

Extremely low-fat diets aren't healthy and can actually raise cholesterol, since about half of the cholesterol in the body is used to make bile to digest fats. However, you need to get the right kinds of fats in your diet.

Unfortunately, most people are eating poor-quality fats, which include margarine, shortening, processed vegetable oils, and animal fat from factory-farm raised raised animals. They tend eat too many omega-6 EFAs (essential fatty acids) and not enough omega-3 EFAs.

Omega-3 EFAs protect against heart disease and benefit the immune system. They help control the chronic inflammation that underlies the development of hardening of the arteries, arthritis, memory loss in aging, and other degenerative disease. The best sources of omega-3 EFAs are wild game, grass-fed beef, eggs and poultry, and deep-ocean fish (not farm raised). Avocados and nuts, especially walnuts, also contain good fats.

Because most people get too many bad fats, and not enough good fats, they can benefit from supplementing their diet with omega-3 EFAs. The best way to get omega-3 EFAs is through fish-oil supplements. While flax seed and hemp seed oil contain omega-3 EFAs, they are shorter-chain fatty acids and must be converted to the longer-chain DHA and EPA. Many people have problems with this conversion.

Medium-chain saturated fats are also important. The best source for these is coconut oil and organic butter from grass-fed cows. You can make a great soft-spread butter by mixing softened butter with flaxseed oil, getting the benefit of all your essential fats at the same time. Use half as much flax seed oil as butter, blend it together well, and refrigerate it. The result is a nice soft-spread butter.

Heavy Metal Cleanse

Heavy metal detoxification is important for anyone who has worked around a lot of chemicals in their job (including painters, beauticians, lab technicians, dry cleaners, carpet cleaners, farmers, and factory workers in many industries). It's also a good cleanse for people suffering from any kind of chronic inflammatory disorder or problem that involves nerve damage. I also recommend it after anyone has had a vaccine containing mercury compounds.

Because the body is naturally exposed to small amounts of heavy metals, even in natural foods, it has defensive mechanisms to help it eliminate these toxic elements, as well as other harmful substances, from our body. By nutritionally supporting these mechanisms while keeping the body's channels of elimination open, one can help the body remove excess heavy metals from the system.

Heavy metals (and many other environmental toxins) are not water-soluble; this means the body uses cholesterol to bind and transport them in the blood. So make sure you are supplementing the diet with good fats when trying to remove heavy

metals from the system. Consider taking cod liver oil, coconut oil, krill oil, or some other good fatty-acid supplement.

Enzyme systems, primarily located in the liver, convert the heavy metals into a water-soluble form. Typically, they are too heavy to be flushed through the kidneys, so the liver eliminates them by binding them to cholesterol in the bile and flushing them out of the gallbladder into the small intestines. Fiber is needed to bind the cholesterol and heavy metals so they will be carried out of the body.

While any kind of fiber helps, a particular form of mucilage known as sodium alginate is especially good at binding heavy metals. Sodium alginate is a mucilaginous fiber derived from kelp. Kelp is a purifier of the oceans because the alginate in it bonds to heavy metals and other toxins to neutralize them. Sodium alginate binds to heavy metals such as lead and mercury in the intestinal tract and carries them out of body with regular bowel movements. Apple pectin can also help bind heavy metals.

If you know or suspect you have heavy metal poisoning it's probably a good idea to work with an experienced doctor, naturopath, or herbalist to custom design a program for your individual needs. However, as a starting point, here's a basic mercury and heavy metal detox program:

One tablespoon of coconut oil twice daily.

A *Heavy Metal Cleansing Formula* twice daily (follow directions on the label).

Two to four algin capsules three times daily or one tablespoon of a *Fiber Blend Formula* in a glass of water or juice twice daily. You can also use the *Gut Healing Fiber Formula*.

Drink half an ounce of water per pound of body weight daily while on the cleanse.

Make certain the bowels are moving at least two to three times per day. If not, you may wish to take *Stimulant Laxative* or *Gentle Laxative Formula*.

If you develop a strong cleansing reaction (rash, diarrhea, nausea, dizziness, weakness, etc.) while on the cleanse, stop taking it for a couple of days. You can use the *Drawing Bath* strategy to help the body detoxify more rapidly. In fact, doing a drawing bath once or twice a week while doing heavy metal cleansing will help you avoid any adverse reactions.

The cleansing programs listed under the condition *Chemical Exposure* have also been shown to increase secretion of heavy metals.

Herbal Back Adjustment

A very effective way to ease tension in the back muscles is to do an herbal back adjustment. This procedure can help the spine to come into better alignment, ease spasms causing back pain, and release tension so the spine can move more freely.

In some cases, this relaxing of the muscles will allow subluxations (misaligned vertebrae) to correct themselves with stretching exercises. At the very least, it will make chiropractic adjustments or other spinal alignment work easier to perform.

Start by mixing lobelia and capsicum extracts in equal parts. Massage them into the muscles on both sides of the spine. Lobelia helps relax muscle spasms, and capsicum draws blood into the area. Both help to ease pain.

After massaging the capsicum/lobelia mixture into the spine, you can follow it up by applying an *Analgesic EO Blend* or a *Topical Analgesic Formula* and massaging it into the back.

For added benefit, soak a towel in hot water (bath temperature) and wring it out until mostly dry. Then lay out the warm, moist towel on the back to further drive the herbs and essential oils into the muscles. You can also apply the *Enzyme Spray Formula* to drive the herbs and oils into the muscles.

This technique can also be done on neck and shoulders or any other part of the body where there is pain associated with muscle tension or spasms. Used on the neck, it can be helpful for relieving headaches. Simply stretch the neck after the procedure.

Hiatal Hernia Correction

Due to stress and repeated bouts of bloating and gas, or chronic nervous tension, the stomach may move up into the diaphragm, creating a hiatal hernia. In a simple hiatal hernia, tension is holding the stomach up. In more severe cases, the stomach may adhere, requiring surgery. Because doctors use muscle relaxants when testing for a hiatal hernia, the simple kind often goes undetected. The instructions here are for the simple hiatal hernia, where there are no adhesions.

A hiatal hernia stresses the stomach by inhibiting the vagus nerve and blood flow to the stomach. Protein digestion is impaired and the resulting lack of essential amino acids causes glandular malfunction, immune system deficiency, poor muscle tone, excessive weight loss or gain, cold limbs, and general physical weakness.

Symptoms of a hiatal hernia include the inability to breathe from the diaphragm, tension in the solar plexus, difficulty swallowing capsules, the sensation of a "lump" in throat, and an over-stimulated thyroid gland (high metabolism). Chronic intestinal gas may occur as the ileocecal valve becomes permanently swollen and irritated and unable to close properly. Most people suffering from general poor health have this condition. This problem can be overcome using a variety of self-help techniques.

Breathing from the Diaphragm

Check your breathing. As a first step in treating the hiatal hernia, perform this simple test to assess your pattern of breathing. Put your hand on your abdomen as you breathe. If your abdomen moves in and out more than your chest, you are probably handling your stress well, or at least you aren't letting stress control you.

If you are breathing from the top of your lungs, just sit back and relax to allow your breathing apparatus to revert to normal abdominal breathing. If it doesn't, then you need to relax the diaphragm. To do this, take lobelia essence or blue vervain in liquid form. Then, practice breathing from the abdomen again. You can also practice abdominal breathing while relaxing in a bath with lavender oil.

Dealing with Stress

Another help for overcoming a hiatal hernia is to find healthy ways to vent your repressed anger and frustration. This releases tension from the diaphragm and will help defuse much of the tension maintaining the hiatal hernia problem. For example, try taking a long, slow deep breath and feel the tension build up in your diaphragm (like you are starting to get angry). Make your hands into fists and raise them up in front of you as if you want to punch somebody. Exhale forcefully with an angry "Huh!" sound while shaking your fists downward like you are hitting something. Do this several times, safely discharging your inner tension and frustrations.

Other methods of dealing with stress include changing your environment, finding new ways to resolve problems, and communicating your thoughts and feelings honestly with others. See the condition *Anger (Excessive)*.

Physical Manipulation

You can also find a chiropractor or a massage therapist who knows how to manually manipulate a hiatal hernia. It usually takes four to six treatments combined with self-help techniques to bring down a hiatal hernia.

As an alternative to having someone work on the problem for you, you can use the following technique.

Drink a pint of warm water first thing in the morning. Next, stand on your toes and drop suddenly to your heels several times. The force of this little jump and the weight of the water helps pull the stomach down in place while the warm temperature of the water relaxes the stomach area. Taking a dropperful of lobelia essence with the water will relax the stomach and make the treatment more effective.

If you're adventurous, jump off a chair or down a short flight of stairs to get the same effect. The idea behind this technique is to get your stomach to "drop" as if you were in an elevator that suddenly started going down.

If this doesn't solve the problem, place both hands under your breastbone in the center of your rib cage. Take a deep breath, press your fingers firmly into the solar plexus area (just under the breastbone). As you forcefully exhale, push your fingers downward and bend forward slightly. Be careful not to push your fingers up under the rib cage. Repeat this action several times. Do this before meals on an empty stomach.

You can find more information on dealing with a hiatal hernia, including two videos demonstrating how to work on the problem, on my website: stevenhorne.com/article/Hiatal-Hernia.

Hydration

Water is the most important nutrient the body needs besides oxygen. Most people can survive for weeks without food, but without water they would only last a few days at best. A loss of 15 to 20 percent of the body's water can be fatal. Adequate intake of pure water is one of the simplest and cheapest health insurance policies one can buy. Water is necessary to properly utilize the food we eat and the supplements we take.

It has been estimated that 75 percent of all Americans are chronically dehydrated. So of all underlying causes of ailments, dehydration is probably the most common and frequently overlooked. In about one-third of all Americans, the thirst mechanism is so weak that it is often mistaken for hunger. In one University of Washington study, a glass of water eliminated hunger in almost 100 percent of all the dieters studied.

Dehydration contributes to a wide variety of ailments, including indigestion, colitis, appendicitis, heart burn, rheumatoid arthritis, back and neck pain, headaches, stress, depression, high blood pressure, asthma, fatigue, memory loss, and allergies. Many people have found that increasing their water intake reduces pain of all kinds, but especially headache, back, and neck pain. Preliminary research indicates that eight to ten glasses of water a day could significantly ease back and joint pain for up to 80 percent of sufferers. Lack of water is the number one trigger of daytime fatigue.

Drinking water can also help to prevent disease. Water is necessary to flush waste products, particularly acid waste products, from the system. There is research to suggest that drinking five glasses of water daily could decrease the risk of colon cancer by 45 percent. Increased water intake could also slash the risk of breast cancer by 79 percent and reduce bladder cancer risk by 50 percent.

The brain is 80 percent water, so proper hydration is essential to its function. A mere 2 percent drop in body water can trigger fuzzy short-term memory, trouble with basic math, and difficulty focusing on the computer screen or on a printed page.

How Much Water Do We Need?

A good rule of thumb to determine how much water you need is to divide your body weight in half and drink that many ounces of water per day. So if you weigh 160 pounds, you need to drink about 80 ounces of water each day. There are 32 ounces in a quart, so this would equate to a little less than three quarts of water per day.

You can develop the habit of drinking more water by picking specific times to drink. Start by drinking a glass of water first thing in the morning; also drink a glass of water about 15-20 minutes prior to meals and again at bedtime. You can also make it a habit to keep a glass or bottle filled with water handy for when you feel thirsty.

If you have trouble drinking plain water, try adding some lemon or lime juice, or putting a few slices of cucumber into it. You can also take a pinch of natural salt, such as Himalayan Pink, Celtic or Redmond salt. The salt will increase your thirst and help your body utilize the water.

When drinking adequate water especially when previously being in a state of dehydration you may need to supply extra minerals and electrolytes. You can do this with just a pinch of natural salt. You can also use commercial rehydration drinks, or make your own. To make your own rehydration drink remember the 8-8-8 rule: eight ounces of water or fruit juice, one-eighth teaspoon salt, and eight teaspoons of sugar mixed together.

If you're only drinking a little water and don't feel thirsty, you really need to drink more water anyway. When sufficiently dehydrated, your thirst mechanism shuts off. This means that senior citizens are at greater risk for dehydration than younger people because their bodies are less effective at letting them know when they need water.

What Type of Water Should We Drink?

It isn't just the amount of water that is important. The kind of water you drink is critical, too. Increasingly, water supplies are being polluted and poisoned with disastrous consequences to good health and well-being. So drink the purest water you can find. Here are some options to consider

Carbon Filtration

Carbon filters are helpful in improving water quality and taste. In particular, they are very effective at removing chlorine and chlorine by-products. Carbon filters can be put on your shower heads or on the intake system for your whole house to remove these types of chemicals from the water you bathe and wash in, as well as drink. Unfortunately, however, there are two major downsides to carbon filters.

First, they do not remove contaminants such as heavy metals, and secondly, they are prone to periodic dumping. That is, unless changed regularly, they can become saturated and dump previously removed contaminants back into your drinking water. Carbon filtration also works better the longer the water is able to be in contact with the carbon, so when water is passed too rapidly through a carbon filter, it is less effective.

However, at the very least, you should use a carbon filter for your drinking water. As long as you change it regularly, it will greatly improve the quality of the water you drink.

Distillation

Distilling water is an effective way to purify drinking water. With the exception of a few volatile chemicals that also evaporate in the distillation process, distilling water removes all contaminants. By running distilled water through a carbon filter after distillation, even these volatile substances can be removed. The major drawbacks to distillation are expense, cleanup, and taste. Distillation is an expensive way of purifying water and requires considerable cleanup. The taste of distilled water is flat, but can be improved through aeration.

Reverse Osmosis

Reverse osmosis (RO) is the all-around best way to treat water for home use. Like distillation, RO removes all contaminants from water except for a few gases like chlorine, which are easily removed by carbon filtration. Reverse osmosis is a very inexpensive way to treat water, too, since it requires no other energy source except for the pressure in the tap. And unlike distilled water, RO water has a fresh, clean taste that makes you want to drink more. Many families have discovered that making RO water reduces their food budget for sodas, juices, and other beverages because the water tastes so good. The only drawback of reverse osmosis is that it does not deal with bacteria, so RO units are suitable for use with treated tap water only.

RO water has a couple of drawbacks. It tends to be slightly acidic, so it is not very good at alkalizing the body. This drawback can be overcome by increasing magnesium and potassium intake. The other drawback is that it is not as healthy a water structure as ionized water. Still, it is a very good choice for cleaning up drinking water at home.

Ozone

Ozone is a natural element created by ultraviolet light. Ozone oxidizes toxic substances. In fact, it destroys microorganisms in water three thousand times faster than chlorine and without chlorine's toxic effects. Ozone even helps to remove chlorine. *E. coli*, salmonella, giardia, cryptosporidium, parasites, bacteria, cysts, molds, and a variety of others pollutants are all neutralized by ozone. In fact, washing produce in ozonated water will help to kill any of these organisms that might be present on your fruits and vegetables.

Ozone water can be very therapeutic, but it does not taste as good as the RO water. It also requires electricity, though it does not use even a fraction of the energy consumed in distillation.

Ozone is already being used in place of chemicals for hot tubs and swimming pools. Someday, this technology may replace the use of chemicals like chlorine in the treatment of municipal water supplies as well. So where bacteria or microorganisms are a concern, such as with well water, ozonation would be the ideal choice.

Ionized Water

Research from Japan has shown that ionized water is by far the healthiest water to drink. Ionized water can be produced at varying degrees of alkalinity, which helps to counteract acid waste in the body. It also has antioxidant properties. Another advantage of properly ionized water is that it has the same structure as glacial runoff water, the healthiest water in the world. This is one of the factors that makes it superior for healing over reverse osmosis water. Carbon filtration is still needed in ionizing units to remove chemicals.

One of the biggest drawbacks of ionized water is the cost of the machines needed to produce it. The machines cost thousands of dollars and do require electricity. Machines that produce ionized water are also highly variable in quality. If you do decide to invest in one of these units, do your research and make sure you get a high-quality unit.

Bottled Water

Bottled water is best saved as a last resort. It is expensive and wasteful and can vary widely in quality. Some bottled water is simply tap water run through a carbon filter, while others are waters bottled from various springs or natural sources. Plastic bottles can also leach chemicals into water, especially if they are left in a warm place. Bottled water can be a good solution for emergencies or traveling when other sources aren't readily available.

Increase Dietary Fiber

Unless you're eating fruits and vegetables every day, including edible skins and seeds, and eating only whole grains, then you probably aren't getting enough fiber.

Fiber has numerous benefits. It absorbs bile from the gallbladder to help reduce cholesterol levels, slows the release of sugar into the blood to regulate hypoglycemia and diabetes, absorbs toxins in the intestinal tract to help detoxify the body, reduces inflammation in the gut, and provides food for friendly bacteria. Fiber also reduces the risk of colon cancer and prevents diverticulitis and hemorrhoids. And of course, it helps ensure regular elimination.

Many people think that cleansing the colon means taking a stimulant laxative. These products just stimulate peristalsis, which is something that is rarely needed. Most people are constipated from lack of fiber, lack of water, and magnesium deficiency. Besides, fiber is what really cleanses the colon, because fiber is what binds the toxins so they can't be absorbed into the bloodstream. So fiber is the one cleansing product that can be taken regularly by most Americans.

The natural way to get more fiber is to eat more fresh fruits and vegetables, beans, and whole grains. Foods like apples, beans, prunes, and figs are especially helpful.

You can also try taking just one heaping teaspoonful of a *Fiber Blend Formula*, first thing in the morning, along with a large glass of water, can make a dramatic difference. The main problem you might run into with fiber is if you don't drink enough water with it. Without water, fiber can actually bind you, so make certain you drink plenty of water when you take fiber.

If you are taking fiber and stop having regular bowel movements, discontinue the fiber and drink plenty of water. You many need to take a *Stimulant Laxative* or a *Gentle Laxative Formula* to get the colon working properly again.

If you have SIBO or severe dysbiosis, fiber can also increase intestinal gas and bloating. If this happens, follow the directions under these conditions to reduce bacterial overgrowth and improve the balance of friendly bacteria in your intestines. Then introduce fiber gradually.

Ketogenic Diet

A ketogenic diet can help to revitalize the function of cellular mitochondria, balancing blood sugar and aiding brain function. It is believed to help to clear the carbohydrate metabolic pathways in the mitochondria and rebalance mitochondrial function. The result is more efficient energy production and less free radical damage.

It is important to understand that the mitochondria don't directly utilize carbohydrates, fats, or proteins. All these potential fuel sources must be converted into a compound called acetyl-CoA. It is acetyl-CoA that is drawn into the mitochondria and converted to energy.

The cells of the brain and nervous system rely primarily on glucose to produce acetyl-CoA. Thus, the brain requires a stable level of glucose (blood sugar) to function properly. This is why blood sugar must be tightly regulated. If there is too much glucose, it can chemically react with proteins and other substances and damage them. So if the blood sugar is too high, the body moves glucose out of the blood using insulin to store it as glycogen or fat.

If blood sugar levels get too low, as happens in starvation or fasting, the brain has a hard time keeping your mind clear and your mood stable. So there is a backup system called ketosis for supplying your brain and nerves with energy. In ketosis, the liver converts fats into ketones to produce acetyl-CoA to supply energy for your brain.

A ketogenic diet severely limits carbohydrate intake, which forces the body into ketosis. Clinical evidence suggests that this is helpful for losing weight, controlling blood sugar levels, improving mental focus, reducing hunger, and increasing energy. Ketogenic diets may also help to reduce cholesterol levels and blood pressure, combat acne and even treat epilepsy. Research suggests they may also be helpful in treating cancer and neurological disorders.

On a ketogenic diet, all sugary and starchy foods are eliminated, including sugary fruits and starchy vegetables like potatoes. The diet consists of meat, high-fat dairy foods, nonstarchy or low-glycemic vegetables (see *low-glycemic Diet* strategy), nuts, seeds, berries, and quality fats like butter and coconut oil.

In a true ketogenic diet, about 70-75 percent of your caloric intake should come from natural (not processed) fats and 20-25 percent from protein, leaving only 5-10 percent of your caloric intake coming from carbohydrates. Modified ketogenic diets where 40 percent of calories come from fat, 30 percent from protein and the remaining 30 percent from fruits and vegetables are also beneficial for regenerating mitochondrial function and normalizing energy production and utilization.

If you need more information, there are many books and websites that can help you with the specifics of a ketogenic diet. These can easily be found by doing an internet search.

Liver Detoxification

Technological society has created a new challenge to our health—environmental toxicity. Each day we are exposed to hundreds of chemicals. When these chemicals enter our body through our lungs, digestive tract, or skin, the body has to break them down and eliminate them to protect our health.

The good news is that the body has systems for doing this. In particular, an amazing organ called the liver has numerous enzyme systems that process various kinds of toxins for elimination. So we can handle a certain amount of chemical exposure and remain healthy. The bad news is that our modern lifestyle puts a great deal of stress on the liver, which means it isn't always able to keep up with its job.

The liver needs nutrients in order to process these toxins. Vitamins, minerals, amino acids, and other nutrients are needed to construct and activate the enzyme systems that break down chemicals in the body. The junk-food diet of many people in modern civilization doesn't provide the raw materials the body needs to get rid of these toxins.

As a result, the liver may be unable to protect the body from these chemicals, which contributes to the development of many forms of disease. For example, some of the ailments that may involve environmental toxins include: allergies, asthma, autism, autoimmune disorders (like lupus, MS, arthritis, etc.), birth defects, cardiovascular disease, cancer, chronic headaches, fatigue, hormonal imbalances, kidney diseases, learning disabilities (ADHD, mental retardation, memory loss, senility, etc.), liver disease, neurological disorders, obesity, and skin disorders (eczema, rashes, and psoriasis). It's a long list, but the truth is that almost all chronic ailments probably involve some irritation to the system from chemical toxicity.

The liver is an amazing organ. It filters everything coming from the digestive tract and plays the dual role of processing nutrients for utilization and processing toxins for elimination. In its detoxification role, the liver deals with normal by-products of metabolism (cholesterol, hormones, cellular waste, etc.), toxins produced by microbial infections, drugs—and other chemicals and toxins that were previously stored in fatty tissue.

To process these toxins, the liver has numerous enzymes, which convert toxins into water-soluble compounds that can be flushed from the system. It does this in two steps: phase 1 detoxification and phase 2 detoxification. In phase 1 detoxification, about fifty different enzymes will create an electrical charge on the toxins by adding or removing an electron. In phase 2, six different detoxification pathways will attach these electrically charged toxins to another compound. These six pathways are acylation, glucuronidation, glutathione conjunction, methylation, sulfation, and acetylation. This six-pathway, phase 2 detoxification system makes the toxin water-soluble so it can be removed from the body via the urine or bile.

When a person has a strong liver, they can drink alcohol, caffeinated beverages, or take medications and the effects of these substances will be relatively short-lived. A person who has sluggish detoxification will find that the effects of these substances is relatively long-lasting. Another sign of sluggish detoxification is having difficulty getting to sleep at night, then waking up with a sort of groggy, "drugged" feeling. One may also experience a bloated and stuffy feeling under the right rib cage or readily experience light-headedness, dizziness, or headaches when smelling chemicals.

Sometimes phase 1 detoxification is working fine, but phase 2 detoxification pathways are sluggish. When this is the case, taking supplements that enhance phase one detoxification can make you feel sick. This is probably the cause of the "healing crisis" that occurs in natural medicine when someone consumes healthy foods and supplements and starts to feel sick. What is happening is that phase 1 detoxification is being increased but phase 2 systems and subsequent elimi-

nation of the toxins via the bowels and kidneys can't keep up with the toxic load.

Part of the problem is that phase 1 detoxification produces free radicals (superoxide radicals, to be precise). The intermediate metabolites produced by phase 1 detoxification can also be free radicals (radical oxygen intermediates). If these compounds are not processed rapidly enough through phase 2, they start causing irritation and inflammation to tissues. This can also happen when the body doesn't have enough antioxidants to neutralize these free radicals. Symptoms of this problem include headaches, stomach pain, nausea, fatigue, dizziness, and "brain fog" during detoxification, fasting, or weight loss. Toxemia during pregnancy is also a sign of sluggish phase 2 detoxification.

Of course, even if you don't have any of the symptoms above, but are regularly exposed to any kind of chemicals in your job, it would be wise to support your liver's ability to detoxify. Examples of people who may wish to consider regular liver support include dry cleaners, painters, construction workers, lab technicians, beauticians, people who handle agricultural chemicals (like farmers and landscapers). and carpet cleaners.

Many factors can inhibit your liver's ability to detoxify. These include certain drugs, low thyroid hormones, liver diseases, insulin resistance (metabolic syndrome and diabetes), and nutritional deficiencies. Fortunately, there are several things you can do to support your liver's detoxification systems. For starters, because both phase 1 and phase 2 detoxification require a variety of vitamins, minerals, and amino acids, attention should be paid to basic good nutrition.

Obviously, a diet of whole, nutrient-rich foods is optimal. Processed foods are not only low in the vitamins and minerals the liver needs to detoxify but also contain chemical additives that contribute to its workload. There are a number of specific herbs and supplements that aid in liver detoxification. Supplements that aid liver detox include alpha-lipoic acid, indole-3-carbinol, N-acetyl-cysteine, and SAMe. Herbs that assist the liver in detoxification include milk thistle, dandelion, bupleurum, and turmeric. B-complex vitamins and vitamin C are also important for aiding liver detoxification.

For people who work around chemicals of any kind, it's a good idea to take an *Hepatoprotective Formula* every day. Be sure to drink plenty of water and take antioxidants to assist the process of liver detoxification.

Low-Glycemic Diet

The single biggest problem with modern diets is the excessive amount of refined carbohydrates in them. There are many problems with large quantities of refined sugars, white flour, and processed grains. The glycemic index is a rough measure of how much insulin is secreted when we eat a food. Refined carbohydrates and highly starchy foods release a lot of insulin, which leads to insulin resistance. This causes metabolic syndrome, which can eventually lead to diabetes.

A low-glycemic food is one that does not trigger high levels of insulin. Starchy foods like potatoes and whole grains have a higher glycemic index than non-starchy vegetables. low-glycemic vegetables include green leafy vegetables, zucchini squash, green beans, cruciferous vegetables (broccoli, cabbage, cauliflower, etc.), tomatoes, onions, asparagus, cucumbers, peppers, and turnips. Fruit juice also has a high glycemic index. Fruits with a lower glycemic indexes include apples, apricots, cherries, grapefruit, lemons, limes, peaches, pears, and plums.

A low-glycemic diet focuses on removing high-glycemic carbohydrates and replacing the with low-glycemic carbohydrates to aid in overcoming blood sugar problems, losing weight and improving overall health. It also focuses on reducing the glycemic load, which is a rough estimate of the glycemic index of foods when they are combined.

For example, adding fat, like butter or sour cream, to a baked potato will lower the amount of insulin released, thus lowering the glycemic load. When looking at prepackaged foods, you can calculate the glycemic load of the food using the following formula. Take the total carbohydrates and subtract the amount of fiber and half of the fat. This gives you the glycemic load. You want to keep this under ten grams.

So for example. If you have a food that has twelve grams of carbohydrates, two grams of fiber and two grams of fat, the glycemic load would be 9. That's 12 minus 2 for the fiber and 1 for the fat.

For a list of low- and high-glycemic foods consult our *Blood Type, pH and Nutrition* charts. You can also search "glycemic index" on the internet to discover which foods are high-glycemic and which ones are low-glycemic.

Lymph-Moving Pain Relief

Many years ago, I learned six techniques for relieving pain and aiding the healing of injures. They are all based on an understanding of the inflammatory process and how moving lymph helps reverse inflammation and heal tissues. These techniques work best when applied immediately after an injury; it typically takes five to twenty minutes to permanently relieve the pain and start the healing process. They also work for chronic pain but must be used consistently, often many times each day, for a period of one to two weeks to start seeing permanent results.

Pressure

It's our first instinct to grab a place where we've been injured. The secret to making this technique work is to not let go until the pain stops. Sure, it hurts to hold the injury, but it's going to hurt anyway, so what have you got to lose? If you squeeze tightly for five to twenty minutes, depending on the severity of the injury, the pain will be permanently gone, and you probably won't develop a bruise or lose a nail. I've seen fingers smashed in doors and drawers, cuts, bumps, and other similar injuries completely reversed in as little as five or ten minutes by simply applying pressure.

Rapid-Light Stroking

If you watch a mother's instinctive reaction to her injured child, you'll note that almost all mothers cuddle and stroke a hurt child. Stroking an injured area moves lymphatic fluid and eases the pain while helping the injury to heal. This fact was demonstrated scientifically in 1981 in a presentation at the International Society of Lymphology convention in Montreal, Canada by Dr. W.L. Olszewski.

Rapid-light stroking is a great technique to use on larger injuries where you simply can't hold the area that's been bumped, banged or injured. When doing rapid-light stroking it isn't necessary to apply any pressure to the skin, simply move your hand back and forth very quickly and rapidly while just barely touching the skin. As pain diminishes you can apply more pressure, but the procedure shouldn't hurt.

Massage

You have probably noticed that sore stiff muscles feel tight and full, kind of puffy. They are full of fluids built up in and around those muscles. These slow-moving fluids are like the stagnant water in a swamp, they collect excessive amounts of waste materials, such as lactic acid and carbon dioxide, which of course, causes those muscle cells to send pain signals asking for help. They need oxygen and nutrients.

So we instinctively massage them, which breaks up the fluid and protein around the cells and helps pump the fluid, and the toxins, into the lymphatic system. As fresh, oxygen-laden fluid moves into the spaces around the cells, the muscles begin to feel better.

It doesn't take massage therapy school to learn how to find these stagnant pockets and massage them until the pain goes away. With a little practice anyone can learn to feel the knots or tight spots that signify swollen and inflamed muscle tissues. Whether this swelling and inflammation is new (resulting from yesterday's overexertion) or has been there for months, or even years, massage still helps to move the fluid and relieve the pain. The only difference is the amount of time that needs to be employed to get the job done.

Deep Breathing

Deep breathing also increases lymphatic flow and oxygenates the tissues, which helps ease pain. I've lead people through deep breathing exercises in a class and at the end of the exercise had people report that headaches and muscle aches were gone. Deep breathing can be used in conjunction with any of the primary pain relief techniques we've already discussed. See the *Deep Breathing* strategy.

Lymphasizing

Another excellent method of moving the lymphatics is to gently bounce up and down on a mini trampoline. Dr. C. Samuel West, one of my early mentors, popularized the use of mini trampolines as a means of improving lymphatic movement. He called the technique lymphasizing. When combined with deep breathing, gentle bouncing moves congested lymphatics in a very powerful way. Combined with massage and stroking, it can do wonders to help ease pain.

When doing the gentle bounce on the mini-trampoline your feet should not leave the mat as you bounce up and down. This is not jumping, just bouncing.

As with the previously mentioned techniques, lymphasizing is something we do instinctively to ease pain and provide comfort to children. Remember the lymphatic system has no pump, so a tiny baby doesn't get a lot of lymphatic movement when they are just lying there. The lymphatic stagnation starts causing the infant pain and discomfort. Mom and dad instinctively know what to do. They pick up the baby and start bouncing or rocking the child.

This same bouncing motion can work to ease pain and distress when older children or even adults are sick. I've held a child with an earache or respiratory congestion in my arms and gently bounced up and down on a mini trampoline to help ease the pain. I've done the same thing for myself when I've been sick. One can even lymphasize a person who can't stand up, such as a person confined to a wheelchair. Simply have the person put their legs on the mini trampoline while another person gently bounces up and down on the mat.

Apply Electrical Energy

When the cells are not getting sufficient oxygen and nutrients (due to excess fluid in the tissue spaces), the cell's electrical field is diminished. This was discussed in the introduction. Fredrick Plogg, M.D., who has worked with lymphatics in Germany, maintains that the diminished electrical effect is what causes the blood proteins to cluster together in the tissue spaces, making it difficult for them to be removed by the lymphatic system. He indicates further that the application of energy, any energy for that matter, into the clustered plasma proteins will cause them to break up, making them easier for the lymphatics to move.

There are many devices on the market today which use electrical stimulation or magnets to help ease pain. Piezo-generated electric spark appliances are good examples. These

devices emit a small static electric shock, like one gets from rubbing one's feet on a carpet. I've had one of these devices for years and have used it to ease headaches, muscle aches. and other pains. I apply the static electric spark to the inflamed area, then follow with stroking, and massage.

I've also tried the use of devices that generate micro electrical currents. They are particularly helpful for easing pain and promoting healing with older injuries and chronic pain. I've also experimented with magnets and found them to be effective as well.

Special Notes on Dealing With Chronic Pain

Working on chronic pain with these techniques takes longer because once tissues have become swollen, they become stretched. Dr. C. Samuel West likened it to repeatedly blowing up the same balloon. Each time the balloon is stretched by being blown up, it becomes easier and easier to blow up because it starts to lose its elasticity. The same thing happens with a chronic injury. The longer the tissues stay swollen, the more they lose structural tone, and the easier it becomes for them to become swollen again.

This is why many people who have had a severe injury in their body will notice that the site of that injury is more prone to inflammation than areas where the tissue was never damaged. Old injuries to knees, ankles, shoulders, etc., often ache after only minor irritations to the body such as weather changes or poor food choices. However, this tendency can be lessened, if not completely corrected.

The key is to understand that sites of chronic inflammation will require many massages over an extended period of time to break up the stagnation and help tissues heal. Dr. West taught that if you could make the pain go away by massaging the area you could get the tissues to heal. The secret, he taught, was to not wait until the pain returned before you massaged the area again.

You see, what most people do is to rub the pain until it eases a little or stops. Then, they wait until the pain comes back before the rub it again. If you massage something until the pain stops, this means you've cleared the stagnation out of the tissues. If you wait until the pain returns before you rub or massage again, you've allowed the tissues to return back to the same stagnant state they were in before. So if you rub and the pain goes away for four hours, then repeat the massaging action every two hours (even when you don't feel the pain) for several weeks. Remarkable pain relief and healing has occurred from following this simple plan. The effect can also be enhanced by using other techniques such as the topical application of herbs and improvements in diet.

For example, I injured my knee and wrist in a moped accident many years ago. For years, my knee ached every time I tried to run or exert it. I started a program of massaging around my knee several times every day, often applying a *Topical Analgesic Formula*. I also tried to eat a healthier diet. Within one month I was able to run without pain for the first time in several years. So I have firsthand experience with the effectiveness of working consistently on old injuries or sites of chronic pain using these techniques.

You can learn more about these techniques and how to apply them to specific types of pain and injury in my *Fundamentals of Natural Healing* course.

Meditation

In 1976 Dr. Herbert Bensen wrote a now-famous book, *The Relaxation Response*. Dr. Bensen documented how using a simple meditation technique can reduce stress levels and stress-related illness. Dr. Benson's contribution was to remove the religious overtones from meditation and document its benefits scientifically. He devised a simple nonreligious meditative technique that anyone can use to reduce stress levels.

There are three steps to doing a nonreligious, physically and mentally relaxing meditation.

First, get into a comfortable position, either sitting or lying down, and consciously allow the muscles of your body to relax.

Second, start breathing slowly and deeply.

Third, create a single point of mental focus so that you can stop the flow of obsessive thoughts in your brain (sometimes referred to as monkey chatter). Dr. Benson simply had the person repeat the word *one* over and over again in their mind. Another simple technique is to count with your breathing. As you breath in and out you think, "In two three four; Hold two three four; Out two three four; Hold two three four;" And repeat this pattern over and over.

Quieting the mind allows the brain to stop signaling the release of stress chemicals through the hypothalamus, resulting in a rapid reduction of stress levels. It can help reduce anxiety and feelings of stress, improve sleep, lower blood pressure, and improve overall mental and emotional health.

Mineralization

Your body is literally composed of minerals (i.e., "the dust of the earth"). Because of this, healthy bodies are connected to healthy soil. If any element is missing from the soil, then it will be missing from the foods you eat, and as a result, you will not be properly nourished.

Unfortunately, commercial methods of agriculture are depleting the soil of trace minerals and destroying the ability of plants to be able to utilize those elements. Hence, food is nutritionally deficient right from the start. To make matters worse, as food is refined and processed, more of its nutri-

tional content is removed. The reasons people are mineral deficient is explained in more detail in the introduction under "healing strategy 3" in the introduction.

Most people need something to supplement their mineral intake. When seeking to obtain minerals, the first source people should be encouraged to use is mineral-rich plants. This is because the minerals in plants are more bioavailable to the body. Consider using *Joan Patton's Herbal Minerals Formula*. Directions for making it can be found in this book.

Another way human beings get minerals is colloidal minerals. Colloidal minerals are made by using a mineral-rich rock that helps form mineral springs, which have long been sought out for their healing benefits. A *Colloidal Minerals Formula* is essentially concentrated mineral water and are a great way to increase trace mineral intake.

Oral Chelation

Hardening of the arteries is a precursor to cardiovascular disease, the leading cause of death in the United States. Intravenous chelation is a controversial but effective therapy many people have used to help reverse hardening of the arteries. Oral chelation is an alternative to intravenous chelation.

The idea that one can reverse arterial plaque with supplements is very controversial. Most medical people think it can't be done. However, there are many people who have experienced dramatic improvement in their circulation (verified by doctors) and major improvements in their health using this procedure.

Oral chelation isn't just for improving circulation, either. It can help a wide variety of health problems, including helping to detoxify the body from heavy metals.

It is very important to start slowly with this program and work up as instructed. Otherwise, symptoms, such as nausea, dizziness, headaches, and skin eruptions, may occur. It is also important to taper off as instructed, or fatigue and temporary nutritional deficiencies may result.

For the first week, take the following with breakfast and dinner:

　　1 tablet of the *Oral Chelation Formula*

　　-1/2 ounce of a *Colloidal Minerals Formula*

Each week increase the dosage of *Oral Chelation Formula* by one tablet. So the second week, take two tablets twice daily, and on the third week take three tablets twice daily. Gradually increase the amount of minerals as well, until you are taking one ounce in the morning and one ounce at night.

A full dose of *Oral Chelation Formula* is four to six tablets twice daily, depending on body weight. Persons over 200—225 pounds should probably take the full six tablets per day. People who weigh less than 125—150 pounds may be able to take only four tablets twice daily. Individuals of average height and weight should find five tablets two times per day (for a total of ten per day) sufficient. When you reach full dose, you will be taking the following with breakfast and dinner:

4-6 tablets of *Oral Chelation Formula*

1 ounce of a *Colloidal Mineral Formula*

You will need to stay on this full dose for a minimum of one month for each ten years of your age. Thus, if you are forty you need to stay on the full dose for at least four months, six months if you are sixty, and so forth. If you have serious problems, you should consider staying on the program for one and a half months for every ten years of your life. That is, six months if you are forty and nine months if you are sixty.

It is important to taper off in a similar manner to building up. On the full program you are taking very large doses of certain vitamins and minerals and the body gets lazy about extracting them from food. Hence, if you quit all at once, your body may experience a sudden drop in nutrient levels until it readjusts to absorbing these vitamins and minerals from food.

Taper off by reducing the amount you take by two tablets each week. So if you were taking five tablets twice daily, then take four tablets twice daily for a week. The next week drop it to three tablets twice daily and so forth until you reach one tablet twice daily. After that, you can either discontinue the program entirely, or stay on a maintenance dose of one tablet twice daily. Many elderly people find that they do well using one or two tablets of the *Oral Chelation Formula* twice daily in place of a multivitamin and mineral supplement.

As the body removes the plaque from the walls of the arteries, the cholesterol level in the blood will temporarily rise. This is normal. The kidneys and liver will remove the calcium, cholesterol, and other impurities from the body. If there are indications that these organs are weak it may be necessary to give them extra support as follows:

For persons with kidney weakness (history of symptoms like arthritis, chronic back pain, urinary infections, etc.), take the *Chinese Water-Increasing Formula* as directed on the bottle. You can also put one-half teaspoon each of *Liquid Kidney Formula* and *Liquid Lymph Formula* into a quart of water and sip this throughout the day.

For persons with liver weakness (history of high cholesterol, skin problems, digestive upset, etc.), take one heaping teaspoon of a *Fiber Blend* in a large glass of water or juice upon arising and again before retiring. Be sure to drink plenty of water when taking fiber. Also take the *Chinese Wood-Decreasing Formula* as directed on the bottle.

You may also wish to add some of the following supplements for special problems. These are suggested full doses.

You can work up gradually on taking these supplements as well.

For heart problems take two hawthorn berries with each meal. Also take 200-400 mg. of Co-Q10 daily.

For senility, Alzheimer's, or other problems with memory, use the *Memory Enhancing Formula* as directed on the bottle.

For varicose veins and high risk of stroke take two butcher's broom with each meal or one *Vein Tonic Formula* twice daily.

For heavy metal detoxification take one *Heavy Metal Cleansing Formula* along with two to three capsules of sodium alginate twice daily.

For dissolving calcium deposits or calcifications, take two hydrangea and 400 mg. of magnesium twice daily.

For high blood pressure consider using the *Nitric Oxide Boosting Formula* daily or taking one capsule of a *Blood Pressure Reducing Formula* three times daily.

The *Cardiovascular Nutritional Program* will offer many of the benefits of the oral chelation formula and can also be used with any of the above products for special needs.

Pleasure Prescription

A pleasurable experience does more good for your body than a stressful experience does harm, so one of the secrets to reducing stress is to make time for relaxation and pleasure. People in modern society tend to be workaholics who are busy twenty-four hours a day, seven days a week. The body heals when we're relaxed, so creating a relaxed peaceful environment is essential for recovery from many illnesses.

Taking one day a week to rest and contemplate the higher meaning of life can be a real blessing. It's also important to get in touch with what you need physically and emotionally and create pleasant, happy, relaxing experiences every day, or preferably several times a day if you're recovering from a serious illness.

People often complain they are too busy to do this, but making this time "sharpens your saw"—meaning it makes you more productive with the rest of your week or day. So the busier you are, the more you need to do this.

Make a list of ten things that bring you physical pleasure and plan time to do at least one of these things every day, or at least three or four times per week. Pleasurable activities to consider include:

Taking a warm bath or soaking in a hot tub

Engaging in crafts or hobbies that you enjoy

Getting a massage

Listening to positive and uplifting music

Engaging in a relaxing sporting activity (such as fishing or golf)

Taking a walk (especially in nature)

Savoring a delicious treat

Sharing affection with your spouse or children

This time could also involve developing your spiritual nature by doing things like the following:

Meditating or praying

Reading or studying Scriptures or other spiritually uplifting books

Contemplating the meaning and purpose of your life and setting positive goals

Poultice

A poultice is a mixture of crushed fresh herbs or dried herbs moistened with water to make a paste. The crushed herbs or paste are applied topically. It is similar to a compress, but plant parts are used rather than a liquid extraction.

To make a poultice with fresh herbs, simply crush, chop, or mash the fresh plant parts and apply them topically. To make a poultice with dried herbs, use a base of mucilaginous herbs like comfrey root, slippery elm, or marshmallow and add other herbs to it. Add enough water to form a thick paste. You can also make a paste of herbs using aloe vera gel. Apply the paste directly to the skin.

Poultices can be covered with a gauze bandage or other dressing. Change the poultice at least once or twice daily. For treating bites and stings, change hourly.

Herbs to Consider for Poultices

Aloe Vera: good for moistening other herb powders in place of water to bind poultice; cooling, moisturizing, anti-inflammatory

Calendula: astringent, cooling, drying, styptic; good for deep/infected wounds

Comfrey leaf: vulnerary, soothing, absorbs, mild astringent; not for deep wounds

Comfrey root: binding and drawing agent; soothing, moistening

Flaxseed: lubricating, emollient, softening, nutritive, warming

Goldenseal: astringent, vulnerary, antiseptic; good for skin ulceration

Lobelia: antipoisonous, stimulates lymphatic drainage, relaxing for spasms and cramps

Lily of the valley: use fresh leaves only; very drawing, pulls slivers and pus, disinfecting

Marshmallow: binding, soothing, cooling, moistening

Pine gum: very drawing, pulls slivers; disinfectant, warming, drying and astringent

Plantain: drawing, anti-inflammatory, mildly astringent; antipoisonous, fresh leaves are one of the best poultices for insect bites; stimulates lymphatic drainage

Psyllium seeds: binding, mildly drawing; absorbs moisture

Slippery Elm: binding and drawing agent; cooling, soothing, nutritive

White Oak bark: astringent, cooling, drying

Yarrow: astringent, drying, stimulating; good for deep/infected wounds; helpful for arresting bleeding

Non-Herbal Items to Consider for Poultices

Clay: drying, drawing and binding; pulls heavy metals and irritants from tissues

Charcoal: draws toxins; helpful for spider bites (mix with aloe vera gel to make sticky and change hourly); helpful for infected wounds, pulls pus and infection

Instant potato flakes: can be mixed with the juice of a fresh herb (plantain juice or fresh plant tincture) for an instant poultice

Reduce Chemical Exposure

In little more than one hundred years our world has been miraculously transformed by advances in technology. This scientific progress has blessed and enriched our lives and part of it has been the creation of hundreds of thousands of new chemicals.

These chemicals keep our clothes wrinkle-free and make our carpets and upholstery stain-resistant. They control insects in our home and garden and kill weeds and insects that would destroy our food supply. They preserve our foods, keep food production facilities sterile, and prevent food from sticking to our pans.

Chemicals are also used to manufacture personal care products (deodorants, toothpaste, shampoo, lotions, make-up), household cleaning products (laundry detergents, dish soap, stain removers) and in the very materials used to make our homes, furnishings, and clothing. A group of chemicals called plastics allow us to create containers for food, beverages, and numerous other products. These plastics also allow manufacturers to create many cheap, useful, and often disposable items and gadgets.

These are just a few examples of the way modern chemistry has transformed our lives. Without it we would not have cars, planes, cell phones, computers, or any of the other conveniences of modern life.

The Toxic Burden of Our Chemical World

Unfortunately, as with many things in life, there is also a downside to our to all of this. These chemicals are now found in our air, water, soil, and food supply throughout the earth, and we are experiencing exposure to chemicals on a scale never before seen in human history. Unfortunately, the health impact of these chemicals is yet to be fully understood. But, with over ninety thousand chemicals in current use and growing signs of their toxicity to human and animal life, we may be facing a global health crisis.

The most vulnerable of our population are children. In one rather-alarming study, blood was taken from the umbilical cords of ten newborn infants. Over 287 toxic chemicals were found in this blood. On average each blood sample contained about 200 environmental toxins. These included dioxins, flame retardants, Teflon, pesticides, and industrial chemicals. These chemicals were stored in the mother's body and crossed the placenta to wind up in the infant's body as it was developing in the womb.

Although the concentrations were small, toxins can have synergistic effects—meaning that small amounts of many toxins can be as large a health risk as larger amounts of a single toxin. Of the 287 chemicals discovered in this blood, 134 are known to cause cancer in lab animals or people, 151 are associated with birth defects, 154 are endocrine disrupters, and 130 were immune system toxins.

Symptoms of the Growing Toxic Burden

The overall chemical burden modern society is experiencing helps explain the sharp increases in many ailments affecting children. For example, acute lymphocytic leukemia has increased in children by 84 percent. Childhood brain cancers have increased 57 percent.

The nervous system seems particularly vulnerable as many chemicals are fat-soluble, which means they are attracted to the fatty tissues of the brain and nervous system. Toxins may be responsible for the growing problems with autism-spectrum disorder which now affects about 1 in 110 children. Other growing neurological problems in children include ADD, ADHD, Tourette's syndrome, stuttering, delayed speech development, dyslexia, and behavioral disorders.

Environmental toxins affect adult nervous systems as well and may be contributing factors in anxiety, depression, insomnia, numbness, tingling, brain fog, sleep apnea, dementia, and mental illness. Because many of these toxins get stored in fat, the inability of many adults to lose weight may be another sign of toxic overload. The body simply does not want to let go of the fat because it can't deal with the toxins stored in it.

Since many of these chemicals are endocrine disrupters, they may also be responsible for increasing reproductive problems in both men and women. Chemicals may cause premature breast development in girls and contribute to PMS, uterine fibroids, tender breasts, and heavy menstrual bleeding in women. Boys may have undescended testicles,

develop breasts, and have delayed onset of puberty due to these chemicals. In adult men, they may cause infertility, prostate problems, and low testosterone levels. See the *Avoid Xenoestrogens* strategy for more information.

Other possible signs our body is overburdened with these chemicals include general fatigue, frequent muscle and joint pain, frequent headaches, chronic, low-grade infections (such as chronic sinus problems), and skin conditions (like eczema, psoriasis, and rosacea, dermatitis, and itchy skin). These toxins may also depress and confuse the immune system, which may contribute to autoimmune disorders and cancer.

Protecting from Chemical Overload

Here are a few basic rules to follow to minimize our exposure to potentially harmful chemicals.

First, drink the purest water you can find. Purchase some kind of water filtration system, such as a reverse-osmosis system coupled with carbon filtration or at the very least some kind of water filter, especially if you live in a heavily industrialized area or in an area where there is a lot of commercial agriculture. You can also buy treated water from most grocery stores using reusable containers. Avoid bottled water, especially in soft plastic bottles, as the plastic leaches chemicals. Water is one of the best, if it's pure, and drinking pure water is also a way to help your body detoxify.

Second, eat organic food or food that has been raised without chemicals wherever possible. Also purchase food that is free of chemical additives, such as preservatives, natural and artificial flavorings, food colorings and artificial sweeteners. Wash produce with natural soap and rinse well before eating it to remove pesticide residues, too.

Third, remember that for most people the number one place they are exposed to environmental toxins is within the walls of their own homes. So select the most natural, non-toxic products you can afford for all household uses. This means using natural laundry soap, dish soap, and other household cleaning products. If you put it on your skin it's going to be absorbed into your body, so also find natural toothpaste, shampoo, deodorants, lotions, and cosmetics. Also use non-toxic methods to control household pests.

Fourth, if you work around any chemicals in the workplace, be sure to follow proper safety protocols. Many people do not think about the fact that they are routinely exposed to chemicals at work, but examples of professions where there is chemical exposure include janitors, carpet cleaners, beauticians, hair dressers, house painters, dry cleaners, auto mechanics, print shop workers, builders, farmers, gardeners, and welders.

Fifth, if you live in an area where there is air pollution invest in a filtration system for your home and/or office.

A good option is the boomerang, which uses a technology developed for NASA (hypoair.com/boomerang/).

To assist the body to detoxify from chemical exposure see the *Detoxification* and *Liver Detoxification* strategies. Also look at the suggestions under the conditions *Chemical Exposure* and *Heavy Metal Poisoning*.

Reduce EMF Exposure

In modern society, we are constantly exposed to electromagnetic frequencies (EMFs) from computers, microwave ovens, radar, TV sets, digital clocks, and other electrical items. Cell phones are another growing source of electromagnetic pollution, and many people in the natural health community are concerned about the potential problems with the new 5G technology. While the research is not yet clear, evidence suggests there may be a link between electromagnetic pollution and cancer. Electromagnetic radiation may also reduce immunity and make one more susceptible to viral infections.

Minimize your exposure to these energy fields by keeping digital clocks and other electronic devices at least three feet away from your head while sleeping, keeping some distance between yourself and computers and TV sets (such as not using a laptop computer on your lap), wearing a headset when using a cell phone, avoiding microwave ovens, not sleeping on electric blankets, and turning off your WiFi at night. Mimize time spent on cell phones and other electrical devices. Also, avoid living near cell phone towers, electrical substations and high voltage power lines.

There are a number of devices in the marketplace that are reported to help reduce the negative effects of electromagnetic pollution, such as Wayne Cook's Diodes, which were the first devices I tried. I've used several other brands as well and have seen positive benefits from their use. Simply carrying a small magnet in your left pocket seems to have a similar effect.

My midwife friend, Joan Patton, claimed that fresh horse chestnut seeds would work as natural diodes. I've tried them and they do seem to work too. You can find a list of natural remedies that help reduce the effects of electromagnetic radiation on your body under the condition *Electromagnetic Pollution*.

Sleep

Getting shortchanged occasionally on your sleep isn't a serious problem, but when it happens night after night, you build up a backlog of needed sleep. This sleep debt adversely affects your mood, health, and safety.

The average person needs around eight and one-half hours of sleep every night. You might need a little less or a little more, but you need this sleep every day, just like you need water and oxygen every day. Losing just one hour of sleep per day (seven hours instead of eight, for instance) builds up a "sleep debt."

It's not just the quantity of sleep that you need; it's also the quality of that sleep. You need several hours of REM (rapid eye movement) sleep every night to be healthy. This is the sleep where you dream. When catching up on sleep-debt, your body will often "compress" sleep patterns to catch up on this much-needed REM sleep.

You also need a certain amount of deep sleep. During the deepest stages of sleep, your body releases growth hormone to stimulate tissue repair and regeneration. This means that if you don't get enough good-quality sleep, it will adversely affect your physical health.

For instance, sleep debt makes you more likely to catch a cold or the flu. In fact, sleep deprivation can actually cause flu-like symptoms without an infection. Sleep debt even makes you more prone to heart disease and stroke.

Lack of sleep also affects your mood and your performance. It makes it harder for you to concentrate, which means you're not as productive at work. Sleep debt can make you irritable or depressed and otherwise affect your mood. You even age more quickly when you don't get enough sleep.

Another major problem with sleep debt is that it causes you to be more accident-prone. About one hundred thousand automobile accidents occur due to sleep deprivation every year, resulting in fifteen hundred deaths and about 12.5 billion dollars in damages. Numerous industrial accidents are also caused by a lack of sleep. The famous Exxon Valdez oil spill in Alaska was not caused by alcohol as most people think. In the trial, it was found that sleepiness was the actual cause. It cost 2 billion dollars to clean up that spill and Exxon was fined 5 billion dollars.

The bad news is that one-half of all Americans suffer from some degree of insomnia, and about one-third suffer from life-disrupting insomnia. So a large percentage of the population is suffering from sleep debt and/or poor-quality sleep.

Many adults in America only get about six to seven hours of sleep, or less. This isn't enough to be healthy. If you want to be healthy, you should try to get about eight to nine hours of sleep each night. You may need more if you're recovering from injuries, stress, or chronic illness. If you have trouble sleeping, see the condition *Insomnia* for information on how to overcome this problem.

Stress Management

It has been estimated that 75—90 percent of all visits to primary care physicians are for stress-related health problems. So learning how to manage stress is a major key to maintaining good health.

When the brain perceives stress, it sends a chemical message to the pituitary via the hypothalamus, which triggers the release of the adrenocorticotropic hormone (ACTH). ACTH causes the adrenals to start producing hormones like epinephrine (adrenaline) and cortisol. Epinephrine is both a hormone and neurotransmitter. It tenses muscles, increases heart rate and blood pressure, dilates the bronchi and speeds up breathing, shuts down digestion and other functions not essential to immediate survival, and otherwise prepares the body for action.

Cortisol reduces inflammation, which helps to deal better with injury and pain. Although it's role in reducing inflammation is important, too much cortisol causes premature aging, depresses immune function, and leads to loss of muscle and weight gain. Stress-related hormones also cause a rise in blood sugar levels and an increase in blood clotting factors.

With this understanding, it's easy to see how chronic, long-term stress can become a factor in numerous health problems, including poor digestive function, constipation, tension headaches, neck and shoulder pain, low back pain, ulcers, high blood pressure, blood clotting, increased risk of infections, asthma, diabetes, excess weight, and even cancer and autoimmune disorders. In fact, it is probable that a large percentage of all the illness has a stress component.

If stress can cause so many health problems, it's obvious that you need to know how to reduce stress to both prevent and heal from these health issues. And while you may not be able to eliminate all the stressful situations in your life, you can reduce the stressful effects these problems cause.

Here are seven keys to reducing the effects of stress on the body.

1. Breathe Deeply

One of the simplest things you can do to reduce your stress level, calm your anxiety, and relieve the tension in your body is to just breathe. If you stop and notice what happens when you are feeling stressed, you will probably notice that you are either holding your breath or breathing very rapidly and shallowly. By concentrating on breathing slowly and deeply, you will activate the parasympathetic nervous system and help reduce your stress levels. You can also try breathing in while thinking, "I am," and out while thinking, "Relaxed." See *Deep Breathing* strategy for more information.

2. Practice Meditation

You can take the breathing a step further by utilizing the simple form of meditation Dr. Herbert Benson dubbed "The Relaxation Response." In 1975, Dr. Benson published his book of that title showing how a simple, non-religious meditation technique could help patients with insomnia, heart problems, high blood pressure and chronic pain. See the *Meditation* strategy for instructions. Taking just 20 minutes a day for this process (or any other form of meditation) will dramatically reduce stress levels.

3. Avoid Caffeine and Sugar

Have you ever noticed how attractive junk food is when you are under stress? Sugar and caffeine may give you a quick pick-up, but they'll let you down just as fast. Even worse, they tend to further stress the adrenal glands, which eventually will tire and give you that burned-out feeling. To reduce stress, avoid sugar-sweetened, high carbohydrate snacks in favor of snacks high in protein and good-quality fats (like nuts, jerky, or organic cheese). If you feel tired without caffeine, consider taking an *Adrenal Glandular, Chinese Qi-Increasing,* or *Chinese Fire-Increasing Formula* to rebuild your adrenals and increase your energy.

4. Hydrate

This may seem strange, but drinking more water can actually make your nerves feel calmer and help you sleep more soundly. Dehydration increases anxiety levels, so drink plenty of purified water when you are under stress. See the *Hydration* strategy for information.

5. Exercise

What are those stress hormones for? They're gearing your body up to take physical action, and that's what makes modern stress such a big problem. The stress hormones gear your body to run, fight, or physically work to combat the problem, but a sedentary lifestyle doesn't burn off these stress hormones in physical activity. Even light exercise, like walking, will help work off those stressful feelings. See the *Exercise* strategy for ideas.

6. Feed Your Nerves and Take Adaptogens

Nerves, like any other part of the body need nutrition. For starters, nerves need good quality fats like butter, coconut oil, nuts, olive oil, flax seed oil and omega-3 essential fatty acids.

Vitamins are also important for nerve functions. Many people have found that B-complex vitamins help them cope with stress more easily. Vitamin C and pantothenic acid are also helpful because they support the adrenal glands. Many people find the *Anti-Stress B-Complex Formula* helpful for counteracting stress.

Silica helps the nerves become more resilient because it strengthens the myelin sheath. It is found in the herbs horsetail and dulse, which are key ingredients in *Watkin's Hair, Skin, and Nails Formula.*

There is a specific class of herbs that has been shown to greatly reduce the impact of stress on your health. These herbs are called adaptogens. Adaptogenic herbs modulate the signals that are sent from the hypothalamus and pituitary glands causing a reduction of adrenal output of adrenaline and cortisol, thus lowering overall stress levels. They help to break the damaging fight-or-flight chain reaction patterns in which the body gets stuck due to chronic stress. By reducing cortisol levels, these herbs also help boost the immune system.

Eleuthero root was the first to be identified as an adaptogen. Russian studies proved it helps increase stamina, endurance and energy, improve concentration and stimulate male hormone production. It also helps the immune system response. Other single herbs that have been identified as possessing adaptogenic properties include gotu kola, American and Korean ginseng, suma, and schizandra berries. Although you can take single adaptagens, for the best effect, try using any of the adaptagen formulas listed in this book, such as the *Adaptogen-Immune*, *Suma Adaptogen*, or *Ashwagandha Complex Formula*.

7. Make Time for Rest and Relaxation

Telling someone to reduce stress is like telling them to avoid death and taxes—it just isn't going to happen. The good news is you don't have to avoid stress to reduce its effects. It turns out that a pleasurable experience causes the release of hormones and neurotransmitters that counteract the effects of stress. And, a pleasurable experience creates more positive benefits than a stressful experience causes harm. So instead of focusing on reducing stress, start deliberately creating pleasure and enjoyment in your life. See the *Pleasure Prescription* strategy.

Part of this is also making sure you are getting a good night's sleep. See the *Sleep* strategy. If you aren't, look up the condition *Insomnia* and follow some of the suggestions there.

Practicing these principles of stress management will not only help you stay healthy, it will also help you heal more quickly if you are sick.

Sweat Bath

Many people in temperate climates the world over have used sweating both to prevent and treat disease. Scandinavians built saunas; Native Americans built sweat lodges. Samuel Thomson would wrap a person sitting in a chair in blankets and place a hot stone in a pail at his feet. By pouring water into the pail, the steam would come up under the blankets until the patient started to perspire.

During his college years Thomas Easley used a hot plate with a pan of water on it. By administering a sudorific formula with extra lobelia and steaming fellow students for about twenty minutes, they were able to knock out all kinds of acute illnesses.

With modern hot running water and bathtubs, inducing perspiration to clear toxins isn't that difficult. Start by drinking plenty of fluids.

Sudorific herbs are herbs that enhance perspiration. They move blood to the surface of the skin and help to open the sweat glands to promote elimination. You can also make a warm tea of any sudorific herb or formula with warm liquids. Some of the best herbs for this purpose include yarrow, capsicum, ginger, catnip, and blue vervain. Helpful sudorific formulas include *Fire Cider*, *Ed Millet's Herbal Crisis*, *Steven Horne's Children's Composition*, or *Herbal Composition*. Dilute these formulas in warm liquids to make a tea.

After drinking the tea, draw a bath as hot as can be comfortably tolerated. Add to the water a couple of tablespoons of ginger powder, a handful of yarrow, rosemary, or mint leaves, or other aromatic herbs. Put the herbs in a cloth bag so the leaves don't get all over in the tub. Another, even easier, sweat bath water treatment is to put about five to ten drops of an essential oil such as lavender, tea tree, eucalyptus, or peppermint in the bath. Dissolve the oils in a little liquid soap before putting them into the bath-water so they will mix with the water and don't just float on the surface.

After getting out of the bath, don't dry off. Wrap up in a cotton sheet and go to bed. Pile on the blankets and allow the sweat to come freely. It's fine to fall asleep. When done, take a cool shower to cleanse the skin and close your pores. Don't allow chilling during the process.

With small children, don't put them into a really hot bath. Use a warm bath, and gently wash the child's body down with some natural soap (such as Dr. Bronners) and a washcloth to make certain the pores are open. Adding just a small amount of lavender essential oil or tea tree essential oil to the bath (again mixed with soap to make sure it dissolves). You can also use a natural soap that has essential oils in it will help to stimulate the circulation and draw the blood to the extremities.

I have found sweat baths to be helpful for all types of acute ailments, especially colds, fevers, flu, sinus congestion, rashes, and earaches. Sweat baths are not recommended for people who are infirm, elderly, or have heart conditions.

Section Four

Conditions

Conditions, Ailments, and Health Problems

This section contains specific conditions, ailments and health problems. Under each condition you will also find the following information.

A list of related health conditions (*See also*): These are other health problems that may be associated with or have similar root causes to the condition you are trying to resolve. Many health problems are interconnected, meaning they arise from the same root causes. So, you may wish to look up the related conditions and read about them, too. If a remedy or strategy shows up under more than one of the conditions you have, it's very likely that it is going to help improve your overall health. Include it in your healing strategy.

A description of the condition and possible natural solutions: After the related conditions (see also) you will find one or more paragraphs talking about the condition. We start by explaining what the condition is and perhaps some basic statistics and information about the problem. Then, we discuss various strategies that can help to resolve that condition.

Where a particular symptom or problem can have many different causes, we've tried to address the most common underlying causes and provide you with information that will help you determine if those causes apply to the person who has this problem. For each potential cause, we list strategies and remedies that may be helpful. Some conditions list many options as possible remedies because there are many possible root causes. Please carefully review this material as it will help you select the right strategies and natural remedies to correct the problem at its roots.

Some conditions are serious and potentially life-threatening. In these cases, self-treatment is not wise. Where we encourage you to seek medical attention, *please do so*. Even if you opt to go the natural route for these problems, you should be monitored by modern medical testing to make sure you're on the right track. You may also want to seek out the help of a qualified herbalist or naturopath for serious health issues.

A list of helpful diet and lifestyle changes and other useful basic *Strategies*: Next we provide a list of strategies that can be helpful in eliminating the root causes of the problem. As explained in the introduction, building your overall health is an important step in getting well. So, before thinking about herbs and supplements, read about the recommended strategies listed under the condition.

Lists of various types of products that may be helpful for the condition: Finally, we give a list of remedies that may be helpful for this condition. We've highlighted our personal favorites in bold. We've also broken down the products into types, so you can get an idea of different kinds of products you might use. Here are the product types:

Formulas: These are formulas that only contain multiple ingredients. Formulas combine several herbs and/or nutrients that deal with a particular problem. This means that a well-chosen formula will often work better than a single herb or nutrient because of the synergy of the ingredients. That's why it is easier for beginners to get results with formulas. Formulas also have a wide margin of safety, so you can safely double or sometimes triple the recommended dose on the label. This should be done for short periods only, and the dose lowered as health improves. Formulas will often help to heal a problem, which means that they will not need to be taken forever.

FDA and FTC regulations make it legally dangerous for us to list the actual trade names of these formulas and the names of companies that sell them. So we have created generic names for them. Look the formulas up in the "Remedies" section and do an internet search for formulas with the listed key ingredients. A formula doesn't have to have all the key ingredients to be effective, just most of them. You can also become a member at stevenhorne.com to get help finding formulas.

Programs: There are some pre-packaged programs which contain multiple formulas, herbs and supplements. These programs are generally even more broad acting than formulas. Where appropriate, consider using one of these programs to balance your body and improve your overall health.

Flower Essence Blends: Where appropriate, we've listed flower essence blends that may be helpful for the condition. Flower essences are emotional remedies. They don't actually work on the physical health issue, but they can help with underlying emotional issues. In the introduction we explain that the first step in your strategy for healing should be dealing with your mental and emotional state. So, where flower essences are recommended, don't overlook this important step in your strategy for healing.

Essential Oil Blends: Aromatherapy has both physical and mental/emotional benefits. Blends of essential oils that may be helpful for the condition will be listed where appropriate. Do not use these blends internally. They are best inhaled or applied topically. Use them as directed on the label. See *Aromatherapy* in the *Strategies Section* for instructions on how to use these essential oils safely.

Herbs: These are often many single herbs that may be helpful for a particular problem. Which herbs will be the most helpful depends on the underlying causes for the condition? So, single herbs work best when the overall energetics and properties of the herb are matched to the overall pattern of health problems in the person. It is often harder for beginners to get consistent results with singles, but single herbs can have wonderful results when they are properly matched to the overall symptoms and constitution of the person.

Supplements: These are single vitamins, minerals, nutrients and phyochemicals that can also help various conditions. Like single herbs, these supplements are more targeted to specific deficiencies. Since the body does not use nutrients in isolation, single nutrients are generally best used temporarily for specific therapeutic purposes. They do not need to be taken forever, only until health improves. For health maintenance purposes, it is generally best to use formulas.

Abrasions/Scratches

See also wounds & sores

An abrasion is an injury caused by the scraping away of a portion of skin or mucous membrane. Scratches are wounds to the skin from sliding contact with sharp or rough objects. Abrasions and scratches can be treated naturally with topical applications (*Poultice* or *Compress or Fomentation* strategy) of the key herbs listed below. If there is a concern about an infection, use an antiseptic essential oil or silver. Vitamin E or a poultice of gotu kola can be applied topically to help prevent scarring. Topical application of plantain can help to draw dirt out of abrasions.

Strategies: Aromatherapy, Compress or Fomentation, Lymph-Moving Pain Relief, and Poultice

Formulas: Healing Salve, Enzyme Spray, Liquid Lymph, **Vulnerary**, CBD Topical Analgesic, and Hemp Oil with Terpenes

Flower Essence Blends: Shock and Injury FE

Herbs: Aloe vera, **calendula**, comfrey, goldenseal, **gotu kola**, honeysuckle, **plantain**, Saint John's wort, and yarrow

Supplements: Collagen, **nanoparticle silver**, vitamin C, vitamin E, and zinc

Essential Oils: Cajeput, helichrysum, lavender, and **tea tree**

Abscesses

See also infection (bacterial)

An abscess is an open sore exuding pus, usually surrounded by inflamed tissue; or a covered cavity containing pus. Abscesses form as a response to infection or other foreign objects. Topical remedies are most effective for abscesses. Apply them with the *Compress or Fomentation* or *Poultice* strategy. My favorite topical remedies would be echinacea, plantain, and garlic. Avoid using comfrey and goldenseal topically; they might heal the abscess from the outside in, trapping the infection beneath the skin.

Internally, you can take an kind of a blood purifier or detoxifying formula. Some of the best herbs to use internally would include echinacea, Oregon grape and red clover.

Strategies: Compress or Fomentation and Poultice

Formulas: Blood Purifier, Liquid Lymph, **Healing Salve**, **Drawing Salve**, Lymphatic Infection, **Detoxifying**, and **Alterative-Immune**

Herbs: Amur cork, burdock, **echinacea**, forsythia, fritillary, oregano essential oil, **Oregon grape**, plantain, polygala, **red clover**, thlaspi, usnea, and yarrow

Supplements: Propolis, vitamin C, and vitamin D

Essential Oils: Bay leaf, chamomile (Roman), lemon, and tea tree

Aches   see *pain*

Acid Indigestion
Heartburn, Acid Reflux, GERD

See also hiatal hernia, SIBO, and low stomach acid

Heartburn occurs when the valve at the top of the stomach allows acid to seep back (reflux) into the esophagus. This acid burns and inflames the esophageal lining and creates a burning sensation in the center of the chest, which is why it is called heartburn. One in every four Americans, or about sixty million people, experiences heartburn at least once a month, and almost fifteen million people have heartburn each day.

Although uncomfortable, occasional heartburn is not a serious condition. If it happens frequently and persistently, the repeated burning and inflammation can result in damage to the esophagus that forms scar tissue. The scar tissue can narrow the passageway and increase the risk of esophageal cancer. Chronic heartburn is called gastroesophageal reflux disease (GERD) or acid reflux for short. GERD is surprisingly common, affecting an estimated 5-7 percent of the American population.

Medical Treatment

The medical approach to acid reflux and GERD is to take antacids or acid blockers. While they can be helpful if there are active ulcers that need a chance to heal, they do not fix the problem and have undesirable side effects. By lowering stomach acid, antacids and acid blockers inhibits the breakdown and absorption of calcium and many other minerals, along with a reduced absorption of folate and other vitamins. Over the long term, this can increase your risk of osteoporosis and bone fractures. It can also increase your risk of heart and kidney disease and make you more susceptible to gastric infections.

Strategies for Healing Acid Indigestion and GERD

Most acid indigestion is not caused by an excess of stomach acid. It is frequently a combination of poor mucosal health from stress, the frequent use of NSAIDS, a lack of stomach acid, and poor peristaltic movement of the small intestines. All this leads to poorly digested foods, which facilitates the overgrowth of bacteria and/or yeast in the small intestines. As these bacteria and yeast break down food stuffs they release acid waste and gas, increasing abdominal pressure, pushing the stomach upwards which forces open the lower esophageal sphincter and causes the symptoms of heartburn. Obesity and pregnancy also increase abdominal pressure, causing heartburn. A hiatal hernia will also cause stress on the valve of the stomach and is frequently involved in GERD (See *Hiatal Hernia Correction* strategy.)

For immediate relief from acid indigestion, take bitter herbs with water. In my experience, goldenseal, yellow dock and dandelion are reliable herbs for immediate symptomatic relief.

For severe burning, calcium supplements, especially calcium carbonate, can offer immediate symptomatic relief. This is not a long-term solution, as calcium carbonate reduces HCl production, which creates a vicious cycle of continuing indigestion.

For long-term relief, start by addressing low stomach acid and/or intestinal dysbiosis (see *low stomach acid and SIBO).* If so, correcting these problems will stop your acid indigestion.

If you don't have these problems, try slowing down and chewing your food better, eating only when relaxed, drinking more water between meals, and eating smaller meals. If these solutions don't prove helpful, keep a food journal and try to figure out if there are any specific foods that trigger acid indigestion. You may have a food sensitivity or allergy. Common foods that cause acid indigestion include onions,

peppermint, chocolate, coffee, citrus fruits, tomatoes, garlic, and spicy foods.

If you have a lot of gas and bloating after meals, you may want to try carminative herbs to help the body expel this gas and relieve the bloating and pressure.

Healing Tissue Damage from GERD

To heal damage to the esophagus and digestive tract due to acid reflux, use soothing, mucilaginous remedies. Three of the best remedies are aloe vera juice, licorice, and slippery elm. Sipping small amounts of aloe diluted in water, or sucking on licorice or slippery elm lozenges, soothes the burning or inflammation in the esophagus. Chewable or powdered deglycerized licorice can also help heal the damage and soothe the irritation.

Strategies: Eat Enzyme-Rich Foods, Eliminate Allergy-Causing Foods, Eliminate FODMAPs, Gut-Healing Diet, Hiatal Hernia Correction, Hydration, and Stress Management

Formulas: Christopher's Carminative, **Children's Colic**, Herbal Bitters, Digestive Support, **Papaya Enzyme**, Betaine HCl, **Natural Antacid**, and Intestinal Soothing

Herbs: Aloe vera, blessed thistle, **catnip**, chamomile, chirata, devil's claw, **gentian**, **goldenseal**, **licorice**, **meadowsweet**, orange (bitter), papaya, red raspberry, safflower, slippery elm, turkey rhubarb, and **yellow dock**

Supplements: Calcium, iron, magnesium, sodium alginate, **sodium bicarbonate**, vitamin B-complex, and zinc

Essential Oils: Lemon and peppermint

Acid pH	**see** *overacidity*
Acid Reflux	**see** *acid indigestion*

Acne
Pimples, Blackheads

See also hypothyroidism and leaky gut

Acne is an inflammatory condition of the skin. The small glands that excrete an oily substance to lubricate the skin become irritated and inflamed. They may also become infected and filled with pus.

There are several underlying causes of acne. It may involve poor fat metabolism and a general need to improve the diet and detoxify the body. It may also be due to hormonal fluctuations, lack of proper skin care and may even involve emotional issues.

The strategy to heal acne should start from the inside. Eat a healthier diet and improve the health of the colon, liver, and lymphatics. In particular, avoid hydrogenated fats and replace them with healthier fats. (See the *Healthy Fats* strategy.)

Blood purifiers and liver cleansing formulas are usually helpful. Both burdock and chickweed are blood purifiers that also aid the body in properly metabolizing fats.

Another therapy to consider is higher doses of fat-soluble vitamins, particularly vitamins A and D, which help keep fats from oxidizing. Oxidation causes fats to become rancid and irritating to the body.

One of the reasons teenagers are so prone to acne is that their hormones are out of balance. For this reason, chaste tree berries have also been beneficial in clearing up teenage acne. Other glandular herbs that might be helpful include sarsaparilla (which is also a blood purifier) for teenage boys and dong quai (also a blood tonic) for teenage girls.

In some cases, low thyroid can contribute to this problem. The thyroid hormones are needed to properly combust fats in the body. (See remedies for *hypothyroidism*.)

Cleansing the skin thoroughly to remove excess oil from the glands and to get rid of unwanted microorganisms is also helpful. After cleaning the skin, try blending antiseptic essential oils like tea tree oil with a little hydrated bentonite and use this as a facial mask. Essential oils can also be mixed with a nanoparticle silver gel and applied topically to control infection.

Strategies: Detoxification, Drawing Bath, Eliminate Allergy-Causing Foods, Gut-Healing Diet, Healthy Fats, Increase Dietary Fiber, and Low-Glycemic Diet

Formulas: Blood Purifier, Essiac Immune Tea, **Detoxifying**, Enzyme Spray, **Ayurvedic Skin Healing**, Skinny, General Glandular, **Female Cycle**, Female Tonic, Drawing Salve, and Probiotic

Herbs: Aloe vera, blue flag, **burdock**, chamomile, chaparral, **chaste tree**, chickweed, dandelion, echinacea, Indian madder, kelp, lomatium, milk thistle, **red clover**, and yellow dock

Supplements: Clay (bentonite), **clay (Redmond)**, lipase, MSM, **nanoparticle silver**, potassium, **vitamin A**, vitamin B-complex, vitamin B_5, vitamin B_6, **vitamin D**, and **zinc**

Essential Oils: Bay leaf, chamomile (Roman), copaiba, cypress, eucalyptus, juniper, lavender, lemongrass, ravintsara, red mandarin, sandalwood, and tea tree

ADD/ADHD
Hyperactivity

See also heavy metal poisoning, hypoglycemia, and leaky gut

ADD (attention deficit disorder) and ADHD (attention-deficit hyperactive disorder) are characterized by inappropriate inattention, impulsivity, and hyperactivity. There is a tendency toward haphazard, poorly organized activity. I

have come to believe that true ADHD involves a weakness of the sympathetic nervous system and a corresponding overactivity of the parasympathetic nervous system. These children tend to have very small pupils, and since the parasympathetic nervous system contracts the pupil while the sympathetic nervous system dilates it, this shows that the parasympathetic nervous system tends to dominate.

Pupil size or tonus also provides a useful clue to what type of remedies the child needs to help them calm down. In my experience, it is the children with small pupils (parasympathetic dominance) who are calmed down by the use of small doses of a stimulant like Ritalin (which is an epinephrine mimic, in the same class of drugs as all speed or uppers like cocaine).

It was once thought that Ritalin changed the faulty brain chemistry in children with ADD/ADHD. New research shows that it has the same action on the brain in children with or without ADD/ADHD. Research also shows that the benefits of Ritalin and other stimulants are short-lived, with a return of behavioral problems within five years. Also, use of these stimulants tends to lead to later problems with drug addiction.

Strategies for ADHD

Most kids with ADHD are undernourished, overstimulated, and sleep-deprived. Before you try anything else, there are a few simple steps to take that often improve the symptoms of ADHD.

Eliminate Sugar

From starting the day with sugary breakfast cereals to candy and soda vending machines at school to stores stocked with candy, pastries and sodas, kids are eating their way not only to high dentist bills but also to wild blood sugar swings that make them overly active and unable to pay attention in school. Many teachers note that when kids return from high-sugar-filled lunches and snacks, they "bounce off the walls." Eliminating juice, soda, pastries, candy, and cereals will improve the energy and focus of most sufferers. See the *Avoid Sugar* strategy.

Eat Healthy

Eating a diet of whole foods provides most of the essential nutrients people need. To speed up the improvements found when people become nutritionally replete, add a multiple vitamin and mineral and a little extra magnesium. See the *Eat Healthy* strategy.

Get Adequate Sleep

Children generally need more sleep than adults, typically nine hours. Many children are not getting adequate sleep and need to make up for sleep debt. See the *Sleep* strategy.

Limit Time on Cell Phones and Computers

Technology over-stimulation is a real problem. The fast pace of computer games, movies, and TV shows decreases attention span. In addition, the blue light from cell phone and computer screens inhibits sleep. Restrict computer, TV, and cell phone time to no more than two hours per day.

Balance the Nervous System

You can determine how much stress is contributing to ADHD symptoms and what remedies to use to correct it by looking at the pupils (as suggested earlier). Enlarged pupils signal an excess of sympathetic nervous system activity, which means that the child is stressed and anxious. In this case, relaxing nervines like lavender and chamomile will be helpful. *Jeannie Burgess's Stress Formula* is a good choice. B-complex vitamins and vitamin C may also be helpful.

If the pupils are small and contracted, then there is an excess of parasympathetic nervous system activity. When this is the case, relaxing herbs like lavender can actually make the child more agitated, while stimulants like caffeine will have a calming effect. If your child has small pupils, consider using *Vandergriff's Energy Booster* or a *Metabolic Stimulant Formula*. Rosemary and lemon balm are great herbs for people that need a little stimulation to focus.

Use Healthy Fats

Essential fatty acids are critical to proper brain function since the brain structure is mostly composed of fat. Children's brains need a lot of good fats, particular fats with omega-3 essential fatty acids, especially DHA. See the *Healthy Fats* strategy.

Ensure Adequate Protein Intake

Protein is also very important, both for balancing blood sugar and creating neurotransmitters. The amino acid L-tyrosine is very important because it is the precursor to epinephrine and norepinephrine. One of its richest sources is red meat.

Feeding children with ADHD a hearty breakfast that includes eggs and red meat often helps them become more focused. Simple carbohydrates (such as sugar-sweetened cereals) should not be eaten for breakfast, as the blood sugar roller coaster which follows contributes to ADHD symptoms.

Use Brain Calming Remedies

There are specific neurotransmitters that calm down excess nervous system reactions. The *Attention-Focus Formula* will help activate these neurotransmitters. The nutritional supplement GABA may also help to calm down the brain.

Avoid Salicylates and Food Additives

Don't substitute artificial sweeteners for sugar. Food additives, including aspartame, can be linked with hyperactivity and other behavioral disorders. Artificial colorings have also been linked with ADHD. Children who have these sensitivities may also react to foods high in salicylates. (See the *Eliminate Salicylates* strategy.)

Drugging children is not the solution to behavioral problems. They need proper nutrition and good parental discipline to develop properly. These are just a few possible solutions that may help children avoid the drugs and perform better at school and life.

Strategies: Avoid Sugar, Blood Type Diet, Eat Healthy, Eliminate Salicylates, Friendly Flora, Healthy Fats, Low-Glycemic Diet, Reduce Chemical Exposure, Sleep, and Stress Management

Formulas: Attention-Focus, **Brain Calming**, Herbal Sleep Aid, Jeannie Burgess' Stress, Hypothyroid, **Vandergriff's Energy Booster**, Suma Adaptogen, Adaptogen-Immune, General Glandular, Anti-Stress B-Complex, **Adrenal Glandular**, Algae, Heavy Metal Cleansing, Antihistamine, **Metabolic Stimulant**, Probiotic, and Stimulating Energy

Essential Oil Blends: Mood Lifting EO and Renewing and Releasing EO

Herbs: Ashwagandha, bacopa, bee pollen, black currant, blue-green algae, chamomile, jujube, **lemon balm**, licorice, **schisandra**, spirulina, tea, and wood betony

Supplements: CBD, **GABA**, krill oil, L-carnitine, **L-glutamine**, lithium, **magnesium**, multiple vitamin and mineral, **omega-3 DHA**, omega-3 EFAs, vitamin B_5, and zinc

Essential Oils: Chamomile (Roman) and lemon

Addictions

See also alcoholism, addictions (tobacco), addictions (coffee, caffeine), addictions (drugs), and addictions (sugar/carbohydrates)

Addictions are all around us, but they are often difficult for people to acknowledge or talk about. An addiction is a dependency that creates a compulsive or habitual need to repeat an experience. The addiction may be mild or severe, socially acceptable or socially unacceptable.

When we think of addictions, we commonly think of socially unacceptable addictions, specifically addiction to drugs, but many addictions are socially acceptable. Two of the most common addictive substances in North America are tobacco and alcohol, and both are widely accepted socially, in spite of their potential dangers. A car is a lethal weapon when the driver is under the influence of alcohol, while smoking damages the lungs not only of smokers but also of people who are inhaling the secondhand smoke.

Alcoholism and cigarette smoking are obvious addictions, but an even more common addiction is caffeine. How many people just can't "get through the day" without a cup of coffee or a caffeinated soda? And what about food? With 70-80 percent of the people in this country being overweight, how many people are suffering from food addictions?

Behaviors can be addictive too. People can become compulsive about sex, gambling, or shopping. What makes a behavior addictive is its compulsive and repetitive nature. The Greeks had a saying about this: "Everything in moderation; nothing in excess." When we can't stop a behavior that is damaging to ourselves and to others, it is addictive.

What causes addiction? It's the desire to feel good! One reason people may become addicted to certain substances or behaviors is that they stimulate the release of neurotransmitters in their brain and nervous system, such as endorphins, dopamine, or epinephrine. Most addictive substances either mimic or trigger the release of these chemicals, all of which elevate mood and help us feel good. The body becomes accustomed to this outside stimulus, which becomes necessary to trigger the release of these chemicals, and the person becomes addicted.

General Strategies for Addictions

Moderation is the key, and it's easier said than done. It's a dilemma that is deeply rooted in human nature, our need for ritual, our love of pleasure, and our cravings. Here are some basic suggestions.

First, it is critical to understand that one does not overcome addictions by willpower. It simply doesn't happen. The instinctive drive for pleasure and self-satisfaction is too strong for us to resist. It easily subverts people's good intentions.

That's why the first thing anyone needs to do to overcome an addiction is to seek outside help. One of the reasons for the remarkable success of organizations like Alcoholics Anonymous (AA) is that they provide a support system that gives people accountability to a power outside of themselves.

Forming groups of people that meet together to support one another in overcoming addictions to drugs, alcohol or even overeating (weight loss) has proved to be one of the most successful models for helping people become free of addictive behaviors. So first, seek assistance from other people who have overcome the addiction you wish to overcome. Allow yourself to be accountable to outside influences, including spiritual sources, so you are not relying on your own willpower.

Secondly, since addictions are motivated by the inner desire we all share to feel good, improving overall health and nutrition will make it much easier to overcome addictions. When our diet contains a proper balance of nutrients, and we are otherwise taking care of the body, it produces the chemicals that make us feel good. This is the healthy way to feel good.

Finally, cleansing the body is very helpful in overcoming addictions, especially in helping a person going through withdrawal. A good general cleanse with a general blood and liver-cleansing formula can help the body flush the toxins created by the addictive substance out of the system.

Strategies: Affirmation and Visualization, Avoid Sugar, Emotional Healing Work, Forgiveness, Pleasure Prescription, and Stress Management

Flower Essence Blends: Self-Responsibility FE

Herbs: Kava kava, rose, and Saint John's wort

Supplements: CBD, L-cysteine, **L-glutamine**, multiple vitamin and mineral, omega-3 EFAs, vitamin B-complex, and vitamin D

Addictions (Coffee, Caffeine)

See also adrenal fatigue, fatigue, insomnia, and addictions

Caffeine is addictive, yet most adults use it nearly every day and freely offer it in various forms to their children. Caffeinated beverages made from caffeine-bearing plants like coffee or cola nuts or the addition of isolated caffeine, are widely used as energy drinks, even though they actually deplete rather than provide energy.

Caffeine works by binding to receptor sites for a chemical messenger in the brain called adenosine. It blocks or inhibits these receptor sites. Adenosine communicates that the body is tired and need to rest. Blocking the message, "You're tired," isn't giving a person energy, it's just interfering with the warning signal that says, "You need to rest."

That's useful if you have to drive late at night and need something to help you stay awake, but when you use it daily it actually stops working because the body overrides the caffeine. The body still needs to communicate it requires rest, so it builds more receptors for adenosine. In other words, it adjusts for the presence of the caffeine and overrides it by up-regulating the adenosine system.

Now, you have a problem. If you stop using caffeine, you have more adenosine receptors than you need. So you feel tired, maybe get a headache or otherwise experience symptoms of withdrawal. During this withdrawal, the body adjusts to the lack of caffeine by down-regulating the adenosine system.

The more a person abuses coffee, tea, cola drinks and energy drinks the more depleted their body's energy reserves become. The adrenal glands weaken and fatigue, anxiety, nervousness, insomnia and other nervous symptoms follow. Caffeine constricts arteries, raising blood pressure, and being a diuretic it also tends to be dehydrating. Excessive use can also disrupt sleep patterns, which results in deeper fatigue and more cravings for the stimulus of caffeine to stay alert. In short, caffeine is not the innocent substance many people seem to think it is.

Although research suggests that there are some health benefits to coffee and green tea, because of their antioxidant qualities, it's wise to limit one's intake of these beverages to one or two cups a day. Cola drinks are worse because they also contain loads of sugar and questionable chemicals. The so-called energy drinks have the highest caffeine content of all and should be avoided completely as they have none of the antioxidant benefits of coffee or green tea.

To overcome caffeine addiction one needs to actively support the adrenal glands, reduce one's stress levels and increase energy production. Adaptogens may be helpful in weaning off caffeine.

B-complex vitamins and vitamin C can help boost energy naturally by supporting the adrenal function. Vitamin B_5 (pantothenic acid) is very helpful if the adrenal glands have become exhausted from excessive consumption of caffeine.

The natural way to increase energy is to rest. If you aren't getting enough sleep, look up remedies for insomnia.

Strategies: Avoid Caffeine, Hydration, Low-Glycemic Diet, Sleep, and Stress Management

Formulas: Adrenal Glandular, Chinese Fire-Increasing, Vandergriff's Energy Booster, Mitochondria Energy, **Brain Calming**, Chinese Qi-Increasing, Stimulating Energy, and Ashwagandha Complex

Flower Essence Blends: Self-Responsibility FE

Herbs: Ashwagandha, cocoa, eleuthero, ginseng (American), ginseng (Asian/Korean), licorice, and **schisandra**

Supplements: N-acetyl cysteine, **vitamin B-complex**, and vitamin C

Addictions (Drugs)
Drug Detox, Drug Withdrawal

See also addictions

In discussing drug addiction we're talking about both illegal (meth, rave, crystal, cocaine, etc.) and prescription drugs (such as pain-killers, stimulants or barbiturates), which can also be addictive. Of course, professional assistance should be sought with drug addiction, but there are natural remedies that can help too. The general strategy withdrawal from drug addiction requires detoxification and nutritional support for the nervous and glandular system.

Drugs of all kinds place a heavy burden on the detoxification systems of the liver. So herbs and nutrients that support liver detoxification are probably central to any nutritional program for drug withdrawal. These can include single herbs milk thistle and schisandra and formulas designed to protect the liver. It is also important to drink lots of pure water to help flush drugs from the system.

Studies have suggested that CBD may assist in withdrawal from a variety of drugs. It is especially helpful for counteracting negative effects of THC-rich marijuana but may also be helpful for withdrawal from nicotine, alcohol, stimulants like cocaine, and opiates like morphine and heroin.

Anyone withdrawing from drugs is going to experience mental and emotional stress. Hence, nervines could be another important component to consider in a drug-withdrawal program. If the person is suffering from post-traumatic stress disorder or adrenal fatigue, an *Adrenal Glandular Formula* can be very helpful. Omega-3 essential fatty acids and L-glutamine can also be helpful for nervous system support.

Specific Nervous System Support

Support for the nervous system depends on the type of drugs one is addicted to. If stimulants are the problem, then use something that's naturally stimulating, such as stimulating adaptogens like eleuthero, schizandra, and ginseng. B-complex vitamins (especially niacin), along with vitamin C, may also be helpful.

Overcoming an addiction to tranquilizers can be aided by herbs that also provide a relaxing effect, such as nervine or sleep formulas. Single herbs like hops, kava kava, licorice root, lobelia, passion flower, Saint John's wort, and valerian may be helpful as well. GABA and L-theanine can also be used to ease anxiety.

For addiction to pain killers, try a milder analgesic, such as lobelia, kava kava, passion flower, or valerian. For opiates, try California poppy or corydalis. The rule of thumb is to find an herbal remedy with a similar but milder effect and use it to transition off the drug.

Strategies: Affirmation and Visualization, Healthy Fats, Hydration, and Stress Management

Formulas: Blood Purifier, **Anti-Stress B-Complex**, Detoxifying, **Adrenal Glandular**, Chinese Qi-Increasing, **Hepatoprotective**, Chinese Fire-Increasing, Ashwagandha Complex, and **Adaptogen**

Flower Essence Blends: Self-Responsibility FE

Herbs: Ashwagandha, California poppy, chamomile, **corydalis**, **eleuthero**, ginseng (Asian/Korean), hops, Indian pipe, kava kava, licorice, lobelia, milk thistle, oat seed (milky), passion flower, Saint John's wort, schisandra, valerian, and **vervain (blue)**

Supplements: CBD, **GABA**, **L-glutamine**, L-threonine, omega-3 EFAs, **vitamin B-complex**, vitamin B_3, and vitamin C

Essential Oils: Grapefruit (pink) and lavender

Addictions (Sugar/ Carbohydrates)

See also diabetes, infection (fungal), metabolic syndrome, hypoglycemia, and addictions

For information on why sugar is so addictive and tips on how to break the sugar habit, see the *Avoid Sugar* strategy. The supplements listed here may aid the process of balancing your blood sugar levels and reducing your cravings for sugar and refined carbohydrates.

To ease cravings, I've had people take two capsules of the *Algae Formula* and two capsules of licorice root at breakfast time. Don't eat any simple carbohydrates for breakfast. Either eat protein-rich foods or use a protein smoothie. Repeat this at lunch. Repeat again in the afternoon if you have an afternoon energy slump. If you have high blood pressure, use bee pollen instead of licorice. You could also use one capsule of the *Chinese Qi-Increasing Formula.*

B-complex vitamins and chromium help the body utilize sugar properly and can be very helpful in overcoming sugar addiction. If you are diabetic, use a *Blood Sugar Formula* to help control blood sugar levels.

Both good fats and fiber help to stabilize blood sugar levels. Good fats reduce sugar cravings and fiber slows the release of sugar into the bloodstream resulting in a more stable blood sugar level.

Sugar cravings can be a symptom of chronic yeast infections. Yeast feed on sugar and produce a chemical that makes the brain crave sugar See *infections (fungal)* for ideas on dealing with this problem.

Strategies: Healthy Fats, Increase Dietary Fiber, Low-Glycemic Diet, Mineralization, and Stress Management

Formulas: **Adrenal Glandular**, Mitochondria Energy, 5-HTP Adaptogen, **Algae**, Chinese Yin-Increasing, Chinese Fire-Increasing, Chinese Qi-Increasing, **Sugar Craving Reducer**, Blood Sugar Control, Probiotic, and Adaptogen

Programs: Yeast Cleansing

Flower Essence Blends: Self-Responsibility FE

Herbs: Bee pollen, eleuthero, **licorice**, and **spirulina**

Supplements: 5-HTP, alpha-lipoic acid, chromium, **L-glutamine**, L-tryptophan, omega-3 EFAs, **vitamin B-complex**, and **xylitol**

Addictions (Tobacco)

See also addictions

Nicotine, the addictive substance in tobacco, is one of the most highly addictive substances known. It is rapidly absorbed into the bloodstream and is present in the brain within about ten seconds after inhalation. Nicotine causes a quick release of dopamine, but its effects dissipate quickly, leading to regular use to maintain the pleasurable feelings and prevent withdrawal. Nicotine also attaches to nicotinic receptor sites in the sympathetic nervous system, mimicking the action of epinephrine.

Lobelia contains lobeline, an alkaloid with a similar structure to nicotine, which also attaches to nicotinic receptors, but has an inhibiting rather than stimulating action. Lobelia has been used to reduce the physical cravings for tobacco in studies going back to the 1930s. While studies haven't shown using lobelia for smoking cessation works long-term, many people find that the feelings of relaxation induced by lobelia can help with the initial irritability of withdrawal.

Smokers generally need to build up their nutrient reserves. Smoking depletes vitamin C levels and B-complex vitamins, which can be supplemented along with relaxing nervines and adaptogens to support people trying to quit smoking.

Withdrawal from tobacco products also requires support to the respiratory system. Since tobacco smoke dries the lungs, the *Chinese Metal-Increasing* Formula, mullein, cordyceps and/or marshmallow can help strengthen and hydrate the lungs and promote healing.

Strategies: Affirmation and Visualization and Stress Management

Formulas: **Anti-Stress B-Complex** and **Chinese Metal-Increasing**

Flower Essence Blends: Self-Responsibility FE

Herbs: Catnip, chamomile, damiana, kanna, **lobelia**, oat seed (milky), **Saint John's wort**, **skullcap**, and valerian

Supplements: **Vitamin B-complex** and vitamin C

Essential Oils: Clove, lemon, and pine

Addison's Disease

See also adrenal fatigue

Addison's disease is an autoimmune condition that results in a severe depletion of the adrenal cortex hormones, primarily cortisol and mineralocorticoids. It results in extreme weakness, loss of weight, low blood pressure, gastrointestinal disturbances, and brown pigmentation of the skin and mucous membranes. It is a life threatening disease and requires medical diagnosis and treatment with prescription medication. In addition to medical care, an *Adrenal Glandular Formula* or adaptogens might be helpful along with appropriate dietary changes and following the *Stress Management* strategy.

Strategies: Gut-Healing Diet, Low-Glycemic Diet, and Stress Management

Formulas: Adrenal Glandular, Suma Adaptogen, Adaptogen-Immune, and Probiotic

Herbs: Codonopsis, cordyceps, eleuthero, **licorice**, maitake, reishi, and rhodiola

Supplements: Magnesium, SAM-e, vitamin B$_5$, and vitamin C

Adenitis

See also congestion (lymphatic)

Also known as lymphadenitis, adenitis is inflammation of a lymph node or gland. Use lymphatic herbs, which improve the flow of lymph and drink plenty of water. To help fight any infection, often the cause of adenitis, consider infection-fighting herbs like echinacea.

Strategies: Drawing Bath, Exercise, Hydration, and Poultice

Formulas: Liquid Lymph, Liquid Kidney, Blood Purifier, Chinese Wind-Heat Evil, and **Lymphatic Infection**

Herbs: Baptisia, cleavers, **echinacea**, lobelia, myrrh essential oil, **red clover**, **red root**, and **stillingia**

Supplements: Vitamin A, vitamin C, vitamin D, and zinc

Adrenal Fatigue
Adrenal Exhaustion, Burnout

See also Addison's disease, fatigue, insomnia, and stress

The concept of Adrenal Fatigue is not a medical one; it's really a description of the later stages of chronic stress, where a person feels mentally and physically exhausted or burned out. It's characterized by severe fatigue, coupled with restless and disturbed sleep, and the feeling that one "just can't take it anymore." Sex drive is typically reduced, and there may be difficulties with short-term memory and concentration.

The adrenals help the body cope with or adapt to stress. Long-term stress, extreme emotional or physical trauma, and loss of sleep can increase the production of adrenal hormones like cortisol and upset the balance in the nervous and endocrine system. Elevated cortisol can create anxiety, muscle tension, poor digestion, poor elimination, reduced immune response (due to cortisol's immune-suppressing effect), high blood pressure, shallow breathing, and a difficulty meeting the challenges of life.

Remedies that reduce stress levels like adaptogens (especially cordyceps and ashwagandha) and relaxing nervines (passion flower, skullcap, kava kava) can help with burnout. It's important to get adequate sleep and take time for rest and relaxation. Getting a massage, meditating or doing anything else that calms the mind and relaxes the body will help.

Two particularly helpful products are an *Adrenal Glandular* and the *Chinese Fire-Increasing Formula*. Vitamin B$_{12}$, pantothenic acid and magnesium are often very helpful as well.

Strategies: Avoid Caffeine, Avoid Sugar, Eat Healthy, Eliminate Allergy-Causing Foods, Emotional Healing Work, Epsom Salt Bath, Low-Glycemic Diet, Pleasure Prescription, Sleep, and Stress Management

Formulas: Adrenal Glandular, Suma Adaptogen, **Anti-Stress B-Complex**, **Chinese Fire-Increasing**, Methyl B12 Vitamin, Methylated B Vitamin, and **Adaptogen**

Herbs: Ashwagandha, borage, cordyceps, kava kava, maca, oat seed (milky), reishi, **skullcap**, and **vervain (blue)**

Supplements: Co-Q10, **magnesium**, multiple vitamin and mineral, **vitamin B$_{12}$**, **vitamin B$_5$**, **vitamin C**, and **vitamin D**

Essential Oils: Chamomile (Roman), geranium, red mandarin, and spruce (hemlock)

Afterbirth Pain

See also pain

After childbirth, there is often discomfort in the abdominal and pelvic regions from the exertion, contractions and stretching that occurred in labor. Baths (particularly sitz baths) using the essential oils of lavender and rose may also be helpful. Using red raspberry during pregnancy may help to prevent this problem. The mineral magnesium may also be helpful. Lobelia may be applied topically to relax the muscles and ease pain.

Formulas: Stan Malstrom's Herbal Aspirin and Anti-Inflammatory Pain

Herbs: Cocoa, lobelia, red raspberry, and valerian

Supplements: Magnesium and potassium

Essential Oils: Jasmine, lavender, and rose

Age Spots

See also free radical damage and sunburn

Also called liver spots or solar lentigo, age spots are pigments on the skin that are usually caused by overexposure to the sun. Age spots are typically treated with methods that cause superficial destruction of the skin, which can leave white spots and occasional scars. They may be reduced or eliminated by using antioxidants and nutrients that heal and protect the skin against free radical damage, such as vitamins A, D, and E.

Strategies: Eat Healthy and Healthy Fats

Formulas: Enzyme Spray, **Antioxidant**, Chinese Wood-Decreasing, and GLA Oil

Herbs: Ginkgo, hawthorn, and rose essential oil

Supplements: Vitamin A, vitamin C, vitamin D, and vitamin E

Essential Oils: Rose

Aging

See also free radical damage and memory/brain function

Many people spend a lot of time and energy saving, investing, and planning for retirement. Most of these people will develop chronic and degenerative health problems as they age, which diminish the quality of life they experience in their senior years. It won't do much good to have a fat bank account if they die of a heart attack or cancer or suffer from crippling arthritis or other conditions that prevent them from enjoying life as they grow older.

When we are planning and preparing for our senior years, we ought to invest some time, effort, and money into improving and maintaining our health at the same time. And remember that government health care programs like Medicare and private health insurance policies don't really ensure good health. All they cover is the cost of disease care and the use of drugs or surgery to treat symptoms of disease after they develop. This is not the same as investing in creating good health.

An investment in good health isn't all that complex. It doesn't even require that much self-discipline. Self-discipline suggests some type of self-deprivation, but caring for your health is the exact opposite of self-deprivation. Instead, it is self-nurturing.

Investing in your health involves forming positive health habits. Once you start making these investments, the physical, mental, and emotional dividends will become obvious. The following are some anti-aging strategies you can use to invest time, energy and money in your health.

Eat Quality Food

Good nutrition is the place to start. The basic investment rule here is simple: avoid putting your money into refined and processed foods and purchase whole, natural, and organically grown foods instead. (See the *Eat Healthy* strategy.)

Food is both the fuel that energizes your body functions and the source of raw materials to produce healthy structures. Eating cheap junk food is no way to save money. It will reduce your energy, weaken your tissues, and you'll wind up spending far more in doctor and hospital bills than you saved by eating low-quality food.

Drink Water and Breathe Deeply

Two things one can do to ensure health are to drink plenty of pure water (*Hydration* strategy) and practice the *Deep Breathing* strategy. These two practices alone can reduce pain and inflammation throughout the body while increasing energy levels and overall health.

Balance Rest and Exercise

It is very important to stay physically active as one grows older. A rigorous exercise program isn't necessary, but some form of moderate physical activity such as walking, swimming, or gentle bouncing on a mini-trampoline is essential to good health. The lymphatic system stagnates when we aren't breathing deeply and moving around. This causes metabolic toxins to accumulate in the system and contributes to chronic inflammation, aging, and degenerative disease. A daily stretching routine can help keep the lymphatic system moving and the structural system balanced.

Balance activity with rest. As we grow older, it's natural to slow down a little. Taking short naps or otherwise resting when tired is good for our health. Getting a sound night's sleep is important, and is something that often becomes a challenge as we get older. If you're having trouble sleeping, see *insomnia* for suggestions on how to improve sleep.

Supplements for Long Lasting Health

Even if you're eating a healthy diet, you can take out some additional health insurance by selecting a few well-chosen supplements. These can be general supplements designed to support overall nutrition, or specific supplements to address common health concerns associated with aging. Various tonic herbs, like ashwagandha, ginkgo, cordyceps, and codonopsis are used in other cultures to help people stay healthier as they age. Here are a few ideas for some basic herbal formulas and supplements to counteract the aging process.

Free radicals and oxidative stress are associated with the aging process. You can supplement with antioxidant formulas or individual antioxidants like alpha-lipoic acid and Co-Q10. Fresh or frozen berries are wonderful antioxidants too.

Herbs and nutrients to protect the brain and memory can also be helpful. See *memory/brain function* for ideas on how to protect your mind.

Elderly people often have diminished digestive function. A *Betaine Hydrochloric Acid Supplement* or *Digestive Support Formula* is often helpful to improve general nutrition as one ages.

Strategies: Avoid Sugar, Deep Breathing, Eat Healthy, Exercise, Healthy Fats, Hydration, Low-Glycemic Diet, Mineralization, and Stress Management

Formulas: Adaptogen-Immune, Brain and Memory Protection, Proanthocyanidins, Suma Adaptogen,

Green Tea Polyphenols, Whole Food Green Drink, **Antioxidant**, **Memory Enhancing**, Mitochondria Energy, Betaine HCl, and **Digestive Support**

Programs: Cardiovascular Nutritional

Herbs: Bacopa, bee pollen, **cordyceps**, ginkgo, **ginseng (American)**, **ginseng (Asian/Korean)**, gotu kola, milk thistle, rehmannia, and tea

Supplements: Alpha-lipoic acid, Co-Q10, DHEA, melatonin, multiple vitamin and mineral, N-acetyl cysteine, selenium, vitamin B_5, vitamin E, and zinc

Essential Oils: Frankincense, lemon, patchouli, sandalwood, and ylang ylang

AIDS
HIV, Acquired Immune Deficiency Syndrome

See also infection (viral)

AIDS (acquired immune deficiency syndrome) is a disease in which the body's immune system is depressed. AIDS is the final stage of infection with HIV (human immunodeficiency virus). One may be HIV positive but not have symptoms of AIDS. Late stages of AIDS include severe susceptibility to infections of all kinds and a general weakening of the body.

In developing a strategy for AIDS it is important to work on overall health and mental attitude. Supporting normal immune function is an important key, but preventing secondary infections is also important. For starters, an immune-boosting blend containing medicinal mushrooms may have a regulating effect in people with AIDS. The *Chinese Wind-Heat Evil Formula* may also be helpful.

Here are some specific things that may be helpful. Swollen lymph nodes and low platelet counts are common in AIDS patients. Red root and echinacea can be helpful here.

Many AIDS patients suffer from systemic yeast infections. Antifungal herbs and formulas are helpful for yeast infections.

Respiratory infections are a common cause of death in people with AIDS. Raw garlic can be very helpful in fighting these infections.

Because of the seriousness of this condition, professional assistance and medical supervision should be sought when designing a natural program to combat AIDS. A professional herbalist or naturopath can help you design a comprehensive program.

Strategies: Affirmation and Visualization, Friendly Flora, Healthy Fats, Mineralization, and Stress Management

Formulas: DHEA with Herbs, **Chinese Wind-Heat Evil**, Suma Adaptogen, **Stabilized Allicin**, Whole Food Green Drink, Mitochondria Energy, Antioxidant, Adaptogen-Immune, **Gut Immune**, and Immune-Boosting

Herbs: Aloe vera, baptisia, barley grass, **bitter melon**, chaga, elder, **garlic**, lomatium, milk thistle, pau d'arco, **red root**, Saint John's wort, shitake, and turkey tail

Supplements: Co-Q10, collagen, DHEA, L-arginine, N-acetyl cysteine, protease, **selenium**, and vitamin B_{12}

Essential Oils: Geranium

Alcoholism

See also hypoglycemia and addictions

While a moderate amount of alcohol (such as a glass of wine with a meal) does not seem to cause any serious health problems, excessive alcohol consumption does. Over-consumption of alcohol damages the liver and brain, destroys personal relationships, and is the number one cause of traffic accidents. Here are some strategies for overcoming alcoholism.

As is stressed under the condition *addictions,* alcoholics need to seek outside assistance to obtain the social and emotional support they need to overcome the habit. Good nutrition can help the process. Cravings for alcohol increase with poor nutrition, so adopting the *Eat Healthy* strategy and controlling blood sugar can be helpful as alcohol acts like refined carbohydrates and contributes to hypoglycemia. B-Complex vitamins, chromium and licorice root can all help stabilize sugar (glucose) levels in the blood and reduce alcoholic cravings.

Some research indicates that evening primrose oil helps reduce the craving for alcohol. Also try one thousand mg of vitamin C a day. Alcohol robs the body of large amounts of magnesium too. To soothe the nerves and resolve headaches try hops, chamomile, or a nervine combination.

Two excellent herbs to aid the recovering alcoholic are kudzu and Saint John's wort. Kudzu is a vine common to the Southern states with the remarkable properties of reducing high blood pressure, relieving pain (analgesic), and relieving cramps (antispasmodic). Studies have demonstrated it also possesses the ability to help control cravings for alcohol.

In laboratory studies, alcoholic golden hamsters voluntarily and significantly reduced their alcohol consumption when given a water extract of kudzu. In clinical practice, some people have reduced (not stopped) their alcohol consumption. The flowers of kudzu have been used to treat alcohol poisoning (hangover). Saint John's wort adds the benefits of bringing the nervous system back into balance and helping to dispel negative emotions associated with alcoholism.

Beer contains a relaxing herb, hops, which might explain its appeal to some people. Hops can be taken to reduce cravings for beer, providing a similar relaxing effect without the negative problems associated with alcohol.

Since the liver works overtime to neutralize alcohol when levels are too high in the blood, the liver itself breaks down after long abuse. The liver can repair itself; all it needs is rest. Milk thistle can be especially helpful for protecting the liver from the effects of alcohol, or in helping the liver to heal. When the liver has suffered severe damage due to alcoholism, milk thistle and SAM-e, along with topical application of helichrysum essential oil over the liver area, will promote healing.

Strategies: Avoid Sugar, Hydration, Low-Glycemic Diet, and Stress Management

Formulas: Adrenal Glandular, Herbal Sleep Aid, Liver Cleanse, Christopher's Nervine, **Anti-Stress B-Complex, Hepatoprotective, Chinese Wood-Increasing**, and Hypoglycemic

Flower Essence Blends: Self-Responsibility FE

Herbs: Chamomile, evening primrose, **hops**, kava kava, **kudzu**, licorice, **milk thistle, Saint John's wort**, spirulina, and valerian

Supplements: Chromium, **L-glutamine, magnesium, SAM-e**, vitamin B-complex, vitamin B_1, vitamin B_3, and vitamin C

Essential Oils: Helichrysum, rose, rosemary, and thyme

Alkalosis   see *overalkalinity*

Allergies, Food
see *food allergies/intolerances*

Allergies, Respiratory
Allergic Rhinitis, Hayfever

See also adrenal fatigue, food allergies/intolerances, congestion (lymphatic), infection (fungal), leaky gut, rhinitis, and methylation (under)

As nature awakes each spring and plants begin to bud and bloom, flowers release their pollen and millions of Americans are suddenly miserable. Most people call this condition hay fever, but technically it is allergic rhinitis, and pollen isn't the only thing that causes it. Rhinitis is an inflammatory condition that affects the sensitive membranes of the nasal and sinus passages, the eyes, and the throat. In allergic rhinitis, the inflammation is caused by allergic reactions. However, rhinitis can have other causes besides allergies.

Respiratory allergies, like allergic rhinitis, are caused by an overly sensitive immune response reacting to environmental substances. In the case of an allergic reaction, the immune system overproduces immunoglobulin E (IgE) antibodies. When antibodies attach to an allergen, it causes your body to release histamine. This causes inflammation and the symptoms associated with rhinitis and respiratory allergies, which can include congestion, sinus discharge, sneezing, watery eyes, itchy eyes, sinus pain and/or pressure, coughing, and/or sore throat. It may even upset the digestive tract, causing bloating, gas, loss of appetite, and abdominal discomfort.

Seasonal allergic rhinitis, which occurs during specific seasons of the year, is always caused by pollen. Tree and grass pollens, as well as pollen from flowers like ragweed, plantain, and dandelion, are common culprits. However, when the rhinitis symptoms occur year-round, the allergic reactions are usually caused by indoor irritants such as dust, dust mites, pet dander, feathers, and mold. The non-allergic rhinitis can be caused by household cleaning agents, cosmetics, perfumes and other chemicals (see *Rhinitis*).

Strategies for Respiratory Allergies

Most of the medical treatments available for these conditions only treat the symptoms but never actually cure the underlying problem. Fortunately, there are natural ways to relieve respiratory allergies and create more permanent relief.

Avoid Respiratory Irritants

It's pretty obvious that the place to start in getting relief from rhinitis is to remove the source of the respiratory irritants, whenever possible. For example, get rid of toxic household cleaning products and chemicals and, if air pollution is a serious problem, purchase an air filtration system. Even if it's pollen you're allergic to, reducing the amount of irritants your sensitive membranes have to deal with will go a long way to easing your problems.

You can also gain relief from rhinitis by dealing with a number of underlying health issues that are often contributing to the problem. These include all the following strategies.

Eliminate Allergy-Causing Foods

Allergic reactions to foods in the intestinal tract will hypersensitize the immune system and make you more susceptible to respiratory allergies. Common food allergies that may be contributing to rhinitis include wheat, corn, dairy, citrus, eggs, peanut butter, shellfish, and soy. Food additives, dyes, and preservatives in processed foods may also be a contributing factor.

There are signs that indicate food allergies may be a contributing factor. If a person experiences any of the following after eating a food, they probably have an allergic reaction to it: dark circles under the eyes; redness of the ears, face or eyes; a glassy look; an increased pulse rate; bloating; fatigue; or mood changes. If a person craves certain foods excessively, they may be allergic to them.

If you suspect food allergies may be contributing to your respiratory allergies, eliminate all suspected allergy-producing foods or do a short fast for two or three days. If symptoms improve, then food allergies are probably an underlying factor. Reintroduce suspected foods one at a time and watch for symptoms or reaction. See the *Eliminate Allergy-Causing Foods* strategy.

Keep Your Body Hydrated

A little-known contributing factor to respiratory allergies is dehydration. Normally, mucus traps irritating particles and allows them to be swept off the surface of the membranes. Tears wash away irritants from the eyes. When a person is dehydrated, their mucous membranes and eyes can be dry. This allows irritants to sit on the membranes. In response, the body creates an inflammatory reaction, driven by histamine, to flush the irritants from the nose, eyes, and throat.

Staying well hydrated by drinking lots of water can greatly reduce allergic reactions. It also helps to take a little natural salt with the water, as mucus and tears are salty. Allergic reactions can often be calmed down rapidly by drinking water and taking a pinch of salt.

Heal the Intestinal Tract

Inflammation in the colon tends to congest the lymphatic system and trigger inflammation in the respiratory tract. If you're eating a standard American diet and have allergies, cleansing the colon will probably help relieve respiratory-allergy symptoms. See the *Detoxification* strategy.

It takes about three to four weeks before you'll start seeing significant results, but this cleaning out the colon and restoring intestinal health with probiotics, enzymes, and anti-inflammatories has helped many people obtain permanent relief from respiratory allergies. See *leaky gut syndrome* and *dysbiosis* for more information.

Also take digestive enzyme supplements. An enzyme from pineapple called bromelain is especially helpful if you have allergies.

Reduce Systemic Inflammation

Since allergies are an inflammatory response, remedies that reduce inflammation may be helpful. Vitamin C is a great antioxidant and anti-inflammatory remedy, with the added benefit that it helps break down histamine. MSM and Co-Q10 are other anti-inflammatory remedies that may calm down allergic reactions.

Correct Specific Nutritional Deficiencies

Nutritional deficiencies may play a role in respiratory allergies. The over sensitivity of the immune system may be due to a lack of essential nutrients needed to regulate the immune response.

For instance, vitamin C and bioflavonoids (especially quercetin) have been shown to reduce histamine reactions.

Deficiencies of calcium and magnesium have also been linked with respiratory allergies. Many Americans are particularly low in magnesium. Omega-3 essential fatty acids help produce compounds that mediate inflammation and reduce inflammatory reactions.

Try Homeopathic Remedies

Homeopathy addresses the hypersensitive reaction of the allergen. By giving diluted doses of remedies that can cause allergy-like symptoms, homeopathic remedies can desensitize the immune system so that it no longer overreacts. Look for an appropriate homeopathic remedy made from the substances that trigger your allergies. Sometimes you can find locally made homeopathic remedies from the pollen of local species known to cause allergic reactions.

Many people with pollen allergies have been able to achieve an effect similar to that of homeopathic remedies by taking locally gathered bee pollen internally, which actually helps diminish allergic reactions to pollen. Start by taking a very small amount (just a few grains) and gradually work up to several capsules a day. Locally grown honey that has not been filtered can also be helpful as it contains small amounts of pollen.

Use Natural Remedies for Symptomatic Relief

There are herbs that desensitize mast cells and calm down allergic reactions. These include blessed thistle, burdock, nettles, eyebright, goldenrod, and ambrosia. Taking these remedies throughout the allergy season won't solve the underlying causes of the allergies, but they can reduce reactions and symptoms.

Symptomatic relief can also be had through using herbs that help to decongest respiratory passages and dry up excessive secretions. Yerba santa, horseradish, marshmallow, and mullein are all good choices for decongesting the airways.

Strategies: Balance Methylation, Blood Type Diet, Detoxification, Eat Healthy, Eliminate Allergy-Causing Foods, Friendly Flora, Gluten-Free Diet, Gut-Healing Diet, and Hydration

Formulas: Jeannie Burgess' Allergy-Lung, Sinus, Seasonal Cold and Flu, Topical Analgesic, **Antihistamine**, Ayurvedic Bronchial Decongestant, Colostrum-Immune Stimulator, Lung Moistening, Pepsin Intestinal, **Anti-Inflammatory Pain**, **Antioxidant**, Christopher's Sinus, **Steven Horne's Anti-Allergy**, Digestive Support, Triphala, Chinese Metal-Decreasing, Herbal Eyewash, and Adrenal Glandular

Programs: Ivy Bridge's Cleansing

Herbs: Baical skullcap, **bee pollen**, bibhitaki, black currant, blessed thistle, blue-green algae, burdock, butterbur, cherry, devil's claw, **eyebright**, feverfew, **goldenrod**, haritaki, holy basil, horseradish, licorice, lobelia, lomatium, maitake, **mangosteen**, marshmallow, mullein, **nettle, stinging**, **orange (bitter)**, osha, picrorhiza, and yerba santa

Supplements: Bromelain, calcium, Co-Q10, colostrum, MSM, omega-3 EFAs, omega-6 CLA, omega-6 GLA, potassium, **quercetin**, selenium, vitamin A, **vitamin C**, and zinc

Essential Oils: Helichrysum, lavender, and tansy (blue)

ALS

Amyotrophic Lateral Sclerosis, Lou Gehrig's Disease

See also autoimmune disorders, multiple sclerosis, and mitochondrial dysfunction

Originally known as Lou Gehrig's disease, because it afflicted the famous baseball player, Lou Gehrig, ALS is a rare, progressive degenerative condition that affects nerves in the brain and spinal cord that control muscles. As the muscles get weaker, it becomes harder for the afflicted person to walk, talk, eat or breathe. It usually begins in middle age and is characterized by increasing and spreading muscular weakness that eventually leads to paralysis. There is currently no medical cure.

Possible causes are neurotoxicity due to overactivation of glutamate. There may also be an autoimmune component, where the immune system is attacking the nerve cells. Mitochondrial dysfunction and oxidative stress may also be involved. Some potential risk factors for developing the disease include exposure to lead or other heavy metals, head injuries, pesticides and exposure to excessive electromagnetic radiation.

Medical assistance is essential, especially in the later stages of this disease. Strategies to adopt that may assist in slowing the progress of the disease or perhaps reversing it would include increasing antioxidants to protect brain tissue, modifying the diet to help improve mitochondrial function (See *mitochondrial dysfunction*) and helping to reduce neuroexcitation by avoiding MSG and all other potential neurotoxins. CBD and other phytocannabinoids may be helpful in calming neuroexcitation in the brain, reducing oxidation and relaxing muscle spasms. Work with a competent herbalist or naturopath to experiment with remedies that may be helpful. (findanherbalist.com)

Strategies: Affirmation and Visualization, Eat Healthy, and Healthy Fats

Formulas: Colloidal Mineral, Ashwagandha Complex, and Digestive Support

Herbs: Ashwagandha, **cannabis**, ginseng (American), ginseng (Asian/Korean), and pau d'arco

Supplements: CBD, **omega-3 EFAs**, vitamin C, **vitamin D**, and vitamin E

Altitude Sickness

Any time you go above eight thousand feet, you can be at risk for altitude sickness as oxygen levels in the atmosphere decrease the higher you go in elevation. It is also called mountain sickness, and symptoms of this problem include shortness of breath, fatigue, difficulty sleeping, loss of appetite, dizziness, headache, muscle aches, nausea. In severe cases, it can result in a buildup of fluid in the lungs, which can be very dangerous and even life-threatening. In the most severe cases it causes edema on the brain, which must be treated medically.

Remedies that aid circulation, such as ginkgo, and help your body adapt to stress, such as cordyceps or eleuthero, may be helpful if you are traveling to higher elevations. Don't overexert yourself and watch for symptoms of altitude sickness if you travel to high elevations.

Strategies: Hydration

Formulas: Nitric Oxide Boosting and Adaptogen

Herbs: Cordyceps, eleuthero, garlic, **ginger**, **ginkgo**, and rhodiola

Supplements: L-arginine

Aluminum Toxicity

See also heavy metal poisoning

Aluminum is one of the most abundant elements in the Earth's crust and a major component of dirt. Normally, aluminum isn't a big problem because it's very poorly absorbed. In modern times, however, it's being created and used in forms and quantities that do allow small amounts to be more easily absorbed. It is used in cookware, some baking powders, antiperspirant deodorants, and medications like antacids. Aluminum, mixed with solvents that make it absorbable, is also replacing mercury in vaccines.

There is also evidence that planes have been spraying nanoparticle aluminum into the upper atmosphere in what are called chemtrails. This may be causing respiratory problems, and the particles may be small enough that they are being absorbed into the bloodstream.

To avoid aluminum toxicity, don't cook in aluminum cookware or foil, especially with high-acid foods like tomatoes. Read labels and avoid products that contain aluminum, such as antacids and baking powder.

High levels of aluminum are found in the brains of people with Alzheimer's disease. It is unknown whether this is the direct cause of the disease or something that happens because of the disease (See *Alzheimer's disease* for more information). We do know that aluminum displaces silica, which is essential to brain function. Other possible symptoms of aluminum toxicity include nervousness, immune weakness, softening of the bones, and muscle weakness.

At this point little is known about specific ways to detoxify aluminum, but the *Heavy Metal Cleanse* strategy will probably help, along with taking extra silica in the form of silica-rich herbs to help displace the aluminum from the body.

Strategies: Heavy Metal Cleanse

Formulas: Watkin's Hair, Skin, and Nails, Algae, and **Heavy Metal Cleansing**

Herbs: Dulse, **horsetail**, and spirulina

Supplements: Silicon

Alzheimer's Disease

See also free radical damage, heavy metal poisoning, memory/brain function, dementia, and aluminum toxicity

Named after the German neurologist Alois Alzheimer, this is a progressive, degenerative disease of the central nervous system. In Alzheimer's abnormal protein deposits form plaques in the spaces between the nerve cells, while twisted fibers of a protein called tau build up inside the cells. These proteins damage and kill nerve cells. The disease begins in the area of the brain responsible for memory and gradually spreads to other parts of the brain.

Initial symptoms involve difficulty remembering newly acquired information. As the disease progresses the person develops more severe memory loss, disorientation and changes in mood and behavior. It can eventually affect motor control causing problems with speaking, swallowing and walking.

The exact cause of Alzheimer's remains unknown, but risk factors include head injuries, low cholesterol, high blood pressure, high blood sugar and advancing age. Currently there is no medical cure.

There is also no way to objectively diagnose Alzheimer's while a person is alive, but doctors are about 90 percent accurate in assessing through symptoms. According to the Alzheimer's Association, the people who are diagnosed with Alzheimer's typically die within four to eight years. This makes Alzheimer's the sixth leading cause of death in America according to the Center for Disease Control (CDC).

It's most common in Western Europe and North America and rare in less developed countries, which suggests it is associated with Western diets and lifestyles.

Research on the connection between aluminum toxicity and Alzheimer's disease started in the 1960s and has remained controversial since the beginning. Studies have shown high levels of aluminum in the brains of some, but not all, Alzheimer's patients. Epidemiological studies have

had mixed results as well, with some showing an association and some showing no association. The current scientific consensus is that while aluminum toxicity is a plausible cause for Alzheimer's, it likely contributes to only a small number of cases. Still, it is wise to limit one's exposure to aluminum (see *aluminum toxicity*).

Recent research into Alzheimer's shows that at least some cases are caused by elevated insulin levels and oxidative damage causing faulty glucose metabolism in the brain. Moderately high insulin levels are associated with increased levels of inflammatory markers and beta-amyloid in cerebrospinal fluid, suggesting a causal link between hyperinsulinemia and Alzheimer's disease. Eliminating refined starches and sugar from the diet is a good step towards prevention.

One of the most promising remedies for helping improve brain function in Alzheimer's is the daily intake of good fats such as coconut oil. There are anecdotal reports that taking two tablespoons of organic, virgin coconut oil two to three times daily has resulted in improvement in Alzheimer's patients. Also consider omega-3 essential fatty acids, especially DHA.

Researchers agree that free radical damage is at work in Alzheimer's. The brain is mostly fat (50 percent by dry weight) and needs adequate amounts of antioxidants (especially fat-soluble vitamins like A, D, E, and K) to protect it from damage. Antioxidant herbs and nutrients like green tea, rosemary, alpha-lipoic acid, and Co-Q10 may be of benefit in both preventing and slowing the progression of Alzheimer's.

To protect the brain, minimize exposure to alcohol, tobacco, and environmental toxins. Eat generous servings of fresh fruits and vegetables every day and stay mentally active. These general tips help to protect against memory loss due to aging, which includes reducing the risk of Alzheimer's. Herbs traditionally used to enhance memory may also be helpful.

Strategies: Avoid Sugar, Eat Healthy, and Healthy Fats

Formulas: Brain and Memory Protection, DHEA with Herbs, **Oral Chelation**, Heavy Metal Cleansing, Attention-Focus, Green Tea Polyphenols, Antioxidant, Brain-Heart, **Memory Enhancing**, and Methyl B12 Vitamin

Herbs: Bacopa, cinnamon, **coconut oil**, **ginkgo**, gotu kola, periwinkle, **rosemary**, tea, and turmeric

Supplements: Alpha-lipoic acid, **berberine**, CBD, Co-Q10, colostrum, curcumin, **huperzine A**, magnesium, **N-acetyl cysteine**, omega-3 DHA, omega-3 EFAs, potassium, resveratrol, vitamin B-complex, **vitamin B$_{12}$**, and vitamin B$_3$

Essential Oils: Clary sage and lemon

Amenorrhea
Lack of Periods

Amenorrhea is a lack of periods or menstrual flow. When periods are scant, infrequent, or absent, it is important to try to identify the cause. The most common causes are extreme diets (especially diets low in fats and protein), excessive exercise, stress, general poor health, thyroid imbalances, and medications. Seek appropriate professional assistance in identifying the cause, but you can also try some basic remedies for balancing hormones.

Herbs that were traditionally used to bring on "delayed menstruation" were called emmenagogues. Some of these herbs are actually abortifacients—meaning they were used to abort the fetus and restart menstruation in early pregnancy. Blue cohosh is one of these herbs and should be avoided if there is a possibility one is pregnant, as it can be very harmful to the fetus.

Strategies: Healthy Fats, Mineralization, and Stress Management

Formulas: Thyroid Glandular, Colloidal Mineral, Women's Aphrodisiac, and Female Tonic

Herbs: **Blue cohosh**, cyperus, **dong quai**, false unicorn, ginger, ligusticum, motherwort, myrrh, peony, and salvia

Supplements: Omega-3 EFAs and vitamin B-complex

Essential Oils: Clary sage, geranium, myrrh, and rose

Amyotrophic Lateral Sclerosis   see ALS

Anal Fistula/Fissure

See also hemorrhoids

An anal fistula is an abnormal passageway in the anal area. To heal an anal fistula, it is important to keep the stool soft. Take an *Irritable Bowel Fiber Formula* and a *Gentle Bowel Cleansing Formula* along with plenty of water to keep the bowels moving without strain. Apply astringent herbs like white oak bark or stone root (collinsonia) topically mixed with a *Healing Salve* or a little aloe vera gel.

You can also take antimicrobial herbs internally. It's impossible to heal a fistula without dealing with the abscess and infection. Nanoparticle silver gel can be applied to prevent infection. Avoid using goldenseal and comfrey topically to prevent sealing the fistula before the infection in gone.

Strategies: Hydration and Increase Dietary Fiber

Formulas: Intestinal Soothing, **Irritable Bowel Fiber**, Healing Salve, **Gentle Bowel Cleansing**, and Stimulant Laxative

Herbs: Butcher's broom, calendula, **collinsonia**, echinacea, horse chestnut, horsetail, plantain, and **white oak**

Supplements: Bioflavonoids, magnesium, and **nanoparticle silver**

Anemia

See also low stomach acid

Anemia indicates that there is a deficiency in red blood cells, hemoglobin (the component in red blood cells that carries oxygen), total blood volume, or a change in size of the red blood cells. This results in fatigue, reduced resistance to illness, and other symptoms. Iron alone is not necessarily the solution, since there are many other nutrients necessary for the utilization of iron and the production of hemoglobin. In working with your doctor, it is important to get all levels of iron measured, not just serum iron. Check transferrin, total iron binding capacity (TIBC) ferritin, B_{12} and folate, along with a CBC panel to evaluate the whole picture.

Iron and B_{12} deficiency anemia is common in vegetarians and vegans from inadequate intake. Iron-deficient anemia is common in premenopausal women because of monthly blood loss. Anemia is also common in severe malabsorption from celiac and Crohn's disease. Iron-deficiency anemia in men is a red flag, and the cause should be investigated by a primary care practitioner.

A nutrient-dense diet should be combined with supplements to correct deficiency. The best food sources of iron are beef liver, beef, and eggs. Red meat from organic, exclusively grass-fed animals is also a good blood-building tonic for anemia.

To supply the body with iron, take a heme iron supplement. Heme iron, from animals is absorbed up to twenty times better than non-heme iron (from plants), and doesn't cause constipation. If you have to supplement with non-heme iron, take it with vitamin C to increase absorption and negative effects.

An *Herbal Iron Formula* can be helpful for iron deficient anemia. Herbs like nettles, yellow dock, dong quai, and alfalfa can help anemia, probably by improving the absorption of iron, or helping free iron stores from the liver. The *Pregnancy Tea Formula* can be helpful in preventing anemia during pregnancy.

Supplements that help the utilization of iron in the body include vitamin C, vitamin A, vitamin B_{12}, folate (not folic acid), vitamin B_6 and zinc. Vitamin B_{12} supplementation is often necessary with SIBO and always necessary with pernicious anemia. A good way to supplement this is to take 5,000 mcg of methyl B_{12} (methylcobalamin) sublingually daily. In severe cases, B_{12} injections may be needed. If you do have anemia, it is best to work with a competent practitioner to figure out the cause.

Megaloblastic anemia (enlarged red blood cells) is caused by a defect in red-cell DNA synthesis and is most often due to vitamin B$_{12}$ and folate deficiency. A good way to get both iron and folate is to eat a lot of dark-green, leafy vegetables like kale and beet greens.

Although it does not contain iron, chlorophyll may be helpful in building up iron poor blood. The absorption of iron also requires hydrochloric acid in the stomach (see *low stomach acid*).

Strategies: Gut-Healing Diet and Mineralization

Formulas: Chinese Wood-Increasing, Pet Supplement, **Christopher's Herbal Iron**, Chinese Fire-Increasing, Whole Food Green Drink, Algae, **Methyl B12 Vitamin**, Methylated B Vitamin, Betaine HCl, and **Pregnancy Tea**

Herbs: Alfalfa, angelica, beet, chicory, dong quai, gentian, **nettle, stinging**, and **yellow dock**

Supplements: Chlorophyll, iron, L-glutamine, manganese, **vitamin B$_{12}$**, vitamin B$_2$, vitamin B$_6$, vitamin B$_9$, vitamin C, and zinc

Essential Oils: Lemon

Aneurysm

An aneurysm is a blood-filled dilation of a blood vessel wall as a result of a blood vessel disease or weakness. Appropriate medical attention should be sought for this condition as it is life-threatening. Herbs like yarrow and capsicum can be administered during transport for medical care. Other listed remedies may aid in recovery.

Herbs: Alfalfa, butcher's broom, capsicum, goldenseal, hawthorn, **horse chestnut**, rose hips, and **yarrow**

Supplements: Bioflavonoids and magnesium

Essential Oils: Frankincense and helichrysum

Anger, Excessive

See also bipolar mood disorder, depression, irritability, and PTSD

While not commonly thought of as a mood disorder like depression or anxiety, excessive anger is harmful both to health and relationships. In traditional Chinese medicine (TCM), excess anger is thought to damage the liver and gallbladder. The liver and gallbladder connection to anger is also found in traditional Western medicine and culture, as shown in the expression "That really galls me" (*gall* being another word for *bile*).

Modern Western medicine recognizes that angry people are at higher risk for cardiovascular problems. Again, our language intuitively recognizes this when we talk about angry and controlling people as being "hard-hearted." Anger and aggression also inhibit elimination, hence the phrase pissed off" suggesting that anger turns off our ability to urinate. Constantly being angry and controlling makes us constipated or tight assed. Phrases like "Venting one's spleen" suggest that anger also affects the digestive organs.

As if the damage to our physical health isn't bad enough, anger also destroys relationships. Constantly venting anger destroys love in marriages, ruins parent-child relationships, and adversely affects other personal and business relationships.

Clearly, we need to learn how to manage anger to preserve both our health and the health of our relationships. Let's begin by understanding two important facts about anger.

Facing and Understanding Anger

Anger is not a bad or negative emotion. Anger is the emotion that allows us to protect and defend ourselves. It only becomes a destructive influence in our lives when we aren't able to express it constructively. Most people only know two ways of dealing with anger. They either vent their anger by attacking and belittling others, or they suppress their anger and let other people have their way to avoid a fight. Both of these approaches are unhealthy.

The second thing we need to understand is that the relationship between anger and our physical health goes both ways. Anger can damage our health, but health problems can make us more prone to being angry and irritable. Just like depression can have physical causes, so can being easily angered.

Because of this, we're going to explore learning how to manage anger from both directions, emotionally and physically. If you have problems with anger, work on it from both directions for best results.

Underlying Causes of Excessive Anger

There are three primary health issues that can lead to excess anger and irritability. They are liver toxicity, blood sugar problems, and stress. We'll look at each of these issues and then talk a little bit about managing anger.

1. Liver Toxicity

Traditional Chinese medicine associates the element of wood with the liver and gallbladder. The element of wood represents our ability to grow, expand, and live. When this ability to flow is disrupted, we feel irritable and angry. To understand this, just imagine that you are driving down the freeway and are running a little late. You are anxious to get to your destination when suddenly you run into a huge traffic jam that grinds traffic to a halt.

If you're normal, this block in your flow probably makes you feel frustrated at the least and angry at the worst. This inhibition of flow is something similar to the concept of constricted liver qi (energy) in TCM. When the liver is congested and toxic, we tend to feel defensive and irritable. This is why excessive anger is associated with an imbalance in the wood element in traditional Chinese medicine.

This is why taking a good liver-cleansing formula, such as a *Blood Purifier*, *Cholagogue* or *Liver Tonic Formula* can help cool down irritable feelings. The Chinese herb bupleurum can be particularly helpful because it is said to remove feelings of anger and sadness from the liver. Bupleurum "dredges" the liver and can stir up unresolved emotions. Be sure that people have the energy to deal with these emotions before giving bupleurum.

In detoxifying the body to reduce anger, you may also want to consider working with the kidneys. The kidneys help to flush toxins processed by the liver, so if your kidneys can't keep up with the toxic load, you may also feel angry and irritable because your ability to piss is off. If you're angry and you're having problems with your kidneys or bladder, use a *Diuretic Formula*.

2. Blood Sugar Problems

Refined carbohydrates cause rapid increases in blood sugar, which overstimulates the brain. If you're a careful observer, you will notice how a relaxed and calm child can suddenly become a little monster after eating a bunch of sugary foods. The same thing happens to adults, who can become agitated and aggressive after consuming lots of sugar and caffeine.

When blood sugar levels rise dramatically, they also tend to fall dramatically, sort of like a blood sugar roller-coaster ride. Later, when the blood sugar drops, one may feel shaky, agitated, defensive, or withdrawn. Barbara Reed, a juvenile parole officer in Upstate New York, found that delinquent teenagers often had serious blood sugar issues. When fed a diet designed to control hypoglycemia (low blood sugar), these kids never got in trouble with the law again. This diet consisted of fresh fruits, vegetables, whole grains, and meat with no sugar, alcohol, and caffeine. Regulating blood sugar helps regulate our mood so we can face the problems of life with a calmer, clearer head. (See the strategy *Avoid Sugar*.)

3. Too Much Stress

The adrenal hormones that pump through the body when we experience stress make our heart beat faster, raise our blood pressure, tense our muscles, and otherwise prime the body for action. This is called the fight-or-flight response because it is preparing us to flee the danger or fight it off.

One of the effects of this response is that the flow of blood to our higher brain (cortex) diminishes, leaving our animal instincts in charge. Since we are primed to fight, one of the reactions we might have is to lash out in anger to protect ourselves. Lashing out in anger often makes the situation worse rather than better, so we need to find a way to calm the stress response.

Sleep is the most important factor in reducing the stress response. Studies have shown that people getting inadequate sleep view the world as a more dangerous place, increasing the chance of a stress response. (See the *Sleep* strategy and *insomnia* condition.)

Managing Anger Constructively

To understand how to use anger constructively, we need to understand a concept called personal boundaries. Our personal boundary separates the things we are in control of from the things we are not. We are responsible (that is, able to respond) to the things inside our personal boundaries, but we are not responsible for what is outside of them or what we have no control over. This means that we are only responsible for our own thoughts, feelings, and choices (actions), as nothing else is in our control.

Problems with anger involve problems with personal boundaries. We are either trying to control something that is not in our control or allowing others to control something inside our personal boundary. When we try to control something not in our control, we vent our anger, using it to threaten, attack, belittle, and manipulate others. When we vent anger, we are trying to solve our problem by controlling other people.

This is impossible, of course, and it is not a positive way to use anger. It is a sign that we have a poor understanding of our personal boundaries and lack responsibility for ourselves. Venting anger pushes other people away, creating feelings of loneliness and isolation, which can lead to heart disease, increased stress, and other health problems.

Another choice we have would be to suppress our anger. This often means we cave in to unreasonable demands and expectations of others, allowing them to control us. This is also not healthy. It weakens our immune system and eventually leads to frustration and resentment, which can also destroy relationships. This is a sign that we are not taking control of our own life, which is also a sign of holes in our personal boundaries.

These two ways of dealing with anger—control or be controlled—are the only two options most people are aware of. However, there is a third option. We can assert our right to control our own life and affirm the right of others to control theirs. This means that we embrace our personal boundaries, we aren't trying to attack others, and we aren't allowing others to push us around. We are standing up for or asserting ourselves. This is the constructive way to deal with anger.

A good anger-management course or book can help you learn to be assertive without being controlling, but here are a few basic tips. When you are feeling angry, train yourself to pause and take a few deep breaths. This is particularly important if you are prone to vent your anger (that is, to attack other people, trying to belittle or control them). Before speaking or acting in anger, first try to understand the real source of your frustration.

If you are trying to control someone else's behavior, take a look at why you feel you have the right to demand that they change for your benefit. Ask yourself, "How do I feel my personal well-being is being threatened?" Then ask, "What could I do about this that doesn't involve trying to attack or control someone else?"

We can communicate that something bothers us without having to make the other person's actions wrong. We can just state that we like or dislike certain things. We can also decide what our course of action is going to be to resolve a problem. In other words, how could we change our own behavior in a way that would make us feel better about something that is causing us to feel angry? All this does not come easy at first, but it is worth the effort.

Finally, anger is a common symptom of other problems, such as anxiety, depression, bipolar depression, and PTSD. If these simple techniques don't help your anger issues, please find a good therapist to identify the causes of your anger.

Strategies: Aromatherapy, Avoid Sugar, Balance Methylation, Blood Type Diet, Counseling or Therapy, Deep Breathing, Emotional Healing Work, Exercise, Forgiveness, Hydration, Low-Glycemic Diet, Sleep, and Stress Management

Formulas: Chinese Wood-Decreasing and Liver Cleanse

Essential Oil Blends: Analgesic EO

Flower Essence Blends: Personal Boundaries FE and **Anger-Reducing FE**

Herbs: Agrimony, bee pollen, **bupleurum**, chamomile, dandelion root, linden flowers, rose petals, and vervain (blue)

Supplements: Chromium, L-glutamine, N-acetyl cysteine, vitamin B-complex, vitamin B_5, and vitamin C

Essential Oils: Chamomile (Roman), helichrysum, lavender, patchouli, rose, tansy (blue), and ylang ylang

Angina

See also cardiovascular disease, gallbladder problems, gas & bloating, and anxiety disorders

Angina is chest pain that can range from mild to severe and is caused by lack of blood flow to the heart muscle. Anxiety, gallbladder problems, or digestive problems like severe abdominal bloating, atypical acid reflux, and esophageal spasms can cause a similar type of pain. Seek appropriate medical attention for a proper diagnosis and then select appropriate remedies based on the cause.

In true angina, which is due to constriction of blood vessels in the heart, magnesium supplements, Co-Q10, L-arginine (five grams daily), and antispasmodic herbs (like lobelia) can ease blood flow to the heart. Where there is no arterial blockage and stress and anxiety are the primary factors, adaptogens and nervine herbs should be helpful. Also consider B-complex vitamins and magnesium.

Strategies: Eat Healthy, Healthy Fats, Hiatal Hernia Correction, and Stress Management

Formulas: Stan Malstrom's Herbal Aspirin, Heart Health, **Chinese Fire-Increasing**, Lung Moistening, Anti-Stress B-Complex, Liquid Kidney, **Brain-Heart**, **Chinese Fire-Decreasing**, Methylated B Vitamin, and **Nitric Oxide Boosting**

Herbs: Arjuna, arnica, black cohosh, black currant, **cramp bark**, ginkgo, gynostemma, **hawthorn**, he shou wu, **khella**, **lobelia**, motherwort, and salvia

Supplements: Bromelain, **Co-Q10**, **L-arginine**, L-carnitine, magnesium, vanadium, vitamin B_9, and vitamin E

Essential Oils: Neroli and orange (sweet)

Anorexia

See also appetite (deficient) and anxiety disorders

Anorexia nervosa is an eating disorder characterized by severe food restriction. It occurs most commonly among teenage women and includes an irrational fear of weight gain and distorted body image. Seek appropriate medical attention, including following the *Counseling or Therapy* strategy, when dealing with this condition.

To stimulate appetite, take small doses of bitter herbs such as gentian, or an *Herbal Bitters Formula*. It is absolutely essential that you taste these herbs as it is the bitter taste that has the effect. Carminative herbs may also stimulate appetite when taken as teas prior to mealtime. Teas with chamomile or peppermint as a primary ingredient would be good choices.

Strategies: Affirmation and Visualization, Counseling or Therapy, Emotional Healing Work, Healthy Fats, Hydration, Mineralization, and Stress Management

Formulas: Anti-Stress B-Complex, Chinese Earth-Increasing, **Chinese Qi and Blood Tonic**, Christopher's Carminative, **Herbal Bitters**, Jeannie Burgess' Stress, Probiotic, Green Tea Polyphenols, Antioxidant, Chinese Fire-Increasing, Colloidal Mineral, Digestive Support, and Hypoglycemic

Flower Essence Blends: Self-Responsibility FE

Herbs: Angelica, blessed thistle, borage flower essence, cardamom, catnip, chamomile, cinnamon, **gentian**, **goldenseal**, licorice, peppermint, picrorhiza, sage, Saint John's wort, and saw palmetto

Supplements: CBD, **multiple vitamin and mineral**, and vitamin B-complex

Essential Oils: Cinnamon, geranium, and grapefruit (pink)

Antibiotic Resistance

See also antibiotic side effects, infection (fungal), infection (bacterial), infection (viral), and infection (mrsa)

There is no question about it: antibiotics are one of the wonders of modern medicine and they have saved countless lives.

These drugs are also commonly prescribed for conditions where they have little or no effect. Antibiotics only work on bacterial infections and are worthless on viral or fungal infections. This means that there is absolutely no reason to take an antibiotic for the common cold or flu. Antibiotics are also ineffective in many, if not most, cases of sore throats, sinus infections, bronchitis, respiratory congestion, and earaches (otitis media).

In spite of these facts, many people run to their doctor and practically insist on getting a prescription for an antibiotic for these types of health problems. What these people don't realize is that using antibiotics in this inappropriate manner will actually harm their health in the long run.

This is partly because antibiotics kill friendly bacteria in the intestinal tract. When these friendly bacteria are destroyed, yeast and infectious bacteria proliferate, causing intestinal inflammation, leaky gut syndrome, and a weakened immune system. This makes the person even more susceptible to future infections.

An even more serious problem created by antibiotic overuse is the development of antibiotic-resistant bacteria, sometimes called superbugs. Here's how this happens: antibiotics never kill all the bacteria, and the few that survive are the ones that are most resistant to the drug. Over time, the process of natural selection gradually creates strains of bacteria that can't be killed by that particular antibiotic.

Antibiotic resistance can develop very quickly. Once penicillin entered regular use following World War II, it only took four years for microbes to develop resistance to penicillin. New antibiotics have to be introduced regularly, and it's a losing battle. Antibiotic resistance is now a worldwide problem, especially in hospitals and medical clinics. Diseases such as tuberculosis, gonorrhea, and childhood ear infections are more difficult to treat now than they were a few decades ago.

Prescribing antibiotics for colds and other viral infections and feeding livestock antibiotics for "prevention" has hastened the development of antibiotic resistance, which is why we need to put a halt to this abuse of antibiotics, especially when there are natural ways to treat most infections. There are many natural remedies that are not only effective against bacterial infections but also work on viral and fungal infections. More importantly, bacteria do not seem to develop resistance to whole plant extracts.

Some alternatives to antibiotics that may be useful for antibiotic resistant infections are listed here. (See the listings for various types of infections for more information on other alternatives to antibiotics.)

Formulas: Antibacterial, **Stabilized Allicin**, and Immune-Boosting

Herbs: **Echinacea**, echinacea, garlic, **goldenseal**, and Oregon grape

Supplements: **Berberine** and **nanoparticle silver**

Essential Oils: Cinnamon, myrrh, oregano, tea tree, and thyme

Antibiotic Side Effects

See also infection (fungal)

Antibiotics destroy good bacteria in the gastrointestinal and female reproductive tracts. This allows yeast, and occasionally pathogenic bacteria, to multiply out of balance with other organisms in the gut and vagina.

After completing a round of antibiotics, it is important to take probiotics and/or eat cultured foods in order to replace the friendly bacteria that have been destroyed. (See the *Friendly Flora* strategy.)

It may also be helpful to take antifungal herbs following antibiotic therapy to knock down yeast. See *infections (fungal)* for more information.

Strategies: Friendly Flora

Formulas: **Probiotic** and Immune-Boosting

Programs: Yeast Cleansing

Herbs: **Barberry**, **black walnut**, garlic, **neem**, oregano, and pau d'arco

Supplements: Colostrum and vitamin B_5

Anxiety Attacks
Panic Attack

See also anxiety disorders

When a person experiences mild to severe apprehension or uneasiness over a present or impending event, with symptoms such as cold sweat, heart palpitations, trembling, faintness, a sense of pressure in the chest over the heart area, and/or dry mouth, he or she is experiencing anxiety. A panic attack occurs when a state of anxiety is so severe that the person begins to breathe in a rapid, shallow manner and becomes tense to the point of cramping and the inability to act.

People with blood type A are more prone to anxiety and panic because they have a harder time breaking down the stress hormones produced by the adrenal glands. Adaptogens can help overcome the tendency to anxiety by reducing the production of stress hormones. Avoid caffeine and other stimulants. Taking B-complex vitamins, particularly B_6, and eliminating refined sugar from the diet will also be helpful. CBD can be helpful for reducing severe anxiety too.

To relieve acute anxiety or panic attacks, it is necessary to calm down the function of the sympathetic nervous system with sympatholytic agents and to increase the activity of the parasympathetic nervous system with parasympathomimetic agents. To do this, try taking ten to fifteen drops of lobelia or kava kava extract every two to three minutes or one capsule of kava kava every ten minutes while concentrating on breathing slowly and deeply. You can also take the *Shock and Injury FE.*

Strategies: Avoid Caffeine, Deep Breathing, Emotional Healing Work, and Stress Management

Formulas: Jeannie Burgess' Stress, **Adrenal Glandular**, Anti-Stress B-Complex, and **Anti-Anxiety**

Essential Oil Blends: Calming and Relaxing EO and Relaxing and Soothing EO

Flower Essence Blends: Shock and Injury FE

Herbs: Haritaki, **kava kava**, **lobelia**, motherwort, and **vervain (blue)**

Supplements: CBD, **GABA**, lithium, and magnesium

Anxiety Disorders

See also adrenal fatigue, anxiety attacks, insomnia, neurosis, stress, OCD, PTSD, phobias, anxiety (situational), and methylation (under)

If you've ever encountered a threatening situation, you're probably familiar with the physical sensations of the fight-flight-or-freeze response that has prepared your body to respond to the danger. Symptoms of the fight-flight-or-freeze response include rapid heartbeat or heart palpitations, muscle tension, trembling, irritability, cold sweats, feeling faint, dry mouth, headaches, and nausea.

The body's response to a threatening situation is a wonderful thing that prepares us to act by shifting blood flow and energy away from our core, toward our muscles in anticipation of the fighting or fleeing to follow.

It's helpful to think of these symptoms as the preparedness response, because they are a manifestation of your body preparing to escape or avoid the threat. The feelings induced by the preparedness response are often a complex combination of apprehension, fear, dread, and worry. It's absolutely normal to have these symptoms and feelings of anxiety when facing difficult or dangerous situations. (See *anxiety, situational*).

The feelings and symptoms that make up anxiety can be abnormally elevated in some people, who will have anxiety that is out of proportion to the stressful situation, lasts after the situation has gone, or appears for no apparent reason when there isn't a stressful situation.

People who experience this level of anxiety are said to have an anxiety disorder. According to the Anxiety and Depression Association of America, anxiety disorders are the most common mental health problem in the US, affecting forty million adults in the United States age eighteen and older. This means that about 18 percent of adults suffer from chronic anxiety.

Generalized Anxiety Disorder (GAD)

If these symptoms and feelings of abnormal anxiety occur regularly, causing you distress and interfering with your day-to-day activities, you might have a condition called generalized anxiety disorder. Symptoms of this problem include the following:

- Feeling continually restless, irritable, tense, worried, and on edge
- Having fears that you know are irrational, but can't be shaken
- Difficulty concentrating, or feeling like your mind has gone blank
- Abnormal fatigue
- Insomnia, normally characterized by having issues falling asleep, not staying asleep
- Belief that danger and catastrophe are around every corner
- Avoiding everyday activities because the activity might cause anxiety
- Surges of overwhelming panic
- Feeling like you are losing control or going crazy
- Trouble breathing or experiencing a choking sensation
- Feelings of being detached or unreal

Other Anxiety Disorders

In addition to generalized anxiety disorder, there are six additional major types of anxiety disorders recognized in modern medicine, each with their own distinct set of symptoms. These are anxiety attacks (panic disorder), obsessive-compulsive disorder, illness anxiety disorder, phobia, social anxiety disorder, and post-traumatic stress disorder (PTSD). For instance, if your anxiety is about a specific thing, like spiders, it's probably a phobia. See related conditions for more information about these disorders.

Strategies for Reducing Anxiety

The following seven strategies can help to reduce anxiety in all types of anxiety disorder, but there are additional steps you might need a practitioner to guide you through if you're dealing with something more than generalized anxiety disorder. (See the related conditions for help with specific anxiety disorders.)

1. Get Counseling or Therapy

It is usually helpful to get help in dealing directly with the thoughts and anxious feelings through following the *Counseling or Therapy* strategy. With mild to moderate anxiety, this may involve a support group, help from a minister or other caring individual. With severe anxiety, professional help is usually necessary. Severe anxiety is often rooted in past trauma and painful memories that have not been processed.

2. Get Adequate Sleep

Adequate sleep is essential for reducing anxiety. If you sleep less than eight to nine hours per night, sleep debt may be contributing to your anxiety. (See *insomnia* for suggestions on solving sleep problems.)

3. Exercise More

The stress response, which causes anxiety, is designed to prepare the body for action. Exercise helps to "burn off" the hormones and neurotransmitters involved in this reaction and help us calm down. That's why simply taking a walk when we are upset often helps us clear our mind and calm down our nerves.

Some forms of exercise like yoga and tai chi not only help you become more active and reduce anxiety, but also have additional benefits, like increasing balance, coordination, and flexibility. Whatever form of physical activity you find enjoyable, do more of it!

4. Correct Basic Nutritional Deficiencies

Most Americans have one or more nutritional deficiencies, and many nutritional deficiencies can contribute to feelings of anxiety. The most common nutrient deficiencies in our clients that have anxiety are magnesium, omega-3 essential fatty acids (EPA/DHA), iron, folate, and vitamin B_{12}. Get counsel on correcting these deficiencies or experiment with some basic supplements to see which ones help you.

5. Try Deep Breathing Exercises

Deep breathing exercises help stimulate the parasympathetic nervous system, reducing sympathetic stimulation and the fight-or-flight response. A number of studies have been conducted on breathing exercises, which show a lowering of cortisol and a decrease in anxiety for those not only with GAD but also phobias and PTSD. One small study found breathing exercises to be as effective as cognitive therapy in anxiety. (See the *Deep Breathing* strategy for instructions on deep breathing.)

6. Practice Mediation

Meditation can be extremely helpful in overcoming anxiety disorders because it not only lowers the body's production of the chemical messengers involved in anxiety but also helps clear a person's mind and allows them to take control of their thoughts. (See the strategy *Meditation* for a simple, non-religious meditation technique.)

7. Use Specific Herbs, Essential Oils, and Nutritional Supplements

Depending on the specific situation there are a variety of other herbs and supplements that can reduce feelings of anxiety and aid the implementation of some of the lifestyle practices mentioned above. Supporting the adrenal glands with an adrenal glandular or adaptogens may be helpful. Relaxing nervines that reduce muscle tension and aid sleep may also be helpful. Various essential oils can also be diffused into the air to promote more calm feelings.

Strategies: Affirmation and Visualization, Aromatherapy, Avoid Caffeine, Avoid Sugar, Balance Methylation, Blood Type Diet, Counseling or Therapy, Deep Breathing, Eliminate Salicylates, Emotional Healing Work, Exercise, Flower Essence, Forgiveness, Healthy Fats, Hydration, Low-Glycemic Diet, Meditation, Mineralization, Pleasure Prescription, Reduce Chemical Exposure, Sleep, and Stress Management

Formulas: Adrenal Glandular, Adaptogen-Immune, Suma Adaptogen, Chinese Fire-Increasing, **Anti-Stress B-Complex**, **Chinese Fire-Decreasing**, **Anti-Anxiety**, **Brain Calming**, Ashwagandha Complex, CBD Brain, and **Adaptogen**

Flower Essence Blends: Self-Responsibility FE and Fear-Reducing FE

Herbs: Ashwagandha, bacopa, bugleweed, California poppy, chamomile, **damiana**, holy basil, hops, **kava kava**, lemon balm, lobelia, **mimosa**, motherwort, oat seed (milky), passion flower, polygala, skullcap, valerian, and **vervain (blue)**

Supplements: CBD, **GABA**, iron, L-theanine, L-threonine, lithium, **magnesium**, omega-3 EFAs, vitamin B-complex, vitamin B_{12}, vitamin B_5, vitamin B_6, vitamin B_9, and zinc

Essential Oils: Frankincense, lavender, lemon, sandalwood, and ylang ylang

Anxiety, Situational

See also anxiety attacks and anxiety disorders

Anxiety is a normal emotion we all experience from time to time. For instance, when faced with a problem at work, when preparing for a test, when in conflict in a personal relationship, or even when having to get up in front of a group to make a presentation, it's normal to feel nervous or anxious. Most of the time we are able to carry through with the task at hand and the anxiety dissipates.

There are a number of useful remedies for situational anxiety. Just taking a few slow deep breaths while saying to yourself, "I am relaxed, everything will be fine," is very helpful. The *Shock and Injury FE* can be taken to help you feel more calm and present. It can also help to take some relaxing nervine herbs like those listed below.

For suggestions on anxiety that is ongoing, and not situationally based, see *anxiety disorders*. For acute anxiety that results in the inability to act, leaving a person feeling frozen, tense, or even paralyzed, see *anxiety attacks*.

Strategies: Aromatherapy, Flower Essence, Good Posture, and Sleep

Formulas: Jeannie Burgess' Stress, **Anti-Anxiety**, **Anti-Stress B-Complex**, Chinese Qi-Regulating, and Thyroid Calming

Flower Essence Blends: Shock and Injury FE

Herbs: Chamomile, hoelen, **kanna**, **kava kava**, linden, and motherwort

Supplements: L-theanine, **magnesium**, and vitamin B-complex

Essential Oils: Anise, atlas cedarwood, chamomile (Roman), clary sage, copaiba, fennel, lavender, lime, neroli, orange (sweet), patchouli, ravensara, ravintsara, rose, spearmint, tansy (blue), and ylang ylang

Apathy

See also adrenal fatigue, depression, and anxiety disorders

Apathy is an "I don't care" attitude that may have its roots in depression, PSTD, and wounds to self-esteem. Severe apathy will probably require the *Counseling or Therapy* strategy, but consider herbal remedies for depression and anxiety. Low thyroid may also be a factor.

Strategies: Aromatherapy, Avoid Sugar, Counseling or Therapy, Emotional Healing Work, and Flower Essence

Formulas: Thyroid Glandular

Essential Oil Blends: Mood Lifting EO

Flower Essence Blends: Fear-Reducing FE and **Personal Boundaries FE**

Herbs: Mimosa, oat seed (milky), peppermint, **rose petals**, and rosemary essential oil

Supplements: SAM-e, vitamin B-complex, and vitamin C

Essential Oils: Frankincense, geranium, jasmine, lavender, lemon, patchouli, peppermint, rose, and rosemary

Appendicitis

Inflammation of the appendix is called appendicitis. It is characterized by swelling and pain in the lower abdomen, just inside the right hip. This is a serious condition! The appendix can rupture and cause a life-threatening infection of the abdominal cavity. Avoid stimulant laxatives and enemas when having an acute episode of appendicitis.

In many countries outside of the United States, appendicitis is treated without surgery by putting the patient on a diet of clear liquids (no solid food) and giving large doses of antibiotics. It is possible that similar results could be achieved with large doses of an *Antibacterial Formula*. However, according to the British Medical Journal, about 20 percent of the time appendicitis that was treated with antibiotics reoccurred within a year.

Due to the seriousness of this condition, appropriate medical attention should be sought before undertaking any course of treatment and that a natural approach only be tried under medical supervision.

Formulas: Stabilized Allicin, Liquid Lymph, and Anti-Inflammatory Pain

Herbs: Baptisia, echinacea, **goldenseal**, thlaspi, and wild yam

Supplements: Vitamin C

Appetite, Deficient

See also anorexia, bulimia, and wasting

A deficient appetite is a lack of desire for food. A loss of appetite is often due to illness, nervous or endocrine system problems, stress, or a congested digestive tract and liver. A short-term loss of appetite when sick is normal and is nothing to worry about. A long-term loss of appetite can result in loss of weight and health.

The appetite can be stimulated by taking an *Herbal Bitters Formula* about 20 minutes prior to eating. The *Emotional Healing Work* strategy may be needed. If these approaches don't work, seek appropriate assistance.

Strategies: Detoxification, Eat Enzyme-Rich Foods, Emotional Healing Work, and Hydration

Formulas: Christopher's Carminative, Chinese Earth-Decreasing, Liver Cleanse, Betaine HCl, 5-HTP Adaptogen, Plant Enzyme, **Herbal Bitters**, **Digestive Support**, and Steven Horne's Horehound Cough

Herbs: Artichoke, asparagus, black pepper, blessed thistle, chamomile, codonopsis, dandelion, fringe tree, **gentian**, hoelen, horehound, **orange (bitter)**, and Oregon grape

Supplements: 5-HTP, copper, multiple vitamin and mineral, vitamin C, and zinc

Essential Oils: Bay leaf, lemon, lime, myrrh, and pine

Appetite, Excessive

See also excess weight

When a person craves food beyond what is nutritionally necessary to sustain life, health, and optimum body weight, there may be a need for substances that curb appetite. Often the problem is related to eating too many empty calories, or foods that have a very low content of vitamins, minerals, and other micronutrients, such as refined sugar and white flour. By supplying the body with the nutrients it requires, the body will crave less food because its nutritional requirements are satisfied.

Supplements that help to curb appetite in this manner include mineral-rich herbs like alfalfa and barley juice powder, and essential fatty acids and good fats. Taking a couple of spoonfuls of coconut oil prior to meals can be helpful. There may also be hormonal or nervous system imbalances that you may need assistance in correcting.

Strategies: Avoid Sugar, Emotional Healing Work, Exercise, Fasting, Healthy Fats, Hydration, Increase Dietary Fiber, Low-Glycemic Diet, Mineralization, and Stress Management

Formulas: Sugar Craving Reducer, Skinny, Metabolic Stimulant, Garcinia Fat-Burning, Chinese Wood-Increasing, Algae, 5-HTP Adaptogen, GLA Oil, Colloidal Mineral, Whole Food Protein, **Chinese Qi-Increasing**, and Whole Food Green Drink

Essential Oil Blends: Mood Lifting EO

Herbs: Barley, black walnut, blue-green algae, chickweed, coffee, **garcinia**, psyllium, and **spirulina**

Supplements: 5-HTP, L-glutamine, L-phenylalaine, multiple vitamin and mineral, and omega-3 EFAs

Essential Oils: Grapefruit (pink), lavender, and ylang ylang

Arrhythmia
Irregular Heart Rate

Arrhythmia is a medical term referring to an irregular heartbeat. Arrhythmias can be benign or very serious and should be assessed and monitored by a primary care provider. In serious cases, drugs may be needed to stabilize the condition. It is sometime congenital (inherited) and in this case cannot be effectively eliminated. Arrhythmias can be diffi-cult to treat with herbs and nutrition, but there are natural therapies that sometimes prove helpful.

Arrhythmias can be a sign of mineral deficiencies. Magnesium in particular is often lacking in the diet and may be helpful as a supplement. Sometimes calcium, potassium, or trace mineral deficiencies may play a role.

Nervine formulas, especially ones containing motherwort, passionflower, lobelia, or valerian may be helpful. When suffering from arrhythmia avoid stimulants like caffeine, tobacco, alcohol, ephedra, licorice root, and peppermint essential oil.

Some of the best herbs for arrhythmia are toxic botanicals available only from a professional herbalist or naturopath. These include lily of the valley and mistletoe. If you decide to try any of these stronger botanicals, do so under the supervision of an herbalist familiar with their contraindications.

Strategies: Hiatal Hernia Correction, Hydration, and Mineralization

Formulas: Heart Health

Herbs: Arjuna, black cohosh, hawthorn, khella, lobelia, **mistletoe**, **motherwort**, **night-blooming cereus**, passion flower, and skullcap

Supplements: Calcium, **magnesium**, and vitamin B_5

Essential Oils: Rose

Arsenic Poisoning

See also chemical exposure and heavy metal poisoning

Arsenic has often been used to poison people (as in the play and movie *Arsenic and Old Lace*), but oddly enough, like mercury, arsenic has been used in medicine. Because of its toxicity, it has been used in pesticides and herbicides as well. So it found its way into water supplies and foods. It's also used in wood preservatives.

Before you get enough to kill you, exposure to arsenic can cause headaches, confusion, convulsions, and stomach pain. It may also contribute to vitamin A deficiency, heart disease, cancer, stroke, and diabetes.

Acute arsenic poisoning should be treated medically. To get arsenic out of the tissues, use the *Heavy Metal Cleanse* strategy or one of the programs under the condition *chemical exposure*. In addition to these general protocols, sulfur helps the body get rid of arsenic. Sulfur-rich foods include garlic, onions, and cruciferous vegetables.

Strategies: Fasting and Heavy Metal Cleanse

Formulas: Stabilized Allicin

Herbs: Garlic

Supplements: Alpha-lipoic acid, iodine, MSM, and selenium

Arteriosclerosis
Atherosclerosis, Hardening of the Arteries

See also cardiovascular disease, cholesterol (high), and free radical damage

Arteriosclerosis, or hardening of the arteries, occurs when there is damage to the lining of the blood vessels from poor diet, infection, or free radical damage. There is a thickening of interior vessel walls, usually by fatty or mineral deposits, that reduces the opening size and obstructs blood flow.

Restricted blood flow prevents tissues from getting oxygen and nutrients, which prevents wounds from healing, causes coldness in the extremities, and affects memory and cognitive function. When a blood clot forms in the circulatory system, it may get lodged in the heart, causing cardiac arrest, or in the brain, causing a stroke.

Although most people believe that high cholesterol causes arteriosclerosis, there is ample research to suggest that cholesterol itself has little to do with the problem. It is mostly due to elevated insulin from high carbohydrate consumption, lack of exercise, chronic inflammation, and general poor nutrition. It may also occur in response to infection.

To reduce your risk of arteriosclerosis, use healthy fats, eliminate refined carbohydrates, and increase your antioxidant and nutrient rich vegetables and fruits. If you have gingivitis, you should work on dental health as there is a link between gum infections and arterial infections and hardening of the arteries. Co-Q10 is a nutrient that can help both the gums and the arteries.

If you have already developed arteriosclerosis the most effective treatment is substantial weight loss. There is limited but profound research showing that medically supervised long-term fasting can reverse arterial plaque. It's likely that fasting for shorter durations can offer benefits.

The *Oral Chelation* strategy has proven beneficial for many people with hardening of the arteries. It requires some commitment as it takes many months, but many people have had major improvements in blood flow after completing it. It may also be helpful to use the *Enhance Nitric Oxide* strategy as this also can help improve blood flow. Also, see related conditions, especially *cardiovascular disease*, for more suggestions on preventing and reversing this condition.

Strategies: Avoid Sugar, Eat Healthy, Enhance Nitric Oxide, Healthy Fats, Heavy Metal Cleanse, Low-Glycemic Diet, Oral Chelation, and Stress Management

Formulas: Circulatory, Stabilized Allicin, **Oral Chelation**, Green Tea Polyphenols, Skinny, Antioxidant, **Heart Health**, **Nitric Oxide Boosting**, and Oral Chelation

Programs: Cardiovascular Nutritional

Herbs: Arjuna, black currant, capsicum, garlic, ginkgo, guggul, **hawthorn**, olive, reishi, rose, and tea

Supplements: Chromium, **Co-Q10**, **L-arginine**, **omega-3 EFAs**, **vitamin B$_3$**, vitamin B$_9$, vitamin C, vitamin D, vitamin E, and zinc

Essential Oils: Grapefruit (pink)

Arthritis
Osteoarthritis

The word arthritis literally means "inflammation of a joint," but there are many different kinds of arthritis and many different causes. When dealing with this disturbingly common disease (more than 20 million Americans are thought to suffer from it) it is necessary to look at its underlying causes and deal with them to achieve any kind of real results.

Most people are familiar with the two most common forms of arthritis, osteoarthritis and rheumatoid arthritis. Osteoarthritis affects more than 15 million Americans and occurs most frequently in older people. In osteoarthritis, the cartilage that coats the ends of the bones in our joints begins to break down, starting a vicious cycle of damage, reduced function and health, leading to more damage. It is not a systemic disease but the result of damage from local wear and tear, trauma, and surgery or infection to a specific joint. It can also result from the effects of other diseases.

The main symptoms of osteoarthritis are: pain in the affected joint(s) after repeated use, especially later in the day; swelling, pain and stiffness after long periods of inactivity, like sleep, that subside with movement and activity; continuous pain, even at rest, with advanced osteoarthritis.

In contrast, rheumatoid arthritis is much more rare, occurring in less than 1 percent of the population. Unlike osteoarthritis, rheumatoid arthritis is an autoimmune disease—meaning the tissues that surround and cushion the joints are attacked by the body's own immune system. This happens throughout the whole body, not just in joints that have been subjected to wear and tear. It usually occurs between the ages of twenty-five and fifty, but it can develop at any age and generally strikes women three times as often as men.

Symptoms of rheumatoid arthritis include: swollen, warm, painful joints, especially after long periods of inactivity; fatigue and occasional fever: symmetrical pattern of inflammation if one wrist is involved, the other will be also, the small joints of the body (hands, fingers, feet, toes, wrists, elbows and ankles) are usually affected first; as the disease progresses, the joints often will become deformed and may freeze in one position, making it difficult to move them.

Other Forms of Arthritis

In addition to these most common forms of arthritis, there are some other recognized forms. Here are a few. Allergic arthritis, as the name implies, is triggered by an allergic reaction. Gonorrheal arthritis is inflammation of the joints resulting from gonorrheal infection. Gouty arthritis was the most widely known variety until the 20th century. Caused by an elevation of uric acid in the blood, it also causes joint inflammation and usually affects one joint at a time.

What all these forms of arthritis have in common is that the joints have been subjected to some kind of stress: mechanical, biochemical, or infectious. Joints are meant to endure a certain amount of wear and tear, but when toxins and inflammation are present, it creates more friction in the joints (just like the dirty oil in a car). When nutrients needed for joint health are absent, repairs can't be made, which makes the joint more easily damaged and inflamed.

Healing Strategies for Arthritis

There are three main things that need to be done to help arthritis to heal. First we need to identify and remove sources of stress, whether they are mechanical, biochemical, or infectious. Secondly, we need to reduce inflammation and tissue toxicity. Finally, we need to supply the nutrients necessary for joint health to aid the body in effecting repairs.

Remove Sources of Irritation

In osteoarthritis, reducing mechanical stress to the joints is an important key. This mechanical stress is often the result of repetitive habits of movement and posture that were not properly balanced. Correcting structural alignment through stretching, yoga, massage, or other forms of bodywork will help to take mechanical stress off joints and allow better blood flow and alignment. If excess weight is putting stress on joints, losing weight will relieve some of that stress. Mild exercise that doesn't put much stress on the joints will improve blood and lymph flow to bring healing energy to the joints. Self-massage (especially using some type of *Analgesic EO Formula*) will also improve blood and lymph flow.

Where there is an infectious cause, the infection will need to be dealt with using whatever remedies are appropriate to that type of infection. Where the cause of stress is biochemical, as in rheumatoid, allergic, or gouty arthritis, improving the diet is a crucial step.

Wheat, dairy (A1 beta-casein), corn, GMOs, and chemicals in our food have been implicated in triggering arthritis. So have nightshade vegetables like eggplant, tomatoes, potatoes, and green peppers. Tobacco, which is also in the nightshade family, also increases the risk of arthritis. Follow the *Eliminate Allergy-Causing Foods* strategy and see if it helps. One could also try the *Fasting* therapy, especially with raw vegetable juices.

Reduce Inflammation

Since arthritis is an inflammatory condition, remedies that reduce inflammatory reactions is another obvious strategy for recovery. Inflammation can be combated nutritionally by cooking with herbs like ginger and turmeric. Oily fish such as salmon, are excellent sources of Omega-3 fatty acids, which also combat inflammation.

Herbs containing salicylates have been used for thousands of years to ease arthritic pain. Salicylates, the forerunners of modern aspirin, reduce joint swelling and inflammation, and ease pain. Plants containing salicylates include willow bark, black cohosh, meadowsweet, and wintergreen.

If massage relieves pain, then massage around sore joints several times a day using a blend of analgesic essential oils. Besides easing pain, this keeps fluid out of the tissue spaces and allows more oxygen and nutrients to reach the tissues better for more effective healing. The use of massage for reducing inflammation and easing pain are part of the *Lymph-Moving Pain Relief Strategy* and are discussed in detail in my *Fundamentals of Natural Healing* course.

Herbal Arthritis Formulas are designed to ease pain and promote healing in arthritic joints. These formulas typically rely on anti-inflammatory herbs (like boswellia, white willow, Devil's claw, turmeric, and yucca), tissue-healing and mineralizing herbs (like alfalfa), and detoxifying herbs (like burdock and sarsaparilla), providing a multi-action relief.

Provide Nutrition to the Joints

Bones and joints aren't static, dead objects; they are composed of living tissue. This makes them capable of growth, change, and repair. To aid this repair one must get the right nutrients in the diet and a good flow of blood and lymph to the tissues (which can be aided by regular massage as described above).

Minerals are extremely critical to aiding joint repair. Silica adds resiliency to joints, so they are less susceptible to damage. It is found in herbs like horsetail and dulse and *Watkin's Hair, Skin and Nails Formula*.

Collagen is a major supportive tissue in the human body. Cartilage, ligaments and tendons are primarily made of collagen. Collagen supplements seem to help regulate the inflammatory response by encouraging the formation of T-Reg cells in the gut. Small clinical trials show benefit in both osteoarthritis and rheumatoid arthritis.

Three other important nutrients that can aid joint repair include MSM, glucosamine, and chondroitin. You can read more about each in the remedies section. All of them are found in the *Joint Healing Nutrients Formula*.

A great way to get the nutrients needed for healthy joints and bones is to make homemade stock. This is done by simmering bones, meat scraps and vegetables in water for a long time. Directions for making stock can be found in the *Bone Broth* strategy.

Additional Remedies

There are many other herbs, nutrients and essential oils that have been used to aid arthritis. It's best to match remedies to the tissue state. Some people needing warming, blood-moving herbs, and others needing cooling, moistening remedies. Solomon's seal is an underutilized cooling and moistening remedy, specific for dry, creaky arthritis. It's also effective for arthritis of the small joints when applied topically as a salve.

Strategies: Affirmation and Visualization, Alkalize the Body, Bodywork, Bone Broth, Compress or Fomentation, Detoxification, Drawing Bath, Eat Healthy, Eliminate Allergy-Causing Foods, Eliminate Salicylates, Enhance Nitric Oxide, Fasting, Healthy Fats, Hydration, Lymph-Moving Pain Relief, and Mineralization

Formulas: Stan Malstrom's Herbal Aspirin, Herbal Calcium, **Colloidal Mineral**, **Joint Healing Nutrients**, Proanthocyanidins, **Watkin's Hair, Skin, and Nails**, **Herbal Arthritis**, Chinese Water-Increasing, Enzyme Spray, **Topical Analgesic**, Gut Immune, Chinese Yang-Reducing, Vulnerary, Skeletal Support, Anti-Inflammatory Pain, **Analgesic Nerve**, General Analgesic, Nitric Oxide Boosting, Joan Patton's Herbal Minerals, **CBD Anti-inflammatory**, **CBD Topical Analgesic**, Hemp Oil with Terpenes, and CBD Joint

Essential Oil Blends: Analgesic EO

Herbs: Alfalfa, amur cork, black currant, borage, **boswellia**, burdock, capsicum, cat's claw, celery seed, chicory, **devil's claw**, dogwood (Jamaican), epimedium, evening primrose, Grape, horsetail, licorice, meadowsweet, nettle, stinging, noni, prickly ash, reishi, safflower, **solomon's seal**, **turmeric**, **willow**, and yucca

Supplements: Boron, **CBD**, **chondroitin**, **collagen**, copper, **curcumin**, **glucosamine**, magnesium, **MSM**, omega-3 DHA, **omega-3 EFAs**, omega-6 GLA, selenium, silicon, and vitamin D

Essential Oils: Camphor, copaiba, eucalyptus, fir, frankincense, helichrysum, jasmine, juniper, lemon, marjoram, menthol, oregano, ravintsara, rosemary, spruce (blue), and **wintergreen essential oil**

Arthritis, Rheumatoid

Rheumatism

See also food allergies/intolerances, arthritis, autoimmune disorders, and leaky gut

Rheumatoid arthritis is a type of arthritis that has an autoimmune component. It is characterized by inflammation and pain in muscles, joints, or fibrous tissues. See *autoimmune disorders* for a detailed approach to working with autoimmune disorders in general. Also read the entry for *arthritis*.

Some specific remedies that may be helpful for rheumatoid arthritis include omega-3 essential fatty acids, CBD, cat's claw, and turmeric. Fasting can be helpful. It's also important to address the health of the bowel and eliminate any potential food allergies and intolerance. Nightshades, in particular, such as tomatoes and potatoes, are problematic for many people.

Strategies: Detoxification, Eliminate Allergy-Causing Foods, Fasting, Gluten-Free Diet, Gut-Healing Diet, Healthy Fats, and Hydration

Formulas: Herbal Arthritis, Joint Healing Nutrients, Antioxidant, and Analgesic Nerve

Herbs: Alfalfa, **aloe vera juice**, ashwagandha, **astragalus**, bladderwrack, blue cohosh, boswellia, **cat's claw**, **celery**, chickweed, couchgrass, **devil's claw**, gravel root, kava kava, meadowsweet, nettle, stinging, noni, prickly ash, **solomon's seal**, **turmeric**, and yucca

Supplements: Bromelain, **CBD**, collagen, **curcumin**, glucosamine, **MSM**, **omega-3 EFAs**, vitamin B_3, and **vitamin D**

Essential Oils: Clove, grapefruit (pink), lemon, marjoram, spruce (blue), and spruce (hemlock)

Asthma

See also adrenal fatigue, food allergies/intolerances, allergies (respiratory), congestion (bronchial), congestion (lymphatic), hiatal hernia, leaky gut, and COPD

Asthma is a condition where the air passages either constrict or become swollen making breathing difficult. It is often unpredictable; and this is what makes it so intimidating. Those who suffer from it experience bouts of breathlessness which can come on suddenly during periods of stress, anxiety, exercise, low blood sugar, laughing, changes in temperature, extremes of dryness or dampness, or exposure to allergens such as dust, animal dander, smoke, mold, or food additives. Asthma attacks can last from minutes to hours and can come daily or annually.

Asthma on the rise, affecting about seventeen million Americans (five million children and twelve million adults). The dramatic increase in asthma appears to be linked to the increase in air pollution and other lung irritants, including chemicals in food such as pesticides, preservatives, sugar in refined foods, and GMOs.

Everyone's lungs will react to irritants by the process of inflammation, swelling, mucus production, and coughing. For the person with asthma these reactions are exaggerated or hyperactive. Swelling and inflammation in the lung tissue trigger emotions that cause spastic reactions in the lungs, which further constrict airways. As air is trapped in the lungs, excess carbon dioxide builds up in the blood creating the suffocating feeling.

Medical Treatment

Asthma is commonly treated with antihistamines (substances which reduce allergic reactions), anti-inflammatories (substances that reduce swelling and inflammation) and bronchial dilators (substances that relax the bronchial passages, allowing air to escape). These therapies are effective for symptomatic relief and can ease attacks and even save lives, but they do not help to relieve any of the underlying causes of this disease.

Strategies for Asthma

If more than symptomatic relief is to be had, you need to identify the causes of the immune imbalance and lung irritation. Here are some of the underlying causes to consider and work on.

Eliminate Allergens

Most individuals who experience asthma notice that it is prompted by substances such as pollen, dander, smoke, or cold air, or even excessive exercise. Environmental allergens like dust, mites, molds, and pet dander can trigger allergies or asthma, but diet is often at the root of the problem. Food allergies or intolerances can be a problem in asthmatics. Dairy products and grains containing gluten are the most common culprits. They, along with refined carbohydrates, promote dysbiosis, which sets the stage for the inflammatory immune reaction that causes asthma. Look for more information under *allergies (respiratory)* and *food allergies and intolerances*.

Avoid Xenoestrogens

Adult asthma tends to be most prevalent in women. Many physicians believe this to be hormonally related. With the rising number of asthma cases, this could be due in part to the influence of xenoestrogens (estrogen-like chemicals such as pesticides and plastics) present in our environment. See the *Avoid Xenoestrogens* strategy.

Manage Stress and Support the Adrenal Glands

Epinephrine (adrenaline) acts as a bronchial dilator. Forms of it can be injected or are used in bronchial inhalers in order to halt asthma attacks. Epinephrine is both an adrenal hormone and a sympathetic neurotransmitter.

Corticosteroid drugs are also used to treat asthma. These drugs are mimics of another adrenal hormone, cortisol, which reduces inflammation in the body.

This suggests a connection between stress and possibly adrenal function in asthma cases. People who have been involved in any type of organized athletics are bound to have met individuals with exercise-induced asthma. A number of nutrients may be helpful here. Vitamin C is important for adrenal function and the production of epinephrine. Licorice root has a cortisol-sparing action and can be helpful in reducing the inflammation associated with asthma, especially in children. An *Adrenal Glandular Formula* is sometimes helpful (see *adrenal fatigue*). It is also wise to avoid refined sugar, and foods and beverages containing caffeine.

Correct Digestive Problems

Many, if not all, asthmatics have digestive issues. A hiatal hernia, which inhibits free movement of the diaphragm, contributes to poor digestion of and the resulting dysbiosis. A common but largely unexplored mechanism of asthma is the irritation of the respiratory mucosa from silent GERD. Food intolerances and diets high in refined carbohydrates often fuel a specific type of dysbiosis called small intestinal bacterial overgrowth (see It these are problems see the appropriate entry for suggestions about natural therapy.). There may also be fungal overgrowth.

When there is an overgrowth of bacteria or fungus in the small intestines, there is increased gas production in the small intestines. This gas increases intra-abdominal pressure and causes malfunction of the lower esophageal sphincter, the valve that keeps stomach acid from rising upward. It also presses the stomach upward causing a hiatal hernia. When acid gases from the stomach rise without causing apparent irritation of the esophagus, it's called silent reflux. These acidic gases can irritate mucosa in the sinuses and lungs and set the stage for allergic responses.

It's possible that most people with chronic sinusitis, chronic ear infections and asthma have undiagnosed silent reflux. FODMAP restriction (see *Eliminate FODMAP* strategy) and remedies for *leaky gut syndrome* and *SIBO* may be helpful.

Cleansing the liver and colon is an effective traditional approach for many respiratory complaints. The benefits probably aren't due to improvements in liver or colon function but are likely due to changes in the gut microbiome and its regulatory effects on the inflammatory process.

Break up Mucus Congestion

Mucus buildup in the lungs may be a contributing factor in asthma. This can occur partly because the epinephrine-based inhalers used to stop asthma attacks have a drying action that tends to dry out mucus secretions in the lungs. Yerba santa, grindelia, mullein, and plantain are particularly good remedies for loosening this mucus in the lungs.

Use Natural Bronchial Dilators

To stop asthma attacks it is necessary to dilate the bronchial passages to let in more air. Lobelia is a very effective bronchial dilator and antispasmodic. It has a long history of successful use in easing asthma attacks. A tincture or extract of lobelia can be administered in doses of three to twenty drops at one-to-two minute intervals, starting at the beginning of the attack until it subsides. Lobelia can also be rubbed onto the chest to relax feelings of tightness and to relieve coughing.

Occasionally, taking lobelia internally will cause a person to vomit. If this happens, don't be alarmed. The asthma attack nearly always subsides as soon as the person vomits.

Asthma is a serious condition yet one that can often be dealt with effectively by natural means. It will take some determination, study, and a commitment to a generally healthier lifestyle. If you have improved your health and asthma symptoms, it's still a good idea to keep an emergency inhaler at hand for unexpected emergencies.

Strategies: Avoid Sugar, Avoid Xenoestrogens, Colon Hydrotherapy, Detoxification, Eat Healthy, Eliminate Allergy-Causing Foods, Enhance Nitric Oxide, Fasting, Gut-Healing Diet, Healthy Fats, Hiatal Hernia Correction, Hydration, and Stress Management

Formulas: Adrenal Glandular, Jeannie Burgess' Allergy-Lung, Ayurvedic Bronchial Decongestant, Chinese Metal-Increasing, **Lung Moistening, Chinese Metal-Decreasing, Antispasmodic**, Nitric Oxide Boosting, and Betaine HCl

Essential Oil Blends: Lung-Supporting EO

Herbs: Amalaki, apricot, asafetida, astragalus, bibhitaki, black currant, butterbur, cherry, chicory, chirata, coleus, **coltsfoot, cordyceps**, cyperus, elecampane, **grindelia**, haritaki, holy basil, honeysuckle, hyssop, **khella**, kutki, licorice, **lobelia**, magnolia, marshmallow, mulberry, mullein, oregano, picrorhiza, skunk cabbage, vervain (blue), and **yerba santa**

Supplements: CBD, Co-Q10, **magnesium**, MSM, N-acetyl cysteine, quercetin, vitamin B-complex, and vitamin B_5

Essential Oils: Anise, eucalyptus, frankincense, helichrysum, lemon, marjoram, menthol, peppermint, pine, red mandarin, rose, spruce (hemlock), tansy (blue), tea tree, thyme, and ylang ylang

Atherosclerosis   *see arteriosclerosis*

Athlete's Foot

See also infection (fungal)

Athlete's foot is a fungal infection of the foot most often between the toes and on the soles of the feet. Symptoms include pain, burning and itching. The problem in treating athlete's foot is that it exists inside the skin where it is difficult to reach via the circulatory system and it is also difficult to eradicate. Use herbs or essential oils with antifungal action topically, consistently for forty-five uninterrupted days. Athletes foot is more common in those with poor circulation and immunity, frequently caused by insulin resistance. Also consider doing a *Yeast Cleansing Program*.

Strategies: Avoid Sugar, Friendly Flora, and Low-Glycemic Diet

Formulas: Standardized Acetogenin and Anti-Fungal

Programs: Yeast Cleansing

Essential Oil Blends: Antifungal EO

Herbs: Black walnut, calendula, garlic, myrrh, **oregano**, pau d'arco, pawpaw, thuja, and usnea

Supplements: Vitamin A, vitamin C, vitamin D, and zinc

Essential Oils: Myrrh, neroli, oregano, tea tree, and thyme

Attention Deficit Disorder   **see** *ADD/ADHD*

Autism
Autism Spectrum Disorder (ASD)

See also heavy metal poisoning and vaccine side effects

Autism, also known as autism spectrum disorder (ASD), is a mental condition of self-centered subjective mental activity (daydreams, fantasies, delusions, hallucinations, etc.) often accompanied by a marked withdrawal from reality. Autism has increased dramatically in the past few decades suggesting it is linked to cultural changes. These could include increasingly poor diets, exposure to environmental toxins and the increased number of vaccines given to children.

Two theories link autism and vaccines. The first theory suggests that the MMR (Mumps-Measles-Rubella) vaccine may cause intestinal problems leading to the development of autism. The second theory suggests that a mercury-based preservative called thimerosal, used in some vaccines, could be connected to autism. The medical community continually refutes these theories, but a very passionate group of parents and researchers continues to disagree. I personally believe that there is a link, but that vaccines are not the only problem (see *vaccine side effects*).

There is some evidence that autism is linked to problems in the immune system. Autistic individuals often have other physical issues related to immune deficiency. Some researchers say they have developed effective treatments based on boosting the immune system.

There is also evidence that allergies to certain foods could contribute to autistic symptoms. Most people who hold to this theory feel that gluten (a wheat product) and casein (dairy) are the most significant culprits.

Strategies for Autism

Because of the complexity and seriousness of this condition, professional assistance and support should be sought. The following may be helpful in getting started.

First, improve the diet in general so children are getting the nutrients they need. For starters, avoid refined carbohydrates (simple sugars and starches) and using more fresh fruits and vegetables. Make sure the child is getting high quality fats and proteins. Eliminate possible food allerges (see *food allergies/intolerances*). Dairy products and grains are often major contributing factors to this condition. The specific carbohydrate diet and the GAPS diet (see *Gut-Healing Diet* strategy) have been successful for many children. Also, heal the intestinal tract, as intestinal inflammation is often a major issue (see *leaky gut syndrome*).

Immune overactivity, specifically antibodies to certain brain proteins, has been found in several small studies. Many children with ASD also have other autoimmune disorders, including celiac and eczema. A general approach of balancing the immune system through diet, nutritional supplements, and herbs has been helpful in many children.

Astragalus, codonopsis and medicinal mushrooms have a balancing action on the immune system and could play a role in natural autism treatment. Some specific nutritional deficiencies that are common with autism include B_{12}, folate, vitamin C, vitamin A, and vitamin D.

Strategies: Avoid Sugar, Eat Healthy, Friendly Flora, Healthy Fats, Heavy Metal Cleanse, and Reduce Chemical Exposure

Formulas: Green Tea Polyphenols, **Heavy Metal Cleansing**, Brain Calming, Methylated B Vitamin, Methyl B12 Vitamin, and Mushroom Immune

Herbs: Astragalus, black walnut, codonopsis, ginkgo, **lemon balm**, linden flowers, mimosa, Saint John's wort, and tea

Supplements: CBD, Co-Q10, **L-glutamine**, **magnesium**, N-acetyl cysteine, omega-3 DHA, **omega-3 EFAs**, protease, vitamin A, **vitamin B-complex**, vitamin B_6, vitamin B_9, vitamin C, and vitamin D

Essential Oils: Frankincense, lavender, and myrrh

Autoimmune Disorders

See also fibromyalgia, Graves' disease, Hashimoto's disease, ALS, lupus, multiple sclerosis, myasthenia gravis, arthritis (rheumatoid), and vaccine side effects

The human immune system is a marvel. Most of the time, it does a wonderful job of protecting us from infections, tox-

ins, and abnormal cells of all kinds. It is able to protect us because it is able to determine which cells and proteins are part of the body and which are not. In other words, it identifies what is self and what is not-self. It is able to tag what is not-self, then destroy and eliminate it.

Unfortunately, the immune system can become confused about what is self and what is not-self. When this happens, the confused immune system starts tagging the body's own tissues and proteins as if they were foreign invaders. This causes the immune system to attack and damage the body's own tissues. Medicine has dubbed the diseases where this happens as *autoimmune*.

Autoimmune disorders have been likened to a problem that occurs in a war when a commanding officer, acting on bad information, attacks and targets his own troops. The military calls this friendly fire. So the root of autoimmune disorders is confusion about who the enemy is, resulting in friendly fire on the part of the immune system.

There are many autoimmune disorders, but they fall into two broad categories. There are conditions where the immune system confusion is confined to a specific organ or tissue, and there are conditions that are systemic in nature—meaning the immune system is attacking tissues throughout the body. Hashimoto's thyroiditis, Graves' disease, myasthenia gravis, Crohn's disease, multiple sclerosis, and vitiligo are examples of organ-specific autoimmune diseases. Systemic disorders include Sjögren's syndrome, scleroderma and rheumatoid arthritis.

What Causes Autoimmune Reactions?

So what causes the confusion in the immune system? Medical science has proposed several theories. One theory is that chronic, low-grade viral and bacterial infections stimulate an excessive immune response, resulting in a dysregulation of the immune system. This may be a factor in autoimmune disease like rheumatoid arthritis, lupus, and Crohn's.

Another theory suggests that foreign substances (antigens), such as gluten from certain grains, are being absorbed into the body and triggering immune reactions. Because these proteins are similar to proteins found naturally in the body, the immune system winds up waging war on both. This is called molecular mimicry. Intestinal dysbiosis and leaky gut syndrome may be at the root of this problem, as the gastrointestinal (GI) tract issues are what allows these substances to be absorbed.

A third theory, called the hygiene hypothesis, suggests that the cause of people's dysbiosis and intestinal problems lies in our over-sterilized living environments. This is a known factor in the increase in the development of allergies, which are another form of immune system dysregulation, where the immune system is overreacting to harmless external influences.

The reason this is a factor is that the friendly microbes that live in our GI tract are part of our immune system and contribute to its regulation. In order to create a healthy gut microflora, we need to be exposed to dirt and the microbes it contains in early childhood, so the immune system can figure out what is a real threat and what is not. Because of this, children growing up on farms have healthier immune systems and fewer incidences of allergies and asthma than kids who grow up in sterile environments.

All these theories are somewhat interconnected and it is probable that autoimmune disorders have more than one cause. What this means to the person suffering from an autoimmune disorder is that there is never going to be a magic pill or specific cure that is going to fix an autoimmune condition. There may be very effective symptom-relieving drugs, but to actually restore normal immune functions, one has to approach the problem from multiple directions.

Strategies for Autoimmune Diseases

What follow are some basic therapies that can be helpful for all autoimmune disorders. These therapies are a good place to start the healing journey. There may also be therapies for specific autoimmune diseases that you can employ in addition to these core therapies, but you'll have to explore those by working closely with your herbalist, naturopath, natural healer, or holistic medical doctor.

Reduce Exposure to Environmental Toxins

There are those who believe that the dramatic rise in autoimmune disorders is linked to environmental influences that are damaging our health. Both vaccinations and environmental toxins may be factors.

One study found that when mice were given a certain number of vaccines, comparable to the schedule given to humans, they developed antibodies associated with autoimmune disease. There are a number of researchers who believe that we may be trading acute infections for autoimmune diseases and allergies by giving too many vaccines (see *vaccine side effects*).

Another potential environmental trigger for autoimmune diseases may be the ever-increasing number of chemicals we are exposed to from air pollution, water pollution, household cleaning supplies, food additives, and agricultural chemicals. It is well-known that many of these chemicals disrupt communications in the glandular system. Is it possible that they could also be disrupting communication in the immune system?

The bottom line is that anyone who has an autoimmune disorder should do their best to minimize their exposure to toxins of all kinds. Switching to natural household cleaning products and eating organic foods are good places to start. (See *Reduce Chemical Exposure* strategy.)

Gently Detoxify the Body

A person with autoimmune disease should do some gentle cleansing to help remove toxins from their body. The cleansing must be gradual and gentle, as strong cleansing programs may exacerbate symptoms in autoimmune diseases. The best herbs to use for detoxification in these cases are alteratives, like red clover and burdock, and *Blood Purifier Formulas* that contain them.

As the body becomes stronger, heavy metal detoxification may be helpful for clearing heavy metals and other toxins from the body. The key is to start slowly, drink plenty of water, and discontinue any cleansing herbs if symptoms get worse.

Heal the Gastrointestinal Tract

Healing the GI tract is a critical, basic strategy for anyone with autoimmune conditions. There several parts to this. First, use digestive enzymes and/or hydrochloric acid supplements to improve digestive function. Most people with autoimmune disorders benefit greatly from these supplements but often require high doses (two to three times the normal dose).

It is also wise for people with autoimmune issues to eliminate all potential allergy-causing foods. It may take some experimentation to find out which foods need to be eliminated (see *Eliminate Allergy-Causing Foods* strategy).

As previously suggested, leaky gut syndrome may be a contributing factor in most, if not all, autoimmune conditions (see *leaky gut syndrome*). Developing and maintaining a healthy intestinal microflora is essential to balancing the immune functions in these problems (see *Friendly Flora* strategy).

Fix Low Grade Infections

As mentioned earlier, chronic low-grade viral and bacterial infections have been implicated in causing immune dysregulation. You may need professional assistance in identifying these infections if they are present. These infections could include Epstein-Barr virus, gingivitis, chronic sinusitis, or ongoing urinary tract infections. In treating these infections, one should follow the same advice as for cleansing. Start with a low dose to make sure the supplement is tolerated, then gradually work up to a larger dose.

Balance the Immune System

With autoimmune disorders, the goal is not to stimulate the immune system but to regulate it. Remedies that balance immune function are known as immune modulators or immune amphoterics. These include herbs like ashwagandha, codonopsis, reishi, and turkey tail. As with other supplements for autoimmune conditions, start with small doses, and if symptoms get worse, discontinue the supplement.

Another way to balance the immune system is to down-regulate inflammatory processes. So a person with an autoimmune condition will benefit from using foods, herbs, and supplements that reduce inflammation. These include turmeric or curcumin, omega-3 essential fatty acids, and licorice root, which also supports adrenal function.

A relatively new supplement for autoimmune disorders is CBD. CBD helps normalize immune responses and is also anti-inflammatory, making it potentially helpful in various autoimmune conditions.

Support Adrenal Function

The adrenal glands produce a hormone called cortisol that reduces inflammatory responses and calms down the immune system. The corticosteroid drugs often used to treat autoimmune disorders are mimics of this hormone, which is also released from the body during stress.

Chronic stress weakens the adrenal glands, which can result in cortisol levels being too low. In my experience, everyone I've seen with an autoimmune disorder has exhausted adrenals, so supporting the adrenal glands and managing stress is another key strategy for these problems. Two herbs that have a cortisol-like action and can be helpful for autoimmune disorders are licorice and yucca. An *Adrenal Glandular Formula* may also be helpful.

In summary, autoimmune disorders are best approached by focusing on an overall program of health improvement. As toxins are eliminated, the health of the GI tract is improved and inflammation is reduced, then the immune system will do a better job of identifying friend from foe. It takes some persistent and patient effort, but it can be done.

Strategies: Affirmation and Visualization, Avoid Sugar, Blood Type Diet, Bone Broth, Eat Healthy, Eliminate Allergy-Causing Foods, Forgiveness, Friendly Flora, Gluten-Free Diet, Gut-Healing Diet, Healthy Fats, Heavy Metal Cleanse, Hiatal Hernia Correction, Hydration, Increase Dietary Fiber, Low-Glycemic Diet, Pleasure Prescription, and Stress Management

Formulas: Adrenal Glandular, Heavy Metal Cleansing, **Plant Enzyme, Whole Food Green Drink,** Adaptogen-Immune, Chinese Yang-Reducing, **Antioxidant, Ashwagandha Complex, Digestive Support,** Blood Purifier, Hemp Oil with Terpenes, Betaine HCl, Probiotic, and Adaptogen

Flower Essence Blends: Personal Boundaries FE

Herbs: Aloe vera, **ashwagandha,** astragalus, **codonopsis,** cordyceps, hydrangea, **licorice,** reishi, solomon's seal, turkey tail, and turmeric

Supplements: Bromelain, CBD, colostrum, curcumin, omega-3 EFAs, omega-6 GLA, potassium, protease, and vitamin D

Backache
Back Pain, Lumbago

See also spinal disks

Problems with the spine are so common that nearly everyone experiences them at some point in their life. Statistics suggest that about 80 percent of the population will experience back pain, and the older you get, the more likely back pain becomes.

Back pain or backache can be caused by many things. The most common form is pain in the lower back, also known as lumbago. Structural imbalances, caused by poor posture, are a common cause. Excess weight, straining the back by lifting heavy things, muscle tension or spasms, and a general lack of physical fitness all contribute to the problem.

Interestingly, 50 percent of people with chronic low back pain have no structural damage and 50 percent of people with a herniated disc have no back pain. This leads many to believe that back pain has more to do with stress and general inflammation than tissue damage. In the natural world, nutritional deficiencies, poor kidney function and even emotional issues, such as fear or depression can contribute to back problems.

Nerves, Emotions and Your Backbone

Your spine is more than just a structural support that lets you stand upright and move; it's also a protective conduit for your nerves. Spinal problems don't just cause backaches; they also interfere with nerve signals, which can create problems throughout the body.

Strategies for Overcoming Back Pain

Here are some ways to avoid back problems and help to reverse them when they occur.

Straighten Up Your Act

Since poor posture is a major contributor to back problems, do things to improve your posture. For example, practice standing straight by standing with your back against a wall. Stretch out your back and try to align your back against the wall. Also practice sitting up straight when working at a computer or desk. Move the computer monitor so it is at eye level to keep your head straight.

Make Sure Your Hips Are Aligned

Check the alignment of your hips by standing in front of a mirror and placing your fingers on the hip bones on both sides of your body. Notice if they are level. If they are not (that is, if one hip is higher than the other), this could be causing your back pain. It can also cause neck and shoulder pain because the pelvis is the foundation for the spine. If the pelvis is out of alignment, then the whole spine will be stressed all the way to the neck.

If your pelvis is out of alignment, bodywork along with exercise and improving your posture will often correct the alignment. Seek out a chiropractor who works with muscles and connective tissue, a well-trained massage therapist who can do deep tissue work, or other bodyworker who can assist you in getting your pelvis and spine in alignment.

Stretch and Move Your Spine

Practice bending and stretching your spine in different directions to keep it flexible. If you work at a desk or sit a lot, try stretching backward, putting your hands on your hips and leaning backwards. If you're really stiff, try the *Herbal Back Adjustment* strategy and get some body work done to help loosen up your back. Chiropractic care, massage therapy, or yoga may be helpful (see *Bodywork* strategy).

Change Your Mood, Change Your Posture

Since the spinal column is closely connected with the nervous system, it makes sense that mood affects the health and function of the spine. A healthy spine is associated with courage and fortitude, as shown by the phrase "Show some backbone." And standing straight and tall is associated with integrity, which is why it is referred to as uprightness.

When you feel discouraged, sad, or depressed, you are more likely to hang your head and slump forward. When you feel confident, happy, and motivated you are more likely to stand tall and hold your head up high.

In traditional Chinese medicine (TCM), this forward-slumping posture due to depression and sadness is called "sagging qi," which could be translated as "sagging energy." A *Chinese Qi-Regulating Formula* can help you stand upright and feel better about yourself.

Interestingly enough, research shows that while mood affects posture, posture also affects mood. When a person stands or sits up straight, plants their feet firmly on the floor, and throws their shoulders back, they will actually feel more confident and positive. Try it and see how you feel.

Strengthen Your Kidney Qi

In TCM, the kidneys are said to build the bones—meaning water and good kidney function are considered essential to a healthy structural system and especially to the bones. Water lubricates the joints and keeps the discs between the vertebrae hydrated. Dehydration thins the discs and stresses the joints. So if you have back pain, make sure you are drinking enough pure water every day.

The kidneys also help to maintain balance between the fluids of the body and the minerals needed for healthy structure.

In TCM, a deficiency of kidney qi (energy) can cause not only back pain but weakness of the legs, knees, and ankles. A *Chinese Water-Increasing Formula* can be used to tonify (or increase) the kidney qi to ease back pain and strengthen the bones and joints in general. Where there is water retention, a *Chinese Water-Decreasing Formula* may be helpful.

Reduce Chronic Inflammation

Since back pain can involve inflammation, it can also be helpful to take anti-inflammatory herbs and remedies if there is heat and some swelling of tissues in the back. Look for a formulas containing herbs like turmeric or curcumin, boswellia, white willow bark, and/or mangosteen pericarp and take it at least twice each day.

Strategies: Alkalize the Body, Bodywork, Good Posture, Herbal Back Adjustment, Hydration, Lymph-Moving Pain Relief, and Mineralization

Formulas: Stan Malstrom's Herbal Aspirin, Herbal Calcium, **Chinese Water-Increasing**, Chinese Water-Decreasing, **Enzyme Spray**, Skeletal Support, Topical Analgesic, Joint Healing Nutrients, Anti-Inflammatory Pain, Chinese Qi-Regulating, **CBD Topical Analgesic**, and CBD Anti-inflammatory

Essential Oil Blends: Analgesic EO

Herbs: Achyranthes, arnica, asparagus, broomrape, **corydalis**, cramp bark, devil's claw, **dogwood (Jamaican)**, eucommia, kava kava, lobelia, mullein root, skullcap, vervain (blue), and wood betony

Supplements: Bromelain, collagen, glucosamine, **magnesium**, **MSM**, vitamin B_3, and vitamin C

Essential Oils: Camphor and wintergreen

Bacterial Infection   see *infection (bacterial)*

Bad Breath   see *halitosis*

Baldness   see *hair loss/thinning*

Bedwetting

See also incontinence

When a child loses bladder control while sleeping and wets the bed, it can be caused by the same problems that cause some adults to wake up during the night to use the bathroom.

Severe stress inhibits urinary function, which may resume when a person is resting at night. Blood sugar problems can cause a child to wet the bed. A protein snack before bedtime (such as a couple of ounces of almond butter, cottage cheese, or jerky) can help reduce blood sugar irregularities and help kids sleep better. Don't feed children high-sugar foods in the evening.

Children who wet the bed may have fears, which can create stress. This stress may be a factor in their bedwetting problem, so the child's fears need to be addressed to correct the problem.

Mineral deficiencies may also play a role in bedwetting, so getting more minerals, especially magnesium, may be helpful. If the problem is a lack of tone in the sphincter of the bladder then uva ursi or another astringent herb might be helpful.

Strategies: Hydration and Low-Glycemic Diet

Formulas: Diuretic, Green Tea Polyphenols, Urinary Support, Liquid Kidney, and Hypoglycemic

Flower Essence Blends: Fear-Reducing FE

Herbs: Licorice, marshmallow, parsley, red raspberry, Saint John's wort, tea, **uva ursi**, and white oak

Supplements: Chromium, **collagen**, **magnesium**, and vitamin B₅

Belching

See also gas & bloating, hiatal hernia, SIBO, and low stomach acid

Belching, gas bubbles from the stomach expelled through the esophagus and mouth, can signal a problem with poor digestion. Digestive problems are likely when a person belches and a foul, rotten-egg odor and taste accompany the belch. A lack of hydrochloric acid often causes this problem. An *Herbal Bitters, Plant Enzyme* or *Digestive Support Formula* may be helpful. If there is a lot of intestinal gas too, a *Carminative Formula* may be helpful. Charcoal can also be used to absorb the gas (see *gas and bloating*).

Strategies: Eliminate FODMAPs and Hiatal Hernia Correction

Formulas: **Chinese Earth-Decreasing**, **Christopher's Carminative**, H. Pylori-Fighting, **Papaya Enzyme**, Children's Colic, **Plant Enzyme**, **Digestive Support**, Betaine HCl, and Herbal Bitters

Herbs: Angelica, catnip, coptis, **fennel**, gentian, **peppermint enteric coated**, and wormwood

Supplements: Charcoal and protease

Essential Oils: Clove, peppermint, red mandarin, and spearmint

Bell's Palsy

See also neuralgia & neuritis

Paralysis of the facial nerve producing distortion on one side of the face is called Bell's palsy. This is a form of neuralgia. There are several conditions that can cause facial paralysis, including Lyme disease, stroke, and a brain tumor. In Bell's palsy, the cause of paralysis is unknown. It is thought to be caused by inflammation of the facial nerve, possibly by latent viral infections or an autoimmune response. It can also be caused by an injury or other irritation to the nerves.

Since Bell's palsy is an inflammatory condition, herbs that reduce inflammation, particularly in the nerves. can be helpful. Essential fatty acids can also be helpful for controlling inflammation.

Strategies: Healthy Fats

Formulas: Anti-Stress B-Complex, **Analgesic Nerve**, Chinese Fire-Decreasing, and **Chinese Wind-Heat Evil**

Herbs: Mullein root, **Saint John's wort**, **vervain (blue)**, and **wood betony**

Supplements: Calcium, **magnesium**, N-acetyl cysteine, omega-3 EFAs, and **vitamin B-complex**

Benign Prostate Hyperplasia   see *BPH*

Bipolar Mood Disorder
Manic Depressive Disorder

See also depression, mania, mitochondrial dysfunction, and methylation (under)

Bipolar disorder, formerly known as manic-depressive disorder, is a psychological condition where a person has dramatic swings between depression and mania. In the depressed phase, the person may sleep a lot; have very little motivation; feel discouraged, anxious, sad or irritable; and have thoughts of suicide. During the manic phase, the person may have grandiose thoughts, insomnia, poor judgment, increased sex drive, and feel like they can do anything. The exact cause of bipolar disorder is not known, but like many other mood disorders it may have its roots in unresolved trauma and abuse from childhood.

Most people with bipolar disorder take medication to control their symptoms. Studies show that people taking medication for bipolar disorder recover much quicker when they are in therapy than those who use medication by itself.

The best nutritional therapy for bipolar disorder is high doses of EPA and DHA from fish oils. DHA specifically seems to reduce brain inflammation, helping improve the depressive phase, and reduce the frequency and severity of the manic phase. People with bipolar disorder need about five thousand mg a day of combined EPA and DHA.

New animal research shows that lithium helps increase DHA in the brain, possibly explaining one of its mechanisms of action. Lithium orotate and citrate are available as supplements but don't have any advantage over prescription lithium carbonate.

Magnesium glycinate can increase the efficacy of prescription mood stabilizers. Start with three hundred mg twice a day and working up to one thousand mg a day, or bowel tolerance. If you develop loose stools, back off the dose. Herbs like turmeric, rosemary, and saffron, which reduce brain inflammation can also be helpful.

This disorder may involve environmental sensitivities and food allergies. Avoid food additives and chemicals and screen for food allergies. Keeping a mood chart along with a food journal can be helpful to identify triggers.

In bipolar disorder you need to avoid herbs and supplements that stimulate dopamine, as they can induce mania. Avoid Sam-e, eleuthero, rhodiola, ginseng, Saint John's wort, and mimosa bark (albizia).

People with the O blood type are more prone to this disorder because they can develop high levels of dopamine (the neurotransmitter that creates the manic feelings) and then have these neurotransmitters rapidly converted to epinephrine and used up, leaving the person depressed. Adequate intake of the amino acid L-tyrosine is essential to maintaining adequate levels of dopamine in the brain. This amino acid is found primarily in red meat. Wheat is also high in this amino acid, but people with the O blood type tend to be allergic to wheat. Excessive consumption of wheat also contributes to the development of hypoglycemia, which further contributes to this problem.

Strategies: Avoid Sugar, Balance Methylation, Counseling or Therapy, Emotional Healing Work, Healthy Fats, Low-Glycemic Diet, Mineralization, and Stress Management

Formulas: Algae, **Chinese Qi-Regulating**, Anti-Stress B-Complex, GLA Oil, and **Colloidal Mineral**

Herbs: **Ashwagandha**, damiana, holy basil, linden flowers, **rosemary**, **skullcap**, and **turmeric**

Supplements: **Lithium**, **magnesium**, omega-3 DHA, **omega-3 EFAs**, and omega-6 GLA

Essential Oils: Clary sage, frankincense, and lemon

Birth Control Side Effects

See also infection (fungal) and leaky gut

Birth control pills contain hormones that can disrupt the body's normal hormonal balance. They may also contribute to yeast overgrowth. These remedies help counter side effects from using birth control pills.

Formulas: Female Tonic and Female Cycle

Herbs: **Chaste tree** and milk thistle

Supplements: L-glutamine, magnesium, **vitamin B-complex**, and vitamin B_6

Birth Control, Natural

Wild yam has been promoted as a natural birth control agent, but the evidence suggests that this isn't effective. I am not aware of any herbs that offer a safe and reliable alternative to birth control pills. There are, however, other methods of avoiding pregnancy naturally.

A fairly effective way to practice natural birth control is to chart the menstrual cycle. On a normal twenty-eight day menstrual cycle, a woman is fertile about fourteen days after the beginning of her period, and this period of fertility lasts between five and seven days. In women with regular cycles there is little risk of pregnancy if unprotected intercourse is limited to the seven days after menstrual flow ceases and the seven days prior to the beginning of the period. Limiting sex to half the month is the biggest deterrent for most people using this method, which unfortunately, also doesn't work well for women who have irregular cycles.

Another natural approach to birth control is the use of lambskin condoms. Lambskin condoms do not interfere with sensation as much as latex condoms do. They are effective at preventing conception, but not sexually transmitted diseases (STDs), so they should only be used in a monogamous relationship where both partners have been tested for STDs.

A less-reliable method of natural birth control is withdrawal, which involves the man withdrawing from the vagina prior to ejaculation. The reason this method is not as reliable is twofold. One, many men do not have the self-control to withdraw early enough, and two, there is a chance sperm can be released in the lubricating solution men release during intercourse. However, this method does dramatically reduce the chances of pregnancy in sex where no other method is used.

Birth Defect Prevention

See also pregnancy, avoid during pregnancy, and methylation (under)

When a woman is pregnant, she needs to get extra nutrition to ensure she has adequate nutrients for the developing child. Many birth defects are caused by toxins and nutritional deficiencies. Women planning to get pregnant should do a cleanse before getting pregnant but should not do cleanses during pregnancy. They should also minimize their exposure to tobacco, alcohol, drugs (including over-the-counter and prescription medications), food additives, and chemicals of all kinds.

Strategies: Avoid Sugar, Eat Healthy, Healthy Fats, Mineralization, Reduce Chemical Exposure, and Stress Management

Formulas: **Prenatal Support**, Whole Food Green Drink, Colloidal Mineral, **Methylated B Vitamin**, **Joan Patton's Herbal Minerals**, and Pregnancy Tea

Herbs: Alfalfa, kelp, nettle, stinging, and **red raspberry**

Supplements: Multiple vitamin and mineral, omega-3 EFAs, and **vitamin B$_9$**

Bites & Stings

There are many herbs that can be applied topically to help heal bites and stings from ants, chiggers, mosquitos, and other insects. These natural remedies reduce swelling and inflammation, relieve itching and ease pain, often very rapidly. My favorites are plantain, lobelia, or any astringent herb that happens to be handy. These herbs should be applied topically by crushing fresh plants, moistening dried powders using the *Poultice* strategy, or using tinctures and extracts in the *Compress or Fomentation* strategy. The *Enzyme Spray* has been reported to ease itching from mosquito and chigger bites.

For poisonous spider bites a poultice of fresh plantain or activated charcoal is often helpful. These should be changed every hour. High doses of vitamin C, about 1,000 mg, can be taken internally every two hours to aid recovery. Medical assistance should be sought in treating poisonous spider bites.

Bites from poisonous snakes may be eased by the use of poultices of herbs like plantain, echinacea, and black cohosh. These treatments should be used en route to the emergency room for medical treatment.

Strategies: Aromatherapy, Compress or Fomentation, and Poultice

Formulas: Enzyme Spray, Vulnerary, **Topical Analgesic**, and Antihistamine

Essential Oil Blends: Analgesic EO

Herbs: Bayberry, **black cohosh**, blackberry, calendula, cyperus, **echinacea**, **grindelia**, lobelia, **plantain**, polygala, purslane, tea, **white oak**, and yarrow

Supplements: Charcoal, quercetin, **sodium bicarbonate**, and vitamin C

Essential Oils: Cajeput, copaiba, fennel, lavender, lemon, lemongrass, patchouli, tea tree, thyme, and ylang ylang

Blackheads   see *acne*

Bladder Infection

See also urinary tract infections

The bladder can easily become infected, especially in women, from fecal bacteria. Infections occur more frequently when the microflora of the intestinal tract has been upset due to the use of antibiotics, birth control pills, and other medications. Bladder infections can result in pain, itching, burning urination, and frequent urgency to void.

To prevent bladder infections, be sure to urinate after sex. Several herbs can help to prevent or treat bladder infections. Uva ursi works best when taken as a tea. Some people swear by cranberry juice, and it works for some, but not for everyone.

Juniper berry is probably the single most effective herb we have for UTIs. It is however very irritating because of the antiseptic volatile oils. Never use juniper if you have a kidney infection, or have a severe bladder infection with intense burning and pain.

Soothing herbs like marshmallow and corn silk, taken as a tea, can relieve symptoms of burning and pain so quickly effectively that they risk masking the infection. You should always follow up an herbal protocol with a home urine test to make sure you've cleared the infection.

An untreated or poorly treated bladder infection can lead to a kidney infection, a serious condition. If after twenty-four hours of natural treatment your symptoms don't improve, you may wish to consult a physician.

Strategies: Friendly Flora and Hydration

Formulas: Diuretic, Chinese Water-Increasing, Urinary Support, **UTI Prevention**, and Urinary Immune

Herbs: Barberry, cranberry, **juniper**, **pipsissewa**, **usnea**, and **uva ursi**

Supplements: Berberine and vitamin C

Essential Oils: Lemongrass

Bladder, Irritable

See also urethritis, urination (burning/painful), urinary tract infections, and urination (frequent)

With an irritable bladder there is a constant urge to urinate, even when there is only a small amount of urine in the bladder. This can be due to mucosal dryness from dehydration or inflammation of the bladder from irritants or infections.

Most people who have this problem drink less water, trying to avoid having to urinate so frequently, but this is the wrong approach as it concentrates irritating compounds excreted from the kidneys even more, causing greater irritation. Drinking more water dilutes the toxins and helps the body flush them more effectively.

Herbs that soothe the urinary passages, like corn silk or marshmallow will be helpful. Kava can numb the bladder, relieving pain from irritation. You should also consider the possibility of a urinary tract infection. If one is present, use formulas for fighting urinary tract infections internally.

Cautions: Juniper and other herbs rich in volatile oils are warming and can irritate the bladder in some people. Do not use these herbs if you are experiencing burning or painful urination. For many people, the alcohol in tinctures can be irritating. If you are sensitive to alcohol use a tea, a glycerite, or an encapsulated herb.

Emotionally, an irritable bladder may be a symptom of unresolved angry feelings, in other words, being pissed off. Dealing with whatever is making you angry can ease the irritation.

Strategies: Hydration and Stress Management

Formulas: Liquid Kidney, Liquid Lymph, Urinary Support, Prostate, and Probiotic

Flower Essence Blends: Personal Boundaries FE

Herbs: Cleavers, **corn silk**, couchgrass, kava kava, **marshmallow**, **pipsissewa**, and uva ursi

Supplements: MSM

Bladder, Ulcerated

See also bladder (irritable)

When bladder tissues become damaged through continuous inflammation, they may become chronically inflamed and sore. Ulcers may develop in the bladder just as they can in the stomach or intestines.

Single herbal remedies that may be helpful here include goldenseal, corn silk, and marshmallow. If there is blood in the urine, consider adding horsetail.

Strategies: Eat Healthy and Healthy Fats

Formulas: Liquid Kidney and Liquid Lymph

Herbs: **Corn silk**, **goldenseal**, horsetail, hydrangea, and marshmallow

Supplements: MSM

Bleeding Gums   see *gingivitis*

Bleeding, External

See also cuts and nosebleeds

To stop bleeding, normally all that's required is a little pressure. Styptic herbs can be applied directly to a bleeding wound that doesn't respond to direct pressure. Two of the best styptics are yarrow and cinnamon. Just about any astringent herb, such as bayberry root bark or white oak bark will also be helpful. Capsicum also works, but it stings when you use it. For any serious bleeding or blood loss, seek appropriate medical attention.

Strategies: Lymph-Moving Pain Relief and Poultice

Herbs: Acacia (Indian), achyranthes, bayberry, **calendula**, capsicum, **cinnamon**, Indian madder, lady's mantle, **tienchi ginseng**, white oak, and **yarrow**

Supplements: Vitamin C

Essential Oils: Rose

Bleeding, Internal
Hemorrhage

See also bleeding (external) and blood in stool

To stop internal bleeding, homeostatic herbs are used. These herbs should be taken internally at frequent intervals (anywhere from every few minutes to every couple of hours, depending on the situation). Two of my favorite homeostatic herbs are yarrow and bayberry.

Vitamin C with citrus bioflavonoids is helpful for strengthening blood vessels and preventing easy bleeding. Horsetail is very helpful for strengthening mucous membranes in the kidneys and lungs for minor bleeding in these organs. For serious bleeding, especially internally, immediately seek appropriate medical attention.

Formulas: **Internal Bleeding** and Watkin's Hair, Skin, and Nails

Herbs: Acacia (Indian), agrimony, bayberry, capsicum, **cinnamon**, horsetail, hyacinth, lady's mantle, periwinkle, **tienchi ginseng**, and **yarrow**

Supplements: Bioflavonoids and vitamin C

Blisters

Blisters are formed by an irritation that causes a bump filled with lymphatic fluid on the skin. Herbs can be applied directly to blisters as a poultice to promote healing. When blisters pop, silver or antiseptic essential oils like tea tree oil can be used to prevent infection and promote healing.

Strategies: Compress or Fomentation and Poultice

Formulas: Healing Salve

Herbs: Calendula, **comfrey**, and yarrow

Essential Oils: Eucalyptus and tea tree

Bloating   see *gas & bloating*

Blood Clot Prevention

See also thrombosis

Blood contains a protein called fibrinogen, which helps to form blood clots when we cut ourselves, an important defense mechanism that protects us from bleeding to death. This same substance can cause our death when a blood clot forms inside the circulatory system and lodges in our heart or brain, resulting in a heart attack or stroke.

When the blood is too thick with fibrin, doctors prescribe blood thinners. There are some natural options to prevent the formation of blood clots in the circulatory system. One of these options is vitamin E, which acts as an antioxidant and helps to thin the blood naturally.

Butcher's broom is an herb most commonly used to treat varicose veins. It also appears to inhibit clot formation in blood vessels without thinning the blood, especially when taken with vitamin E. Many other herbs traditionally used for the cardiovascular system have mild blood-thinning properties, including alfalfa and ginkgo.

The enzyme nattokinase, found in the fermented soy product natto, shows promise as an aid to preventing blood clots. It breaks down the fibrin mesh that forms blood clots. Research has demonstrated that taking nattokinase may prevent blood clots from forming in the circulatory system and may even dissolve blood clots that have already formed.

If you're on blood-thinning medications, seek professional assistance before using herbs or nutrients that help to thin the blood.

Strategies: Blood Type Diet, Eat Healthy, Healthy Fats, and Hydration

Formulas: Oral Chelation, Blood Pressure Reducing, and Nattokinase Enzyme

Programs: Cardiovascular Nutritional

Herbs: Butcher's broom, capsicum, garlic, and **ginkgo**

Supplements: Omega-3 EFAs, protease, and **vitamin E**

Blood in Stool

See also inflammatory bowel disorders

Blood in the stool can be caused by something simple like hemorrhoids or can be a sign of severe intestinal inflammation, ulcers, injuries in the colon or rectum, or cancer. Appropriate medical diagnosis should be sought to determine the exact nature of the problem before determining what remedies to use. To help stop bleeding while seeking medical attention, use herbs with styptic or hemostatic properties. You can also soothe intestinal irritation by using the *Intestinal Soothing Formula*.

Strategies: Eat Healthy, Friendly Flora, and Mineralization

Formulas: Internal Bleeding, Green Tea Polyphenols, **Intestinal Soothing**, Irritable Bowel Fiber, and Intestinal Soothing

Herbs: Aloe vera, **bayberry**, capsicum, coptis, white oak, and **yarrow**

Supplements: L-glutamine and **MSM**

Blood in Urine

See also bleeding (internal)

Blood in the urine can be caused by severe irritation and inflammation in the kidneys or bladder. It can also be caused by tumors or other serious problems. Appropriate medical diagnosis should be sought to determine the exact nature of the problem before determining what remedies to use.

Horsetail is a good herb for strengthening the urinary system to reduce bleeding in the urine by toning the tissues. Astringents may be helpful, especially if they have affinity for the urinary system.

Strategies: Eat Healthy

Formulas: Watkin's Hair, Skin, and Nails, Chinese Water-Increasing, and Internal Bleeding

Herbs: Agrimony, bayberry, coptis, gardenia, **horsetail**, marshmallow, tienchi ginseng, uva ursi, **white oak**, and yarrow

Supplements: Bioflavonoids and vitamin C

Blood Poisoning

Sepsis

See also infection (bacterial) and wounds & sores

Sepsis or blood poisoning is a disease caused by the spread of bacteria or toxins in the bloodstream. The immune response to sepsis triggers inflammation in the blood system, which leads to blood clots and leaky vessels. This results in impaired blood flow, which damages the body's organs by depriving them of nutrients and oxygen. Initial symptoms of sepsis include chills, fever, and weakness. Severe cases of sepsis can cause multiple organ failure and death. Seek appropriate professional assistance for sepsis.

The combination of baptista and echinacea is one of the best herbal treatments I know of for a serious infection of this nature. To prevent blood poisoning, treat wounds with silver or antiseptic essential oils. You can also use the *Poultice* or *Compress or Fomentation* strategy with herbs like echinacea or goldenseal. Activated charcoal also works as a poultice to draw out infection.

Strategies: Compress or Fomentation, Hydration, and Poultice

Formulas: Blood Purifier, **Stabilized Allicin**, Chinese Yang-Reducing, **Lymphatic Infection**, and Detoxifying

Essential Oil Blends: Disinfectant EO

Herbs: Baptisia, dandelion, **echinacea**, garlic, isatis, lobelia, pau d'arco, red clover, thuja, and usnea

Supplements: Charcoal, MSM, **nanoparticle silver**, SAM-e, and vitamin C

Blood Pressure, High   see *hypertension*

Blood Pressure, Low   see *hypotension*

Bloodshot Eyes   see *eyes, bloodshot*

Body Building

See also exercise (recovery)

When trying to gain muscle mass, it helps to get adequate protein and make sure digestion is working properly. Adaptogens have been shown to improve athletic performance, so they may also be helpful for body-builders. When you overexert yourself, a tea made of safflowers helps to reduce lactic acid buildup in the muscles and ease muscle aches.

Strategies: Avoid Xenoestrogens, Eat Healthy, and Hydration

Formulas: Adrenal Glandular, **Whole Food Green Drink**, and **Whole Food Protein**

Herbs: **Cordyceps**, **eleuthero**, ginseng (American), ginseng (Asian/Korean), and safflower

Supplements: **Collagen**, MSM, and multiple vitamin and mineral

Body Odor

When there is an excessively offensive odor associated with sweat, it can be an indication of a need for better hydration and lymph movement. Antiperspirant deodorants, although popular, are not good for health because sweating is used as a means of detoxifying the body and inhibiting sweat inhibits that detoxification.

Chlorophyll acts as a natural deodorizer when taken internally. You can also find a good natural deodorant that doesn't act as an antiperspirant. The *Enzyme Spray Formula* has been used as a natural deodorant. It works better when you add essential oils to it. It may also help to do some detoxification (see *Detoxification* and *Fasting* strategies).

Strategies: Detoxification, Fasting, and Hydration

Formulas: **Enzyme Spray**, Whole Food Green Drink, Detoxifying, and Liquid Lymph

Herbs: Parsley, pau d'arco, and sage

Supplements: **Chlorophyll**, vitamin B-complex, vitamin B_{12}, and zinc

Essential Oils: Eucalyptus, lavender, neroli, and tea tree

Boils

A boil is an infection of a skin gland resulting in localized swelling and inflammation, having a hard central core often filled with pus and/or watery fluid. Boils are best treated by using remedies internally that cleanse the blood and help drain the lymphatics. Antiseptic essential oils or infection-fighting herbs like echinacea or goldenseal can also be applied topically as using the *Compress or Fomentation* or *Poultice* strategies.

Strategies: Compress or Fomentation and Poultice

Formulas: **Ayurvedic Skin Healing**, Enzyme Spray, Liquid Lymph, **Detoxifying**, **Drawing Salve**, and Alterative-Immune

Herbs: Amur cork, baptisia, black walnut, burdock, chickweed, **echinacea**, polygala, and red clover

Essential Oils: Bay leaf, lemon, rose, and **tea tree**

Bone Spurs   **see** *calcium deposits*

BPH
Benign Prostate Hyperplasia

See also prostatitis

This is a nonmalignant, abnormal growth of the prostate tissue. The severity is measured in stages I to IV (mild to serious), which refers to the size of the growth (walnut-size to grapefruit-size) and the impact this enlargement has on the quality of life.

The enlargement of prostate tissue can cause partial or complete obstruction of the urethra, leading to urinary hesitancy, painful urination, frequent urination, and increased risk of urinary tract infections. Having BPH can elevate the PSA test, but fortunately, BPH doesn't lead to an increased risk of cancer.

There are several theories as to the cause of BPH. Some research suggests that an excess of a special form of testosterone called dihydrotestosterone (DHT) is to blame, while other research indicates that elevated estrogens and venous stagnation is the cause.

A popular key herb in the treatment of BPH is saw palmetto. In several clinical trials, saw palmetto has been shown to be at least as effective in treating BPH as the most common prescription drug Proscar. Saw palmetto works not only to inhibit DHT, one of the possible causes of BPH, but also, it seems to balance estrogen and testosterone. It takes large doses of saw palmetto to help the prostate, so go for concentrated extracts and fluid extracts over standard tinctures or capsules. Other herbs that have beneficial effects on BPH include nettle root and pygeum.

Equol binds to DHT and prevents it from binding to the prostate and stimulating growth. It can be very helpful in improving urinary function and other symptoms of BPH.

The mineral zinc, long known for its beneficial effects on the male prostate, has been found to be a potent inhibitor of 5a-reductase, which converts testosterone into DHT. A reasonable dose of zinc for inhibiting BPH would be fifty mg daily with an added two mg of copper, which could easily be supplied by drinking an ounce of liquid chlorophyll.

Excess estrogen, or an imbalance of estrogens and androgens, is implicated in BPH. Estrogen production naturally increases as fat stores increase. (See *Avoid Xenoestrogens*.)

Cruciferous vegetables contain sulfur compounds that help the liver to break down excess estrogens, and exercise can help decrease estrogen as well. Avoid grapefruit as this inhibits estrogen breakdown. Beer should also be avoided, as the hops in beer is also estrogenic.

Recent research has focused on venous stagnation as a cause of BPH. Enlargement of the prostate is associated with a sedentary lifestyle and is more common in men with desk jobs and those who sit for long periods, like truck drivers. Regular physical activity, sitz baths, and pelvic floor exercises (Kegel exercises) can help stimulate pelvic circulation.

Strategies: Avoid Xenoestrogens, Detoxification, Exercise, and Healthy Fats

Formulas: Chinese Water-Increasing, Phytoestrogen Breast, and **Prostate**

Herbs: Collinsonia, damiana, **nettle, stinging root**, pomegranate, pumpkin seed, pygeum, saw palmetto, and **white sage**

Supplements: Equol, indole-3-carbinol, omega-3 EFAs, and **zinc**

Brain Fog   see confusion and cloudy thinking

Breast Infection   see mastitis

Breast Lumps

See also body odor, cancer, and cystic breast disease

If you have a lump in your breast, obtain an appropriate medical diagnosis to find out if you are dealing with benign breast lumps or breast cancer. If the lumps are cancerous, see *Cancer.* If the lumps are benign, then the following information may be useful.

Start by eliminating caffeine, as this is a major cause of breast lumps (see *cystic breast disease*). Since lumps are usually a sign of too much estrogen stimulation, check out the strategy *Avoid Xenoestrogens* and use the *Phytoestrogen Breast Formula* to block their action. Indole-3 carbinol also helps detoxify xenoestrogens.

Topical application of frankincense essential oil has helped some women get rid of breast lumps. This should ideally be done along with herbs to help the lymphatic system drain better. Poke oil or castor oil packs have also been applied topically to help get rid of lumps. See the *Castor Oil Pack* strategy.

Avoid using antiperspirant deodorants. They inhibit detoxification of the lymphatics in the breast area. See *body odor* for alternatives.

Strategies: Avoid Xenoestrogens, Castor Oil Pack, Detoxification, and Eat Healthy

Formulas: Phytoestrogen Breast, Liquid Lymph, **Enzyme Spray**, and Detoxifying

Herbs: Asparagus, black currant, **chaste tree**, and evening primrose

Supplements: Indole-3-carbinol and vitamin E

Essential Oils: Frankincense

Breast Milk   see *nursing*

Breast Milk, Surplus

See also nursing

These remedies can help dry up breast milk when stopping nursing. They should be avoided while nursing.

Herbs: Parsley, **sage**, and white sage

Essential Oils: Clary sage

Breasts (Swelling/Tenderness)

See also PMS Type H

Tenderness or pain in the breast tissue may be due to lymphatic congestion. Hormonal imbalances may also cause breast swelling and tenderness.

Herbs that improve the flow of lymph are often helpful when used with plenty of water. Diuretic herbs can also be used if the swelling occurs in other tissues of the body. Poultices with herbs like mullein, comfrey, and burdock have also eased this problem (see *Poultice* strategy).

When associated with PMS, this problem may be due to elevated aldosterone. Vitamin B_6, magnesium, vitamin E, omega-3 fatty acids, evening primrose oil, and the essential oils of frankincense and lemon are all remedies that may help.

Strategies: Avoid Xenoestrogens, Compress or Fomentation, Hydration, and Poultice

Formulas: Female Tonic, **Liquid Lymph**, Chinese Water-Decreasing, Lymph Cleansing, **Liquid Kidney**, and Chinese Metal-Decreasing

Herbs: Black cohosh, black currant, burdock, calendula, **chaste tree**, cleavers, comfrey, dong quai, evening primrose oil, **mullein**, parsley, polygala, and red clover

Supplements: Magnesium, omega-3 EFAs, vitamin B_6, vitamin B_6, and vitamin E

Essential Oils: Frankincense, geranium, and lemon

Breasts, Undersized

Certain phytoestrogens in plants appear to encourage breast development. Saw palmetto, in particular, has been reported helpful for this purpose, but the effect is temporary and only lasts while taking the herb.

One way to enhance breast appearance (and health) is exercise. Exercises such as push-ups, swimming and arm swings can add inches to a woman's bustline, but more importantly, such exercises can keep breasts firmer and healthier.

Strategies: Exercise

Herbs: Saw palmetto

Essential Oils: Clary sage and ylang ylang

Broken Bones
Fractures

Broken bones will heal better if one has good nutrition. A good mineral supplement such as the *Skeletal Support Formula* will be helpful. Vitamins D_3 and K_2 are also helpful for speeding the healing of broken bones.

Herbal remedies can also aid the healing of broken bones. Two remedies that may be helpful include the *Herbal Minerals* and *Watkin's Hair, Skin and Nails Formulas*. In cases where it is possible to apply herbs topically, you can also use the *Poultice* or *Compress or Fomentation* strategies with herbs like mullein or comfrey.

Strategies: Bone Broth, Compress or Fomentation, Mineralization, and Poultice

Formulas: **Herbal Calcium**, Enzyme Spray, **Watkin's Hair, Skin, and Nails**, **Skeletal Support**, Vulnerary, **Colloidal Mineral**, **Joan Patton's Herbal Minerals**, and Hemp Oil with Terpenes

Herbs: **Comfrey**, drynaria, horsetail, **mullein**, and rehmannia

Supplements: Boron, calcium, collagen, magnesium, MSM, silicon, vitamin C, **vitamin D**, and **vitamin K**

Bronchial Congestion
see *congestion (bronchial)*

Bronchitis
See also congestion (bronchial)

Bronchitis is an inflammation of the small tubes of the lungs, usually as a result of a respiratory infection. Expectorants and decongestants can help bronchitis when taken with plenty of water. One of the best remedies providing these actions is the *Ayurvedic Bronchial Decongestant Formula*.

To reduce chronic bronchial irritation try taking cordyceps, licorice, and/or marshmallow. For infection use silver, echinacea, or garlic. It can also help to put a few drops of essential oils into a pan of boiling water and inhale some of the steam. Essential oils can also be diffused or inhaled directly from the bottle.

Strategies: Eat Healthy and Hydration

Formulas: **Jeannie Burgess' Allergy-Lung**, **Ayurvedic Bronchial Decongestant**, Lung Moistening, Chinese Metal-Increasing, Stabilized Allicin, and Chinese Metal-Decreasing

Essential Oil Blends: Disinfectant EO and **Lung-Supporting EO**

Herbs: Asafetida, astragalus, bibhitaki, cherry, chirata, cinnamon, clove, coleus, **cordyceps**, **echinacea**, elecampane, garlic, grindelia, **horehound**, horseradish, khella, **licorice**, lobelia, loquat, **marshmallow**, mullein, oregano, **osha**, pine, plantain, reishi, skunk cabbage, thyme, vervain (blue), and **yerba santa**

Supplements: MSM, N-acetyl cysteine, nanoparticle silver, **vitamin A**, and vitamin D

Essential Oils: Atlas cedarwood, camphor, clary sage, clove, cypress, eucalyptus, fir, helichrysum, marjoram, **menthol**, myrrh, neroli, oregano, peppermint, pine, ravensara, ravintsara, rose, rosemary, sandalwood, spruce (hemlock), tea tree, and thyme

Bruises
See also easily bruised

Bruises are caused by an injury to the tissues where stagnation sets in, causing the area to turn a purplish black color. Homeopathic arnica is particularly helpful in treating bruises both topically and internally. You can also use the *Poultice* or *Compress or Fomentation* strategy to help bruises heal.

Strategies: Compress or Fomentation, Lymph-Moving Pain Relief, and Poultice

Formulas: Enzyme Spray, **Topical Analgesic**, Antioxidant, **Vein Tonic**, CBD Topical Analgesic, and Hemp Oil with Terpenes

Essential Oil Blends: Topical Injury

Herbs: Angelica, **arnica**, bilberry, butcher's broom, comfrey, horse chestnut, horsetail, tienchi ginseng, **yarrow**, and yerba santa

Supplements: Bioflavonoids and **MSM**

Essential Oils: Helichrysum, marjoram, and rose

Bulimia
See also anorexia and anxiety disorders

Bulimia is a disorder characterized by binge eating followed by self-induced vomiting and the use of laxatives, fasting, or diuretics to prevent weight gain. Herbs and supplements may help with appetite or nerves, but this disorder is psychologically based and requires counseling. (See *Counseling or Therapy* strategy.)

As an adjunct to professional assistance you can use an *Herbal Bitters Formula* to stimulate appetite and *Digestive Enzyme Formulas* to improve digestion. Avoid cleansing programs and herbal laxatives.

Strategies: Counseling or Therapy, Emotional Healing Work, Healthy Fats, Mineralization, and Stress Management

Formulas: Chinese Earth-Increasing, **Herbal Bitters**, and Digestive Support

Flower Essence Blends: Shock and Injury FE

Herbs: Ashwagandha, bee pollen, eleuthero, and gentian

Supplements: Lithium, magnesium, and multiple vitamin and mineral

Bunions

A localized swelling at a joint in the foot caused by an inflammation of the bursa is called a bunion. Anti-inflammatory and analgesic remedies can ease the pain and aid healing. You can also apply herbs topically using the *Poultice* or *Compress or Fomentation* strategy.

Strategies: Compress or Fomentation and Poultice

Formulas: Anti-Inflammatory Pain and Herbal Arthritis

Herbs: Arnica, burdock, Saint John's wort, and **solomon's seal**

Supplements: MSM

Burning Feet/Hands

See also anemia, circulation (poor), diabetes, metabolic syndrome, inflammation, and peripheral neuropathy

Burning hands and feet are caused by an abnormal nervous system signal and medically classified as peripheral neuropathy. This can be caused by many conditions, including alcoholism, diabetes, nutrient deficiencies, autoimmunity, infections, and some medications. You have to identify the cause of the neuropathy to be able to address it properly.

Burning, tingling, or pain in the hands can be caused by nerve compression in the cervical spine, and those sensations in the feet can be caused by nerve compression in the lower back, but it's not common for the symptoms to occur on both sides of the body. If it's on one side only, you may wish to consult a chiropractor or other bodyworker.

If you're experiencing burning, tingling or pain in both feet, or both hands the cause is likely systemic. Here are some suggestions for relief.

The most common cause of peripheral neuropathy is elevated blood sugar. Even if your fasting blood sugar is okay, you can have blood sugar spikes after meals high enough to damage nerves. Try to keep your fasting glucose below 100 and your one hour post meal glucose below 145 to prevent nerve damage. The *Chinese Yin-Increasing Formula* may be helpful if the problem is blood sugar related. See *diabetes* and *metabolic syndrome* for more information on controlling blood sugar.

Peripheral neuropathy can be caused by anemia from a B_{12} or folate deficiency. In alcoholics or those with severe malabsorption, thiamine deficiency can cause burning feet. It can also be caused by deficiencies of vitamins B_3, B_6, and iron and copper. It's not a bad idea to take a high-quality multivitamin and a B-complex while getting to the bottom of the cause. Because inflammation is involved, an *Antioxidant Formula* and omega-3 essential fatty acids may also be helpful in reducing the burning sensations.

Strategies: Avoid Sugar, Healthy Fats, Hydration, and Low-Glycemic Diet

Formulas: Chinese Yin-Increasing, Anti-Stress B-Complex, GLA Oil, **Chinese Yang-Reducing**, Analgesic Nerve, **Oral Chelation**, **Methyl B12 Vitamin**, and **Antioxidant**

Herbs: Capsicum, ginger, prickly ash, and Saint John's wort

Supplements: Alpha-lipoic acid, copper, iron, multiple vitamin and mineral, **omega-3 EFAs**, **vitamin B-complex**, vitamin B-complex, vitamin B_1, **vitamin B_{12}**, vitamin B_6, and **vitamin B_9**

Burnout   **see** *adrenal fatigue*

Burns & Scalds

See also sunburn

Burns and scalds can be very painful. Minor burns (*first-degree*) involve normal symptoms of inflammation—redness, pain and swelling. More severe burns (*second-degree*) can result in blisters and the most severe burns (*third-degree*) can have permanent skin damage that prevents skin regeneration and can threaten life due to infection or fluid loss if the area is extensive. The remedies here are primarily for first- and second-degree burns. Third-degree burns, especially if over a large area of the body, should be treated medically.

Running the burned area under cold water to cool the heat is very helpful for pain. Effective topical remedies for burns include aloe vera gel, lavender essential oil, real vanilla extract, raw honey, and plantain leaf and can be applied using the *Poultice* or *Compress or Fomentation* strategies. Two of these remedies, honey and vanilla, are available in most kitchens. Vitamin E can be applied once the pain is gone from the burn to prevent scarring and speed tissue repair. Zinc and vitamin C, taken internally, help to speed the healing of burns.

Strategies: Aromatherapy, Compress or Fomentation, Lymph-Moving Pain Relief, and Poultice

Formulas: Enzyme Spray

Flower Essence Blends: Shock and Injury FE

Herbs: Aloe vera, marshmallow, nopal, plantain, and **vanilla extract**

Supplements: MSM, **vitamin C**, vitamin E, and zinc

Essential Oils: Lavender, peppermint, rose, and tea tree

Bursitis

See also arthritis

Bursitis is an inflammation of the connective tissue capsule of joints, resulting in pain and inflammation. It is treated naturally in a similar manner to arthritis, but some of the more specific remedies that can be helpful for it are listed here.

Strategies: Eliminate Allergy-Causing Foods, Healthy Fats, and Hydration

Formulas: Herbal Arthritis, **Topical Analgesic**, Chinese Yang-Reducing, Gut Immune, Anti-Inflammatory Pain, CBD Topical Analgesic, Hemp Oil with Terpenes, and CBD Joint

Essential Oil Blends: Topical Injury

Herbs: Boswellia, burdock, devil's claw, pleurisy, Saint John's wort, **solomon's seal**, teasel, turmeric, and willow

Supplements: Curcumin, magnesium, and **MSM**

Cadmium Toxicity

See also chemical exposure and heavy metal poisoning

Cadmium levels have dramatically increased in the environment due to the introduction of rechargeable nickel-cadmium batteries, which are rarely recycled. It is also used in electroplating and found in some paints and fertilizers. Cigarette smoke is the biggest way to be exposed to cadmium, but you can also be exposed to it from drinking water, foods, and plastics. Cadmium is known to damage the kidneys. It displaces zinc in the body. When inhaled it causes respiratory illness. It is also known to contribute to osteoporosis and cancer.

Acute cadmium toxicity should be treated medically. For getting low levels of cadmium out of the body one can follow the general programs for detoxifying chemicals and heavy metals found under the strategy *Heavy Metal Cleanse* and the condition *chemical exposure*, adding specific supplements to help the body expel cadmium. Since it displaces zinc, supplementing with zinc and other cadmium antagonists like calcium and copper should be helpful.

Strategies: Heavy Metal Cleanse

Formulas: Heavy Metal Cleansing and Algae

Herbs: Chlorella

Supplements: Alpha-lipoic acid, calcium, copper, manganese, sodium alginate, vitamin C, and **zinc**

Calcium Deficiency

See also osteoporosis

A deficiency of calcium does not necessarily mean the diet doesn't contain enough calcium. The calcium in the diet may be poorly absorbed due to a deficiency of hydrochloric acid, for example. It may be poorly utilized because the diet lacks fat-soluble vitamins, particularly D_3 and K_2. Silica, magnesium, boron, copper and zinc are a few of the many mineral co-factors necessary to help calcium affix into the bones. So besides calcium supplements, consider some of the following herbs and supplements, many of which can help the body assimilate and utilize calcium more efficiently.

Strategies: Mineralization

Formulas: Watkin's Hair, Skin, and Nails and Herbal Calcium

Herbs: Alfalfa, horsetail, kelp, nettle, and stinging

Supplements: Calcium, copper, **magnesium**, omega-3 EFAs, silicon, **vitamin D**, **vitamin K**, and zinc

Calcium Deposits
Calcification, Bone Spurs

See also kidney stones

In the presence of mineral imbalances and a vitamin K_2 deficiency, calcium can come out of solution and form kidney stones, hardened tissue, or bone spurs. Calcium deposits often signal a lack of magnesium or other nutrients used in conjunction with calcium.

Herbs that have lithotriptic properties can help bring calcium back into solution in the body. These include hydrangea, gravel root and stone breaker. Since lemon juice is also lithotriptic, adding freshly squeezed lemon to water and drinking several glasses a day can be helpful as well.

If you have been taking calcium supplements, discontinue their use and take five hundred to one thousand mg of magnesium each day. If you feel you still need a calcium supplement try using *Herbal Calcium* or *Joan Patton's Herbal Minerals Formula*.

Strategies: Mineralization

Formulas: Herbal Arthritis, Oral Chelation, Chinese Water-Increasing, **Watkin's Hair, Skin, and Nails**, Joan Patton's Herbal Minerals, Herbal Calcium, and Kidney Stone

Herbs: Blessed thistle, gravel root, **hydrangea**, and lemon juice

Supplements: Krill oil, magnesium, omega-3 EFAs, and vitamin K

Cancer

See also cancer treatment side effects, leukemia, and lymphoma

Anyone who has ever had cancer, or had a loved one with cancer, knows the feelings of fear, anxiety, worry, and often hopelessness that this very serious illness can bring. This is understandable, considering cancer is the second leading cause of death in civilized nations. Furthermore, conventional treatments, such as chemotherapy, radiation, and surgery, are often dangerous in and of themselves. So it's little wonder that cancer generally causes intense emotional distress in everyone involved. However, one should always believe that there is hope, even when orthodox medicine offers none. As long as the body has life, there is hope.

Of course, the subject of cancer is far too involved to adequately address in this book. I can acquaint you with some important information about cancer from a natural healing perspective and give you some ideas about options you may not be familiar with. However, I strongly encourage you to seek professional help when dealing with cancer. You need competent health-care professionals helping you with your program and monitoring your progress, but you should also do some study on your own and learn about things you can do for yourself.

Understanding Cancer

Cancer is a disease involving cells that have undergone a genetic mutation so they are no longer responsive to messages from the body that regulate cell metabolism and growth. Some of these mutations are believed to be the result of free radical damage that causes the cells to develop an anaerobic metabolism and turn cancerous. Other mutations seem to be genetic or caused by cellular injuries from infection or chemicals. Normal cells have an aerobic metabolism, which means they produce energy by means of oxygen and oxidation. Anaerobic cells produce energy without oxygen via a process of fermentation.

This is important to know because if the body is highly oxygenated, the environment for cancer does not exist. In fact, in 1931, Dr. Otto Warburg won a Nobel Prize for proving that whenever any cell is denied 60 percent of its oxygen requirements, it can become cancerous. So conditions that deprive cells of oxygen (such as chronic inflammation, buildup of toxins or problems with red blood cells or circulation) increase the risk of cancer. Cancer creates a low-oxygen, acidic environment to encourage its growth.

Another important thing you should know is that cancer cells are forming in the body regularly. Very likely, you have a few inside you right now. Don't worry, the immune system normally recognizes these deviant cells and destroys them.

Therefore, in order for you to develop cancer, two factors must exist. First, your body has to have a toxic, low-oxygen environment that encourages the development of anaerobic cancer cells, and second, your immune system must be weakened so that it is not able to recognize and destroy these cells.

Holistic Strategies for Cancer

Killing cancer cells (the goal of conventional cancer therapy) is an important part of treating cancer, but it does not fix the underlying problems that created the cancer in the first place. This is the weakness of the standard medical approach to cancer. An effective protocol for cancer should do more than just destroy cancer cells; it should try to restore a normal, healthy environment in the body and rebuild the immune system. Even if one chooses to use orthodox cancer therapies, they would be wise to consider doing natural therapy both to restore the body's state of health and to prevent the cancer from reoccurring. Here are the basic principles of natural cancer therapy.

Increase Oxygen Levels

As noted, cancer cells are anaerobic. They get their energy by metabolizing nutrients, notably sugars and carbohydrates, without oxygen via a fermentative process. Cancer cells cannot survive in a high-oxygen environment, so keeping the body well oxygenated inhibits cancer. Do this by getting plenty of fresh air and exercise. Practice the *Deep Breathing* strategy. If you smoke, quit.

Liquid chlorophyll is a great way to enhance oxygen transport. It helps the blood carry more oxygen to the tissues, and research has shown that it reduces the risk of cancer. The natural way to get more chlorophyll is to consume dark-green, leafy vegetables, wheat grass, barley grass and other green plant foods.

If you have problems with the lungs, herbs like astragalus or cordyceps can also be helpful in restoring lung function and aiding the immune system at the same time. You can also consider a *Chinese Metal-Increasing Formula*.

Increase Nutrient Intake From High Quality Foods.

Eat large quantities of fresh, preferably organic, fruits and vegetables every day. This is well-recognized as one of the best ways of decreasing your risk of cancer, but unfortunately, its benefit in helping people recover from cancer is often ignored. Fresh fruits and vegetables not only have vitamins, minerals, and phytonutrients that are anti-cancerous, they also strengthen immunity, aid detoxification, and provide antioxidants. See the *Eat Healthy* strategy.

A lack of hydrochloric acid leads to excess lactic acid in the body and poor digestion and absorption of nutrients, which sets the stage for cancer. An *Herbal Bitters Formula* can be taken before meals to stimulate appetite and increase hydrochloric acid production. You may also want to use the *Enzyme Supplement with Betaine HCl* to improve digestion.

Strengthen the Immune System

As previously noted, a healthy immune system recognizes and destroys cancer cells. When the immune system is unable to recognize these deviant cells or is too weak to destroy them, the disease we call cancer develops.

Immune Stimulant and *Mushroom Immune Blend Formula*s are principal immune-boosting remedies that are helpful with natural cancer therapy. A high-quality colostrum may also be helpful in fighting cancer. These supplements can be used in conjunction with medical cancer therapy as well.

Fu Zheng therapy is a combination of herbs from China that strengthen the immune system and help with the side effects of chemotherapy. It has been found to substantially decrease the immune suppression associated with chemotherapy, and it increases survival time. Fu Zheng therapy uses a combination of astragalus, ligustrum, ginseng, codonopsis, atractylodes and reishi (ganoderma). The *Chinese Qi and Blood Tonic Formula* has many of these herbs and is used in a similar manner to strengthen the body and help it resist the negative impact of chemotherapy and radiation.

Cannabinol (CBD) may be helpful in getting the immune system to recognize and destroy cancer cells. It may also be helpful in combating the side effects of conventional cancer therapy.

Detoxify

The human body is bombarded with toxins, heavy metals, chlorine, and thousands of chemicals that we breathe in, consume in our diet, or absorb through our skin. These all cause the release of the free radicals that contribute to the environment of cancer. Avoiding these toxins is part of both cancer prevention and holistic cancer therapy. In particular, avoid or eliminate refined and processed foods (especially foods raised with pesticides, antibiotics, or steroids), toxic cleaning products (such as laundry detergents, skin care items, fluoridated toothpaste, etc.), and chlorinated and fluoridated water. Also, avoid microwaved or irradiated foods and protect yourself from electrical equipment. (See *Reduce Electromagnetic Exposure* strategy.)

It is also helpful to assist the body in detoxifying from these substances using blood purifiers like burdock, red clover, and sheep sorrel. These have all been used in traditional herbal remedies for cancer. The *Essiac Immune Tea* and *Alterative-Immune Formulas* contain herbs like these, as do many *Detoxifying Formulas*.

Use Antioxidants

Our need for oxygen exceeds the demand for any nutrient, even water, because we need oxygen for normal energy production in the cells. However, oxygen can also produce free radicals that can damage normal cells and cause cancer. Antioxidant nutrients protect the body from this free radical damage, thereby reducing cancer risk. Antioxidants can also be used in a treatment program for cancer because they help protect the body from harmful side effects of radiation and chemotherapy. So adding an *Antioxidant Formula* can be helpful for cancer recovery, whether a person is using a natural approach or a medical approach.

Some antioxidants to consider here include green tea extract, mangosteen, and turmeric. Green tea contains polyphenols called catechins, powerful antioxidants that protect cells from cancer and kill cancer cells. One of these catechins is epigallocatechin gallate (EGCG), which was shown in several lab studies to kill cancer cells without harming healthy tissue.

Mangosteen contains xanthones, powerful antioxidants that have been shown in numerous studies to inhibit cancer cells and aid in tumor reduction. These compounds cause apoptosis (preprogrammed cell death) in cancer cells. Xanthones exert cytotoxic (cancer cell killing) effects against human hepatocellular carcinoma cells and have been shown to inhibit the growth of human leukemia HL60 cells. Xanthones have also been shown to be effective against human breast cancer SKBR3 cells.

Turmeric, a spice commonly used in Indian food, also has powerful anticancer and antioxidant properties. In one study, curcumin (an active constituent in turmeric) induced apoptosis in cancer cells without cytotoxic effects on healthy cells. In an animal study, curcumin inhibited the growth of cancer cells in the stomach, liver, and colon as well as oral cancers.

Kill Cancer Cells

For those diagnosed with cancer, it is important to kill the cancerous cells. The problem is that chemotherapy and radiation also cause damage to healthy cells. Killing cancer cells also produces toxins that the body must eliminate.

There are some natural compounds that can help kill cancer cells too. Two of these remedies are graviola (*Annona muricata*) and the American pawpaw tree (*Asimina triloba*). These plants contain compounds called acetogenins that have been shown in scientific studies to cause apoptosis in cancer cells by inhibiting their energy production. It's best to use the *Standardized Acetogenin Formula* as the amount of acetogenins in the herbs varies widely.

Other possible cancer-destroying remedies include mistletoe, Venus fly trap, bloodroot, chaparral, and poke root.

Some of these plants are potentially toxic and should only be used under the guidance of a skilled professional herbalist. You will probably need to locate a professional herbalist to even obtain most of them (findanherbalist.com).

Increase Joy and Pleasure

One German study shows the commonality that all cancer patients experienced a trauma and an unresolved psychological issue shortly before the cancer developed. Stress is a big component of cancer because psychological stress creates physical stress that dramatically reduces immune function.

Reducing stress should be a stress-free task. That's why the goal here is not to reduce stress, but rather to deliberately seek out joy and pleasure. A pleasurable, happy experience has a more positive effect on the immune system and healing than a stressful experience.

So seek out pleasurable experiences. Follow the *Pleasure Prescription* strategy. Find things that make you laugh. Spend time with family, friends or pets. Take a walk in the fresh air and sunshine. Surround yourself with pleasing colors, smells, and sounds. Listen to your favorite music; get up and dance. Listen to calming, meditative music. Take a hot bath in Epsom salts and lavender oil. Treat yourself to a massage, take a mini-vacation, or go to a spa for the day.

You can also reduce stress by taking adaptogens or nervines to help you relax. B-complex vitamins and vitamin C will also help reduce feelings of stress. They will also help with detoxification and have antioxidant properties.

Forgive

I have found that many people who have cancer are being eaten alive with resentment. Often they martyr themselves taking care of other people, while failing to take care of themselves. This is why increasing joy and pleasure is so important in recovery, but it is also why forgiveness is important for people with cancer. Carefully read and follow the *Forgiveness* strategy, as it is an essential part of a holistic approach to this disease.

Cancer is a difficult disease to work with, but many people have successfully recovered from cancer using both natural therapies and conventional therapies, or a combination of the two. Seek out professional assistance in designing the holistic program that's right for you. Remember, there is hope!

Strategies: Affirmation and Visualization, Alkalize the Body, Avoid Sugar, Avoid Xenoestrogens, Colon Hydrotherapy, Counseling or Therapy, Deep Breathing, Detoxification, Eat Healthy, Emotional Healing Work, Epsom Salt Bath, Forgiveness, Hydration, Pleasure Prescription, and Stress Management

Formulas: Colostrum-Immune Stimulator, **Essiac Immune Tea**, **Digestive Support**, Proanthocyanidins, **Immune-Boosting**, **Standardized Acetogenin**, Betaine HCl, **Gut Immune**, Green Tea Polyphenols, Probiotic, **Antioxidant**, **Whole Food Green Drink**, **Chinese Qi and Blood Tonic**, Detoxifying, **Mushroom Immune**, and **Alterative-Immune**

Herbs: Aloe vera, apricot, asparagus, asparagus (Chinese), **astragalus**, barberry, bitter melon, boswellia, **burdock**, cannabis, **cat's claw**, chaga, **chaparral**, codonopsis, **cordyceps**, echinacea, eleuthero, garlic, ginseng (American), ginseng (Asian/Korean), kelp, **maitake**, **mangosteen**, neem, noni, pau d'arco, **pawpaw**, red clover, **reishi**, shitake, suma, sweet annie, tea, turkey tail, **turmeric**, **venus fly trap**, and yellow dock

Supplements: Berberine, beta-glucans, **CBD**, chlorophyll, Co-Q10, **colostrum**, indole-3-carbinol, N-acetyl cysteine, potassium, **protease**, vitamin B-complex, and vitamin B_9

Essential Oils: Frankincense, geranium, lavender, myrrh, rosemary, and sandalwood

Cancer Prevention

See also cancer, cancer treatment side effects, and methylation (under)

Cancer is the leading cause of death during middle age (forty-five to seventy-five), while heart disease is the leading cause of death in old age (after seventy-five). In people between the ages of thirty-five and forty-five and beyond age seventy-five cancer is the second leading cause of death. So if you're interested in a long and healthy life, you should be interested in preventing cancer.

Cancer is largely a disease of modern civilization. Environmental toxins are probably major factors in the development of cancer.

Most experts agree that increasing intake of antioxidants and other nutrients by eating five to nine one-half cup servings of fresh fruits and vegetables daily (ideally organic, or at least washed to remove chemical residues) is the best way to prevent cancer. Eating organic food, using natural personal care and household cleaning products, and otherwise avoiding chemicals will help reduce the risk of cancer.

Since it is impossible to avoid all toxins, it also helps to take nutrients and herbs that help your body break down toxins, especially if you are exposed to chemicals regularly in your work. Besides eating the recommended fruits and vegetables, you should probably consider using both an *Antioxidant* and a *Hepatoprotective Formula* on daily.

To reduce the risk of estrogen-dependent cancers like breast, uterine, and prostate cancer it is also important to follow the *Avoid Xenoestrogens* strategy. Foods rich in phytoestrogens, like beans, green leafy vegetables, and whole grains may also be helpful.

Keeping the immune system healthy is also important to avoiding cancer. Consider taking a *Mushroom Immune Formula* to tonify the immune system. The *Chinese Qi and Blood Tonic* may also be helpful if you have a weak immune system (that is, you catch contagious diseases easily).

There is research that suggests that major stresses in life can trigger tumor growth. Since stress can weaken the immune system, the *Stress Management* strategy is a major part of preventing cancer and many other diseases. The bad news is that none of us can avoid stress. The good news is that we don't have to. Make time for pleasure and recreation by following the *Pleasure Prescription* strategy.

Strategies: Alkalize the Body, Avoid Sugar, Avoid Xenoestrogens, Balance Methylation, Deep Breathing, Eat Enzyme-Rich Foods, Eat Healthy, Healthy Fats, Increase Dietary Fiber, Reduce Chemical Exposure, Reduce EMF Exposure, Sleep, and Stress Management

Formulas: **Phytoestrogen Breast**, Proanthocyanidins, **Antioxidant**, **Hepatoprotective**, Mushroom Immune, Chinese Qi and Blood Tonic, and Jeannie Burgess' Thymus

Flower Essence Blends: Personal Boundaries FE

Herbs: Açaí, astragalus, chlorella, cordyceps, Grape, maitake, mangosteen, **milk thistle**, pomegranate, red clover, **reishi**, shitake, and **turmeric**

Supplements: Chlorophyll, curcumin, equol, **indole-3-carbinol**, iodine, lycopene, omega-3 EFAs, resveratrol, **selenium**, **vitamin A**, **vitamin C**, **vitamin D**, and **zinc**

Cancer Treatment Side Effects

See also cancer, chemical exposure, and radiation

The chemotherapy and radiation commonly administered in cancer treatments have side effects that can be eased by the use of herbs and supplements. Although they are reasonably safe to use in conjunction with standard cancer treatment, people may need to find a doctor who will cooperate with their wishes. Some cancer doctors forbid their patients from using herbs or supplements because it creates reactions in the body that are different from what they expect. With this in mind, here are some helpful tips.

Chemotherapy Side Effects

Chemotherapy is the administration of poisons in an attempt to kill cancerous cells. Cancer cells are generally weaker than normal body cells, so the trick is to give enough poison to kill the cancer but not the patient. This overall poisoning of the body is very destructive, and the symptoms and side effects can be widespread, severe, and varied.

Many chemotherapy agents target rapidly growing cells. Since the cells that line the digestive tract, white blood cells, and skin and hair cells all grow rapidly, these cells often take the brunt of chemotherapy. This is why it is common to have digestive upset, loss of hair, and a lowering of the immune response associated with standard chemotherapy.

Digestive Upset

The digestive tract of patients on chemotherapy can be soothed using mucilant herbs to absorb irritants and reduce inflammation. Aloe vera juice, slippery elm, or marshmallow are good options.

If appetite is poor, take an *Herbal Bitters Formula* prior to meals. Also consider the *Digestive Support Formula* to help the body break down food. Taken between meals, these same enzymes or protease enzymes by themselves will also help the body fight the cancer.

Where nausea and vomiting are a problem, try taking some ginger to settle the stomach. Peppermint or chamomile tea, or a drop of peppermint essential oil in a cup of warm water, can be sipped slowly to ease nausea too.

CBD may also be helpful for nausea and vomiting due to chemotherapy. It also enhances the immune system.

Countering Toxicity

A number of nutrients can support this detoxification, particularly in the liver. This helps the body break down chemotherapy agents faster to avoid damage to healthy tissues. These include B-complex vitamins, magnesium, and MSM.

Overcoming Drug Resistance

Cancer patients who have a relapse after a few years often have drug resistant cancer cells. The *Standardized Acetogenin Formula* can be used to restore the effectiveness of chemotherapy. In addition to having anticancer activity of its own, it also has the ability to inhibit a pumping mechanism in the membranes of cancer cells that enables them to purge toxic drugs and become drug resistant.

Radiation Side Effects

Radiation causes free radical damage and can actually turn healthy cells cancerous. Antioxidants can help protect healthy cells from radiation. Organically grown fresh fruits and vegetables should be used freely and may be supplemented with *Antioxidant Formulas*. Particularly helpful is an intracellular antioxidant called glutathione. N-acetyl cysteine and alpha-lipoic acid can enhance glutathione production, thus protecting healthy cells from damage. High doses of vitamin C can also be helpful.

General Support for Both Cancer Therapies

There are also things one can do to support the body's ability to resist harmful effects of both chemotherapy and radiation. Some of these things can be used to actually enhance the effectiveness of the treatment as well.

Adaptogens

Adaptogens are also helpful for improving the body's ability to resist radiation. They also enhance the function of the immune system. The *Chinese Qi and Blood Tonic* is particularly helpful for many people. It helps strengthen the system against the harmful effects of both radiation and chemotherapy.

Building the Immune System

Mainstream cancer treatments tend to depress immune function, and since the immune system tends to be deficient in people with cancer in the first place, it is very important to build immune function. *Mushroom Immune* and *Immune Stimulating Formulas* can be helpful for raising white blood cell counts and helping the body rebuild between chemotherapy sessions.

Supporting Detoxification

Toxins are part of the reason people get cancer in the first place, and fighting cancer results in an increase of toxins, partly due to the drugs and partly because of the die-off of cancer cells. Most traditional anticancer formulas are based on herbs that act as blood purifiers, meaning they have a gentle detoxifying action. It is very helpful to do detoxification therapy to help the body get rid of this waste. It can be helpful to alternate cleansing and building during therapy too.

Start by drinking plenty of water (one-half ounce or more per pound of body weight daily). *Fiber Blends* and *Detoxifying Formulas* are helpful, along with regular enemas or colonics. This can also help to ease pain in cancer.

Cancer die-off sometimes causes lymphatic congestion and swelling. This can be eased by adding one teaspoon each of the *Liquid Kidney* and *Liquid Lymph Formulas* into a quart of water and sipping it throughout the day. In severe cases you can add a drop or two of poke tincture to this mixture. You could also take a *Lymph Cleansing Formula* and drink lots of water.

Easing Pain

Pain can be a problem in cancer. Remedies that relax tension and/or relieve pain like kava kava, lobelia, corydalis, or California poppy are helpful. A good nervine for this purpose is cannabis, which is legal for medical use in some states but illegal in most. CBD may also be helpful and does not have the same legal issues.

Eating a very clean diet with lots of fresh, raw, organic produce and drinking lots of water also eases pain. Echinacea is also helpful for easing pain in cancer. It also boosts the immune system and aids detoxification.

Strategies: Affirmation and Visualization, Eat Healthy, Epsom Salt Bath, Friendly Flora, Healthy Fats, Increase Dietary Fiber, and Pleasure Prescription

Formulas: Antioxidant, **Chinese Qi and Blood Tonic**, Adaptogen-Immune, Herbal Bitters, Digestive Support, **Mushroom Immune**, **Immune-Boosting**, Fiber, Detoxifying, Essiac Immune Tea, Probiotic, Gut Immune, Intestinal Soothing, **Standardized Acetogenin**, and **Adaptogen**

Herbs: **Aloe vera juice**, ashwagandha, **astragalus**, bayberry, blackberry root, butcher's broom, **cannabis**, cat's claw, chamomile, codonopsis, **cordyceps**, corydalis, **echinacea**, **eleuthero**, ginger, **gynostemma**, horse chestnut, kava kava, maitake, mangosteen, marshmallow, noni, pau d'arco, **pawpaw**, peppermint, red raspberry, **reishi**, rhodiola, schisandra, shitake, and **slippery elm**

Supplements: Alpha-lipoic acid, **CBD**, charcoal, Co-Q10, magnesium, MSM, multiple vitamin and mineral, N-acetyl cysteine, **protease**, **vitamin B-complex**, vitamin C, **vitamin D**, and vitamin E

Candida Albicans/Candidiasis
see *infection (fungal)*

Canker Sores
Mouth Ulcers, Stomatitis

A small painful ulcer usually in the mouth is called a canker sore. It has a grayish-white base surrounded by a red inflamed area.

A few drops of a tincture of goldenseal, myrrh, or propolis applied directly to the canker sore a few times will help them heal quickly. It may burn a little when you apply it, but this rapidly subsides. A drop of *Topical Analgesic* essential oils or tea tree oil, applied topically to the sore, will relieve the pain within minutes. It will also sting a little at first.

In several small studies, supplementing with vitamin B_{12} and folate has decreased canker sore occurrence by 75 percent. L-lysine is an amino acid that some have reported helps to prevent canker sores. Where canker sores are frequent and severe, the *Chinese Wind-Heat Evil Formula*, taken regularly, will help to prevent them.

Formulas: **Topical Analgesic**, **Chinese Wind-Heat Evil**, Chinese Fire-Decreasing, Methyl B12 Vitamin, and **Methylated B Vitamin**

Herbs: Achyranthes, echinacea, gardenia, **goldenseal**, myrrh, and prickly ash

Supplements: L-lysine, multiple vitamin and mineral, **propolis**, vitamin B-complex, vitamin B_{12}, and vitamin B_9

Essential Oils: Lemon, myrrh, and tea tree

Capillary Weakness

See also bruises and spider veins

Capillaries are the smallest of blood vessels that allow the passage of nutrients and oxygen from the bloodstream to the cells of the body. Some are so small that red blood cells must pass through them in single file. Nutritional deficiencies can cause these thin walls to become fragile and prone to rupture, causing bleeding and bruising. Rose hips and vitamin C are also helpful, as are astringent herbs and *Vein Tonic Formulas.*

Strategies: Eat Healthy and Healthy Fats

Formulas: Watkin's Hair, Skin, and Nails, Antioxidant, and **Vein Tonic**

Herbs: Bilberry, **butcher's broom**, hawthorn, horse chestnut, lemon, **rose hips**, and yarrow

Supplements: Bioflavonoids, omega-3 EFAs, and **vitamin C**

Essential Oils: Geranium and lemon

Carbuncles

See also infection (bacterial)

A carbuncle is a deep-seated infection of the skin, usually arising from several hair follicles that are close together. Because it is a bacterial infection, silver gel, echinacea, or other antibacterial remedies will help. You can also apply antiseptic essential oils over the area.

Strategies: Compress or Fomentation and Poultice

Formulas: Ayurvedic Skin Healing

Essential Oil Blends: Disinfectant EO

Herbs: Coptis, **echinacea**, honeysuckle, purslane, and thlaspi

Supplements: Nanoparticle silver

Essential Oils: Tea tree

Cardiac Arrest
Heart Attack

See also cardiovascular disease

A cardiac arrest or heart attack is caused by an acute episode of insufficient blood supply to the heart muscle often resulting in damage to the heart and possibly even death. This lack of blood supply to the heart is triggered by a blood clot or dislodged plaque. Prompt medical treatment is essential.

When a person is having a heart attack, capsicum and lobelia extracts or powders placed under the tongue can help support the heart and may save the person's life. Large doses of vitamin E (400 IU every ten to twenty minutes) can also be helpful. These remedies should be administered while awaiting an ambulance and/or en route to the emergency room.

After a heart attack, high doses of Co-Q10 (one hundred mg or more) will help the body repair the damage. Other supplements that may support recovery from a heart attack include hawthorn, magnesium and formulas that support the heart and circulation.

Strategies: Stress Management

Formulas: Heart Health and Brain-Heart

Flower Essences: Broken and Hardened Hearts FE

Herbs: Capsicum, **hawthorn**, and **lobelia**

Supplements: Co-Q10, magnesium, potassium, and vitamin E

Cardiovascular Disease
Heart Disease

See also arteriosclerosis, blood clot prevention, hypertension, cholesterol (high), hypothyroidism, and anger (excessive)

Cardiovascular disease is still the leading cause of death in Western civilization. One out of two people die from it. It makes sense, then, to do what we can to reduce our risk of becoming one of the one-in-two statistic. Unfortunately, much of the information in the popular media about reducing one's risk of heart disease is based on outdated research.

For instance, most people believe that high cholesterol causes heart disease and that the lower your cholesterol level, the less risk you have of dying of heart disease. This simply isn't true. More recent research shows that chronic inflammation (not cholesterol) is the major cause of heart disease and that having your cholesterol get too low is more dangerous to your health than having high cholesterol.

Most people also believe that fats cause heart disease and that low-fat diets will prevent heart disease. This is partially true, because the wrong kinds of fats (such as margarine and partially hydrogenated vegetable oils) do contribute to the development of heart disease. However, it's also true that good fats (such as olive oil, omega-3 essential fatty acids, and the medium-chain saturated fats found in coconut oil and organic butter from grass fed cows) actually protect your heart and reduce your risk of heart disease. Foods marketed as fat-free or low-fat often contain high amounts of refined sugars that actually increase inflammation and heart disease risk, which means they are not good for heart health.

Eating refined carbohydrates is far worse for your heart than eating fats. This is because sugar, white flour, and other empty-calorie carbohydrates spike insulin levels. High insulin levels are a bigger risk factor for heart disease than high cholesterol or high blood fats (triglycerides). If this information comes as a surprise to you, it's time to update your knowledge a little.

Evaluating Your Risk of Heart Disease

Most people feel that heart disease strikes without warning, but the truth is that there are many subtle clues that demonstrate the heart needs help long before a person has a heart attack. Besides high blood pressure and high cholesterol, here are some things to consider.

Gum Disease. There is a high correlation between inflammation of the gums and the risk of dying of a heart attack. If your gums are inflamed, so are your arteries.

Varicose Veins and Hemorrhoids. These problems are reflections of sluggish circulation and poor blood vessel tone.

Weakness. Fatigue and shortness of breath, feeling no desire for physical activity, getting winded with minor exertion, and feelings of pressure or pain in your chest are early warning signs that your heart may need some help.

Facial Clues. A red, bulbous tip on the nose, spider veins in the nose, and a vertical crease in the left earlobe are all early warning signs that your heart may need help. A bright-red tip and pointed tongue is also an indicator of heart stress.

Iridology. If you know an iridologist or are familiar with iridology, markings in the heart area of the iris, having a spleen heart transversal, and/or having a lipemic diathesis (lipid ring) are all indicators of a genetic tendency to heart disease.

Blood Tests. If you are concerned about your heart and circulation, get blood tests for homocysteine, fibrinogen, C-reactive protein, hemoglobin A1C, fasting insulin, fasting blood glucose, Lp(a), and ferritin (iron). These tests can be more revealing of heart disease risk than cholesterol or triglycerides alone. Work with a holistic practitioner to interpret the results and determine what your body needs to reduce your risk of heart disease.

Strategies for Preventing Heart Disease

If you show signs of needing help with your heart, take action now. Waiting until you have a heart attack or stroke is too late. Here are some steps to take.

Reduce Inflammation and Free Radical Damage

Oxidative stress and the inflammation that accompanies it is what allows cholesterol and minerals to stick to our arteries, forming arterial plaque. This lessens blood flow to the heart, brain, and other parts of the body, increasing the risk of heart attack, stroke, and other arterial blockages.

That's why the single most important thing you can do to reduce your risk of heart disease is to obtain adequate amounts of antioxidant and anti-inflammatory nutrients. If you're one of the millions of Americans who aren't eating enough fresh fruits and vegetables, start now! Get the extra antioxidants you need either from foods like blueberries, blackberries, and raspberries, or from supplements. This is one of the best things you can do to reduce your risk of heart disease, as well as cancer, dementia, and other degenerative diseases associated with aging. You can also consider using *Antioxidant* or *Cardiovascular Antioxidant Formulas.*

When it comes to protecting your heart, one of the best antioxidants is Co-Q10. It reduces blood pressure, aids recovery from heart attacks, keeps LDL cholesterol from oxidizing, and improves energy production in the heart muscle. Statin drugs deplete Q-10, so this supplement should always be taken by people using statin drugs to lower cholesterol.

Get an Oil Change

For a long time we've heard the dogma that high-fat diets contribute to heart disease, and that margarine and vegetable oils are healthier for us than butter, coconut oil, or animal fats. In response to this propaganda, many people have adopted low fat diets, avoiding eggs, whole milk, and red meat in an effort to stay healthier. Unfortunately, this hasn't reduced deaths from heart disease.

The fact is that fatty acids are the preferred fuel of the heart. In other words, the heart needs fats to be healthy, but not just any kind of fats; it needs good fats. In particular, you need omega-3 essential fatty acids, which can be obtained through dietary changes or supplements. See the *Healthy Fats* strategy. You should also reduce (or completely eliminate) your intake of margarine, shortening, processed vegetable oils, and most deep-fat-fried foods. If your cholesterol level is high (over 250 mg/dl.) see *cholesterol (high)* for suggestions on how to reduce it.

If You Smoke, Quit

Tobacco smoke contains almost five thousand different chemicals, many of which damage and inflame the artery walls, starting a cascade of damage-inflammation-plaque buildup that ultimately leads to atherosclerosis, or a narrowing of artery walls. In addition, nicotine constricts blood vessels, increasing blood pressure and forcing the heart to work harder. And the carbon monoxide in cigarette smoke replaces some of the oxygen in the bloodstream—meaning your heart has to work harder just to get the same amount of oxygen to the heart and other tissues.

The good news is that people who quit smoking start to get significant benefits immediately. Their risk of heart disease drops dramatically within one year of quitting.

Get Physically Active

Regular exercise has almost the opposite effect of smoking; it increases blood flow to the heart and strengthens the heart so that it pumps more blood with less effort. It also controls weight and reduces fat—a big gain if you consider that one pound of fatty tissue contains *one mile* of capillaries that the heart has to pump blood through. Exercise also can reduce your chances of developing other conditions that may put strain on your heart, such as high blood pressure and diabetes. And finally, exercise can reduce stress, which is generally considered a contributor to high blood pressure. See the *Exercise* strategy.

Control Your Temper

Anger damages the heart. It is well documented that angry people are more prone to heart disease. If you have a problem with your temper, learn how to manage your anger and develop closer relationships. Having loving relationships reduces your risk of heart disease. See the condition *anger (excessive)*.

Use Appropriate Supplements to Support Heart Health.

In addition to Co-Q10 and omega-3, here are some of the most important herbs and nutritional supplements that can help to both prevent and reverse heart disease.

L-carnitine for heart energy. This important amino acid, found primarily in red meat, transports fatty acids to be metabolized for energy in the mitochondria. It improves energy production and oxygen utilization in the heart and can be very helpful for improving heart health.

Magnesium to prevent spasms. About half of all Americans are deficient in magnesium, a critical mineral for heart health. Magnesium helps the heart and blood vessels to relax properly, which reduces stress on the heart, helps protect the heart against spasms, and helps lower blood pressure. Magnesium is also essential for energy production in the heart.

Hawthorn and other herbs to strengthen the heart. Cardiac Tonic Formulas are built around hawthorn berries and other key herbs for strengthening the heart. They may also enhance peripheral circulation. The *Brain-Heart Formula* is another option, which helps protect both the brain and the heart. It's a safe, effective preventative that elderly people at risk for heart disease or dementia can take every day.

Herbs and nutrients to lower blood pressure. If your blood pressure is high, consider using a *Hypotensive Formula* (see *blood pressure, high*). Another possibility is the *Nitric Oxide Boosting Formula*. It also aids general circulation and can reduce inflammation and plaque formation (see the *Enhance Nitric Oxide* strategy).

Don't be one of the statistics. Alter your lifestyle and start using some of the many supplements that can keep your heart healthy.

Strategies: Avoid Sugar, Blood Type Diet, Deep Breathing, Eat Healthy, Enhance Nitric Oxide, Exercise, Healthy Fats, Hydration, Low-Glycemic Diet, Sleep, and Stress Management

Formulas: Brain-Heart, **Oral Chelation**, Garcinia Fat-Burning, Nattokinase Enzyme, Blood Pressure Reducing, Antioxidant, Heart Health, **Cardiovascular Antioxidant**, **Nitric Oxide Boosting**, and Cholesterol-Regulating

Flower Essence Blends: Anger-Reducing FE

Flower Essences: Broken and Hardened Hearts FE

Herbs: Açaí, **arjuna**, capsicum, cocoa, cordyceps, evening primrose, **ginkgo**, ginseng (American), ginseng (Asian/Korean), gynostemma, **hawthorn**, holy basil, kelp, mangosteen, night-blooming cereus, **orange (bergamot)**, and **prickly ash**

Supplements: Alpha-lipoic acid, berberine, choline, chromium, Co-Q10, curcumin, **krill oil**, **L-arginine**, lycopene, **magnesium**, **omega-3 EFAs**, potassium, resveratrol, selenium, vitamin B_9, **vitamin C**, and **vitamin E**

Essential Oils: Lavender, lemon, rose, rosemary, and ylang ylang

Carpal Tunnel

Carpal tunnel syndrome is a narrowing of the bony passage in the wrist, which constricts blood vessels and nerves passing to and from the hand, causing pain and disturbances of sensation in the hand. Repetitive movements such as constant typing cause carpal tunnel syndrome.

Vitamin B_6 has helped many people with carpal tunnel syndrome. *Topical Analgesic Formulas* may also be helpful when combined with massage and stretching exercises to keep the wrists flexible. Chiropractors and other body workers can also make adjustments to the wrists to support healing.

Strategies: Lymph-Moving Pain Relief

Formulas: Antioxidant and **Topical Analgesic**

Herbs: Boswellia and **solomon's seal**

Supplements: Magnesium, MSM, vitamin B-complex, vitamin B_2, and **vitamin B_6**

Essential Oils: Lavender and marjoram

Cartilage Damage

See also arthritis

Cartilage is a spongy material that cushions the ends of bones at the joints. Cartilage has no blood supply, so it's entirely dependent upon synovial fluid for nutrients for repair. A lack of essential nutrients, a lack of synovial fluid, or a lack of synovial fluid movement can exacerbate normal wear and tear. Synovial fluid movement is dependent upon physical activity, so the more sedentary you are, the less repairs can take place.

Bone broth, gelatin, and collagen supplements can be helpful for repairing cartilage. Reducing the systemic inflammatory process is also essential to joint healing.

Strategies: Bone Broth, Eat Healthy, Lymph-Moving Pain Relief, Mineralization, and Poultice

Formulas: Vulnerary, Herbal Arthritis, **Joint Healing Nutrients**, Gut Immune, and Enzyme Spray

Herbs: Boswellia, **burdock**, cat's claw, **solomon's seal**, spirulina, and turmeric

Supplements: **Collagen**, **MSM**, multiple vitamin and mineral, and vitamin C

Cataracts

See also free radical damage

Any clouding of the lens in the eye is called a cataract. Cataracts usually develop from age-associated free radical damage, but they may also be caused by injury. Symptoms include hazy vision, glare, trouble focusing, rapid eye fatigue, and double vision. Cataracts are the number 1 cause of blindness in the elderly worldwide. Cigarette smoking greatly increases the risk of cataracts.

A diet high in antioxidants (fruits and vegetables) and low in refined sugars reduces cataract risk. Because cataracts are due to damage from the sun, wearing sunglasses in bright light can also be helpful.

In traditional Chinese medicine there is a connection between eye and liver health. Both the eyes and the liver require large quantities of antioxidants. Lutein and zeaxanthin are important antioxidant nutrients that help protect eye health and may be helpful in preventing cataracts. If you are concerned about developing cataracts, you can reduce your risk by increasing an *Antioxidant Eye Formula* with these nutrients along with omega-3 essential fatty acids, particularly DHA.

Large doses of vitamin C may be helpful for cataracts. Some people have reported benefits from using N-acetyl cysteine eye drops, but this does not seem to be a very dependable approach to reversing cataracts. In most cases, surgery is the only way to get rid of cataracts once they are formed. However, some people report that using the *Herbal Eyewash Formula* daily (as an eye wash, not internally) for a period of several months has helped.

Strategies: Eat Healthy and Healthy Fats

Formulas: Antioxidant, Oral Chelation, Antioxidant Eye, Methylated B Vitamin, and Herbal Eyewash

Herbs: **Bilberry**, chicory, elder berry, and eyebright

Supplements: L-carnitine, **lutein**, N-acetyl cysteine, **omega-3 EFAs**, vitamin A, vitamin B_1, vitamin B_2, vitamin B_3, vitamin B_9, vitamin C, vitamin E, **zeaxanthin**, and zinc

Cavities see *dental health*

Celiac Disease

See also autoimmune disorders and inflammatory bowel disorders

Celiac disease is an autoimmune disorder, primarily of the small intestines, but symptoms can occur elsewhere. It involves an inflammatory immune response to gliadins and glutenins, compounds in wheat, barley, and rye, which cause damage and shortening of the villi in the small intestines. This can lead to malabsorption, multiple nutrient deficiencies, and anemia.

This disease requires avoiding grains containing gluten. Some people have a gluten intolerance, but this is not as serious as celiac disease. In either case, besides avoiding gluten, one can use probiotics and herbs that soothe and heal the intestinal system such as the *Intestinal Soothing* or *Irritable Bowel Fiber Formula*. A *Digestive Support Formula* may also be helpful.

Strategies: Eat Healthy, Eliminate Allergy-Causing Foods, Friendly Flora, Gluten-Free Diet, and Gut-Healing Diet

Formulas: Irritable Bowel Fiber, **Probiotic**, **Intestinal Soothing**, Digestive Support, Gentle Bowel Cleansing, H. Pylori-Fighting, and Betaine HCl

Herbs: **Aloe vera**, calendula, chamomile, **marshmallow**, plantain, slippery elm, and yarrow

Supplements: Lipase, **magnesium**, MSM, protease, and **vitamin B_{12}**

Cellulite

See also fatty tumors/deposits and excess weight

Cellulite is made of fatty deposits trapped by collagen that give the skin a dimpled, orange peel look. It tends to develop most on the thighs, hips and buttocks.

It is a fallacy to think that certain remedies specifically target cellulite. Some herbs traditionally used to help the body metabolize fats and release toxins, such as chickweed and burdock, might help to burn cellulite and excess fats in general. See more information under *weight loss* and *fatty tumors/deposits*.

Strategies: Healthy Fats and Low-Glycemic Diet

Formulas: **Skinny** and Metabolic Stimulant

Herbs: Burdock and **chickweed**

Supplements: L-carnitine and omega-3 EFAs

Essential Oils: Atlas cedarwood, grapefruit (pink), lemon, patchouli, and rosemary

Cervical Dysplasia

Cervical dysplasia occurs when abnormal squamous cells develop on the surface of the cervix. It results from a chronic infection of HPV. Women are at a higher risk of HPV causing cervical dysplasia if they smoke, have diabetes, are immunodeficient, give birth before sixteen years of age, or have a poor diet and nutrient deficiencies.

In the earlier stages of this disease, the body's immune system has a 50-70 percent chance of resolving the problem on its own. Supporting the immune system with adequate nutrition, antiviral herbs, and immune stimulant herbs will help.

Many women have reversed their cervical dysplasia by supplementing with high doses of folate (5-MTHF) or folinic acid. Folate does inhibit viral replication, but at high doses it's potentially a double-edged sword, with small studies showing a slight increase in cancer risk for people taking folate. Supplementing with 400-800 mcg of folate is likely to be helpful and not harmful.

Formulas: **Standardized Acetogenin**, Detoxifying, and Chinese Wind-Heat Evil

Programs: Chinese Balanced Cleansing

Herbs: Baptisia, **echinacea**, elder berry, isatis, and pawpaw

Supplements: Indole-3-carbinol, multiple vitamin and mineral, vitamin A, vitamin B_{12}, **vitamin B_9**, vitamin C, and zinc

Essential Oils: Clove and lemon

Chemical Exposure

See also heavy metal poisoning

Many people work at jobs that expose them to chemicals daily. Examples include carpet cleaners, dry cleaners, painters, auto mechanics, and beauticians. If you have to work around chemicals or you have one of the many health problems associated with chemical poisoning (see the *Reduce Chemical Exposure* strategy) eating a nutrient dense diet helps ensure you'll have the raw materials your liver needs to detoxify adequately.

You can also take a *Fiber Blend* and do a periodic cleanse. The *Chinese Balanced Cleaning Program* and *Ivy Bridge's Cleansing Program* are two excellent cleanses to do once or twice each year. You can also take milk thistle or a *Hepatoprotective Formula* on a daily basis.

Antioxidants, as found in fresh fruits and vegetables and herbal *Antioxidant Formulas,* are important for helping the

liver deal with chemicals. Nutritional supplements like N-acetyl cysteine, alpha-lipoic acid, and SAM-e are all helpful for some stages of liver detoxification.

For acute chemical poisoning it is best to consult a poison control center for advice. Massive doses of activated charcoal are often given to absorb many kinds of poisons after they have been ingested, but ask the poison control center for specific instructions. Acute cases of chemical poisoning should be treated medically, with herbal and nutritional therapies used for backup support.

Strategies: Balance Methylation, Detoxification, Drawing Bath, Eat Enzyme-Rich Foods, Eat Healthy, Fasting, Heavy Metal Cleanse, Hydration, Liver Detoxification, and Reduce Chemical Exposure

Formulas: Fiber, Heavy Metal Cleansing, Detoxifying, Probiotic, Chinese Wood-Decreasing, **Hepatoprotective**, Gut-Healing Fiber, and Nitric Oxide Boosting

Programs: Ivy Bridge's Cleansing and **Chinese Balanced Cleansing**

Herbs: Milk thistle, red clover, reishi, and schisandra

Supplements: Alpha-lipoic acid, **charcoal**, **N-acetyl cysteine**, omega-3 EFAs, and SAM-e

Chest Pain

See also acid indigestion, angina, gallbladder problems, pain, and pleurisy

Chest pain can have several causes, including a gallbladder attack, heartburn or acid reflux, inflammation in the pleura, muscle tension, or angina. Get a proper diagnosis and see appropriate related conditions.

Strategies: Avoid Caffeine, Emotional Healing Work, and Forgiveness

Formulas: Nitric Oxide Boosting and Chinese Fire-Increasing

Herbs: Black cohosh, capsicum, and **lobelia**

Supplements: Magnesium

Chicken Pox

See also itching, infection (viral), and shingles

Chicken pox is an acute, contagious infection of the *varicella zoster* virus. The immune response to this infection creates a low-grade fever and oozing, itching sores almost anywhere on the surface of the body. They may even occur on mucous membrane surfaces such as the throat. If sores are scratched or picked, they can leave scars.

Chicken pox is treated naturally by enhancing the immune system's ability to expel the virus from the body. This is accomplished by taking small, frequent doses (every two to four hours) of alterative or blood purifying herbs, along with plenty of water. Oregon grape, burdock, and yellow dock are good options.

Sudorific formulas, like *Steven Horne's Children's Composition Formula* or yarrow tea with peppermint added for flavoring, can be used to help reduce fever and inflammation. Aspirin is not recommended because it suppresses the body's ability to eliminate the virus, which causes problems with shingles later in life.

Remedies used to ease topical itching may be helpful as well. These include using the *Drawing Bath* or *Compress or Fomentation* strategies with herbs like burdock, goldenseal, chickweed, or Oregon grape.

Antiviral herbs may also be helpful for chicken pox. Safflowers, Saint John's wort, lemon balm, and lomatium are some of the herbs that may be helpful for chicken pox. The *Chinese Wind-Heat Evil Formula* may also be helpful.

Strategies: Compress or Fomentation, Drawing Bath, and Hydration

Formulas: **Chinese Wind-Heat Evil**, Blood Purifier, Detoxifying, Chinese Yang-Reducing, and **Steven Horne's Children's Composition**

Herbs: Burdock, chickweed, goldenseal, lemon balm, lobelia, lomatium, olive, **Oregon grape**, safflower, **Saint John's wort**, vervain (blue), yarrow, and **yellow dock**

Supplements: Clay (bentonite), clay (Redmond), and vitamin E

Essential Oils: Bergamot, lavender, and tea tree

Childbirth
see *labor & delivery* **and** *pregnancy*

Chills

Chills are usually associated with an increased internal body temperature during a fever but can also be present in severe blood loss or shock. Mild, chronic feelings of cold, especially in the extremities, is usually caused by anemia, poor circulation, or low thyroid. The hypothalamus regulates the body temperature and opens and closes the vents or pores in the skin to help regulate the body temperature. It's important to identify the cause of the chills before taking herbs.

Formulas: Circulatory, Chinese Qi and Blood Tonic, and Chinese Yang-Reducing

Herbs: Capsicum, cinnamon, forsythia, garlic, and ginger

Essential Oils: Cinnamon

Cholera
See also diarrhea

Cholera is an acute infection caused by the bacterium *Vibrio cholerae*. It generally causes diarrhea and dehydration. Since it is a bacterial condition, use antibacterial herbs like goldenseal, echinacea, and/or berberine. You can also take large doses of nanoparticle silver (two to four ounces per day). In severe cases, however, it may be best to seek medical treatment and get an antibiotic.

The big issue with cholera is severe dehydration. Staying hydrated will allow the infection to run its course without serious complications in most cases. You can use commercial rehydration salts or make you own using the following recipe from Thomas Easley, which uses the 8-8-8 rule: eight ounces of boiled water or fruit juice, eight teaspoons of sugar and one-eighth teaspoon of salt mixed together.

You can also help the diarrhea by taking fiber or activated charcoal. See *diarrhea* for additional ideas.

Strategies: Hydration

Formulas: Fiber and **Stabilized Allicin**

Herbs: Echinacea, garlic, **goldenseal**, marshmallow, and slippery elm

Supplements: **Berberine**, **charcoal**, and nanoparticle silver

Essential Oils: Rosemary

Cholesterol, High
See also cholesterol (low) and hypothyroidism

High cholesterol is a symptom of metabolic imbalance, not a root cause of any health problem. The lab ranges for cholesterol have been artificially reduced due to pressure from the pharmaceutical industry in order to sell more highly profitable statin drugs. Normal cholesterol ranges should probably be 150 to 250 mg/DL, with the optimal range between 180 and 230 mg/DL.

Cholesterol plays a very important role in the body. The primary use of cholesterol (60-80 percent) is to make bile for the digestion of fats. Cholesterol is also used to make adrenal and reproductive hormones and to sequester toxins in the body.

Cholesterol below 150 is too low and can cause serious health risks, including infertility, depression, increased risk of cancer, and a higher tendency toward death from a heart attack (see *cholesterol, low*). The following strategies can help lower cholesterol when it is too high.

Fiber. Fiber in the diet helps to reduce cholesterol levels. Fiber binds toxins in the gut and to cholesterol being released in the bile to prevent it from being reabsorbed. If you want to lower your cholesterol naturally, start by increasing fiber in your diet and/or taking a *Fiber Blend* and drinking lots of water.

Cholagogue herbs. Herbs like artichoke leaf, milk thistle, fringetree, and barberry promote the flow of bile, which eliminates excess cholesterol from the liver. When there is adequate fiber in the intestinal tract to bind this cholesterol, it can't be reabsorbed.

Healthy fats. Cholesterol can be lowered by consuming adequate quantities of high-quality fats. Taking several tablespoons of olive oil or coconut oil daily will actually help lower cholesterol because more bile has to be produced to emulsify the fats. Again, this strategy works best if you are taking plenty of fiber and drinking lots of water. Essential fatty acids in omega-3 supplements may also help lower cholesterol.

Low thyroid. A lack of thyroid hormones may be a cause of high cholesterol. If your thyroid is low, work on the thyroid to get your cholesterol down (see *hypothyroidism*).

Other remedies. There are a number of herbs and nutrients that help maintain normal cholesterol levels. These include niacin, garlic, and guggul. Red yeast rice is the natural alternative to statin drugs; both work by blocking the synthesis of cholesterol in the liver. However, both also block the synthesis of Co-Q10, so anyone taking them should supplement with Co-Q10.

Strategies: Eat Healthy, Gallbladder Flush, Healthy Fats, and Increase Dietary Fiber

Formulas: Cholesterol-Regulating, Fat-Absorbing Fiber, Skinny, Chinese Wood-Increasing, Garcinia Fat-Burning, Christopher's Gallbladder, **Fiber, Cardiovascular Antioxidant**, and Mushroom Immune

Programs: Cardiovascular Nutritional and Chinese Balanced Cleansing

Herbs: Acacia, **artichoke**, barberry, chaga, flax seed, fringe tree, garcinia, garlic, guar gum, **guggul**, gynostemma, maitake, milk thistle, myrrh, orange (bergamot), psyllium, psyllium, **red yeast rice**, reishi, turmeric, and yellow dock

Supplements: Berberine, charcoal, Co-Q10, omega-3 DHA, **omega-3 EFAs**, sodium alginate, **vanadium**, vitamin B$_3$, and **vitamin B$_3$**

Essential Oils: Clary sage, helichrysum, lemon, and myrrh

Cholesterol, Low

See also adrenal fatigue, fat metabolism (poor), gallbladder problems, and hyperthyroid

A cholesterol level below 175 mg/DL should be considered low. Low cholesterol increases one's risk of death from cardiovascular diseases and cancer. In fact, the lower the cholesterol, the higher the risk of cancer. Low cholesterol also interferes with glandular function, especially the adrenal and reproductive hormones. It may be a cause of infertility and depression. Low cholesterol is also linked with increased risk of suicide.

There are many possible causes of low cholesterol, which include taking statin drugs, low thyroid, lack of bile flow or production, low fat diets, low protein diets, poor fat or protein metabolism, and adrenal fatigue. Remedies will depend on the cause, so talk to a holistically-minded practitioner who understands this problem to help you determine an appropriate approach.

Many people are not eating enough good fats because they have been led to believe that all fats are "bad." If a person is on a low fat diet, they need to add good fats back into the diet in the form of olive oil, coconut oil, butter from grass-fed cows, avocados, nuts, and/or deep ocean fish.

Cholesterol is a lipoprotein, meaning it is a combination of fat and protein, so low-protein diets and/or problems with protein metabolism may also contribute to low cholesterol. If this is the case, increase intake of protein foods and/or take protease enzyme supplements and hydrochloric acid supplements to aid protein metabolism.

If cholesterol is low, it's also good to eat cholesterol-rich foods, like eggs, red meat, and butter. If one is taking statin drugs and has low cholesterol, they should consider discontinuing the drugs with the help of a holistic practitioner.

Strategies: Healthy Fats

Formulas: Thyroid Glandular, Adrenal Glandular, Methylated B Vitamin, and Betaine HCl

Herbs: Black walnut, chickweed, dulse, kelp, and Oregon grape

Supplements: Iodine, L-carnitine, lipase, manganese, MSM, omega-3 EFAs, protease, SAM-e, vitamin B-complex, vitamin B$_{12}$, and vitamin B$_9$

Chronic Fatigue Syndrome
see *Epstein-Barr virus*

Chronic Obstructive Pulmonary Disorder
see *COPD*

Circulation, Brain

See also Alzheimer's, memory/brain function, and dementia

The following suggestions should help improve circulation to the brain, which can help with senility and cognitive functions as a person ages. Regular exercise, like walking, helps pump more blood to the brain too. This is why walking often helps to clear a person's mind.

Strategies: Flower Essence and Oral Chelation

Formulas: Oral Chelation, Brain and Memory Protection, Nitric Oxide Boosting, and **Brain-Heart**

Programs: Cardiovascular Nutritional

Herbs: Blessed thistle, **ginkgo**, **gotu kola**, and **rosemary**

Essential Oils: Rosemary

Circulation, Poor

See also anemia, cardiovascular disease, and hypothyroidism

Poor circulation is characterized by a variety of symptoms. It may result in cold hands and feet, fatigue, loss of memory, wounds or sores that won't heal in the extremities, loss of eyesight, swelling in the legs, and tingling sensations in the arms, hands, legs, and feet.

Poor circulation is most commonly caused by insulin resistance and sedentary lifestyles, but can be related to dehydration and nutritional deficiencies. Cardiovascular herbs like capsicum, garlic, prickly ash, or ginkgo help to stimulate circulation and can be good symptomatic remedies while working on the root cause. Capsicum, in particular, tends to normalize blood flow throughout the body. The *Enhance Nitric Oxide* strategy relaxes blood vessels and improves blood flow too.

Strategies: Enhance Nitric Oxide, Exercise, Hydration, and Oral Chelation

Formulas: **Circulatory**, Stabilized Allicin, **Brain-Heart**, Heart Health, **Oral Chelation**, Vein Tonic, Male Performance, Vandergriff's Energy Booster, **Nitric Oxide Boosting**, and Cholesterol-Regulating

Programs: Cardiovascular Nutritional

Herbs: **Capsicum**, cinnamon, dong quai, garlic, **ginger**, ginkgo, guggul, hawthorn, **prickly ash**, and salvia

Supplements: Omega-3 DHA, omega-3 EFAs, vitamin B$_3$, and vitamin E

Essential Oils: Anise, cajeput, cinnamon, fir, neroli, pine, rose, rosemary, and thyme

Cirrhosis of the Liver

See also autoimmune disorders, hepatitis, and fatty liver disease

Cirrhosis is an end-stage, degenerative liver disease associated with functional failure of liver tissues and, if left untreated, eventual liver failure. The liver tissue becomes scarred from viral infections, alcoholism, reactions to drugs, and exposure to environmental toxins. The disease can result in the need for a liver transplant. Cirrhosis is a severe disease; seek appropriate medical assistance, and the help of an experienced herbalist or natural healer (findanherbalist.com).

To address cirrhosis, you must address the cause of the cirrhosis. Chronic alcoholism is the leading cause of cirrhosis in the US, and alcohol must be completely given up in cirrhosis (including herbal tinctures).

Modern medicine now has very effective antivirals for hepatitis B and C, the second leading cause of cirrhosis. Antiviral and immune-stimulating herbs can be helpful adjuncts to pharmaceutical antivirals. Herbs can also be used to combat the side effects of antivirals.

Herbs and nutrients like SAM-e, N-acetyl cysteine, schisandra, milk thistle are specific remedies that are useful for cirrhosis of the liver. Helichrysum essential oil and the *Castor Oil Pack* strategy applied over the liver area are traditional therapies to promote healing. Licorice root, MSM, and dandelion are also potentially useful supplements here.

Strategies: Castor Oil Pack, Eat Healthy, Gut-Healing Diet, and Hydration

Formulas: **Hepatoprotective** and Chinese Wood-Increasing

Flower Essence Blends: Anger-Reducing FE and Broken and Hardened Hearts FE

Herbs: **Dandelion**, goldenseal, licorice, **milk thistle**, picrorhiza, schisandra, and yellow dock

Supplements: MSM, N-acetyl cysteine, **SAM-e**, and vitamin B-complex

Essential Oils: Frankincense, helichrysum, and myrrh

Cloudy Thinking

See also adrenal fatigue, hypoglycemia, insomnia, and SIBO

When a person's thinking is cloudy, they are having a difficult time concentrating, remembering, or thinking clearly. We sometimes say the person has brain fog. There are a number of reasons this may be happening. It is important to determine the cause in order to find an effective therapy, but here are some helpful strategies.

Dehydration will interfere with clear thinking; so make sure you stay properly hydrated (see the *Hydration* strategy).

Low blood sugar (hypoglyecemia) makes it hard to think clearly too. If you crave sweets and caffeine you may need to get your blood sugar under control. Adopt the *Low-Glycemic diet* strategy and follow the instructions for dealing with *hypoglycemia*.

If you've been under a lot of stress and are feeling tired and not sleeping well, you may be suffering from nervous and glandular fatigue. Adaptogens may be helpful in this case, such a the *Chinese Fire-Increasing* or *Ashwagandha Complex Formula*. See *adrenal fatigue* and *nervous exhaustion* for more ideas.

If you have a lot of indigestion, gas and bloating, you may have small intestinal bacterial overgrowth. Use the *Detoxification* strategy and perhaps the *Gut-Healing Diet* strategy. See *SIBO* for more information.

The *Memory Enhancing Formula* can aid brain function as can rosemary and bacopa. Peppermint can be helpful to improve mental alertness as a tea, essential oil, or flower essence, especially for people with digestive problems.

Strategies: Avoid Sugar, Detoxification, Hydration, and Low-Glycemic Diet

Formulas: Adaptogen-Immune, **Attention-Focus**, Oral Chelation, **Chinese Fire-Increasing**, Anti-Stress B-Complex, Blood Sugar Control, **Ashwagandha Complex**, Brain and Memory Protection, **Memory Enhancing**, and Digestive Support

Herbs: Bacopa, ginkgo, ginseng (American), gotu kola, peppermint, and **rosemary**

Supplements: L-glutamine, L-tyrosine, and vitamin B-complex

Essential Oils: Eucalyptus, lime, **peppermint**, pine, and spearmint

Cold Hands/Feet

See also anemia, circulation (poor), hiatal hernia, hypoglycemia, hypothyroidism, and stress

Mild, chronic feelings of cold, especially in the extremities, can be a symptom of several different health problems. Seek appropriate assistance to determine the cause before embarking on a course of therapy. Here are a few of the more common causes of cold hands and feet.

Thyroid. Low thyroid is a common cause and taking remedies like *Hypothyroid Formulas* can resolve the problem. In some cases thyroid medication may be needed (see *hypothyroidism*).

Anemia. Any of the common forms of anemia can cause cold hands and feet, but it's most common with iron-deficiency anemia (see *anemia*).

Circulation. Another common cause is poor circulation to the extremities. Try taking herbs that stimulate circulation and get more exercise (see *circulation, poor*).

Stress. Chronic stress can cause a constriction of peripheral blood vessels, leading to cold extremities. If stress, anxiety, or insomnia are present use relaxing nervines and adaptogens (see *stress*).

Digestion. Poor digestion may also be a factor in cold hands and feet. People with a hiatal hernia are often pale and cold (see *hiatal hernia*).

Blood Sugar. Low blood sugar may trigger sudden feelings of cold in the hands, feet or nose (see *hypoglycemia*).

Strategies: Exercise

Formulas: Brain-Heart, **Chinese Qi and Blood Tonic**, **Chinese Wood-Increasing**, Circulatory, **Oral Chelation**, **Thyroid Glandular**, and Nitric Oxide Boosting

Programs: Cardiovascular Nutritional

Herbs: Capsicum, garlic, **ginger**, ginkgo, hawthorn, prickly ash, skullcap, and vervain (blue)

Supplements: Omega-3 EFAs and vitamin B_3

Cold Sores
Fever Blisters

See also herpes

A cold sore is an infection of the *Herpes simplex* virus that causes a painful, oozing group of blisters usually located around the lips. They turn into a scabby sore. Cold sores are also known as fever blisters.

The *Chinese Wind-Heat Evil Formula* is especially helpful for herpes infections. Lemon balm, black walnut, self heal, and Saint John's wort are also potential remedies, topically and internally, for cold sores. Some people find supplementation with large doses of L-lysine helpful (10,000 mg). L-arginine is contraindicated with this condition. Since outbreaks are often stress-related, the *Stress Management* strategy may be helpful in reducing the frequency of outbreaks.

Strategies: Friendly Flora and Stress Management

Formulas: Topical Analgesic, **Chinese Wind-Heat Evil**, and Probiotic

Herbs: Black walnut, lemon balm, and Saint John's wort

Supplements: Chlorophyll, **L-lysine**, omega-3 EFAs, vitamin B-complex, and zinc

Essential Oils: Bergamot, peppermint, and tea tree

Colds

See also chills, congestion, fever, infection (viral), and cough

Colds are a group of acute, contagious infections characterized by malaise, fever, chills (thus the name), and respiratory congestion. The goal in working with colds should be to help the body eliminate the toxins it is trying to expel from the body.

Although echinacea or formulas with goldenseal and echinacea are commonly used for colds, these are not the most effective cold remedies, especially during the early stages of a cold. They are more helpful in the latter stages of a cold, when there is thick, discolored mucus.

During the early stages of a cold, when mucus is thin and clear or pale white, the best herbal remedies are aromatic or pungent herbs, taken every hour or two with plenty of fluids. Examples of aromatics that are helpful for colds include yarrow, peppermint, chamomile, and catnip. These work best when taken as hot teas. Pungent herbs include capsicum, ginger, garlic, and horseradish. These are often easier to take as capsules or extracts and should also be taken with warm or hot liquids.

Some really great do-it-yourself formulas for colds and flu use aromatic and pungent herbs. These include *Ed Millet's Herbal Crisis*, *Fire Cider* and *Children's Composition Formula*. All work best taking in small, frequently repeated doses while fasting and drinking lots of water.

Using the *Colon Hydrotherapy* and *Sweat Bath* strategies to improve elimination and stimulate perspiration is a highly effective way to rapidly recover from a cold. Taking aromatic and pungent herbs every two to four hours after these procedures usually clears colds in less than twenty-four hours.

Essential oils can often be rubbed on the chest or throat to help get rid of colds. When doing this, it's best to dilute them with a fixed vegetable oil like olive oil. You can also breathe in these aromatic vapors, which helps to open airways and clear congestion. Putting a few drops into hot water and inhaling the steam can be very effective.

When you have a cold, stop eating. The famous saying "Feed a cold, starve a fever" means that "if you feed a cold, you'll have to starve a fever." If you are hungry when you have a cold, drink some fresh fruit or vegetable juices or a little soup or broth. Avoid grains, animal proteins, nuts, beans, and other heavier foods when sick. Use the more specific cold listings that follow to deal with more specific types of cold symptoms.

Strategies: Colon Hydrotherapy, Fasting, Hydration, and Sweat Bath

Formulas: Paavo Airola's Cold, Flu and Vomiting, Seasonal Cold and Flu, **Cold Lozenges**, Immune-Boosting, Chinese Yang-Reducing, **Jeannie Burgess' Allergy-Lung**, Chinese Metal-Decreasing, Herbal Composition, **Ed Millet's Herbal Crisis**, **Steven Horne's Children's Composition**, and **Fire Cider**

Herbs: Acerola, **andrographis**, asparagus, astragalus, **boneset**, capsicum, catnip, chamomile, cinnamon, clove, echinacea, **elder berrberry & flower**, garlic, ginger, holy basil, horseradish, hyssop, lemon, lobelia, **osha**, peppermint, polygala, rosemary, siler, thyme, usnea, vervain (blue), and yarrow

Supplements: Vitamin A, vitamin C, vitamin D, and zinc

Essential Oils: Menthol and ravintsara

Colds (Antiviral)

See also infection (viral)

These are remedies that may have antiviral activity that makes them potentially beneficial for colds and flu.

Strategies: Aromatherapy

Formulas: Immune-Boosting, **Elderberry Cold and Flu**, and **Children's Elderberry Cold and Flu**

Essential Oil Blends: Disinfectant EO

Herbs: Astragalus, echinacea, **elder berry & flower**, garlic, olive, and yarrow

Essential Oils: Cinnamon, helichrysum, jasmine, lemon, marjoram, myrrh, pine, and thyme

Colds (Decongestant)

These are remedies that can help to break up respiratory congestion associated with colds, flu, and other acute illness. See *Aromatherapy* for ideas on how to use essential oils as an inhalation to break up congestion.

Strategies: Aromatherapy

Formulas: Topical Analgesic, Sinus, **Jeannie Burgess' Allergy-Lung**, Seasonal Cold and Flu, and Damp Cough Syrup

Essential Oil Blends: Disinfectant EO

Herbs: Eyebright, garlic, lobelia, and perilla

Essential Oils: Clove, **eucalyptus**, **pine**, rosemary, tea tree, and thyme

Colds With Fever

See also fever

The following remedies are for colds accompanied by fever.

Strategies: Colon Hydrotherapy and Hydration

Formulas: Chinese Yang-Reducing, Stabilized Allicin, and Steven Horne's Children's Composition

Herbs: Angelica, **chrysanthemum**, garlic, honeysuckle, sage, and **yarrow**

Colic, Adults

See also gas & bloating

Colic involves acute abdominal pain, characterized by cramping and gas. It is common in infants, but adults can have this problem too. These remedies help to relax colon muscles and/or expel intestinal gas.

Formulas: Herbal Bitters, **Christopher's Gallbladder**, **Herbal Composition**, **Ed Millet's Herbal Crisis**, Fire Cider, and Digestive Support

Herbs: Angelica, calamus, chamomile, hops, **lobelia**, passion flower, and **wild yam**

Essential Oils: Bergamot, fennel, **peppermint**, sandalwood, thyme, and ylang ylang

Colic, Children

See also gas & bloating, irritable bowel, and colon (spastic)

Colic involves acute abdominal pain, characterized by cramping and gas. The combination of catnip and fennel is a tried-and-true remedy for colic in infants and children. Giving the child probiotics, especially bifidophilus, will also help.

A midwife once told me that a magnesium-deficient mother will produce a colicky baby. Cramps are often a sign of magnesium deficiency. Nursing mothers should consider supplementing with magnesium if their baby is colicky. Some of the remedies that aid breast milk will also make the mother's milk less prone to cause colic (see *nursing*).

Mother's milk has a 2:1 ratio of calcium to magnesium. Infant formulas tend to have more calcium and less magnesium and may produce colic. This may be why some infants get colicky from being fed baby formulas. Raw goat's milk is usually better than infant formulas, but if a child is getting an infant formula, consider giving them a small amount of magnesium with it.

Yeast infections can also cause colic. If the mother has a history of vaginal yeast infections, the baby make pick up yeast in passing through the birth canal. Try rubbing some highly diluted (40:1) antifungal essential oils like lavender and cajeut on the infant's belly once daily.

Strategies: Friendly Flora

Formulas: Children's Colic

Essential Oil Blends: Antifungal EO

Herbs: Anise, **catnip**, chamomile, **fennel**, lemon balm, lobelia, peppermint, and safflower

Supplements: Magnesium

Essential Oils: Anise, cajeput, lavender, marjoram, peppermint, red mandarin, and **spearmint**

Colitis

See also inflammatory bowel disorders

Colitis is inflammation of the colon and small intestine. Some helpful strategies and remedies are listed here, but colitis is discussed in more detail under the heading *inflammatory bowel disorders*.

Strategies: Eat Healthy, Eliminate Allergy-Causing Foods, Fasting, Friendly Flora, Gut-Healing Diet, Increase Dietary Fiber, and Stress Management

Formulas: Intestinal Soothing, **Irritable Bowel Fiber**, Vulnerary, Jeannie Burgess' Stress, **Gentle Bowel Cleansing**, **Gut-Healing Fiber**, Betaine HCl, and Probiotic

Herbs: Aloe vera, amalaki, cat's claw, **catnip**, chamomile, coptis, licorice, **marshmallow**, **plantain**, and slippery elm

Supplements: L-glutamine, omega-3 DHA, and omega-3 EFAs

Essential Oils: Cinnamon, helichrysum, and thyme

Colon, Atonic

See also constipation (adults) and diverticulitis

An atonic colon is one that has lost muscular tone and balloons, lacking sufficient peristaltic strength to push material forward. This is the less-common form of constipation and results in very slow but regular, bowel movements. This is where *Stimulant Laxative Formulas* are the most useful, especially if taken with *Fiber Blends*.

For a long-term solution, *Triphala Formula*, an Ayurvedic blend of three fruits, can slowly help restore tone and function to the colon. It is part of the *Gentle Bowel Cleansing Formula*.

Strategies: Friendly Flora and Mineralization

Formulas: Stimulant Laxative, **Gentle Bowel Cleansing**, Fiber, **Probiotic**, and **Triphala**

Herbs: Black walnut, buckthorn, **butternut**, cascara sagrada, psyllium, senna, **turkey rhubarb**, and white oak

Supplements: Vitamin C

Colon, Spastic

See also irritable bowel and stress

A spastic colon is caused by muscle spasms in the colon that inhibit peristalsis. It is characterized by irregular bowel movements and constipation that is aggravated by stress. Most adults and children who are constipated have a spastic bowel condition. Stimulant laxatives can aggravate a spastic bowel condition. The more modern term for a spastic bowel is *irritable bowel syndrome (IBS)*.

Strategies: Eliminate Allergy-Causing Foods and Stress Management

Formulas: Intestinal Soothing, **Gentle Bowel Cleansing**, **Irritable Bowel Fiber**, and **Triphala**

Herbs: Amalaki, **catnip**, chamomile, lobelia, and wild yam

Supplements: Magnesium

Concentration, Poor

See also adrenal fatigue, ADD/ADHD, circulation (poor), memory/brain function, and stress

Poor concentration is often due to anxiety, PTSD, depression, lack of sleep, stress, and blood sugar imbalances. Figuring out the cause is essential to finding the proper remedies. See related conditions for more specific remedies.

In general, nourishing adaptogens and nerve tonics will help improve concentration when the problem is due to chronic stress. As a person ages, herbs like ginkgo, bacopa, and gotu kola may also be helpful for keeping the mind clear and focused. When the problem is associated with ADD, you need to use remedies to calm the brain.

Inhaling peppermint oil can stimulate the mind and aid concentration and focus. Other essential oils that may help stimulate the mind and improve concentration are rosemary, pine, and eucalyptus.

Strategies: Deep Breathing, Eliminate Salicylates, Healthy Fats, Low-Glycemic Diet, and Sleep

Formulas: Brain-Heart, Brain Calming, Oral Chelation, **Chinese Fire-Increasing**, Topical Analgesic, **Attention-Focus**, and **Adrenal Glandular**

Essential Oil Blends: Renewing and Releasing EO and Analgesic EO

Herbs: Bacopa, bee pollen, ginkgo, **gotu kola**, holy basil, peppermint, **rosemary**, and skullcap

Supplements: GABA, magnesium, **omega-3 DHA**, omega-3 EFAs, and vitamin B-complex

Essential Oils: Eucalyptus, marjoram, **peppermint**, pine, and rosemary

Concussion   **see** *traumatic brain injury*

Confusion
Brain Fog

See also adrenal fatigue and hypoglycemia

Transient confusion is often a sign of low blood sugar (see *hypoglycemia*). Confusion can also occur from lack of sleep or excessive stress. It can occur in the elderly from common infections like UTIs. Poor intestinal health may make concentration difficult too. Confusion can also occur from many other diseases, including liver disease, kidney disease, heart disease, Alzheimer's, severe anemia, PTSD, anxiety disorders, depression, and more. Figure out the cause before selecting appropriate remedies.

Strategies: Deep Breathing, Emotional Healing Work, Hydration, Low-Glycemic Diet, Reduce Chemical Exposure, Sleep, and Stress Management

Formulas: Chinese Fire-Increasing, **Adrenal Glandular**, Algae, Attention-Focus, Anti-Stress B-Complex, Hypoglycemic, and Adaptogen

Essential Oil Blends: Renewing and Releasing EO, Refreshing and Cleansing EO, and Analgesic EO

Herbs: Bacopa, ginkgo, gotu kola, **peppermint**, **rosemary**, and thyme

Supplements: Chromium, magnesium, MSM, multiple vitamin and mineral, omega-3 EFAs, and potassium

Essential Oils: Frankincense, geranium, grapefruit (pink), helichrysum, lavender, lemon, patchouli, peppermint, pine, rosemary, and thyme

Congestion

See also congestion (bronchial), congestion (lungs), congestion (lymphatic), congestion (sinus), and COPD

Excessive mucus collected in the nasal or lung passages causes congestion, which can interfere with breathing. The lymphatics can also become congested from the same irritants that caused the respiratory congestion, resulting in swollen lymph nodes, earaches, and sore throats. Decongestant and expectorant herbs can be used to break up and expel mucus from the body.

It is important to understand that expectorant and decongestant remedies won't necessarily dry up the sinuses. Since they promote breakup of congestion and the expulsion of mucus, they may cause a temporary increase in drainage as the lungs and sinuses clear out irritants. This is normal. Just keep drinking plenty of water.

The long-term solution to many people's congestion issue involves normalizing the intestinal tract, as there is a strong connection between the mucous membranes of the digestive system and the respiratory system. *Herbal Bitters* and *Digestive Support Formulas* will improve digestion, often resulting in less congestion. The *Detoxification* and *Colon Hydrotherapy* strategies may also be helpful.

See other headings for dealing with specific types of congestion, such as sinus and lymphatic congestion.

Strategies: Colon Hydrotherapy, Detoxification, Fasting, Friendly Flora, Hydration, Increase Dietary Fiber, and Sweat Bath

Formulas: Chinese Earth-Decreasing, Sinus, **Liquid Lymph**, Topical Analgesic, **Jeannie Burgess' Allergy-Lung**, Dry Cough Syrup, Herbal Bitters, and Digestive Support

Herbs: Acacia (Indian), balloon flower, cleavers, elecampane, fenugreek, garlic, **lobelia**, marshmallow, mullein, **red clover**, rosemary, thyme, typhonium, and **yerba santa**

Supplements: N-acetyl cysteine, protease, and vitamin C

Essential Oils: Anise, bay leaf, cajeput, cinnamon, **eucalyptus**, **pine**, rosemary, and **thyme**

Congestion, Bronchial

See also bronchitis and COPD

The following remedies may be helpful when the bronchial passages are inflamed, swollen, congested with mucus, or constricted due to stress. When inflammation is the cause, the condition is known as bronchitis. When chronic mucus congestion is the cause, it is classified as COPD (chronic obstructive pulmonary disorder).

Strategies: Detoxification, Hydration, and Stress Management

Formulas: Jeannie Burgess' **Allergy-Lung**, **Ayurvedic Bronchial Decongestant**, Antihistamine, **Chinese Metal-Decreasing**, and Steven Horne's Horehound Cough

Essential Oil Blends: Lung-Supporting EO

Herbs: Anise, cherry, elecampane, grindelia, khella, licorice, **lobelia**, **mullein**, and yerba santa

Supplements: L-cysteine, MSM, **N-acetyl cysteine**, and vitamin B$_5$

Essential Oils: Camphor and menthol

Congestion, Lungs

See also congestion, cough (damp), pneumonia, and cough

When the lungs are congested, it can be very difficult to breath. Decongestant and expectorant herbs can be used to break up and help the lungs expel excess mucus. One can also inhale essential oils directly or drop them into boiling-hot water and inhale the steam to help clear the lungs. (See *Aromatherapy* strategy.)

Remedies for a damp cough will also be helpful. When the mucus is hardened and difficult to expel, grindelia and plantain are good herbs to loosen it. Elecampane and yerba santa also help relieve deep-seated congestion in the lungs. Drink plenty of water to thin the mucus secretions.

Strategies: Aromatherapy, Eliminate Allergy-Causing Foods, and Hydration

Formulas: Jeannie Burgess' Allergy-Lung, Ayurvedic Bronchial Decongestant, **Stabilized Allicin**, Steven Horne's Horehound Cough, Damp Cough Syrup, and Dry Cough Syrup

Flower Essence Blends: Grief and Sadness FE

Herbs: Angelica, asparagus, **elecampane**, **garlic**, ginger, grindelia, **horehound**, horseradish, lomatium, mullein, oregano, plantain, thyme, and yerba santa

Supplements: L-cysteine and vitamin A

Essential Oils: Eucalyptus, fennel, menthol, and **pine**

Congestion, Lymphatic

See also swollen lymph glands

Most people aren't aware that the body has a drainage system. The lymphatic system works hand in hand with the circulatory system to keep the various tissues and organs alive and healthy. It's the lymphatic system's job to make sure the fluid around the cells in the body doesn't become stagnant. Sometimes the lymphatic system becomes congested, and like a clogged or sluggish drain, an unhealthy stagnation of fluids occurs. Without proper lymphatic drainage, the tissues in the body become like a stagnant swamp. conditions.

Lymphatic congestion contributes to swollen lymph nodes, earaches, sore throats, chronic sinus and respiratory congestion, tonsillitis, lumps and tumors, lymphatic cancers, and other health problems. Here are some strategies to clear lymphatic congestion.

The *Deep Breathing* strategy, combined with any form of exercise, is the key to pumping the lymph and keeping it moving. Exercise increases lymph flow as much as five to fifteen times. A popular form of lymphatic exercise is gentle bouncing on a mini trampoline, called rebounding.

If a person is unable to stand on the mini trampoline, he or she can still obtain benefit by sitting in a chair next to the trampoline, with his or her feet on the trampoline. Another person stands on the trampoline and gently bounces up and down to passively move the lymphatics as the seated person's legs move with the motion of the trampoline.

If you don't have a mini trampoline, walking and breathing deeply will greatly enhance lymphatic circulation, as will any other form of moderate exercise. Lymphatic drainage massage, done by a trained massage therapist, can be really helpful in cases of severe lymphatic congestion.

The *Hydration* strategy is another second key to reducing lymphatic sluggishness. Even moderate dehydration will contribute to poor lymphatic drainage.

Dietary change may also be helpful. Certain foods seem to clog up the lymphatic system more than others. For many people, dairy products are major culprits. Wheat and other gluten-bearing grains are another lymphatic congestant for many people. Any food that creates allergic reactions for a person may contribute to lymphatic stagnation.

There are many herbs that improve lymphatic function, but my favorites are echinacea, red root, cleavers, and red clover. There are also essential oils, which when appropriately diluted and applied topically, can also break up lymphatic congestion.

Strategies: Aromatherapy, Bodywork, Deep Breathing, Exercise, and Hydration

Formulas: Lymphatic Infection, **Liquid Lymph**, **Lymph Cleansing**, Essiac Immune Tea, Chinese Water-Decreasing, **Alterative-Immune**, Chinese Metal-Decreasing, and Chinese Qi-Regulating

Herbs: Chaparral, cleavers, **echinacea**, garlic, lobelia, mullein, **red clover**, **red root**, and **stillingia**

Essential Oils: Cajeput, fennel, geranium, grapefruit (pink), **helichrysum**, juniper, lavender, lemon, lemongrass, and thyme

Congestion, Sinus
Runny Nose

See also allergies (respiratory), leaky gut, polyps, headache (sinus), and sinus infection

When sinuses are congested, the first and most obvious remedy to try is a *Sinus Formula*. The mixture of fenugreek and thyme is especially helpful for breaking up sinus congestion. You can also inhale various essential oils either straight from the bottle or in steam.

Using a neti pot to wash the sinuses with salt water can help to cleanse the sinuses. If infection is present, silver, natural salt, or goldenseal and echinacea can be diluted and for use in the neti pot or squirted into the sinus passages with a nasal syringe. You can also sniff some of the *Steven Horne's Sinus Snuff*.

When sinus problems are chronic, it is usually a sign of poor diet and chronic problems with digestion and the gastrointestinal tract. Start by following the *Eliminate Allergy-Causing Foods* strategy. Then improve digestive function. In many cases, generalized dysbiosis and leaky gut syndrome may be a factor and the *Gut-Healing* strategy may be helpful.

Strategies: Aromatherapy, Detoxification, Fasting, Gut-Healing Diet, and Hydration

Formulas: Jeannie Burgess' Allergy-Lung, **Sinus**, **Christopher's Sinus**, Anti-Snoring, **Topical Analgesic**, Seasonal Cold and Flu, Antihistamine, Ed Millet's Herbal Crisis, and **Steven Horne's Sinus Snuff**

Essential Oil Blends: Lung-Supporting EO

Herbs: Bayberry, **fenugreek**, goldenseal, **horseradish**, orange (bitter), and **thyme**

Supplements: Bromelain, L-theanine, vitamin A, and vitamin D

Essential Oils: Camphor, eucalyptus, **pine**, ravensara, ravintsara, and wintergreen

Congestive Heart Failure

See also cardiovascular disease

Congestive heart failure is a decline in the function of the heart due to damage of the heart muscle, normally from ischemic heart disease. Appropriate medical assistance should be sought for this condition.

Hawthorn or arjuna may be helpful, along with nutritional supplements like Co-Q10, magnesium, L-arginine, and L-carnitine. Some of the bests botanical remedies for congestive heart failure are toxic botanicals like lily of the valley and arnica that require the assistance of a professional herbalist (findanherbalist.com).

Strategies: Eat Healthy, Emotional Healing Work, and Healthy Fats

Formulas: Liquid Kidney, Liquid Lymph, Nitric Oxide Boosting, and **Heart Health**

Herbs: Arjuna, arnica, asparagus, astragalus, coleus, **hawthorn**, khella, night-blooming cereus, Oregon grape, and pleurisy root

Supplements: Berberine, **Co-Q10**, **L-arginine**, **L-carnitine**, **magnesium**, **omega-3 EFAs**, and **vitamin B$_1$**

Conjunctivitis
Pink Eye

See also sty

Conjunctivitis is inflammation that causes redness in the whites of the eyes. It may be due to allergic reactions or infections such as pink eye (a contagious viral condition). A sty is a closely related condition that is caused by a staph infection in the eyelid.

Conjunctivitis and sties can be treated naturally using teas of herbs like chamomile, eyebright, or goldenseal. Soak a cotton ball or a clean, soft cloth in a warm (not hot) tea of the herbs and apply over the closed eye as a compress for about fifteen minutes (see *Compress or Fomentation* strategy). Or submerge a tea bag in warm water just long enough to moisten it and apply the tea bag over the closed eyelid. You can do this several times a day until the infection clears up.

You can apply vitamin A topically by poking a hole in a gel capsule and rubbing the liquid on the closed eyelid and eye socket. A solution of nanoparticle silver can be dropped directly into the eye as an antiseptic. Avoid putting any herbs directly into the eye.

Strategies: Compress or Fomentation

Formulas: Herbal Eyewash

Herbs: Barberry, calendula, **chamomile**, chrysanthemum, eyebright, and **goldenseal**

Supplements: Nanoparticle silver, **vitamin A**, and vitamin D

Constipation (Adults)

See also infection (fungal), gallbladder problems, inflammatory bowel disorders, parasites, and colon (spastic)

Constipation is a lack of normal bowel movement. Many people are slightly constipated and don't know it.

Ideally, the stool should move two to three times a day, depending on the number of meals consumed, and should be soft and easy to pass. It should come out in long "banana-like" pieces. Hard, round balls that are difficult to pass are a sign of dehydration and a form of constipation.

A slow colon transit time could also be considered constipation. Colon transit time is the time it takes for food materials to move through the length of the entire gastrointestinal tract. A great way to check colon transit time is to eat red beets or take liquid chlorophyll and see how long it takes to pass the red or green color of these substances in the stool.

It should take less than twenty-four hours for this material to show up in the stool and it should be cleared from the system in less than thirty-six hours. The average colon transit time of most people is forty-eight to seventy-two hours, which is too long and a sign of constipation.

Strategies for Constipation

Taking a laxative, even an herbal one is only a temporary solution to chronic constipation. It's important to look deeper and figure out why you are constipated. Here are some things to consider.

Water. Dehydration is the main cause of constipation in adults. So start by drinking plenty of pure water. (See the *Hydration* strategy.) If drinking water isn't hydrating you, try the *Chinese Yin-Increasing Formula.*

Fiber. Lack of sufficient dietary fiber is the second main cause of constipation. Increasing fibrous foods in the diet (like vegetables, fruits, beans and whole grains) helps keep the colon healthy. You can also take a *Fiber Blend* once or twice daily. Always drink plenty of water when taking fiber. (See the *Increase Dietary Fiber* strategy.)

Dysbiosis. Long-term constipation is often due to intestinal inflammation and disruption of the friendly microbes living in the intestines. Probiotics and enzyme supplements are very important to long-term bowel health in these cases.

Triphala. This is a blend of three fruits used in Ayurvedic medicine to tone the bowel and is a good tonic for long-term bowel problems. It reduces intestinal inflammation, tones the bowel, and has a gentle laxative action. It is one of the main ingredients in the *Gentle Bowel Cleansing Formula.* I've also mixed *Triphala Formula* with equal parts with psyllium hulls and freshly ground flaxseeds to make a gut-healing fiber blend that lubricates and tones the bowels.

Magnesium. A deficiency in this mineral is a common cause of constipation. Most people will start to get diarrhea if they take too much, but about 70 percent of North Americans do not get enough magnesium. It is part of the *Gentle Bowel Cleansing Formula*, but you can take more magnesium with it to increase its effectiveness. Start with 200 mg per day and increase the dose by another 200 mg every couple of days. When the stool starts to get too loose back off the dose.

Vitamin C. This vitamin also has a bowel tolerance. If you start with 1000 mg and increase the dose by 500 mg every few days until the stool gets loose, then you can back off and you'll have the correct amount for toning the colon. I've done this along with magnesium and it's a good way to break dependence on stimulant laxatives.

Stress. Constipation can also be stress-related. If the bowel is spastic, antispasmodic herbs like lobelia can have a mild laxative action (see *colon, spastic*).

Bile Secretion and Gallbladder Health. The bile from the liver also has a laxative action, so cholagogue herbs like burdock, milk thistle, and yellow dock may also be helpful for some cases of constipation.

Stimulant Laxatives. Temporary constipation can be relieved by the use of various stimulant laxatives based on herbs like cascara sagrada, buckthorn, and senna. These herbs contain anthraquinone glycosides that hold moisture in the stool and decrease colon transit time.

These herbs are fine for an occasional cleanse but should not be used regularly as they tend to deplete the tone of the bowel. They also cause the colon to become stained, which can alarm doctors who give colonoscopies. There is no evidence this harms the bowel, but it is still not the best approach to long-term bowel health.

It's also a good idea to do a cleanse of some kind once or twice a year. This will help clean and tone the colon, as well as detoxify the body in general.

Strategies: Colon Hydrotherapy, Detoxification, Eat Healthy, Fasting, Friendly Flora, Gallbladder Flush, Gut-Healing Diet, Hiatal Hernia Correction, Hydration, and Increase Dietary Fiber

Formulas: Chinese Yin-Increasing, Irritable Bowel Fiber, Probiotic, **Stimulant Laxative**, Intestinal Detoxification, Christopher's Gallbladder, **Gentle Bowel Cleansing**, **Fiber**, **Probiotic**, and **Triphala**

Programs: Ivy Bridge's Cleansing and **Chinese Balanced Cleansing**

Herbs: Acacia, aloe vera, amalaki, apricot, asparagus (Chinese), biota, broomrape, **buckthorn**, burdock, **butternut**, **cascara sagrada**, **flax seed**, guar gum, haritaki, ligustrum, milk thistle, ophiopogon, **psyllium**, senna, **turkey rhubarb**, and yellow dock

Supplements: Magnesium

Essential Oils: Lemon and orange (sweet)

Constipation (Children)

Children, like adults, can suffer from constipation and sluggish colon transit time. It is not wise, however, to use stimulant laxatives with children in most cases, except for very mild laxative herbs like yellow dock.

A little prune juice or fresh apple juice is often enough to overcome constipation in children. Children with constipation may also be magnesium deficient. Flaxseeds and slippery elm make good bulk laxatives for children.

Like adults, children may need enzymes and probiotics for bowel health. Papaya is a good source of enzymes for children, and cultured dairy products like yoghurt and kefier can supply probiotics. (Just make sure they aren't loaded with refined sugar, which feeds dysbiosis and yeast overgrowth.)

Children are often constipated due to stress, so if a child seems stressed, give them some relaxing nervine herbs along with extra water or fresh fruit and vegetable juices to help their colon move normally.

Strategies: Eat Enzyme-Rich Foods, Friendly Flora, Healthy Fats, and Hydration

Formulas: Gentle Bowel Cleansing, Probiotic, and Triphala

Herbs: Flax seed, haritaki, licorice, papaya, slippery elm, and yellow dock

Supplements: Magnesium and omega-3 EFAs

Convalescence

After a prolonged illness, the body is often in a debilitated state and needs special nutritional support to aid in rebuilding and recovering good health. This period of recovery from debility is called convalescence.

Adaptogens are good basic remedies for convalescence. The *Chinese Qi and Blood Tonic* is very good for strengthening the body both during and after prolonged illness.

If the illness has involved the intestines (intestinal infection, diarrhea, flu, nausea and vomiting) a round of probiotics should be taken to aid recovery. *Bacillus coagulans* is a good probiotic to consider. Aloe vera, slippery elm, and marshmallow have also been eaten after illness of this type to rebuild digestive health.

After a bout of long-term contagious disease or cancer, it may be helpful to fortify the immune system with medicinal mushrooms such as cordyceps or the *Mushroom Immune Formula*. The *Whole Food Green Drink Powder* and the *Algae Formula* are also helpful for supplying nutrition during recovery.

Strategies: Eat Healthy

Formulas: Algae, **Whole Food Green Drink**, Suma Adaptogen, **Chinese Qi and Blood Tonic**, Colostrum-Immune Stimulator, Chinese Metal-Increasing, Chinese Wood-Increasing, Mitochondria Energy, Chinese Earth-Increasing, **Mushroom Immune**, Colloidal Mineral, Ashwagandha Complex, Digestive Support, Jeannie Burgess' Thymus, and Adaptogen

Herbs: Alfalfa, aloe vera, **ashwagandha, astragalus**, barley, bee pollen, blue-green algae, borage, chlorella, **codonopsis, cordyceps**, Grape, Irish moss, marshmallow, **slippery elm**, spirulina, and vervain (blue)

Supplements: Bacillus coagulans, Co-Q10, multiple vitamin and mineral, omega-3 EFAs, and pancreatin

Essential Oils: Clary sage and lavender

Convulsions   see *epilepsy* **and** *seizures*

COPD
Chronic Obstructive Pulmonary Disease

See also addictions (tobacco), allergies (respiratory), asthma, bronchitis, grief & sadness, and hiatal hernia

COPD (chronic obstructive pulmonary disease) is a slow-developing disorder that causes chronic obstruction in the lungs, making breathing difficult. COPD can involve asthma, chronic bronchitis, or emphysema. Symptoms include cough with mucus, shortness of breath, fatigue, frequent respiratory infections, and wheezing.

Medical treatment for this disorder is to use inhalers, like those used in asthma, to open airways. Corticosteroid drugs and antibiotics are often used during flare-ups, and oxygen therapy may be used in severe cases.

It is important to avoid smoking and breathing very cold air. Reducing air pollution by getting an in-house air filtration system may be helpful. It is also important to eat a nutrient dense diet with plenty of fresh fruits and vegetables for their inflammation-reducing phytochemicals.

There are several categories of herbal remedies that may be helpful here. Lung and respiratory tonics like astragalus, cordyceps, licorice, and mullein can be used to strengthen the lung tissue and reduce risk of infection. Anti-inflammatory herbs can be used to reduce tissue swelling and make breathing easier. Bronchiodilator herbs like lobelia will help to open airways and make breathing easier.

There is a big connection between the health of the mucous membranes of the digestive tract and the mucous membranes of the lungs. Digestive enzymes, probiotics, fiber, and other supplements that improve gastrointestinal health will often help respiratory conditions clear up as well.

Some people with asthma or COPD have a hiatal hernia. Correcting this can greatly improve lung function and breathing capacity. See the *Hiatal Hernia Correction* strategy. There may be deep-seated, unresolved grief in chronic lung problems too. (See the condition *grief & sadness*.)

Strategies: Detoxification, Eat Healthy, Eliminate Allergy-Causing Foods, Enhance Nitric Oxide, Fasting,

Forgiveness, Hiatal Hernia Correction, Hydration, and Increase Dietary Fiber

Formulas: Chinese Metal-Increasing, Nitric Oxide Boosting, Jeannie Burgess' Allergy-Lung, Digestive Support, Probiotic, and Dry Cough Syrup

Flower Essences: Broken and Hardened Hearts FE

Herbs: Astragalus, cherry, coltsfoot, **cordyceps**, horsetail, khella, **licorice**, **lobelia**, **mullein**, reishi, and thyme

Supplements: Magnesium, **N-acetyl cysteine**, and omega-3 EFAs

Essential Oils: Eucalyptus, frankincense, and sandalwood

Copper Toxicity

See also mental illness and anger (excessive)

Copper is an essential nutrient, but if a person gets too much copper in their body, it will increase levels of norepinephrine and decreases levels of dopamine in the brain. Possible symptoms of copper overload include hyperactivity, ringing in the ears, high anxiety, sleep problems, hemochromatosis, low thyroid, rheumatoid arthritis, and emotional meltdowns.

Copper levels are regulated tightly by proteins, the most important being metallothionein (MT). Some people have a genetic inability to regulate copper, which means they need to avoid nutritional supplements containing copper. This includes liquid chlorophyll, which contains sodium copper chlorophyllin.

Zinc is a copper antagonist, so taking zinc can help bring down copper levels. Pumpkin seeds are naturally high in zinc. MSM is a supplement that helps the liver flush excess copper. If a person tends to have copper overload, it also helps to drink plenty of water and do things to relax the overstimulated sympathetic nervous system.

Strategies: Heavy Metal Cleanse

Formulas: Anti-Stress B-Complex

Herbs: Gardenia

Supplements: MSM, potassium, vitamin B-complex, vitamin C, vitamin E, and **zinc**

Corns

Corns are a lesion of the skin formed between two toes as a result of pressure between them. The surface of the skin is macerated and yellowish in color. Remedies can be applied topically for relief. Mix essential oils with a little coconut oil or aloe vera gel.

Strategies: Compress or Fomentation and Poultice

Formulas: Enzyme Spray

Herbs: Aloe vera, celandine, chamomile, and garlic

Supplements: Vitamin E

Essential Oils: Clove, peppermint, and **tea tree**

Cough

See also cough (damp), cough (dry), and cough (spastic)

Under normal conditions, the lungs and sinuses secrete a thin protective layer of mucus that traps dust and other particles in the air. Thin, hair-like projections called cilia sweep this mucus to the back of the throat (from the sinuses) or to the top of the throat (from the lungs). When the mucus gets trapped in the lungs and the cilia are unable to move it out of the lungs, this creates an involuntary, explosive expulsion of air from the lung in an attempt to expel the mucus and irritants from the lungs.

All over-the-counter cough medicines contain cough suppressants that suppress the cough reflex. This does not help the body eliminate the irritants.

Decongestant herbs help thin the mucus so that it can move more freely, and expectorants stimulate the cilia to move it out of the system. Expectorant herbs help activate the cilia to move the mucus out of the lungs. In general, the best way to treat a cough is to take a formula that has both expectorants and decongestants with plenty of water. Once the irritants have been removed from the lungs, the cough will stop.

One can also inhale decongestant and expectorant essential oils. These can be rubbed on the chest, diffused in the air, or inhaled in steam.

When coughing becomes excessive, antitussive remedies may help to calm it down so a person can sleep. These include lobelia, licorice, and coltsfoot.

Also look at the specific types of coughs listed in this book for more specific cough remedies.

Strategies: Eliminate Allergy-Causing Foods and Hydration

Formulas: Jeannie Burgess' Allergy-Lung, **Stabilized Allicin**, Topical Analgesic, Lung Moistening, and Steven Horne's Horehound Cough

Herbs: Amalaki, anemarrhena, asafetida, asparagus (Chinese), cherry bark, **coltsfoot**, cordyceps, elecampane, **garlic**, **horehound**, horseradish, **lobelia**, marshmallow, mullein, oregano, pine bark, quince (Asian), red clover, rosemary, **thyme**, and **yerba santa**

Supplements: Vitamin C

Essential Oils: Anise, atlas cedarwood, cajeput, **eucalyptus**, fennel, fir, myrrh, **pine**, ravensara, ravintsara, rosemary, spruce (hemlock), tea tree, and wintergreen

Cough, Damp

See also congestion (lungs), pneumonia, and cough

A damp cough is a cough that produces a lot of phlegm. There is excess mucus production and fluid in the lungs. Remedies that help to tone mucous membranes and reduce excess secretions are helpful for damp coughs. My favorite herbs for damp cough are pine bark, wild cherry bark, horehound, and yerba santa. I also find inhaling eucalyptus and pine oil helpful.

Strategies: Eliminate Allergy-Causing Foods

Formulas: **Jeannie Burgess' Allergy-Lung**, Ayurvedic Bronchial Decongestant, Stabilized Allicin, **Chinese Metal-Decreasing**, Ed Millet's Herbal Crisis, Steven Horne's Horehound Cough, and **Damp Cough Syrup**

Essential Oil Blends: Disinfectant EO

Herbs: Apricot, balloon flower, **bayberry**, **cherry bark**, chirata, cordyceps, couchgrass, elder, **garlic**, ginger, **horehound**, horseradish, hyssop, magnolia, mulberry, **osha**, **pine bark**, polygala, rosemary, tangerine (Mandarin), thyme, and **yerba santa**

Supplements: Vitamin C and vitamin D

Essential Oils: Clove, **eucalyptus**, jasmine, and **pine**

Cough, Dry

See also cough

When a cough is unproductive (dry and hacking) so that there is little mucus production, the lungs are dehydrated. Moistening expectorants and decongestants, like astragalus, licorice, mullein, and marshmallow, are needed.

Strategies: Hydration

Formulas: Chinese Yin-Increasing, **Lung Moistening**, **Chinese Metal-Increasing**, and **Dry Cough Syrup**

Herbs: Aloe vera, angelica, astragalus, cordyceps, fenugreek, flax, **fritillary**, Irish moss, **licorice**, loquat, lycium, **marshmallow**, **mullein**, ophiopogon, plantain, **pleurisy root**, schisandra, slippery elm, stillingia, and yam (Chinese)

Essential Oils: Lemon, **sandalwood**, and thyme

Cough, Spastic

See also croup and pertussis

A spastic cough is one in which there is muscle constriction in the bronchi. This can come as a result of muscle exhaustion after an extended period of coughing. Coughs that have a whooping sound or constricted quality to them need remedies with an antispasmodic action. Pertussis and croup are diseases that typically have spastic coughs as part of their symptomology.

When there is a spastic cough, use the appropriate general remedies for coughs along with antispasmodics like lobelia or khella to help relax the bronchi and calm the cough. One can also inhale relaxing essential oils like lavender and sandalwood.

Herbs: Black cohosh, coltsfoot, dogwood (Jamaican), **khella**, **lobelia**, rosemary, skunk cabbage, thyme, and vervain (blue)

Supplements: Vitamin C

Essential Oils: Lavender, rosemary, **sandalwood**, and **thyme**

COVID-19

See also infection (viral)

COVID-19 is a new virus in the coronavirus category of viral diseases. Many cold viruses are also coronaviruses. While this disease is of too recent discovery to have any definitive treatments for it as yet, there are many nutrients that help the body defend itself against all viral infections. The suggestions found here are basic suggestions of nutrients and herbs that might be helpful for preventing and treating this disease in the early stages based on what other natural healers are reporting helpful.

Strategies: Affirmation and Visualization and Eat Healthy

Formulas: Chinese Wind-Heat Evil

Herbs: Cordyceps, mullein, and yarrow

Supplements: Vitamin C, **vitamin D**, and **zinc**

Cradle Cap

See also eczema

Cradle cap is a skin condition affecting the scalp of babies. It is characterized by large oily yellow flaking from the baby's scalp. It is a form of dermatitis and is related to eczema. It may involve yeast infections. Often, babies who have this are severely deficient in essential fatty acids, most likely due to a deficiency in the mother's diet during pregnancy. Vitamin E and aloe vera gel make good topical applications for cradle cap.

Strategies: Healthy Fats

Formulas: Probiotic and GLA Oil

Herbs: **Aloe vera**, black walnut, calendula, and pau d'arco

Supplements: Nanoparticle silver, **omega-3 EFAs**, and **vitamin E**

Cramps & Spasms

See also tension

A cramp is a painful, involuntary spasmodic contraction of a muscle. A spasm is an involuntary and abnormal contraction of a muscle that can be extremely painful. Muscles expend energy to contract and must regenerate energy in order to relax again. A muscle that cramps is low in energy. Stretching exercises help to rebuild energy charges in muscles and promote relaxation of cramps, as does the *Deep Breathing* strategy.

Cramps are often signs of magnesium and potassium deficiencies. The *Epsom Salt Bath* strategy can help relax and recharge cramped or tense muscles. Antispasmodic herbs can taken internally or applied topically. Relaxing essential oils can also be diluted in a carrier oil and rubbed into cramping muscles.

Strategies: Aromatherapy, Bodywork, Deep Breathing, Epsom Salt Bath, and Lymph-Moving Pain Relief

Formulas: Antispasmodic, Herbal Potassium, **Fibromyalgia**, and Chinese Earth-Increasing

Herbs: Black cohosh, black haw, **cramp bark**, **dogwood (Jamaican)**, hops, **kava kava**, ligusticum, **lobelia**, quince (Asian), siler, **skullcap**, skunk cabbage, valerian, wild yam, and wood betony

Supplements: **Magnesium**, potassium, vitamin B_5, and zinc

Essential Oils: Clary sage, **copaiba**, helichrysum, lavender, lemon, **marjoram**, wintergreen, and **ylang ylang**

Cramps, Leg

See also cramps & spasms

Cramps in the legs are usually a sign of magnesium and/or potassium deficiencies. Stress can be a contributing factor. In addition to supplementation with magnesium and potassium, antispasmodic herbs (like lobelia) or essential oils (like marjoram) can be applied topically.

Strategies: Lymph-Moving Pain Relief

Formulas: **Herbal Potassium**, Skeletal Support, Watkin's Hair, Skin, and Nails, and **Antispasmodic**

Herbs: Cramp bark, hops, kava kava, lobelia, and valerian

Supplements: **Magnesium**, **potassium**, vitamin B-complex, and vitamin B_6

Essential Oils: Lavender, **marjoram**, and ylang ylang

Cramps, Menstrual

See also cramps & spasms, dysmenorrhea, PMS Type P, and estrogen dominance

Menstrual cramps are cramping pains that occur during menstruation. They are one form of dysmenorrhea (painful periods). They often signal a lack of magnesium and/or vitamin B_6 in the diet. They may also be due to excess estrogen. Antispasmodic herbs may be helpful. Relaxing essential oils can also be diluted and massaged into the cramping areas for relief.

Strategies: Avoid Xenoestrogens, Healthy Fats, Lymph-Moving Pain Relief, Mineralization, and Stress Management

Formulas: **Antispasmodic**, Analgesic Nerve, Female Tonic, **Female Cycle**, and Herbal Potassium

Herbs: **Angelica**, **black cohosh**, black haw, blue cohosh, butterbur, chaste tree, **cramp bark**, dong quai, **khella**, motherwort, muira puama, peony, thyme, and **wild yam**

Supplements: DHEA, **magnesium**, omega-3 EFAs, potassium, **vitamin B_6**, and vitamin E

Essential Oils: **Clary sage**, **jasmine**, and red mandarin

Crohn's Disease
see *inflammatory bowel disorders*

Croup

See also cough (spastic)

A spasmodic laryngitis, especially in infants, is called croup. Symptoms include difficulty breathing and a hoarse, metallic cough. Antispasmodic herbs may be helpful. Relaxing essential oils may diluted and rubbed onto the throat and chest for added relief, but should be diluted with olive oil (or another vegetable oil) at least 40:1 when applied to infants.

Strategies: Hydration

Formulas: Jeannie Burgess' Stress

Essential Oil Blends: Lung-Supporting EO and Renewing and Releasing EO

Herbs: **Catnip**, echinacea, **fenugreek**, **lobelia**, mullein, pine, rosemary, thyme, and **vervain (blue)**

Supplements: Omega-3 EFAs, vitamin D, vitamin E, and zinc

Essential Oils: Eucalyptus and rosemary

Cushing's Disease

Cushing's disease is characterized by elevated adrenal glands—meaning that the adrenal glands are overactive and overproducing adrenal hormones. Symptoms include excess cortisol, low blood sugar, poor wound healing, lowered immune response, thinning hair, muscle wasting, abdominal fat, and high blood pressure. This is a serious illness requiring competent medical help.

In this disease, licorice root and other supplements that enhance adrenal function should be avoided. Adaptogens may help to calm down elevated adrenal function. B-complex vitamins, kava kava, and blue vervain may also be beneficial.

Strategies: Affirmation and Visualization and Stress Management

Formulas: Suma Adaptogen, Anti-Stress B-Complex, and **Cortisol-Reducing**

Herbs: Chamomile, **eleuthero**, **holy basil**, hops, kava kava, passion flower, and vervain (blue)

Supplements: Magnesium, **vitamin B-complex**, and vitamin B_5

Essential Oils: Chamomile (Roman) and lavender

Cuts

See also bleeding (external)

Cuts are breaks in the skin that create bleeding. Pressure helps stop bleeding. Most cuts will heal without any external help, but you can use antiseptic herbs, essential oils, or nanoparticle silver to prevent infection. Styptics like calendula, capsicum, and yarrow can be used topically to help stop bleeding in more serious cuts.

Strategies: Lymph-Moving Pain Relief and Poultice

Formulas: Healing Salve, Vulnerary, and Topical Analgesic

Herbs: Bayberry, **calendula**, capsicum, goldenseal, grindelia, honeysuckle, uva ursi, white oak, **yarrow**, and yerba santa

Supplements: Nanoparticle silver and vitamin E

Essential Oils: **Helichrysum**, lavender, and tea tree

Cystic Breast Disease

See also breast lumps

The formation of benign fluid-filled sacs in the breast tissue is called cystic breast disease. If you have lumps in the breast they should be tested to determine if they are benign or malignant before choosing a course of therapy.

If the lumps are benign, start by following the *Avoid Caffeine* strategy. Caffeine contributes to this problem and all forms should be avoided.

There is a need to improve lymphatic drainage from the breast tissue, so use herbs to support the lymphatic system. Frankincense essential oil can be massaged into the breasts to help lumps. A few drops of poke oil can also be massaged into the breasts, but this should be done under the supervision of a qualified professional herbalist (findanherbalist.com) or naturopath.

A colon and liver cleanse can be helpful. These will also help to improve lymphatic drainage and reduce fluid-filled sacs.

There may also be a problem with low thyroid and a lack of iodine. In this case, seaweeds or iodine supplements may be helpful.

Excess estrogens and xenoestrogens, in particular, can contribute to cystic breast disease. Use the strategy *Avoid Xenoestrogens*. Since the liver breaks down excess estrogens, supplements that enhance liver detoxification, especially indole-3-carbinol, may also be helpful.

Strategies: Avoid Caffeine and Avoid Xenoestrogens

Formulas: Blood Purifier, Phytoestrogen Breast, **Liquid Lymph**, **Enzyme Spray**, Lymph Cleansing, **Lymphatic Infection**, and Digestive Support

Herbs: Chamomile, evening primrose, **false unicorn**, gentian, hydrangea, and Oregon grape

Supplements: **Indole-3-carbinol**, iodine, magnesium, omega-3 EFAs, vitamin A, vitamin C, vitamin D, **vitamin E**, and zinc

Essential Oils: Frankincense

Cystic Fibrosis

Cystic fibrosis is a hereditary disease that appears in early childhood and involves a generalized disorder of the exocrine glands. Symptoms include faulty digestion due to a deficiency of pancreatic enzymes, difficulty breathing, and excessive loss of salt in the sweat.

Natural remedies may not offer a cure, but they can ease symptoms. For starters, high-quality, nutrient-packed foods need to be eaten (see *Eat Healthy* strategy and consider adopting a *Gut-Healing Diet* strategy). Also consider the *Eliminate Allergy-Causing Foods* and *Detoxification* strategies. Increase antioxidants and good fats. *Digestive Support Formulas* and N-acetyl-cysteine will help to improve digestive function and thin mucus. For additional natural help one should work with a qualified alternative health practitioner.

Strategies: Detoxification, Eat Healthy, Eliminate Allergy-Causing Foods, Gut-Healing Diet, Healthy Fats, and Mineralization

Formulas: **Digestive Support**, Papaya Enzyme, Betaine HCl, Colloidal Mineral, and **Probiotic**

Herbs: Alfalfa, black currant, cordyceps, evening primrose, fenugreek, juniper, marshmallow, mullein, papaya, spirulina, thyme, and **vervain (blue)**

Supplements: MSM, **N-acetyl cysteine**, **protease**, vitamin B-complex, and vitamin B_{12}

Cystitis   see *interstitial cystitis*

Cysts

Cysts are closed sacs with distinct membranes that are usually fluid filled. They form abnormally in a cavity or other structure of the body. Detoxification is essential for eliminating cysts. General cleansers like lymphatic herbs and blood purifiers can be taken internally. The *Poultice* strategy using a blend containing plantain can help to break up cysts. The *Castor Oil Pack* strategy is also good for breaking up cysts.

Strategies: Aromatherapy, Castor Oil Pack, Detoxification, and Poultice

Formulas: Enzyme Spray, Liquid Lymph, **Detoxifying**, and **Drawing Salve**

Herbs: Burdock, chickweed, corn silk, gentian, kelp, **plantain**, **red clover**, red root, safflower, saw palmetto, and yellow dock

Supplements: Protease, vitamin A, and vitamin D

Essential Oils: Helichrysum, peppermint, and tea tree

Dandruff

See also infection (fungal) and leaky gut

Dandruff is caused by extreme dryness of the scalp, which results in white flakes. Coconut oil may also be applied to the scalp. Increase intake of essential fatty acids.

Adding tea tree, rosemary, or other essential oils to one's shampoo to stimulate circulation to the scalp can also relieve dandruff. Dandruff can be related to stress, so B-complex vitamins and nervine herbs may be helpful. In some cases, dandruff may be linked to yeast overgrowth in the intestinal tract or intestinal inflammation and leaky gut syndrome.

Strategies: Aromatherapy, Healthy Fats, and Stress Management

Formulas: Watkin's Hair, Skin, and Nails, Enzyme Spray, Anti-Stress B-Complex, GLA Oil, and Digestive Support

Herbs: Aloe vera, **black walnut**, evening primrose, kelp, pau d'arco, and rosemary

Supplements: Omega-3 EFAs, selenium, vitamin B-complex, vitamin E, and zinc

Essential Oils: Lavender, **rosemary**, and **tea tree**

Deafness

Hearing Loss

See also mitochondrial dysfunction

Deafness is partial or complete loss of hearing. Some people have reported using the *Antispasmodic Ear Formula* as ear drops has been helpful. These remedies can help to prevent or slow the progress of deafness, or correct problems with the ears causing a temporary loss of hearing. They will not reverse complete deafness.

Formulas: Antispasmodic Ear and Methylated B Vitamin

Herbs: Lobelia and Saint John's wort

Essential Oils: Helichrysum

Debility

See also convalescence

Debility is a general weakness of the body brought on by prolonged illness or general poor health. The following remedies help overcome debility by strengthening the body overall.

Formulas: Digestive Support, **Chinese Qi and Blood Tonic**, Antioxidant, Chinese Earth-Increasing, Chinese Qi-Increasing, **Whole Food Green Drink**, **Algae**, and Colloidal Mineral

Herbs: Asparagus, **bee pollen**, chirata, chlorella, cocoa, **cordyceps**, ginseng (American), ginseng (Asian/Korean), Grape, slippery elm, and **spirulina**

Supplements: Co-Q10, colostrum, omega-3 EFAs, and pancreatin

Dehydration

See also diabetes

Dehydration is a lack of water in the tissues of the body. Although water needs to be consumed to overcome dehydration, sometimes water is not being properly taken up and utilized by the tissues. When this happens, the person drinks water, urinates excessively, and is still thirsty. This can be an early warning sign of diabetes and other blood sugar problems.

Licorice root and the *Chinese Yin-Increasing Formula* can help the body stay more hydrated. If the problem is related to blood sugar, then *Blood Sugar Reducing Formulas* may help. If these remedies don't help, medical diagnosis should be sought to determine if diabetes is a factor.

Mineral electrolytes like sodium and potassium help the body hold onto moisture. These can be lost during exercise. The *Electrolyte Drink Powder* can be taken to restore mineral balance and help the body recover from moisture lost during exercise.

Strategies: Hydration and Low-Glycemic Diet

Formulas: Herbal Potassium, **Chinese Yin-Increasing**, Chinese Fire-Increasing, and Electrolyte Drink

Herbs: Kelp, **licorice**, and nopal

Supplements: Magnesium, potassium, and vitamin B$_{12}$

Dementia

See also Alzheimer's, memory/brain function, and Parkinson's disease

Dementia is a loss of cognitive and intellectual function, without the loss of perception. It is a syndrome rather than a disease, which means it can have multiple causes. Symptoms include disorientation, impaired memory and judgment, and a loss of intellectual capacity.

Alzheimer's and Parkinson's disease are the most common causes of dementia. It can also be caused by infections, cardiovascular disease, strokes, and drug use.

One can reduce the risk of dementia by adopting the *Eat Healthy* strategy. In particular, avoiding sugar and getting adequate amounts of omega-3 essential fatty acids are helpful. The *Antioxidant* and *Brain and Memory Protection Formulas* may also help to prevent dementia or slow the deterioration. It also helps to stay physically and mentally active. See related conditions for more detailed suggestions.

Strategies: Avoid Sugar, Eat Healthy, Enhance Nitric Oxide, Exercise, Healthy Fats, Low-Glycemic Diet, and Oral Chelation

Formulas: Oral Chelation, **Brain and Memory Protection**, **Memory Enhancing**, Nitric Oxide Boosting, and Antioxidant

Herbs: Bacopa, coconut, **ginkgo**, gotu kola, periwinkle, **rosemary**, and sage

Supplements: Alpha-lipoic acid, **huperzine A**, krill oil, L-arginine, **magnesium**, **N-acetyl cysteine**, **omega-3 DHA**, **omega-3 EFAs**, and **vitamin B-complex**

Essential Oils: Frankincense, peppermint, and rosemary

Dental Health
Cavities, Tooth Decay

Tooth decay affects just about everyone living in modern society. Modern dentistry teaches us that this is all the fault of bacteria in the mouth and the only way to prevent the problem is through brushing, flossing, and using mouthwash, coupled with dental visits for cleanings and other treatments. On top of the problem of cavities, numerous teenagers have malformed bites and misplaced teeth requiring orthodontic work. Many adults also have serious problems with gum disease. Is all of this just an inevitable part of life?

Dr. Weston Price, who was appointed as the first director of the National Dental Association, which would later become the American Dental Association, believed that nutrition had a lot to do with dental health. He spent many years traveling the world seeking out native people who were resistant and even immune to tooth decay. He found that indigenous people living on traditional diets had bacteria in their mouth, but did not get tooth decay until they were exposed to modern, refined foods. His conclusion? "Tooth decay is not only unnecessary, but an indication of our divergence from Nature's fundamental laws of life and health."

He discovered that nutritional deficiency was the root cause of all dental problems, including cavities, impacted wisdom teeth, improperly formed bites and displaced teeth requiring orthodontic work, and gum disease. Dr. Price also observed that good dental health went along with good physical and mental health. He concluded that improved nutrition, not better cleaning of the teeth and gums, is the ultimate answer to our modern dental problems.

Diet and Dental Health

Dr. Price found that indigenous groups with the highest immunity to tooth decay ate at least two of the following three kinds of food daily: dairy products from grass-fed animals, fish and shellfish, and the organ meats of land animals. What these foods all have in common is that they are very high in good fats and fat-soluble vitamins.

Dr. Price found that on average, traditional diets had ten times more fat-soluble vitamins than modern diets. He also noted they had four times more water-soluble vitamins and three to four times more calcium and phosphorus. Remember that this was in the 1930s and people's diets are much worse today.

To build healthy bodies, including healthy bones and teeth, Dr. Price recommended supplementing the diet with one-fourth teaspoon of cod liver oil and one-fourth teaspoon of high-vitamin butter oil two to three times daily with a meal. Today these nutrients can be supplemented by taking omega-3 essential fatty acids, vitamin D_3 and vitamin K_2.

Dr. Price also recommended liberal consumption of organ meats from wild or grass-fed animals. These can be difficult foods to find, but organ meats (if you can find them) are generally cheaper cuts of meat and a great way to save money in today's economy.

Stock is also helpful for bone and dental health. It is made by simmering bones and meat scraps (sometimes with vegetables as well). This extracts minerals and other nutrients needed for healthy bones, teeth and bodies. See the *Bone Broth* strategy.

For more information on Dr. Price's dietary recommendations and discoveries, get the book *Nourishing Traditions* by Sally Fallon. It provides excellent nutritional information and recipes based on indigenous diets.

Supplements for Dental Health

In addition to diet, one might also consider using mineral supplements to improve dental health. These include *Colloidal Minerals, Skeletal Support,* and *Joan Patton's Herbal Minerals Formula.* I've had a number of parents use the herbal minerals formula along with vitamins A and D_3 (or fish oil containing them) and report their kids had a reduction of tooth decay and an overall improvement in general health.

Natural Dental Hygiene

Xylitol is one of our allies in helping to prevent tooth decay and gum disease. Using xylitol candy and gum has been shown to reduce tooth decay because the cavity-causing bacteria that thrive on sugar can't survive on xylitol. You can also get a xylitol mouthwash.

Herbal Tooth Powders can also strengthen tooth enamel and improve gum health. Use a separate toothbrush from the one you use for your toothpaste, as this powder stains the toothbrush. (It won't stain your teeth, however, it will make them whiter.)

Strategies: Avoid Sugar, Bone Broth, Healthy Fats, and Mineralization

Formulas: Herbal Calcium, **Colloidal Mineral**, **Watkin's Hair, Skin, and Nails**, **Joan Patton's Herbal Minerals**, **Herbal Tooth Powder**, and **Skeletal Support**

Herbs: Alfalfa, **black walnut**, elecampane, **horsetail**, **myrrh**, **neem**, tea, thyme, and **white oak**

Supplements: Krill oil, omega-3 EFAs, **vanadium**, vitamin B-complex, vitamin B_6, **vitamin D**, **vitamin K**, **xylitol**, and xylitol

Essential Oils: **Cinnamon** and myrrh

Denture Sores

Denture sores are abrasions or ulcerations on the gums or gingiva as a result of improperly fitted dental appliances. Aloe vera, chamomile, and vitamin E are all remedies that can be applied directly to the gums to reduce inflammation and promote healing.

Formulas: Enzyme Spray

Herbs: **Aloe vera**, **chamomile**, clove, and turmeric

Supplements: **Nanoparticle silver** and vitamin E

Essential Oils: Clove and tea tree

Depression

See also grief & sadness, hypothyroidism, inflammatory bowel disorders, postpartum depression, seasonal affective disorder, PMS Type D, and methylation (under)

Everybody feels down once in a while, but clinical depression is more than just feeling sad or discouraged. A severely depressed person loses interest in life. They may overeat or lose interest in food, feel worthless, helpless and pessimistic, withdraw socially, suffer from extreme fatigue, and experience disturbed sleep. They may also start to think about dying or committing suicide. A depressed person can't just pull themselves together and get better. They need outside help to regain interest in life.

About 7 percent of the American population has a major depressive episode each year. About 10 percent of all doctor and hospital visits are about depression.

Causes of Depression

Most of the time, the cause of depression isn't physical. People get depressed when they suffer extreme loss and are in deep grief. They can also become depressed due to excessive stress that overwhelms their ability to cope.

However, depression can have physical causes and it isn't really a disease, but rather a symptom. One has to identify the mental, emotional and/or physical causes and address them to get over it. But, before we lay out some natural strategies for depression, let's talk about the use of drugs to treat it.

Drug Treatment of Depression

The most common category of antidepressant medications drugs is selective serotonin reuptake inhibitors (SSRIs). SSRIs were developed in the 1980s. They work by inhibiting nerve cells releasing serotonin from reabsorbing it. Blocking the reuptake of serotonin is believed to increase the activity of serotonin in the brain, but the body tends to counteract external regulation of neurotransmitters when a drug like this is used, which means the body adapts to the drug. This can cause both side effects and severe withdrawal symptoms if the drug is discontinued.

Although they do appear to relieve feelings of severe depression, SSRIs, like other drugs, are not without side effects. A 2009 study of seven hundred patients taking SSRIs found the following side effects in the group: 56 percent experienced decreased sexual functioning, 53 percent drowsiness and 49 percent gained weight. Less common side effects were dry mouth (19 percent), insomnia (16 percent), fatigue (14 percent), nausea (14 percent), light-headedness (13 percent) and tremor (12 percent).

These side effects might be worth the risk for someone who is severely depressed, but there are more issues with SSRIs than those listed in this study. The FDA itself issued a black box warning, which is the strictest warning the agency can give, in 2004. They warned that SSRIs were associated with suicidal thoughts and behaviors. The warning was updated in 2007 to specify that the highest risk was for young adults between the ages of eighteen and twenty-four as well as children under eighteen.

This is important to know as suicide rates have dramatically increased in recent years. Rates have gone up 30 percent in the past two decades. Suicide is now the tenth leading cause of death in the United States and the second leading cause of death among young people age fifteen to twenty-one. Obviously, it's a bad idea for young people who are depressed to be taking SSRIs if it increases suicide risk.

Other known side effects of SSRIs include mania, increased aggression and violent behavior, and psychosis. People on SSRIs are more likely to fight with spouses, bosses and even police, causing problems with work, marriage, and other conflicts. To understand why we need to understand the nature of serotonin neurons.

Understanding Serotonin

The nerve cells that release serotonin are located at the base of the skull. They serve to connect nerves in the spinal column with the brain, thus forming a link between mind and body.

They fire steadily when a person is awake, slow down when we sleep, and stop firing when we dream. Interestingly, LSD causes hallucinations by blocking serotonin receptors, causing the brain to enter an ungrounded dream-like state.

Research shows that serotonin neurons are involved in the drive for status and achievement. People who have achieved a high degree of status in life have higher levels of serotonin. Psychologist Dr. Jordon Peterson says this is even true for lobsters. When a dominant lobster is defeated by a stronger lobster, the loser suffers a loss of serotonin. Given SSRIs, the losing lobster may return and fight again.

This explains why people given SSRIs may become more aggressive and violent. Having felt defeated in life, they may begin to fight back, but not necessarily in constructive ways.

Given these neurons are located at the base of the skull, it's interesting to note that we slump forward and hang our head when we feel defeated. But what's even more interesting is that by throwing our shoulder's back, lifting our head and determining to do something worthwhile in life, we automatically increase our serotonin levels.

Enhancing Serotonin Naturally

Serotonin is produced from the amino acid tryptophan. Serotonin levels in the brain and directly linked with levels of tryptophan. Oddly enough, tryptophan was withdrawn from the US market as a supplement, due to problems created by a contaminated batch of the supplement (not a problem with the supplement itself), shortly before the introduction of SSRIs.

Fortunately, a derivative of tryptophan, 5-hydroxytryptophan or 5-HTP for short, was discovered that can be taken to naturally boost serotonin levels in the brain. Taking 5-HTP is a natural alternative to SSRIs but should not be taken while a person is on an SSRI.

When it gets dark, the pineal gland coverts serotonin to melatonin, which aids sleep, so taking 5-HTP about one hour before bedtime may help some people get to sleep. It also helps some people with carbohydrate cravings.

Saint John's wort has also been shown to modulate serotonin and research suggests it can help relieve mild to moderate depression. Saint John's wort does much more than affect serotonin. It also modulates levels of dopamine, GABA, and other neurotransmitters involved in anxiety and depression. It helps regulate digestion and reduces inflammation.

Saint John's wort is especially good for depression associated with digestive upset and anxiety. However, like 5-HTP it should not be taken with SSRIs or other drugs that modulate serotonin levels.

Weaning Off Antidepressant Drugs

People taking antidepressant drugs like SSRIs should not discontinue them abruptly. This can be very dangerous. The FDA has warned that abrupt changes in the dose (whether increasing or decreasing it) can produce hostility and psychosis and increase the risk of suicide. The brain adjusts to the presence of these chemicals, which means that the balance of the neurotransmitters is abruptly changed when the dose is altered.

The daily dose should be reduced slowly over the course of many months, or even years. This is done by shaving very small amounts off the pills, as opposed to trying to cut them. This should be done, ideally, under professional supervision, over the course of many months. If a person has been on SSRIs or other antidepressants for more than five years, it's a good idea to spend a year weaning off them.

While transitioning, it's important to work on one's general health and follow some of the basic strategies for depression listed below. For more information on weaning off of SSRIs go to https://www.drugawareness.org/icfda-warning/

Strategies for Overcoming Depression

Here are some of the strategies you can use for depression. We'll begin with the general strategies and then discuss specific remedies for specific kinds of depression.

Get Counseling or Other Help

Professional counselors, pastors, ministers, and even good friends may be able to help a person find their way through their difficulties. Counseling, in fact, has about the same success rate as SSRIs in overcoming depression, without the potential side effects. So start by reaching out for help.

Take Care of Yourself

One of the first steps to overcoming depression is to simply start taking better care of oneself. Unfortunately, when a person is feeling depressed they usually don't take the good care of ourselves. They binge out on junk food, eat too much, or lose their appetite and don't eat enough. They often don't sleep well or exercise either.

Oddly enough, high carbohydrate meals temporarily stimulate dopamine and serotonin, which causes a brief elevation of mood. Unfortunately, this is followed by an even larger emotional let down, as rapid fluctuations in blood sugar also adversely affect mood.

When a depressed person has been eating a lot of sugar and other refined carbohydrates, they will benefit from taking *Anti-Stress B-Complex Vitamins* or just a B-complex vitamin with vitamin C. Simple carbohydrates deplete these vitamins, which are needed for neurotransmitter synthesis in the brain.

Exercise has been shown to lift depression. Just walking for thirty to sixty minutes a day in the fresh air and sunshine will help. It also helps to get a good night's sleep.

Reduce Inflammation

Recent research suggests that there is a link between chronic inflammation and depression. While the inflammation is not the direct cause of depression, it appears that in many people, reducing chronic inflammation eases depression.

Where depression is associated with chronic inflammation, a person may experience general aches and pains, have a dark red or purplish colored tongue, and high levels of C-reactive protein. If this is the case you might try an *Antioxidant Formula*, turmeric or curcumin, omega-3 essential fatty acids, or other anti-inflammatory remedies.

Basic Remedies for Depression

In addition to Saint John's wort and 5-HTP mentioned earlier, the *Chinese Qi-Regulating Formula* is a good basic herbal remedy that works on many underlying causes of depression. It's a good formula to consider if you are trying to wean off drugs for depression (see cautions above). It's actually designed to raise your energy so you stand more erect, and to work on underlying issues with the digestion and liver that contribute to depression.

Dealing with Specific Causes of Depression

Recognizing the cause of one's depression is important in being able to permanently resolve it. Here are some of the major causes of depression, some information on how to recognize them, and remedies that will work for each.

Depression Caused by Grief and Sadness

When depression is due to a recent tragedy in one's life, such as the death of a loved one, breakup of a relationship, loss of a job, or other difficulties, it is a natural part of the grieving process. There are five recognized stages of grieving. These are (1) denial and isolation, (2) anger, (3) bargaining, (4) depression, and finally (5) acceptance.

Although not everyone experiences all five stages, nor do they occur in any particular order, depression is a common part of this process and should not be viewed as a disease. Instead, it's a sign that a person needs emotional help and support, as well as time to go through their grieving process.

There are a few essential oils that can help to lift the spirits of a grieving person. Rose helps to heal depression brought on by grief by opening the heart to the experience of love again. The oils of pine, bergamot or helichrysum may also help with the grieving process. The *Grief and Sadness FE Blend* can also help the person emotionally release what they have lost.

Stress-Related Depression

Stress can bring us down and make us feel tired and overwhelmed. If a person's depression is related to stress, it will be accompanied by anxiety and nervousness. There may also be severe fatigue, a loss of interest in life, and the feeling of "I just can't cope anymore!"

If this fits you, try the *Anti-Stress B-Complex Vitamins* along with the *Chinese Fire-Increasing Formula*. If the stress has been intense enough to cause post traumatic stress disorder, an *Adrenal Glandular Formula* may be helpful.

Disturbed Methylation

Disturbed methylation may be involved in depression, anxiety, and even mental illness. Signs of undermethylation include high levels of homocysteine and histamine in the blood, a tendency toward seasonal allergies, and depression that responds favorably to SSRIs.

If you have symptoms of undermethylation, try taking SAM-e. Studies suggest SAM-e can be effective for mild to moderate depression. It helps the body produce more mood-enhancing neurotransmitters such as dopamine and serotonin, and acts as a natural reuptake inhibitor for these neurotransmitters. It also aids liver detoxification, which aids the next cause of depression. You might also take methylated vitamin B_{12} (methylcobalamin), methylated folic acid (methylfolate), or *Methylated B Vitamin Formula*.

Toxicity and Depression

Depression was once called melancholia and was thought to be an accumulation of black bile. Today we'd consider black bile an accumulation of toxins.

More serotonin is produced in the gut than in the brain, and gut health has been directly linked with mood problems, like anxiety and depression. The liver also breaks down excess hormones and neurotransmitters, so when the liver isn't detoxifying well one can become irritable, anxious or depressed.

Doing *Ivy Bridge's Cleansing Program*, *Chinese Balanced Cleansing Program* or any similar colon cleansing program can help a person feel lighter, have more energy, and reduce feelings of heaviness. See the *Detoxification* strategy.

Seasonal Depression

Many people get depressed in winter, a condition known as seasonal affective disorder. One of the causes of this may be a lack of vitamin D_3, which is produced in the skin in response to sunlight. Taking 2000 IU of vitamin D_3 daily can cause significant improvement in seasonal depression. Saint John's wort may also helpful for seasonal depression, as can the use of full-spectrum lights.

Age-Related Depression

As a person ages, they may become depressed. This may be associated with dementia or the early stages of Alzheimer's disease. Ginkgo has been helpful for this type of depression. Ginseng and gotu kola may also be helpful.

Depression and Sex Hormones

Depression associated with PMS, pregnancy, the aftermath of childbirth, and menopause is typically hormonally related. An herb that is often helpful in these cases is black cohosh. It is also a good antidepressant for women who feel trapped or anyone who feels like they are wrestling with darkness, like the cartoons with the black cloud following a person around.

Low testosterone can cause depression in men (see *testosterone, low*), in which case ginseng, maca or DHEA may be helpful. Damiana is also mood elevator that can ease depression in both men and women when it is caused by low reproductive hormones.

Depression and the Thyroid

The thyroid plays an important role in mood regulation. Hypothyroidism is often overlooked as a possible cause of depression. If you have fatigue, problems losing weight, dry skin, low body temperature, and/or high cholesterol levels, low thyroid may be a contributing factor to your depressed feelings. If this is a problem, consider taking a *Thyroid Glandular Formula* or otherwise boosting thyroid hormones (see *hypothyroidism*).

If you need help identifying the cause of your depression, consider working with a competent herbalist or naturopath (findanherbalist.com or americanherbalistsguild.com).

Strategies: Affirmation and Visualization, Balance Methylation, Blood Type Diet, Detoxification, Eliminate Salicylates, Emotional Healing Work, Exercise, Forgiveness, Friendly Flora, Good Posture, Pleasure Prescription, Reduce Chemical Exposure, Sleep, and Stress Management

Formulas: 5-HTP Adaptogen, Adrenal Glandular, **Chinese Qi-Regulating**, Anti-Stress B-Complex, Chinese Wood-Increasing, Chinese Fire-Increasing, **Thyroid Glandular**, Methyl B12 Vitamin, Methylated B Vitamin, **Ashwagandha Complex**, Nitric Oxide Boosting, Probiotic, and Testosterone

Essential Oil Blends: Mood Lifting EO

Flower Essence Blends: Personal Boundaries FE and **Grief and Sadness FE**

Herbs: Ashwagandha, **black cohosh**, black walnut, bupleurum, calendula, cocoa, **damiana**, dulse, eleuthero, ginkgo, ginseng (American), ginseng (Asian/Korean), gotu kola, kanna, kava kava, **lemon balm**, **mimosa**, motherwort, muira puama, oat seed (milky), passion flower, **Saint John's wort**, **turmeric**, and yellow dock

Supplements: 5-HTP, berberine, CBD, curcumin, iron, L-glutamine, L-phenylalaine, L-threonine, L-tryptophan, lithium, **magnesium**, omega-3 DHA, omega-3 EFAs, omega-6 CLA, **SAM-e**, **vitamin B-complex**, **vitamin B_{12}**, vitamin B_3, vitamin B_6, vitamin B_9, and vitamin D

Essential Oils: Bay leaf, cinnamon, frankincense, helichrysum, jasmine, lemon, lime, neroli, orange (sweet), patchouli, pine, ravensara, red mandarin, rose, **rosemary**, and ylang ylang

Dermatitis

See also diaper rash, eczema, poison ivy/oak, and rashes & hives

Inflammation of the skin is known as dermatitis. This problem may be the result of the skin being exposed to an irritant (such as poison ivy). Identification and removal of the irritant is the first step in healing.

Blood purifying herbs are traditional remedies for dermatitis. They can be used internally or in baths, compresses, lotions, or other topical applications.

Internally, essential fatty acids like omega-3 or gamma linolenic acid (GLA) can be helpful. You can also mix soothing essential oils with GLA, aloe vera, or vitamin E for topical use. CBD can also be applied topically to reduce inflammation and itching.

When dermatitis is chronic it is called eczema. See *eczema* for more recommendations.

Strategies: Aromatherapy, Detoxification, Eat Healthy, Healthy Fats, Reduce Chemical Exposure, and Stress Management

Formulas: Blood Purifier, Enzyme Spray, **Antihistamine**, GLA Oil, **Ayurvedic Skin Healing**, and Probiotic

Herbs: Aloe vera, **burdock**, chamomile, coptis, **dulse**, gotu kola, grindelia, milk thistle, nettle, stinging, **Oregon grape**, **pau d'arco**, red clover, Saint John's wort, wild yam, and **yucca**

Supplements: CBD, lipase, MSM, **omega-3 EFAs**, **omega-6 GLA**, vitamin A, vitamin B$_{12}$, vitamin B$_5$, vitamin C, vitamin D, vitamin E, and zinc

Essential Oils: Chamomile (Roman), geranium, helichrysum, jasmine, lemon, **rose**, and thyme

Diabetes

See also cardiovascular disease, metabolic syndrome, and mitochondrial dysfunction

Diabetes is a problem with insulin, a hormone produced by the pancreas that enables the cells of the body to utilize glucose or blood sugar. There are two types of diabetes.

In type 1 (insulin dependent) diabetes, the pancreas has been damaged or destroyed and doesn't produce the necessary insulin. It is believed that this damage is the result of an autoimmune response. Insulin production may be as low as four units (versus the normal thirty-one) in this type of diabetes.

People with Type I diabetes must have regular insulin shots and constant monitoring of insulin levels to keep them as close to the normal thirty-one as possible. Supplements that reduce insulin resistance can reduce the need for insulin in this type of diabetes, but they will not restore normal pancreatic function.

In type 2 (insulin resistant) diabetes, the pancreas has no trouble producing insulin. The problem is that the cells of the body develop resistance to insulin, so the pancreas produces more insulin in order to overcome the cells' resistance. Insulin levels may exceed one hundred units. Type 2 develops slowly, over the course of years. It is begins as metabolic syndrome.

Strategies for Diabetes

Although type 2 diabetes is said to be incurable, many people have managed to completely control their diabetes through diet, lifestyle changes and supplements. The strategies for type 2 diabetes will also lower insulin requirements for type 1.

Change the Diet

In both types of diabetics, a person should adopt the *Low-Glycemic Diet* and *Avoid Sugar* strategies. To get blood sugar under control rapidly go on a temporary diet of nothing but low-glycemic or non-starchy vegetables, while taking a *Blood Sugar Control Formula*. Once blood sugar levels have stabilized, one can start to gradually introduce high-quality fats and animal proteins back into the diet.

After a few months on this diet it may be possible to reintroduce whole grains, whole fruits and starchy vegetables back into the diet, but all refined sugars and grain products should continue to be strictly avoided. To help transition away from sugar you can use stevia and xylitol as sweeteners.

Exercise and Weight Loss

Regular exercise reduces insulin resistance and enhances insulin utilization. It also aids circulation. Circulation problems are a common side effect of diabetes. Losing weight will also help.

Remedies to Overcome Insulin Resistance

There are a number of herbs that can reduce insulin resistance. These include bitter melon, nopal, devil's club, huckleberry, cinnamon, gymnema, and jambul can reduce insulin resistance. Although there is no guarantee that the pancreas can be rejuvenated in type 1 diabetes, two of the above herbs may be helpful, particularly in the early stages. They are gymnema and bitter melon.

I've also found the green fruits (cones) of Chinese arborvitae helpful for type I diabetes. They are not commercially available. You will have to harvest them yourself. Along with CBD they might help stop or reverse the autoimmune destruction of the pancreas. At the vary least, these herbs may reduce the need for insulin or other medications.

There are also a number of nutrients that help overcome insulin resistance. Chromium, zinc, and vanadium are all important minerals in blood sugar regulation. Omega-3 essential fatty acids help membranes become more permeable to insulin and sugar. alpha-lipoic acid has also been helpful in lowering insulin resistance in diabetics.

Diabetes is a serious disorder. So seek appropriate medical assistance and monitor the condition regularly. You may wish to work with a professional herbalist or naturopath (findanherbalist.com or americanherbalistsguild.com).

Strategies: Affirmation and Visualization, Avoid Sugar, Eat Healthy, Enhance Nitric Oxide, Exercise, Healthy Fats, Increase Dietary Fiber, Ketogenic Diet, and Low-Glycemic Diet

Formulas: Blood Sugar Control, Chinese Fire-Increasing, Whole Food Protein, and Nitric Oxide Boosting

Herbs: Amalaki, anemarrhena, astragalus, bilberry leaf, **biota**, **bitter melon**, **cinnamon**, cordyceps, fenugreek, garlic, ginseng (American), ginseng (Asian/Korean), goldenseal, **gymnema**, holy basil, jambul, maitake, noni, **nopal**, **stevia**, suma, trichosanthes, uva ursi, velvet bean, and yam (Chinese)

Supplements: Alpha-lipoic acid, **berberine**, CBD, **chromium**, Co-Q10, DHEA, L-carnitine, **magnesium**, MSM, omega-3 DHA, omega-3 EFAs, omega-6 GLA, resveratrol, **vanadium**, vitamin B$_{12}$, vitamin B$_3$, vitamin B$_6$, **vitamin D**, xylitol, and zinc

Essential Oils: Ylang ylang

Diabetic Retinopathy

See also diabetes

Diabetic retinopathy is caused by damage to the retina due to complications of diabetes. Antioxidants can help to prevent and possibly heal this condition. Some of the best remedies to consider include bioflavonoids and vitamin C, alpha-lipoic acid, proanthocyanidins, and bilberries. Good fats, especially DHA, may also be helpful. Some people have found the *Oral Chelation* strategy helpful.

Strategies: Avoid Sugar, Healthy Fats, and Low-Glycemic Diet

Formulas: Oral Chelation, Antioxidant Eye, and Antioxidant

Herbs: Bilberry and ginkgo

Supplements: Alpha-lipoic acid, bioflavonoids, **omega-3 EFAs,** and **vitamin C**

Diaper Rash

See also dermatitis

Diaper rash is a form of contact dermatitis (inflammation of the skin) that is common in infants and young children, where there is prolonged exposure to urine-soaked or soiled diapers and the chemicals found in disposable diapers.

Apply a healing salve when changing diapers to prevent diaper rash. You can also soothe diaper rash by applying aloe vera gel to the rash or sprinkling slippery elm powder into the fresh diaper when changing. Be sure to change diapers promptly after a child wets or soils them.

A fiery-looking diaper rash is typically caused by yeast infections. The infant may also have thrush. Probiotics are beneficial in this case. Open the capsules and put the sweet-tasting powder into the baby's mouth. Probiotic powder can also be sprinkled in the diaper to help prevent this type of diaper rash.

Strategies: Friendly Flora

Formulas: Enzyme Spray, **Healing Salve,** and **Probiotic**

Herbs: Aloe vera, calendula, chickweed, corn silk, and **slippery elm**

Supplements: Chlorophyll

Essential Oils: Lavender

Diarrhea
Dysentery

See also giardia, infection (bacterial), inflammatory bowel disorders, and parasites

Excessively loose, watery, and frequent bowel movements are a sign that the bowels are trying to eliminate toxic irritants. Dysentery is a severe form of diarrhea characterized by frequent watery stools, often with blood and mucus. Symptoms include pain, fever, and dehydration.

The best approach to treating these conditions naturally is to use agents that absorb toxins in the digestive tract, such as activated charcoal or a *Fiber Blend*. For severe diarrhea, activated charcoal is the best choice, but be careful not to use too much activated charcoal as it is so effective it can actually cause constipation. For diarrhea in infants and young children, slippery elm or marshmallow are good choices.

When diarrhea is extremely watery, astringents may be needed to tone bowel tissue and halt fluid loss. Some of the herbs that can be used for this purpose include blackberry root, bayberry, and white oak bark, although almost any astringent may help.

For diarrhea caused by infectious organisms, goldenseal, berberine, garlic, or silver are good antimicrobial remedies that can be helpful.

Diarrhea may also be due to parasites or giardia. So if diarrhea develops after foreign travel or drinking possibly contaminated water, get checked for parasites. If this is a problem look up what to do for parasites.

Probiotics can be helpful for both treating and preventing diarrhea from infectious microbes. When traveling, taking digestive enzyme supplements and probiotics can help prevent diarrhea. Take three to four times the normal dose of the probiotics.

Constant diarrhea is a symptom of inflammation in the bowels (see *inflammatory bowel disorders*).

After a bout with diarrhea it is always good to take probiotics as well as minerals (such as the *Electrolyte Drink Powder* or *Herbal Potassium Formula*) to replace lost mineral electrolytes. If diarrhea is severe or persistent, seek medical attention.

Strategies: Friendly Flora and Gut-Healing Diet

Formulas: Irritable Bowel Fiber, **Fiber, Probiotic,** Chinese Earth-Decreasing, Intestinal Soothing, Chinese Earth-Increasing, **H. Pylori-Fighting,** Electrolyte Drink, Herbal Potassium, and Colloidal Mineral

Herbs: Acacia (Indian), agrimony, alisma, **andrographis,** asparagus, atractylodes, **bayberry root bark, blackberry root,** boswellia, **cinnamon,** clove, codonopsis, cyperus, dodder, drynaria, galangal, garlic, ginger, **goldenseal,** honeysuckle, hyacinth, Irish moss, jambul, kudzu, lady's mantle, lotus, marshmallow, myrrh, pau d'arco, psyllium, quince (Bengal), **red raspberry, slippery elm,** tangerine (Mandarin), white oak, yam (Chinese), yarrow, and yellow dock

Supplements: Bromelain, **charcoal,** clay (bentonite), **nanoparticle silver,** potassium, and zinc

Essential Oils: Cinnamon, clove, fennel, geranium, lemon, myrrh, orange (sweet), peppermint, and sandalwood

Dieting   see *excess weight*

Digestion, Poor

See also hiatal hernia and wasting

Poor digestion leads to an inability to properly break down food into usable nutrients. Symptoms include pain, bloating, gas, cramping, and/or heartburn. This is usually due to a deficiency of stomach acid or digestive enzymes. When poor digestion becomes chronic and severe, it can lead to weight loss, an inability to develop muscle mass, wasting, pallor, and fatigue.

It is also a good idea to start by trying to stimulate the body's natural digestive secretions with *Herbal Bitters Formulas*. If a person is not producing enough hydrochloric acid (see *Low Stomach Acid*) they need a *Betaine HCL Formula*. They may also need a *Digestive Support* or *Plant Enzyme Formula*.

When a person is elderly, herbs like American ginseng, saw palmetto, licorice root, and astragalus can help to restore good digestion. The *Chinese Earth-Increasing Formula* is particularly helpful for elderly people with poor appetite and poor digestion.

Chronically poor digestion may be caused by a hiatal hernia. This is a mechanical and stress-related problem that needs to be fixed before digestive powers can be restored (see *hiatal hernia*).

It takes water to digest food, especially proteins, so if you are dehydrated digestion will be poor. Try drinking two glasses of water and taking a pinch of salt twenty to thirty minutes prior to meals.

Strategies: Blood Type Diet, Eat Enzyme-Rich Foods, Hiatal Hernia Correction, and Hydration

Formulas: Herbal Bitters, Papaya Enzyme, **Chinese Earth-Increasing**, Chinese Earth-Decreasing, **Plant Enzyme**, **Digestive Support**, **Betaine HCl**, Christopher's Carminative, and Probiotic

Herbs: Astragalus, atractylodes, chamomile, couchgrass, **dandelion**, **gentian**, ginseng (American), goldenseal, horehound, horseradish, marshmallow, **Oregon grape**, **papaya**, quince (Bengal), rosemary, safflower, saw palmetto, turmeric, and vervain (blue)

Supplements: Amylase, bromelain, lipase, magnesium, pancreatin, and protease

Essential Oils: Anise, cajeput, clary sage, clove, copaiba, fennel, grapefruit (pink), helichrysum, juniper, lemon, lemongrass, orange (sweet), **peppermint**, red mandarin, rose, spearmint, and thyme

Diphtheria

See also contagious disease prevention

Diphtheria is an infectious disease caused by the bacteria *Corynebacterium diphtheria*. *C. diphtheria* produces a toxin that causes degeneration of the nerves, heart, and other tissues. If you have diphtheria, seek medical attention. Diphtheria can cause anemia and fatigue if left untreated. A steam inhalation with essential oils for the respiratory system, such as pine or eucalyptus, may be helpful. It is important to stay hydrated to flush toxins.

Strategies: Hydration and Sweat Bath

Formulas: Stabilized Allicin

Herbs: Black cohosh, cordyceps, **echinacea**, **garlic**, lobelia, and vervain (blue)

Supplements: Nanoparticle silver

Essential Oils: Eucalyptus, helichrysum, marjoram, and **pine**

Dislocation

A dislocation is the displacement of a body part, such as an internal organ or the bones in a joint, from its proper position. Dislocations should be mechanically corrected by a professional therapist, but herbs and nutrients to support tissue healing or relieve pain can be helpful. If the area is accessible to topical applications, you can use the *Poultice* or *Compress or Fomentation* strategies, or apply essential oils diluted with a fixed oil (see the *Aromatherapy* strategy).

Strategies: Aromatherapy, Compress or Fomentation, and Poultice

Formulas: Herbal Calcium, **Watkin's Hair, Skin, and Nails**, Vulnerary, Topical Analgesic, Analgesic Nerve, **Anti-Inflammatory Pain**, **CBD Anti-inflammatory**, and CBD Topical Analgesic

Herbs: Boswellia, lobelia, mullein, **solomon's seal**, and turmeric

Supplements: CBD, **curcumin**, and **MSM**

Essential Oils: Camphor, **copaiba**, helichrysum, marjoram, and wintergreen

Dissociative Identity Disorder

See also mental illness and PTSD

Dissociative identity disorder, or DID (previously known as multiple personality disorder), is a severe form of dissociation, where a person appears to have more than one disconnected personality. It appears to be associated with severe trauma in childhood in the form of extreme and repetitive sexual, physical, and/or emotional abuse. Psychologists believe that the person compartmentalizes their personality to shut themselves off from memories that are too painful to process.

An alternative explanation, one that is more spiritually based, is that a person's spirit leaves their body during the abuse to avoid the pain, which leaves the body open for possession by other spiritual entities (personalities) to take control. Later, when something triggers the memories of the trauma, the person disassociates again, leaving them open for these spirit entities to take control again.

I have personally worked with people where I saw evidence that this was what was happening. I once knew a psychologist who also believed this and worked to overcome this problem in people by having them gradually reconnect with and take charge of their body. I have used this technique successfully myself.

It works like this: You have the person breathe deeply and then ask them to feel (or turn their awareness onto) the various parts of their body. If they encounter painful memories, have them breathe through them and acknowledge the pain. If they need to cry or express anger or tremble, you allow this to happen.

I also attended a workshop where an herbalist had discovered, by accident, that barberry helped reintegrate a person with DID. We watched videos of them slowly pulling their personality together over several sessions. He said other people had done testing with homeopathic barberry and found it helpful in similar circumstances.

There are some flower remedies which might be helpful. These include the following:

Arnica, which is for disassociation from shock and trauma

Manzanita, which is for people who are not fully integrated into their body

Shooting star, which helps embody a person

Purple monkeyflower, which helps people who have been victims of ritualistic or cult abuse

Golden ear drops, which helps people get in touch with an integrate painful childhood memories

The *Counseling or Therapy* strategy is needed for this problem. See the *Emotional Healing Work* strategy for additional techniques I have used for problems like DID.

Strategies: Counseling or Therapy, Emotional Healing Work, and Flower Essence

Herbs: Barberry

Diverticulitis
Diverticula

See also inflammatory bowel disorders

Diverticula are abnormally formed pockets in the bowel. When they become inflamed, the afflicted person has diverticulitis.

Fiber can be very helpful for diverticula. Very soft fibers like marshmallow and slippery elm are preferred over fibers like bran and psyllium. Make sure to drink plenty of water and stay well hydrated while taking the fiber.

When diverticula are inflamed (diverticulitis) it is best to avoid fiber and use gentler remedies to relieve the inflammation and tone the colon. These include chamomile, licorice, cat's claw, and black walnut.

The *Gentle Bowel Cleansing Formula* or *Triphala Formula* may be used to help keep the stool soft and moving properly, but stimulant laxatives with herbs like cascara sagrada or senna should be avoided when diverticula are inflamed.

Strategies: Hydration and Increase Dietary Fiber

Formulas: Intestinal Detoxification, **Intestinal Soothing**, **Gut Immune**, Vulnerary, Gentle Bowel Cleansing, **Irritable Bowel Fiber**, Probiotic, and **Triphala**

Herbs: **Black walnut**, **cat's claw**, chamomile, couchgrass, ginger, **marshmallow**, **slippery elm**, and wild yam

Supplements: Clay (bentonite) and omega-3 EFAs

Dizziness
Vertigo

See also circulation (poor), earache, and hypoglycemia

A loss of the sense of balance, associated with vertigo or dizziness, can be caused by an ear infection or damage to the inner ear. Other possible causes include poor circulation, low blood sugar, and nerve damage. Seek professional help to determine the cause before selecting remedies, as the remedies that help will depend on the cause.

Strategies: Low-Glycemic Diet and Stress Management

Formulas: Chinese Wood-Increasing, Chinese Water-Decreasing, Chinese Metal-Increasing, Chinese Qi-Regulating, Chinese Fire-Decreasing, Chinese Water-Increasing, Chinese Qi and Blood Tonic, Chinese Yang-Reducing, Chinese Wind-Heat Evil, Brain-Heart, **Antispasmodic Ear**, Methyl B12 Vitamin, Methylated B Vitamin, and Hypoglycemic

Herbs: Alisma, amalaki, black cohosh, chrysanthemum, cordyceps, dodder, eleuthero, gastrodia, **ginger**, **ginkgo**, gotu kola, hawthorn, he shou wu, **licorice**, ligustrum, linden, mistletoe, peppermint, and periwinkle

Supplements: L-glutamine, manganese, omega-3 EFAs, vitamin B-complex, vitamin B_{12}, and vitamin B_9

Essential Oils: Peppermint

Down Syndrome

See also pregnancy

Down syndrome is a genetic defect characterized by slow physical development and moderate to severe mental retardation. I am not aware of any specific cure for Down syndrome, but some of the basic supplements and therapies that promote better overall health will likely help.

One important factor to consider is that there is excessive oxidative stress in Down syndrome, which suggests that antioxidants might be beneficial. This also appears to be tied into disturbed methylation. Possible remedies to help here include methylated B_{12} and B_9, alpha-lipoic acid and melatonin.

Deterioration of the brain like that in Alzheimer's disease is part of the problem. Curcumin may help slow the inflammation involved in this process.

Good prenatal care may help to prevent Down syndrome. Folic acid (vitamin B_9), for example, is known to reduce the risk of genetic defects in babies.

I recommend you do your research and use remedies based on the child's specific symptoms. Experiment a little, starting with small doses of any new supplement. Carefully observe for signs of improvement or worsening of symptoms and discontinue or increase the dose depending on your observations.

Strategies: Eat Healthy, Friendly Flora, and Mineralization

Formulas: GLA Oil, Methylated B Vitamin, Methyl B12 Vitamin, and Probiotic

Herbs: Ashwagandha, black currant, evening primrose, ginkgo, and kelp

Supplements: 5-HTP, alpha-lipoic acid, Co-Q10, **curcumin**, L-carnitine, **melatonin**, **omega-3 EFAs**, vitamin B-complex, vitamin B_{12}, **vitamin B_9**, vitamin D, vitamin K, and **zinc**

Dropsy   see *edema*

Drug Detox/Withdrawal
see *addictions (drugs)*

Duodenal Ulcers

See also ulcers

An ulceration of the first part of the small intestine. See *ulcers* for more suggestions.

Strategies: Increase Dietary Fiber

Formulas: H. Pylori-Fighting and Intestinal Soothing

Herbs: Aloe vera and **licorice**

Dysbiosis

See also infection (fungal) and SIBO

Dysbiosis is an imbalance in the bacteria and yeast living in the intestinal tract, which are collectively known as the microbiome. (See *Friendly Flora* strategy.) It can be a factor in many health problems, including chronic sinus problems, frequent colds and flu, earaches, swollen lymph nodes, fatigue, reduced immunity, brain fog, various types of yeast infections, and leaky gut syndrome.

Dysbiosis occurs primarily because of overuse of antibiotics and other drugs such as birth control pills, NSAIDs, and chemotherapy agents, which upset the balance of intestinal microflora by killing the friendly bacteria. Other substances that have negative effects on intestinal flora include refined sugar, glycophosphate weed killers, certain GMO foods, alcohol, chlorinated drinking water, MSG, nitrates, and sulfates.

When friendly flora are disrupted, yeast or harmful strains of bacteria can proliferate, which can weaken the immune system. When the bacteria or yeast grows out of control, it secretes substances that weaken the integrity of the intestines, resulting in intestinal inflammation and leaky gut syndrome. These substances are then absorbed into the bloodstream, weakening the immune system and the body in general. Both yeast and bacteria feed on sugar and when they get out of balance in the body, they release chemicals that make a person crave sugar, thereby perpetuating the environment that sustains their existence.

Here are four important strategies for correcting dysbiosis and restoring intestinal health. It is important to adopt each of these strategies in the order they are given.

Step 1: Modify the Diet

Yeast and bacteria love carbohydrates, especially simple sugars. Eliminate all simple sugars, refined grain products, and alcohol from your diet for two weeks. Sugars and refined grains are added to most packaged foods; read labels carefully. If you have severe dysbiosis, you may need to avoid whole grains, most fruit, and even starchy foods like potatoes. However, severely restricting carbohydrates can cause ketosis, and candida prefers ketones over sugar, so be sure to include fruits and vegetables in your diet so you obtain sugar through complex carbohydrates. See the *Avoid Sugar* and *Low-Glycemic Diet* strategies.

Step 2: Take Digestive Enzymes

Yeast and bacteria can get out of control when the environment becomes conducive to their growth. To get them back under control, change the environment of the digestive tract. Normally, the hydrochloric acid and enzymes found in the stomach help keep these microbes in check. Consider taking a *Digestive Support Formula* and/or a *Betaine HCl Formula*. Taking protease enzyme supplements between meals will help to regulate digestive microbes. Digestive secretions can be stimulated by taking *Herbal Bitters Formulas* with water twenty minutes before meals. Bitters will also help relieve the gas and bloating that commonly occurs with dysbiosis.

Step 3: Use Antifungal and Antimicrobial Agents

After cutting off their food supply, you can take steps to reduce the overgrowth of unfriendly microorganisms. Some good remedies for doing this include cinnamon, cat's claw, and berberine. You can also use berberine-containing herbs like barberry or goldenseal. Enteric coated peppermint oil is especially helpful for dysbiosis. You can add a drop of peppermint oil to a tablespoon of coconut oil and take it internally to obtain similar effects to enteric coated peppermint oil.

Step 4: Repopulate with Friendly Bacteria

The final strategy in correcting dysbiosis is to repopulate the intestines with friendly bacteria or probiotics. This can be done with food and/or supplements. See the *Friendly Flora* strategy.

Inulin-rich herbs like dandelion or chicory can help to feed friendly flora and improve the intestinal biome. High quality colostrum may also help.

Strategies: Avoid Sugar, Eat Enzyme-Rich Foods, Friendly Flora, and Low-Glycemic Diet

Formulas: Betaine HCl, Digestive Support, H. Pylori-Fighting, **Gut Immune**, **Probiotic**, and Herbal Bitters

Programs: Yeast Cleansing and Chinese Balanced Cleansing

Essential Oil Blends: Antifungal EO

Herbs: Barberry, **bee balm**, **cat's claw**, chicory, **cinnamon**, coconut, dandelion, **goldenseal**, nopal, oregano, and **pau d'arco**

Supplements: Berberine and colostrum

Essential Oils: Lavender and **peppermint enteric coated**

Dysentery   see *diarrhea*

Dysmenorrhea
Painful Menstruation

See also cramps (menstrual) and PMS

Painful menstruation or pain during menses is called dysmenorrhea. Minor discomfort is common, but when the pain is excessive it is a sign of imbalances in the body. Here are a few strategies to consider for easing the discomfort.

As a general remedy for menstrual problems consider using a *Female Tonic Formula* or a *Chinese Wood Formula*. Also follow the *Avoid Xenoestrogens* and Hydration strategies.

When pain is dull, it is probably congestive pain caused by a lack of good blood flow in the pelvic region. Pelvic decongestants will help. Two of the best herbs for this purpose are ginger and yarrow. The *Castor Oil Pack* strategy can be used over the lower abdomen to ease congestive pain.

When the pains are sharp and cramping, they are probably due to muscle spasms. Antispasmodics such as black cohosh, lobelia, and wild yam can be helpful. Magnesium is also helpful for menstrual cramping. Essential oils like peppermint, clary sage, and lavender can be applied topically over the abdomen to help relax spastic pain.

Chronic dysmenorrhea can also be due to unresolved emotional trauma such as rape, sexual abuse, or shame surrounding menstrual functions. If this is the case, it is important to address these issues with the *Counseling or Therapy* and/or *Emotional Healing Work* strategies.

Strategies: Avoid Xenoestrogens, Castor Oil Pack, Counseling or Therapy, Eat Healthy, and Emotional Healing Work

Formulas: Antispasmodic, Female Cycle, Chinese Wood-Decreasing, Chinese Wood-Increasing, and **Female Tonic**

Herbs: Achyranthes, angelica, **black cohosh**, black haw, blue cohosh, capsicum, chaste tree, **cramp bark**, cyperus, **dogwood (Jamaican)**, dong quai, false unicorn, **ginger**, ginseng (Asian/Korean), Indian madder, kava kava, **lobelia**, milk thistle, partridge berry, passion flower, peppermint essential oil, salvia, **wild yam**, and **yarrow**

Supplements: Boron, bromelain, **magnesium**, and SAM-e

Essential Oils: Chamomile (Roman), clary sage, cypress, geranium, lavender, myrrh, and peppermint

Dyspepsia
See also gastritis, indigestion, and SIBO

Impaired gastric function due to some disorder of the stomach is called dyspepsia. Symptoms include pain and sometimes nausea or burning. Drinking more water and taking a *Plant Enzyme Formula* will often help. These symptoms are part of the pattern of excess earth in Chinese medicine, so a *Chinese Earth-Decreasing Formula* may be helpful. A *Papaya Enzyme Formula* is helpful for both children and adults. *Herbal Bitters Formulas* are also helpful for this condition and should be taken fifteen to twenty minutes prior to meals with one or two large glasses of water.

Strategies: Eat Enzyme-Rich Foods, Hiatal Hernia Correction, and Hydration

Formulas: Plant Enzyme, Probiotic, Digestive Support, Papaya Enzyme, Pepsin Intestinal, Children's Colic,

Natural Antacid, **Chinese Earth-Decreasing**, **Herbal Bitters**, Chinese Wood-Decreasing, Betaine HCl, and Christopher's Carminative

Herbs: Aloe vera, amalaki, angelica, **catnip**, chamomile, cyperus, **fennel**, fenugreek, garlic, ginger, goldenseal, jambul, kutki, **papaya**, picrorhiza, thyme, and velvet bean

Supplements: Calcium, magnesium, and vitamin B-complex

Essential Oils: Grapefruit (pink), neroli, orange (sweet), **peppermint**, red mandarin, and thyme

Earache
Ear Infection, Otitis Media

See also food allergies/intolerances, infection (fungal), and swollen lymph glands

An earache occurs as the result of inflammation, often due to infection in the ear. The irritation or infection can happen in the outer ear canal (otitis externa or swimmer's ear), in the middle ear behind the eardrum (otitis media), or in the inner ear (otitis interna). An inner ear infection causes the sudden onset of vomiting, vertigo, and loss of balance. Children are more prone to earaches than adults because their ear passages are small, so an amount of fluid that would not cause a problem in an adult can cause severe problems in a child. Here are some strategies to employ with earaches or infections.

Check for Allergies

Earaches are often allergy-induced. The allergy is usually to cow's milk or infant formula, but wheat is another common allergen. If a child has frequent ear infections, check for the possibility of food allergies. Allergies can cause irritation to the mucous membranes, which results in swelling and constriction of the eustachian tube, the tube that goes between the middle ear and the throat. The eustachian tube allows for equalization of pressure on both sides of the eardrum and for drainage of fluid from the inner ear. When it is swollen, pressure builds up in the inner ear and causes pain.

Antibiotics are usually used to treat ear infections. They are often ineffective and contribute to problems in the intestinal tract that weaken the immune system and create lymphatic stagnation, perpetuating the tendency toward earaches. There is no scientific evidence that antibiotics do anything for 99 percent of people with ear infections. In 1 percent of the population, antibiotics shorten the duration of pain and infection.

Natural Remedies for Infection

There are some effective natural infection fighters that do work well for ear infections. Garlic oil is very effective for ear infections. Warm the oil to body temperature and place a few drops in the ear. Allow it to remain there for a few minutes. You can rub some of the oil down the side of the neck to improve lymphatic drainage. There are also *Ear Drop Formulas* that are very effective.

Essential oils like lavender, thyme, and tea tree can be diluted in olive oil (one drop of essential oil to twenty drops of olive oil) and used as ear-drops. Lobelia extract can be used as an ear drop to reduce pain. The *Antispasmodic Ear Formula* has also been used as ear drops. Make sure that anything you put in the ear is warmed to body temperature first.

For adults or older children, cut a clove of raw garlic, put a little olive oil on it, and place it on the outside of the ear where an external hearing aid would be placed. This will help eliminate infection, stimulate lymphatic drainage, and relieve the pain.

Another treatment is to bake or steam an onion and place a few drops of the cooled onion juice in the ear. Or cut the cooked onion in half and place it over the ear while it is still warm. In most cases, the onion will rapidly relieve the pain, as well as helping to fight any infection that may be present.

Opening the Eustachian Tubes

Eyebright is the herbal equivalent of ear tubes: it can prevent the eustachian tubes from swelling and open them after they are swollen. It works best as a tincture of the fresh plant, but large doses of the dried powder may also be effective. Osha has been used to reduce the allergic reactions that cause earaches, and open the eustachian tubes, especially when the allergy is due to dairy products. Osha is endangered in many areas, so be cautious about where you obtain it. Gently massaging under the ear to increase lymphatic drainage can also help to open the eustachian tubes.

Strategies: Aromatherapy, Eliminate Allergy-Causing Foods, and Gluten-Free Diet

Formulas: Jeannie Burgess' Allergy-Lung, **Antispasmodic Ear**, **Chinese Yang-Reducing**, Liquid Lymph, Lymphatic Infection, **Ear Drop**, and Chinese Metal-Decreasing

Herbs: Andrographis, echinacea, **eyebright**, **garlic oil**, hyacinth, **lobelia**, **mullein flowers**, osha, quince (Bengal), Saint John's wort, and spilanthes

Supplements: L-glutamine and **nanoparticle silver**

Essential Oils: Eucalyptus, fennel, helichrysum, lavender, **tea tree**, and thyme

Ears, Itchy   see *itchy ears*

Ears, Ringing   see *tinnitus*

Easily Bruised

See also bruises, capillary weakness, and circulation (poor)

If a person bruises easily, this is a sign of fragile capillaries and poor circulation. Remedies are needed to reduce oxidative stress and improve venous circulation and capillary tone.

Formulas: Antioxidant, **Vein Tonic**, and Proanthocyanidins

Herbs: Bilberry, **butcher's broom**, ginkgo, hawthorn, mangosteen, noni, **rose hips**, and yarrow

Supplements: Bioflavonoids and **vitamin C**

Eczema

See also itching, dermatitis, psoriasis, rashes & hives, and skin problems

Eczema is chronic dermatitis. It involves a rash, itching, redness, and flaking of the skin. In eczema, the skin is repeatedly irritated and inflamed, which causes the upper layer of the skin (epidermis) to thicken as skin cells multiply rapidly. This creates a scaly effect on the surface of the skin. Oil glands become obstructed, and the skin becomes dry.

The scaly skin inhibits elimination through the skin, causing toxins to become trapped under the skin. This causes itching, which leads the person to scratch. Scratching breaks the epidermal layer so the skin develops a broken and cracked appearance.

Eczema is caused by the body being hypersensitive to certain irritants, so it is closely related to allergic asthma, hay fever and food allergies. Children are extremely prone to eczema. Almost 30 percent of all newborn babies develop this condition. It often occurs on the scalp or the cheeks, but can spread over other parts of the body, making children itchy and miserable.

Although 75 percent outgrow this condition by their mid-teens, adults who had eczema as children will remain prone to dry skin in later years and to occasional flare-ups of skin inflammation. Eczema can be difficult to get rid of because it has multiple causes, but here are some of the strategies that can be helpful.

Eat a Clean, Healthy Diet

Diet can be very important in treating eczema. Start by identifying and eliminating allergy-causing foods and food intolerances (see the *Eliminate Allergy-Causing Foods* strategy). Adopt the *Eat Healthy* strategy too.

Eliminate Chemical Irritants

It also helps to reduce exposure to chemical irritants. Use natural laundry detergents as well as natural skin care products. (See the *Reduce Chemical Exposure* strategy)

Enhance Fat Metabolism

There may be problems with fat metabolism in eczema. Fat-soluble vitamins like A and D are often helpful along with eating healthy fats and avoiding bad fats. (See the *Healthy Fats* strategy.)

Herbs like burdock and chickweed can aid fat metabolism in the body and have been helpful for eczema in some people. Sometimes the thyroid is involved because the thyroid hormones are essential to fat metabolism. Seaweeds like kelp and dulse or a *Thyroid Glandular Formula* may be helpful. Seaweeds can also be used in baths or topical lotions to ease itching and lubricate the skin.

Reduce Inflammation

Eczema is sometimes treated medically with corticosteroid drugs that mimic the anti-inflammatory action of the adrenal hormone cortisol. People with eczema often suffer from adrenal exhaustion (with a corresponding deficiency in the production of cortisol). This helps explain why excessive inflammation is present and why eczema can flare up under stress, as stress depletes the adrenals.

Herbs with an anti-inflammatory or cortisol-like action can be helpful. These include yucca, licorice, and turmeric. An *Adrenal Glandular Formula* may also be useful for people with eczema.

CBD is a promising new aid for eczema. It modulates immune responses and can be used both topically and internally to calm the inflammation in the skin.

Use Blood Purifiers

Blood Purifier or *Detoxifying Formulas* are a traditional herbal approach to conditions like eczema. Look for blood purifiers that contain herbs like burdock, chickweed, dandelion, gotu kola, pau d'arco, and red clover. These herbs have also been used in baths or lotions to help soothe the skin and ease itching.

Moisten the Skin

When the skin is dry, topical application of coconut oil, olive oil, or a natural lotion will help ease dryness and itching. Vitamin E and appropriate essential oils can be mixed with the oil or lotion. Good choices are sandalwood, frankincense, helichrysum, and chamomile.

Manage Stress

Eczema can have roots in the nervous system. Too much intellectual activity in the head, without enough engaging in artistic or physical activities can make one's neurosensory system overstimulated, a condition known as neurodermatitis. If eczema isn't responding to physical treatments, consider using the *Flower Essence, Meditation* or *Emotional Healing*

Work strategies to help heal unresolved emotional wounds. See *skin care (general)* for more information on the connection between the nervous system and the skin.

Strategies: Drawing Bath, Eat Healthy, Eliminate Allergy-Causing Foods, Friendly Flora, Healthy Fats, and Reduce Chemical Exposure

Formulas: Detoxifying, Antihistamine, Ayurvedic Skin Healing, Blood Purifier, Anti-Stress B-Complex, GLA Oil, **Adrenal Glandular,** Enzyme Spray, Watkin's Hair, Skin, and Nails, Betaine HCl, Colloidal Mineral, Digestive Support, and Probiotic

Programs: Chinese Balanced Cleansing

Herbs: Acacia (Indian), aloe vera, amur cork, baical skullcap, barley, black currant, black walnut, blue flag, borage, **burdock, chickweed,** coptis, **dandelion,** dulse, echinacea, evening primrose, flax, gotu kola, grindelia, Irish moss, kelp, licorice, myrrh, nettle, stinging, pau d'arco, pleurisy, **red clover,** turmeric, and yucca

Supplements: CBD, omega-3 EFAs, omega-6 GLA, **vitamin A,** vitamin B-complex, vitamin B_5, vitamin D, vitamin E, and zinc

Essential Oils: Bergamot, cajeput, chamomile (Roman), clary sage, **frankincense,** geranium, **helichrysum,** jasmine, juniper, lavender, lemon, myrrh, rose, **sandalwood,** tansy (blue), and tea tree

Edema
Dropsy, Water Retention, Swelling

See also congestive heart failure

Edema is water trapped in the body's tissues causing swelling. It may occur in any part of the body. Generally speaking, it indicates poor lymphatic drainage and/or a lack of kidney function. It may also be due to heart problems and inflammation.

Start by using a *Diuretic Formula* or single diuretic herbs. You can use stimulating diuretics like juniper, buchu, and uva ursi or more gentle nourishing diuretics like nettles, goldenrod, dandelion leaf, and corn silk. The former should not be used if the kidneys are inflamed. The later are better for burning urination.

In addition diuretics, you can use herbs that aid lymphatic drainage. These include cleavers and red clover or a *Lymph Cleansing Formula.* It may also help to take potassium. Believe it or not, drinking more water with a pinch of natural sea salt may actually help to relieve edema in some cases.

Essential oils can be diluted with a fixed oil or lotion and massaged into the skin over swollen areas. This helps move fluid out of the tissues.

Edema can also be the result of congestive heart failure. In this case, medical assistance should be sought (see *congestive heart failure*).

Strategies: Exercise, Hydration, and Mineralization

Formulas: Diuretic, Chinese Water-Decreasing, Liquid Kidney, Liquid Lymph, Urinary Support, UTI Prevention, Herbal Potassium, Heart Health, Chinese Metal-Decreasing, and Lymph Cleansing

Herbs: Alisma, asparagus, baical skullcap, **buchu,** cleavers, coffee, corn silk, **dandelion leaf, goldenrod,** hoelen, horsetail, **juniper,** mulberry, **nettle, stinging, parsley,** polygala, prickly ash, purslane, red clover, trichosanthes, **uva ursi,** and zhu-ling

Supplements: Potassium

Essential Oils: Geranium, grapefruit (pink), juniper, lavender, lemon, lemongrass, and patchouli

Electromagnetic Pollution

If you are exposed regularly to electromagnetic radiation, see tips for reducing exposure under the strategy *Reduce EMF Exposure*. Also make sure you get plenty of antioxidant nutrients, especially in the form of raw fruits and vegetables. You can also use single herbs like bee pollen, cordyceps, and barley grass or the *Chinese Qi and Blood Tonic*. These remedies seem to boost the body's ability to deal with electromagnetic pollution.

Strategies: Eat Healthy and Reduce EMF Exposure

Formulas: Antioxidant, **Chinese Qi and Blood Tonic,** Algae, and **Adaptogen**

Herbs: Barley grass, bee pollen, blue-green algae, **chlorella,** cordyceps, and spirulina

Supplements: Vitamin C

Essential Oils: Frankincense and myrrh

Emotional Sensitivity
See also adrenal fatigue, anxiety attacks, PTSD, and estrogen dominance

When people are emotionally sensitive, getting angry, sad, or anxious over small, insignificant things, it is often due to being tired, exhausted from chronic stress, or emotionally fragile from previous trauma or abuse.

When the emotional sensitivity is coupled with feelings of fatigue, mental confusion, restless sleep, disturbed dreams, and/or a loss of sex drive it probably indicates a high level of stress or anxiety. This may also make a person feel shaky inside and unable to cope with life. They may even tremble (that is, have trembling hands). There may be a feeling, "I just can't take it anymore." If you have these symptoms, see *adrenal fatigue.*

If the person has been traumatized in the past from war, tragedy, abuse, or other traumatic incidents, they may have post traumatic stress disorder (see *PTSD*).

People with highly sensitive nervous systems, who are easily thrown off balance in life, may benefit from herbs that act as nerve tonics (like milky oat seed or skullcap), increased mineral intake (particularly calcium, magnesium, and potassium), and including good fats in the diet (see *Healthy Fats* strategy). If little things bother you a lot and you tend to fidget, fuss over details, worry about the small stuff, and feel nervous a lot, use these nerve-enhancing remedies.

When there is a high state of anxiety, kava kava is an excellent single herb, especially when a person has a lot of muscle tension. Chamomile is a good remedy for emotionally sensitive children (and adults) who make a lot of fuss over small things.

Women who are delicate and extremely sensitive may have excess estrogen (see *estrogen dominance*). Pulsatilla is often used as a homeopathic remedy for this problem.

Emotional sensitivity may be linked to feelings of excessive fear or the inability to stand up for oneself. Often this is linked to being abused as a child, which makes one hypervigilant and always on the alert for danger. The *Emotional Healing Work* strategy and the *Broken and Hardened Hearts* or *Fear-Reducing FE Blends* may be helpful in working on these unresolved emotional wounds.

Strategies: Avoid Sugar, Counseling or Therapy, Emotional Healing Work, Flower Essence, Healthy Fats, Low-Glycemic Diet, Sleep, and Stress Management

Formulas: Chinese Fire-Increasing, Anti-Stress B-Complex, Chinese Fire-Decreasing, Chinese Qi-Regulating, **Adrenal Glandular,** and Anti-Anxiety

Essential Oil Blends: Calming and Relaxing EO

Flower Essence Blends: Fear-Reducing FE

Herbs: Ashwagandha, chamomile, eleuthero, **kava kava, oat seed (milky),** and skullcap

Supplements: Calcium, CBD, DHEA, **magnesium,** omega-3 EFAs, and **potassium**

Essential Oils: Chamomile (Roman) and jasmine

Emphysema

See also addictions (tobacco) and COPD

Emphysema is a chronic lung condition and one form of chronic obstructive pulmonary disorder (see *COPD*). It involves a loss of elasticity of the alveoli, the tiny air sacs in the lungs. The alveoli eventually collapse, causing drowning in lung fluid. Symptoms include labored breathing, wheezing, and a husky cough. Smoking is one of the most common causes of emphysema. This is a serious condition requiring appropriate medical assistance.

In addition to following a general program for improving health, a number of specific herbs may be helpful in emphysema. Mullein is helpful when taken in doses of about six capsules per day for at least six months. It has a slow, cumulative effect in helping the lungs become more moist and supple. Horsetail can also be used to help restore elasticity to lung tissue. Astragalus and cordyceps are Chinese herbs that are also very nourishing to the lungs and supportive of this condition.

Since there is a lot of structural damage to lung tissue in this condition, it may also be helpful to use remedies that help soothe and moisten tissue while promoting healing. Look for herbal formulas that contain slippery elm, marshmallow, plantain, horsetail, and/or nettles.

Antioxidants and good fats are also important for this condition. Try an *Antioxidant Formula*. Also consider omega-3 supplements and the fat-soluble vitamins A and D, and follow the *Healthy Fats* strategy.

Strategies: Affirmation and Visualization, Eat Healthy, Healthy Fats, Heavy Metal Cleanse, and Stress Management

Formulas: Chinese Metal-Increasing, Lung Moistening, Antioxidant, and Dry Cough Syrup

Herbs: Coltsfoot, cordyceps, fenugreek, garlic, **grindelia, horsetail, licorice,** lobelia, marshmallow, **mullein,** plantain, and thyme

Supplements: Chlorophyll, Co-Q10, **N-acetyl cysteine, omega-3 EFAs,** vitamin A, and vitamin D

Endometriosis

See also estrogen dominance

A common cause of pelvic pain, endometriosis is a disorder where endometrial tissue is found outside of the uterus. This tissue responds to hormonal changes in the menstrual cycle just like the uterine lining. It falls apart at the same time the uterine lining sheds, causing menstruation. This can cause internal bleeding that causes surrounding tissues to become swollen and inflamed. It may even cause scar tissue.

Medical treatment for endometriosis can range from using nonsteroidal anti-inflammatory drugs (NSAIDs, like ibuprofen) to ease the pain of surgically removing the endometrial tissue or undergoing a complete hysterectomy. Medical treatment can also involve using birth control pills or other synthetic progestins (progesterone mimics) to counteract the estrogen stimulation of these tissues.

About 10 to 20 percent of adult women have endometriosis. No one is sure why this uterine tissue is growing outside the womb, but some researchers believe the high incidence of it may be due to the influence of xenoestrogens. This excess estrogen stimulation promotes the growth of estrogen-sensitive tissues such as the uterine lining and breasts. So the first thing women with endometriosis should do is follow the *Avoid Xenoestrogens* strategy.

Fat cells make estrogen, so if you are overweight, get on a program to lose weight. This will also reduce estrogen production. See *estrogen dominance* for remedies that reduce excess estrogen and balance hormones.

Because progesterone and estrogen compete for receptor sites (which is why synthetic progesterone is used by the medical community to treat endometriosis), women with endometriosis could try using progesterone creams to enhance progesterone levels. False unicorn also has a progesterone-like effect.

Endometriosis is often painful. In Chinese medicine, pain is a symptom of blocked qi, and in this case it may also be thought of as blocked blood or blood stagnation. A good strategy for easing the pain and breaking up the stagnation is the *Castor Oil Pack*. This topical application of castor oil boosts the immune system; reduces inflammation, pain, and swelling; and can help the body detoxify.

Because there is inflammation associated with endometriosis, herbs that reduce pain and inflammation may be helpful. A Canadian herbalist shared with me an effective program that combines the *Chinese Yang-Reducing Formula*, which reduces inflammation, with the *Standardized Acetogenin Extract*, which reduces abnormal cell growth. It has proven helpful for many women.

Medical science believes that endometriosis is incurable without surgery, but many women have found relief from this problem naturally by adopting a healthier diet, using appropriate supplements, and working with their emotions and stress. Symptoms of endometriosis will disappear naturally with menopause, so even if natural means don't offer a complete cure, they may allow a woman to be symptom-free and maintain the integrity of her reproductive organs by avoiding drugs and surgery.

Strategies: Avoid Xenoestrogens, Castor Oil Pack, Detoxification, Eat Healthy, and Healthy Fats

Formulas: **Standardized Acetogenin**, **Chinese Yang-Reducing**, GLA Oil, and Female Tonic

Herbs: Alfalfa, bayberry, **false unicorn**, gentian, pau d'arco, and **pawpaw**

Supplements: **Indole-3-carbinol**, **omega-3 EFAs**, vitamin A, **vitamin D**, and vitamin E

Endurance, Lack Of

See also adrenal fatigue, anemia, fatigue, hypothyroidism, and nervous exhaustion

A lack of stamina and endurance can result from glandular imbalances such as low thyroid or adrenal weakness.

It can also be due to anemia, stress, lack of sleep, and poor metabolism.

Strategies: Alkalize the Body, Eat Healthy, Hydration, and Low-Glycemic Diet

Formulas: Suma Adaptogen, **Adrenal Glandular**, **Vandergriff's Energy Booster**, Chinese Qi and Blood Tonic, Colloidal Mineral, and Digestive Support

Herbs: Ashwagandha, bee pollen, cordyceps, **eleuthero**, epimedium, **ginseng (American)**, **ginseng (Asian/Korean)**, and licorice

Supplements: Multiple vitamin and mineral

Energy, Lack Of   see *fatigue*

Enervation   see *nervous exhaustion*

Enteritis

See also inflammatory bowel disorders

Enteritis is an inflammation of the intestines, often the ileum, marked by diarrhea. See *inflammatory bowel disorders* for more information about dealing with this problem.

Formulas: **Intestinal Soothing**, Anti-Inflammatory Pain, Probiotic, and Irritable Bowel Fiber

Herbs: Slippery elm

Enuresis   see *incontinence*

Environmental Pollution

See also chemical exposure and heavy metal poisoning

Pollutants from the environment are a growing health concern. People who work in polluted areas or with toxic chemicals of any kind (dry cleaners, beauty salons, labs, etc.) should consider taking remedies to protect their body from these pollutants. Follow the strategy *Reduce Chemical Exposure*. Hepatoprotective herbs like milk thistle and schizandra will help the liver process these chemicals and protect the body from them. *Fiber Blends* can also be taken to bind toxins in the digestive tract for elimination. It is also important to drink adequate amounts of pure water. A periodic cleanse (once or twice a year) is also helpful. See *chemical exposure* for additional suggestions.

Strategies: Detoxification, Eat Healthy, Friendly Flora, Healthy Fats, Hydration, Increase Dietary Fiber, and Liver Detoxification

Formulas: **Detoxifying**, Antioxidant, **Hepatoprotective**, Gut-Healing Fiber, Probiotic, and Adaptogen

Programs: Chinese Balanced Cleansing

Herbs: Lycium, **milk thistle**, quince (Bengal), schisandra, and turmeric

Supplements: Alpha-lipoic acid, N-acetyl cysteine, and omega-3 EFAs

Epilepsy

See also seizures

Epilepsy refers to disorders marked by disturbed electrical rhythms of the central nervous system. Episodes of excess firing in the neurons may create convulsions or a clouding of consciousness. Appropriate medical help should be sought for this condition.

If there has been a blow or other trauma to a person's head, a cranial adjustment may be helpful. This can relieve pressure on the brain. (See *Bodywork* strategy.)

GABA is an inhibitory neurotransmitter that calms brain activity. It may be helpful in some cases of epilepsy. CBD has been helpful in reducing seizures in many people. (See *Seizures* for more information.) Good fats are also important for healthy brain function. Follow the *Healthy Fats* strategy. The *Ketogenic Diet* strategy has also proven beneficial for many people.

Strategies: Healthy Fats and Ketogenic Diet

Formulas: Hypothyroid, Brain Calming, Attention-Focus, GLA Oil, **Methyl B12 Vitamin**, and Antispasmodic

Herbs: Black currant, blue cohosh, **cannabis, coconut**, evening primrose, gastrodia, gotu kola, hops, lobelia, passion flower, siler, **skullcap**, and vervain (blue)

Supplements: **CBD, GABA, magnesium, omega-3 EFAs**, omega-6 GLA, **vitamin B-complex**, and **vitamin B**$_{12}$

Essential Oils: Lavender

Epstein-Barr Virus

See also chronic fatigue syndrome

The Epstein-Barr virus is one of the most common viruses. It is spread through bodily fluids, primarily saliva. Epstein-Barr does not cause any symptoms in many people. In others it can cause mild symptoms such as fever and sore throat. In some cases Epstein-Barr causes a chronic infection that creates severe lack of energy, lymphatic swelling, muscle aches, and sleep disturbances.

If you have been diagnosed with Epstein-Barr, start by strengthening your immune system by adopting good general health practices. Follow the *Healthy Diet* strategy and make time for adequate rest and relaxation. The *Stress Management* strategy can help you relax and give the body time to heal. Antiviral herbs may help the body get rid of the viral component. You can also use formulas to boost the immune system, particularly the *Chinese Wind-Heat Evil Formula*.

Strategies: Affirmation and Visualization, Eliminate Allergy-Causing Foods, Healthy Fats, and Stress Management

Formulas: **Chinese Qi and Blood Tonic, Chinese Wind-Heat Evil**, Liquid Lymph, Lymphatic Infection, Antioxidant, Suma Adaptogen, Immune-Boosting, **Gut Immune**, Digestive Support, Probiotic, and Fibromyalgia

Herbs: Ashwagandha, black walnut, **cat's claw**, echinacea, elder, eleuthero, licorice, **lomatium**, maca, mullein, olive, and pau d'arco

Supplements: Magnesium, MSM, and potassium

Erectile Dysfunction
Impotency

See also arteriosclerosis, hypertension, diabetes, metabolic syndrome, and testosterone (low)

Erectile dysfunction (ED) is the inability to get and keep an erection firm enough for sex. Formerly known as impotency, this problem afflicts an estimated thirty million men in the United States. ED can be caused by both physical or psychological issues. It may also be a side effect of some drugs. Here are some possible causes and strategies for recovery.

Check Medications and General Health

Start by checking all medications for warnings, as many medications can cause ED as a side effect. ED is common in men with Parkinson's disease, multiple sclerosis, and Peyronie's disease. Tobacco use, sleep disorders, treatments for prostate cancer, and surgeries or injuries that affect the pelvic area or spinal cord may also cause ED. If you have any of these problems you will need to work on these issues to address the cause. Seek professional advice and assistance before discontinuing or altering the dose of prescription medications.

Increase Testosterone and Avoid Xenoestrogens

Adequate testosterone levels are essential to achieving an erection. Low testosterone has become quite common in Western society. See *testosterone (low)* for more information.

A possible contributing factor in ED is the influence of endocrine disruptors like xenoestrogens, which can compete with testosterone for receptor sites. See the *Avoid Xenoestrogens* strategy.

Avoid Fluoride

Fluoride from water, toothpaste, and dental treatments may also be interfering with testosterone (https://www.ncbi.nlm.nih.gov/pubmed/23654100). So avoid fluoridated water and toothpaste. Iodine, which you can get from seaweeds, like kelp or dulse, can help detoxify fluoride because they are both halogens and displace each other chemically.

Improve Circulation

Erections are dependent on a strong supply of blood to the penis. Anything that interferes with blood flow into the penis, such as high blood pressure and atherosclerosis, can make getting an erection difficult. The popular performance-enhancing drug Viagra® works by enhancing the action of nitric oxide, a chemical messenger that relaxes blood vessels, improving blood flow. Natural substances that have a similar effect include the amino acid L-arginine and the herbs yohimbe and horny goat weed. Using the *Male Performance Formula* or the *Nitric Oxide Boosting Formula* can be helpful. You can also use herbs and nutrients that help to manage blood pressure (see *hypertension*).

Balance Blood Sugar

A hidden cause of ED is metabolic syndrome, a condition where sugar and insulin levels in the blood are elevated. It is the precursor to diabetes. Metabolic syndrome increases inflammation throughout the body while reducing circulation and energy production. Stabilizing blood sugar levels and reducing inflammation can improve libido and stamina (see *metabolic syndrome*).

Deal with Emotional Issues

There are also emotional factors in ED. When a man is unable to perform he may start to experience anxiety about sex, which adds to his difficulty in maintaining an erection. Stress plays a role in diminishing sex drive and may also contribute to ED. Being unable to perform creates greater feelings of anxiety, which can start a vicious cycle that makes the problem worse, even if the cause was originally physical and has been corrected.

Communication is very important in dealing with this aspect of ED. The female partner needs to be reassured that she is desirable and the male partner needs to relax and focus on the pleasure of foreplay without feeling rushed or pressured about intercourse.

Strategies: Avoid Sugar, Avoid Xenoestrogens, Counseling or Therapy, Enhance Nitric Oxide, Exercise, Flower Essence, and Stress Management

Formulas: DHEA with Herbs, Chinese Water-Increasing, Oral Chelation, Chinese Fire-Increasing, **Male Performance**, Prostate, **Nitric Oxide Boosting**, and **Testosterone**

Programs: Cardiovascular Nutritional

Herbs: Ashwagandha, asparagus, broomrape, cordyceps, **damiana**, dodder, eleuthero, **epimedium**, eucommia, false unicorn, ginkgo, ginseng (American), ginseng (Asian/Korean), he shou wu, maca, **muira puama**, nettle, stinging root, noni, pomegranate, rhodiola, suma, velvet bean, and **yohimbe**

Supplements: Chromium, DHEA, **L-arginine**, L-citruline, **magnesium**, **omega-3 EFAs**, vitamin E, and **zinc**

Essential Oils: Cinnamon, rose, and sandalwood

Estrogen Dominance

See also cystic breast disease, endometriosis, fibroids (uterine), menorrhagia, and PMS Type A

Although women can have low estrogen, it's very common for women in modern society to have too much estrogen. This is partly due to the effect of xenoestrogens, environmental chemicals that mimic estrogen. See the *Avoid Xenoestrogens* strategy for more information.

Taking prescription estrogen during menopause can also overstimulate estrogen. Excess estrogen can also be caused by a lack of liver health, as the liver breaks down excess estrogens.

High estrogen is the cause of the most prevalent type of PMS, known as PMS type A, which is characterize by anxiety, irritability, anger, mood swings, and nervous tension. Too much estrogen increases adrenaline, noradrenaline, and serotonin levels, which make a woman feel more nervous, angry, and aggressive. It's a genuine physical problem and not the result of some character flaw.

Besides PMS type A, symptoms of estrogen dominance include heavy menstrual bleeding, headaches (especially migraines), panic attacks, and an irregular menstrual cycle. Too much estrogen coupled with too little progesterone will cause pregnant women to miscarry and may also cause spotting between periods. Excess estrogen also contributes to health problems like uterine fibroids, ovarian cysts, endometriosis, fibrocystic breast disease, and breast cancer.

Besides avoiding xenoestrogens you can take herbs and supplements to help balance hormones. First, the liver removes excess estrogens from the body. The *Chinese Wood-Decreasing Formula* can aid liver function, especially in women who are prone to PMS type A. Indole-3-carbinol activates metabolic pathways in the liver that break down excess estrogen too. It is found in cruciferous vegetables like cabbage and broccoli.

Second, you can use herbs that help to restore the balance of estrogen and progesterone. One of the best is chaste tree. It can help balance out a woman's monthly cycle when it is irregular, reduce the excess hormones in teenagers that produce acne, and aid hormonal balance during menopause. Wild yam and false unicorn may also help. Look for a *Female Cycle Formula* containing these herbs as primary ingredients.

Strategies: Avoid Xenoestrogens

Formulas: Internal Bleeding, Female Cycle, and **Chinese Wood-Decreasing**

Herbs: Chaste tree, **false unicorn**, and wild yam

Supplements: Indole-3-carbinol

Estrogen, Low

See also PMS Type D

Estrogen is the hormone that dominates in the female body, just like testosterone dominates in men. The word estrogen is derived from the Latin *oestrus* and Greek *oistros*, words that refer to the time of the month when a female is fertile and ready to mate. *Gen* means to generate or produce, so the word estrogen refers to a compound that makes a woman ovulate and become fertile.

What most women don't understand is that estrogen isn't a single compound. There are, in fact, many forms of estrogen.

For starters, a woman's body produces three primary forms of estrogen: estrone (E1), estradiol (E2), and estriol (E3). There are also phytoestrogens (estrogen-like compounds found in plants) and xenoestrogens (chemical pollutants that have estrogenic effects).

Estrogens are involved in a lot more than just ovulation. There are over three hundred tissues in the body with estrogen receptor sites, and estrogens play a role in four hundred functions of the body. These include bone density, mood, eye health, muscle strength, energy production, temperature regulation, intestinal function, libido, and even brain and nervous system function (which is why men and women think differently and even have different sensory perceptions).

Estradiol (E2)

Estradiol is the strongest estrogen and the main form of estrogen produced by a woman's body during her childbearing years. Estradiol is produced in the ovaries under the influence of the follicle-stimulating hormone (FSH) from the pituitary. FSH causes an egg-bearing follicle to mature, producing E2.

E2 is the estrogen that stimulates breast development, so it is increased E2 that causes many of the changes a woman experiences during puberty. After menopause, when eggs are no longer maturing, the ovaries stop producing E2. The decline in levels of E2 causes many of the changes associated with menopause.

E2 helps absorption of minerals (which help to build bone). E2 also decreases LDL cholesterol, increases HDL cholesterol, and balances triglycerides, which reduces a woman's risk of heart disease. It also makes tissues more insulin-sensitive, which reduces the risk of diabetes. Low levels of E2 can cause fatigue, problems sleeping, memory problems, increased risk of blood clots, and depression.

Estrone (E1) and Estriol (E3)

E1 is the main form of estrogen produced after menopause. It can be formed in the adrenal glands, liver, and fat cells, as well as the ovaries. During a woman's fertile years the ovaries convert E1 to E2. After menopause this conversion stops.

E3 is a milder estrogen that does not stimulate the breast tissue or uterine lining like E1 and E2 do. Because of this E3 protects the intestinal tract, vaginal lining, and the breasts. E3 is even used to treat breast cancer in other countries. Asian and vegetarian woman have higher levels of E3 and lower rates of breast cancer.

Remedies for Low Estrogen

When a woman's estrogen levels are low, herbs may help to balance her hormones. These herbs and foods may contain phytoestrogens or they may help boost the production of E1 and E3. Foods with phytoestrogens include soy, other beans and legumes, green leafy vegetables, and whole grains.

Remedies that contain phytoestrogens (estrogen-like compounds), like flax seeds, hops, and soybeans, can help with low estrogen levels. Other herbs helpful for low estrogen include black cohosh and licorice root. Essential oils like geranium, clary sage and pink grapefruit also appear to stimulate estrogen.

Formulas: Chrisopher's Menopause, Hot Flash, Phytoestrogen Breast, and **DHEA with Herbs**

Herbs: Black cohosh, flax, hops, **licorice,** and red clover

Supplements: DHEA and vitamin B_6

Essential Oils: Clary sage, geranium, and grapefruit (pink)

Excess Weight
Obesity, Overweight

See also metabolic syndrome, hyperthyroid, hypothyroidism, and sugar cravings

The best approach excess weight is to adopt a healthier lifestyle. Don't go on a diet because 90% of the people who lose weight in this manner simply gain it back. In fact, diets often backfire, causing people to gain more weight than they lost. Here's why.

Appetite, metabolism, and mood are all controlled by messenger chemicals in the body. When you restrict calories, the cells of the body assume that there is a famine going on. In response, cells send chemical messengers that elevate cortisol, causing thyroid hormone to become inactive, which reduces metabolism (the rate at which you burn calories). This conserves the body's energy during the famine.

Because your metabolism is lower, your energy is reduced, so you become less physically active. Your mood also changes because you feel deprived, so your body is attracted to foods that enhance mood—particularly carbohydrates. When food is available, other chemical messengers are released to stimulate appetite and program the body to store energy (fat) in preparation for the next famine. Thus, a vicious cycle of "feast" and "famine" ensues.

In addition, fat itself acts like a gland, secreting its own chemical messengers. One of these is a hormone called leptin. Leptin is supposed to increase your metabolism and reduce your appetite. However, inflammation blocks the action of leptin. Weight can also cause leptin resistance, much like insulin resistance causes type 2 diabetes.

It is evident, then, that unless one changes the type of chemical messages being sent by the cells, one is fighting a losing (alternating with "gaining") battle. Conversely, by getting our cells to send the right chemical messages, we can increase energy, reduce appetite, burn fat, enhance mood, and have a better functioning immune system at the same time.

Strategies for Weight Loss

There are four basic strategies to achieving this goal, as follows.

1. Start with an Attitude Adjustment

There is a simple but powerful principle—whatever we focus our mental energy on, we tend to create. Most people hate certain things about themselves and their bodies. For instance, they may not like their stomach or their thighs or their complexion.

Mentally and emotionally, we associate being "wrong" with the need to be "punished." So negative attitudes about the body make us want to punish the body for being "wrong." This is why many people are driven to unhealthy diet or exercise regimens in trying to achieve the ideal image of weight and beauty. Real beauty comes from health and inner happiness. It radiates from within as a glowing complexion, sparkling, clear eyes, and a happy countenance.

If you stop and think about it, the biggest reason people pig out on junk food (or acquire any other bad habit) is that they are unhappy. Being unhappy sends the wrong chemical messages to your cells. So "beating yourself up" mentally and emotionally for being overweight is only going to perpetuate the problem.

Conversely, it has been scientifically documented that pleasurable experiences (such as loving relationships, laughter, enjoyable activities, time spent in nature, etc.) cause the body to send out chemical messages that reduce inflammation, enhance immunity, promote healing, improve metabolism, and otherwise improve health and well-being. In fact, the biggest single factor in having a long and healthy life isn't your weight, diet, or exercise level—it's your attitude. People who experience pleasure in life live longer, healthier lives.

So instead of being hard on yourself, be gentle with yourself and find ways to experience pleasure in your life. Do things that help you find joy and fulfillment. Practice the *Pleasure Prescription* strategy.

This includes enjoying your food! Make a decision to enjoy whatever you decide to eat (even if it isn't the healthiest food). This means taking time to notice the color, aroma, texture, and taste of each bite. It also means eating your food slowly and chewing it thoroughly. A good way to train yourself to do this is to put your fork or spoon down after each bite and take some nice deep breaths while chewing. If you just do this, you'll automatically eat less and feel more satisfied.

Remember that all healing, including losing weight, is inherently about love and nurturing, not fear and deprivation. So if your self-talk is negative, start changing it. A good way to do that is to keep a journal and write down your feelings about yourself and your body. Then, start affirming that you love yourself, that you are loving and caring for your body.

2. Focus on Healthy Food

The single biggest reason why so many Americans are overweight and sick is because we are eating refined and processed foods. These foods are lacking in vitamins, minerals, enzymes, and other phytonutrients the body is looking to obtain from food. When we eat these foods, we may be getting enough calories, but we still feel hungry because the body is still looking for the nutrition it needs.

Refined sugars (e.g. sucrose, high fructose corn syrup), white flour, polished rice, processed vegetable oils, margarine, shortening, and most processed and packaged foods fall into this category. If you want to lose weight and be healthy, you must start eliminating these foods from your diet and replacing them with whole, natural, nutrient-rich, unprocessed foods. When you do so your body will get the nutrition it needs and stop telling you it is hungry.

Of course, if you focus on the negative (what you shouldn't be eating) you'll never succeed. The way to succeed is to start incorporating more whole, natural foods into your diet. Eat plenty of fresh vegetables and fruits (with a greater emphasis on vegetables that are not starchy). Choose good sources of protein for your blood type and eat high quality protein and vegetables as your primary food source. Go easy on grains (bread, pasta, etc.) and only use whole grains when you do eat them. Eat high quality fats too. Eat the foods that are good for you first and your body will start craving the good foods while your desire for the "junk" foods will diminish. See the *Eat Healthy* and *Low-Glycemic Diet* strategies.

3. Eat Small, Regular Meals

Here is a surefire recipe for gaining weight, even on good food. Skip breakfast and eat a big meal right before going to bed. This puts your blood sugar on a roller coaster and results in a daily famine-feast cycle. You aren't hungry in the morning, so you don't eat. Your body, thinking it is starving, sends messengers to lower your metabolism and energy level throughout the day. By night, your body is starving and you eat too much. However, since you are inactive (going to sleep), the body stores the excess calories for tomorrow's "famine."

To change this cycle, always "break your fast" by eating something for breakfast. Start the day with some quality fat and protein. For example: avocado, eggs, meat or whole milk yogurt with fruit and nuts. You can also try taking a couple of teaspoons of coconut oil. This sets your metabolism to start burning fat instead of storing it.

When you eat carbohydrates for breakfast, you raise insulin levels, which prompts the body to store fat. Starting off with a meal that contains fat and protein, not just carbs, kicks a hormone called glucagon into action and mobilizes stored sugars.

Then, whenever you feel a little bit hungry during the day, eat a healthy snack such as nuts, fruit, organic cheese, fresh vegetables, tuna, a salad, etc. By eating small regular meals, your body realizes there's no more famine and will start adjusting your appetite accordingly. You won't be so hungry at night and won't overeat at bedtime. You will feel better, and these meals will help you lose weight.

4. Get Physically Active

Forty-eight million Americans are considered sedentary, which contributes directly to obesity. Being sedentary means one doesn't get enough exercise to maintain health.

Almost every system of the body is affected by exercise. Exercise tones the heart, which is a muscle and needs exercise as much as other muscles do. It also increases the body's ability to use oxygen, raises the amount of blood pumping through the body, decreases blood pressure, lubricates the joints, and makes the body function better in the use and storing of calories. That means better health and less excess body fat.

Don't worry—this doesn't mean you have to go to the gym. Choose physical activities that you enjoy, such as swimming, riding a bike, playing a sport, gardening, or hiking. Just getting out and taking a walk every day is helpful. You can also consider yoga or tai chi, as these exercises also help reduce stress. Resistance exercise (such as weight lifting) helps increase weight loss, because muscle tissue burns more calories than fat. So consider doing at least a little bit of weight lifting.

Underlying Health Problems

Part of the secret to dealing with excess weight is to identify specific underlying issues and correct them with appropriate supplements and lifestyle changes. You may want to consult a natural health professional to help identify them, but here are a few of the most important problems to consider.

Low Thyroid

The body burns fat in order to stay warm, and the gland that sends the chemical messages to burn that fat is the thyroid. Low thyroid levels of thyroid hormones are extremely common, especially among women, and can result in weight gain, fatigue, depression, cold hands and feet, and dry skin. If you have any of these symptoms, consider supporting your thyroid. If lab tests show you have normal levels of thyroid hormones, but you still exhibit symptoms of hypothyroidism, you may have a problem with conversion of T4 (the inactive form of the thyroid hormone) to T3, the active form. *The Target Mineral Thyroid Formula* can boost your thyroid to help with weight loss.

Toxic Overload

Toxins contribute to weight gain in two ways. First, toxins cause inflammation, and inflammation causes fluid retention in the tissues. The rapid weight loss most people experience at the beginning of any diet program or cleanse is typically due to a reduction of inflammation and fluid retention.

The second reason toxins contribute to weight gain has to do with the fact that many toxins we're exposed to are fat-soluble. So if the body can't break them down, it stores them in fat. It may also increase cholesterol levels to transport them. The body won't release the fat if it can't deal with the toxins.

This is why learning to eat natural foods is critical to weight loss. Not only are natural foods free of the chemical additives found in processed foods, but they also contain more vitamins and minerals to break down toxins. It also explains why a cleanse can help a person lose weight.

The *Weight Loss Cleansing Program* is a great way to start any weight loss program. Be aware that most of the weight lost on a cleanse is not fat; it is simply water retained in the tissues from inflammation. It is not uncommon for people to lose five to ten pounds after a cleanse, but the loss of fat proceeds more slowly (about one to two pounds per week).

Adding fiber to the diet is another way to increase weight loss. Fiber binds toxins for removal and results in a feeling of fullness that reduces appetite. Be sure to take fiber supplements with plenty of water.

Stress

Stress and unresolved emotional issues can also contribute to weight gain. Many people eat to feed emotional needs. Stress also releases hormones from the adrenals like cortisol, which causes a breakdown of muscle tissue and can contribute to creating fat deposits. Stress can also cause a release of other chemicals that create food cravings and otherwise upset the body's biochemistry.

Keeping an emotional journal where you can write down your feelings when you are having the desire to eat junk food, or otherwise fail to take care of your body, can help you identify and fulfill your real emotional needs. Cravings for sugar and sweets often signal a lack of joy or "sweetness" in one's life. Finding ways to bring more joy into your life can help fulfill those emotional needs in more constructive ways.

Supplements that help you deal with stress more effectively, such as the *Corisol-Reducing Formula* or the *Ashwagandha Complex Formula* may help reduce stress levels and inhibit excess cortisol production. This can be particularly helpful where there is abdominal fat due to stress.

Depression may also be involved in weight problems and food cravings; 5-HTP can help increase serotonin levels, which can reduce appetite and improve mood. Remember that cortisol is also released in response to chronic inflammation, so a supplement with antioxidant and anti-inflammatory properties can also help to reduce cortisol output. Reducing inflammation also increases metabolism and helps leptin, the fat-burning hormone, work more efficiently.

Food Cravings

Sometimes it seems that food cravings are our worst enemy when trying to change our diet. Therefore, supplements that reduce appetite or specific food cravings may also be helpful as part of a weight loss program. Cravings for sugar are signs of blood sugar problems and usually indicate that the diet is lacking fat and protein. Try an *Appetite Reducer* or a *Sugar Craving Reducer Formula*.

Poor Fat Metabolism

If you eliminate simple sugars and starches in the diet by adopting the *Low-Glycemic* or *Ketogenic Diet* strategies while increasing physical activity, your body will start burning fats instead of carbohydrates, which will help you start burning off fat reserves. You can boost this process using the *Garcinia Fat-Burning Formula*. Guggul and berberine also helps this process.

Strategies: Affirmation and Visualization, Avoid Sugar, Blood Type Diet, Detoxification, Eat Enzyme-Rich Foods, Eat Healthy, Emotional Healing Work, Exercise, Fasting, Healthy Fats, Hydration, Increase

Dietary Fiber, Ketogenic Diet, Low-Glycemic Diet, Pleasure Prescription, Sleep, and Stress Management

Formulas: 5-HTP Adaptogen, Fat-Absorbing Fiber, **Garcinia Fat-Burning**, Skinny, Target Mineral Thyroid, Hypothyroid, Cortisol-Reducing, Chinese Qi-Increasing, **Whole Food Protein**, Sugar Craving Reducer, Metabolic Stimulant, Ashwagandha Complex, and Digestive Support

Programs: Weight Loss Cleansing and Ivy Bridge's Cleansing

Herbs: Acacia, bee pollen, black currant, bladderwrack, chia, **chickweed**, coconut, coffee, cyperus, dulse, garcinia, ginseng (American), **guggul**, gymnema, Irish moss, kelp, licorice, psyllium, and **tea**

Supplements: 5-HTP, **7-keto**, **berberine**, **collagen**, colostrum, **L-carnitine**, **L-glutamine**, L-phenylalaine, L-tryptophan, omega-3 EFAs, omega-6 CLA, sodium alginate, and vanadium

Essential Oils: Grapefruit (pink) and lemon

Exercise (Performance)

When you're exercising you can use herbs and nutrients to help you get better results. The *Enhancing Nitric Oxide* strategy is a very useful strategy for people who are having trouble exercising. It enhances endurance and stamina.

Adaptogens have also been shown to improve athletic performance and stamina, so consider using some adaptogenic herbs when exercising. When exercising, it's important to stay well hydrated and to get adequate amounts of mineral electrolytes which can be lost due to sweat.

Strategies: Enhance Nitric Oxide, Hydration, Low-Glycemic Diet, and Mineralization

Formulas: Adaptogen-Immune, Mitochondria Energy, **Vandergriff's Energy Booster**, Algae, Antioxidant, Chinese Qi-Increasing, **Electrolyte Drink**, Chinese Wood-Increasing, Whole Food Protein, **Nitric Oxide Boosting**, and **Adaptogen**

Herbs: Cordyceps, **eleuthero**, ginseng (American), ginseng (Asian/Korean), rhodiola, and schisandra

Supplements: Colostrum, multiple vitamin and mineral, N-acetyl cysteine, omega-6 CLA, and selenium

Exercise (Recovery)

See also body building

Boosting nitric oxide aids exercise recovery. See the *Enhancing Nitric Oxide* strategy and take the *Nitric Oxide Boosting Formula* prior to exercise. Try using the *Electrolyte Drink Powder* with plenty of water after exercise. A number of adaptogenic herbs, like eleuthero and cordyceps, have also been shown to help improve athletic performance.

A tea made with safflower will help to neutralize lactic acid buildup and ease sore muscles. You can make this tea using 4 capsules or 1 teaspoon safflower in a quart of water. Drink the entire quart to ease muscle soreness. Sore muscles can also be massaged with a *Topical Analgesic Formula* or *Analgesic EO Blend*.

Strategies: Bodywork, Enhance Nitric Oxide, Hydration, Low-Glycemic Diet, Lymph-Moving Pain Relief, Mineralization, and Sleep

Formulas: Colloidal Mineral, **Topical Analgesic**, Joint Healing Nutrients, CBD Topical Analgesic, Male Performance, Nitric Oxide Boosting, **Electrolyte Drink**, and Adaptogen

Essential Oil Blends: Analgesic EO

Herbs: Barley, bee pollen, beet, **cordyceps**, **eleuthero**, rhodiola, and **safflower**

Supplements: **L-arginine**, omega-3 EFAs, omega-6 CLA, and potassium

Essential Oils: Wintergreen

Eye Health

See also cataracts, conjunctivitis, glaucoma, macular degeneration, sty, and diabetic retinopathy

Eye health is not isolated from general health. In fact, most eye diseases are signs of deeper health problems, such as stress, free radical damage, diabetes, and circulatory disorders. To maintain healthy eyes and/or improve eyesight consider the following strategies.

Use Antioxidants

Certain antioxidants called carotenoids are particularly critical to eye health. One of these is beta-carotene, which is a precursor to the formation of vitamin A. Two other carotenoids are also essential for healthy eyes. These are lutein and zeaxanthin. Lutein is found in the macula (the center of the retina) and has been shown to counteract free radical damage caused by blue and ultraviolet light. It protects against macular degeneration and inhibits the formation of cataracts (the number one cause of blindness in the elderly). Zeaxanthin also protects the macula from light damage and inhibits cataract formation.

Several antioxidant vitamins are also essential to eye health, including vitamins A, E, and C. Vitamin A is extremely critical to eye health. In fact, another name for vitamin A is retinol (showing its relationship to protecting the retina of the eye). Vitamin A keeps fats in the eye from oxidizing and prevents the eye from dehydrating by helping with tear formation. A deficiency is known to cause blindness. Carrots are high in beta-carotene, a precursor to vitamin A, which explains why they have a reputation for aiding the eyes.

Vitamin E is found in both the retina and the lens. Adequate intake of this fat-soluble vitamin reduces the risk of cataract formation. It also works with bioflavonoids to inhibit macular degeneration.

Vitamin C is also critical to eye health because it helps protect the capillaries nourishing the eye tissue. It reduces pressure in glaucoma (the second leading cause of blindness), reduces cataract formation, and helps rebuild the cornea when it has been damaged.

Eat Healthy Fats

The eyes, like the brain, need good fats to be healthy too. Omega-3 essential fatty acids, especially DHA, are critical to eye health. DHA helps with communicating information from the eyes to the brain. Good fats also lubricate the eyes and keep them from drying out. See the *Healthy Fats* strategy.

Prevent Eyestrain

Poor nutrition isn't the only reason eyesight deteriorates. Eyes need exposure to natural sunlight, and artificial lighting plays a part in our diminishing eye health. Stress, and, more particularly, eye-strain, also plays a big role in vision problems.

In fact, the major reason myopia (nearsightedness) is becoming increasingly common is the amount of time people are spending doing close-up work like reading and working on computers. Constantly staring at these nearby objects strains the eyes, which need to regularly shift their focus from looking at nearby objects to objects in the distance, to stay relaxed. The eye-strain caused by working at computer terminals and other close-up work creates muscle tension that inhibits the eyes from relaxing and seeing in the distance.

Taking a periodic break to relax the eyes and allow them to see into the distance helps prevent eyestrain. There are also exercises which can be done to improve vision. You can do an internet search and find information about these exercises if you wish to improve your eyesight.

Protect the Eyes from Injury

A final, but extremely important aspect of general eye health is protecting the eyes from injury. It is very important when working with chain saws, weed trimmers, and other power tools to wear protective eye gear. About two thousand cases of eye injury occur daily, and most of these could be prevented with protective eye-wear.

Strategies: Compress or Fomentation, Eat Healthy, Healthy Fats, and Hydration

Formulas: Oral Chelation, **Antioxidant Eye**, and Herbal Eyewash

Herbs: Bilberry, eyebright, and lycium

Supplements: Lutein, omega-3 DHA, **vitamin A**, **vitamin C**, vitamin E, and **zeaxanthin**

Eye Infection   see *conjunctivitis* **and** *sty*

Eyes, Bloodshot

See also conjunctivitis and eyes (red/itching)

Bloodshot eyes are eyes with many red blood vessels showing in the whites of the eyes. This may be caused by fatigue, stress, irritation, or an infection. Herbs can be used topically to reduce irritation to the eyes in the form of a wash or a compress. Tea bags are great for eye compresses: Dip a tea bag (chamomile or green tea works great) into hot water for a second or two just to get the herbs damp. Let the bag cool until it is safe to put on the skin. Close your eye and lay the warm tea bag over your closed eyelid for an instant compress. An *Antioxidant Eye Formula* can also be taken internally.

Strategies: Compress or Fomentation and Hydration

Formulas: Antioxidant Eye

Herbs: Bilberry, **chamomile**, eyebright, and **tea**

Supplements: Vitamin C

Eyes, Red/Itching

See also allergies (respiratory) and rhinitis

Eyes can become red due to stress or irritation. When they are red and itchy, it is typically an allergic reaction. An *Herbal Eye Wash Formula* can be used topically to ease the redness. The alkaloids in goldenseal were once used in a popular over-the-counter eye-drop that promised to take the redness away from tired and sore eyes. A chamomile or green tea bag can be used as a compress. For allergy-related problems, see *rhinitis or allergies (respiratory)*.

Strategies: Compress or Fomentation, Eat Healthy, Hydration, and Stress Management

Formulas: Jeannie Burgess' Allergy-Lung, Antihistamine, Antioxidant, and **Herbal Eyewash**

Herbs: Chamomile, chickweed, chicory, chrysanthemum, eyebright, **goldenseal**, marshmallow, and tea

Supplements: Vitamin A and vitamin C

Failure to Thrive

Failure to thrive is a problem when infants don't gain weight and develop properly. If a child is not gaining weight properly you should have them checked by a medical doctor.

If there are no serious health issues, try changing the mother's diet (if nursing) or the infant's formula can be helpful. It may also help to mix a small amount of plant enzymes with food. A little bit of black-strap molasses and some gruel made with slippery elm may also be beneficial.

Strategies: Eat Enzyme-Rich Foods

Formulas: Plant Enzyme, Whole Food Green Drink, and Algae

Herbs: Flax seed, marshmallow, and slippery elm

Supplements: L-lysine, omega-3 DHA, and omega-3 EFAs

Fainting

Fainting happens when a person suddenly feels weak or as if they are about to lose consciousness. This may be caused by a variety of factors, including anemia, poor circulation, low blood pressure, low blood sugar, or shock. Persistent fainting should be checked by a medical doctor to determine the cause. The following remedies may be helpful, depending on the cause.

Formulas: Brain-Heart and Hypoglycemic

Flower Essence Blends: Shock and Injury FE

Herbs: Anemarrhena, capsicum, and **licorice**

Essential Oils: Lavender

Fat Cravings

See also fat metabolism (poor) and gallbladder problems

The body needs good fats, and contrary to popular opinion, good fats are essential to health. Good fats include organic butter from grass-fed cows, coconut oil, olive oil, avocados, flaxseeds, chia seeds, hemp seeds, walnuts, macadamias, deep-ocean fish, and fat from grass-fed animals.

When a person craves fats constantly, they is probably not getting enough essential fatty acids in their diet or not digesting and metabolizing fats correctly. Lipase enzymes and cholagogue herbs that activate bile flow may help. These include herbs like barberry, dandelion, and fringetree. See *fat metabolism (poor)* for more information.

Strategies: Gallbladder Flush and Healthy Fats

Formulas: GLA Oil, Chinese Wood-Decreasing, Christopher's Gallbladder, **Lipase Enzyme**, and Digestive Support

Herbs: Barberry, black currant, burdock, chickweed, dandelion, evening primrose, **fringe tree**, gentian, milk thistle, and turmeric

Supplements: Bile salt, krill oil, **lipase**, and **omega-3 EFAs**

Fat Metabolism, Poor

See also gallbladder problems, hypothyroidism, and fatty liver disease

If you have a problem digesting fats, start by taking lipase enzymes and/or bile salts or a formula that contains both. You may also need cholagogue herbs like artichoke, fringetree, dandelion, or barberry to stimulate gallbladder function.

The inability to properly or adequately digest and assimilate lipid or fat-containing foods is common in individuals who have had their gallbladders removed. If this is the case, ox bile and pancreatin taken in supplement form, such as the *Digestive Support Formula*, may help. Lipase enzymes may also be helpful.

Problems utilizing fats in the body may be due to problems with the liver, thyroid, spleen, prostate, or uterus. If you have low thyroid, or have had your uterus or prostate removed, consult with a professional herbalist for suggestions (findanherbalist.com or americanherbalistsguild.com).

Strategies: Gallbladder Flush

Formulas: Skinny, Thyroid Glandular, Digestive Support, Chinese Wood-Decreasing, Christopher's Gallbladder, and **Lipase Enzyme**

Herbs: Artichoke, **barberry**, burdock, chickweed, dandelion root, and **fringe tree**

Supplements: Bile salt, L-glutamine, **lipase**, omega-6 CLA, and pancreatin

Essential Oils: Orange (sweet)

Fatigue

See also adrenal fatigue, anemia, depression, Hashimoto's disease, hypoglycemia, hypothyroidism, insomnia, tension, and mitochondrial dysfunction

Fatigue is a symptom that something is wrong with energy production in the body. Many systems are involved in energy production, so it is important to identify which systems need support. So consider all the related conditions listed above. Here are some strategies to help you regain energy if you are excessively fatigued.

Don't Use Stimulants

Stimulants like caffeine and even many adaptogens don't actually increase energy. Instead, they cause the body to dip into its energy reserves, which means that over time, they deepen fatigue. It then takes more and more of the stimulant to have an effect. So if you're tired, avoid stimulants and figure out what's causing the lack of energy and correct it.

Get Adequate Sleep

One of the major causes of fatigue is a simple lack of sleep. The body rebuilds its energy reserves through rest. If we do not get eight to nine hours of sleep each night, we can wind up with a sleep debt that results in low energy levels. The person suffering from a lack of sleep further depletes their energy by using stimulants and a vicious cycle of energy loss ensues. Read about the *Sleep* strategy and look up remedies for *insomnia*.

Check Your Thyroid and Adrenals

Another major cause of fatigue is low thyroid. When low thyroid is the problem, the person may be cold, have difficulty losing weight, and have problems with dry skin. *Hypothyroid Formulas* may be of help, but this problem may require other remedies. Also read about *hypothyroidism and hashimoto's disease*.

When the adrenals are involved in the fatigue, the person may have symptoms like a quivering tongue, dark circles under their eyes, and restless sleep. *Adrenal Tonic* or *Adaptogen Formulas* should be helpful (see *adrenal fatigue*).

Balance Your Blood Sugar

Low blood sugar will cause fatigue in the afternoons or sudden fatigue a few hours after eating. The nose or limbs will suddenly go cold and the person may have difficulty concentrating. Licorice root or *Energy-Boosting Formulas* may be of benefit here. Dehydration will also cause fatigue and increase the craving for sugary foods (see *hypoglycemia*).

Check for Anemia

Anemia may also be a cause of fatigue. If you are pale and get cold or tired easily, try an *Iron Formula*. Approximately 60 percent of Americans have a mild to severe B_{12} deficiency. This can create fatigue, insomnia, tingling in the fingers and toes, and poor digestion. So also take vitamin B_{12}. See *anemia* for more information.

Other Possible Causes

Fatigue can be associated with depression, poor digestion, having a toxic body, exposure to excessive electromagnetic radiation, micochondrial dysfunction, and not getting enough exercise. Check out these related conditions for more information. You may also want to find an herbalist or naturopath that can help you sort out the underlying cause of your fatigue (findanherbalist.com or americanherbalistsguild.com).

Strategies: Alkalize the Body, Balance Methylation, Eat Healthy, Hydration, Low-Glycemic Diet, Reduce Chemical Exposure, Reduce EMF Exposure, and Sleep

Formulas: Adaptogen-Immune, Adrenal Glandular, Chinese Wood-Increasing, **Mitochondria Energy,**

Vandergriff's Energy Booster, Christopher's Herbal Iron, Chinese Qi-Regulating, **Chinese Fire-Increasing**, Suma Adaptogen, Target Mineral Thyroid, **Chinese Qi and Blood Tonic**, Algae, **Chinese Qi-Increasing**, Metabolic Stimulant, Stimulating Energy, **Methyl B12 Vitamin**, Hypothyroid, and **Ashwagandha Complex**

Essential Oil Blends: Balancing EO, Renewing and Releasing EO, Refreshing and Cleansing EO, and Analgesic EO

Herbs: Ashwagandha, **bee pollen**, capsicum, cinnamon, cocoa, **codonopsis**, coffee, cordyceps, **damiana**, dulse, **eleuthero**, epimedium, ginseng (American), ginseng (Asian/Korean), gotu kola, guarana, jujube, kelp, **licorice**, **maca**, muira puama, oat, rhodiola, **spirulina**, suma, vanilla, and yerba maté

Supplements: Chlorophyll, Co-Q10, **iron**, L-carnitine, L-glutamine, magnesium, multiple vitamin and mineral, **vitamin B-complex**, **vitamin B_{12}**, vitamin B_3, vitamin B_5, vitamin B_6, and vitamin C

Essential Oils: Cinnamon, fir, jasmine, lemon, lime, peppermint, pine, ravensara, rosemary, thyme, and ylang ylang

Fatty Liver Disease

The accumulation of fat in the liver of people who drink little or no alcohol is called nonalcoholic fatty liver disease. It is common and, in most people, causes no signs or symptoms.

For some people, however, it can lead to inflammation, scarring of the liver, and eventually liver failure. It is probably related to a diet high in refined carbohydrates and processed oils. Essential fatty acid supplements should be avoided by people with fatty liver disease.

Some herbs that may be helpful in getting rid of fat in the liver include chickweed, milk thistle, and burdock. Take these herbs with lipase enzyme supplements and a *Fiber Blend*. Also adopt the *Low-Glycemic Diet* strategy.

Strategies: Avoid Sugar, Fasting, Forgiveness, Gallbladder Flush, Gut-Healing Diet, Increase Dietary Fiber, Liver Detoxification, and Low-Glycemic Diet

Formulas: **Skinny**, **Hepatoprotective**, Fat-Absorbing Fiber, Fiber, **Lipase Enzyme**, and Digestive Support

Herbs: Burdock, chickweed, and **milk thistle**

Supplements: **Choline**, iodine, **L-carnitine**, L-threonine, and lipase

Essential Oils: Geranium

Fatty Tumors/Deposits

See also fat metabolism (poor), hypothyroidism, and fatty liver disease

These are abnormal growths that are mostly composed of lipid or fatty material. Herbs that have been used historically to break up these deposits include burdock, chickweed, and red clover. Guggul lipids may also be helpful.

Low thyroid could also contribute to the development of these deposits. Seaweeds, like kelp, dulse, and bladderwrack, have been used historically both to aid the thyroid and to shrink swollen masses in the body. So taking an *Herbal Thyroid Formula* containing these seaweeds might help. Iodine supplements may also be helpful.

Strategies: Gallbladder Flush

Formulas: **Skinny**, Garcinia Fat-Burning, and Hypothyroid

Herbs: **Bladderwrack**, burdock, **chickweed**, dulse, garcinia, **guggul**, Irish moss, and **kelp**

Supplements: **Iodine** and lipase

Essential Oils: Geranium

Fear

See also adrenal fatigue, hypoglycemia, and anxiety disorders

Fear is the emotion we feel when situations arise that we perceive have a great potential for pain or loss. Fear can arise from potentially painful or traumatizing situations, but it can also arise in positive situations where there is a lot at stake (such as starting a new relationship or a new business).

Fear strongly affects the systems that regulate body functions, such as the glandular system (particularly the adrenal glands and thyroid) and the nerves. It activates the parasympathetic nervous system and the adrenal glands to produce a heightened state of energy and tension. This response primes the body to be ready for optimal action, not just to "fight or flee," but to be able to physically perform to the best of our abilities.

In dangerous situations, fear is a useful emotion. It can prompt us to be alert and careful and help us make choices that keep us safe.

However, some fears have no basis in any real danger. Children are born with only a few natural fears. Most fears are learned from parents and other adults. That is, children sense when their parents are afraid of something, and they adopt the same fear. Many fears are rooted in experiences that wounded the person emotionally. For example, many adults are afraid of making mistakes because past mistakes caused them pain. Children have no such fear.

Overcoming Irrational Fears

Any fear that is not based in an actual danger—that is, something that can cause you actual physical or psychological harm—is not a healthy fear. If other people are able to do something safely and it frightens you, then the fear is likely based in emotional wounds or unrealistic thought processes. These are the fears that people need to overcome if they want to improve their lives.

What overcomes these unhealthy fears is the ability to take action in spite of them. When the energy produced by the fear response is channeled into action, it fulfills its purpose and fuels us for maximum performance. Courage is the ability to take action in spite of our fear. Both the hero and the coward feel fear on the battlefield, but the hero is able to do what he needs to do in spite of his fear. Courage is the ability we have to allow our mind to override the anxiety and stress we feel, make the best choice we can, and then take appropriate action.

When the energy of fear is channeled into constructive action through exercising courage, it builds excitement and self-confidence. People who are able to overcome their fears and take calculated risks develop strong "wills" instead of "won'ts." These people develop the confidence that they can handle what life brings to them and rise above it. This allows them to lead more exciting lives, achieving the status of the "hero." Those who are unable to take action in the face of fear are allowing cowardice to keep them stuck in mediocrity.

Strategies for Reducing Fear

The *Fear Reducing FE* and individual flower remedies like aspen, mimulus, and borage can help a person deal with fear. Essential oils like bergamot, frankincense, sandalwood, and ylang-ylang can also be helpful in calming fear.

Keeping blood sugar stable with the *Low-Glycemic Diet* strategy also reduces fear. Interestingly, traditional systems of medicine associate fear with the kidneys. In Traditional Chinese medicine, the water element is associated with fear and is connected to the kidneys, urinary bladder, and adrenal glands. The *Chinese Water-Decreasing* or *Chinese Water-Increasing Formulas* may be helpful for fear. Following the *Hydration* strategy can help a person feel more relaxed in difficult circumstances, as dehydration interferes with brain function.

Because the adrenal glands are involved in fear, an *Adrenal Glandular* or *Adaptagen-Immune Formula* may also help to reduce fears. B-complex vitamins and vitamin C also support the adrenal glands and can help to reduce feelings of stress and fear. So you could also try the *Anti-Stress B-Complex Formula*.

Strategies: Affirmation and Visualization, Aromatherapy, Counseling or Therapy, Emotional Healing Work, Flower Essence, Hydration, Low-Glycemic Diet, Meditation, Sleep, and Stress Management

Formulas: Chinese Water-Increasing, **Adrenal Glandular**, Chinese Fire-Decreasing, Chinese Water-Decreasing, Anti-Anxiety, Chinese Earth-Increasing, **Chinese Fire-Increasing**, Adaptogen-Immune, and **Anti-Stress B-Complex**

Essential Oil Blends: Balancing EO

Flower Essence Blends: Shock and Injury FE and **Fear-Reducing FE**

Herbs: Black currant, chamomile, eleuthero, ginseng (American), licorice, **reishi**, Saint John's wort, and schisandra

Supplements: Amber (succinum), GABA, vitamin B-complex, and vitamin C

Essential Oils: Bergamot, chamomile (Roman), eucalyptus, **frankincense**, jasmine, lavender, lemon, myrrh, neroli, **sandalwood**, and **ylang ylang**

Fever

See also infection (bacterial) and infection (viral)

Most of the time fevers are generated by the immune system as part of its effort to fight infection. Unless the fever is very high (104 or higher) or lasts more than a day or two, it is not a cause for serious concern.

In my experience, especially with children, fever will go down as soon as the bowel is cleared. An herbalist, who used to be a nurse many years ago, told me that hospitals once administered enemas to people with fevers because it helped to bring the fever down. Obviously this isn't done anymore, but it still works.

A solution of herbal tea or a liquid herbal product added to water will make the enema more effective. Catnip, yarrow, elderflower, peppermint, chamomile, and garlic make good enema solutions.

The other strategy for bringing down fever is to induce perspiration. Herbs that do this are called sudorifics or diaphoretics, and were traditionally used to fight acute infections. Some useful diaphoretics include yarrow, peppermint, chamomile, catnip, ginger, and capsicum. Ideally, these should be taken as warm teas or as extracts taken with warm water.

Yarrow is particularly helpful for serious fevers when taken in the form of a hot tea, but it tastes better when combined with peppermint and other more pleasant-tasting herbs as it is in the *Children's Composition Formula*.

Boneset is a good herb for fever associated with the flu, where the bones ache. Garlic (especially raw garlic) is another herb that can help with fevers, especially when caused by bacterial infection or respiratory infection.

Generally speaking, sour herbs like lemon, lycium (gogi or wolfberries), acai, mangosteen, and elderberries contain antioxidants that will reduce fever and inflammation in the body. Historically, white willow bark was used for fever and inflammation. However, I do not recommend using willow to reduce fevers as this is actually suppressing immune activity that is fighting the infection.

Essential oils like chamomile, lemon, lavender, peppermint, rosemary, and thyme, can be used topically as an aromatherapy application for fevers. Dilute them in lukewarm water, then moisten a washcloth with the aromatic water and gently sponge off the fevered person.

If a fever is high, or doesn't respond to natural remedies within a day or two, seek appropriate medical attention.

Strategies: Colon Hydrotherapy, Hydration, and Sweat Bath

Formulas: **Chinese Yang-Reducing**, **Antioxidant**, Stabilized Allicin, Elderberry Cold and Flu, Herbal Composition, Ed Millet's Herbal Crisis, and **Steven Horne's Children's Composition**

Herbs: Anemarrhena, baical skullcap, bamboo, **boneset**, borage, bupleurum, capsicum, catnip, chamomile, chicory, chirata, devil's claw, echinacea, **elder flowers**, **feverfew**, forsythia, **gardenia**, garlic, ginger, honeysuckle, horehound, isatis, lemon balm, lobelia, lycium, ophiopogon, osha, pau d'arco, peppermint, pleurisy root, purslane, rose hips, rosemary essential oil, sweet annie, thyme essential oil, turmeric, vanilla, **vervain (blue)**, willow, and **yarrow**

Supplements: Nanoparticle silver

Essential Oils: Bay leaf, cajeput, chamomile (Roman), fir, fir, jasmine, lavender, lemon, lemongrass, lime, peppermint, ravintsara, rose, rosemary, and spearmint

Fever Blisters   see *cold sores*

Fibroids, Uterine

See also fibrosis and estrogen dominance

Fibroids are abnormal growths of connective tissue, usually benign, that are found in the uterus or breast. Symptoms of uterine fibroids include heavy menstrual bleeding, abdominal bloating, menstrual cramps, and spotting between periods. Anemia may result from loss of blood, and there may be abdominal pain, pain during intercourse, painful urination, or constipation. Since symptoms are often obscure, it is important to get an accurate medical diagnosis. Once you have a proper diagnosis, you can employ some of the follow strategies to get rid of uterine fibroids.

Balance Hormones

Excess levels of estrogen in the body usually cause fibroids. High levels of estrogen are often the result of xenoestrogens. (See the *Avoid Xenoestrogens* strategy and the condition *estrogen dominance* for more information.) Herbs that help balance estrogen and progesterone like chaste tree and false unicorn may also be helpful.

Decongest the Liver

Fibroids can be related to congestion in the liver, so a cleanse of the liver and colon may be of help. Use a *Detoxifying Formula* and a *Fiber Blend* or follow the *Detoxification* strategy. Indole-3-carbinol helps break down excess estrogens. It is found naturally in cruciferous vegetables.

Adopt a Healthier Lifestyle

Factors that increase the risk of uterine fibroids are too much caffeine, too much of the wrong kinds of fats in the diet, deficiencies of essential fatty acids, hormone imbalances, underactive thyroid, birth control pills, and X-rays. Obesity and family history of fibroids further increase the tendency for them to develop. Follow the *Eat Healthy* strategy and adopt a healthier lifestyle in general to reduce these risk factors.

Try Some Herbal Remedies

Yarrow has been helpful in breaking up fibroids in many cases. It is also a good herb for arresting the heavy bleeding that sometimes accompanies uterine fibroids. The *Internal Bleeding* or *Female Tonic Formula* may also be helpful.

Protect The Uterus

The uterus helps the body metabolize fats and having it removed can cause permanent problems with fat metabolism, which can lead to weight and heart problems. The uterus serves many important functions, and if possible, should not be removed. Using some of the remedies described here, it is possible to get rid of uterine fibroids without having a hysterectomy.

Strategies: Avoid Xenoestrogens, Detoxification, Eat Healthy, and Reduce Chemical Exposure

Formulas: **Internal Bleeding**, Female Tonic, Detoxifying, and Digestive Support

Herbs: **Chaste tree**, dong quai, false unicorn, and **yarrow**

Supplements: **Indole-3-carbinol**, iodine, lecithin, omega-3 EFAs, and vitamin E

Essential Oils: Frankincense and helichrysum

Fibromyalgia

See also autoimmune disorders, Epstein-Barr virus, and SIBO

Fibromyalgia syndrome (FMS) can cause severe pain and impair deep sleep. It is a stress-related autoimmune disorder, and many of the symptoms mimic those of chronic fatigue syndrome (CFS) and arthritis.

Symptoms of fibromyalgia include painful, tender, and recurrent aches in various points all over the body. There is a persistent, but diffused pain in the structural system (bones and muscles), accompanied by fatigue, headaches, general weakness, irritable bowel, poor sleep patterns, digestive problems, and nervous system problems (depression and anxiety).

Modern medicine hasn't identified the cause of FMS, but it is likely caused by diet and lifestyle factors, as evidenced by the fact that many people have experienced relief from FMS by making diet and lifestyle changes. While there is no magic bullet formula or secret recipe of things to do to cure FMS, working on the suspected causes will probably bring relief, if not complete recovery. Here are the basic strategies.

Adopt a Healthy Diet

Nutrition should be a person's first concern in overcoming FMS. A mild food diet consisting primarily of fresh vegetables with some fruits has led to a reduction in joint stiffness and pain in many FMS suffers. Sugar, refined carbohydrates, processed vegetable oils, shortening, margarine, and processed, packaged foods should be avoided. See the *Eat Healthy*, *Gut-Healing Diet* and *Avoid Sugar* strategies.

Take Iodine and/or Black Walnut

Iodine is an essential nutrient for the thyroid gland and many FMS sufferers also have a dysfunctional thyroid. Dr. David Brownstein, author of *Iodine: Why You Need It, Why You Can't Live Without It*, claims that iodine supplements alone have cured fibromyalgia. You can get iodine from seaweeds or an iodine supplement.

Several natural healers independently discovered that black walnut was helpful for FMS. Black walnut, especially concentrated black walnut, helps the thyroid and is also antimicrobial, antiparasitic, and mildly detoxifying.

Take Magnesium

Magnesium is essential for the synthesis of adenosine triphosphate (ATP), the energy powerhouse for cells. Deficiencies of magnesium causes cells to resort to using anaerobic pathways to produce energy, which leads to lactic acid formation and pain in the muscles. Magnesium ions are also essential to helping muscles relax, so deficiencies lead to muscle stiffness.

Supplements containing magnesium with malic acid have been beneficial for FMS. This combination aids in the production of ATP in the muscles and helps reduce muscle pain and stiffness. It also helps reduce fatigue in people suffering from FMS.

Eat Healthy Fats

Omega-3 essential fatty acids are essential for the health of nerve fibers and aid in the production of chemical messengers resulting in reduced inflammation and pain. Most modern diets are deficient in omega-3 fatty acids, so supplements containing them may also be helpful. See the *Healthy Fats* strategy for more information.

Heal the Gut

One of the biggest contributing factors to FMS and its related conditions may an unhealthy GI tract. See *SIBO* and *dysbiosis* for more information. If these conditions apply, you may wish to take supplements to alter your intestinal microflora and adopt a *Gut-Healing Diet*.

In addition, people who suffer from FMS tend to be low in enzymes and may need enzyme supplements. In many cases, FMS sufferers also have a hiatal hernia that needs to be corrected.

Detoxify, but Gently

FMS sufferers may need to detoxify, but they need to do so slowly and gently. For instance, they may wish to take just one capsule per day of a *Detoxifying* or *Hepatoprotective Formula* along a small amount of a *Fiber Blend* and plenty of water. If you suspect heavy metals may be involved, try using just one capsule of a *Heavy Metal Cleansing Formula* per day along some fiber or algin to bind the heavy metals.

Manage Stress

FMS is most common in hardworking perfectionists. K. P. Khalsa, RH(AHG), has noted that FMS sufferers are usually high-achieving women who are burning the candle at both ends and in the middle too. From this point of view, FMS can be considered a health collapse related to chronic stress.

Chronic stress depletes the adrenal glands, which makes it difficult for the body to control pain and inflammation. See *adrenal fatigue* for more information about this.

People suffering from FMS should learn to pace themselves by setting realistic goals and balancing work with rest and recreation. Taking breaks when one is tired, getting a good night's sleep, and allowing time in one's life for relaxing activities is a must. Consider stretching, meditation, yoga, tai chi, relaxing baths, or long walks in nature. See the *Pleasure Prescription* strategy.

Many people with FMS have found relief through natural healing, but recovery can take time and dedication to lifestyle changes. You will probably want to consult with a qualified professional herbalist or naturopath to help you customize a program for FMS (findanherbalist.com or americanherbalistsguild.com).

Strategies: Affirmation and Visualization, Avoid Sugar, Bodywork, Eat Healthy, Gut-Healing Diet, Healthy Fats, Heavy Metal Cleanse, Hiatal Hernia Correction, Hydration, Increase Dietary Fiber, Pleasure Prescription, and Stress Management

Formulas: Fibromyalgia, Mitochondria Energy, Detoxifying, Plant Enzyme, **Digestive Support**, Antioxidant, **Probiotic**, Hepatoprotective, Fiber, and Adaptogen

Herbs: Ashwagandha, **black walnut**, cannabis, cat's claw, kava kava, kudzu, licorice, lobelia, and yucca

Supplements: 5-HTP, **CBD**, colostrum, indole-3-carbinol, iodine, L-tryptophan, **magnesium**, MSM, omega-3 DHA, omega-3 EFAs, protease, and SAM-e

Essential Oils: Copaiba

Fibrosis

See also fibroids (uterine)

Fibrosis is the abnormal formation of fibrous tissue in a part of the body, such as the lungs, breast, or uterus. Protease enzyme supplements, taken between meals, can help to break down this fibrous tissue. Vitamin E may also be helpful. Castor oil packs may be used to break up fibrosis.

Strategies: Castor Oil Pack

Formulas: Hypothyroid, Thyroid Glandular, and Digestive Support

Herbs: Black currant, devil's claw, evening primrose, licorice, mullein, plantain, and red clover

Supplements: Protease and **vitamin E**

Fingernail Biting

See also nervousness and parasites

Nail biting may be due to nervousness, parasites, or mineral deficiencies. Horsetail, colloidal minerals, or *Watkin's Hair Skin and Nails Formula* can supply minerals that correct deficiencies behind the urge to bite nails. See the *Mineralization* strategy.

If stress and nervous tension are the primary cause try the *Anti-Stress B-Complex Vitamins*. The *Chinese Mineral Qi Adaptogen Formula* will help both stress and mineral deficiencies (see *nervousness*).

Doing a *Parasite Cleansing Program* can help to remove parasites causing deficiencies (see *parasites*).

Strategies: Mineralization and Stress Management

Formulas: Watkin's Hair, Skin, and Nails, Herbal Calcium, **Anti-Stress B-Complex**, Antiparasitic, and **Colloidal Mineral**

Programs: Parasite Cleansing

Herbs: Horsetail

Supplements: Vitamin B-complex

Fingernails, Weak/Brittle

Weak or brittle fingernails are a sign of a lack of silica and other trace minerals. *Watkin's Hair, Skin, and Nails* or *Colloidal Mineral Formula* may be of help. Using the *Bone Broth* strategy is one of the best ways to get these extra minerals naturally.

Strategies: Bone Broth and Mineralization

Formulas: Pet Supplement, **Watkin's Hair, Skin, and Nails**, Herbal Calcium, **Colloidal Mineral**, and Digestive Support

Herbs: Horsetail and **kelp**

Supplements: Collagen, manganese, and **silicon**

Flatulence   see *gas & bloating*

Fleas

Essential oils may be helpful for fleas on pets. A few drops of any of the listed essential oils may be blended with the *Enzyme Spray Formula,* or with water mixed with a few drops of natural soap, and applied topically as a repellant. The powder of the *Standardized Acetogenin Formula* can be added to a shampoo and used to give the animal a bath to help kill fleas.

Formulas: Enzyme Spray and Standardized Acetogenin

Herbs: Pawpaw

Essential Oils: Eucalyptus, lemon, **lemongrass**, pine, **rosemary**, and tea tree

Floaters

Floaters are small black specks that appear to dance or float across the visual field. Possible causes include an unhealthy diet, excessive eyestrain, and inadequate rest. A generally good diet is helpful, along with extra doses of vitamin A, zinc, vitamin C, and magnesium.

An eyewash or compress over the eyes using a tea made from eyebright or chamomile may also be helpful. You can also dip tea bags in warm water to moisten them and place them over the eyes as a compress.

Strategies: Compress or Fomentation and Eat Healthy

Herbs: Bayberry, **chamomile**, **eyebright**, and goldenseal

Supplements: Magnesium, protease, **vitamin A**, **vitamin C**, vitamin D, and zinc

Flu

Influenza

See also colds and contagious disease prevention

Also known as influenza, the flu refers to viral infections accompanied by nausea, vomiting, diarrhea, fever, malaise, body pain, and respiratory symptoms. The media is constantly warning people about flu epidemics to scare people into getting vaccines, but the truth is that most of the people who die of the flu are elderly or have compromised immune systems and die from secondary infections after getting the flu.

There are numerous effective natural remedies for the flu. For prevention, simply wash hands frequently and use a nanoparticle silver gel as a natural hand disinfectant. Take something to boost the immune system, such as elderberry; vitamins A, C, and D; and zinc when the flu is "going around." You can also take an *Immune-Boosting* or *Mushroom Immune Formula* for prevention.

If you do get the flu try taking a good antiviral remedy, such as the *Elderberry Cold and Flu, Children's Composition*, or *Ed Millet's Herbal Crisis Formula*. For settling the stomach flu, two of the best remedies are ginger and peppermint. For flu with aches and fever try yarrow, boneset, or andrographis. Drink plenty of liquids and try the *Colon Hydrotherapy* and/or the *Sweat Bath* strategy, both of which can bring about very rapid recovery.

- **Strategies:** Colon Hydrotherapy, Fasting, Hydration, and Sweat Bath
- **Formulas: Flu and Vomiting**, Chinese Yang-Reducing, **Elderberry Cold and Flu**, Immune-Boosting, Children's Elderberry Cold and Flu, Herbal Composition, **Ed Millet's Herbal Crisis**, **Steven Horne's Children's Composition**, Fire Cider, **Mushroom Immune**, and Seasonal Cold and Flu
- **Essential Oil Blends:** Disinfectant EO
- **Herbs: Andrographis**, angelica, astragalus, **boneset**, capsicum, catnip, cinnamon, echinacea, **elder berry and flower**, garlic, **ginger**, hyssop, isatis, lemon, lemon balm, **osha**, **peppermint**, pleurisy, spilanthes, thyme, usnea, and **yarrow**
- **Supplements: Vitamin A**, **vitamin D**, and **zinc**
- **Essential Oils:** Cajeput, cinnamon, jasmine, lemon, menthol, peppermint, pine, **ravensara**, rosemary, spearmint, tea tree, and thyme

Food Allergies/Intolerances

See also autoimmune disorders, leaky gut, SIBO, and dysbiosis

There's an old saying that "one man's meat is another man's poison," which is especially true in the case of food allergies and food sensitivities. Normal foods can be nourishing for some people while causing illness and discomfort to others. Food sensitivities, also known as food intolerances, are especially important to understand because they can be hard to identify. Let's start by explaining the difference between allergies and intolerances.

Food Allergies

Food allergies are immune reactions involving mast cells. Mast cells, which are found in the mucous membranes of the lungs and intestines, trigger inflammatory reactions to certain substances via the release of histamine. This happens when a particular protein structure binds to IgE antibodies on the surface of the mast cell. This initiates an immune reaction, which treats the substance as an invader and seeks to flush it from the body.

Food allergies can cause extremely severe reactions to certain foods. The most common foods causing serious allergic reactions are cow milk, eggs, soy, peanuts, tree nuts, wheat, fish, and shellfish. Reactions to these foods can occur within a few minutes and be severe enough to be life-threatening.

If you have a true food allergy, even a tiny amount of the allergy-causing food can trigger a reaction. Food allergies often affect young children and require parents and guardians to carefully monitor the child's diet. People with severe food allergies can get injectable epinephrine to use if they accidentally ingest an allergy-causing food.

Food Intolerances

Food intolerances are much more subtle problems. First, the negative reactions to the food are typically more delayed, starting an hour or so after eating or perhaps even a day or more later. Tests for food allergies do not detect food sensitivities because there are no immune factors (antibodies) to detect. Food intolerances can produce allergy-like symptoms; it's just not an immune reaction.

Symptoms of food intolerances may show up as problems with the skin, respiratory tract, and/or the gastrointestinal tract. Skin reactions can include hives and rashes, dermatitis, eczema, and itchy skin. Respiratory symptoms can include congestion, sinusitis, asthma, and an unproductive cough. Digestive symptoms can include irritable bowel syndrome, mouth ulcers or canker sores, gas, bloating, nausea, constipation, occasional diarrhea, and intestinal cramping.

If you suspect food allergies or intolerances are causing some of your health problems, adopt the following strategies in the order given.

1. Identify Allergies and Intolerances

There are several ways to identify if you have hidden food allergies or intolerances. First, look at the most common allergy-causing foods, which were listed earlier. See the *Eliminate Allergy-Causing Foods* strategy.

In the search for possible food intolerances, you could also start with the foods that are incompatible with your blood type (O, A, B, or AB). Tree of Light has *Blood Type, pH and Nutrition* charts for each of the four blood types that can help you in addition to Peter D'Adamo's *Eat Right for Your Type* books.

You can also create a food journal. Each day, write down everything you eat and the time you eat it. Also write down any symptoms you feel throughout the day (digestive upset, moodiness, low energy) and note the time you started experiencing them. After a week or two you should start to see correlations between eating various foods and symptoms you may be experiencing.

2. Do a Test Elimination Diet

Once you create your list of suspect foods, eliminate *all* of them for a week. If you can't go a full week, then eliminate them for at least three days. If your health problems are linked to food sensitivities, you should notice an improvement in your energy, mental clarity, mood, and symptoms.

If you do notice an improvement, you can determine which foods are causing you problems by doing a challenge test. Add just one of the suspect foods back into your diet and notice how you feel during the next twenty-four to forty-eight hours. If symptoms return, that food is probably causing your problems. You can optionally repeat the challenge test more than once to verify that the food is actually a problem.

3. Heal the GI Tract

To reduce food intolerances and allergies, one needs to start with restoring gut health. You can read about this by looking up the conditions *dysbiosis, leaky gut syndrome* and *sibo*. You should also follow the *Gut-Healing Diet* strategy.

4. Use Appropriate Supplements

You can reduce the body's reaction to many foods by making sure you have adequate enzymes and hydrochloric acid to break food down properly. Try taking *Digestive Enzymes* or *Plant Enzymes* with meals. There are herbs, like nettles and osha, that can reduce food reactions. An *Antihistamine Formula* may also help.

Strategies: Blood Type Diet, Detoxification, Eat Enzyme-Rich Foods, Eat Healthy, Eliminate Allergy-Causing Foods, Emotional Healing Work, Friendly Flora, Gut-Healing Diet, Hiatal Hernia Correction, and Hydration

Formulas: Digestive Support, Antihistamine, Liver Cleanse, Chinese Wood-Decreasing, Gut Immune, **Lactase Enzyme**, **Plant Enzyme**, GLA Oil, Pepsin Intestinal, Jeannie Burgess' Allergy-Lung, Chinese Earth-Increasing, Herbal Bitters, Gut-Healing Fiber, Steven Horne's Anti-Allergy, Joan Patton's Herbal Minerals, **Betaine HCl**, and Probiotic

Programs: Ivy Bridge's Cleansing and Parasite Cleansing

Herbs: Aloe vera, barley, **black walnut**, burdock, **cat's claw**, devil's claw, ginger, goldenrod, goldenseal, nettle, stinging, osha, and plantain

Supplements: Berberine, clay (bentonite), Co-Q10, colostrum, MSM, omega-3 EFAs, omega-6 CLA, and protease

Food Poisoning

Consuming contaminated food can create severe symptoms of food poisoning, which include nausea, vomiting, and diarrhea. In severe cases, medical attention should be sought.

Lobelia can be used to induce vomiting, to expel the toxic material more quickly from the body. If lobelia isn't available, ipecac is an alternative. Other herbs that may help induce vomiting include boneset, blue vervain, and yellow mustard. After throwing up, peppermint tea or essential oil can be used to settle the stomach.

To absorb irritants in the digestive tract and ease diarrhea, activated charcoal is a good remedy. Alternatives include slippery elm and psyllium. Taking probiotics at three to four times the normal dose can help prevent food poisoning when traveling. You can also use natural antibiotics like nanoparticle silver, goldenseal, and echinacea to fight the infection.

Formulas: Probiotic and **Antibacterial**

Herbs: Aloe vera, echinacea, garlic, **goldenseal**, **lobelia**, milk thistle, peppermint, psyllium, slippery elm, and vervain (blue)

Supplements: Bacillus coagulans, **charcoal**, clay (bentonite), and **nanoparticle silver**

Essential Oils: Peppermint

Foot Odor

Severe foot odor is a good indication of the need to do some cleansing. Improve the diet, do the *Detoxification* strategy, and perhaps the *Drawing Bath* strategy. You can even soak your feet in a pan containing water and Epsom salts. You can also use the *Enzyme Spray Formula* on shoes, socks or feet to reduce odor. Adding a few drops of essential oils to it makes the enzyme spray even more effective.

Strategies: Detoxification, Drawing Bath, and Epsom Salt Bath

Formulas: Enzyme Spray

Supplements: Chlorophyll

Essential Oils: Lemongrass, pine, and tea tree

Fractures   see *broken bones*

Free Radical Damage

See also aging

Experts suggest that about 50-80 percent of all chronic and degenerative diseases, including heart disease, cancer, diabetes, arthritis, macular degeneration, Alzheimer's, and dementia are caused by oxidative stress, also known as free radical damage. Free radical damage also causes the cosmetic problems we associate with aging, dry skin, wrinkles, age spots, and so forth. It is also closely tied in with chronic inflammation.

The best way to prevent free radical damage is to minimize exposure to environmental toxins and eat five to seven helpings of fresh fruits and vegetables daily. Dark chocolate is an excellent antioxidant. You can also take antioxidant supplements like those listed here.

Strategies: Eat Healthy

Formulas: Green Tea Polyphenols, Proanthocyanidins, and **Antioxidant**

Herbs: Açaí, barley grass, bilberry, cocoa, ginkgo, Grape, **lycium**, **mangosteen**, rosemary, and tea

Supplements: Alpha-lipoic acid, chlorophyll, Co-Q10, L-carnitine, lutein, lycopene, vitamin A, **vitamin C**, **vitamin D**, **vitamin E**, zeaxanthin, and zinc

Frigidity   see *sex drive (low)*

Frostbite Prevention

Sprinkle tiny amounts of capsicum in socks or gloves to prevent frostbite.

Herbs: Capsicum

Frozen Shoulder

This is a condition where inflammation in the shoulder inhibits movement. It is often linked with stress or minor injuries. Reducing the inflammation aids recovery, as do gentle stretching exercises.

Strategies: Lymph-Moving Pain Relief

Essential Oil Blends: Topical Injury

Herbs: Black cohosh and **Saint John's wort**

Fungal Infection   see *infection (fungal)*

Gallbladder Problems

See also gallstones

Sluggish activity of the gallbladder will result in poor digestion of fats. It will also make it difficult for the body to eliminate excess cholesterol. Clay-colored or greasy stools that float are symptoms of sluggish gallbladder function.

Herbs that stimulate gallbladder function are called cholagogues and taking them before meals or when one feels bloated or stuffy under the right rib cage can be helpful. Lipase enzyme and bile salts are also helpful for problems with digesting fats. These remedies are also helpful for someone who has had their gallbladder removed.

Strategies: Gallbladder Flush

Formulas: Christopher's Gallbladder, Liver Cleanse, Hepatoprotective, **Chinese Wood-Decreasing**, **Lipase Enzyme**, Digestive Support, and Cholesterol-Regulating

Herbs: Artichoke, **barberry**, blue flag, buckthorn, burdock, cascara sagrada, celandine, **dandelion**, **fringe tree**, gentian, jambul, milk thistle, **turmeric**, **wild yam**, and yellow dock

Supplements: Bile salt, curcumin, **lipase**, and SAM-e

Essential Oils: Geranium and helichrysum

Gallstones

Deposits, resembling small rocks, that form in the gallbladder are called gallstones. They are usually composed primarily of cholesterol. If they are large or numerous enough, they may cause severe abdominal pain. The *Gallbladder Flush* strategy has helped many people with gallstones. Fringetree, barberry, and turmeric taken regularly with plenty of water and dietary fiber can also be helpful.

Strategies: Gallbladder Flush and Hydration

Formulas: Liver Cleanse, Hepatoprotective, Christopher's Gallbladder, Chinese Wood-Decreasing, Digestive Support, and Cholesterol-Regulating

Herbs: Barberry, celandine, chicory, **fringe tree**, khella, lemon juice, milk thistle, **turmeric**, and **wild yam**

Supplements: Curcumin, lipase, and magnesium

Essential Oils: Lemon

Gangrene

Gangrene is localized death of the skin and underlying soft tissue due to lack of blood supply. This is a serious illness, and medical attention should be sought. However, the following natural remedies may be helpful.

Nanoparticle silver gel have been proven in scientific studies to halt the progression of gangrene and often prevent the need for amputation. Apply the gel topically and liberally several times a day.

One can also dilute antispetic essential oils in a carrier oil and apply them topically. Internally, echinacea, baptista, thuja, and usnea are some of the stronger antimicrobials that may prove helpful.

This problem often develops because of poor circulation due to complications of diabetes. When this is the case, do the *Oral Chelation* strategy and take alpha-lipoic acid.

An interesting natural therapy is to use for gangrene on the feet is alternating soaks with ice water and warm water to stimulate circulation. Make two pans, one with ice water and the other with warm water. You can add a few drops of an antiseptic essential oil or a tincture of antimcirobial herbs to the warm water. Have the person put their feet in the ice water for about thirty to sixty seconds, then put them in the warm water for two or three minutes. Repeat this several times. This can be done once a day to bring blood flow to the afflicted area.

Strategies: Eat Healthy and Oral Chelation

Formulas: Oral Chelation, Stabilized Allicin, and Antibacterial

Herbs: Baptisia, capsicum, **echinacea, garlic (raw)**, goldenseal, **thuja**, and **usnea**

Supplements: Alpha-lipoic acid, MSM, **nanoparticle silver**, and **vitamin C**

Essential Oils: Lavender and tea tree

Gas & Bloating

Flatulence

See also belching, hiatal hernia, ileocecal valve, lactose intolerance, and SIBO

Intestinal gas is created by the action of friendly flora on foods we eat. Some amount of gas production is normal. Bloating is an abnormal feeling of fullness in the gastrointestinal tract caused by excessive gas that builds up pressure in the abdomen. Bloating puts pressure on the stomach and contributes to the development of a hiatal hernia. It may even cause stress on the heart. Where bloating is frequent, the ileocecal valve is probably swollen and inflamed and needs to be closed (see *ileocecal valve*).

Excessive gas and bloating can also be caused by an overgrowth of bacteria in the small intestines (see *SIBO*). When this is the case taking fiber supplements and probiotics may make the gas and bloating worse. It may also signal problems digesting certain foods. In this case, *Digestive Support, Betaine HCL,* or *Plant Enzyme Formulas* will help reduce intestinal gas.

Herbs used to relieve gas and bloating are called carminatives. They can be taken as part of an *Herbal Bitters* or *Carminative Formula* or used as warm herbal teas. Catnip, chamomile, fennel, ginger, and peppermint are all good carminatives. Peppermint oil is a powerful carminative. Put one or two drops in some warm water and sip it slowly.

If gas and bloating occurs after consuming dairy products, it is a sign of lactose intolerance. In this case probiotics and a *Lactase Enzyme Formula,* which contains the lactose digesting enzyme lactase, will help. Where bloating is severe and accompanied by foul belching, there is putrefaction taking place in the digestive tract. Activated charcoal can be very helpful for relieving this condition.

Strategies: Aromatherapy, Avoid Sugar, Colon Hydrotherapy, Detoxification, Eat Enzyme-Rich Foods, and Eliminate FODMAPs

Formulas: Chinese Earth-Decreasing, Christopher's Carminative, Intestinal Detoxification, **Children's Colic, Digestive Support**, Papaya Enzyme, **Betaine HCl**, Lactase Enzyme, **Plant Enzyme**, Triphala, Chinese Earth-Increasing, and Herbal Bitters

Essential Oil Blends: Digestive Settling EO

Herbs: Angelica, anise, asafetida, **barberry**, black pepper, blessed thistle, bupleurum, calamus, cardamom, catnip, **chamomile**, cilantro/coriander, cinnamon, clove, coleus, fennel, garlic, **gentian, ginger**, kava kava, orange (bitter), papaya, **peppermint**, perilla, rosemary, safflower, and **thyme**

Supplements: Amylase, Bacillus coagulans, and **charcoal**

Essential Oils: Anise, bay leaf, cajeput, chamomile (Roman), clary sage, clove, **fennel**, lemon, myrrh, neroli, orange (sweet), oregano, patchouli, **peppermint**, ravensara, red mandarin, rosemary, **spearmint**, wintergreen, and ylang ylang

Gastritis

See also acid indigestion, indigestion, leaky gut, and SIBO

Gastritis is an inflammation of the stomach. It is caused by a combination of factors, including stress, rapid eating, alcohol and tobacco use, NSAIDs, and dehydration. It can also be caused by an overgrowth of bacteria in the small intestines giving rise to excessive gas and pressure on the stomach. Headaches and constipation are also commonly associated with gastritis. A person may feel dull and drowsy after eating but have difficulty falling asleep at bedtime.

To correct gastritis, the diet should be simple, consisting primarily of meat and vegetables. Simple sugars and starchy foods should be avoided (especially if there is gas and bloating). *Digestive Support* and *Betaine HCl Formulas* may be helpful to take with meals.

Taking an *Herbal Bitters Formula* about fifteen to twenty minutes prior to meals along with a glass or two of water, then avoiding liquids with meals, can also be helpful. Dehydration decreases downward motility of the digestive organs, but liquids should primarily be consumed between meals.

Soothing, mucilaginous herbs like aloe, licorice, marshmallow, and slippery elm can also soothe stomach irritation. An *Intestinal Soothing Formula* is often helpful. Meadowsweet not only helps to neutralize acid burning, it also eases pain and inflammation.

Strategies: Gut-Healing Diet and Hydration

Formulas: H. Pylori-Fighting, Pepsin Intestinal, **Digestive Support**, **Betaine HCl**, **Herbal Bitters**, Digestive Support, and **Intestinal Soothing**

Herbs: **Aloe vera**, amalaki, cat's claw, chaga, **goldenseal**, **licorice**, **marshmallow**, **meadowsweet**, olive, **peppermint**, red raspberry, Saint John's wort, and slippery elm

Supplements: Calcium

Essential Oils: Geranium, peppermint, sandalwood, and thyme

Gastroesophageal Reflux Disease
see *acid indigestion*

Generalized Anxiety Disorder
see *anxiety disorders*

Giardia
See also parasites

Giardia is a single-cell organism that is the most common cause of waterborne disease in the United States. It is transmitted by drinking contaminated water. Giardia form cysts in water that cannot be destroyed by chlorination. Water can be disinfected by heating it to a rolling boil for one minute, or by using a special filter.

Symptoms of giardia infection include diarrhea, gas, stomach cramps, nausea, and greasy stools that tend to float. Symptoms usually appear seven to fourteen days after exposure. Goldenseal is considered an official remedy for giardia in some countries. You can also try taking berberine. Activated charcoal can be helpful for the diarrhea. Drink plenty of water and replace electrolytes by taking a pinch of table salt and

some *Herbal Potassium Formula* or *Electrolyte Drink Powder*. If symptoms are severe, seek medical attention.

Strategies: Hydration

Formulas: Antibacterial, Lymphatic Infection, Probiotic, Electrolyte Drink, and Herbal Potassium

Herbs: **Andrographis**, black walnut, echinacea, **goldenseal**, and thuja

Supplements: Berberine, **charcoal**, and potassium

Gingivitis
Bleeding Gums, Gum Disease, Pyorrhea
See also cardiovascular disease

When bacteria get into the space between the teeth and the gums, they can cause inflammation (gingivitis) and a breakdown of the gum tissue. This leads to bleeding of the gums. Pyorrhea is an advanced form of periodontal disease associated with a discharge of pus and loose teeth.

A thorough cleaning by a dental hygienist can prevent and treat gingivitis. Teeth should be brushed and flossed at least two times a day in between cleanings.

After brushing your teeth with toothpaste, you can brush with an *Herbal Tooth Powder Formula*. Leave some of the powder on your gums for five minutes or even overnight and then rinse. These herbs fight infection, strengthen tooth enamel and gums, and contract tissues to stop bleeding.

Xylitol will inhibit the growth of the bacteria involved in gingivitis. You can also apply a nanoparticle silver gel directly to the gums to kill the bacteria and promote healing. Herbs that can be applied topically to the gums to help infection include cloves, myrrh, and spilanthes.

Using a *Colloidal Minerals Formula* as a mouth wash will also help to stop bleeding. You can also use the *Enzyme Spray Formula* as a mouthwash. It is even more effective if you add a few drops of antimicrobial essential oils to the enzyme spray. Good oils to consider are clove and myrrh.

Internally, Co-Q 10 helps reduce gum inflammation. It also helps reduce inflammation in the cardiovascular system, which is important because gingivitis is an early warning sign of developing heart disease. Vitamin C is also helpful for healing the gums.

Strategies: Avoid Sugar, Eat Healthy, Low-Glycemic Diet, and Mineralization

Formulas: Chinese Yang-Reducing, Colloidal Mineral, Anti-Inflammatory Pain, Enzyme Spray, and **Herbal Tooth Powder**

Herbs: Acacia, achyranthes, amalaki, bayberry root bark, **black walnut**, calendula, clove, echinacea, goldenseal, **myrrh**, **neem**, **spilanthes**, usnea, and **white oak**

Supplements: Co-Q10, **nanoparticle silver**, **propolis**, vitamin B₉, **vitamin C**, vitamin D, vitamin K, and zinc

Essential Oils: Cinnamon, **clove**, helichrysum, lemon, **myrrh**, rose, and tea tree

Glaucoma

See also free radical damage and eye health

Glaucoma is a serious eye disease characterized by abnormally elevated fluid pressure within the eye. This is caused by a tiny mesh in the eye that allows fluid to drain becoming clogged. The clogging is usually due to free radical damage causing debris in the lymph. Untreated, this pressure can damage the retina and destroy the optic nerve, resulting in loss of vision or blindness. In fact, glaucoma is the most common cause of blindness.

Risk factors for this disease include people of African ancestry, people with diabetes, high blood pressure, severe myopia (nearsightedness) or a family history of glaucoma, and those taking corticosteroid preparations. Other contributing factors include diabetes, food allergies, excess caffeine, adrenal exhaustion, liver and thyroid problems, and arteriosclerosis. Coffee should be eliminated from the diet along with other sources of caffeine, including chocolate and soft drinks.

To prevent glaucoma, eat plenty of fresh fruits and vegetables to get antioxidants in the diet. You can also supplement with nutrients that aid the eyes, especially vitamins and lutein and zeaxanthin. See *Eye Health* for more information.

It also helps to avoid too much bright sunlight. Shade your eyes and wear sunglasses when out in the bright sunlight.

If you have glaucoma, seek medical attention. Remedies listed here are things you can use in addition to medical treatment.

Remedies that relax the eye and allow the drain to open may be helpful. One such remedy is cannabis, which is legal in only a few states. It temporarily reduces ocular pressure, but isn't a cure. CBD might be helpful too, but it is the THC in cannabis itself that appears to lower the pressure. It is possible that CBD could be used with kava kava or lobelia to create a similar effect, but this should not be done in place of medical treatment.

The famous herbalist John Christopher reported that his herbal eye wash formula was helpful, but I don't have any personal experience with this. If you want to try it, I'd add a relaxing herb like lobelia or chamomile to the formula.

Strategies: Avoid Caffeine, Enhance Nitric Oxide, and Stress Management

Formulas: **Antioxidant Eye**, Oral Chelation, **Antioxidant**, Nitric Oxide Boosting, and Herbal Eyewash

Herbs: Bilberry, coleus, eyebright, ginkgo, kava kava, **lobelia**, and spirulina

Supplements: Alpha-lipoic acid, CBD, Co-Q10, lutein, **magnesium**, N-acetyl cysteine, **vitamin A**, **vitamin C**, vitamin D, vitamin E, and zeaxanthin

Goiter

See also Graves' disease, Hashimoto's disease, and hypothyroidism

An enlargement of the thyroid gland that can be seen as a swelling in the neck is a goiter. This results from insufficient intake of iodine or an immune attack on the thyroid called Hashimoto's thyroiditis. See related conditions for more detailed suggestions.

Formulas: **Thyroid Glandular** and **Hypothyroid**

Herbs: Black walnut, bladderwrack, **dulse**, Irish moss, and **kelp**

Supplements: Iodine

Gonorrhea

See also infection (bacterial)

Gonorrhea is a sexually transmitted bacterial infection that causes inflammation of the genital mucous membranes. Symptoms of gonorrhea in men include painful urination and a thick discharge from the penis. Women may have no initial symptoms, or they may have painful urination, vaginal discharge, and abnormal menstrual bleeding. In advanced stages, gonorrhea can cause fever, muscle aches, and inflamed joints. It can also cause infertility.

Seek medical attention for gonorrhea. You can use antibacterial herbs along with antibiotics. Repopulate the colon with probiotics when you have finished taking the antibiotics.

Formulas: Antibacterial and Probiotic

Herbs: Baptisia, echinacea, garlic, and goldenseal

Essential Oils: Lemon

Gout

See also arthritis

Gout is a metabolic disease characterized by excessive amounts of uric acid in the blood and deposits of uric acid crystals in the joints. Uric acid is a byproduct of protein and fructose metabolism and is filtered from the blood by the kidneys.

Animal protein consumption should be reduced, and when it is consumed, a *Betaine HCl Formula* should be taken with it. Soda pop, and any drink sweetened with fructose, should be eliminated. Make sure you are drinking sufficient amounts of pure water to flush metabolic waste from the body.

Complex carbohydrates such as fresh fruits, dark-green vegetables, and other antioxidant foods should be increased in the diet. Black cherry juice and lemon water are also helpful for flushing the acid out of the system. Nettle leaf is particularly good for flushing acid waste from the system, but other alteratives like alfalfa, red clover, cleavers, and dandelion can also be helpful.

Strategies: Eat Healthy and Hydration

Formulas: Herbal Arthritis, **Chinese Water-Increasing**, Liquid Kidney, and **Betaine HCl**

Herbs: Alfalfa, amalaki, barley, burdock, celery seed, chickweed, chicory, couchgrass, dandelion, devil's claw, Grape, **gravel root**, kava kava, lemon juice, **lemon juice, nettle, stinging**, red clover, safflower, and uva ursi

Supplements: Chlorophyll, L-glutamine, magnesium, omega-3 DHA, omega-3 EFAs, and potassium

Essential Oils: Cajeput, fennel, lemon, and pine

Graves' Disease
Hyperthyroid

See also adrenal fatigue, autoimmune disorders, and Hashimoto's disease

Graves' disease is the most common hyperthyroid disease. In Graves' disease the immune system attacks enzymes that break down the thyroid hormone, causing levels to elevate. There are other forms of hyperthyroid diseases and the information here may help them as well.

A hyperthyroid over-stimulates metabolism. You can think of this as having the thermostat set too high or racing the engine on your car. As a result, fuel burns too quickly, which results in weight loss, intolerance to heat, hyperactivity, and restlessness. Some of the specific symptoms associated with Graves' disease include bulging eyes, rapid pulse rate (90-160), heart palpitations, tremors, restlessness and anxiety, lack of periods, muscle weakness, and impaired sleep.

Hyperthyroid disorders are a serious medical condition and need proper medical attention. The rapid heartbeat can over stress the heart and circulation, resulting in life-threatening effects. This is why it is essential that a physician monitor someone with a hyperthyroid condition, even if the patient is opting to try a natural approach. Medication may be needed to lower the heart rate and inhibit the thyroid while you work on removing the underlying health problems.

While it is important to have proper medical monitoring of a hyperthyroid condition, the most common medical treatments for hyperactive thyroid conditions leaves much

to be desired. The treatment is to irradiate the thyroid with radioactive iodine to destroy thyroid cells and then put the person on thyroid medication for the rest of their life.

Clearly, this should be the last option if other remedies fail to bring the condition under control. So here are some strategies to overcome hyperthyroid conditions naturally.

Use Herbs That Calm Thyroid Function

There are herbs that contain substances known to bind to TSH receptor sites in the thyroid, inhibiting them and thereby reducing thyroid output. The most well known are bugleweed and lemon balm. They are the primary ingredients in *Thyroid Calming Formulas*. Cruciferous vegetables like cabbage and broccoli have a mild thyroid inhibiting effect, so they can also be consumed freely.

Use Herbs to Calm the Heart

Two other herbs that can be helpful for calming the rapid heartbeat associated with hyperthyroid are motherwort and mistletoe. Motherwort is often found in *Thyroid Calming Formulas*.

Remedies can be also taken to help protect the heart. Hawthorn has a cooling (anti-inflammatory) effect and Co-Q10, l-carnitine, and magnesium can also help. Magnesium will help calm the heart rate and reduce high blood pressure.

Balance Immune Activity

In Graves' Disease, the underlying problem is the immune attack on the thyroid. See *autoimmune disorders* for suggestions on how to calm and balance the immune naturally.

Manage Stress

People with Graves' disease and hyperthyroid disorders are often under a lot of stress. They may tend to "burn the candle at both ends." It is very important with this condition to relax as much as possible. One should not push themselves or take on too much. In Chinese medicine, hypothyroidism is linked with excess fire and is treated with herbs like those in the *Chinese Fire Reducing Formula*.

Support Adrenal Function

The adrenals tend to work with and balance the thyroid. People with hyperactive thyroid function also tend to have adrenal problems. The stress hormone, cortisol, is an anti-inflammatory, so hyperthyroidism may be a sign of excess stress, accompanied by adrenal weakness. In this case, the immune calming effect of the adrenal hormone, cortisol, is reduced. Adaptogens, licorice root, or even an *Adrenal Glandular Formula* can sometimes be helpful. I've also found the *Chinese Fire-Increasing Formula* helpful.

Support Iodine Utilization

Hyperthyroid patients may not be properly utilizing iodine. This may be due to a deficiency in selenium or zinc. There may be some link between the use of chemical iodine (such as iodized salt) and hyperstimulation of the thyroid. So avoid any chemical iodine supplements.

However, here's an interesting idea to contemplate. In order to protect the body from radioactive iodine released by nuclear accidents, people are given iodine supplements to saturate the body with iodine to prevent the uptake of the radioactive iodine. The fact that the body uptakes the radioactive iodine suggests the person may not have enough iodine.

So taking a small amount of seaweed, like kelp or dulse, might be helpful, but one has to monitor the situation to make sure they don't over stimulate the person. I used a modification of this strategy with one client who had opted for the radiation treatment. I had him take large amounts of seaweed (about twelve capsules per day) for two weeks prior to the procedure. The theory was that this would protect his thyroid from being completely destroyed.

This appears to have worked. After the procedure, his levels of thyroid hormone dropped down into normal ranges, but didn't go below this. The medical doctors were puzzled, but he did not have to start taking thyroid medication. Whether this would work for others, or not, I don't know, but I offer it as something to consider.

Adopt a Healthy Diet

Diet can also play a role in helping to balance an overactive thyroid. High-carbohydrate diets, coupled with low protein and/or fat intake, tend to elevate thyroid function. So a properly balanced diet with correct proportions of fats, proteins, and low-glycemic carbohydrates is helpful. Many of the same dietary therapies that are helpful for Hashimoto's disease can also be helpful for Graves' disease.

If you're going to try a natural approach to a hypothyroid disorder like Graves, it would be wise to work with an experienced herbalist or naturopath (findanherbalist.com or americanherbalistsguild.com).

> **Strategies:** Avoid Caffeine, Eat Healthy, Low-Glycemic Diet, Pleasure Prescription, and Stress Management
>
> **Formulas:** Chinese Yang-Reducing, **Chinese Fire-Increasing**, Suma Adaptogen, **Chinese Fire-Decreasing**, Adrenal Glandular, Anti-Anxiety, Betaine HCl, and **Thyroid Calming**
>
> **Herbs: Bugleweed**, eleuthero, hawthorn, hops, **lemon balm**, licorice, mistletoe, and **motherwort**
>
> **Supplements:** CBD, Co-Q10, L-carnitine, **magnesium**, **selenium**, vitamin B-complex, vitamin B_5, and zinc

Essential Oils: Spruce (blue)

Grief & Sadness

See also shock (medical)

Everyone experiences the pain of loss and heartbreak at some point in their life. When we lose someone or something that brought us joy and pleasure, we experience grief. Grief begins as a shock to the system. In shock, the blood retreats from the skin and moves into the internal organs. In the grieving process, this creates a swelling sensation in our chest we call heartbreak. If the pain is intense enough, it actually feels like our heart is going to burst.

If you've ever seen a person go into shock, you'll see the color drain from their face, making them look pale. They also feel cold. Their eyes glaze over, and they feel numb. They become cold and clammy. This is exactly the opposite energetic state to that of being in love, which causes blood to flow more readily to the surface of the skin, making the person rosy, warm, and radiant. Love opens us up to greater connection. Shock is a state of being withdrawn and closed down.

When a grieving person is able to acknowledge their pain, they will start sobbing. Sobbing is more than just shedding tears; it involves the whole body. The convulsive shaking of the body associated with sobbing can also lead to wailing, moaning, or even screaming. These actions empty the lungs (which causes a release of endorphins which help the person feel better). It also forces redistribution of the blood so a person can feel again.

The emptying of the lungs is symbolic of the letting go associated with grieving. Grieving is a releasing of what we have lost, a breaking of the attachment or desire we felt. Sighing (which also involves a long, slow exhale) is a milder form of the same energy.

Grieving can also involve anger. Feeling deeply hurt often brings out feelings of anger. The grieving person may be mad at the person who left them or even blame God for taking the person away from them.

Grief and the Lungs

When a person is unable to fully grieve and let go, they can become congested, particularly in the lungs. In traditional Chinese medicine, it was recognized that prolonged sorrow damages the energy of the lungs. A person who is unable to fully grieve may cough because they need to get something off their chest. Their lungs may fill up with fluid, resulting in pneumonia, or they may shed tears internally in the form of post nasal drip. This is why formulas that support the respiratory system, such as a *Chinese Metal-Decreasing Formula*, may be helpful for the grieving person.

Healthy grief is an expression of love. It is healthy to express grief when we have lost someone or something important to us. Grieving helps us to accept our loss, to rediscover peace and joy, and then to move forward.

During a time of loss, people will often reach out to the grieving person, offering comfort and help. This is a wonderful thing, but it cannot replace the grieving process. One still has to go through the process of releasing pain and letting go of that which has been lost. The *Grief and Sadness FE Blend* is very helpful for this process. Two of the flower essences in it, bleeding heart and California wild rose, I have consistently found helpful for people who are grieving. I've also found rose essential oil and lemon balm helpful for grieving.

In other words, receiving help is good, but a person still needs to experience the sighing, sobbing, or wailing that allows the pain to be released from the body. When a person doesn't allow themselves to do this, they may become addicted to the comfort and sympathy of others, seeking it like an addict seeks a drug. This places responsibility for their healing outside of themselves, which means they become perpetually stuck in seeking sympathetic allies to try to heal their grief.

Softening a Hardened Heart

Sometimes the suffering a person feels leads them to conclude that it is dangerous to experience love and vulnerability. So they close down their hearts to avoid feeling close to anyone or anything, hoping to avoid experiencing future grief or sorrow.

Unfortunately, closing oneself off to pain also closes one off to the joy that comes from love and connection. It causes one to become hard of heart and experience a lack of empathy and compassion for others. A person with a closed heart will become inflexible, rigid, and judgmental.

Heart problems, such as hardening of the arteries, high blood pressure, and heart attacks can all be signs of a person who has closed their heart to try to avoid having to feel grief or pain. A closed heart not only prevents one from experiencing loving connections with others, but also reduces one's ability to experience joy, happiness, and pleasure in one's life. Diabetes and blood sugar problems can also be signs of a closed heart and the inability to experience the sweetness of love.

Seeking counseling or assistance from a minister or a friend may be necessary when one has undergone a lot of grief. Make sure, however, that you work with someone who isn't afraid of allowing people to express their grief as described above.

Strategies: Aromatherapy, Counseling or Therapy, Emotional Healing Work, Flower Essence, Pleasure Prescription, and Sleep

Formulas: Chinese Metal-Decreasing, Jeannie Burgess' Allergy-Lung, and Chinese Metal-Increasing

Essential Oil Blends: Mood Lifting EO and Lung-Supporting EO

Flower Essence Blends: Grief and Sadness FE

Flower Essences: Broken and Hardened Hearts FE

Herbs: Bupleurum, **lemon balm**, **mimosa**, night-blooming cereus, and oat seed (milky)

Supplements: Vitamin B-complex and vitamin C

Essential Oils: Eucalyptus, frankincense, helichrysum, lemon, marjoram, myrrh, pine, and **rose**

Gum Disease   see *gingivitis*

Hair Loss/Thinning
Baldness

See also hair care, Hashimoto's disease, and hypothyroidism

Loss of hair or baldness may be caused by hormonal imbalances such as low thyroid, lack of protein in the diet, stress, and poor circulation to the scalp. Appropriate remedies depend on the underlying causes.

One of the most common causes (especially in women) is low thyroid. In this case, an iodine supplement, kelp, or other thyroid supporting remedies may be helpful. See *hashimoto's disease* and *hypothyroidism* for ideas on how to work with this condition. For men who are experiencing balding, try using maca, muira puama, or other male tonics to balance your hormones.

Lack of adequate protein in the diet or difficulty in digesting and assimilating protein is another common cause. If your diet is low in protein, increase consumption of protein-rich foods. If you have a hard time digesting them, a *Digestive Support* and/or *Betaine HCL Formula* may help.

Minerals can also aid hair growth. Consider using mineral rich herbs like horsetail, nettles, rosemary and sage or the *Watkins Hair, Skin, and Nails Formula*. These remedies have all proven helpful for improving the health of hair, along with skin and fingernails.

Stress can cause hair to thin. If you are under a lot of stress, try using adaptogens to ease your stress. The *Chinese Mineral Qi Adaptagen Formula*, listed as one of the *Colloidal Mineral Formulas*, provides both minerals and herbs to help reduce your stress level.

Sage and rosemary essential oils can also be used topically on the scalp to encourage circulation to the scalp. Simply add a few drops to your shampoo.

These are basic suggestions. Each case must be evaluated individually to determine the underlying cause.

Strategies: Mineralization

Formulas: Watkin's Hair, Skin, and Nails, Hypothyroid, **Thyroid Glandular**, **Betaine HCl**, Adrenal Glandular, **Digestive Support**, and Colloidal Mineral

Herbs: Dulse, eleuthero, he shou wu, **horsetail**, kelp, khella, maca, muira puama, nettle, stinging, noni, **rosemary**, and sage

Supplements: Co-Q10, iodine, iron, protease, **silicon**, vitamin B_{12}, and zinc

Essential Oils: Lavender, rosemary, and ylang ylang

Hair, Graying

Gray hair is associated with aging and is typically the result of mineral deficiencies, as minerals like copper and zinc help to add color to the hair. It can also be a sign of declining hydrochloric acid production (resulting in poor protein digestion and mineral absorption). A lack of B-complex vitamins may also contribute to this problem. He shou wu has a reputation in China as an herb that can prevent or reverse graying if taken regularly.

Strategies: Mineralization

Formulas: Chinese Water-Increasing, **Betaine HCl**, and **Colloidal Mineral**

Herbs: He shou wu and sage

Supplements: Copper, manganese, selenium, vitamin B-complex, vitamin B_5, and **zinc**

Halitosis
Bad Breath

See also belching and sinus infection

Halitosis is a bad odor from the mouth. Sinus infections, oral diseases, cigarette smoking, and poor digestion can all contribute to halitosis. Start by cleaning the teeth.

Essential oils like myrrh, clove, and peppermint can be added to water and used as a mouthwash. Propolis can also be used as a mouthwash and helps to fight infection.

If the bad odor is caused by foul belching, use remedies to aid digestion. Colon cleansing may also be helpful. Chlorophyll is a very good natural deodorizer and can reduce body odor in general, including bad breath.

Strategies: Detoxification

Formulas: Plant Enzyme, **Digestive Support**, **Chinese Earth-Decreasing**, and Christopher's Carminative

Programs: Chinese Balanced Cleansing

Herbs: Cardamom, coptis, licorice, parsley, and peppermint

Supplements: Chlorophyll, **propolis**, and vitamin B_3

Essential Oils: Clove, lemon, **myrrh**, **peppermint**, and spearmint

Hangover

See also alcoholism and hypoglycemia

A hangover is a set of acute symptoms such as headache, nausea, and/or vomiting as a result of recent excessive consumption of alcohol. Alcohol is dehydrating and causes blood sugar swings (hypoglycemia). One can reduce the negative effects of alcohol by consuming about twice the amount of water as alcoholic beverages and by using alcohol with meals so that there are proteins and fats available to keep blood sugar stable. Herbs and supplements that aid liver detoxification, like milk thistle, kudzu, and N-acetyl-cysteine, can help the liver detoxify the alcohol and reduce the tendency for hangovers.

Strategies: Hydration and Liver Detoxification

Formulas: Chinese Wood-Decreasing, Liver Cleanse, and **Hepatoprotective**

Herbs: Borage, **kudzu**, licorice, **milk thistle**, nopal, and Saint John's wort

Supplements: N-acetyl cysteine, vitamin B-complex, and vitamin B_{12}

Hardening of the Arteries
see *arteriosclerosis*

Hashimoto's Disease
Thyroiditis

See also autoimmune disorders, hyperthyroid, leaky gut, and dysbiosis

Hashimoto's disease is the most common cause of hypothyroidism (low thyroid activity). It is an autoimmune disease in which the immune system attacks the tissue that produces the thyroid hormone. Since 90 percent of the people who have been diagnosed with low thyroid hormones have antibodies to thyroid tissue in their blood, this is the most common cause of low thyroid hormones.

Conventional medicine has no effective treatments for this disease other than to replace the hormones that are not being made because of the damage to the thyroid. Most herbalists simply try to strengthen the thyroid with iodine or iodine-rich herbs. However, none of this is effective because Hashimoto's is not a disease of the thyroid; it is a disease of the immune system.

If you have low thyroid, you may wish to have your antibodies checked to see if you have Hashimoto's. If you do, here are some strategies that may help correct this problem. These strategies came from Thomas Easley, who co-authored *Modern Herbal Dispensary* with me.

Avoid Gliadin (Gluten)

Several studies have shown a link between autoimmune thyroid disorders and gluten intolerance. The molecular structure of gliadin in gluten closely resembles that of the thyroid gland. When gliadin passes the protective barrier of the gut and enters the bloodstream, the immune system tags it for destruction. These antibodies to gliadin (and possibly the other one hundred protein structures in wheat) also cause the body to attack thyroid tissue by molecular mimicry.

Avoid all gluten bearing grains. You need to be very strict about this. It may also help to avoid all other grains and legumes for a few months while the gut heals. See the *Gluten-Free Diet* strategy.

Heal the Gut

The thyroid hormone helps gut integrity and a loss of gut integrity contributes to autoimmune disorders. So it's important to heal the gut. See the *Gut-Healing Diet* strategy, but more importantly read about correcting *dysbiosis* and *leaky gut syndrome*. Since thyroid hormones play a big role in regulating the tight junctions of the intestinal membrane you may need a prescription thyroid medication (like Armour Thyroid) temporarily while the gut is healing.

Supplement with Selenium

The exacerbation of Hashimoto's disease by iodine almost always occurs in the presence of a selenium deficiency. Selenium by itself has been shown in several studies to reduce thyroid antibodies, showing a lessening of the immune attack on the thyroid. Take one capsule a day of a selenium supplement that supplies 200 mcg of selenium preferably in the form of L-selenomethionine, sodium selenate, selenodiglutathione and Se-methyl L-selenocysteine. This can improve thyroid function and balance immune excess.

Supplement with Vitamin D

Vitamin D is produced from cholesterol when your skin is exposed to the sun. Vitamin D deficiency is very common and most people don't have adequate levels. People with Hashimoto's should try to slowly increase their blood level to the therapeutic level of 70 ng/ml. Vitamin D also works best when balanced with vitamins K, E, and A.

Iodine

Dr. David Brownstein published the theory that supplemental iodine in large doses might help Hashimoto's disease. Iodine loading test show that about 70 percent of the people coming to Dr. Brownstein do have a mild iodine deficiency. After you have been taking selenium and vitamin D for two weeks, you can start taking herbs or herbal formulas that contain iodine, or an iodine supplement. I'd recommend trying one to two drops of liquid dulse as a source of iodine and gradually increase the dose by one or two drops each week. Monitor how you are feeling, if symptoms get worse, stop taking the iodine.

Use Botanicals that Balance Immune Function

Astragalus and ashwagandha have a strong balancing action on the immune system and the thyroid. Since this is an autoimmune disorder, avoid immune stimulants. See *Autoimmune Disorders* for more information.

Use Armour Thyroid If Needed

If your thyroid tests show function is low, you may need a *Thyroid Glandular Formula*. If that isn't enough, you may need to take Armour Thyroid. Armour Thyroid is the most well known brand of desiccated porcine thyroid. It is available by prescription only. You should never take any form of desiccated porcine thyroid without doctor's supervision and regular blood testing. Unfortunately, many doctors are resistant to prescribing Armour Thyroid because of misinformation by pharmaceutical representatives promoting Synthroid. You may have to hunt around for a doctor who will be willing to write a prescription for you.

You may wish to work with a professional herbalist or naturopath (findanherbalist.com or americanherbalistsguild.com).

Strategies: Affirmation and Visualization, Blood Type Diet, Friendly Flora, Gluten-Free Diet, Gut-Healing Diet, and Stress Management

Formulas: Thyroid Glandular, **Chinese Yang-Reducing**, Adaptogen-Immune, Stan Malstrom's Herbal Aspirin, Anti-Inflammatory Pain, **Betaine HCl**, Adrenal Glandular, Hypothyroid, and Ashwagandha Complex

Herbs: Ashwagandha, **astragalus**, black walnut, dulse, eleuthero, gotu kola, **he shou wu**, licorice, lobelia, milk thistle, and saw palmetto

Supplements: Co-Q10, iodine, lecithin, **selenium**, **vitamin D**, vitamin E, vitamin K, and zinc

Hay fever
see *allergies (respiratory)*
and *rhinitis (allergic)*

Headache

See also headache (tension), headache (migraine), pain, stress, headache (sinus), and headache (cluster)

Headaches are a symptom of an imbalance in the body, or some type of interference with normal body processes. While an analgesic can temporarily suppress the pain, if you want long-term relief from chronic headaches, you need to start identifying what might be throwing your body out of balance.

Before we begin suggesting remedies, let's discuss two basic types of headaches, Most migraines are vasodilative and feel like the head is pounding or exploding. Other headaches are vasoconstrictive in nature. In vasoconstrictive headaches, the head feels like it is in a vice or being squeezed. Most of the tips under *headache (migraine)* work for vasodilative headaches, while suggestions under *headache (tension)* work for vasoconstrictive headaches.

Here are some strategies to consider for all headaches.

Stay Hydrated

Dehydration can cause headaches. Bathed in a saline solution, the brain is the most hydrated organ in the body. Even a slight decrease in the water level of the brain affects neurotransmitters that can trigger headaches. This may be why caffeine, alcohol, and exercise trigger headaches; they all increase water loss. See the *Hydration* strategy for more information.

Ease the Eye and Neck Strain

Many people get headaches from working too much at the computer. As people strain to look at the screen, their head leans forward, causing the muscles in their upper back and neck to strain trying to hold the head up against the weight of gravity. This creates upper back, shoulder, and neck tension, which can ultimately result in a "splitting" headache. Eye strain can also cause headaches.

Here are some ways to eliminate this type of headache. Be aware of your posture and try to keep your head erect. Put your monitor at eye level so you look straight ahead to see the screen. Take breaks from close work, letting your eyes look up and focus across the room every fifteen minutes. At the same time, stretch the neck and shoulders backwards to help relax the muscles. Make sure your work or reading area is well lit. Have your eyes checked regularly and wear glasses if needed.

Ease Neck and Shoulder Tension

Tension in the neck and shoulders is a common cause of many types of headaches. I've relieved many headaches with massage. Applying remedies topically to help the muscles in the shoulders and neck while massaging them. These include lobelia, liquid magnesium, analgesic essential oils or *Analgesic EO Blends*, and *Antispasmodic Extracts*. Laying down and practicing the *Deep Breathing* strategy after doing this self-massage will increase its effectiveness.

You may find that the services of a massage therapist or chiropractor helpful too. Chiropractors often relieve headaches by adjusting the vertebrae in the upper back and neck to release pressure on nerves. You can also try some of the techniques in the *Lymph-Moving Pain Relief* strategy.

Eliminate Allergy-Causing Foods

Many headaches are triggered by allergies. Histamine, a neurotransmitter released in allergic reactions, can affect the brain and cause headaches. If you suffer from frequent headaches, especially migraines, it may be helpful to keep a food journal. Record what you eat throughout the day and the time you eat it. Also, record the times when you experience headaches. This can help you identify food triggers that may be making your head ache. See the *Eliminate Allergy-Causing Foods* strategy for more ideas.

Use Herbal Remedies to Ease Pain

Try using some analgesic herbal remedies to take the edge off the pain while working on the root causes. Kudzu can help headaches caused by tension in the neck. Black cohosh can also be helpful for these types of headaches. Willow bark has also been traditionally used to ease the pain of headaches. If you're under a lot of stress, take some supplements to help your body relax more, such as kava kava. See *stress* for more information.

You can also look up remedies for specific types of headaches such as migraines, tension headaches, cluster headaches, and sinus headaches. If you suffer from persistent headaches you may wish to consult with a medical doctor to make sure that there are no serious underlying medical causes for your headaches.

Strategies: Alkalize the Body, Aromatherapy, Deep Breathing, Eliminate Allergy-Causing Foods, Emotional Healing Work, Good Posture, Herbal Back Adjustment, Hydration, Lymph-Moving Pain Relief, Reduce Chemical Exposure, and Stress Management

Formulas: Chinese Yang-Reducing, **Topical Analgesic**, **Stan Malstrom's Herbal Aspirin**, Anti-Inflammatory Pain, **Analgesic Nerve**, General Analgesic, CBD Topical Analgesic, and Antispasmodic

Essential Oil Blends: Analgesic EO and Calming and Relaxing EO

Herbs: Black cohosh, capsicum, chrysanthemum, **dogwood (Jamaican),** forsythia, kava kava, kudzu, ligusticum, linden, **lobelia,** mulberry, sage, siler, thyme, and **willow**

Supplements: 5-HTP, **CBD, magnesium,** potassium, and **vitamin B-complex**

Essential Oils: Copaiba, helichrysum, lavender, lemon, neroli, rose, spearmint, and **wintergreen**

Headache, Cluster

See also headache

Cluster headaches are severe and often occur after a person falls asleep. The burning, sharp pain typically occurs on one side of the head, often around the eye. There is often swelling under or around the eye (or eyes), tearing, red eyes, runny nose, and a flushed face.

Cluster headaches may be due to a lack of oxygen from congested sinuses or other problems. They may also be a sign of problems with the hypothalamus, hormonal imbalances, digestive disorders, nerve dysfunction, structural issues, or stress. If you have problems with cluster headaches, work with your natural health care advisor to try to identify the underlying causes and try some of the basic remedies listed under *headache*.

Strategies: Detoxification, Eliminate Allergy-Causing Foods, and Hydration

Formulas: Topical Analgesic

Essential Oil Blends: Analgesic EO

Herbs: Barberry, capsicum, celandine, chicory, and **skullcap**

Supplements: Iron, **magnesium,** and vitamin B$_{12}$

Essential Oils: Peppermint and rosemary

Headache, Migraine

See also food allergies/intolerances, anemia, leaky gut, headache, SIBO, and mitochondrial dysfunction

A migraine is a recurrent, moderate to severe headache often accompanied by visual disturbances, nausea, and vomiting. Migraines affect about twenty-eight million Americans. People experiencing a migraine typically have an intense unilateral headache, with one half of their head in pain of a pulsating nature. Migraines can last from two to seventy-two hours and can cause nausea, vomiting, increased sensitivity to light and/or sound, with pain normally exacerbated by physical activity.

Migraines are typically associated with a dilation of the cranial blood vessels, as opposed to the constriction of cranial vessels with common tension headaches. Migraines are also associated with the release of the neurotransmitter serotonin from affected nerve endings.

The most used class of migraine medications are triptans (i.e., Imitrex, Maxalt, and Zomig), which carry an increased risk of stroke and can cause high blood pressure, vascular spasms, and birth defects. Triptans and common OTC analgesics like Tylenol, aspirin, and ergotamine are all associated with rebound migraines, thus perpetuating the pain. None of these medications will stop you from getting migraines. To end them you need to identify and remove the cause.

This can be tricky because there are many factors that contribute to migraines. However, here are some of the most common causes to check for and the natural therapies that can help.

Check for Food Allergies and Chemical Triggers

Migraines often have food allergy triggers, including chocolate, citrus, alcohol, and aged or cured foods. An exaggerated immune response is correlated with migraines. For example, people with celiac disease, an immune attack on the intestinal tract from a gluten allergy, are ten times more likely to have migraines! People with any autoimmune disorder are also much more prone to migraines.

Common foods that may cause this reaction include: chocolate, processed and pickled foods, smoked fish, chicken livers, figs, avocados, bananas, citrus fruits, nuts, peanut butter, onions, dairy products, and gluten-bearing grains like wheat, oats, barley, and rye. Certain chemicals, both manmade and some found in nature, are also known to trigger migraines. So you want to reduce chemical exposure by avoiding aspartame, MSG (monosodium glutamate), nitrates (in deli meats), and sulfites (found in wine, dried fruit, and some foods in salad bars). See the *Eliminate Allergy-Causing Foods* strategy and the *food allergies/intolerance* condition for ideas on screening out allergy-causing foods.

Take Magnesium

Many people with migraines have magnesium deficiency. If your migraines are accompanied by muscular tension or cramping (anything that feels too tight), constipation, heart palpitations, anxiety, insomnia, and/or fatigue, this may be a factor. Start with 200-400 mg per day and see if this helps. You can work up to a higher dose (800-1,000 mg per day) if you're severely deficient.

Check for and Correct Anemia

There are many causes of anemia, but no matter the cause, anemia reduces oxygen to the brain. Insufficient oxygen to the brain means headaches. The migraine-related symptoms of anemia include general weakness, fatigue even when rested, malaise, poor concentration, pale tongue and gums, the compulsive consumption of non-food items like ice, soil, paper, wax and grass (pica), restless legs, and twitching muscles. Anemia is easy to test for because it causes lowered hemoglobin and hematocrit on a CBC panel. If anemia is an issue, see the suggestions under *anemia*.

Check for and Correct Hypothyroidism

Symptoms that low thyroid may be a factor in migraines include depression, weight gain, cold intolerance, fatigue, anxiety, cold hands and feet, chronic muscle pain, constipation, and dry skin. If these symptoms accompany migraines, see the suggestions under *Hashimoto's Disease* and *Hypothyroidism*.

Check for and Correct Hormonal Imbalances

If migraines are accompanied by PMS with bloating, fluid retention, breast tenderness, menstrual cramps, and/or heavy or irregular menstrual cycles, hormonal imbalances may be a factor. Birth control pills can be an issue. If symptoms or hormone saliva testing indicates imbalances in progesterone and estrogen levels, supplements to balance estrogen or progesterone may be helpful. See *estrogen (low)* or *progesterone (low)* for suggestions.

Heal the Gut

If you have intestinal bloating and gas, frequent indigestion, mood swings or abdominal discomfort of any kind, you probably need to heal your intestines and improve the balance in your friendly flora. Leaky gut syndrome and SIBO are major underlying causes of migraines. Follow the *Gut-Healing Diet* strategy and the recommendations under *leaky gut syndrome* and *SIBO*.

Take Herbal Bitters

Migraines are often liver related and respond well to bitter herbs that help to detoxify the liver. In most migraines, it seems like too much blood and energy is flowing upward into the head. Bitters draw blood and energy downward into the digestive tract and eliminative organs. So it may also be helpful to take an *Herbal Bitters Formula* prior to meals and when one is having a migraine. Where migraines are liver related, the *Chinese Wood-Decreasing Formula* or the *Chinese Balanced Cleansing Program* may help reduce their frequency and intensity.

One of the most popular bitter herbs used to relieve migraines is feverfew. Studies have shown that feverfew can reduce both the symptoms and the severity of migraines in many people when taken regularly. Feverfew is a bitter, which is part of the reason it helps. It is important to understand that feverfew is not very effective at easing a migraine once it has started. It needs to be taken regularly to help prevent migraines.

Improve Mitochondrial Function

Improving mitochondrial function may help to reduce the inflammatory response involved in migraines. Try taking:

400 mg vitamin B_2 (riboflavin) twice a day

200 mg a day of Co-Q10

See *mitochondrial dysfunction* for more information.

Release Burdens and Tense Muscles

I've done massage on the neck and shoulders many times to relieve migraine pain and it does so about 90 percent of the time. I've observed that migraine sufferers tend to carry a lot of burdens emotionally, feeling overly responsible for other people. This results in tense shoulder muscles, which often give the shoulders a rounded appearance.

Rub a small amount of *Topical Analgesic Formula* along with some lobelia extract or tincture into your neck and shoulders while doing the massage to ease the tension. Do this nightly to prevent the headaches from occurring. You may find that the services of a massage therapist or chiropractor will be helpful too.

Additional Remedies

A single herb that has proven helpful for some migraine sufferers is butterbur. CBD has also been helpful for some people. You may wish to consult with a qualified herbalist or naturopath to find and remove the cause of your migraines (findanherbalist.com or americanherbalistsguild.com).

Strategies: Bodywork, Detoxification, Eliminate Allergy-Causing Foods, Eliminate Salicylates, Good Posture, Gut-Healing Diet, and Hydration

Formulas: Topical Analgesic, **Chinese Wood-Decreasing**, Antihistamine, **Herbal Bitters**, and **Headache**

Programs: Chinese Balanced Cleansing

Herbs: Butterbur, cannabis, coffee, **dogwood (Jamaican)**, dong quai, **feverfew**, ginger, ginkgo, linden, lobelia, periwinkle, siler, and wood betony

Supplements: CBD, **Co-Q10**, L-arginine, L-tryptophan, lithium, **magnesium**, SAM-e, **vitamin B_2**, and vitamin B_3

Essential Oils: Helichrysum, marjoram, peppermint, and ylang ylang

Headache, Sinus

See also congestion (sinus)

Sinus headaches are the result of sinus infections and are felt in the sinus areas (below and above the eyes). Not all headaches felt in this area are related to the sinuses, however. It is only a sinus headache when there is infection present.

Fenugreek and thyme have proved beneficial for decongesting the sinuses in these situations. You should also use echinacea and goldenseal for the infection.

Strategies: Detoxification

Formulas: Sinus, Anti-Snoring, Jeannie Burgess' Allergy-Lung, **Topical Analgesic**, Steven Horne's Sinus Snuff, and Chinese Metal-Decreasing

Herbs: Echinacea, **fenugreek**, **goldenseal**, Saint John's wort, **thyme**, and wood betony

Supplements: Vitamin A and **vitamin D**

Headache, Tension

See also headache

If you have a tension headache, it is generally felt equally on both sides of the head. The pain may be dull or squeezing, with a sensation that the head is in a tight band or a vice. You will also typically have tension and even soreness in your neck and shoulders.

The quickest way to ease a tension headache is to drink a lot of water and massage your neck and shoulders as described under the general condition *headaches*. Anything that helps your body relax is going to help you ease the pain of a tension headache, such as kava kava, passionflower, lavender, valerian, or hops. Emptying the contents of a magnesium capsule onto your tongue is another way to relax tension quickly.

Tension headaches may arise from the digestive system and from being constipated. If you've got digestive upset, acid indigestion, or your bowels aren't moving regularly, take something to clear out your gastrointestinal tract, like a *Stimulant Laxative* or a *General Detoxifying Formula*. Often the headache will go away as soon as the digestive tract is clear. If you suffer from frequent tension headaches, try following the *Detoxification* strategy.

Strategies: Aromatherapy, Bodywork, Deep Breathing, Detoxification, Herbal Back Adjustment, Hydration, Lymph-Moving Pain Relief, Sleep, and Stress Management

Formulas: Christopher's Nervine, **Analgesic Nerve**, Chinese Fire-Decreasing, **Topical Analgesic**, and Headache

Essential Oil Blends: Balancing EO, Mood Lifting EO, and Calming and Relaxing EO

Herbs: Black cohosh, California poppy, eleuthero, gynostemma, hops, **kava kava**, khella, lobelia, mistletoe, passion flower, periwinkle, **skullcap**, skunk cabbage, typhonium, valerian, **vervain (blue)**, wild lettuce, and wood betony

Supplements: L-arginine, **magnesium**, and vitamin B-complex

Essential Oils: Jasmine and lavender

Hearing Loss

See also earache, free radical damage, and tinnitus

Hearing loss is common among the elderly and middle-aged folks, but today's youth are starting to experience hearing problems that used to belong only to the older generation. Ear-buds, exotic car audio systems, and high-output home theater components crank out tunes at unprecedented volume levels, and most people are completely unaware of the damage they are inflicting on their delicate ears. Hearing specialists say they're also seeing more people in their thirties and forties who suffer from pronounced tinnitus, an internal ringing, whooshing, or humming in the ears.

Of all the factors contributing to hearing loss, loud noise is generally the most common. Fortunately, this is something over which we have a lot of control. Noise levels are measured in decibels, or *dB* for short. The higher the decibel level, the louder the noise. Our hearing system can be injured not only by a loud blast but also by prolonged exposure to high noise levels. Sounds of 85 to 90 decibels and higher can cause permanent hearing loss.

To get an idea of the decibel level of various sounds, here are a few examples: sounds over 120 decibels can be acutely painful, such as a jet plane taking off or a siren (120 decibels), a jackhammer (130 decibels), firearms (140 decibels) and fireworks at three feet (150 decibels). Prolonged exposure to the following extremely loud sounds can also create hearing problems: a passing motorcycle (90 decibels), a hand drill (100 decibels), small gas engines like lawn mowers and snow blowers (106 decibels) and a chain saw (110 decibels). 110 dB is the maximum output of most MP3 players.

In contrast, a vacuum cleaner or busy traffic is only 70 decibels, and most kitchen appliances and hair dryers are between 80-90 decibels. A typical conversation is only 60 decibels.

If you have to raise your voice to be heard, can't hear someone three feet from you, have difficulty discerning speech after leaving a noisy area, or have pain or ringing in your ears after exposure to noise, your hearing has probably been damaged, so get your ears checked.

Nutrition and Hearing

The ear is often referred to as the most energy-hungry organ of the body. All parts of the ear require high quantities of nutrients to function properly and to avoid degenerative problems such as hearing loss or tinnitus. Only if the right minerals and enzymes are present can the nerves successfully fire the precise signals at millisecond intervals required to accurately transmit sound.

The delicate balance of the hearing system can be upset by

- insufficient oxygen due to poor circulation in the inner ear,
- a deficiency in the trace minerals needed for enzyme activity,
- a toxic overload being carried by the body, and
- excessive free radical activity.

The electrical stability of the cochlea depends on the presence of minerals such as magnesium and calcium, as well as a correct balance of necessary enzymes, fatty acids, and amino acids. The tiny hair-like cells called cilia are the final stage of sound transmission before the charge is relayed to the auditory nerve. Slight disturbances in the equilibrium of enzymes can lead to the death of some of the cilia.

Strategies for Hearing Loss

Based on this information, here are some natural strategies that may help your hearing. First, antioxidants protect your ears, just like they protect your eyes. See *free radical damage* for a list of antioxidant remedies.

Second, trace minerals are critical to hearing. *Colloidal Mineral Formulas* may aid hearing and help restore ear health.

Third, loud noises cause tiny muscles on the bones in the ear to contract tightly, which limits sound transmission. Using remedies as eardrops that help these muscles relax can be helpful for hearing. These include lobelia, the *Antispasmodic Ear Formula,* and *Ear Drop Formulas* that contain Saint John's wort. Magnesium taken internally may also help.

Fourth, where there is nerve damage, Saint John's wort can be taken internally and helichrysum EO can be diluted (10:1) and used as eardrops. All eardrops should be warmed to body temperature before being used in the ear.

Strategies: Eat Healthy, Hydration, and Mineralization

Formulas: Antispasmodic Ear, Colloidal Mineral, and Ear Drop

Herbs: Dogwood (Asian), **ginkgo**, lobelia, periwinkle, and **Saint John's wort**

Supplements: Calcium, **magnesium**, manganese, and vitamin B_9

Essential Oils: Helichrysum

Heart Attack   see *cardiac arrest*

Heart Disease   see *cardiovascular disease*

Heart Fibrillation/Palpitations

See also hiatal hernia

Rapid, irregular contractions of the heart muscle are called heart palpitations or fibrillations. Symptoms can include an irregular or rapid heart rate, skipped heartbeats, shortness of breath, and chest discomfort. They may be congenital—meaning the person has them as part of a lifelong, perhaps genetic, pattern but they may also be acute problems caused by anxiety, lack of exercise, high blood pressure, diabetes, hyperthyroid, or other problems.

If the heart palpitations are associated with extreme stress or burnout, then the *Chinese Fire-Increasing Formula* may help. If they are associated with a high strung personality that finds it difficult to relax, the *Chinese Fire-Decreasing Formula* may help.

One of the best natural solutions is to make sure the person has adequate amounts of minerals, especially magnesium, potassium, and calcium. These minerals help to regulate heart rhythm.

A hiatal hernia can sometimes put stress on the heart and cause palpitations. See the *Hiatal Hernia Correction* strategy.

You may need to consult with a professional herbalist or naturopath (findanherbalist.com or americanherbalistsguild.com) to find the right remedies to help this problem. You should also have the condition monitored by a medical doctor.

Strategies: Affirmation and Visualization, Emotional Healing Work, Hiatal Hernia Correction, and Stress Management

Formulas: Chinese Fire-Decreasing, Herbal Potassium, Methyl B12 Vitamin, and Chinese Earth-Increasing

Flower Essences: Broken and Hardened Hearts FE

Herbs: Asparagus, astragalus, biota, bugleweed, California poppy, capsicum, cherry, eleuthero, **hawthorn**, hoelen, lemon balm, ligustrum, linden, **motherwort**, night-blooming cereus, passion flower, polygala, salvia, and valerian

Supplements: Amber (succinum), calcium, chlorophyll, Co-Q10, iron, L-carnitine, **magnesium**, **potassium**, vitamin B-complex, vitamin B_{12}, and vitamin E

Essential Oils: Marjoram, neroli, orange (sweet), and ylang ylang

Heart Rate, Irregular   see *arrhythmia*

Heart Rate, Rapid   see *tachycardia*

Heart Valves

Heart valve problems may be present at birth or can be caused by infections, heart attacks, or some other damage to the heart. There are three basic problems that can occur. First, the valve may not close tightly, allowing blood to leak back through the valve. This is called regurgitation. Second, if the valve doesn't open wide enough to allow for normal blood flow, this is called stenosis. The third and most common heart valve problem occurs in the mitral valve. Sometimes it doesn't close tightly, allowing regurgitation. This is called mitral valve prolapse.

Heart valve conditions should be monitored by a medical doctor. There are some herbs and nutrients that may be helpful too. For instance, night blooming cereus is a particularly good remedy for mitral valve prolapse and other valvular problems. Hawthorn and magnesium can also helpful for valvular insufficiency. Problems with heart valves require medical attention. For help with natural remedies seek out a qualified herbalist or naturopath (findanherbalist.com or americanherbalistsguild.com).

Strategies: Mineralization

Formulas: Brain-Heart

Herbs: Ginkgo, **hawthorn**, and **night-blooming cereus**

Supplements: Magnesium

Essential Oils: Marjoram

Heart Weakness

See also cardiac arrest, cardiovascular disease, and congestive heart failure

When the heart has been stressed or weakened by disease, there are herbs and nutrients that can be used to strengthen it. Cardiac formulas containing herbs like hawthorn, arjuna, night-blooming cerus, and lily of the valley can encourage a stronger heartbeat and improve cardiac function. Good fats and nutrients like magnesium, l-carnitine, and Co-Q10 may also be helpful. Consult with a qualified herbalist or naturopath (findanherbalist.com or americanherbalistsguild.com) to help determine which supplements would be best.

Strategies: Eat Healthy, Healthy Fats, and Oral Chelation

Formulas: Heart Health, **Chinese Fire-Increasing**, Brain-Heart, Steven Horne's Horehound Cough, and **Nitric Oxide Boosting**

Flower Essences: Broken and Hardened Hearts FE

Herbs: Arjuna, astragalus, capsicum, coffee, eleuthero, ginkgo, **hawthorn**, night-blooming cereus, and passion flower

Supplements: Co-Q10, L-carnitine, **magnesium**, omega-3 EFAs, and vitamin B_1

Heartburn   **see** *acid indigestion*

Heavy Metal Poisoning

See also chemical exposure, lead poisoning, mercury poisoning, and aluminum toxicity

The term *heavy metal* refers to a group of elements that have metallic properties and a high molecular weight. This includes mercury, arsenic, lead, and cadmium, all of which have no nutritional value and are toxic. In natural healing circles, we often include aluminum in this discussion, even though it is not technically a heavy metal.

There are also metallic elements that are needed in small amounts, which become toxic in large quantities or in the wrong forms. These include copper, vanadium, chromium, tin, nickel, and even iron. The following discussion is about dealing with heavy metals in general. You can look up individual metals for additional suggestions.

Heavy metals occur naturally in the earth's crust. So everyone is exposed to small amounts of them regularly. Fortunately, these elements are hard to absorb in their natural forms, and if they do get absorbed, the body is equipped with detoxification mechanisms to get rid of them.

Unfortunately, the Industrial Revolution involved mining, concentrating, and using heavy metals in industry, agriculture, and medicine. These modern industrial processes create higher concentrations of these substances, increasing risk of exposure. This is compounded by the fact that the detoxification mechanisms for eliminating them require nutrients and many people in modern society are on nutrient-deficient diets.

The result is that heavy metals have become a serious health concern in modern times. Many of these metals are particularly harmful to the nervous system because of its high fat content and many are known to cause neurological disorders. They also tend to disrupt immune function and may contribute to autoimmune diseases and cancer, as well as increased inflammation.

Acute heavy metal poisoning is best diagnosed and handled by medical professionals. The concern for people who simply want to preserve their health is the constant exposure to low doses of these substances. The effects of this are more subtle.

Reducing Exposure

The most important thing to do is to reduce your exposure to heavy metals. Here are a few important strategies for doing this.

Purify your water. Heavy metals can enter municipal water supplies through industrial and consumer waste, acid rain, or even from pipes. You can remove heavy metals from the water you drink with a reverse osmosis water purification system or distallation, but carbon filters are ineffective.

Eat organic food as much as possible. Eating organic foods minimizes your exposure to all chemicals, including heavy metals.

Reduce Exposure to Aluminum. Avoid cooking with aluminum. Acidic foods like tomatoes and citrus are particularly problematic as they leech aluminum into the food. Use aluminum-free baking powder and avoid aluminum-based antiperspirant deodorants.

Educate yourself about vaccines. Make an informed choice about what vaccines, if any, you will allow. Vaccines can contain both mercury and aluminum.

Limit intake of fish with a high mercury content. Look for fish that are not harvested from contaminated waters.

Have amalgam fillings replaced with composites. This should be done by a dentist who knows how to remove them safely.

Reduce Chemical Exposure. Avoid using chemical pesticides, herbicides, and other toxic products and replace them with nontoxic natural alternatives. If you work around chemicals pay attention to safety precautions. Wear appropriate protective clothing.

Testing for Heavy Metals

Assessing whether low-grade exposure to heavy metals may be a factor in a person's health problems can be difficult. Blood tests to determine levels of heavy metals can be run, but these are best at detecting acute heavy metal poisoning. A low level of a heavy metal in the blood does not necessarily mean that excessive exposure has not occurred, because heavy metals do not stay in the blood for very long.

Another way to detect possible heavy metal toxicity is through hair analysis. High levels of heavy metals in your hair are a possible indicator that there may be heavy metals in your body. However, heavy metals in the hair may not be coming from inside the body but from outside exposure.

Even without this kind of analysis, people who work around chemicals (i.e., painters, beauticians, lab technicians, dry cleaners, carpet cleaners, farmers, and factory workers) who are developing neurological or immune problems may benefit from taking herbs or supplements periodically that aid heavy metal detoxification. People with autism, cancer, neuralgia, memory loss, chronic inflammation, and autoimmune disorders may also benefit from a heavy metal detoxification program.

Read the *Heavy Metal Cleanse* strategy for a basic heavy metal detoxification program and seek assistance from a competent herbalist or naturopath (findanherbalist.com or americanherbalistsguild.com). You can also look up specific protocols for mercury, lead, arsenic, cadmium, and aluminum.

Strategies: Drawing Bath, Epsom Salt Bath, Heavy Metal Cleanse, Liver Detoxification, and Oral Chelation

Formulas: Intestinal Detoxification, **Heavy Metal Cleansing**, **Oral Chelation**, Hepatoprotective, Fiber, and **Gut-Healing Fiber**

Programs: Ivy Bridge's Cleansing

Herbs: Blue-green algae, chaparral, chlorella, cilantro/coriander herb, **milk thistle**, and psyllium

Supplements: **Alpha-lipoic acid**, clay (bentonite), **clay (Redmond)**, iodine, L-methionine, **N-acetyl cysteine**, omega-3 EFAs, and **sodium alginate**

Hemochromatosis

When a person has too much iron in the blood, the condition is commonly known as hemochromatosis. Primary hemochromatosis refers to accumulating too much iron because of a genetic mutation. Secondary hemochromatosis is iron overload from any other (nongenetic) causes like excessive iron consumption, multiple blood transfusions, lack of iron binding capacity, and zinc deficiencies.

Zinc is particularly important because zinc and iron, like many minerals, have an antagonistic relationship. Low levels of zinc can contribute to higher levels of iron and vice versa. Thus, supplementing with zinc will often help to reduce the levels of iron.

Other nutrients that help the body utilize iron better may also be helpful, including folate, vitamin B_6 and vitamin B_{12}. Another option may be taking formulas with iron-rich herbs, as the nutritional cofactors in iron-rich herbs can sometimes help the body utilize iron more efficiently. Medically, giving blood transfusions can be helpful.

Formulas: Chinese Wood-Decreasing, Watkin's Hair, Skin, and Nails, Methyl B12 Vitamin, Methylated B Vitamin, and **Christopher's Herbal Iron**

Herbs: Alfalfa, nettle, stinging, and yellow dock

Supplements: Chlorophyll, **vitamin B_{12}**, **vitamin B_6**, **vitamin B_9**, vitamin C, and **zinc**

Hemorrhage
see *bleeding (external)* **and** *bleeding (internal)*

Hemorrhoids
Piles

See also varicose veins

A hemorrhoid is a mass of dilated veins in the rectum that causes painful bowel elimination. It is important to keep the stool soft with a *Fiber Blend* and plenty of water and to keep the bowels moving using a some kind of herbal laxative (*Stimulant Laxative* or *Gentle Bowel Cleansing Formulas*) for a short period (such as two weeks).

A good natural treatment is to mix white oak bark, collinsonia, or any good astringent herb into a *Healing Salve* or some coconut oil and apply the mixture topically.

Hemorrhoids are in indication that blood vessels, in general, need toning. It is common for an individual with hemorrhoids to have other varicosities like varicose veins. Taking a *Vein Tonic Formula* internally and eating more berries can help to tone veins. Vitamin C with bioflavonoids is also helpful for toning veins.

Strategies: Eat Healthy, Hydration, Increase Dietary Fiber, and Sitz Bath

Formulas: Irritable Bowel Fiber, **Fiber**, **Vein Tonic**, Gentle Bowel Cleansing, **Healing Salve**, Stimulant Laxative, and Chinese Earth-Increasing

Herbs: Acacia (Indian), amalaki, bilberry, butcher's broom, chickweed, **collinsonia**, goldenseal, **horse chestnut**, horsetail, hyacinth, marshmallow, psyllium, slippery elm, **white oak**, and yellow dock

Supplements: Bioflavonoids, **vitamin C**, and vitamin E

Essential Oils: Cypress

Hepatitis

Hepatitis is inflammation of the liver. Hepatitis A is an infectious hepatitis that can be transmitted through poor sanitary conditions, such as food handlers or child-care workers not washing their hands. Hepatitis B or serum hepatitis is passed through a blood transfusion or other contact with blood. Hepatitis C is also infectious and viral in nature. Hepatitis can also be caused by chemicals, poor diet, and other lifestyle factors that damage the liver. Seek appropriate medical assistance when dealing with hepatitis, as it is a very serious condition.

Natural remedies that may be helpful include herbs with hepatoprotective properties such as milk thistle and schizandra. SAM-e and vitamin C can be helpful taken internally. Since most cases are viral-related, antiviral herbs may also aid in recovery. Helichrysum essential oils can be massaged into the area over the liver. CBD may also help reduce inflammation in the liver.

To allow the liver to rest when recovering from hepatitis, fast or eat only mild foods and drink plenty of water. Avoid spices, alcohol, caffeine, and all chemicals such as food additives and preservatives.

Strategies: Avoid Caffeine, Eat Healthy, Fasting, Forgiveness, and Hydration

Formulas: Chinese Wood-Increasing, **Chinese Wood-Decreasing**, Liver Cleanse, **Hepatoprotective**, Chinese Wind-Heat Evil, and Betaine HCl

Flower Essence Blends: Anger-Reducing FE

Herbs: Aloe vera, **andrographis**, asparagus (Chinese), astragalus, **bupleurum**, cordyceps, dandelion, elder, kutki, lycium, **milk thistle**, olive, Oregon grape, **picrorhiza**, rehmannia, **reishi**, schisandra, shitake, spirulina, and yellow dock

Supplements: CBD, **N-acetyl cysteine**, **SAM-e**, and vitamin C

Essential Oils: Frankincense, **helichrysum**, myrrh, and rosemary

Hernias

See also hiatal hernia

The protrusion of an organ through connective tissue or the wall of a cavity by which it is normally enclosed is called a hernia. There are many types of hernias, depending on where the weakness in the abdominal cavity occurs. Medical attention should be sought, but *Vulnerary Formulas* may help strengthen the connective tissue to aid in the healing of a hernia. I've also seen red raspberry help tone abdominal tissue to aid the healing of hernias.

Strategies: Mineralization

Formulas: Chinese Earth-Increasing, Herbal Calcium, and **Vulnerary**

Herbs: Red raspberry

Supplements: Manganese

Essential Oils: Clove

Herniated Disks   see *spinal disks*

Herpes

See also chicken pox and cold sores

Herpes is a name for any of several inflammatory viral diseases characterized by blister-like sores. *Herpes simplex* can cause cold sores or fever blisters around the mouth or genital herpes. *Herpes zoster* is responsible for chicken pox and shingles. Once a herpes virus has occurred in the body, it can lay dormant for years before flaring up again.

Antiviral herbs can help treat herpes infections. Black walnut and propolis can be applied topically to outbreaks. Cat's claw and isatis can also be used. The *Chinese Wind-Heat Evil Formula* was specifically developed by a Chinese herbalist Dr. Wenwei Xi and clinically tested to be effective at an American university. Taken regularly for six to twelve months it appears to help clear the virus from the system.

Research suggests that L-lysine is involved in the immune system and its ability to fight the herpes simplex virus. L-lysine only works if the diet is low in arginine, which is found in legumes, nuts and shellfish.

Enhancing the immune system in general by supplementing with probiotics and using a *Mushroom Immune Formula* may help prevent outbreaks. Stress tends to weaken the immune system and promote outbreaks; managing your stress can reduce outbreaks.

Strategies: Friendly Flora and Stress Management

Formulas: Gut Immune, **Chinese Wind-Heat Evil**, **Standardized Acetogenin**, Mushroom Immune, and Probiotic

Herbs: Bitter melon, **black walnut**, cat's claw, isatis, **lemon balm**, **Saint John's wort**, shitake, and spilanthes

Supplements: L-lysine, **nanoparticle silver**, propolis, and zinc

Essential Oils: Bergamot, eucalyptus, grapefruit (pink), helichrysum, lavender, lemon, myrrh, peppermint, ravensara, rose, and tea tree

Hiatal Hernia

See also ileocecal valve and SIBO

In a hiatal hernia the stomach pushes upward through the opening in the diaphragm for the esophagus. This can cause acid reflux, put stress and pressure on the heart, create poor digestive function, and generally weaken the body. The instructions for dealing with this problem are found under the *Hiatal Hernia Correction* strategy. The remedies listed here may also be helpful.

Strategies: Deep Breathing, Hiatal Hernia Correction, and Stress Management

Formulas: Chinese Earth-Increasing and **Digestive Support**

Flower Essence Blends: Personal Boundaries FE

Herbs: Catnip, **lobelia**, and slippery elm

Hiccups

Hiccups are involuntary, spasmodic contractions of the diaphragm, causing a quick inhalation of air that makes a strange sound. Antispasmodic herbs like lobelia may relax the spasms associated with hiccups.

Herbs: Blessed thistle, catnip, **cramp bark**, **lobelia**, and magnolia

Supplements: Magnesium and vitamin B_5

Essential Oils: Clove and red mandarin

High Blood Pressure   see *hypertension*

High Cholesterol   see *cholesterol (high)*

HIV   see *AIDS*

Hives   see *rashes & hives*

Hoarseness   see *laryngitis*

Hodgkin's Disease   see *lymphoma*

Hormone Replacement   see *estrogen (low)*, *hypothyroidism,* **and** *testosterone (low)*

Hot Flashes

See also menopause

Hot flashes are a complex symptom associated with menopause and the most common menopausal problem. There is an initial feeling of discomfort followed by a sensation of heat moving toward the head. The face becomes red, which is followed by sweating and fatigue. Night sweats are simply hot flashes that occur at night and cause heavy perspiration.

Although the exact cause of hot flashes is not fully understood, there is some evidence that hot flashes occur via the hypothalamus, a part of the brain that sends signals to the pituitary gland to activate various hormones. The hypothalamus also regulates the body temperature.

When the hypothalamus senses there is a need for more estrogen, it sends the gonadotropin-releasing hormone (GNRH) to the pituitary. GNRH stimulates the release of the follicle-stimulating hormone (FSH). During a woman's childbearing years, FSH stimulates the development of an egg follicle, which releases estrogen. The hypothalamus senses the increased estrogen level and stops producing GNRH.

During menopause, when there is no viable egg to develop, there is no estrogen response from the ovaries. So the hypothalamus increases production of GNRH to try to increase estrogen. The low estrogen can cause epinephrine to release from the adrenals, which stimulates the hypothalamus and resets the body's internal thermostat. This doesn't just create the sensations of heat; it can also cause the heart to speed up, resulting in feelings of anxiety and a pounding sensation in the chest.

After a while, the hypothalamus learns to adjust to lower levels of estrogen and stops trying to stimulate the ovaries. But until this happens, hot flashes may be a problem.

Fortunately, there are ways to help balance hormones to reduce the severity of hot flashes, if not eliminate them entirely. Different women will respond to different remedies, so if the first thing you try doesn't work, don't be discouraged. Try some other approaches.

For starters, heat and substances that dilate arteries (coffee, chili, and alcohol) can all aggravate hot flashes, as can smoking and sugar consumption. Stress and adrenal fatigue also contribute to increased problems with hot flashes. Establishing basic health practices, like a good diet, exercise, and adequate sleep is important to minimizing problems with hot flashes.

You can also use herbs like black cohosh and chaste tree to help regulate hormones. The *Hot Flash Formula* containing black cohosh and dong quai has helped many women, while others have been helped by an *Herbal Menopause Formula* or the *Menopause Support Pack*.

Since the adrenal glands produce estrogens, adrenal exhaustion may be a factor in hot flashes and other menopausal symptoms. Pantothenic acid and/or an *Adrenal Glandular Formula* may also be helpful. Adaptogens like eleuthero root or ashwagandha may also help.

Essential oils with estrogen-stimulating effects can also be helpful. These include clary sage, pink grapefruit, and geranium. Lavender essential oil can also be helpful for hot flashes because of its relaxing effects. Make a hydrosol spray by mixing a few drops of these oils with a little water in a small spray bottle and mist this around your face when you are having a hot flash. Essential oils directly affect the hypothalamus via the sense of smell, so this can help to instantly reset your body thermostat and cool you down.

Increasing your intake of good fats containing omega-3 and omega-6 essential fatty acids can also be helpful. Evening primrose oil is frequently used for female problems like hot flashes.

Strategies: Avoid Xenoestrogens, Eat Healthy, Healthy Fats, Low-Glycemic Diet, and Stress Management

Formulas: Chrisopher's Menopause, **Hot Flash**, Chinese Yin-Increasing, General Glandular, Female Tonic, **Adrenal Glandular**, and Chinese Fire-Increasing

Programs: Menopause Support

Essential Oil Blends: Menopause Support EO

Herbs: Ashwagandha, **black cohosh**, **chaste tree**, **damiana**, eleuthero, licorice, motherwort, and peony

Supplements: Equol, omega-3 EFAs, and **vitamin B$_5$**

Essential Oils: Clary sage, cypress, geranium, grapefruit (pink), lavender, lemon, peppermint, and rose

Huntington's Disease

This is a progressive neurodegenerative disease believed to be genetic in nature. It affects motor coordination, causing involuntary jerking movements. It also leads to dementia and disability. At present there is no known cure.

Although there is no known cure, adopting a healthy diet, exercising, and keeping the mind active can slow the progression of the disease and improve quality of life. Reducing inflammation in the nervous system would also be helpful. Some patients have reported that high doses of CBD (200 mg or more) or CBD-rich cannabis have slowed progression of the disease and eased symptoms.

Additionally, a dietary flavonoid called fisetin, which is found naturally in strawberries and other fruits and vegetables, may help slow the onset of motor issues and delays caused by Huntington's disease.

Herbs: Cannabis

Supplements: CBD, Co-Q10, omega-3 DHA, omega-3 EFAs, resveratrol, and **vitamin E**

Hyperactivity   see ADD/ADHD

Hyperinsulinemia see *metabolic syndrome*

Hypertension
High Blood Pressure

See also arteriosclerosis, cardiovascular disease, edema, metabolic syndrome, and excess weight

When there is excessive arterial tension, the heart has to pump harder in order for blood to reach the extremities of the body. This results in high blood pressure.

High blood pressure is not a disease, per se, but rather a symptom that has many different causes. This is why taking a high blood pressure medication doesn't fix the problem. It is only treating the symptom. To cure high blood pressure you have to identify and remove the cause.

Understanding Blood Pressure

To understand strategies for fixing high blood pressure we first need to understand what blood pressure is all about. Blood pressure consists of the systolic pressure and the diastolic pressure. The systolic is the pressure exerted by the contraction of the heartbeat moving blood through the blood vessels. The diastolic is the resting pressure, the pressure remaining in the blood vessel in between heartbeats.

Blood pressure is expressed with the systolic reading first, followed by the diastolic reading. Normal blood pressure is considered 90/60 to 130/90, but research shows that 115–125/70–80 is optimal for health and longevity.

The dynamics of blood pressure are fairly straightforward. Your body has about one hundred thousand miles of blood vessels. The larger vessels have muscular walls that can expand and contract to increase or decrease the diameter of the blood vessels. The diastolic pressure is the pressure needed to maintain full blood vessels. In other words, the blood vessel is like a pipe carrying liquid, which must expand or contract to match the volume of liquid it is carrying.

If air pockets get into the water pipes of your home, water doesn't flow freely to your faucet; instead, it sputters and spurts. Likewise, if the diameter of the blood vessel "pipes" were allowed to be bigger than the volume of blood they were carrying, then pockets would form and disrupt circulation. Thus, the body has a built-in system of pressure regulation to keep its "pipes" full.

If the blood vessels contract or get smaller in diameter, the diastolic pressure will rise. This also means that the heart has to increase its pressure to push the blood through the smaller pipes so there will be a corresponding rise in the systolic pressure.

This increase in pressure has negative consequences on health. It forces the heart to work harder, which wears it out faster. It increases the risk of forming blood clots in the circulatory system, which increases the risk of myocardial infarction, strokes, and thrombosis. It can cause blood vessels to blow from the pressure, causing an aneurism. It can also damage the kidneys, eyes, brain, and other organs.

Furthermore, arterial plaque never forms in veins (which are areas of low pressure). Arterial plaque only forms in areas of the circulatory system subject to high pressures. In fact, plaque formation may be a protective mechanism to shore up blood vessels so they can handle the higher pressure.

High blood pressure is virtually unknown in undeveloped areas of the world where people are living on their traditional diets. For example, high blood pressure is not found in Africa among natives living a traditional lifestyle, even among the elderly. This means that it is a problem associated with Western diet and lifestyle. In fact, about eighty percent of all hypertension cases involve mild to moderate symptoms and can be effectively managed with dietary and lifestyle changes and maybe a few herbs and/or supplements.

Strategies for Hypertension

Here are some strategies for reducing high blood pressure. Experiment and find which ones work best for you.

Properly Hydrate Your Body

In his book *You're Not Sick, You're Thirsty*, Dr. F. Batmanghelidj, MD, explains how dehydration causes an increase in blood pressure. In fact, it's fairly easy to see if you understand that the diastolic pressure is dependent on the volume of blood in the circulatory system. If a person becomes dehydrated, it reduces the volume of blood in their blood vessels, which causes them to contract and increases the pressure.

The reduced amount of water in the blood makes the sodium level in the blood higher, which is why medical doctors often recommend a reduction in salt intake. Many people have discovered that drinking more water (and using a natural form of salt like Real Salt, Celtic Salt, or Himalayan Salt) reduces the sodium level in their blood and their blood pressure (see the *Hydration* strategy).

Improve Kidney Function

When the tissues of the body are filled with fluid, this will put pressure on the blood vessels, again constricting blood flow. Oddly enough, according to Dr. Batmanghelidj this can actually be caused by dehydration. As the body becomes increasingly dehydrated, it tries harder to hang onto salt and water, which causes people to develop edema. Unfortunately, people are given diuretics to try to flush out the water, which reduces their potassium levels and stresses their kidneys.

Furthermore, the kidneys also have an influence on the heart, so problems with the kidneys can also cause the blood pressure to rise. Kidney issues are often an undiagnosed issue behind blood pressure problems. So improving kidney function with non-irritating herbal diuretics (which often supply potassium) sometimes helps bring down blood pressure. See *edema* for more information.

Lose Weight

Excess weight alone can increase blood pressure simply because there are blood vessels the heart has to pump blood through. There is also a link between excess insulin production, which contributes to excess weight and imbalances in messenger chemicals that cause arterial constriction. If you have excess weight, losing it will help reduce your blood pressure. See *excess weight* for suggestions.

Relax Blood Vessels

As mentioned above, major blood vessels have muscular walls that can either tense or relax. When we feel stressed, the body pumps out epinephrine, which attaches to adrenergic receptors. The beta-adrenergic receptors contract arteries to contract and the heart to beat harder, raising blood pressure. Perhaps you've heard of beta-blockers. These are drugs that block these beta-adrenergic receptors, which helps to lower blood pressure.

There are herbs that can do the same thing. One of them is lobelia, which contains lobeline, a natural beta-blocker. Combined with a little capsicum and black cohosh it will reduce cardiac stress and angina, improve circulation to the heart, and lower blood pressure caused by tension. Other nervines like linden flowers, passion flower, and mistletoe may also help relax blood vessels.

Take Magnesium

When muscles contract, calcium ions flow into the muscle cells; as the muscle relaxes, there is an exchange of magnesium for calcium. In other words, calcium helps muscles contract and have tone, while magnesium helps muscles relax.

This is why calcium channel blockers are sometimes used to lower blood pressure. These drugs block calcium from entering the muscle tissues, causing them to be more relaxed. Taking extra magnesium usually produces the same result. It helps blood vessels relax and increases blood flow.

Enhance Nitric Oxide

Recent research has discovered that nitric oxide (NO) acts as a neurotransmitter to dilate arteries and improve blood flow. The nitroglycerine pills used for angina create a release of NO, which is why they work. L-arginine and natural nitrates found in beets and other vegetables help to increase NO levels. Enhancing NO with a *Nitric Oxide Boosting Formula* is a good way reduce blood pressure and improve overall circulation. See *Enhance Nitric Oxide* strategy for more information about NO.

Heal the Endothelial Lining

All the thousands of miles of blood vessels in your body are coated with a lining, just one cell thick, known as the endothelial lining. The endothelial cells make the NO we just discussed. This is why Dr. Sherry A. Rogers, MD, author of *The High Blood Pressure Hoax!*, believes that dysfunction of the endothelial lining is a primary factor in high blood pressure.

The fat-soluble vitamins A, D, E, and K are all essential for the function of the endothelial lining and protecting cardiovascular health. It isn't regular dietary cholesterol that sticks to your arteries; it's oxidized cholesterol that winds up forming arterial plaque. Fat-soluble vitamins keep cholesterol from oxidizing and fats from turning rancid, which protects the endothelial lining.

There are also herbs that help the endothelial lining and create vasodilation. Hawthorn and ginkgo have both been found to dilate peripheral blood vessels and improve blood flow to the extremities, thus reducing hypertension. Numerous studies have also shown that garlic can reduce blood pressure ten to fifteen points when taken regularly. Besides having a vasodilative effect, it also decreases blood cholesterol and triglycerides. Onions also have this effect, as do many pungent spices and herbs, which can all be safely consumed as part of the regular diet.

Reduce Arterial Plaque

Arterial plaque creates obstructions in the blood vessels. Like hard water deposits in a water pipe, these deposits reduce the size of blood vessels and restrict blood flow. As a result, more force is needed to get the blood through the narrower pipes. The *Oral Chelation* strategy can be helpful in reducing and perhaps reversing the formation of arterial plaque. For more suggestions see *arteriosclerosis*.

Balance Blood Sugar

High insulin levels in the blood due to the consumption of refined carbohydrates causes inflammation in the blood vessels, which constricts blood flow. Simple sugars also react with proteins to reduce elasticity, causing blood vessels to lose flexibility. Eliminating simple carbohydrates from the diet can be very helpful for preventing and reversing high blood pressure. See *metabolic syndrome* for more information.

Avoid Caffeine and Other Stimulants

Caffeine stimulates the sympathetic nervous system and causes the release of more epinephrine. So excessive caffeine consumption increases stress responses and raises blood pressure. Other substances that trigger a sympathetic nervous reaction and stress response include alcohol, tobacco, chocolate, cheese, sugar, alcoholic beverages, and cured pork products such as ham and sausages. All these substances can contribute to hypertension and should be avoided or severely restricted in the diet if you have high blood pressure (see the *Avoid Caffeine* strategy).

Reduce Stress

In response to stress, real or perceived, the sympathetic nervous system becomes more active and the body tenses. We've all felt the results of this fight-or-flight response when someone suddenly startled us and adrenaline started pumping. The heart started beating harder and blood pressure rose as the body went on red alert.

Adaptogens can modulate the output of stress hormones and may be very helpful for stress related hypertension. So if you have hypertension and feel like you're under a lot of stress, try using some adaptogens like eleuthero.

It also helps to breathe deeply and learn to manage stress better. I've taken a person's blood pressure down twenty points by just having the do a five minute deep breathing exercise. See the *Stress Management* and *Deep Breathing* strategies.

Other Lifestyle Improvements

Exercise improves blood flow and can help to reduce blood pressure. It also helps to get adequate sleep.

If you're taking high blood pressure medications, it is important to not discontinue them abruptly. This can cause a rapid rebound effect that sends your blood pressure skyrocketing. Try using appropriate herbs, supplements, and lifestyle changes in conjunction with blood pressure medications. As your blood pressure improves, you can work with your doctor to gradually reduce the dose and possibly eliminate the need for the medication entirely. For more information on how to do this safely, consult with a qualified herbalist or naturopath (findanherbalist.com or americanherbalistsguild.com).

Strategies: Avoid Caffeine, Avoid Sugar, Blood Type Diet, Deep Breathing, Eat Healthy, Emotional Healing Work, Enhance Nitric Oxide, Healthy Fats, Hydration, Low-Glycemic Diet, Oral Chelation, Sleep, and Stress Management

Formulas: Blood Pressure Reducing, **Circulatory**, Stabilized Allicin, Heart Health, Chinese Wood-Increasing, Chinese Fire-Decreasing, Oral Chelation, Mushroom Immune, **Nitric Oxide Boosting**, Male Performance, and Adaptogen

Programs: Cardiovascular Nutritional

Herbs: Arjuna, astragalus, **beet**, **black cohosh**, capsicum, chaga, **coleus**, cordyceps, cyperus, eleuthero, eucommia, **garlic**, **ginkgo**, ginseng (American), ginseng (Asian/Korean), guggul, **hawthorn**, khella, kudzu, **linden**, lobelia, maitake, **mistletoe**, **motherwort**, nopal, olive leaf, passion flower, periwinkle, reishi, and vervain (blue)

Supplements: Alpha-lipoic acid, berberine, calcium, chromium, **Co-Q10**, colostrum, **L-arginine**, L-citruline, L-theanine, **magnesium**, N-acetyl cysteine, omega-3 EFAs, omega-6 GLA, potassium, selenium, vitamin B_3, vitamin C, vitamin D, and vitamin E

Essential Oils: Grapefruit (pink), lemon, marjoram, rose, wintergreen, and ylang ylang

Hyperthyroid　　　　**see** *Graves' disease*

Hypochondria

See also fear

A hypochondriac is a person with abnormal or excessive interest in diseases, who fears they have conditions that they do not have. This may actually be a sign of moderate liver disfunction, which presents itself as many vague and fleeting symptoms and a general feeling that a person is not well. Both the *Chinese Wood-Increasing* and *Wood-Decreasing Formulas* may help here, depending on the other symptoms present.

If a person has a fear of infection, they can infuse essential oils like oregano, peppermint, rosemary, tea tree and thyme into their home, which kills airborne germs. They could also consider some nervines or adaptogens to calm their feelings of stress and anxiety. If the person feels a sense of nervous exhaustion, milky oat seed is particularly helpful. *Affirmation and Visualization* strategy, where the person affirms or pictures themselves as healthy, whole, and protected would also be helpful.

Strategies: Affirmation and Visualization

Formulas: Adrenal Glandular, **Chinese Wood-Increasing**, **Chinese Wood-Decreasing**, Anti-Anxiety, and Anti-Stress B-Complex

Herbs: Oat seed (milky)

Supplements: Vitamin B-complex

Essential Oils: Jasmine, marjoram, oregano, peppermint, rosemary, tea tree, and thyme

Hypoglycemia

See also addictions (sugar/carbohydrates) and metabolic syndrome

Hypoglycemia is low blood sugar. When blood sugar gets low, it results in dizziness, weakness, inability to concentrate, cold nose or fingers, irritability, mood swings, and fatigue. The hypoglycemic person tends to experience an energy slump in the middle of the afternoon. There also tends to be a constant craving for sugar and simple carbohydrates. Hypoglycemia is one of the symptoms of hyperinsulinemia.

Start by following the *Low-Glycemic Diet* strategy. Start the day by eating a good breakfast with protein and good fats (like eggs). Do not eat carbohydrates (breakfast cereals, pastries, bread, etc.) for breakfast. Eat small, regular meals containing some protein and a little high-quality fat (like some nuts) throughout the day. Eating small meals with some protein in them throughout the day is very beneficial.

A program I've found very effective is too capsules of the *Algae Formula* and two capsules of licorice root for breakfast, again at lunch, and again in the afternoon around three or four o'clock if the person experiences an energy slump. If a person has high blood pressure, they can replace the licorice root with bee pollen.

Strategies: Avoid Sugar, Healthy Fats, and Low-Glycemic Diet

Formulas: Chinese Wood-Increasing, Chinese Wood-Decreasing, **Algae**, Whole Food Protein, Digestive Support, and **Hypoglycemic**

Herbs: Bee pollen, beet, **blue-green algae**, burdock, chlorella, cinnamon, eleuthero, garcinia, he shou wu, **licorice**, safflower, **spirulina**, and stevia

Supplements: Alpha-lipoic acid, chromium, L-glutamine, **omega-3 EFAs**, and vanadium

Hypotension
Low Blood Pressure

See also adrenal fatigue

While not as readily recognized as high blood pressure, low blood pressure can also be a serious problem. Low blood pressure can result in fatigue, fainting, or dizziness. Low blood pressure may be the result of blood loss, but can also be due to glandular problems, particularly adrenal fatigue. An *Adrenal Glandular Formula* or licorice root will often help this problem.

Capsicum and garlic tend to normalize blood pressure, reducing high blood pressure and increasing low blood pressure. Many adaptogens also help to normalize blood pressure. Shepherd's purse is one of the best vasoconstrictive herbs for tightening blood vessels.

Formulas: Adrenal Glandular, Circulatory, Heart Health, and Adaptogen

Programs: Cardiovascular Nutritional

Herbs: Capsicum, garlic, **ginseng (American)**, ginseng (Asian/Korean), gynostemma, hawthorn, **licorice**, nettle, stinging, and **shepherd's purse**

Supplements: Omega-3 EFAs and vitamin B-complex

Essential Oils: Clove, lavender, lemon, and rosemary

Hypothyroidism

See also Graves' disease and Hashimoto's disease

Hypothyroidism is a problem where the thyroid is not producing enough thyroid hormones. About twenty-seven million Americans (two hundred million worldwide) have some form of hypothyroid disease. It has been estimated that up to 60 percent of the people who have a thyroid problem don't even know it.

One of the reasons for this is that the TSH testing most doctors rely on to diagnose thyroid problems isn't 100 percent reliable in determining thyroid problems. Many people have multiple symptoms of thyroid problems but have been told by their doctor that they don't have a thyroid problem.

TSH levels can vary throughout the day and may not show up as out of range when the test was done, even though the thyroid is struggling. Furthermore, many experts believe that the lab ranges are too broad and need to be adjusted. To really understand the health of the thyroid it's important to look at the big picture.

Symptoms of Thyroid Imbalance

The primary symptoms of low thyroid are being easily chilled and/or fatigued. Your thyroid regulates your mitochondria, which produce heat and energy for your body. If your thyroid is low, you won't be producing enough heat to stay warm, and your body temperature will be too low. You will also not have the energy you need for muscle and brain function, which can result in physical and mental fatigue (brain fog).

A simple way to test for this is to take your temperature first thing in the morning, before getting out of bed, for five days in a row. If your average body temperature is consistently lower than 97.8 degrees, you may have a thyroid problem. (Women should not perform this test during ovulation.)

Other symptoms that could be associated with low thyroid include high cholesterol and weight problems, dry skin, hair loss, depression, infertility, migraines, anxiety, memory problems, and menstrual irregularities. Because every cell in the body has receptors for the thyroid hormone, low thyroid affects the entire body which means additional health problems may be associated with a thyroid problem.

Hashimoto's Disease

The most common cause of modern thyroid problems isn't low iodine. It's Hashimoto's disease, an autoimmune disorder. Since 90 percent of all hypothyroid problems in modern society are due to this autoimmune condition, try the therapies listed under *Hashimoto's Disease* first.

If Hashimoto's is not the cause of the low thyroid (that is, a person tests negative for TPO and thyroglobulin antibodies), the first thing to try is increasing one's intake of dietary iodine.

Iodine and the Thyroid

Iodine is essential to the production of thyroid hormones. This nutrient, while found in abundance in sea foods, is not found in high concentrations in plants or animals raised inland. Furthermore, fluoride, chlorine, and bromide are all found in the same group on the periodic table of elements as iodine. This means they can displace iodine in the body. So the chlorination or fluoridation of water supplies and other forms of exposure to these chemicals can disrupt iodine metabolism.

The safest way to get iodine, and to flush other halogens out of the body, is to consume seaweeds, such as kelp or dulse. If a person is severely deficient they can take an iodine supplement like Iodoral® or Lugol's solution.

Healing the Thyroid

There are also herbs that don't contain iodine that can improve thyroid function. The three I think are most helpful are ashwagandha, nettle leaf, and black walnut. These herbs seem to help rebuild the thyroid itself. Many people also respond well to a *Thyroid Glandular Formula*.

Deficiencies of selenium and zinc can also cause problems with iodine utilization. Cruciferous vegetables and soy have a thyroid inhibiting effect, but it is very mild, so eating these foods in moderation should have little effect. But, if you have low thyroid you may wish to avoid them.

Functional Hypothyroidism

Even if levels of thyroid hormones are normal, one can still have thyroid problems if the liver and other tissues are not converting the inactive thyroid hormone (T4) into active form (T3) properly. This conversion takes place mostly in the liver, so supporting the liver may aid thyroid function. Weak adrenals may contribute to this problem, so *Adrenal Tonic Formulas* or licorice root may have indirect benefits to the thyroid by supporting the adrenal glands.

Strategies: Emotional Healing Work

Formulas: Target Mineral Thyroid, **Thyroid Glandular**, Adrenal Glandular, **Hypothyroid**, Ashwagandha Complex, and Betaine HCl

Herbs: **Ashwagandha**, **black walnut**, bladderwrack, coconut, coleus, **dulse**, he shou wu, **kelp**, licorice, **nettle, stinging**, and saw palmetto

Supplements: 7-keto, **iodine**, L-tyrosine, MSM, N-acetyl cysteine, omega-3 EFAs, SAM-e, **selenium**, and **zinc**

Essential Oils: Myrrh

Hysteria

See also adrenal fatigue, hypoglycemia, and nervous exhaustion

Hysteria is a neurotic condition where there is no recognizable organic disease, but there can be symptoms mimicking various diseases. The person is calm but aloof and may become very emotional (laughing or crying) for no apparent reason. This emotional state is almost like a second personality and there may be a forgetting of what happened in this other state when the normal personality reasserts itself. There is emotional instability with a marked craving for sympathy.

Hysteria may be a sign of adrenal or nervous exhaustion due to chronic stress. The *Stress Management* strategy, along with *Adrenal Tonic* or *Nerve Tonic Formulas* may be helpful. It may also be a sign of unresolved trauma requiring the *Emotional Healing Work* and *Flower Essences* strategies. Low

blood sugar (*see hypoglycemia*) can also be a cause of mood swings, like those found in hysteria.

Strategies: Counseling or Therapy, Flower Essence, and Stress Management

Formulas: **Chinese Fire-Increasing**, Anti-Anxiety, Adrenal Glandular, and Antispasmodic

Herbs: Aloe vera, **black cohosh**, blue cohosh, chamomile, lemon balm, passion flower, peppermint, rosemary, **skullcap**, and thyme

Supplements: Vitamin B-complex

Essential Oils: Chamomile (Roman), jasmine, lavender, neroli, peppermint, and rosemary

IBS   see *irritable bowel*

Ileocecal Valve

See also hiatal hernia

The ileocecal valve is the valve between the small intestine and the large intestine. This valve may become irritated and inflamed and not shut properly. This causes a leakage of material from the colon back into the small intestine which weakens the body. It often causes serious gas and bloating.

Massage to the area helps. To locate the ileocecal valve, draw an imaginary line from your navel (belly button) to the right hip. The ileocecal valve is located about halfway along that line. Massage the area in a clockwise motion to close the valve.

Fiber may be helpful, especially with soothing, mucilaginous herbs like aloe vera and slippery elm. The *Intestinal Soothing Formula* is usually helpful. Digestive enzymes may also be helpful, as can carminative herbs. Problems with the ileocecal valve are often found with a hiatal hernia and a video demonstration of how to work on this valve is included in the hiatal hernia videos found at stevenhorne.com/article/Correcting-a-Hiatal-Hernia and youtube.com/herbaleducation.

Strategies: Increase Dietary Fiber

Formulas: **Intestinal Soothing**, Chinese Earth-Increasing, Plant Enzyme, Chinese Earth-Decreasing, and **Digestive Support**

Herbs: Aloe vera, chamomile, marshmallow, peppermint, and slippery elm

Impetigo

See also infection (bacterial)

Impetigo is an inflammatory skin disease caused by a contagious staph or strep infection. It is characterized by isolated pustules, usually around the nose and mouth, that become crusted and rupture. *Antibacterial Formulas* can be helpful, especially if applied topically. You can also apply antiseptic essential oils like tea tree oil or single herbs like black walnut, echinacea, and goldenseal using the *Compress or Fomentation* strategy.

Strategies: Compress or Fomentation

Formulas: Blood Purifier, Lymphatic Infection, and **Antibacterial**

Herbs: Black walnut, **echinacea**, goldenseal, and usnea

Supplements: Vitamin A and vitamin D

Essential Oils: Geranium, lavender, myrrh, patchouli, peppermint, and tea tree

Impotency   see *erectile dysfunction*

Incontinence
Enuresis

Incontinence is the inability to retain urine through the loss of sphincter control in the bladder. Increasing mineral intake in order to improve muscle tone may be helpful. Stay well hydrated in order to keep urine diluted so it doesn't irritate the bladder. Herbs for the kidneys with an astringent or tonic action, such as agrimony, horsetail, and uva ursi are particularly helpful. Also consider the *Chinese Water-Increasing Formula*. Kegel exercises, which strengthen the pelvic floor, can be helpful, as can the *Sitz Bath* strategy using astringent herbs in the bathwater.

Strategies: Hydration, Mineralization, and Sitz Bath

Formulas: Urinary Support, **Chinese Water-Increasing**, and **UTI Prevention**

Herbs: Agrimony, buchu, corn silk, couchgrass, cranberry, **horsetail**, juniper, noni, Saint John's wort, and **uva ursi**

Supplements: Co-Q10

Indigestion

See also acid indigestion and gastritis

Indigestion is simply a dysfunction of the digestive process that leaves food incompletely digested. This can cause discomfort in the stomach, a heavy feeling in the stomach after meals, gas, bloating, belching, and bad breath. Generally speaking, indigestion is a need for more digestive enzymes, such as a *Digestive Support* or *Plant Enzyme Formula*, and/or a *Betaine HCl Formula*.

In addition to supplements that supply enzymes, *Herbal Bitters Formulas* can be taken 15-20 minutes prior to meals to stimulate digestive secretions. These herbs not only stimulate digestive secretions but also promote downward motility of the digestive tract (to ease belching and reflux) and ease gas and bloating. They should be taken with a large glass of water.

A small pinch of natural salt, taken with water prior to meals, can also be helpful in stimulating digestion. Chamomile or peppermint tea are good for settling the stomach when one has indigestion, as is chewing tablets of a *Papaya Enzyme Formula*.

Strategies: Eat Enzyme-Rich Foods and Hydration

Formulas: Christopher's Carminative, **Chinese Earth-Decreasing**, Children's Colic, **Digestive Support**, Flu and Vomiting, Christopher's Gallbladder, **Papaya Enzyme**, **Betaine HCl**, Pepsin Intestinal, Chinese Earth-Increasing, **Plant Enzyme**, and **Herbal Bitters**

Essential Oil Blends: Digestive Settling EO

Herbs: Alfalfa, aloe vera, artichoke leaf, asafetida, asafetida, blessed thistle, bupleurum, calamus, capsicum, cardamom, catnip, **chamomile**, clove, **dandelion**, devil's claw, fennel, galangal, **gentian**, ginger, lemon balm, papaya, peppermint, quince (Bengal), rosemary, safflower, sage, slippery elm, thyme, vanilla, vervain (blue), and wood betony

Supplements: Pancreatin

Essential Oils: Clove, **fennel**, lavender, lime, **peppermint**, rose, rosemary, **spearmint**, and ylang ylang

Infection Prevention

Contagious diseases occur when infectious organisms like viruses and bacteria breach the immune system and start causing problems. There are two primary strategies for preventing the spread of contagious diseases: practice good hygiene and improve the body's natural resistance.

Practice Good Hygiene

As just about everyone knows, it is important to wash your hands, cover your mouth when you cough, make sure your environment is clean, and practice other methods of modern sanitization to prevent the spread of germs. However, it's counterproductive to sterilize everything because it weakens your immune system and has an adverse effect on your friendly flora.

You can also use a nanoparticle silver gel as a natural hand sanitizer. It actually lasts longer than many commercial, alcohol-based products. You can also make your own disinfectant soap by adding essential oils like eucalyptus, myrrh, sandalwood, thyme or other disinfectant essential oils to a natural liquid soap. Both of these options are less likely to have an adverse effect on your friendly flora.

Another way to prevent the spread of germs is to diffuse essential oils into a room to kill airborne pathogens. You can also make an aerosol spray using water and essential oils to use when traveling. See the *Aromatherapy* strategy for more information on using essential oils.

Wearing a mask can decrease oxygen levels, which can reduce your immunity. They are ineffective in preventing the spread of viral diseases because viruses readily pass through fabrics. Mostly they prevent you from coughing or sneezing on people or surfaces. If you are required to wear them, you can take liquid chlorophyll to help your blood carry more oxygen. Periodically, take a break so you can remove the mask and practice the *Deep Breathing* strategy.

Build Your Natural Resistance

It's equally important to improve the body's natural resistance by paying attention to good health (eating a healthy diet, getting adequate rest and exercise, and drinking enough water). Here are some specific suggestions for building your immune system.

Take Herbs and Nutrients

Echinacea, astragalus, and many medicinal mushrooms will boost the immune system to fight off infections to which the body is exposed. Astragalus, for instance, is widely used in China to ward of wintertime colds and flu. Any *Immune Stimulant Formula* containing these herbs will be helpful. The *Mushroom Immune Formula* is also a good tonic for keeping the immune system strong.

When colds are going around, you can take the *Elderberry Cold and Flu Formula* or give the *Children's Elderberry Cold and Flu Formula* to your children. For people with weak respiratory systems, astragalus or the *Chinese Metal-Increasing Formula* can be used, especially during the winter months.

Deficiencies of vitamins A and D are associated with an increased risk of colds and flu. Vitamin C and zinc also help to strengthen the immune system against infection. Take these nutrients during cold and flu season or when contagious diseases are going around.

Maintain Healthy Gut Flora

Keeping a good balance of friendly microbes (probiotics) in the intestinal tract helps to prevent contagious diseases too. For instance, taking two to four times the normal dose of probiotics when traveling can help to prevent diarrhea and other diseases. See the *Friendly Flora* strategy.

Reduce Stress and Stay Positive

Stress decreases immune responses, so managing stress will help keep the immune system healthy. In fact, keeping a positive attitude and not buying into the fear and hysteria that surrounds the discovery of a new infectious disease will greatly reduce your chances of catching it. See the strategies *Affirmation and Visualization* and *Stress Management*. Always reassure yourself that you are protected from disease and that your body is strong and health.

Strategies: Affirmation and Visualization, Avoid Sugar, Eat Healthy, Eliminate Allergy-Causing Foods, Friendly Flora, Reduce EMF Exposure, and Stress Management

Formulas: Chinese Qi and Blood Tonic, Chinese Metal-Increasing, **Elderberry Cold and Flu**, **Children's Elderberry Cold and Flu**, Colostrum-Immune Stimulator, **Mushroom Immune**, **Immune-Boosting**, Jeannie Burgess' Thymus, and Probiotic

Essential Oil Blends: Disinfectant EO

Herbs: Astragalus, **cordyceps**, **echinacea**, **elder berry**, eleuthero, garlic, maitake, myrrh, reishi, shitake, and thyme

Supplements: Bacillus coagulans, **beta-glucans**, nanoparticle silver, **vitamin A**, **vitamin C**, **vitamin D**, and **zinc**

Essential Oils: Cajeput, copaiba, eucalyptus, **frankincense**, **lemon**, lemongrass, myrrh, oregano, pine, **rosemary**, tea tree, and **thyme**

Infection, Bacterial

See also antibiotic resistance, carbuncles, conjunctivitis, diphtheria, gingivitis, gonorrhea, impetigo, lyme disease, pertussis, staph infections, strep throat, syphilis, tetanus, and tuberculosis

There are many herbs and natural remedies that can be very helpful for fighting bacterial infections. They work best when taken regularly at fairly frequent intervals (two to four hours) until the infection subsides. Here are some of my favorite antibacterial remedies.

Crushed raw garlic is an extremely powerful antibacterial agent against most infection-causing bacteria. Simply crush raw garlic cloves and ingest them anyway you can. I've eaten slices of raw garlic on crackers with a little bit of butter or cheese to make them more palatable. I've also swallowed small pieces of cut up garlic cloves. However, it's more pleasant to take the *Stabilized Allicin Formula*. Powdered garlic in capsules is ineffective.

Herbs containing berberine can be helpful for bacterial infections. These include barberry, goldenseal, Oregon grape, and coptis. They work best for infections on the skin or mucus membraines. Berberine can also be taken as a standardized extract.

Echinacea contains a number of substances that help the body both contain and fight bacterial infections. For more severe bacterial infections, echinacea combines well with herbs like wild indigo, usnea, and thuja. I've found the combination of equal parts echinacea and wild indigo helpful for more serious bacterial infections.

Silver can be very helpful for bacterial infections, but it has to come in contact with the microbes to work. Gargle with it, spray it up the sinuses, or apply it topically to the skin where possible. You can also use a nebulizer to inhale it into the lungs. For internal infections I find taking two to four ounces daily for a couple of days works best. For every serious infections, including antibiotic-resistant infections, people have obtained good results by taking four to eight ounces daily for about a week.

Good antibacterial essential oils include cajeput, tea tree, thyme, and myrrh. These can be applied topically or diluted properly for internal use and used for short periods of time (usually three to four days). Read the instructions in the *Aromatherapy* strategy for safe use of essential oils.

See specific bacterial infections for more information. Some bacterial infections can be hard to treat. You may wish to consult with a professional herbalist or naturopath (findanherbalist.com or americanherbalistsguild.com) or, if the infection doesn't respond to the herbs, consult with a medical doctor.

Strategies: Aromatherapy, Compress or Fomentation, Enhance Nitric Oxide, Friendly Flora, and Poultice

Formulas: Drawing Salve, **Antibacterial**, **Stabilized Allicin**, **Immune-Boosting**, Lymphatic Infection, Nitric Oxide Boosting, Urinary Immune, Digestive Support, and **Probiotic**

Essential Oil Blends: Disinfectant EO

Herbs: Baptisia, barberry, chaparral, coptis, **echinacea**, **garlic**, **goldenseal**, myrrh, neem, oregano, **Oregon grape**, reishi, rosemary, spilanthes, **thuja**, thyme, and **usnea**

Supplements: Berberine, propolis, vitamin A, vitamin C, and vitamin D

Essential Oils: Cajeput, cinnamon, eucalyptus, lemon, **myrrh**, oregano, **tea tree**, and **thyme**

Infection, Fungal
Yeast Infections, Candida albicans, Candidiasis

See also athlete's foot, jock itch, thrush, vaginal discharge, and SIBO

Yeast microorganisms are a type of fungus, like mushrooms. They are present in the soil and part of the mix of microbes needed for soil health. Yeasts are also included in the dozens of species of microorganisms that inhabit our intestines. These gut microbes are known collectively as the intestinal microflora and are critical to health. So yeast can be very beneficial under the right conditions.

Under the wrong conditions, however, yeast can create problems, such as thrush, vaginal yeast infections, athlete's foot, jock itch, and nail fungus. Saying someone has *Candida albicans* or a candida infection is often used as a catchall diagnosis for imbalances in the intestinal microflora (see *dysbio-*

sis) because the symptoms are vague and the medical testing is not very accurate.

Specific herbs that help with yeast infections in general include pau d'arco, usnea, and spilanthes. The *Yeast Cleansing Program* is very helpful for correcting dysbiosis in general, not just yeast infections. It not only helps balance the microflora, it contains an enzyme packet, which taken between meals also helps break down the intestinal biofilm that allows harmful microbes to hide.

Antifungal essential oils include tea tree, lavender, thyme, clove, and oregano. These can be diluted and applied topically or they can be highly diluted and used internally for a period of no more than 7-10 days. See the *Aromatherapy* strategy to learn how to use essential oils safely.

For more tips on overcoming specific yeast infections, see the associated conditions.

Strategies: Aromatherapy, Colon Hydrotherapy, Detoxification, Friendly Flora, and Increase Dietary Fiber

Formulas: Standardized Acetogenin, **Anti-Fungal**, **Probiotic**, Antiparasitic, **Betaine HCl**, and Digestive Support

Programs: Yeast Cleansing

Essential Oil Blends: Antifungal EO

Herbs: Barberry, bee balm, black walnut, chaparral, coconut, garlic, neem, olive, **oregano**, **pau d'arco**, pawpaw, spilanthes, thuja, **usnea**, and yarrow

Supplements: Berberine, protease, and xylitol

Essential Oils: Bay leaf, clove, **lavender**, neroli, oregano, patchouli, peppermint, **tea tree**, and thyme

Infection, Viral

See also chicken pox, colds, Epstein-Barr virus, herpes, measles, mumps, and shingles

When most people think of treating infections, they think of antibiotics. But antibiotics only work against bacterial infections. Most common infections, like colds and flu, are viral, and antibiotics have no effect on viruses. Most coughs, sinus problems, ear infections, sore throats, and other common contagious diseases are also viral in nature, so it's a waste of time and money to treat them with antibiotics.

Viruses don't just cause colds and flu. Chicken pox, mumps, and measles are also acute viral infections. There are also chronic viral infections like herpes and more serious viral infections, such as smallpox, hepatitis C, Epstein-Barr, SARS, COVID-19, AIDS, and Ebola.

The reason serious viral infections raise concerns is that modern medicine has very few effective antiviral drugs. Most drugs only relieve the symptoms of viral infections. So when it comes to viral infections, modern medicine focuses its efforts primarily on trying to create immunity to them through vaccines.

Fortunately, the plant kingdom does have remedies that help the body deal with viral infections. These remedies primarily work by enhancing your body's immune responses. And what's great is that immune-enhancing herbs are often helpful for other types of infections as well.

Understanding Viruses

It's important to understand that a virus is very different from a bacteria or fungus. A bacteria, fungus, or yeast is a single-cell organism. It feeds and grows, then divides to reproduce. However, viruses aren't cells. They are pieces of genetic material, DNA or RNA, wrapped in a protein coat, having none of the structures or processes that cells have. So there is some debate about whether viruses are alive or not.

That's because outside of a living cell, a virus is inert. In order to replicate itself, a virus must enter a living cell and hijack cellular mechanisms that make copies of the DNA or RNA. So a virus has no "life" outside of another cell. It doesn't grow or metabolize nutrients or perform other functions that cellular organisms do. This means you can't "kill" viruses in the way you can kill a bacteria or fungal cell.

How the Body Deals with Viruses

Your body combats viruses in several ways. First, the innate immune system, found primarily in the membranes of the digestive and respiratory system, is designed to destroy foreign material (like viruses) to prevent them from ever entering the body. So a healthy intestinal and respiratory system forms a protective barrier against most viral infections.

If a virus is able to get past the innate immune system, then the adaptive immune system takes over. It produces substances called antibodies that attach themselves to a virus and render it inert so it can't enter cells and disrupt their normal functions.

The adaptive immune system also recognizes cells that are infected with viruses because some of the viral proteins can show up on the surface of the cell membrane. If a specialized cell, called a T cell, recognizes a suspicious viral fragment on another cell, it can destroy the host cell and stimulate the production of more T cells to look for that specific virus.

Viruses, Vaccines, and Antiviral Drugs

The ability of the immune system to create antibodies that bind specific viruses is the basis for vaccines. A vaccine contains viral proteins or viruses that have been weakened or live-attenuated. A healthy immune system recognizes these viruses or viral fragments and produces antibodies so that whenever the person encounters that virus the antibodies to render it inert are already present.

One of the problems with vaccines that contain attenuated or weakened viruses is that they can backfire if the immune system is compromised. In other words, they can actually cause a viral infection that doesn't produce the same symptoms as a normal viral infection. Just as shingles can arise from chickenpox viruses that were never eliminated from the body, some researchers believe that these low-grade viral infections can flare up and cause autoimmune reactions and other forms of chronic disease.

Flu vaccines are perhaps the most controversial vaccines of all, simply because there are thousands of viruses that cause the flu and they mutate very rapidly. In any given year, flu vaccine manufacturers can only select a few strains of viruses they think will be the most problematic that year. This means a flu shot might cause your body to develop immunity to a few strains, assuming you have a healthy immune system, but you are still unprotected from thousands of other strains of the flu.

There are no broad-spectrum antiviral drugs, so most remedies for viral infections like colds and flu are designed only to relieve symptoms. Despite being ineffective, antibiotics are frequently prescribed for viral conditions. Drugs that do exist for viral infections target specific types of viruses by inhibiting their entry into the cell, inhibiting their replication, or other similar mechanisms.

Natural Antiviral Remedies

Because you can't kill viruses, there are no broad-spectrum antiviral drugs or herbs. Herbs that have broad-acting activity against viral infections are those that support natural immune function. They boost production of white blood cells and antibodies, strengthen mucous membranes, and increase white blood cell activity. This helps the body fight infections of all kinds—viral, bacterial, and fungal. This is one way herbal remedies have a huge advantage over pharmaceutical drugs.

There are also herbs that work against specific types of viral infections, probably by inhibiting replication or entry into the cell of those viruses. Some of the better antiviral herbs for acute viral infections like colds and flu include elderberry, yarrow, andrographis, and astragalus. For more chronic viral infections herbs like lemon balm, Saint John's wort, olive leaf, and medicinal mushrooms like maitake, turkey tail, and shiitake are better choices.

Even though an antiviral remedy is effective against the cold or flu doesn't mean it will work against smallpox, hepatitis C, COVID-19, or Ebola. In fact, anyone who makes claims about natural cures for viral infections like Ebola is only guessing about what might work, because there isn't enough practical experience to know what is and isn't effective. That's why it's best to focus on maintaining a strong immune system and preventing the spread of viral infections (see *infection, prevention*).

Strategies: Aromatherapy and Blood Type Diet

Formulas: Chinese Wind-Heat Evil, Standardized Acetogenin, Stabilized Allicin, **Elderberry Cold and Flu**, **Immune-Boosting**, Children's Elderberry Cold and Flu, **Mushroom Immune**, Steven Horne's Children's Composition, Fire Cider, Circulatory, and Jeannie Burgess' Thymus

Essential Oil Blends: Disinfectant EO

Herbs: Aloe vera, andrographis, **astragalus**, chaparral, chrysanthemum, echinacea, **elder berry & flower**, **garlic**, lemon, **lemon balm**, **maitake**, olive, oregano, osha, **Saint John's wort**, shitake, thuja, thyme, turkey tail, and yarrow

Supplements: L-lysine, propolis, **vitamin A**, **vitamin C**, vitamin D, and **zinc**

Essential Oils: Helichrysum, **lemon**, **lemongrass**, oregano, and thyme

Infertility

See also cholesterol (low)

The inability to conceive a baby may be due to multiple factors, so it is wise to seek professional help to determine the exact cause of the problem. Poor general health, a lack of essential nutrients, and excessive stress can all be contributing factors.

Start by eating a healthy diet, including getting adequate amounts of vitamins, protein, minerals (especially trace minerals), and essential fatty acids. It may be a good idea to take a *Colloidal Minerals Formula* along with a multiple vitamin and mineral. During times of high stress, reproductive functions shut down to prevent babies from being born during times when there are not enough resources to care for them. So if you're under a lot of stress, practice the techniques listed under the *Stress Management* strategy.

Low cholesterol can be a factor in infertility in both men and women. A low percentage of body fat can also be a factor, especially in women. Extreme athletic training has been known to cause periods to stop in women too.

In men, low sperm count can be caused by exposure to xenoestrogens. Herbs like ginseng, maca, horny goat weed, and tribulus have been helpful for increasing sperm counts, sperm health, and/or general fertility in men. A *Testosterone Formula* may be helpful.

In women, low thyroid, irregular periods, and hormonal imbalances can be a factor. Herbs like dong quai, maca, false unicorn, and partridge berry have been helpful for balancing hormones and regulating periods. For women, a *Female Tonic Formula* may be helpful.

Strategies: Avoid Xenoestrogens, Healthy Fats, Low-Glycemic Diet, and Stress Management

Formulas: Chrisopher's Menopause, Chinese Water-Increasing, Female Tonic, Male Performance, Women's Aphrodisiac, **Colloidal Mineral**, **General Glandular**, **Whole Food Green Drink**, and Testosterone

Essential Oil Blends: Menopause Support EO

Herbs: Broomrape, chicory, cordyceps, **damiana**, dodder, dong quai, eleuthero, epimedium, false unicorn, **ginseng (American)**, ginseng (Asian/Korean), he shou wu, **maca**, partridge berry, and velvet bean

Supplements: L-arginine, L-carnitine, **multiple vitamin and mineral**, omega-3 EFAs, and vitamin E

Essential Oils: Geranium

Inflammation

See also diabetes, free radical damage, metabolic syndrome, and methylation (under)

Every time your body is injured, it responds to the damage with inflammation. It doesn't matter how the injury happened; whether it got cut, punctured, twisted, banged, smashed, scraped, burned, frozen, infected, or poisoned, the response is the same. This means that all disease begins with an inflammatory process, which must be reversed before healing can take place.

The classic signs of inflammation, recognized from ancient times, are heat, swelling, redness and pain. In Latin the appearance of these four symptoms was called "itis," which is why many traditional names for diseases end with this suffix. The disease name simply tells you the part of the body that has been damaged and is now inflamed.

Thus, when the appendix is inflamed you have appendicitis; when the tonsils are inflamed, you have tonsillitis, and so forth. When you consider all the "itises" there are—arthritis, bronchitis, tendonitis, colitis, dermatitis, gingivitis, conjunctivitis, diverticulitis, sinusitis, to name a few—it's already clear that inflammation is involved in a lot of diseases.

However, what isn't widely recognized is that if the inflammatory process is never reversed it leads to other states of disease. In fact, many researchers now believe that all chronic and degenerative diseases begin with inflammation.

The Benefits of Acute Inflammation

There is nothing wrong with the acute inflammatory process. It is not a disease; instead, it is a protective mechanism of the body. It sequesters the damaged area. It's the same thing police and fire personnel do when they arrive on the scene. They set up a perimeter to keep criminals from escaping and to keep bystanders from being injured.

If there is infection, inflammation helps contain it. If it is a poisonous insect bite, inflammation slows the spread of the toxins.

The pain signals from inflammation alert you to the fact you've been injured and your body needs help. If there were no pain signals, you might not even realize you were injured and you might continue to do things that cause even greater damage and injury to your body. Feeling pain helps you avoid additional damage because you'll be motivated to protect the damaged area and avoid using it.

Chronic Inflammation

While acute inflammation is a good thing, chronic inflammation is not. Once white blood cells have completed their clean-up of the area, a healing phase is supposed to be initiated. A new set of chemical messengers is released that tighten the capillary pores. The excess fluid and plasma proteins are removed from the area via the lymphatic system, and a regenerative cycle begins as these new chemical messengers stimulate tissue growth and repair. In chronic inflammation, the body has been unsuccessful in reversing the process and initiating healing. It remains stuck in the inflammatory state.

Strategies for Reversing Chronic Inflammation

There are several things you can do to reverse the problem of chronic inflammation and help the body move into a healing phrase.

Detoxify Your Life

One of the reasons inflammation never reverses is that the irritant that caused the damage in the first place is never removed. It's like having a splinter that isn't pulled out. A prime example of this is smoking. Cigarettes are constantly irritating and inflaming the lung tissue, which is why smoking is the number one cause of chronic obstructive pulmonary disorder (COPD) and lung cancer. The tissues can't heal because they are continually being damaged.

So to get rid of chronic inflammation you must minimize your exposure to tobacco, alcohol, drugs, pesticides, food additives, toxic household cleaning products and personal care products, and chemicals in general. The less irritants you expose your body to, the less inflammation you will experience. It also helps to follow the *Detoxification* strategy once or twice each year or take supplements to help detoxify the body to remove irritants.

This includes taking care of chronic infections. Infections in the teeth and gums, for example, are linked with increased risk of cardiovascular disease. So maintain good dental health. Be careful with root canals as they are often sources of ongoing infection.

Control Your Blood Sugar

Sugar is a two-edged sword in the body. On the one hand, it is used for fuel, but it is also proinflammatory. High blood sugar, found in metabolic syndrome and diabetes, directly contributes to increased inflammatory processes in the cardiovascular system, brain, and other tissues. This is why the body tries to maintain blood sugar levels within a narrow range. It's also why high blood sugar is a big risk factor for other chronic and degenerative diseases, including cancer and heart disease. If your blood sugar is high, see *metabolic syndrome or diabetes* to learn how to bring it down.

Make an Oil Change

A major dietary problem that increases inflammatory responses and prevents healing is an over-abundance of omega-6 essential fatty acids coupled with a deficiency of omega-3 fatty acids. Many of the chemical messengers that mediate inflammation and healing are made from these fatty acids.

In the absence of sufficient omega-3 fatty acids, there is a tendency to have too many pro-inflammatory chemical messengers. Higher levels of omega-3 help the body produce the chemical messengers that reverse the inflammatory process and start the healing process. Many people have discovered they have less pain, clearer thinking, better mood, and increased overall health by reducing vegetable oils and processed fats in their diet, while taking a high quality omega-3 essential fatty acid supplement (see *Healthy Fats* strategy).

Cool the "Fire" with Antioxidants

Inflammation and oxidative stress are closely linked. There is a great deal of free radical activity at inflammatory sites that must be cooled with antioxidant nutrients. They are like the "fire hoses" that help to cool the heat of inflammation.

Antioxidant vitamins like A, C, and D_3 are helpful, along with zinc, alpha-lipoic acid, carotenoids, and other free radical scavengers can help to cool inflammation and promote the healing response. For example, wounds won't heal without adequate reserves of vitamin C and zinc.

Promote Healing with Anti-Inflammatory Herbs

There are many herbs that help to reverse inflammation and promote healing in the body. If you have any kind of chronic pain or inflammation, willow bark, bowsellia, mangosteen pericarp, and turmeric, taken either as singles or as part of an an *Antioxidant* or *Anti-Inflammatory Pain Formula,* may be helpful.

Keep Cool by Managing Stress

The brain is involved in mediating inflammation and pain, as well as healing. Inflammation and pain increase under the influence of the sympathetic nervous system, which is activated under stress. Healing is activated under the parasympathetic nervous system, which is why rest has always been associated with healing. If you don't allow for down-time when you need to heal the inflammatory process will continue. This is why managing stress, making time for rest and relaxation, and adequate sleep are all essential to controlling chronic inflammation. CBD modulates both stress and pain and can be very beneficial as part of a program for relieving chronic inflammation.

Improve Lymphatic Drainage

One of the major effects of inflammation is the pooling of lymphatic fluid in the spaces around the cells. The only way this fluid can be removed is via the lymphatic system. This is one of the little-known secrets to reducing chronic inflammation. The lymph system has no pump, so moderate exercise (walking, swimming, bouncing up and down on a mini trampoline, etc.) and deep breathing are needed to encourage lymphatic drainage and reduce inflammation. When lymph glands are congested, a *Liquid Lymph* or *Lymph Cleansing Formula* will also improve lymph drainage.

Support the Adrenal Glands

The adrenals produce the hormone cortisol, which keeps inflammation in check. Corticosteroid drugs mimic this hormone. Chronic stress and excessive use of caffeine and sugar will exhaust these important glands and reduce their ability to control inflammation. A *Chinese Fire-Increasing* or *Adrenal Glandular Formula* can help rebuild the adrenal glands and keep chronic inflammation in check. Also, yucca and licorice root are two herbs which have a cortisol-like action, which can be helpful in reduce chronic inflammation.

Strategies: Avoid Caffeine, Avoid Sugar, Balance Methylation, Blood Type Diet, Detoxification, Eat Healthy, Enhance Nitric Oxide, Gut-Healing Diet, Healthy Fats, Liver Detoxification, Low-Glycemic Diet, Lymph-Moving Pain Relief, and Stress Management

Formulas: Herbal Arthritis, Enzyme Spray, Stan Malstrom's Herbal Aspirin, Green Tea Polyphenols, **Chinese Yang-Reducing**, **Analgesic Nerve**, **Antioxidant**, **Anti-Inflammatory Pain**, General Analgesic, Nitric Oxide Boosting, **CBD Anti-inflammatory**, **CBD Topical Analgesic**, **Hemp Oil with Terpenes**, and Myelin Sheath

Essential Oil Blends: Relaxing and Soothing EO

Herbs: Aloe vera, amur cork, **boswellia**, bupleurum, cannabis, **chamomile**, chia, **devil's claw**, feverfew, goldenseal, gotu kola, Grape seed, holy basil, licorice, **mangosteen**, marshmallow, myrrh, noni, pau d'arco, pomegranate, purslane, rose, Saint John's wort, solomon's seal, tea, teasel, **turmeric**, wild yam, yarrow, and **yucca**

Supplements: Alpha-lipoic acid, bromelain, **CBD**, Co-Q10, curcumin, glucosamine, krill oil, **MSM**, N-acetyl cysteine, omega-3 EFAs, omega-6 CLA, and zinc

Essential Oils: Bay leaf, chamomile (Roman), frankincense, geranium, helichrysum, menthol, myrrh, and wintergreen

Inflammatory Bowel Disorders
Colitis, IBD, Crohn's Disease

See also celiac disease, colitis, Crohn's disease, and leaky gut

The term inflammatory bowel disease (IBD) is a broad term referring to any disease characterized by inflammation in the gastrointestinal tract. The two most common types of these diseases are Crohn's and ulcerative colitis. Both of these conditions can make your life miserable with symptoms such as diarrhea, abdominal cramps, rectal bleeding, fever, joint pain, loss of appetite, and fatigue, not to mention fistulas and complications that can require surgery to remove a part of or all the colon. The Centers for Disease Control (CDC) estimates that about 1.4 million Americans suffer from IBD, and 10 percent of those are children.

The main difference between Crohn's disease and ulcerative colitis is the location and nature of the inflammation. Crohn's can affect any part of the gastrointestinal tract, from mouth to anus, although most cases start in the ileum. Ulcerative colitis is restricted to the colon and the rectum. Microscopically, ulcerative colitis is restricted to the epithelial lining of the gut, while Crohn's disease affects the entire wall of the bowel.

People who live in Western countries have a higher risk for developing IBD than people in other countries. However, as countries industrialize and adopt Western diets and lifestyles, IBD increases. So there is definitely a lifestyle cause.

Smokers are at higher risk of developing Crohn's disease, whereas they are at lower risk of developing ulcerative colitis. Research has linked long-term oral contraceptive use to a higher risk of both ulcerative colitis and Crohn's. Other drugs, such as isotretinoin (Accutane), could also play a role. Pain-relieving NSAIDs (like ibuprofen) can worsen IBD symptoms but are not thought to increase the risk of getting the disease initially.

Studies report a possible link to over-consumption of foods high in omega-6 polyunsaturated fatty acids, which suggests a lack of omega-3 essential fatty acids may be involved.

A big factor may be the balance of bacteria in the gastrointestinal tract. Healthy intestines contain trillions of good bacteria or friendly flora. These organisms play a role in digesting certain foods (especially dairy), protecting the body from infection and regulating the immune responses.

Antibiotics and other drugs can disrupt the balance of these intestinal bacteria, as can infections with harmful bacteria, such as salmonella and campylobacter. Both of these bacteria have been associated with IBD. They are ingested in contaminated food and are responsible for thousands of cases of food poisoning each year.

Since stress can trigger these bowel disorders, it's possible they may have emotional triggers too. Adrenal fatigue results in lower levels of cortisol, which controls inflammation. Also, stress can be a factor in the regulation of the immune system, which may aggravate the autoimmune factor in intestinal inflammation.

The following five strategies have helped many people bring Crohn's disease and ulcerative colitis under control.

1. Adopt a Healthy Diet

It is also important to avoid eating refined sugars of all kinds and may even be helpful to eliminate honey, maple syrup, and sugary fruits. In addition, people with IBD should avoid products sweetened with manitol, sorbitol, and xylitol. The *Gut-Healing Diet* strategy can be very helpful.

2. Use Anti-Inflammatory Herbs and Supplements

Consuming soothing, mucilaginous herbs has proven helpful in treating all types of inflammatory bowel disorders. A few good remedies to consider are aloe vera, slippery elm, and marshmallow. The *Intestinal Soothing Formula* has proven very effective for many people. Others have found drinking aloe vera juice to make a difference.

You can also try making slippery elm gruel. Combine one teaspoon of the powder with one teaspoon of honey and two cups of boiling water. Stir well. Flavor with cinnamon and drink one or two cups twice a day. Bulk slippery elm may also be blended with juice or nut milks if honey can't be tolerated.

3. Manage Stress

Stress often acts as a trigger for IBD, IBS and Celiac disease. This is why nervine herbs, like *Jeannie Burgess' Stress Formula,* can also help to manage them. In fact, the *Intestinal Soothing Formula* and *Jeannie Burgess' Stress Formula* work very well together in reducing intestinal inflammation.

Coffee, cola drinks, energy drinks, black tea and other sources of caffeine should be avoided. See the *Avoid Caffeine* strategy.

Learn the skills listed under the *Stress Management* strategy. Practice breathing exercises to relax. You may even want to consider using the *Counseling or Therapy* strategy to work on emotional conflicts that can exacerbate symptoms.

4. Use Probiotics

A healthy digestive system contains thousands of species of friendly bacteria and people who live closer to the earth tend to have more species than people living in more sterile environments. It is very likely that the disruption of the friendly flora has a lot to do with the development of Crohn's, Celiac, colitis, and IBS. See the *Friendly Flora* strategy.

5. Take Omega-3 Fatty Acids

Some studies have found that omega-3 fatty acids may reduce inflammation in people with ulcerative colitis. fat-soluble vitamins may also be helpful. See the *Healthy Fats* strategy.

Additional Tips

A high-fiber diet may also be beneficial for some, but during the active stages of the illness, raw fruits, vegetables, seeds, and nuts will irritate the digestive system. An *Irritable Bowel Fiber Blend*, which is based primarily on slippery elm and marshmallow, could be beneficial. Enzyme supplements to improve digestion may be helpful too.

Strategies: Avoid Caffeine, Avoid Sugar, Bone Broth, Eat Healthy, Fasting, Friendly Flora, Gut-Healing Diet, Healthy Fats, and Stress Management

Formulas: Chinese Yang-Reducing, **Intestinal Soothing**, **Irritable Bowel Fiber**, Fiber, Plant Enzyme, Digestive Support, Pepsin Intestinal, **Probiotic**, **Jeannie Burgess' Stress**, Gentle Bowel Cleansing, **Anti-Inflammatory Pain**, **Triphala**, and CBD Anti-inflammatory

Herbs: **Aloe vera juice**, amalaki, black walnut, **boswellia**, **calendula**, **cat's claw**, catnip, **chamomile**, coptis, kudzu, licorice, **marshmallow**, **plantain**, Saint John's wort, **slippery elm**, wild yam, and yellow dock

Supplements: Bromelain, CBD, chondroitin, MSM, omega-3 EFAs, protease, and vitamin B-complex

Influenza   see *flu*

Injuries

See also abrasions/scratches, broken bones, burns & scalds, cuts, ligaments (torn/injuried), sprains, and wounds & sores

Many herbs can promote faster healing of injuries. Some of my favorites are calendula, comfrey, yarrow, and arnica. Many essential oils, including lavender and tea tree oil, also help injuries heal more quickly. These remedies work well using the *Lymph-Moving Pain Relief* strategy, which both eases pain and helps reverse the injury.

These remedies can be applied topically using the *Compress or Fomentation* or *Poultice* strategies, which is one of the best ways to use them. The *Shock and Injury FE Blend* or the *Enzyme Spray* can be applied topically to aid injured tissues, as well.

Besides topical remedies nutrients like vitamin C, zinc, and/or *Colloidal Mineral Formulas* can be taken internally to speed healing. For pain, try a *Topical Analgesic* or the *Anti-Inflammatory Pain Formula*. See specific types of injuries for more specific ideas.

Strategies: Bodywork, Compress or Fomentation, Flower Essence, Lymph-Moving Pain Relief, Mineralization, Poultice, and Sleep

Formulas: Joint Healing Nutrients, Healing Salve, Watkin's Hair, Skin, and Nails, **Enzyme Spray**, Analgesic Nerve, Antioxidant, **Topical Analgesic**, **Anti-Inflammatory Pain**, **Vulnerary**, General Analgesic, CBD Topical Analgesic, Hemp Oil with Terpenes, Colloidal Mineral, and CBD Anti-inflammatory

Essential Oil Blends: Disinfectant EO and Topical Injury

Flower Essence Blends: Shock and Injury FE

Herbs: Arnica homeopathic, bayberry, **calendula**, collinsonia, **comfrey**, goldenseal, marshmallow, mullein, quince (Asian), white oak, and **yarrow**

Supplements: Bromelain, **collagen**, MSM, vitamin C, and zinc

Essential Oils: Helichrysum and tea tree

Insect Bites   see *bites & stings*

Insect Repellant

See also bites & stings

Aromatherapy can be used as a natural-method insect repellant. Mix oils with a massage lotion or fixed oil and apply topically. Frequent applications are usually necessary. Garlic, taken internally, also helps to repel insects. A diet of natural foods, low in sugar, also makes one less prone to insect bites.

Strategies: Aromatherapy

Formulas: Stabilized Allicin

Herbs: Garlic raw and neem

Supplements: Vitamin B$_1$

Essential Oils: Chamomile (Roman), clove, **geranium**, lavender, lemon, **lemongrass**, patchouli, pine, **rosemary**, tansy (blue), tea tree, and thyme

Insomnia

See also adrenal fatigue, hypoglycemia, sleep (restless/disturbed), stress, tension, and sleep apnea

Insomnia involves difficulty sleeping. This could be trouble falling asleep or trouble staying asleep. If you have difficulty sleeping, it's important to examine your lifestyle and determine what you can do to get the sleep you need. You may even need to experiment a little to determine what will help you get the sleep you need. To get you started, here are some strategies for getting a better night's sleep. Pick one or two to work on at a time and see if they make a positive difference in your sleep patterns.

Schedule Sleep

Your body has an internal clock that helps engage periods of sleep and wakefulness. If you can get on a schedule that allows you to get to bed at roughly the same time each night and wake up at the same time each morning, it will ease both falling asleep and waking up. When your sleep schedule is thrown off (such as during international travel), you can help to reset this biological clock by taking melatonin at bedtime to help you get a new sleeping rhythm.

Get to Bed Early

In Chinese medicine, it is believed that certain meridians (or energy flows) are active at certain times of the day. According to this theory, the gallbladder and liver meridians are active from around 11:00 p.m. to 1:00 a.m. and 1:00 a.m. to 3:00 a.m. respectively. This is the peak time for your body to detoxify if you are asleep by 11:00 p.m. If you are not asleep when the gallbladder meridian becomes active, you may get a surge of nervous energy that inhibits sleep. This will be followed by feeling sluggish and tired the next morning.

Generally speaking, if you can get to bed by about ten thirty, you'll sleep more soundly and wake more refreshed. If you regularly stay up late and have a hard time getting out of bed in the morning, consider taking a *Hepatoprotective* or *Liver Tonic Formula* to support the health of your liver. The *Chinese Wood-Decreasing Formula* may also help.

Avoid Late Night Stimulation

In the evening, avoid activities that get your adrenaline pumping. This includes watching exciting TV shows or movies, listening to loud and stimulating music, or even reading thrilling novels. It's also not a good idea to exercise right before bedtime. Instead, pick evening activities that help you wind down, such as listening to relaxing music, reading uplifting books, or sharing a massage with your partner.

Create a Relaxing Atmosphere

Seek to make your bedroom a place that is conducive to rest, not work or recreation. Remove TVs, computers, cell phones, and other distractions from your sleep area and keep your bedroom uncluttered. Most importantly, don't work or keep work materials in your sleep area. Also, keep electrical equipment, including digital clocks at least three feet away from your bed to minimize electromagnetic influences while you sleep.

If you have a hard time relaxing at night, try taking some nervine herbs in the evening. Kava kava is a good herb to use if your body is tense and you suffer from anxiety. Magnesium taken before bed can also help your muscles relax. Passionflower is good if you can't make your brain stop thinking. skullcap is one of the best for just calming your nerves. Choose a good *Sleep Support* or *Herbal Sleep Aid Formula* that combines a number of herbs and nutrients that help you sleep. You'll typically want to take the remedy about thirty to sixty minutes before bedtime.

Don't Eat Late

It is hard for your body to fall asleep when it is digesting a heavy meal, so try to eat dinner at least two hours and preferably four hours before bedtime. Don't eat sugary snacks before sleeping, as this creates blood sugar problems that can wake you up at night. Also, avoid all stimulants, including spicy foods, in the evening. They interfere with quality of sleep. It is okay to eat a small snack of nut butter, cheese, or some other high protein food before bed if you suffer from hypoglycemia.

Make Your Sleep Area Dark

The natural way to fall asleep is for your body to convert a neurotransmitter called serotonin into melatonin. Melatonin puts you to sleep. Your pineal gland starts converting melatonin to serotonin when it gets dark. Even the LED lights from electric clocks or "on" lights from electronic equipment will inhibit this process and help contribute to keeping you awake.

Unfortunately, with the advent of electric lights, we extend our "day" into the evening hours. This prevents us from falling asleep naturally. Watching TV, staring at a computer screens, and artificial light all inhibit sleep. So make your bedroom as dark as possible and as the time for sleep approaches, turn off the TV and computer and get into a darkened room. You may even want to try wearing a sleep mask.

You can also try taking melatonin or 5-HTP at bedtime. 5-HTP is a precursor to serotonin. Serotonin is converted to melatonin when you turn out all the lights and make your bedroom as dark as possible. Melatonin is useful for helping to reset your biological clock so you fall asleep when you're supposed to, especially if you're suffering from jet lag or have to work night shifts. Some *Sleep Formulas* also contain these ingredients.

Breathe Deeply

Oxygen is very important to sound sleep. Many people find that cracking a window open to let in a little fresh air results in a better night's sleep. If you snore at night, it's a sign that you have constricted airways that are inhibiting the amount of oxygen you are getting while you are sleeping. So snoring not only contributes to insomnia in anyone who sleeps with you, but it also interferes with the quality of your own sleep.

If you snore really loudly, you may have a problem with sleep apnea. See *sleep apnea* for more information.

Quiet Your Mind

If you're one of those people who lie awake at night unable to get your mind to shut up so you can go to sleep, here are some suggestions for quieting your mind for a better night's sleep. First, before going to bed, get a pad of paper and write down your to-do list for the next day. This helps you "get it off your mind" so you can relax. It may also help to have a journal that you write in each evening, allowing you to express things on paper so you can let go of them.

A second technique to quiet your mind is to breathe deeply as you lie in bed and focus on relaxing your body. Starting with your toes and working your way up to your head, tense your muscles and then let them relax. Imagine them sinking into the bed. Focus your mind on your breathing or mentally recite a positive statement, such as "I am relaxed" or "All is well."

If you're still having trouble getting your mind to quiet down, GABA or passion flower may be helpful. Take these supplements about one hour before bedtime. If you are easily distracted by small things (such as a dripping faucet or other small noises), try taking about 400 mg of magnesium. It's best to empty a magnesium capsule or two under your tongue or use a magnesium supplement in liquid form. Let the magnesium sit in your mouth for ten to fifteen seconds before swallowing it.

Reduce Your Stress Level

Since stress is a major factor in sleep problems, reducing your stress level during the day can help you sleep better at night. If you are tired during the day but have poor quality of sleep at night, you may be suffering from adrenal exhaustion. Symptoms of tired adrenals include fatigue, mental confusion, and emotional sensitivity during the day, followed by restless sleep with disturbing dreams. You may also need to wake up frequently to urinate.

In this situation, the *Chinese Fire-Increasing Formula* taken during the day may be helpful. In more serious cases, such as post-traumatic stress disorder, an *Adrenal Tonic Formula* may be helpful.

In addition, it is very important for people suffering from too much stress to avoid sugar and caffeine, as these make the problem worse. You may need to reduce your workload or at least make more time for rest and relaxation.

A good strategy for people who are under a lot of stress is using the *Epsom Salt Bath* strategy. Lavender, bergamot, rose, ylang ylang, and patchouli are good essential oils to use with this strategy. Light a few candles, put on some relaxing music and turn out the lights, then soak in the warm bath for 15-20 minutes. This can really reduce nervous stress and prepare you for a better night's sleep.

Balance Your Blood Sugar

If you wake up in the middle of the night thinking about your problems and unable to get back to sleep, this can be a sign of blood sugar problems. What is happening is that your blood sugar is dropping too low in the middle of the night, and your adrenal glands are firing off stress hormones (adrenaline and cortisol) to elevate your blood sugar. Avoiding sugar, white-flour products, alcohol, and caffeine will help. Eat a small protein-rich snack at bedtime, such as a couple of tablespoons of almond butter, peanut butter, cottage cheese, or a few raw walnuts.

Bed-wetting in children can often be a sign of blood sugar problems or dehydration. If you have a child with bed-wetting problems, try keeping them away from refined carbohydrates and giving them licorice root to stabilize their blood sugar levels. Magnesium and corn silk may also be helpful for bed-wetting.

Stay Hydrated

Not drinking enough water can make you feel anxious and tense. Proper hydration calms the brain and promotes better sleep. Try drinking at least half an ounce of pure water per pound of body weight per day. In other words, two quarts (sixty ounces) is the right amount of water for a 128-pound person.

If you have a problem with waking up to urinate, drink more water during the day, but not a lot of water in the evening. You may also need to take something to strengthen your kidneys, such as a *Kidney Tonic Formula* or work on your adrenals and blood sugar.

Be Physically Active

A sedentary lifestyle will also cause problems with sleep. We need physical activity and rest, so if you work at a desk job and then watch TV when you get home, you may need to become more physically active in order to sleep better. Take a walk, dance, swim, ride a bike, lift weights or otherwise engage your muscles fifteen to twenty minutes per day to improve your sleep. Just don't exercise right before bedtime.

If you need help determining which of these strategies will work for you, talk to a professional herbalist or naturopath (findanherbalist.com or americanherbalistsguild.com).

Strategies: Avoid Caffeine, Avoid Sugar, Balance Methylation, Blood Type Diet, Eliminate Allergy-Causing Foods, Emotional Healing Work, Enhance Nitric Oxide, Epsom Salt Bath, Hydration, Low-Glycemic Diet, Meditation, Reduce Chemical Exposure, Sleep, and Stress Management

Formulas: 5-HTP Adaptogen, Adrenal Glandular, **Herbal Sleep Aid**, **Chinese Wood-Decreasing**, Chinese Qi-Regulating, **Chinese Fire-Increasing**, Anti-Stress B-Complex, Chinese Fire-Decreasing, **Brain Calming**, Nitric Oxide Boosting, **CBD Relaxing**, Hepatoprotective, and **Sleep Support**

Essential Oil Blends: Calming and Relaxing EO

Herbs: Biota, **California poppy**, cannabis, catnip, **chamomile**, cocoa, coleus, **corydalis**, eleuthero, gardenia, gynostemma, hoelen, **hops**, kanna, **kava kava**, lemon balm, ligustrum, linden, lobelia, mimosa, motherwort, oat seed (milky), **passion flower**, polygala, reishi, Saint John's wort, salvia, **skullcap**, **valerian**, vervain (blue), and wild lettuce

Supplements: 5-HTP, amber (succinum), calcium, **GABA**, **L-theanine**, L-tryptophan, lithium, **magnesium**, **melatonin**, potassium, vitamin B-complex, vitamin B$_9$, **vitamin C**, and vitamin D

Essential Oils: Chamomile (Roman), jasmine, **lavender**, marjoram, neroli, orange (sweet), rose, and ylang ylang

Interstitial Cystitis

See also bladder (ulcerated), bladder (irritable), and urinary tract infections

Interstitial cystitis is chronic inflammation of the urinary bladder. This can be caused by infectious organisms. See *urinary tract infections* for more information. Remedies to reduce inflammation and soothe irritation in the urinary passages are helpful. Use soothing urinary herbs like marshmallow, corn silk, horsetail, and parsley. Avoid stimulating diuretics like juniper and uva ursi. Be sure to drink plenty of water to dilute toxins in the urine, thus reducing irritation to the bladder.

Strategies: Hydration

Formulas: Urinary Support, **Liquid Kidney**, UTI **Prevention**, Anti-Inflammatory Pain, **Chinese Water-Increasing**, Diuretic, and Probiotic

Herbs: Agrimony, celery, cleavers, **corn silk**, damiana, garlic, gravel root, **horsetail**, hydrangea, Irish moss, **kava kava**, **licorice**, **marshmallow**, mullein, **parsley**, **pip-**

sissewa, red raspberry, shepherd's purse, slippery elm, spilanthes, and uva ursi

Supplements: Colostrum, L-arginine, **MSM**, nanoparticle silver, omega-3 EFAs, quercetin, and zinc

Essential Oils: Sandalwood and thyme

Irregular Heart Rate   see *arrhythmia*

Irritability

See also hypoglycemia and anger (excessive)

Irritability is the tendency to be easily annoyed and angered, often over insignificant things. Irritability can be related to congestion in the liver, blood sugar problems like hypoglycemia, or hormonal imbalances.

The *Chinese Wood-Decreasing Formula* has been helpful for many people in reducing feelings of irritability, as irritability and excessive anger and aggressiveness are signs of an excess of wood energy in the Chinese system. Chamomile is a specific remedy for people who tend to be peevish and irritable. It can help as an herb, flower essence, or essential oil.

The *Anger-Reducing FE Blend* is also helpful. Lavender and rose essential oils can also ease irritability. Mimosa is also a calming herb that softens the heart and reduces irritability.

Strategies: Affirmation and Visualization, Avoid Caffeine, Avoid Sugar, Counseling or Therapy, Detoxification, Eliminate Salicylates, Emotional Healing Work, Flower Essence, Hydration, Liver Detoxification, and Sleep

Formulas: Children's Colic, **Chinese Wood-Decreasing**, Chinese Fire-Decreasing, Detoxifying, Anti-Anxiety, Anti-Stress B-Complex, CBD Relaxing, and Adaptogen

Flower Essence Blends: Anger-Reducing FE

Herbs: Aloe vera, anemarrhena, **chamomile**, cherry, gardenia, ginkgo, **mimosa**, polygala, Saint John's wort, salvia, skunk cabbage, and vervain (blue)

Supplements: Iron, magnesium, potassium, SAM-e, vitamin B$_5$, and vitamin C

Essential Oils: Chamomile (Roman), clary sage, frankincense, grapefruit (pink), **lavender**, marjoram, orange (sweet), and **rose**

Irritable Bowel

IBS

See also inflammatory bowel disorders, leaky gut, and SIBO

Irritable bowel syndrome (IBS) is characterized by digestive symptoms like painful cramping, bloating, gas, mucus in the stool, diarrhea, and constipation. It has also been called a spastic colon. Unlike inflammatory bowel disease (IBD),

the bowel shows no signs of physical damage like inflammation or ulcerations. However, many of the same therapies that work on IBD may be helpful for IBS. So see *inflammatory bowel disorders* for more ideas on how to improve bowel health.

The symptoms of IBS are quite common and may affect as many as one in five people. This chronic condition is usually not severe enough to require medical attention and can be managed with diet and lifestyle changes, along with appropriate herbs and supplements. Symptoms that something more severe is happening that may require medical attention are rectal bleeding, severe abdominal pain at night, and weight loss.

There are several major factors to consider when trying to improve bowel function in IBS. First, IBS is most likely caused by small intestinal bacterial overgrowth (see *SIBO*) and the leaky gut syndrome that accompanies it. Secondly, stress is often a big factor in IBS. Finally, there may be underlying food allergies or intolerances.

Start by making dietary changes. If you get a lot of gas and bloating, eliminate all sugary and starchy foods; vegetables like cabbage, broccoli, and cauliflower; and legumes like beans and peanuts. Many people experience relief of symptoms by eliminating gluten too. A FODMAP diet where one eliminates carbohydrates that are easily fermented by intestinal flora may also be helpful. See the *Gut-Healing Diet* and *Eliminate FODMAP* strategies for more information.

You can also try some of the therapies suggested for the conditions *SIBO* and *leaky gut*, such as stimulating hydrochloric acid production with *Herbal Bitters Formula* or even supplementing with a *Betaine HCL* or *Digestive Support Formula*. Using herbs and supplements to reduce bacterial overgrowth in the small intestines (such as enteric-coated peppermint oil or berberine) may also be helpful. Supplements to soothe and tone intestinal membranes such as black walnut and marshmallow, or an *Intestinal Toning Formula* may also help. The *Bone Broth* strategy is very helpful for healing the GI tract.

Other possible aids depend on symptoms. For diarrhea, try taking a *Fiber Blend Formula*. Antispasmodic remedies such as lobelia, catnip, or wild yam can reduce feelings of cramping and bloating. For constipation consider a *Gentle Laxative* or *Triphala Formula*. Triphala both tones the intestinal membranes and helps to ease constipation and may be very helpful for normalizing bowel function.

Strategies: Bone Broth, Eliminate Allergy-Causing Foods, Eliminate FODMAPs, Eliminate Salicylates, Gut-Healing Diet, Hydration, and Stress Management

Formulas: **Intestinal Soothing**, Antispasmodic, Hepatoprotective, Pepsin Intestinal, **Gentle Bowel**

Cleansing, Betaine HCl, **Digestive Support**, and **Triphala**

Herbs: Black walnut, **cat's claw**, **catnip**, chamomile, cramp bark, licorice, lobelia, marshmallow, **peppermint enteric coated**, and wild yam

Supplements: Bacillus coagulans, berberine, and magnesium

Itching

See also chicken pox, poison ivy/oak, and rashes & hives

Itching is an irritating sensation on the surface of the skin that compels one to scratch the area affected. It is common in allergic reactions and is a sign of irritants affecting the skin.

To ease itching and prevent scarring when a person is itching due to rashes, exposure to poison ivy or oak, chicken pox, or other afflictions of the skin, the afflicted person use the *Drawing Bath* or *Compress or Fomentation* strategies using herbs like burdock, comfrey, yellow dock, chickweed, and Oregon grape. Baking soda or clay are also good in drawing baths to soothe itching. Another option is oatmeal. Just put a handful of uncooked oatmeal into a cheesecloth bag and put the bag into a hot bath. This prevents the oatmeal from clogging the drain. Seaweeds can be used in a similar manner.

Mixing tea tree oil with vitamin E, one can make a topical application for pox and other irritations. Aloe vera gel and black walnut tincture can also be applied topically to soothe itching. nanoparticle silver applied topically will help prevent open sores from becoming infected and may decrease the itching and speed healing time.

A *Blood Purifier* or *Detoxifying Formula* can be taken internally to ease itching. The *Antihistamine Formula* may be used internally or topically for itching caused by allergic reactions.

Strategies: Compress or Fomentation, Drawing Bath, Eat Healthy, Healthy Fats, and Poultice

Formulas: **Antihistamine**, Blood Purifier, **Enzyme Spray**, Detoxifying, and Chinese Wood-Increasing

Herbs: **Aloe vera**, burdock, **chickweed**, comfrey, dulse, goldenseal, **grindelia**, Irish moss, kelp, linden, Oregon grape, **pau d'arco**, and **yellow dock**

Supplements: **CBD**, clay (bentonite), **clay (Redmond)**, MSM, sodium bicarbonate, vitamin B-complex, vitamin B$_5$, and vitamin E

Essential Oils: Lavender, menthol, and tea tree

Itching, Rectal   **see** *hemorrhoids* **and** *parasites*

Itching/Red Eyes   **see** *eyes (red/itching)*

Itchy Ears

See also food allergies/intolerances and infection (fungal)

An irritating sensation of the ears that compels one to scratch is often a sign of food allergies or intestinal dysbiosis. If you have itchy ears, start by eliminating allergy-causing foods. You may want to do the *Yeast Cleansing Program*.

Strategies: Eliminate Allergy-Causing Foods

Formulas: Stabilized Allicin and **Probiotic**

Programs: Yeast Cleansing

Herbs: Garlic and pau d'arco

Supplements: L-glutamine

Essential Oils: Tea tree

Jaundice (Adults)

See also hepatitis

Jaundice is caused by a buildup of bilirubin in the blood. This causes a yellowing of the skin. Several blood or liver disorders can cause jaundice, including hepatitis. Seek medical attention for an accurate diagnosis and treatment. Herbs and herbal formulas for the liver may be helpful, but hey should be used under professional supervision and after a diagnosis has been made.

One helpful remedy may be activated charcoal, which helps absorb irritants from the liver. A *Hepatoprotective Formula* may also be helpful.

Strategies: Eat Healthy, Fasting, and Increase Dietary Fiber

Formulas: Chinese Wood-Increasing, Blood Purifier, Christopher's Gallbladder, Liver Cleanse, and **Hepatoprotective**

Herbs: Alfalfa, amur cork, artichoke, butcher's broom, **dandelion**, fringe tree, gardenia, gotu kola, kutki, lemon, **milk thistle**, Oregon grape, picrorhiza, safflower, Saint John's wort, trichosanthes, wild yam, and yellow dock

Supplements: **Charcoal**, **SAM-e**, and vitamin C

Essential Oils: Geranium and lemon

Jaundice (Infants)

It is common for newborn infants to have a small amount of jaundice. Exposure to five to ten minutes of sunlight per day is helpful. Safflower tea or activated charcoal mixed with water can also be given to infants to help clear up jaundice.

Herbs: Safflower

Supplements: Charcoal

Jet Lag

See also fatigue and insomnia

Fatigue and irritability after a long flight on an airplane is called jet lag. It is especially a problem when a person crosses several time zones, creating a disruption of the circadian rhythms of the body. Melatonin is a good remedy for helping a person get to sleep after time zone changes. An *Herbal Sleep Aid* or *Sleep Support Formula* may also be helpful. To help with fatigue, try using adaptogens like eleuthero or an *Adrenal Glandular Formula* to ease the stress of jet travel.

Strategies: Reduce EMF Exposure

Formulas: Adrenal Glandular, Chinese Fire-Increasing, Herbal Sleep Aid, and **Sleep Support**

Flower Essence Blends: Shock and Injury FE

Herbs: Ashwagandha, bee pollen, **eleuthero**, ginseng (Asian/Korean), licorice, and spirulina

Supplements: Co-Q10 and **melatonin**

Jock Itch

See also infection (fungal)

Jock itch is a fungal infection that affects the folds of the skin around the groin. Symptoms of jock itch are persistent itching and eruptions of small red bumps or flaking skin. It occurs more commonly in men than in women.

*Antifungal Formula*s or herbs like pau d'arco may be applied topically to the affected areas. Essential oils like tea tree or lavender can be diluted in olive oil and carefully applied. It can help to take probiotics and *Antifungal Formula*s internally. Fungi love damp, warm environments; keep the skin around the groin dry.

Strategies: Friendly Flora, Low-Glycemic Diet, and Sitz Bath

Formulas: Probiotic and Anti-Fungal

Programs: Yeast Cleansing

Essential Oil Blends: Antifungal EO

Herbs: Garlic, **pau d'arco**, and thuja

Essential Oils: Cajeput, lavender, and tea tree

Kidney Infection

See also infection (bacterial)

An infection in the kidneys themselves is much more serious than a urinary tract infection (UTI), in which the bladder or urinary passages are infected. Kidney infections usually cause severe acute symptoms such as fever, chills, pain in the lumbar region, and foul-smelling urine that may include some blood. There may be inflammation present that can be felt as a warm area in the back where the kidneys are located. There may also be nausea, vomiting, and abdominal pain.

Herbs like buchu, goldenseal, pipsissewa, and uva ursi can be used for kidney infections, but avoid juniper berries. Stay well hydrated and eat a plain diet without heavy proteins or simple sugars. A short, one to two days of fasting can take the stress off the kidneys. In serious infections, medical attention should be sought.

Strategies: Fasting and Hydration

Formulas: Liquid Lymph, Chinese Water-Increasing, **UTI Prevention**, and Urinary Support

Herbs: Buchu, cranberry, **echinacea**, **goldenseal**, kava kava, **pipsissewa**, **uva ursi**, and yarrow

Kidney Stones

Deposits resembling small rocks that form in the kidneys are called kidney stones. If they are large or numerous enough, they may cause severe back pain or blood in the urine or interfere with the elimination of urine. Most (80 percent) of kidney stones are made of calcium oxalate and are the result of minerals solidifying out of too-concentrated urine.

People in primitive societies rarely develop kidney stones. So modern diets and lifestyles contribute to this problem. If you are prone to kidney stones, start by drinking more water. This helps keep the minerals in the urine well-diluted so they don't precipitate. You should also avoid foods that increase urinary oxalate significantly, including nuts, chocolate, tea, and peanuts. Caffeine, carbonated beverages, table salt, and animal protein all increase the risk of forming kidney stones.

Magnesium and vitamin B_6 help the body to convert oxalate into other substances. Calcium supplements should be avoided by persons with a history of kidney stones. People who consume plenty of fiber and potassium have a lower risk of forming kidney stones. Fruits and vegetables are high in fiber and potassium.

Several herbs have been used traditionally to aid the passing and inhibit the formation of kidney stones. These include gravel root, hydrangea, nettles, and lemon.

Fresh lemon juice in pure water is very helpful in dissolving and passing stones. One very useful folk remedy for passing kidney stones is to juice four fresh lemons and put the juice in one gallon of distilled water. Fast, drinking only the lemon water, until the stones have passed.

This program can be even more effective when hydrangea or gravel root are taken along with the lemon water, as both of these herbs will help dissolve the stones. At the very least, they help to dissolve the rough edges of the stones so they will pass more easily.

Marshmallow root can also be taken to soothe urinary passages, thus helping the stones to pass. Antispasmodic herbs such as lobelia or kava kava can be taken, especially when there is severe pain, as they will relax urinary passages and help the stones pass more easily. Agrimony also helps with the pain and high doses of magnesium (2,000 to 3,000 mg) can also aid passing stones.

Here's a sample program for helping to pass kidney stones. The exact supplements and amounts required will vary from person to person and from situation to situation. This is only a general guideline. These supplements should be taken while fasting and drinking lemon water as described above:

Hydrangea: 1-2 capsules every two hours

Magnesium: 400 mg capsules every two hours

Marshmallow: 1 capsule every two hours

Kava Kava: 1 capsule every two hours

These measures are effective and have worked for many people. However, always seek medical attention for kidney stones, as this can be a potentially serious condition if the stone blocks a urinary passage for an extended period.

Strategies: Avoid Caffeine and Hydration

Formulas: Chinese Water-Decreasing, Diuretic, and **Kidney Stone**

Herbs: Achyranthes, asparagus, bitter melon, couchgrass, goldenrod, **gravel root**, **hydrangea**, Indian madder, juniper, **kava kava**, khella, **lemon juice**, lobelia, marshmallow, parsley, and uva ursi

Supplements: Magnesium, potassium, and vitamin B_6

Essential Oils: Geranium, juniper, and lemon

Kidney Weakness/Failure

As the kidneys become progressively weak, they become unable to perform their functions effectively. Progressive kidney failure may not produce any symptoms in the initial stages, but as the kidneys become progressively weaker, they stop being able to regulate water and electrolyte balances, clear waste products from the body, and promote red blood cell production.

This may result in weakness, lethargy, edema, anemia, fatigue, loss of appetite, and shortness of breath. The body becomes increasingly acidic and rising levels of urea in the blood will harm the brain and heart. This can lead to congestive heart failure, arrhythmia, tachycardia, and fibrillation. As symptom manifest a person may be placed on dialysis or scheduled for a kidney transplant.

There are herbs that can promote kidney health and increase kidney function. Eucommia, goldenrod, and nettle leaf are examples of kidney tonic herbs that can strengthen renal function. A *Chinese Water-Increasing Formula* may help. Nettle *seed*, not the leaf, is a specific for progressive renal failure. Enhancing nitric oxide may also be helpful for preventing kidney failure.

Strategies: Enhance Nitric Oxide

Formulas: Nitric Oxide Boosting, Urinary Support, and **Chinese Water-Increasing**

Herbs: Cleavers, dandelion leaf, drynaria, eucommia, **goldenrod**, nettle, stinging leaf, **nettle, stinging seed**, noni root, and teasel root

Supplements: Co-Q10

Knees, Weak   **see** *weak knees*

Labor & Delivery

See also pregnancy and avoid during pregnancy

There are a number of herbal remedies that can ease labor and delivery. Using the *Pregnancy Tea* or *Joan Patton's Herbal Minerals Formula*, or just plan red raspberry leaf, can strengthen the uterus and prepare the woman's body for childbirth. The *Prebirth Formula* can be taken starting about five or six weeks before the due date to further prepare the body for childbirth.

During labor, antispasmodic herbs such as lobelia and black cohosh have been taken during labor to reduce the pain from contractions. Taking adequate magnesium during labor also helps ease muscle pain during labor.

Blue cohosh has been used to help induce labor and to strengthen contractions during labor. However, it should never be used during pregnancy, and there are some concerns about it's safety even during labor. Consult with a professional herbalist or midwife skilled in the use of this plant before using.

A mixture of bayberry and capsicum extracts in a little apple cider vinegar has been used to help stop bleeding after the birth. Shepherd's purse has also been used for this purpose.

Be sure to look at *pregnancy (remedies to avoid)*. Consult with a midwife or professional herbalist (findanherbalist.com or americanherbalistsguild.com) for assistance in selecting herbs and supplements appropriate for pregnancy, labor, and delivery.

Formulas: Prebirth, General Glandular, **Pregnancy Tea**, and **Joan Patton's Herbal Minerals**

Herbs: Bayberry, **black cohosh**, blue cohosh, capsicum, chamomile, dong quai, lobelia, partridge berry, **red raspberry**, and shepherd's purse

Supplements: Chlorophyll, **magnesium**, and vitamin C

Essential Oils: Clove and jasmine

Lactose Intolerance

See also gas & bloating

Lactose intolerance results in bloating and gas after eating dairy products due to the inability to break down the lactose or milk sugar in dairy products that have not been cultured. Lactase is the enzyme that helps break down this sugar. The best remedy is to take lactase enzyme supplements and probiotics. One can also take carminative herbs for the gas.

Strategies: Friendly Flora and Gut-Healing Diet

Formulas: **Lactase Enzyme**, Christopher's Carminative, and **Probiotic**

Herbs: Fennel, ginger, and peppermint

Laryngitis

Hoarseness

See also sore throat

Laryngitis is inflammation of the larynx or voice box that causes a complete or partial loss of voice. Sage and licorice tea, sipped slowly or used as a gargle is a good remedy. One can also apply capsicum and lobelia topically to the throat and follow this up with a *Topical Analgesic Blend*. Collinsonia is good for laryngitis brought on by straining the voice and is a useful remedy for singers and public speakers. Sucking on tablets of the *Cold Lozenges Formula*, which contains zinc and vitamin C is also helpful.

Strategies: Emotional Healing Work

Formulas: Lung Moistening, **Cold Lozenges**, Anti-Inflammatory Pain, and Topical Analgesic

Herbs: Capsicum, **collinsonia**, kava kava, **licorice**, lobelia, marshmallow, **sage**, white sage, and yerba santa

Supplements: Zinc

Essential Oils: Clove, frankincense, jasmine, pine, tea tree, and thyme

Lead Poisoning

See also heavy metal poisoning

Lead is one of the most toxic metals known. It's been many years since our society was made aware of the damage that exposure to lead-based paints was doing to our health,

especially to young children, who suck on and chew anything they can get their hands on.

When the lead reaches toxic levels in the body, it can damage the kidneys, liver, heart, and nervous system. The body can't tell the difference between lead and calcium, so pregnant women, children, and other people who are deficient in calcium absorb lead more easily, with infants and children affected most severely. Possible symptoms of lead poisoning include anxiety, arthritis, confusion, chronic fatigue, behavioral problems, juvenile delinquency, hyperactivity, learning disabilities, metallic taste in the mouth, tremors, mental disturbances, loss of memory, mental retardation, impotence, reproductive disorders, infertility, liver failure, and death.

Exposure to lead can come from food that is grown near roads or factories, lead-based paint, hair products, food from lead-soldered cans, imported ceramic products (especially from Mexico and China), lead crystal glassware, ink on bread bags, batteries in cars, bone meal, insecticides, tobacco, lead pipes, and lead solder in the water pipes. If you suspect you could have lead pipes or lead solder in your water system, have the water tested.

Seek medical assistance if you think you have lead poisoning. Remedies that can help eliminate lead from the body include N-acetyl-cysteine, sodium alginate (algin), lobelia and *Heavy Metal Cleansing Formulas*. See *heavy metal poisoning* for additional suggestions.

Strategies: Heavy Metal Cleanse and Oral Chelation

Formulas: **Oral Chelation**, Stabilized Allicin, and **Heavy Metal Cleansing**

Herbs: Garlic, kelp, and **lobelia**

Supplements: **Alpha-lipoic acid**, clay (bentonite), iodine, **N-acetyl cysteine**, sodium alginate, and **zinc**

Leaky Gut

See also infection (fungal), inflammatory bowel disorders, parasites, SIBO, and dysbiosis

Leaky gut is a by-product of inflammatory bowel disorders or SIBO, an overgrowth of bacteria in the small intestines. Leaky gut isn't a medical diagnosis yet, but research is mounting that it exists and that it contributes to numerous health problems. The research suggests that leaky gut may be involved in all of the following:

Frequent gas, bloating, diarrhea, constipation and irritable bowel syndrome

Allergies, asthma, and chronic sinus problems

Autoimmune diseases, including psoriasis, Hashimoto's thyroiditis (the most common cause of low thyroid activity), rheumatoid arthritis, and lupus

Fibromyalgia and chronic fatigue

Depression, anxiety, attention deficit disorder, and hyperactivity

Chronic skin conditions like acne, rosacea, and eczema

Yeast infections

Multiple food allergies, sensitivities. or intolerances

Arthritis, joint or muscle pain

So if you have any of these problems, healing your gut may be an important key to recovering your health.

Understanding Leaky Gut

When the cells lining the intestinal tract are healthy, they are tightly packed, forming a barrier that only allows molecules of completely digested food to be absorbed. These nutrients include simple sugars (monosaccharides), amino acids from protein, fatty acids and glycerol (from fats), and vitamins and minerals. Other materials are blocked from being absorbed.

If the gaps between these cells widen, things that shouldn't be absorbed can enter the blood and lymph. These can pass between the gaps (pancellular) or through the damaged intestinal cells (transcellular).

These larger molecules include partially digested proteins or large protein fragments. These proteins act as allergens, and the immune system reacts to them as foreign invaders. Inflammation is triggered, and antibodies are produced to tag the foreign proteins for destruction. The antibodies prime the immune system to react to these proteins in the diet, creating allergic reactions or food sensitivities.

The enlarged gaps also allow pathogens (viruses, bacteria, yeast, and maybe even some parasites) to get past the intestinal lining. This further triggers immune reactions and inflammation. The inflammation can further damage the intestinal lining and increase its permeability.

The end result is pain, allergic reactions, chronic inflammation, and autoimmune reactions in various tissues. In short, a breakdown of the intestinal lining adversely affects the health of the body as a whole, something natural healers have known for centuries.

Triggers for Leaky Gut

Researchers discovered that a hormone called zonulin is responsible for determining how wide the gaps are between intestinal cells. Zonulin opens the gaps to allow nutrients to pass through. It also opens the gaps when infection or parasites are present so white blood cells can move in to fight the invaders. Researchers have discovered that two key factors increase the release of zonulin.

First, more zonulin is released when there is an overgrowth of bacteria or yeast in the small intestines or an imbalance in the type of microbes in the gut. This condition, known as dysbiosis, will trigger more zonulin production. This leads to a widening of the gaps, allowing white blood cells to move into the intestines to fight the infection.

Second, zonulin is released by a protein called gliadin, which is found in grains that contain gluten, such as wheat, rye, and barley. It's long been known that people with celiac's disease are genetically unable to handle gluten as it inflames and destroys their intestinal lining, but recently many people who don't have celiac's disease have started becoming intolerant of gluten.

As people's intestines become more irritated, they become more gluten intolerant because it aggravates leaky gut and increases autointoxication. Elevated zonulin levels have been confirmed in people suffering from inflammatory bowel diseases, asthma, multiple sclerosis, type 1 diabetes, and Crohn's disease.

Strategies for Leaky Gut

Traditional colon cleansing was primarily focused on increasing elimination via the bowels using fiber and herbal laxatives. This may be a useful first step in healing the intestinal tract, but it is no longer sufficient to restore gut health. Here is a complete strategy for reducing leaking gut and gut inflammation, healing the intestinal membranes and ultimately improving overall health and well-being. Follow these strategies in the order given for best results.

1. Improve Elimination

If your colon transit time is slow, you need to start by improving elimination. Colon transit time is the time it takes for the waste material from the food you eat to exit the body. A healthy transit time is about eighteen to twenty-four hours. This means that in twenty-four hours or less, your body should eliminate what it didn't absorb from a meal.

You can check your colon transit time by taking a few ounces of liquid chlorophyll or eating some red beets and checking how long it takes for the green (chlorophyll) or the red (beets) color to show up in your stool. If it takes longer than twenty-four hours, or if you have less than one bowel movement per day, you should start your gut healing program with one of the prepackaged detoxification programs mentioned in the *Detoxification* strategy.

2. Eliminate Irritants

For reasons I've already pointed out, grains containing gluten, such as wheat, rye, and barley should be avoided while trying to heal leaky gut, but there are other substances that you should avoid as well. Refined sugars, like white table sugar and high-fructose corn syrup, should be avoided as they feed bacterial and yeast overgrowth.

One should also avoid substances that disrupt the friendly flora or can potentially increase intestinal inflammation. These include a variety of drugs (antibiotics, birth control pills, NSAIDs and chemotherapy agents), pesticides, food additives, and genetically modified foods (GMOs). It's also wise to eliminate any food allergens. See the *Eliminate Allergy-Causing Foods* strategy.

3. Balance Gut Flora

If you have a lot of belching, bloating, intestinal gas or IBS, you probably need to balance your gut flora. The *Anti-Fungal Formula* or *H. Pylori-Fighting Herbal Formula* can also be helpful. See *dysbiosis* for more information on balancing gut flora.

4. Nourish the Intestines

There are a number of herbs and nutrients that can help to heal the gut lining after transit time is improved, irritants are eliminated and the gut flora is balanced. For starters, L-glutamine is an amino acid that is extremely helpful in healing leak gut. Although it's found in plant and animal proteins, glutamine is especially plentiful in bone broth, grass fed beef, spirulina, and whey protein. You also can take L-glutamine as part of the *Gut-Healing Fiber Formula*. Some herbs that are helpful for leaky gut include cat's claw, black walnut, pau d'arco, turmeric, and kudzu. The *Triphala Formula* is also very helpful.

Fat-soluble vitamins are helpful for protecting mucous membranes in both the GI and respiratory tract. Vitamin A has been shown to regulate the growth and differentiation of intestinal cells. Lower levels of vitamin A result in a reduced ability for intestinal membranes to resist infections. A lack of vitamin D may also contribute to leaky gut.

There is some research suggesting zinc may be helpful for leaky gut. Zinc is important for the immune system and wound healing and is a common nutritional deficiency, especially in men. Iodine is also important for gut health and seaweeds like kelp and dulse, which are naturally rich in iodine and other minerals, have been used to improve GI tract health as well.

Strategies: Avoid Sugar, Bone Broth, Detoxification, Eliminate Allergy-Causing Foods, Eliminate FODMAPs, Fasting, Friendly Flora, Gut-Healing Diet, and Increase Dietary Fiber

Formulas: Irritable Bowel Fiber, **Gentle Bowel Cleansing**, Anti-Fungal, **Plant Enzyme**, H. Pylori-Fighting, Chinese Wood-Decreasing, Intestinal Soothing, **Probiotic**, **Gut Immune**, Hepatoprotective, **Gut-Healing Fiber**, **Digestive Support**, Pepsin Intestinal, **Betaine HCl**, and **Triphala**

Programs: Ivy Bridge's Cleansing, **Chinese Balanced Cleansing**, and Weight Loss Cleansing

Herbs: Acacia, aloe vera, bee balm, bee balm, **black walnut**, **calendula**, **cat's claw**, chamomile, **kudzu**, licorice, plantain, Saint John's wort, and wild yam

Supplements: Collagen, **colostrum**, **L-glutamine**, magnesium, omega-3 EFAs, and vitamin C

Leg Cramps   see *cramps (leg)*

Leprosy

Leprosy is a chronic infection caused by *Mycobacterium leprae*. It usually affects the skin, peripheral nerves and testes. The following herbs have been reported in historical literature or modern research to help with leprosy; however, this is a condition requiring medical attention.

Herbs: Gotu kola, slippery elm, and yellow dock

Supplements: Nanoparticle silver

Essential Oils: Myrrh

Lesions

See also abscesses, acne, boils, wounds & sores, and moles

A lesion is an area of pathologically altered tissue such as an injury, abscess, boil, mole, pimple, rash, or wound. Look up the specific type of problem for suggested remedies.

Leucorrhea
Vaginal Discharge

See also vaginitis

Leucorrhea is a whitish discharge from the vaginal area and uterus, usually the result of an estrogen imbalance or chronic bacterial or fungal infection. It is associated with inflammation of the vagina (vaginitis). If bacterial in nature try a 10 percent solution of povidone iodine in water as a douche or dilute silver and use it as a douche. One can also take garlic or an *Antibacterial Formula* internally.

For fungal issues, consider pau d'arco or the *Yeast Cleansing Program*. Supplementing with probiotics may be helpful. They can also be mixed with water and used as a douche to restore a balance of friendly microbes to the vaginal area. One can also douche with a tea made of calendula or pau d'arco.

Strategies: Douche, Friendly Flora, and Sitz Bath

Formulas: Stabilized Allicin, GLA Oil, Probiotic, Antibacterial, and Anti-Fungal

Programs: Yeast Cleansing

Herbs: Amalaki, calendula, evening primrose, false unicorn, garlic, hyacinth, kava kava, lady's mantle, lotus, **pau d'arco**, and zhu-ling

Supplements: Iodine, nanoparticle silver, vitamin A, and vitamin D

Essential Oils: Bergamot, clove, and tea tree

Leukemia

See also cancer

Leukemia is a cancer involving a proliferation of abnormal white blood cells (leukocytes). In addition to the general protocols listed under cancer, it is important to use remedies that add herbs that support the lymphatic system. Seek medical attention for this serious health problem.

Strategies: Eat Healthy, Heavy Metal Cleanse, and Reduce Chemical Exposure

Formulas: Chinese Wood-Increasing, **Immune-Boosting, Lymph Cleansing**, and **Essiac Immune Tea**

Herbs: Aloe vera, **baptisia**, burdock, cleavers, pau d'arco, red clover, and red root

Supplements: Protease, vitamin C, and vitamin D

Lice

The following have been used to control head lice, an insect that can infest hair. Mix essential oils or the contents of the *Standardized Acetogenin Formula* capsules with shampoo and wash the hair, leaving the shampoo in the hair for about five to ten minutes before rinsing. It may also be helpful to add essential oils to a shampoo and wash in a similar manner.

Formulas: Standardized Acetogenin

Herbs: Black walnut, false unicorn, and pawpaw

Essential Oils: Cinnamon, **eucalyptus**, oregano, rosemary, **tea tree**, and thyme

Ligaments, Torn/Injuried

See also sprains

A torn ligament is similar to a sprain, but more serious. Torn ligaments cause severe swelling, bruising, and pain, and may require surgical intervention. So seek medical assistance.

Herbs that help tissues to heal, such as arnica, comfrey, and calendula, can all be helpful applied topically using the *Compress or Fomentation* or *Poultice* strategies. Increasing mineral intake and taking supplements that speed the healing of tissues can also be helpful.

Strategies: Compress or Fomentation, Lymph-Moving Pain Relief, Mineralization, and Poultice

Formulas: Herbal Calcium, Vulnerary, Topical Analgesic, and Joan Patton's Herbal Minerals

Essential Oil Blends: Topical Injury

Herbs: Arnica, calendula, **comfrey**, plantain, and **solomon's seal**

Supplements: Collagen, MSM, and vitamin C

Liver Spots   **see** *age spots*

Liver, Fatty   **see** *fatty liver disease*

Lockjaw   **see** *tetanus*

Lou Gehrig's Disease   **see** *ALS*

Low Stomach Acid
Hypochlorhydria

See also hiatal hernia and stress

Many people suffer from low stomach acid, which becomes more common as people age. If you're over fifty and have digestive problems, you may have this problem, which is known medically as hypochlorhydria. Symptoms include gas or bloating shortly after meals, a sense of fullness after eating with food sitting in the stomach for a long time, nausea after taking supplement, weak or cracked nails, and dilated capillaries in the cheeks and nose.

A lack of hydrochloric acid (HCl) may be due to a lack of any of chloride, zinc, and thiamine. These are primary nutritional factors required for the synthesis of hydrochloric acid. It may also be due to stress or a hiatal hernia.

Bitters, like gentian, dandelion root, and artichoke, not only stimulate HCl secretion, but also stimulate pancreatic enzymes and bile from the gallbladder and tend to be mildly antibacterial as well. An *Herbal Bitters Formulas* should be taken fifteen to twenty minutes prior to meals with one to two large glasses of water. A small pinch of a natural salt can also be taken at the same time, as this also helps stimulate HCl production by providing chloride.

Bitters are contraindicated if you have digestive atrophy. So if you have dry mucous membranes, as evidenced by a dry and withered-looking (or shriveled) tongue, don't take bitters, because they dry the mucous membranes.

Many people benefit by taking a *Betaine HCL Formula*. To determine how much you need, you can do a hydrochloric acid challenge test, but do not perform this test if you have an active ulcer or a history of ulcers.

To do the test, take a 400 to 500 mg capsule of betaine HCl prior to a meal. If you notice no burning, increase to two capsules the next meal. Proceed until you notice a mild burning sensation, then immediately reduce your dose to the number of capsules that preceded the burning or heat sensation. Most people find a comfortable dose between 400 and 1,500 mg per meal (two to three capsules).

If one or two capsules cause burning, you either don't have low stomach acid or you have a hiatal hernia or acid reflux that is so severe that you won't be able to take HCl until you get it under control. Also, remember that the more protein you eat with a meal, the greater the need for HCl, so you can vary the dose with the size and content of your meals. Also, if you have severe digestive problems, you may also wish to take the *Digestive Support Formula*, which combines betaine HCl and digestive enzymes.

Within three to six months most people feel a warmth in their stomach with the same dose they have been taking. When this happens it is time to decrease your dose and start weaning off of betaine HCl.

Strategies: Blood Type Diet, Hiatal Hernia Correction, and Stress Management

Formulas: Betaine HCl, Digestive Support, and **Herbal Bitters**

Herbs: Angelica, **artichoke**, dandelion root, **gentian**, goldenseal, and orange (bitter) peel

Lumbago   see *backache*

Lung Congestion   see *congestion (lungs)*

Lupus

See also autoimmune disorders

Lupus is a chronic inflammatory and autoimmune disease that attacks multiple organs. It affects the skin in many people, creating a butterfly rash over the face. Immune stimulants should be avoided, and general therapies for autoimmune diseases should be applied. This is a serious illness, and professional assistance should be sought.

There are a number of natural remedies that may be helpful, however. For starters, levels of DHEA tend to be low in people with lupus. You can supplement with DHEA and/or strengthen the adrenal glands with *Adrenal Tonic Formulas*. It is also useful to calm stress levels with *Adaptogen Formulas*. Licorice root, wild yam, and yucca are single herbs that may help to ease pain and inflammation.

Follow the general strategies for *autoimmune disorders*, paying close attention to the health of the digestive tract, a diet high in antioxidant nutrients, and the *Hydration* strategy.

Strategies: Eat Healthy, Gut-Healing Diet, Hydration, and Low-Glycemic Diet

Formulas: Chinese Wood-Increasing, **DHEA with Herbs**, Herbal Arthritis, **Adrenal Glandular**, Joint Healing Nutrients, GLA Oil, **Probiotic**, Proanthocyanidins,

Antioxidant, Stan Malstrom's Herbal Aspirin, **Analgesic Nerve**, Anti-Inflammatory Pain, and **Betaine HCl**

Herbs: Aloe vera, **astragalus**, black currant, black walnut, chaste tree, cordyceps, garlic, licorice, wild yam, and **yucca**

Supplements: 7-keto, CBD, colostrum, DHEA, indole-3-carbinol, MSM, **omega-3 EFAs**, protease, vitamin B-complex, vitamin C, **vitamin D**, and zinc

Lyme Disease

Lyme disease is a bacterial infection caused by the bacterium *Borrelia burgdorferi* and possibly other related species (like *B. mayonii*). It is transmitted primarily through tick bites. Several days after the bite, the person typically develops a bulls eye-like rash, fever, headache, and fatigue. Most cases of acute Lyme disease can be treated successfully with a few weeks of antibiotics.

According to the Center for Disease Control (CDC) 10 to 20 percent of people treated for Lyme disease develop ongoing symptoms, a condition that has been called post treatment Lyme disease syndrome (PTLDS). It has also been called chronic Lyme disease.

Symptoms of PTLDS can include chronic fatigue, pain (especially migrating joint and muscle pain), restless or disturbed sleep, swelling in the knees, shoulders, elbows, and other large joints, decreased short-term memory, difficulty concentrating (brain fog), and speech problems. Other symptoms can include eye pain, tooth pain, muscle twitching, dizziness, tremors, chest pain, irregular heartbeat, shortness of breath, headaches, and chronic flu-like symptoms. These symptoms last more than 6 months and can sometimes last for many years.

It has been estimated that about 300,000 Americans are infected with Lyme disease each year. Many of these people become ill but don't know why as many medical doctors aren't trained to recognize PTLDS. So if you've ever been bitten by ticks and are suffering from symptoms like those listed above, you should consider the possibility of that you have PTLDS. That's true even if you didn't notice any acute symptoms after the tick bite, as some people with PTLDS didn't experience the acute symptoms of Lyme disease.

Herbal Remedies for Lyme

The ineffectiveness of orthodox medicine in treating PTLDS has caused many people to natural medicine for answers. A study conducted at John Hopkins Bloomberg School of Public Health and published in the peer-reviewed *Journal Frontiers in Medicine* found seven herbs with potential benefit against the *Borrelia* bacteria in test tubes. The top performers were cryptolepsis, Japanese knotweed, black walnut, sweet wormwood, cat's claw (uña de gato), rock rose, and Chinese skullcap.

Stephen Harrod Buhner, author of the book *Healing Lyme* and recognized authority Lyme's disease, has a protocol that includes many of those top performers: Japanese knotweed (or it's extract resveratrol), cat's claw, and Chinese skullcap. In addition to these he also uses andrographis, ashwagandha, eleuthero root, licorice root, red sage, and sometimes echinacea. He also recommends bone broth for collagen support and many other supplements depending on the different body systems the PTLDS is affecting.

Another protocol, based partly on Buhner's, is that set forth by Dr. William Rawls, MD, in his book *Unlocking Lyme*. His list includes most of the remedies Buhner uses, but he also recommends garlic with stabilized allicin, sarsaparilla, cordyceps, reishi, hawthorn and milk thistle. Nutrients he recommends include glutathione, n-acetyl-cysteine, alpha-lipoic acid, Co-Q10, vitamin D_3, and omega-3 essential fatty acids.

Strategies for Chronic Lyme Disease

The exact protocol for PTLDS needs to be adapted to each individual, but based on the experience of these and other experts, here are three key categories of remedies to consider. Other remedies would be added based on the organs affected by PTLDS. For example, if the heart is affected remedies like hawthorn and Co-Q10 would be helpful. I recommend working with an experienced herbalist or other natural health care provider to determine the best remedies for you, but here are the basic strategies.

Take Antimicrobial Herbs to Fight Infection

One of the best remedies is andrographis, which is widely regarded as helpful for acute and chronic infections. For PTLDS a dose of about 200 to 800 mg per day is suggested. Another potentially helpful remedy for PTLDS is cat's claw. It enhances lymphocytes and natural killer (NK) cells, including a specific NK cell that is deficient in PTLDS. The recommended dose is 400-800 mg daily.

Buhner recommends taking astragalus daily to prevent infection from ticks. He recommends 1,000 mg (about two capsules) throughout the year and 3,000 mg (about six capsules) during the tick season, if you live in an area where Lyme disease is prevalent. Resveratrol, extracted from Japanese knotweed, is a primary remedy for *Borrelia* in typical Lyme protocols. It is helpful against other infectious organisms that can be transmitted by ticks, such as *Bartonella* and mycoplasma and helps with candida (yeast) infections from antibiotics. The recommended dose is 200 to 800 mg per day.

Another herb worth mentioning is sarsaparilla, which binds endotoxins from dying bacteria and was traditionally used as a remedy for syphilis, another spirochete bacterial infection. Additional antimicrobial remedies to consider would include Chinese skullcap, black walnut, cryptolepsis, and sweet annie.

Use Immune Modulators to Balance Immune Reactions

Cordyceps has proven to be a valuable remedy for many people with PTLDS. It decreases inflammatory cytokines, while aiding NK cells and macrophage activity to help fight infection. It is a general tonic to the body, but also helps to protect the heart. The recommended dose is 1,000 to 3,000 mg (about two to six capsules daily).

Another medicinal mushroom that may be helpful is reishi (or ganoderma). It improves immune responses, but also reduces inflammatory cytokines. It also helps the nervous system and protects the heart. The recommended dose here is 1,000 to 2,000 mg. Eleuthero root is an adaptogen which aids basic immune responses and improves resistance to stress. It can be a helpful immune modulator where fatigue is one of the symptoms, but a relatively low dose is needed. One capsule per day is plenty. ashwagandha is another helpful immune modulator that can also aid sleep. Dose would be one to two capsules per day.

Use Restorative Remedies to Support Healing

Since collagen is the prime target of stealth microbes like *Borrelia* and mycoplasma, increasing collagen intake can aid with recovery. This may be done by making and drinking bone broth on a regular basis or by taking a collagen supplement. The dose for collagen is 6,000 mg or more per day.

The silica in horsetail can help with collagen support. If you're experiencing joint or muscle pain as part of PTLDS you could take horsetail or *Watkin's Hair, Skin and Nails Formula* daily. The dose for either is one to two capsules three times daily. For pain and sleep problems CBD may be helpful. CBD also helps modulate the immune system, which is important in recovery from PTLDS.

A multiple vitamin and mineral would probably be helpful, but specific nutrients that may help support recovery from PTLDS include vitamin C, vitamin D_3, zinc, and selenium. Omega-3 essential fatty acids also modulate immune responses and may be helpful for supporting nerve and joint function with chronic Lyme disease. An *Anti-Inflammatory Pain Formula* may also be helpful if you have joint or muscle pain.

Strategies: Gut-Healing Diet and Stress Management

Formulas: Gut Immune, Adrenal Glandular, Herbal Potassium, and Adaptogen

Herbs: Andrographis, black walnut, boneset, **cat's claw**, echinacea, garlic, isatis, lomatium, **sweet annie**, **teasel**, and usnea

Supplements: Multiple vitamin and mineral, vitamin A, vitamin B$_6$, vitamin C, **vitamin D**, and zinc

Lymphatic Congestion
see *congestion (lymphatic)*

Lymphoma
Hodgkin's Disease

See also cancer

Lymphoma is a type of cancer involving cells of the immune system called lymphocytes. There are many different types of lymphomas, including Hodgkin's lymphoma. The lymphocytes become cancerous and travel through the lymph system, causing swelling of the lymph nodes. They may also collect in other organs such as the spleen. Professional assistance should be sought for this serious condition.

Herbs that encourage lymphatic drainage, including mullein, red clover, and red root have all been used to aid in the recovery from lymphomas. Digestive enzyme supplements taken between meals on an empty stomach may also be helpful. Since this is a form of cancer, look under *cancer* for additional suggestions.

  Strategies: Detoxification
  Formulas: **Lymph Cleansing**, Liquid Lymph, **Digestive Support**, Alterative-Immune, and Chinese Metal-Decreasing
  Herbs: Mullein, red clover, **red root**, and **venus fly trap**
  Supplements: Vitamin A, **vitamin C**, and **vitamin D**

Macular Degeneration

See also free radical damage

The macula is the center of the retina, and when this part of the retina starts to deteriorate, a person experiences a loss of central vision in one or both eyes. This degeneration of the macula is also caused by inflammation and free radical damage. High blood pressure and hardening of the arteries increase the risk of developing macular degeneration.

As with other eye diseases, increasing dietary antioxidants is an important step to preventing macular degeneration. Avoid cigarette smoke and protect the eyes from UV radiation with hats or sunglasses.

Antioxidant supplements can help to prevent and possibly even reverse macular degeneration. Consider using an *Antioxidant Eye Protecting Formula*. Some people have found the *Oral Chelation Formula* helpful too.

  Strategies: Eat Healthy and Healthy Fats

Formulas: **Antioxidant Eye**, **Oral Chelation**, Proanthocyanidins, **Antioxidant**, and Methylated B Vitamin
Programs: Cardiovascular Nutritional
Herbs: Bilberry and **ginkgo**
Supplements: **Lutein**, **omega-3 EFAs**, **vitamin A**, vitamin B$_9$, **vitamin C**, **vitamin D**, **zeaxanthin**, and **zinc**

Malaria

See also parasites

Malaria is an acute or chronic disease caused by parasites that invade the red blood cells. It is transmitted from an infected person to an uninfected person by the bite of a mosquito. Symptoms include chills, fever, mass destruction of red blood cells, and the parasitic release of toxic substances. Artemisinin, which is an extract of sweet Annie, and the herb cinchona have been used to treat malaria. Malaria is a serious disease, and medical attention should be sought.

Formulas: Probiotic and **Antiparasitic**
Herbs: **Andrographis**, echinacea, and **sweet annie**
Supplements: Vitamin A
Essential Oils: Bay leaf and lemon

Mania

See also bipolar mood disorder

When a person has an abnormally elated mental state, characterized by euphoria, risk-taking, setting unreasonable goals and expectations for themselves, and exaggerated feelings of self-importance, they are exhibiting mania. This can be accompanied by excessive talkativeness, impatience, hyperactivity, and a loss of sleep. In severe cases, mania can have psychotic features. When mania alternates with depression, a person has bipolar mood disorder, also known as manic-depressive disorder.

No one knows the cause of mania, but it may be the result of imbalances in neurotransmitters (serotonin, dopamine, etc.) or unresolved emotional wounds. From a natural point of view, there are many things we can do to help someone who gets manic from time to time.

One of the first steps to maintaining a stable mood is to maintain a stable blood sugar level. When blood sugar goes high, we tend to get more manic because our brain is over stimulated. Following the *Low-Glycemic Diet* strategy and avoiding stimulants, like caffeine, can be helpful.

It is important to start the day with protein for breakfast and to obtain adequate protein from the diet to keep the brain stable. L-tyrosine, an amino acid found in red meat, is often very helpful. It can be taken as a supplement or obtained naturally in the diet by consuming some type of grass-fed, organic red meat daily (preferably for breakfast). Spirulina or an *Algae Formula* can also supply amino acids to help stabilize mood. Feeding the brain and nerves with the *Anti-Stress B-Complex* may also be helpful.

Lemon balm is a particularly useful herb for balancing mania and depression, as it helps stabilize the mood. The *Counseling or Therapy* strategy can be used to help people work through the underlying traumas that contribute to mood swings.

Strategies: Avoid Caffeine, Counseling or Therapy, Emotional Healing Work, Flower Essence, and Low-Glycemic Diet

Formulas: Anti-Stress B-Complex, Memory Enhancing, and Algae

Herbs: Blue-green algae, chlorella, lemon balm, and **spirulina**

Supplements: L-tyrosine and **vitamin B-complex**

Essential Oils: Clary sage, lavender, and lemon

Manic Depressive Disorder
see *bipolar mood disorder*

Mastitis
Breast Infection

See also breasts (swelling/tenderness)

Mastitis is a staph infection in the breast that usually occurs during breast-feeding, causing inflammation and tenderness. ^ of slippery elm, plantain, mullein, or echinacea can be helpful (see *Poultice* strategy). One can also massage a few drops of poke oil diluted in olive oil into the breasts. Do not put poke oil on the nipples if you are nursing as you don't want the nursing baby taking it internally.

Lymphatic herbs and formulas, taken internally, can improve lymphatic flow in the breasts, and echinacea or an *Antibacterial Formula* can be used to fight the infection. If the problem does not clear up in a day or two, seek medical assistance.

Strategies: Hydration and Poultice

Formulas: Liquid Lymph, Anti-Inflammatory Pain, Lymphatic Infection, and **Antibacterial**

Herbs: Baptisia, chicory, **echinacea**, gardenia, lobelia, mullein, red clover, slippery elm, and trichosanthes

Measles
See also contagious disease prevention and infection (viral)

Measles is an acute contagious viral disease that begins with inflammation of mucous membranes, conjunctivitis, and cough. This is followed on the third or fourth day by an eruption of distinct circular red spots.

Internally, Oregon grape, burdock, or a *Blood Purifier Formulas* can help to speed recovery. Yarrow is helpful if there is a fever. In children less than two years old supplementing with 200,000 IU of vitamin A two days in a row can reduce the risk of mortality. The *Drawing Bath* strategy can be used to ease itching and discomfort.

Strategies: Drawing Bath

Formulas: Essiac Immune Tea, **Chinese Wind-Heat Evil**, Steven Horne's Children's Composition, and Blood Purifier

Herbs: Black cohosh, burdock, catnip, goldenseal, **isatis**, **Oregon grape**, pleurisy, and **yarrow**

Supplements: Clay (Redmond) and **vitamin A**

Memory/Brain Function
See also Alzheimer's, dementia, and mitochondrial dysfunction

If you want to keep your mind sharp and your memory efficient, it's important to take good care of your brain. Here are some strategies for maintaining good brain and memory function.

Stay Hydrated

Your brain is 70 percent water and is very sensitive to dehydration. A mere 2 percent drop in body water can trigger problems like fuzzy short-term memory and trouble with basic math. Dehydration can also make it difficult for you to focus on a printed page or a computer screen. See the *Hydration* strategy for more information.

Eat Good Fats

If you remove the water from the brain, over 50 percent of what is left is fat. So good fats are very important to your brain. Children who receive plenty of good fats in the womb and earlier childhood have better brain development. Low fat diets aren't healthy for the brains of children or adults. Omega-3 essential fatty acids, especially DHA, are helpful for brain health. See the *Healthy Fats* strategy for more information.

Get Adequate Protein

Brain cells talk one another by sending messages via chemicals called neurotransmitters. All neurotransmitters are built from amino acids, the building blocks of protein.

So low protein diets aren't good for the mind either. Studies have shown that children who start the day with a traditional breakfast that contains high-protein foods like eggs or a protein smoothie perform better in school than children who eat sugar-sweetened breakfast cereals. It's the same for adults. A great way to get more amino acids for your brain is to take an *Algae Blend*.

Take B Vitamins

Synthesizing neurotransmitters from amino acids takes other nutrients, particularly B vitamins. They are found naturally in most complex carbohydrates, like fruits, vegetables, and whole grains. They are missing, however, from refined carbohydrates, like white sugar, white flour, and white rice, which is why most Americans aren't getting enough Bs to keep their brains working at the A+ level. Try taking a B complex supplement or an *Anti-Stress B-Complex Formula*.

Avoid Sugar

If you want a clear, sharp mind, it's best to avoid refined carbohydrates like refined sugar and white-flour products. These foods spike your blood sugar and then allow it to drop dramatically a couple of hours later. This is bad for the brain, since the amount of sugar reaching your brain affects your memory, focus, and mental clarity.

When your blood sugar is too high, your brain is over-stimulated, which will make you hyperactive and irritable. You'll feel agitated, excitable, and restless, but have difficulty concentrating. When your blood sugar is too low, your brain won't function properly. You'll feel sluggish and lethargic or angry and irrational. See the *Avoid Sugar* and *Low-Glycemic Diet* strategies.

Herbs for the Brain

Besides basic good nutrition, there are some specific herbs that have been shown to help your brain function better. These include ginkgo, gotu kola, bacopa, rosemary, and sage. *Brain and Memory Tonic Formulas* typically combine herbs like these and can be helpful for enhancing learning and slowing memory loss in aging.

Improve Blood Flow

Hardening of the arteries will impair blood flow to the brain and reduce cognitive function. People with reduced blood flow to the brain often get sleepy when they sit for long periods and have problems with being absent minded. I've seen the *Oral Chelation* strategy help these people. It also helps to get regular exercise.

Avoid Toxins

Toxins can seriously damage the brain, especially fat-soluble toxins (such as petrochemical solvents) and metals like mercury, aluminum, and lead. In addition, drugs and alcohol do serious damage to the brain. So to keep your mind clear and active avoid as many chemicals as possible, don't use drugs, and minimize the consumption of alcohol. Follow the *Reduce Chemical Exposure* strategy.

Strategies: Avoid Sugar, Eat Healthy, Enhance Nitric Oxide, Healthy Fats, Hydration, Low-Glycemic Diet, Oral Chelation, and Reduce Chemical Exposure

Formulas: Brain and Memory Protection, Brain-Heart, Chinese Fire-Increasing, **Algae**, Chinese Qi and Blood Tonic, **Oral Chelation**, GLA Oil, Watkin's Hair, Skin, and Nails, Attention-Focus, **Anti-Stress B-Complex**, Antioxidant, **Memory Enhancing**, Methyl B12 Vitamin, Methylated B Vitamin, and **Ashwagandha Complex**

Herbs: Ashwagandha, **bacopa**, blessed thistle, chlorella, cordyceps, **ginkgo**, **gotu kola**, hawthorn, **holy basil**, lemon balm, pomegranate, rhodiola, **rosemary**, and sage

Supplements: Choline, L-theanine, magnesium, MSM, **omega-3 DHA**, **omega-3 EFAs**, **vitamin B-complex**, vitamin B_1, **vitamin B_{12}**, and vitamin B_9

Essential Oils: Clove and peppermint

Ménière's Disease

See also tinnitus

Ménière's disease affects the inner ear. The cause of Ménière's remains unknown. It usually begins between the ages of thirty and fifty. In Ménière's disease, a part of the inner ear called the endolymphatic sac becomes swollen. This disrupts a person's sense of balance.

A person with Ménière's disease will often have a combination of hearing loss, dizziness (vertigo), ringing in the ear (tinnitus), and sensitivity to loud sounds. This type of hearing loss should be managed by a doctor and audiologist. Some people with Ménière's disease report mild or transient symptoms, but for others the symptoms are more severe and permanent.

There is no specific natural therapy for Ménière's disease, but ginkgo biloba and bergamot may be helpful. Some people find the *Antispasmodic Extract*, used as eardrops helpful. For more suggestions, see *tinnitus*.

Strategies: Oral Chelation

Formulas: Antispasmodic Ear, Brain-Heart, Oral Chelation, Herbal Potassium, and Chinese Wind-Heat Evil

Herbs: Bee balm and ginkgo

Supplements: Krill oil and potassium

Meningitis

Meningitis is inflammation of the membranes that surround the brain and spinal cord. It is often caused by a bacteria or virus but may also be caused by adverse reactions to vaccines. Meningitis is a serious condition. Seek medical attention. Herbs can be used as complementary therapies with professional guidance.

Formulas: Immune-Boosting, Antioxidant, Proanthocyanidins, Anti-Inflammatory Pain, and Chinese Wind-Heat Evil

Herbs: Echinacea, goldenseal, gotu kola, **isatis,** Saint John's wort, and yarrow

Supplements: Vitamin C

Menopause

See also aging, hot flashes, and osteoporosis

Menopause has been called the "change of life," It occurs when the ovaries stop producing the high levels of estrogen or progesterone released during childbearing years. This causes periods to cease.

Besides the cessation of periods, common menopausal symptoms include hot flashes, night sweats, vaginal dryness, breast tenderness, and mood swings. It's also common for many women to experience some bone loss (osteoporosis), thinning of hair and the development of more facial hair, and some weight gain.

Emotional changes can also occur with menopause, including irritability, depression, or anxiety. There may be difficulty concentrating, mental confusion, and memory lapses.

Medical Approaches to Menopause

In modern times, doctors began to routinely prescribe synthetic hormone replacement for women going through menopause to ease menopausal symptoms. However, these drugs are not without their side effects.

In July 2002, a study of sixteen thousand women on a common hormone-replacement drug, Prempro®, revealed some serious side effects. There was an increased risk of breast cancer and heart attack in women taking these hormones. Specifically, the stroke rate was 41 percent higher, breast cancer was 26 percent higher, and the rate of blood clots doubled. So although the synthetic hormones do reduce the rate of hip fractures and reduce symptoms of menopause, the increased risks in other areas made routine use of these medications unwise.

These synthetic hormones have other side effects too. The side effects of synthetic progesterone can include weight gain, hair loss, low energy, depression, water retention, migraine headaches, reduced sex drive, and skin problems. In fact, it has been reported that one-half of all women who take synthetic hormone replacement quit after one year because they are unable to tolerate the side effects.

Balancing Estrogen After Menopause

Many of the symptoms women experience after menopause are the result of declining levels of estrogens. There are three primary forms of estrogen in the body: estrone (E1), estradiol (E2), and estriol (E3). You can read more about them under *Estrogen (Low)*. During menopause, the ovaries stop producing E2 but a woman still continues to produce other forms of estrogen through the adrenals, liver, and fat cells. So here are three natural ways a woman can enhance her estrogen after menopause.

For starters, the body has a natural way of storing estrogen to ease the transition to menopause, increasing fat cells. It is common for women to experience a slight weight gain (five to ten pounds) just prior to entering menopause. This is nature's way of storing extra estrogen to be prepared for the hormonal shift. So ladies, don't fight it or worry about it; accept it gracefully because it will make menopause easier.

Secondly, since the adrenal glands are a major source of estrogens after menopause, having healthy adrenal glands is vital to having a trouble-free change of life. Unfortunately, many women enter menopause suffering adrenal fatigue from sugar and caffeine consumption and chronic stress. Remedies that support the adrenals, like an *Adrenal Glandular Formula*, pantothenic acid, and B-complex vitamins, can help to build the adrenals and reduce menopausal discomfort.

Finally, many natural foods and herbs contain plant-based estrogens called phytoestrogens. Women whose diets contain phytoestrogen-rich foods have fewer menopausal problems. Beans (not just soybeans) are great sources of phytoestrogens, as are whole grains and dark green leafy vegetables.

Women of all ages who want to protect their health should avoid xenoestrogens, another type of estrogenic compound. Xenoestrogens can contribute to mood swings, cramps or heavy bleeding, thinning hair, hot flashes, and weight gain. See the *Avoid Xenoestrogens* strategy.

Balancing Progesterone

Progesterone is made by the ovaries before menopause and by the adrenal glands after menopause. This hormone helps to lay down new bone, relieve depression, enhance sex drive, and support thyroid function. Because it competes with estrogen for receptor sites, it also helps prevent over-stimulation of estrogenic processes, reducing the risk of fibrocystic breasts, breast cancer, and other estrogen-dependent cancers.

After menopause, women also experience a decline in progesterone production. Increasing progesterone levels after menopause can help balance blood sugar levels, prevent blood clotting and maintain bone health. Adrenal health is important here just like it is with estrogen. Two herbs that are good at enhancing progesterone and helping to balance estrogen and progesterone levels are chaste tree berries and false unicorn.

Other Factors to Consider

Besides working to balance hormones, taking care of one's overall health will aid the transition of menopause. Here are a few important strategies to consider.

In a culture that places such high value on youthfulness (and often views menopause as a "tragedy"), it's understandable that many women feel sadness, grief, or stress at the onset of a transition that's often seen as the end of that youthfulness. This is coupled with other stresses of middle-aged life—children growing up and becoming more independent, health challenges, and difficulties with finances and career. All of these stresses serve to exacerbate these hormonal imbalances and aggravate the symptoms of menopause. *Flower Essence, Aromatherapy* and *Stress Management* strategies may help.

A major lifestyle issue is a lack of exercise. Studies done at Harvard Medical School, as well as in Scandinavia, showed that women who engaged in regular exercise experienced fewer and less-intense hot flashes. Exercise is very important for maintaining bone health too. See the *Exercise* strategy.

It also follows that a healthy diet will make menopause easier. In many cultures women don't experience any serious menopausal symptoms. Follow the *Eat Healthy* strategy.

A good general program for menopause is the *Menopause Support Program*, which contains several supplements helpful for balancing hormones and aiding the transition of menopause. A *Menopause Support Formula* may also be helpful. See related conditions for additional suggestions on dealing with specific problems like hot flashes and osteoporosis.

Strategies: Aromatherapy, Avoid Xenoestrogens, Eat Healthy, Exercise, Flower Essence, Healthy Fats, and Stress Management

Formulas: Chrisopher's Menopause, Hot Flash, Female Tonic, Female Cycle, **Adrenal Glandular**, **GLA Oil**, Chinese Qi-Regulating, Skeletal Support, Herbal Calcium, Watkin's Hair, Skin, and Nails, and Digestive Support

Programs: Menopause Support

Essential Oil Blends: Menopause Support EO

Herbs: Aloe vera, **black cohosh**, chamomile, **chaste tree**, cordyceps, dong quai, evening primrose, false unicorn, **red clover**, Saint John's wort, and suma

Supplements: Boron, DHEA, equol, L-glutamine, omega-3 EFAs, omega-6 GLA, **vitamin B-complex**, vitamin B$_5$, **vitamin D**, and vitamin E

Essential Oils: Bergamot, chamomile (Roman), clary sage, fennel, geranium, lavender, orange (sweet), peppermint, rose, and ylang ylang

Menorrhagia
Heavy Menstrual Bleeding

See also fibroids (uterine)

Excessive menstrual bleeding or menorrhagia is often caused by excess estrogens or xenoestrogens. It may be due to uterine fibroids too. Get an appropriate medical diagnosis if the problem is persistent and doesn't respond to natural remedies. If the problem is fibroids, look under that section for more assistance.

Yarrow, tienchi ginseng, shepherd's purse, cinnamon, and bayberry are all possibilities for reducing the bleeding. You can take them internally or use them as a douche. The *Heavy Menstrual Bleeding Formula* may help. It often works better when taken with one or two capsules of yarrow.

Chaste tree or false unicorn may help to increase progesterone and reduce estrogens. Nettles are nourishing to make up for the loss of blood. *Christopher's Herbal Iron* and the *Chinese Wood-Increasing Formula* can also be helpful for this too.

Strategies: Affirmation and Visualization, Avoid Xenoestrogens, Eat Healthy, Healthy Fats, Hydration, Low-Glycemic Diet, Mineralization, Reduce Chemical Exposure, and Stress Management

Formulas: Internal Bleeding, **Chinese Wood-Increasing**, Colloidal Mineral, **Christopher's Herbal Iron**, and Vulnerary

Herbs: Bayberry, blue cohosh, calendula, capsicum, **chaste tree**, **cinnamon**, false unicorn, lady's mantle, nettle, stinging, rehmannia, shepherd's purse, white oak, and **yarrow**

Supplements: Iron

Essential Oils: Frankincense and geranium

Menstrual Cramps
see *cramps (menstrual)* **and** *dysmenorrhea*

Menstrual Irregularity

See also PMS

When a woman's menstrual cycle does not follow the normal twenty-eight day pattern (too long, too short, irregular, etc.) herbs can often be helpful in normalizing periods. The easiest place to start is with a *Female Cycle Formula*. There are also specific single herbs that may help more specific problems. For example, chastetree or vitex helps to regulate the menstrual cycle via the pituitary gland and hypothalamus when taken over a period of several months. False unicorn can be helpful when progesterone levels are too low and estrogen levels are too high. The *Chinese Wood-Increasing Formula* contains herbs frequently used in China for women during their childbearing years to build the blood and reduce PMS problems. Consult with a professional herbalist or naturopath (findanherbalist.com or americanherbalistsguild.com) who can help you select the specific remedies that may be helpful for you.

Strategies: Stress Management

Formulas: Chinese Wood-Increasing, **Female Cycle**, GLA Oil, Hepatoprotective, and Thyroid Glandular

Herbs: Angelica, black cohosh, **blessed thistle**, **chaste tree**, dong quai, evening primrose, **false unicorn**, ligusticum, and milk thistle

Supplements: DHEA and omega-3 EFAs

Essential Oils: Clary sage, peppermint, and rosemary

Menstruation (Heavy Bleeding)

see *menorrhagia*

Menstruation, Painful   see *dysmenorrhea*

Menstruation, Scant

The following can help when menstruation is abnormally light. This can be a sign of an imbalance in estrogen and progesterone. Many of these remedies tip the balance more toward estrogen. Some of the remedies that help scant menstruation may cause miscarriage, which means they should be avoided if one is trying to get pregnant.

Formulas: Chinese Qi and Blood Tonic

Herbs: Achyranthes, black cohosh, blue cohosh, motherwort, and red raspberry

Essential Oils: Clary sage, marjoram, and rose

Mental Illness

See also autism, bipolar mood disorder, heavy metal poisoning, hypoglycemia, memory/brain function, schizophrenia, OCD, PTSD, trauma, mitochondrial dysfunction, dysbiosis, and methylation (under)

A mental illness is a medical condition that disrupts a person's thinking, feeling, mood, ability to relate to others and daily functioning. Examples of mental illnesses include severe depression, schizophrenia, bipolar disorder, obsessive compulsive disorder (OCD), panic disorder, autism spectrum disorders, and post-traumatic stress disorder (PTSD).

Unlike problems with mood (such as mild anxiety or depression), which everyone experiences from time to time, mental illness profoundly affects the way a person behaves and interacts with others. It can cause a great deal of stress in people who associate with the mentally ill person, but it is vitally important that people who have to deal with a mentally ill person understand that a person does not choose to be mentally ill. It is not a sign of weakness, lack of character or poor upbringing. Like any other health problem, it needs to be viewed with compassion and understanding.

Medical Approaches

It is now generally accepted by the medical community that most mental disorders involve imbalances in or altered functioning of neurotransmitters. Neurotransmitters are the chemical messengers nerve cells use to talk to one another. This approach has given rise to the development of drugs designed to alter levels of these neurotransmitters. Unfortunately, these drugs do not correct the underlying chemical imbalances in the body and have numerous side effects.

The medical approach does not take in nutritional deficiencies, poor diet or the traumatic triggers that contribute to this problem. In fact, mental illness remains one of the most misunderstood of all medical maladies. It's time for the general public to adopt a different view of mental illness, and perhaps it's time to consider alternative approaches to recovery as well. Here are some strategies to consider when working with mental illness.

Resolving Trauma

Although there appears to be a genetic basis for the biochemical imbalances that cause mental illness, there is usually a triggering event—involving some kind of trauma or abuse—that begins the illness. Genes are regulated by the epigenome, which regulates the expression of a person's genetics. These stressful events may trigger changes in the person's epigenetics, triggering the biochemical errors that create imbalances in brain chemistry.

This is why counseling, emotional healing, work or other techniques that help to release the trauma may be helpful. In his book, *Toxic Psychiatry*, Peter R. Breggin, MD, points out that many people who are labeled mentally ill are simply in emotional and spiritual crisis. Their language is metaphoric and "crazy" sounding because people can't hear what the person is really trying to communicate. Delusions of grandeur ("I'm God" or "I'm Napoleon," for example) can indicate that a person is struggling with their sense of importance. Because they have been unable to express their feelings logically, this symbolic language is the only way they can communicate their suffering to others.

Dr. Breggin stresses that incarcerating, drugging, and shocking these people doesn't help them work through their inner crises or resolve their repressed emotional pain. He also suggests that drugs (which include medications, alcohol, tobacco, and illegal street drugs) only act to chemically lobotomize the brain and numb a person to their inner pain.

Thus, a holistic approach to mental illness would involve application of the *Counseling or Therapy* strategy to help a person deal with previous trauma and abuse, while supporting the body with appropriate nutrients and supplements to balance their biochemistry. The *Emotional Healing Work* and *Flower Essence* strategies can be helpful in this process too.

Adopt a Healthier Diet and Lifestyle

The neurotransmitters drug medications are trying to alter depend on nutrients for their synthesis. In my experience, people with mental illness often have very poor diets and a generally unhealthy lifestyle.

When the nutrients needed to produce the various neurotransmitters are not present in the diet, levels may be too low for proper brain function. For instance, DHA deficiency has been associated with depression, ADHD, schizophrenia, bipolar disorder, and dementia.

It is very important to adopt a generally healthy diet and to ensure adequate intake of protein and good fats. See the *Healthy Fats* and *Eat Healthy* strategies. Balancing blood sugar has also helped to stabilize people with mental illness. See the *Low-Glycemic Diet* strategy.

Correct Specific Issues with Supplements

In his groundbreaking book *Nutrient Power*, Dr. William J. Walsh summarizes the history of mental health treatment and makes a convincing case for change. "Today's emphasis on psychiatric drugs will not stand the test of time. Recent advances in epigenetics and the molecular biology of the brain have provided a road map for the development of effective, natural, drug-free therapies that do not produce serious side effects," he declares.

Thanks to the work of researchers like Dr. Walsh, effective, nutrient-based therapies for mental illness are being developed and tested. In fact, nutrient-based therapies have already helped thousands of people to recover from mental illness. This modality makes a lot of common sense as compared to the use of psychiatric drugs, because it is aimed at a true normalization of the brain chemistry.

Here we'll address some of the major nutritional imbalances that may be present in mental illness. This information is presented merely as an introduction to the subject. People with serious mental health issues should seek out professional assistance in designing a nutrient-based approach.

The exact nutrients needed to balance the brain in a person suffering from mental illness will vary widely from one person to the next, but here are a few major nutritional imbalances that may underlie many mental disorders. Ideally, medical tests should be run to determine which of these factors are present in any individual; however, symptoms and clues for each of these problems are included for those willing to experiment with supplements or use intuitive forms of assessment.

Reduce Copper Overload

Copper is an essential nutrient, but if a person gets too much copper in their body it will increase levels of norepinephrine and decreases levels of dopamine in the brain. Other possible symptoms of copper overload include hyperactivity, ringing in the ears, high anxiety, sleep problems, hemochromatosis, low thyroid, rheumatoid arthritis and emotional meltdowns.

Copper levels are regulated tightly by proteins, the most important being metallothionein (MT). Some people have a genetic inability to regulate copper, which means they need to avoid nutritional supplements containing copper. This includes liquid chlorophyll, which contains sodium copper chlorophyllin.

Zinc is a copper antagonist, so taking zinc can help to bring down copper levels. Molybdenum, sulfur, manganese, selenium, B vitamins, and vitamins C and E are also copper antagonists. If a person tends to have copper overload, it also helps to drink plenty of water and do things to relax the overstimulated sympathetic nervous system. There may be a mild worsening during the first ten days of starting a program to reduce copper levels. This is followed by clear improvement during weeks 3 and 4 and full effectiveness after three to four months.

Correct Zinc Deficiency

Research has shown that more than 90 percent of people with depression, behavioral disorders, ADHD, autism, and schizophrenia have depleted levels of zinc in their blood. Zinc deficiency is associated with poor immune function, poor wound healing, learning problems, anxiety, epilepsy, and problems controlling one's temper. Frequent infections, poor growth during puberty, the tendency to sunburn easily, premature graying of hair and a preference for spicy foods are clues that zinc deficiency might be a problem.

Zinc is important for the brain for many reasons. First, zinc metallothionein is part of the blood-brain barrier which keeps harmful chemicals out of the brain. Zinc also helps protect brain tissue from free radical damage to the brain. Free radical damage to the brain is believed to cause Alzheimer's, Parkinson's, and dementia.

Zinc is needed for the synthesis of the neurotransmitters serotonin, dopamine, and GABA. Low levels of these neurotransmitters are associated with depression, anxiety, insomnia, and difficulty concentrating.

Using Zinc as a supplement, little improvement is seen during the first two weeks, but there is gradual improvement thereafter. Full effectiveness of improving zinc levels is seen after sixty days.

Correct Vitamin B$_6$ Deficiency

Severe deficiencies of vitamin B$_6$ have been associated with irritability, depression, loss of short-term memory, and psychosis. Low B$_6$ levels can cause nervousness, insomnia, muscle weakness, and PMS. Brain levels of this nutrient are one hundred times higher than blood levels, which is required for producing serotonin, dopamine, and GABA, the same neurotransmitters zinc is necessary to form.

There are several forms of this vitamin. Pyridoxine is the most common, but a form called P5P is the most active. Some people do not react well to B$_6$, but react better to P5P. If a person gets too much B$_6$ they may develop neuropathy or have troubling dreams, but these symptoms go away after reducing the dose. Supplementation with Vitamin B$_6$ usually results in noticeable improvement during the first week, with full effectiveness after one month.

Correct Imbalances in Methylation

Methylation is a critical process in many body processes. It is the major liver detoxification pathway for breaking down neurotransmitters. Folic acid (or folate) increases methylation.

Disturbed methylation and folate metabolism is common in people suffering from schizophrenia, bipolar disorder, depression, anxiety, certain behavioral disorders, and Alzheimer's disease. Both undermethylation and overmethylation can cause problems. Dr. Walsh believes that genetic or acquired imbalances in methyl and folate may be responsible for more than 50 percent of all mental illness.

People who are undermethylators may benefit from taking SAM-e, a methyl donor. SAM-e is a natural reuptake inhibitor for serotonin, dopamine, and norepinephrine and can be helpful for some cases of depression. People who are overmethylators will respond well to folic acid, but not to SAM-e.

Knowing which direction to go may require medical testing, but clues that a person may be an overmethylator include low libido, low motivation, high anxiety, obsessive thoughts without compulsive actions, hallucinations, excessive body hair, being talkative and noncompetitive, and having adverse reactions to SAM-e and SSRI antidepressants.

Signs that a person may be an undermethylator include obsessive-compulsive tendencies and ritualistic behaviors, sparse body hair, high libido, being a perfectionist, being strong-willed and highly competitive in games, phobias, and bad reactions to folic acid supplements, but good reactions to SSRI antidepressants.

Although it would be wise to seek professional assistance in determining what supplements to use, overmethylators generally respond well to folic acid or folate supplements. Undermethylators will respond to SAM-e. Taking SAM-e can result in gradual improvement over the course of several months, while folic acid will show no improvement for several weeks, followed by gradual improvement thereafter. To learn more read the *Balance Methylation* strategy.

Reduce Oxidative Stress

Oxidative stress (also known as free radical damage) occurs when there are more free radicals than the body's antioxidant systems can handle. Oxidative stress affects receptors for glutamate, known as NMDA receptors. Glutamate is a neurotransmitter involved in long-term memory. Disruption of these receptors is believed to be present in epilepsy and autism.

Certain people have a genetic tendency to pyrrole overload. When levels of this natural chemical are too high, a person will experience low levels of zinc and B$_6$, which are bound and removed from the body by pyrroles. They will also have high levels of oxidative stress. There is a higher incidence of pyrrole disorder among people with mental health issues like autism, depression, bipolar disorder, and schizophrenia. These people require supplementation with zinc, B$_6$ and antioxidants.

Antioxidant supplements can help reduce oxidative stress, which can aid brain function. Possible choices would be alpha-lipoic acid, vitamin C and the fat-soluble vitamins A and D.

Supplement with Specific Amino Acids

Since neurotransmitters are synthesized from amino acids, specific neurotransmitters may be enhanced by using specific amino acid supplements. For example, 5-HTP, a metabolite of tryptophan, can boost serotonin levels, L-tyrosine helps with dopamine levels, and L-glutamine can aid GABA production. Generally speaking, however, making certain a person has adequate protein intake, rather than supplementing with amino acids, is helpful. Protein is very important to mental health and many people with mental illness tend to be carbohydrate junkies and lack sufficient protein and good fats in their diets.

Detoxification and Gut Health

There are many other issues that can be involved in mental health. One is heavy metals and another is environmental toxins. Metals like mercury, lead and aluminum may all affect brain function. See *heavy metal poisoning* and the *Heavy Metal Cleanse* strategy. Also look at the *Reduce Chemical Exposure* strategy.

The health of the intestinal tract also plays a role in stabilizing brain function. Dysbiosis can lead to mental and emotional imbalances. Consider the *Gut-Healing Diet* and the recommendations under *dysbiosis*.

Strategies: Affirmation and Visualization, Aromatherapy, Balance Methylation, Bodywork, Counseling or Therapy, Eat Healthy, Emotional Healing Work, Flower Essence, Forgiveness, Gut-Healing Diet, Healthy Fats, Heavy Metal Cleanse, Low-Glycemic Diet, Mineralization, Reduce Chemical Exposure, and Stress Management

Formulas: Chinese Fire-Decreasing, **Anti-Stress B-Complex**, Chinese Qi-Regulating, **Chinese Fire-Increasing**, **Adrenal Glandular**, Brain and Memory Protection, Antioxidant, Heavy Metal Cleansing, **Anti-Anxiety**, **Methylated B Vitamin**, Colloidal Mineral, and Hypoglycemic

Flower Essence Blends: Shock and Injury FE

Herbs: Bacopa, barberry, ginkgo, licorice, oat seed (milky), schisandra, and **skullcap**

Supplements: 5-HTP, **alpha-lipoic acid**, calcium, chromium, GABA, L-cysteine, **magnesium**, **omega-3 DHA**, **omega-3 EFAs**, SAM-e, vitamin A, **vitamin B-complex**, vitamin B_3, **vitamin B_6**, **vitamin B_9**, vitamin C, vitamin D, and **zinc**

Mercury Poisoning

See also heavy metal poisoning and multiple sclerosis

Mercury is one of the most toxic substances we can be exposed to, and we are exposed to it fairly regularly. It is found in fungicides, pesticides, dental fillings, contaminated seafood, thermometers, and a host of products, including cosmetics, fabric softeners, inks, tattoo ink, latex, medications, paints, plastics, polishes, solvents, and wood preservatives.

Mercury can be absorbed through the skin or inhaled. It passes through the blood-brain barrier and is attracted to and absorbed by nerve endings. This neurotoxin lodges inside neuron cells, disrupting cellular communication. It can cause autoimmune disorders, arthritis, blindness, candidiasis, depression, dizziness, fatigue, gum disease, hair loss, insomnia, memory loss, muscle weakness, multiple sclerosis, lateral sclerosis (ALS), Alzheimer's, Parkinson's, paralysis, lupus, food and environmental allergies, menstrual disorders, miscarriages, behavioral changes, depression, irritability, hyperactivity, allergic reactions, asthma, metallic taste in the mouth, loose teeth, and more.

A number of nutrients and herbs may be helpful in helping get mercury out of the body. See the *Heavy Metal Cleanse* strategy. The *Heavy Metal Cleansing Formula* is often helpful. The *Drawing Bath* strategy using clay can also be helpful.

Strategies: Drawing Bath, Healthy Fats, Heavy Metal Cleanse, and Increase Dietary Fiber

Formulas: Stabilized Allicin, **Heavy Metal Cleansing**, Algae, Oral Chelation, Hepatoprotective, **Gut-Healing Fiber**, and Nitric Oxide Boosting

Herbs: Bee pollen, **cilantro/coriander**, echinacea, eleuthero, garlic, lobelia, **milk thistle**, and red clover

Supplements: **Alpha-lipoic acid**, clay (bentonite), **clay (Redmond)**, L-methionine, **N-acetyl cysteine**, omega-3 DHA, omega-3 EFAs, **sodium alginate**, and vitamin C

Metabolic Syndrome
Hyperinsulinemia, Syndrome X

See also diabetes, excess weight, mitochondrial dysfunction, and polycystic ovarian syndrome

Metabolic syndrome, which also known as syndrome X or hyperinsulinemia is a metabolic imbalance that contributes towards obesity and numerous chronic and degenerative diseases. It is a precursor to type 2 diabetes.

The easiest way to determine if you have metabolic syndrome is to check your waste/hip ratio. Grab a tape measure and check your circumference at the navel and also at the widest part of your hips. In men, if your waist measurement is larger than your hips, you've probably got metabolic syndrome. In women, the waist should be less than 80 percent of the hip measurement.

Another indicator of metabolic syndrome is your triglyceride and HDL levels. If your triglyceride level is greater than 150 or your HDL level is less than 35, you're having problems with excess insulin production and insulin resistance.

Metabolic syndrome can cause depression, polycystic ovarian syndrome, diabetes, thyroid problems, reduced immune responses, increased risk of cancer and heart disease, and many other health issues.

If you have metabolic syndrome, correcting it will improve your overall health and reduce your risk of many types of disease. Here are some strategies for overcoming metabolic syndrome.

Improve Your Diet

The primary cause of metabolic syndrome is a high-carbohydrate, low-protein diet and a lack of good dietary fats.

This causes the pancreas to produce large amounts of insulin. High insulin is a risk factor for cardiovascular disease and chronic low-grade inflammation. Since the excess carbohydrates are converted to fats and stored, it is also a major cause of obesity. So using the *Avoid Sugar* and *Low-Glycemic Diet* strategies is the major way to combat this problem.

Exercise

Resistance exercise trains muscles to take up glucose without the need for insulin, thereby decreasing insulin requirements. After just five days without exercise, insulin resistance increases. Exercise like weight lifting done to the point that it makes muscles burn a little is causing muscle tissue to take up sugar without insulin. Thus, a program of muscle-building exercise at least three times per week will reduce insulin levels. See the *Exercise* strategy.

Eat Healthy Fats

Consuming too many omega-6 essential fatty acids in the diet, with insufficient omega-3, also contributes to metabolic syndrome. See the *Healthy Fats* strategy. Taking a couple of teaspoons of coconut oil before meals three times daily also helps metabolic syndrome, and reduces sugar cravings.

Take Supplements

Deficiencies of zinc, manganese, vanadium, B-vitamins, and vitamin A may also be involved in metabolic syndrome. Herbs that regulate blood sugar are also helpful, especially cinnamon. Berberine is also helpful in controlling blood sugar levels. You can also try taking a *Blood Sugar Control Formula* and following some of the general guidelines for diabetes.

- **Strategies:** Avoid Sugar, Blood Type Diet, Exercise, Healthy Fats, and Low-Glycemic Diet
- **Formulas: Chinese Yin-Increasing**, **Blood Sugar Control**, Algae, Nitric Oxide Boosting, and Adaptogen
- **Herbs: Bitter melon**, blue-green algae, chia, **cinnamon**, **coconut oil**, dandelion, fenugreek, ginseng (American), ginseng (Asian/Korean), goldenseal, juniper, licorice, nopal, orange (bergamot), stevia, and turmeric
- **Supplements: Alpha-lipoic acid**, **berberine**, **chromium**, **magnesium**, manganese, **omega-3 EFAs**, omega-6 CLA, vanadium, vitamin A, vitamin B-complex, vitamin C, and zinc
- **Essential Oils:** Cinnamon

Methylation, Over

See also ADD/ADHD, depression, insomnia, and OCD

Methylation is a chemical process that takes place in the body and contributes to numerous body processes. See

Balance Methylation strategy to learn more. The following are indications for overmethylation.

Physical: Lower levels of homocysteine and histamine, food and chemical sensitivities but not responding well to antihistamines, sleep disorders, restless legs, dry eyes and mouth, hairy body (hirsutism), low libido

Mental and Emotional: Obsessive thoughts without compulsive actions, ADHD, hyperactivity, low motivation in school, non-competitiveness, being talkative; having high artistic ability, having high anxiety, depression that gets worse with SSRIs

Nutritional: Responding poorly to methyl donors like SAM-e, but respond favorably to folate supplements.

Strategies for Overmethylation

When experimenting with supplements to balance methylation, it's best to start with small doses and see how you react. If you react favorably, you can gradually increase the dose. If you suspect you are overmethylating or have genetic issues that cause methylation problems, here are some strategies that may help reduce excessive methylation.

Take vitamin B_6. Vitamin B_6 helps convert homocysteine (HYC) to cysteine, thus lowering levels of this proinflammatory compound. B_6 plays many other roles in the body and deficiencies can also cause dermatitis, seizures, inflammation of the tongue, cracked lips, carpal tunnel syndrome, and anemia. Vitamin B_6 will decrease methylation by converting HYC into cysteine rather than methionine, which can be helpful for overmethylators.

Take zinc. Zinc is involved in the proteins that turn genes on and off. In fact, it's a cofactor for a critical enzyme in DNA regulation known as DNA methyltransferase. Along with vitamin B_6, zinc also helps lower homocysteine by converting it to cysteine, which means it can be helpful for overmethylators. It also aids in the process of methylating homocysteine back into methionine with the aid of betaine.

Avoid methyl donors. Avoid supplements that act as methyl donors if you are an overmethylator. These include SAM-e and methylated folic acid and B_{12}.

- **Strategies:** Balance Methylation
- **Supplements: Vitamin B_6** and **zinc**

Methylation, Under

See also bipolar mood disorder, cancer prevention, depression, schizophrenia, and anxiety disorders

Methylation is a chemical process that takes place in the body and contributes to numerous body processes. See the

Balance Methylation strategy to learn more. The following are indications for undermethylation.

Physical: High levels of homocysteine and histamine; a greater tendency to inflammatory diseases (including heart disease); a greater tendency to seasonal allergies, but not food allergies; responding well to antihistamines; sparse body hair; high fluid production (saliva, tears); frequent headaches

Mental and Emotional: Obsessive-compulsive, ritualistic behaviors, high libido, having a strong will, being competitive in games and sports, being a perfectionist; tendency toward rumination about the past, tendency toward phobias and addiction, depression that responds positively to SSRIs

Nutritional: Responding well to methyl donors like SAM-e, but don't respond as favorably to folate supplements

Strategies for Undermethylation

When experimenting with supplements to balance methylation it's best to start with small doses and see how you react. If you react favorably, you can gradually increase the dose. If you suspect you are undermethylating or have genetic issues that cause methylation problems here are some remedies that may help enhance methylation.

Take SAM-e. This supplement is a methyl donor used in the methylation cycle. It has many potential benefits for people who are undermethylators, but is contraindicated for overmethylators.

Increase intake of choline. Choline is an amino acid that is powerful methyl donor because it contains three methyl groups. Organ meats, like liver, are rich in choline, which is also found in butter, eggs, peanut butter, potatoes, and whole-wheat bread. One of its forms, phosphatidylcholine helps transport fats and cholesterol, as well as serve as a precursor for the production of acetylcholine.

Take betaine HCl: Betaine is a methylated version of the amino acid glycine. It is part of betaine hydrochloric acid (HCl), which is taken as a nutritional supplement to aid protein digestion. Beets and spinach contain large amounts of betaine if they are grown properly. It's also found in seafood.

Supplement with folic acid or folate. This vitamin is very important in methylation because it's used by enzymes that manufacture methyl groups. It's also a common vitamin deficiency. When taken in the form of methylfolate, it acts as a methyl donor. Folates are better supplements than straight folic acid. Green leafy vegetables are a great source of folates.

Take vitamin B_{12}. With the help of methylfolate, vitamin B_{12} helps to convert homocysteine back into methionine. A *Methylated B Vitamin Formula* containing a combination of methylated B_{12} (methylcobalamine) and methylfolate is a great supplement for enhancing methylation.

Take zinc. Zinc is involved in the proteins that turn genes on and off. In fact, it's a cofactor for a critical enzyme in DNA regulation known as DNA methyltransferase. Along with vitamin B_6, zinc also helps lower homocysteine by converting it to cysteine, which means it can be helpful for overmethylators as well as undermethylators. It also aids in the process of methylating homocysteine back into methionine with the aid of betaine.

Strategies: Balance Methylation

Formulas: Methyl B12 Vitamin, **Methylated B Vitamin**, and Betaine HCl

Supplements: Choline, **SAM-e**, vitamin B_{12}, vitamin B_6, vitamin B_9, and **zinc**

Migraine   see *headache (migraine)*

Miscarriage Prevention

See also pregnancy

The body has to maintain a higher level of progesterone than estrogen during pregnancy. If this balance is upset, bleeding can occur and miscarriage will eventually result. This is not the only cause of miscarriage, but one of the more common ones. Follow the strategy *Avoid Xenoestrogens* to reduce the chance of miscarriage.

Taking red raspberry during pregnancy can help to prevent miscarriages. You can also try the *Pregnancy Tea* or *Herbal Minerals Formula*.

If a woman starts spotting during pregnancy, the miscarriage can sometimes be prevented by taking two capsules or about sixty drops of the tincture of false unicorn every two to four hours along with black haw or cramp bark. A small amount (about ten drops each) of lobelia and capsicum tinctures may also help.

Strategies: Avoid Xenoestrogens

Formulas: Joan Patton's Herbal Minerals and Pregnancy Tea

Herbs: Baical skullcap, **black haw**, capsicum, **cramp bark**, **false unicorn**, lobelia, red raspberry, and wild yam

Supplements: Magnesium and vitamin E

Mitochondrial Dysfunction

See also autoimmune disorders, bipolar mood disorder, diabetes, endurance, fatigue, fibromyalgia, ALS, lupus, multiple sclerosis, Parkinson's disease, deafness, Huntington's disease, and neurodegenerative diseases

Inside the cells of every plant, animal, and human being you will find small structures called mitochondria. These rod-shaped organelles (cellular organs) are the power plants for cells. Their job is to convert the calories from carbohydrates, fats, and proteins into energy the cells can use. They provide every cellular process with the energy it needs to function using a cyclic process known as the Krebs cycle.

Researchers are now discovering that mitochondria do more than produce energy. They also play a role in the synthesis of fatty acids, the regulation of cellular levels of amino acids and enzyme cofactors, balancing levels of heme (the iron compound that forms the basis of hemoglobin), calcium balance, neurotransmitter synthesis, and insulin secretion.

Mitochondria also produce reactive oxygen species (free radicals) that can damage their own structures as well as other structures in the cell if there aren't enough antioxidants present to regulate them. They also play a role in apoptosis, which is the mechanism that triggers cells to die. Apoptosis is the process by which the body gets rid of virally infected cells and cancer cells. Without apoptosis, multicellular organisms can't protect themselves from cells that have started to malfunction.

As all this research is coming forth, science is discovering that mitochondrial dysfunction is involved in numerous degenerative diseases. First, since mitochondria produce energy, anyone who has serious, long-lasting fatigue probably has mitochondrial dysfunction. Mitochondrial problems are also involved in diabetes, deafness, and neuropathy. It's also being proposed that health conditions such as cancer, diabetes, fibromyalgia, and serious mental illnesses (such as schizophrenia and bipolar disease) may result from mitochondrial dysfunction, although the research on the role mitochondria play in all these diseases isn't clear yet.

An article in *Integrative Medicine* in August of 2014 suggested that mitochondrial dysfunction may be occurring in "—neurodegenerative diseases, such as Alzheimer's disease, Parkinson's disease, Huntington's disease, amyotrophic lateral sclerosis, and Friedreich's ataxia; cardiovascular diseases, such as atherosclerosis and other heart and vascular conditions; diabetes and metabolic syndrome; autoimmune diseases, such as multiple sclerosis, systemic lupus erythematosus, and type 1 diabetes; neurobehavioral and psychiatric diseases, such as autism spectrum disorders, schizophrenia, and bipolar and mood disorders; gastrointestinal disorders; fatiguing illnesses, such as chronic fatigue syndrome and Gulf War illnesses; musculoskeletal diseases, such as fibromyalgia and skeletal muscle hypertrophy/atrophy; cancer; and chronic infections." [https://www.ncbi.nlm.nih.gov/pmc/articles/PMC4566449]

Mitochondria require enzymes that depend on nutrients to function. Vitamins like C, D, E, thiamine, and riboflavin and minerals like magnesium, manganese, calcium, and phosphorus are needed to sustain both the Krebs cycle and the processes that feed fuel into the mitochondria.

The primary cause of mitochondrial dysfunction in most people is a diet loaded with refined carbohydrates. Refined carbohydrates have been stripped of the nutrients mitochondria need to efficiently process sugars into energy. Mitochondria simply cannot handle massive amounts of sugar without the accompanying nutrients found in the whole foods.

This is why it is important to avoid refined carbohydrates to correct mitochondrial dysfunction. The *Ketogenic Diet* strategy, which limits carbohydrate intake, along with appropriate nutritional supplements can help to restore mitochondrial function and aid recovery from many chronic ailments. This should followed by the *Low-Glycemic Diet* strategy.

B-Complex vitamins are extremely important to the health of the mitochondria. Since vitamin C is also helpful, the *Anti-Stress B-Complex Formula* may be especially helpful. There are a number of other nutrients that can improve mitochondrial function. Some of the best to consider are alpha-lipoic acid, Co-Q10, and magnesium. The *Mitochondrial Energy Production Formula* is specifically designed to aid energy production in the mitochondria.

Strategies: Avoid Sugar, Balance Methylation, and Ketogenic Diet

Formulas: Mitochondria Energy and Anti-Stress B-Complex

Supplements: Alpha-lipoic acid, calcium, **Co-Q10**, **magnesium**, manganese, N-acetyl cysteine, **vitamin B-complex**, **vitamin B$_1$**, **vitamin C**, vitamin D, vitamin E, and zinc

Mitral Valve

The mitral valve is the valve between the left atrium and left ventricle of the heart. It prevent blood from flowing backward. When the valve slips back into the left atrium, it creates a problem called mitral valve prolapse. When the valve is stiff and constricted, the problem is called mitral valve stenosis.

Nearly eight million people in the U.S. have mitral valve prolapse. It is a common cause of heart murmer. Many cases are symptom free and cause no health problems. The most common symptom is chest pain, but this is not serious and does not increase the risk of heart attack or other heart problems. It is bothersome and often frightening, however. Sometimes mitral valve problems are associated with symptoms like heart palpitations, shortness of breath (especially after exercise), dizziness, fainting, anxiety, or numbness and tingling in the hands and feet.

If blood flows backward through the mitral valve, it's called mitral regurgitation. Moderate or severe mitral regurgitation can cause other heart problems overtime by weakening the heart.

Medical treatment for mitral valve prolapse includes exercise, regular check-ups and relaxation and stress reduction. People with mitral valve problems should avoid caffeine and other stimulants. Medications may also be used to calm the heart rate when people with mitral valve problems experience rapid heartbeat, or tachycardia.

Some natural remedies that may help the mitral valve include magnesium, hawthorn, and Co-Q10. Herbalists also consider night-blooming cereus to be a specific remedy for this condition. Work on this condition under medical supervision. You may wish to consult with a qualified herbalist or naturopath as well (findanherbalist.com or americanherbalistsguild.com).

Strategies: Avoid Caffeine and Stress Management

Formulas: Anti-Stress B-Complex and Heart Health

Herbs: Hawthorn and **night-blooming cereus**

Supplements: Co-Q10, L-carnitine, **magnesium**, and vitamin B-complex

Mononucleosis

See also Epstein-Barr virus

Mononucleosis (mono) is an infectious viral disease that causes an increase in a specific type of white blood cell. Mono is usually linked to the Epstein-Barr virus (EBV) but can also be caused by other viruses, such as cytomegalovirus (CMV). Mono is transmitted through bodily fluids, including saliva, and is often called the kissing disease. Mono causes fever, sore throat, fatigue, and swollen lymph glands, especially in the neck. The *Chinese Wind-Heat Evil Formula* or herbs to boost the immune system and strengthen the lymphatics may be helpful, along with general good health practices.

Strategies: Eat Healthy and Hydration

Formulas: Liver Cleanse, **Chinese Wind-Heat Evil**, Probiotic, **Immune-Boosting**, and Mushroom Immune

Herbs: Andrographis, astragalus, baptisia, **echinacea**, elder berry, isatis, lomatium, red clover, and **red root**

Supplements: L-lysine

Mood Swings

See also adrenal fatigue, hypoglycemia, and stress

Mood swings are abnormal and often-rapid changes in one's state of mind or predominant emotions. They may be caused by mental attitudes, unresolved trauma, stress, hypoglycemia, liver issues, or hormonal imbalances. Start by adopting the *Low-Glycemic Diet* strategy to balance blood

sugar levels. Licorice root or *Paavo Airola's Hypoglycemic Formula* can help to stabilize blood sugar levels. For more suggestions see *hypoglycemia*.

Good fats are especially important for the nervous system in helping to keep moods stable. Include good fats in the diet and consider taking some fatty acid supplements such as DHA or omega-3 essential fatty acids.

Practice the techniques found in the *Stress Management* strategy and use adaptogens, like eleuthero or cordyceps, to help reduce the output of stress hormones. If mood swings are accompanied by fatigue and restless, disturbed sleep try the *Chinese Fire-Increasing Formula* or an *Adrenal Glandular*. See *Stress* and *Adrenal Fatigue* for more ideas.

If mood swings include periods of depression, try using SAM-e to support the liver function. The *Chinese Wood-Decreasing Formula* or Saint John's wort may also be of benefit.

Strategies: Counseling or Therapy, Emotional Healing Work, Flower Essence, Healthy Fats, Low-Glycemic Diet, and Stress Management

Formulas: Chinese Wood-Increasing, Chrisopher's Menopause, Algae, **Chinese Wood-Decreasing**, **Chinese Fire-Increasing**, Adrenal Glandular, Hypoglycemic, and Adaptogen

Herbs: Cordyceps, **eleuthero**, **licorice**, **mimosa**, Saint John's wort, **skullcap**, and spirulina

Supplements: Omega-3 DHA, omega-3 EFAs, and SAM-e

Essential Oils: Bergamot, geranium, grapefruit (pink), helichrysum, jasmine, lemon, neroli, patchouli, and ylang ylang

Morning Sickness

See also pregnancy

Morning sickness is mild to severe nausea, often accompanied by vomiting, that occurs in pregnancy, usually only in the early stages, but in some cases throughout pregnancy. Although common upon rising in the morning, hence the name, it can occur during any part of the day or night.

Some of the simplest remedies to try include ginger, peppermint, or red raspberry. These are best taken as a tea. The *Pregnancy Tea Formula,* which contains alfalfa and peppermint is often very helpful.

Many women also find morning sickness is reduced by taking B-complex vitamins. Morning sickness is often related to liver function. A small dose of a *Liver Cleanse Formula* or the *Chinese Wood-Decreasing Formula* may help.

Formulas: Christopher's Carminative, Chinese Wood-Increasing, **Chinese Wood-Decreasing**, Liver Cleanse, and **Pregnancy Tea**

Herbs: Alfalfa, false unicorn, **ginger**, goldenseal, **peppermint**, and **red raspberry**

Supplements: Vitamin B-complex and vitamin B_6

Essential Oils: Peppermint

Motion Sickness

See also nausea & vomiting and vertigo

Nausea usually caused by travel in a vehicle such as a car, ship, or plane is called motion sickness. Studies have suggested that ginger can be very effective in preventing motion sickness when taken prior to travel. A drop of the *Digestive Settling EO Formula* or peppermint oil on the back of the tongue may also be helpful.

Formulas: Flu and Vomiting and Topical Analgesic

Essential Oil Blends: Digestive Settling EO

Herbs: **Ginger** and peppermint

Supplements: Charcoal, L-glutamine, and vitamin B_6

Essential Oils: **Peppermint** and spearmint

Mouth Ulcers/Sores   see *canker sores*

Mucus   see *congestion*

Multiple Personality Disorder
see *dissociative identity disorder*

Multiple Sclerosis
MS

See also autoimmune disorders

Multiple Sclerosis is an autoimmune disease that attacks the insulating coverings (myelin sheath) of the nerves and brain cells. Symptoms often include weakness, fatigue, debility, and numbness and occur in varied regions of the body depending on the nerves affected. This is not an easy condition to treat, and there are not quick fixes, so professional assistance should be sought. There are, however, some basic natural remedies to consider.

Start by following the general therapy for *autoimmune disorders*. This includes using digestive enzyme supplements, supporting the adrenal function, and reducing stress.

Fats are very important for the myelin sheath. So make sure to include plenty of healthy fats in the diet by following the *Healthy Fats* strategy. It may be helpful to supplement with fat-soluble vitamins such as A, D, and E, which help protect fatty tissues.

Another important component of the myelin sheath is silica. Horsetail is rich in this nutrient and *Watkin's Hair, Skin and Nails Formula* is a great formula to get more silica for the

nerves. It also contains rosemary, which is a good antioxidant that helps protect the nerves.

Other antioxidant nutrients may also help to protect the myelin sheath from damage. So consider taking an *Antioxidant Formula*.

One possible cause of MS is mercury poisoning. Some MS patients have improved after having all metal fillings removed from their mouth, followed by a mercury detoxification program. N-acetyl cysteine, cilantro, and *Heavy Metal Cleansing Formulas* may all be helpful. See the *Heavy Metal Cleanse* strategy for suggestions on mercury detoxification.

Strategies: Affirmation and Visualization, Eat Healthy, Gut-Healing Diet, Healthy Fats, Heavy Metal Cleanse, Increase Dietary Fiber, and Mineralization

Formulas: Herbal Calcium, **Watkin's Hair, Skin, and Nails**, Analgesic Nerve, GLA Oil, **Heavy Metal Cleansing**, Methyl B12 Vitamin, Antioxidant, Colloidal Mineral, Digestive Support, and **Myelin Sheath**

Herbs: **Ashwagandha**, astragalus, black currant, cannabis, cilantro/coriander leaf, coconut, codonopsis, evening primrose, ginkgo, horsetail, psyllium, reishi, and **rosemary**

Supplements: **CBD**, N-acetyl cysteine, **omega-3 DHA**, omega-3 EFAs, omega-6 GLA, vitamin A, **vitamin B-complex**, vitamin B_1, **vitamin B_{12}**, **vitamin D**, and vitamin E

Mumps

See also contagious disease prevention

Mumps is an acute contagious viral disease marked by fever and the swelling of lymph nodes, causing the cheeks to appear swollen and puffy. Herbs that enhance lymphatic drainage, such as burdock, lobelia, mullein, and red root, can be helpful in treating mumps. Infection-fighting herbs like garlic and yarrow can also be helpful. Drink plenty of water and use the *Sweat Bath* strategy to flush the system.

Strategies: Hydration and Sweat Bath

Formulas: Liquid Lymph, **Lymph Cleansing**, **Stabilized Allicin**, and Steven Horne's Children's Composition

Herbs: Burdock, catnip, clove, **echinacea**, garlic, garlic, lobelia, mullein, peppermint, **red root**, and yarrow

Supplements: **Vitamin A** and **vitamin D**

Essential Oils: Clove and peppermint

Muscle Cramps/Spasms
see *cramps & spasms*

Muscle Tone

The following remedies can help improve muscle tone.

Formulas: Chinese Metal-Increasing, **Chinese Earth-Increasing**, Whole Food Green Drink, and **Whole Food Protein**

Herbs: Red clover

Supplements: Co-Q10, iron, and vitamin E

Muscle Twitch   see *twitching*

Muscular Dystrophy

Muscular dystrophy is a disease that progressively destroys muscle tissue. Since it is a genetic disorder, it does not have a cure. However, attention to basic good health habits may ease symptoms and improve one's quality of life. I recommend seeking professional help and assistance.

Strategies: Gut-Healing Diet

Herbs: Licorice and saw palmetto

Supplements: Co-Q10, potassium, **vitamin B-complex**, and vitamin E

Myasthenia Gravis

See also autoimmune disorders

Myasthenia gravis is a disease of progressive weakness and exhaustion of the voluntary muscles of the body without any wasting. It is caused by a defect at nerve and muscle junctions and is considered an autoimmune disease. You should start by following the general guidelines for *autoimmune disorders*. Seek professional assistance. Improved general health habits, such as increasing antioxidants, using good fats, and supplementing with minerals and digestive enzymes will be helpful.

Strategies: Eat Healthy, Healthy Fats, and Heavy Metal Cleanse

Formulas: Chinese Wood-Increasing, Blood Purifier, General Glandular, Antioxidant, Colloidal Mineral, and Digestive Support

Herbs: Gotu kola, licorice, red raspberry, Saint John's wort, **skullcap**, valerian, vervain (blue), yellow dock, and yucca

Supplements: Lecithin, **magnesium**, **omega-3 EFAs**, vitamin B-complex, vitamin B_1, vitamin B_2, vitamin C, and vitamin E

Narcolepsy

See also adrenal fatigue, fatigue, and hypoglycemia

Narcolepsy is a sleeping disorder that causes an overwhelming need to sleep during the day. This can happen very suddenly, and attempts to stay awake will fail. It is caused by damage to the nerves that control sleep and wakefulness.

Strengthen the nerves using nerve tonics like ashwagandha and milky oat seed. Also consider the possibility of adrenal exhaustion and use remedies like the *Adrenal Glandular Formula* or adaptogens to increase stamina and energy.

Eliminating food allergens has helped in some cases. Very low blood sugar has also been known to cause people to pass out, so make sure the blood sugar stays balanced with the *Low-Glycemic Diet* strategy.

Other possible remedies include B-complex vitamins, chromium, and magnesium to aid cellular energy production. Since there is no simple answer to this problem, professional help should be sought.

Strategies: Eliminate Allergy-Causing Foods and Low-Glycemic Diet

Formulas: Anti-Stress B-Complex and **Adrenal Glandular**

Herbs: **Ashwagandha**, damiana, eleuthero, ginkgo, gotu kola, **oat seed (milky)**, **prickly ash**, sage, Saint John's wort, and schisandra

Supplements: Calcium, chromium, Co-Q10, L-glutamine, magnesium, omega-3 EFAs, **vitamin B-complex**, and vitamin E

Nausea & Vomiting

See also morning sickness

Nausea is a queasiness in the stomach that makes one resist food and have the urge to vomit. Vomiting is disgorging the contents of the stomach through the mouth. Nausea and vomiting can be processes used to expel irritating substances from the body, which means they are sometimes helpful in recovering from problems like food poisoning.

When one needs to settle the stomach and ease nausea and the urge to vomit, carminative herbs like ginger, lavender, lemon balm, and peppermint can be used. They are best taken as warm teas and sipped slowly. Essential oils can also be used. Simply add a drop of an essential oil like peppermint or clove to a glass of hot water and sip it slowly.

Strategies: Aromatherapy

Formulas: Chinese Wood-Increasing, **Flu and Vomiting**, Paavo Airola's Cold, and Chinese Earth-Decreasing

Essential Oil Blends: Digestive Settling EO

Herbs: Alisma, aloe vera, **anise**, bamboo, blessed thistle, chirata, cinnamon, clove, galangal, **ginger**, hyacinth, kutki, **lemon balm**, magnolia, **peppermint**, red raspberry, and tangerine (Mandarin)

Supplements: Manganese, vitamin B-complex, and vitamin B_6

Essential Oils: Cinnamon, clove, grapefruit (pink), lavender, lemon, **peppermint**, red mandarin, and spearmint

Nephritis

See also inflammation

Nephritis is inflammation of the kidney. Juniper berry and other kidney stimulants should be avoided. You should use non-irritating diuretics for this problem like the ones highlighted in the list below. These herbs have a more soothing and cooling action on the kidneys. The *Hydration* strategy is essential to working with any kidney disorder. Nephritis should be monitored by a medical doctor.

Strategies: Avoid Sugar, Eat Healthy, Healthy Fats, and Hydration

Formulas: Female Tonic, **Antioxidant**, Chinese Yang-Reducing, Anti-Inflammatory Pain, and Urinary Support

Herbs: Asparagus, astragalus, **cleavers**, **cordyceps**, **corn silk**, dandelion, echinacea, goldenseal, horsetail, and marshmallow

Supplements: Magnesium and omega-3 EFAs

Nerve Damage

When nerves have been damaged, there are a number of nutrients that can maximize their ability to repair. Those include good fats (DHA, omega-3 EFA), magnesium, potassium, silicon, and B-complex.

Saint John's wort is particularly helpful for stimulating nerve repair. It can be used internally, topically or as a homeopathic. In homeopathic form, it has been called the "arnica of the nervous system" because of its ability to stimulate nerve healing after injuries. An oil made from the flowers can be applied topically to aid nerve healing after injuries.

Helichrysum essential oil can also be diluted and applied topically in areas where nerves are damaged. CBD may also be helpful, both internally and topically.

Strategies: Epsom Salt Bath and Healthy Fats

Formulas: **Anti-Stress B-Complex**, GLA Oil, **Watkin's Hair, Skin, and and Nails**

Essential Oil Blends: Topical Injury

Herbs: Horsetail, prickly ash, **Saint John's wort**, skullcap, and wood betony

Supplements: CBD, magnesium, omega-3 DHA, **omega-3 EFAs**, potassium, silicon, and **vitamin B-complex**

Essential Oils: Helichrysum

Nervous Disorders
see *nervousness* **and** *anxiety disorders*

Nervous Exhaustion
Enervation

See also adrenal fatigue

Closely related to adrenal exhaustion, enervation occurs after long periods of stress where the nervous system becomes depleted. The person feels shaky, tired, and "on edge." They have a hard time holding their hands steady. So trembling hands are a good indication for this. So is a quivering tongue.

It is usually important to support the adrenal glands when treating nervous exhaustion. This is done using adaptogens and other therapies discussed under *Adrenal Fatigue*.

Supporting the nerves with B-complex vitamins is usually necessary. Herbs that have a tonic effect on the nervous system are also indicated, and include milky oat seed, blue vervain, skullcap, damiana, and sage. Potassium and magnesium may also be helpful.

The *Epsom Salt Bath* strategy with essential oils like lavender or rose can also do wonders for helping relaxed nerves that feel "frayed." So can staying well hydrated and using healthy fats.

In the long run, following the techniques listed in the *Stress Management* strategy, getting a good night's sleep, and practicing the *Deep Breathing* strategy will all help. *Emotional Healing Work* may be needed in some cases. The *Flower Essence* strategy using the flower essences of olive, oak, and elm can be helpful too.

Strategies: Aromatherapy, Avoid Caffeine, Counseling or Therapy, Deep Breathing, Emotional Healing Work, Epsom Salt Bath, Healthy Fats, Hydration, Pleasure Prescription, and Stress Management

Formulas: Adrenal Glandular, Mitochondria Energy, Antispasmodic, **Chinese Fire-Increasing**, **Anti-Stress B-Complex**, Jeannie Burgess' Stress, **Anti-Anxiety**, Sleep Support, and **Adaptogen**

Flower Essence Blends: Shock and Injury FE

Herbs: Ashwagandha, **cocoa**, **cordyceps**, **damiana**, kava kava, muira puama, noni, **oat seed (milky)**, **olive flower essence**, reishi, rose essential oil, rosemary flower essence, sage, schisandra, **skullcap**, vervain (blue), and white oak flower essence

Supplements: Magnesium, multiple vitamin and mineral, omega-3 EFAs, potassium, **vitamin B-complex**, and vitamin B$_5$

Essential Oils: Bergamot, clary sage, grapefruit (pink), lavender, patchouli, pine, rose, and ylang ylang

Nervousness
Restlessness
See also stress and anxiety disorders

When a person feels on edge all the time and suffers from an excessive sense of nervousness and restlessness, they are in a hypervigilant mode. This means that the hormones and neurotransmitters that trigger their fight-or-flight response are over stimulated and they are having a hard time returning to a state of relaxation. On a physical level, they need to calm down their sympathetic nervous system and activate their parasympathetic nervous system. They also need to calm down the release of stress hormones from the adrenal glands. On an emotional level, they often need to heal from previous traumas and stressful experiences using a strategy involving *Counseling or Therapy*.

To calm down the sympathetic nervous system, use nervines, such as California poppy, chamomile, kava kava, and lavender. These are common ingredients in various nervine formulas.

If one's hands are shaky, one may also need some milky oat seed or magnesium. Using the *Epsom Salt Bath* strategy will also be helpful.

To support the adrenal glands, one can use adaptogens like eleuthero, ashwagandha, and schisandra berries. It is also important to avoid stimulants like caffeine and to stay well hydrated. Good fats and B-complex vitamins are also helpful in calming down the nerves.

Strategies: Aromatherapy, Avoid Caffeine, Avoid Sugar, Counseling or Therapy, Deep Breathing, Emotional Healing Work, Epsom Salt Bath, Flower Essence, Good Posture, Healthy Fats, Hydration, and Stress Management

Formulas: **Anti-Stress B-Complex**, **Jeannie Burgess' Stress**, **Adrenal Glandular**, **Chinese Fire-Increasing**, **Anti-Anxiety**, Methyl B12 Vitamin, Chinese Qi-Regulating, Thyroid Calming, Sleep Support, and **Adaptogen**

Herbs: **Ashwagandha**, **California poppy**, chamomile, cherry, **eleuthero**, haritaki, hoelen, **kava kava**, **motherwort**, **oat seed (milky)**, ophiopogon, schisandra, and skunk cabbage

Supplements: **Magnesium**, omega-3 EFAs, **vitamin B-complex**, vitamin B$_{12}$, and vitamin D

Essential Oils: Bergamot, chamomile (Roman), lavender, patchouli, pine, rose, and ylang ylang

Neuralgia & Neuritis
See also diabetes

Neuralgia is a pain that radiates along the course of one or more nerves. In neuralgia, irritated nerves cause severe pain in the body. Neuritis is inflammation of the nerves, similar to neuralgia, except there may not be any pain. There may also be degeneration of the nerves.

There are many reasons nerves can become irritated or inflamed, so it is important to search for and deal with the cause. Pressure on the nerve from mechanical misalignment of body structures may be a factor, so the *Bodywork* strategy (massage, chiropractic, etc.) may be helpful.

Diabetes is often involved in nerve inflammation and should be brought under control. Infection, a lack of good fats in the diet, heavy metals and environmental toxins, and unresolved emotional issues are additional factors to consider.

Nerves can become inflamed from deficiencies of vitamins B$_{12}$, B$_1$ (thiamine), and B$_3$. So B-complex vitamins may be helpful.

If the person has been exposed to a lot of chemicals or metals, some cleansing therapies may be helpful. Try using the *Detoxification* or *Heavy Metal Cleanse* strategies to eliminate toxins that may be irritating the nerves.

Try using nervines like blue vervain, Saint John's wort, or wood betony to ease pain. Herbs that may help reduce inflammation in the nerves include yucca, wild yam, and Devil's claw.

Strategies: Avoid Sugar, Bodywork, Counseling or Therapy, Detoxification, Eat Healthy, Healthy Fats, and Heavy Metal Cleanse

Formulas: Herbal Arthritis, GLA Oil, **Analgesic Nerve**, **Anti-Inflammatory Pain**, **Antioxidant**, and **Methyl B12 Vitamin**

Herbs: Black cohosh, devil's claw, dogwood (Jamaican), evening primrose, linden, passion flower, **Saint John's wort**, valerian, **vervain (blue)**, wild yam, wood betony, and **yucca**

Supplements: Lecithin, omega-3 DHA, **omega-3 EFAs**, omega-6 GLA, **vitamin B-complex**, **vitamin B$_{12}$**, and vitamin B$_5$

Essential Oils: Cajeput, chamomile (Roman), lavender, marjoram, and neroli

Neurodegenerative Diseases
See also Alzheimer's, ALS, Parkinson's disease, Huntington's disease, and mitochondrial dysfunction

Neurodegenerative diseases involve a progressive deterioration of the central nervous system, which results in cognitive decline, problems with motor control, and other nervous system problems.

Reducing inflammation in the nervous system is important in both preventing and slowing the progress of neurodegenerative diseases. A diet low in sugar, high in fresh fruits and vegetables, as well as good fats and fat-soluble vitamins is helpful. Maintaining physical and mental activity is also helpful. CBD helps regulate nerve functions and inflammation and has shown promising results in helping people with neurodegenerative diseases.

See specific neurodegenerative diseases for further suggestions.

Strategies: Affirmation and Visualization, Eat Healthy, Healthy Fats, Liver Detoxification, and Low-Glycemic Diet

Formulas: Mitochondria Energy, Antioxidant, and CBD Brain

Herbs: Cannabis and **coconut**

Supplements: Alpha-lipoic acid, **CBD**, Co-Q10, **omega-3 DHA**, omega-3 EFAs, and vitamin E

Neurosis see *anxiety disorders* **and** *trauma*

Night Blindness
Night Vision

Night blindness is a difficulty in seeing at night. Bilberry and vitamin A may be helpful for improving night vision.

Formulas: Antioxidant Eye and Antioxidant

Herbs: Bilberry

Supplements: Vitamin A

Night Sweating

See also perspiration (excessive)

When there is profuse perspiration during sleep, the problem is often due to an imbalance in the hypothalamus or adrenals. For women going through menopause it can be a hot flash taking place at night. Remedies that have been helpful for reducing night sweats include sage (drunk as a cold tea), astragalus, and schisandra, all of which help the body hold onto moisture.

Formulas: Chinese Yin-Increasing, Chinese Fire-Increasing, Electrolyte Drink, Adrenal Glandular, and **Hot Flash**

Essential Oil Blends: Menopause Support EO

Herbs: Asparagus, astragalus, black cohosh, peony, **sage**, and **schisandra**

Essential Oils: Clary sage

Nightmares
See also restless dreams and trauma

Nightmares are often a sign of a toxic liver, blood sugar problems, or adrenal fatigue. Use the *Low-Glycemic Diet* strategy and have a protein snack (e.g. nut butter, cheese) at bedtime. Take an *Adaptogen Formula* if stressed, or an *Adrenal Tonic Formula* if suffering from fatigue. Chaparral or Saint John's wort flower essences may be helpful for nightmares, especially in children. Also consider emotional factors such as past trauma or abuse or a highly stressed state of mind.

Strategies: Detoxification, Emotional Healing Work, Flower Essence, Healthy Fats, Low-Glycemic Diet, and Stress Management

Formulas: Chinese Fire-Increasing, Adrenal Glandular, Hepatoprotective, and Chinese Wood-Decreasing

Herbs: Milk thistle

Supplements: Omega-3 EFAs

Essential Oils: Frankincense, myrrh, and sandalwood

Nocturnal Emission
Wet Dreams

Nocturnal emissions, also known as wet dreams, are an involuntary release of semen by males during sleep. This is often accompanied by erotic dreams. There is nothing harmful about this but if it occurs excessively, some of the remedies listed here may help.

Formulas: Sleep Support, **Chinese Water-Increasing**, and Female Cycle

Herbs: Chaste tree, dodder, false unicorn, lotus, wild yam, and yam (Chinese)

Nosebleeds

Nosebleeds are not a serious issue and are generally easy to treat at home. To prevent nosebleeds, you need to look at the underlying causes. A major cause of nosebleeds is dryness of the nasal membranes. This can be caused by dehydration, smoking, dry weather, and the use of cold and allergy medications that dry mucous membranes. So start by keeping your sinus cavities moist by following the *Hydration* strategy. If you live in a dry climate, running a humidifier may help.

Picking your nose can damage membranes, as can rubbing or blowing your nose too hard. Low levels of vitamin C and bioflavonoids also make capillaries more fragile and prone to bleeding. Taking a vitamin C supplement with bioflavonoids or taking remedies like rose hips can strengthen the capillaries. Horsetail can also reduce capillary fragility. Styptic herbs may also be used internally to help stop bleeding.

Strategies: Hydration

Formulas: Internal Bleeding and Steven Horne's Sinus Snuff

Herbs: Achyranthes, bayberry, bilberry, **capsicum**, coptis, eyebright, gardenia, horsetail, **rose hips**, shepherd's purse, wood betony, and **yarrow**

Supplements: Bioflavonoids and **vitamin C**

Essential Oils: Geranium

Numbness

See also nerve damage

Sensations of numbness and tingling in the extremities are often helped by enhancing circulation to the extremities with remedies like capsicum, ginkgo, hawthorn, and prickly ash. Numbness and tingling in the extremities are also signs of B_{12}, folate, and B_1 deficiency.

Numbness and tingling may also involve irritation or pressure on nerves, which may be corrected by chiropractic care or any of the other *Bodywork* strategies. Saint John's wort stimulates nerve regeneration and repair where the problem is caused by bruised or damaged nerves. It can be taken internally or used topically as an oil. When the numbness is due to an injury, a topical application of arnica and Saint John's wort oil can be helpful in reducing swelling and promoting healing and sensation.

Strategies: Bodywork

Formulas: **Brain-Heart**, **Oral Chelation**, Chinese Yin-Increasing, **Anti-Stress B-Complex**, Methyl B12 Vitamin, and **Methylated B Vitamin**

Herbs: Arnica, capsicum, ginkgo, hawthorn, he shou wu, **prickly ash**, and **Saint John's wort**

Supplements: Vitamin B-complex, vitamin B_1, **vitamin B_{12}**, and **vitamin B_9**

Nursing

Nursing is one of the best ways to build a healthy immune system in an infant. Ideally, mothers should nurse their children for one year and longer, if possible. Breast milk not only contains the right ratios of nutrients needed for healthy children but also passes immune factors from mother to child and enhances mother-infant bonding.

Women who are pregnant or nursing need extra nutrition to provide for their own needs and the needs of their offspring. Just as in pregnancy, a good multivitamin or whole food supplement along with a good diet are very important while nursing.

Nursing also helps to develop a healthy gut flora in an infant, which contributes to lifelong immunity in the child. However, mom has to have the friendly bacteria in her own body before she can pass them on to her offspring, so probiotic supplements or eating cultured foods may also be helpful while nursing, particularly if mom has a history of bowel disorders or yeast infections.

Nursing mothers also need extra water and should pay attention to their stress levels. Staying calm and relaxed while nursing aids baby's digestion and helps the child develop a sense of well-being.

There are a number of herbs that can increase the flow of and/or enrich breast milk. These include blessed thistle, marshmallow, nettles, and milk thistle. The *Herbal Mineral Formula* can also help to enrich breast milk and develop healthy bones, teeth, and nerves in developing infants.

When it comes time to stop nursing, parsley and sage can be used to help dry up breast milk.

Strategies: Healthy Fats, Hydration, and Stress Management

Formulas: Herbal Calcium, **Lung Moistening**, Joan Patton's Herbal Minerals, and Probiotic

Herbs: Alfalfa, anise, **blessed thistle**, **fenugreek**, **marshmallow**, **milk thistle**, nettle, and stinging

Supplements: Chlorophyll and vitamin E

Essential Oils: Anise and fennel

Obesity   see *excess weight*

Obsessive Compulsive Disorder   see *OCD*

OCD
Obsessive Compulsive Disorder

See also mental illness, anxiety disorders, and trauma

Obsessive-compulsive disorder (OCD) is an anxiety disorder that is characterized by involuntary thoughts that cause the sufferer to develop a dread that something bad will happen. This makes them feel compelled to perform involuntary, irrational, and time-consuming behaviors. Symptoms range from repetitive hand-washing to preoccupation with sexual, religious, or aggressive impulses.

This condition typically requires the *Counseling or Therapy* strategy, because it is usually rooted in unhealed abuse and trauma. The process of clearing this past trauma and abuse can be aided, however, by using the general principles for working with anxiety disorders. The *Emotional Healing Work* strategy and the *Flower Essence* strategy using the flower essences of vervain, white chestnut, or red chestnut may also be helpful. See *anxiety disorders and trauma* for more suggestions.

Strategies: Affirmation and Visualization, Avoid Sugar, Balance Methylation, Blood Type Diet, Counseling or

Therapy, Emotional Healing Work, Flower Essence, Healthy Fats, and Low-Glycemic Diet

Formulas: Adrenal Glandular, Chinese Fire-Increasing, Anti-Anxiety, Ashwagandha Complex, and Brain Calming

Flower Essence Blends: Shock and Injury FE and **Self-Responsibility FE**

Herbs: Ashwagandha, bacopa, **eleuthero**, kava kava, and schisandra

Supplements: Magnesium, omega-3 EFAs, vitamin B-complex, **vitamin B$_6$**, and **zinc**

Oral Surgery

See also surgery (recovery)

Goldenseal, myrrh, oak, and plantain may help the mouth to heal after oral surgery. These can be used as mouth rinses or applied topically to damaged areas. The *Anti-Inflammatory Pain Formula* can reduce pain and speed healing, as well.

Strategies: Lymph-Moving Pain Relief

Formulas: Colloidal Mineral, Liquid Lymph, Antioxidant, and **Anti-Inflammatory Pain**

Herbs: Goldenseal, myrrh, **plantain**, and white oak

Essential Oils: Myrrh

Osteoarthritis   see *arthritis*

Osteoporosis

See also menopause

Osteoporosis is a decrease in bone density that causes skeletal weakness. Recent estimates suggest that at least ten million people in the US have osteoporosis. Osteoporosis didn't exist in many native cultures and the greatest problems exist in the US and Europe. For example, the Chinese have a very low incidence of osteoporosis, and they don't consume diary products, take calcium supplements, or use hormone replacement therapy. So like many other health problems, bone weakness is a result of dietary and lifestyle choices.

Bones are neither solid nor static; they are living tissue that is continually being renewed. Bone building consists of an array of complex biochemical reactions that maintain a balance between breaking down old and injured bone and building new strong but flexible bone. Old bone is constantly being dissolved and reabsorbed, and new bone is constantly being laid down in its place. Bones weaken when the breaking-down process occurs more rapidly than the building-up process.

If you have osteoporosis or want to prevent it you should start by adopting a healthy diet and lifestyle. You can also try some of the following strategies.

Take the Right Kind of Calcium

The common belief is that we aren't getting enough calcium in our diets. However, if that were actually the case, then all the dairy products, calcium-fortified foods, calcium-based antacids, and calcium supplements we consume would be fixing the problem. The fact is, that this increased calcium intake doesn't make the problem better. It is true that calcium is both the most abundant mineral in the body and the most abundant mineral in bones, but bones are made of much more than calcium. So find a calcium supplement that contains other nutrients needed for bone health like the *Skeletal Support Formula*.

When taking a calcium supplement at least make sure it contains magnesium. The ratio of calcium to magnesium for humans should be 2:1, and it has been established that more people are deficient in magnesium than calcium.

Supplement with Trace Minerals

Bones contain other macro minerals such as magnesium, phosphorus, sodium, chloride, potassium, and sulfur. They also need trace minerals such as silica, iron, molybdenum, copper, zinc, fluoride, selenium, chromium, manganese, iodine, and cobalt. So consider using *Colloidal Minerals* or *Watkin's Hair, Skin and Nails Formula* to get more of these trace elements.

Take Vitamins C, D$_3$ and K$_2$

Vitamin C is important for bone health, but even more important are the fat-soluble vitamins D$_3$ and K$_2$. These vitamins are absolutely essential for building bone, including utilizing the calcium in your diet. The majority of the population, and especially the elderly, are not getting enough of these important vitamins.

Exercise

When astronauts spend long periods in outer space, they suffer a loss of bone mass. This is because their bodies are not having to work against gravity. Bone is built in response to the body's need for structural support. This is why weight-bearing exercise helps keep bones healthy. See the *Exercise* strategy.

Make Sure You Have Adequate HCl

Stomach acid is essential for being able to absorb calcium and other minerals. Many people develop low stomach acid as they age, which can cause acid indigestion from fermentation of the food they eat. As a result they take antacids, which further lower stomach acid. This greatly increases the risk of developing osteoporosis. If you have poor digestion consider taking a *Betaine HCl Formula*.

Balance Hormones

There are a number of hormones involved with the breakdown and rebuilding of bone. So health of the glandular system is important to bone health. However, it's not as simple as just using estrogen or progesterone supplements, because many other glands are involved in bone health.

Parathyroid hormone stimulates the kidneys to convert vitamin D to its active form. It also acts to dissolve calcium and other alkaline minerals out of the bone into the bloodstream to neutralize excess acid in the body. Glucocortical adrenal hormones and the sex hormones estrogen and androgen play a role in remodeling bone as well as calcitonin and thyroxine from the thyroid, insulin from the pancreas, and growth hormone from the pituitary.

So you may need to work with your herbalist or naturopath to support the health of various glands to keep your bones healthy (findanherbalist.com or americanherbalistsguild.com).

Strategies: Alkalize the Body, Bone Broth, Eat Healthy, Exercise, Healthy Fats, and Mineralization

Formulas: Chrisopher's Menopause, **Chinese Water-Increasing**, **Betaine HCl**, **Skeletal Support**, **Watkin's Hair, Skin, and Nails**, and Colloidal Mineral

Programs: Menopause Support

Herbs: Alfalfa, ashwagandha, **black cohosh**, **horsetail**, nettle, stinging, and oat straw

Supplements: Boron, calcium, copper, DHEA, krill oil, magnesium, manganese, omega-3 EFAs, **silicon**, vitamin B$_3$, vitamin C, **vitamin D**, **vitamin K**, and zinc

Ovarian Cysts   see *cysts*

Ovarian Pain

See also cysts, endometriosis, and pain

Ovarian pain should be checked out by a doctor to determine the cause. It could be due to cysts, endometriosis, or other causes. Potentially helpful herbs include chastetree, false unicorn, and black cohosh.

Formulas: Female Cycle

Herbs: Black cohosh, **chaste tree**, **false unicorn**, and wild yam

Supplements: Magnesium

Essential Oils: Frankincense

Overacidity
Acid pH

See also overalkalinity

If urine and saliva testing reveals that the pH of the body is too acidic (see the *Alkalize the Body* strategy) it means there is not enough energy for the body to heal. This can result in chronic pain, low grade inflammation and fatigue. It is also the environment in which cancer cells form and thrive. If

you want to alkalize your system, here are various herbs and supplements that can help you raise your pH to a healthier, more alkaline state.

Start with a more alkaline diet consisting of fruits and vegetables, with smaller portions of animal proteins, grains, beans, and nuts. Also increase your intake of antioxidants and minerals.

When the body is acidic, it is a good indication that you aren't getting enough calcium, magnesium, and/or potassium. Try supplementing with magnesium or calcium and magnesium in a 1:1 or 1:2 ratio of calcium to magnesium. *Epsom Salt Baths* can also be helpful. If you need to alkalize the system quickly, a teaspoon of baking soda (sodium bicarbonate) dissolved in a little water will rapidly alkalize the system.

Many people find that an *Antioxidant Formula* not only protects them against free radicals, it also gives them an energy pick-up, reduces chronic inflammation and pain, and improves their overall health. Combining chlorophyll with a liquid *Antioxidant Formula* (like the *Antioxidant Mangosteen Formula*) provides quick, caffeine-free, alkalizing energy pick up.

You can also drink more water and take the *Chinese Water-Increasing Formula* to help you kidneys flush acid waste more efficiently. If you have respiratory problems, taking cordyceps or a *Chinese Metal-Increasing Formula* will strengthen the ability of your lungs to buffer pH.

Strategies: Alkalize the Body

Formulas: Whole Food Green Drink, Skeletal Support, **Chinese Water-Increasing**, Herbal Potassium, Herbal Bitters, **Colloidal Mineral**, **Antioxidant**, Chinese Metal-Increasing, and Digestive Support

Herbs: Açaí, alfalfa, astragalus, cordyceps, dandelion, lycium, mangosteen, noni, turmeric, and yucca

Supplements: Calcium, **chlorophyll**, **magnesium**, potassium, protease, and **sodium bicarbonate**

Overalkalinity
Alkalosis

See also overacidity

When urine and saliva tests reveal overalkalinity, several things may be happening. First, the person may have very poor digestion. Second, their kidneys may not be working efficiently. Third, the person may be extremely overacid and is creating ammonia as an emergency buffering system. Understanding this, here are some basic suggestions for dealing with an over-alkaline system.

Vegans (vegetarians who eat no animal protein whatsoever) often wind up with overalkaline readings. In many cases, they believe this is healthy, but it is not. Usually, these people have a hard time digesting protein, which is why they feel better when they avoid it. They often need a *Digestive Support* and/or *Betaine HCl Formula* to help their body assimilate protein. They should include some high-quality animal protein in their diet (at the very least some eggs, goat cheese, and/or fish). If a person are unwilling to do this, have them reduce their intake of starches and increase protein from legumes, nuts or protein powders.

If saliva readings are acid and urine readings are alkaline, the kidneys are not doing their job. Drinking more water and taking the *Chinese Water-Increasing Formula* can help the kidneys flush the acid out the tissues. Nettles are also effective at increasing the ability of the kidneys to flush acid.

In cases where the persons smells of ammonia, their system is highly acidic. They need to drink more water, support kidney function, and take supplements with alkalizing minerals (particularly calcium, magnesium, and potassium). They may also benefit by taking a little baking soda (sodium bicarbonate) in water and using the *Epsom Salt Bath* strategy.

Vitamin C may be helpful in cases of over alkalinity. Supplements with acid-forming minerals like sulfur, such as MSM, glucosamine sulfate, and garlic) may also be helpful.

For a more complete understanding of the role of pH in health, read the *Alkalize Your Body* strategy.

Strategies: Alkalize the Body and Epsom Salt Bath

Formulas: Probiotic, Plant Enzyme, **Digestive Support**, Mitochondria Energy, **Betaine HCl**, and Chinese Water-Increasing

Herbs: Garlic and **nettle, stinging**

Supplements: Glucosamine sulfate, MSM, protease, and **vitamin C**

Pain

See also arthritis, inflammation, headache (migraine), overacidity, and headache

Pain is the primary and nearly universal symptom of all our human afflictions, whether they are physical or emotional. Pain is why we seek help when we are sick. If illness didn't cause dis-ease ("lack of ease" or pain), we would not be motivated to avoid doing things that damage the body.

So no matter how much we dislike it and want to make it go away, pain is not an enemy. Pain is a form of communication. It is how the body tells us it is having a problem. It is the "911 system" that the cells of our body use to call for help. Pain is also the teacher that motivates us, if we let it, to not abuse our body and pursue a healthy lifestyle.

Modern pain-relieving drugs are wonderful things. They enable us to undergo necessary surgery or dental work without pain. They can also be of great relief to the person who is suffering because of a serious accident or illness.

Unfortunately, pain-relieving medications allow people to disconnect from taking responsibility for their health. Instead of asking "why" they are getting headaches, upset stomachs, muscle aches, or other pain, they simply pop a painkiller. Thus, they never make the connection that their pain is originating from their diet, lifestyle, and stress and usually don't make the necessary changes they need to make to be healthy.

We need to stop seeing pain as an enemy that needs to be killed. We need to see pain as a teacher that is giving us a "wake-up call" that we need to change the way we are treating our body.

Let's take headaches for example. Headaches have causes. The cause may be as simple as dehydration. Drinking more water has greatly reduced the number of headaches some people have. A headache can also be a sign of an overacid system, of poor bowel elimination, or of excess stress and tension.

Taking pain killers may relieve today's headache, but it won't stop us from having another one tomorrow. When we start "listening" to the headache's message, we can actually learn to stop having headaches altogether. Headaches are a normal part of most people's lives only because the average person has bad health habits.

When we just keep taking painkillers without changing our bad health habits, we keep doing small things that damage our health. After twenty years of failing to heed these little warnings that something is wrong, we get a bigger "wake-up call" in the form of a heart attack, cancer, diabetes, or some other serious illness. Then we wonder, "How could this happen to me?"

Besides, painkillers themselves are toxic drugs. Sure, they're okay for occasional relief of pain, but when used frequently, they can damage the liver, kidneys, nerves, and other organs. They can even increase the risk of heart disease and other serious health problems.

Identifying the Source of Pain

Since pain has a cause, you need to try to identify the source of your pain. When you suffer an acute injury such as a burn, cut, or bruise, it's usually pretty easy to see what caused it. When you experience more long-lasting, chronic pain, it's often more difficult to see what is causing the damage. In fact, you may have to search and experiment a little to discover what is causing your pain, but the reward will be worth it. Here are six sources of pain and how to alleviate them.

Lack of Oxygen

At a cellular level, the primary cause of pain is lack of oxygenation to the tissues. The sharp pain of acute injuries is caused by the inflammatory process depriving cells of oxygen. When cells are chronically deprived of oxygen, you'll get chronic dull pain. Many people have experienced a great deal of relief from chronic pain just by practicing deep breathing. So if you are in chronic pain, start practicing the *Deep Breathing* strategy. The results may amaze you.

Dehydration

Accumulation of toxins in the tissues is another underlying cause of pain. Dehydration inhibits oxygen transport and allows toxins to accumulate. Another simple, but highly effective strategy for reducing chronic pain is to increase your water intake. This simple practice can greatly reduce the frequency of headaches, constipation, indigestion, and muscle aches. See *Hydration* strategy.

Lymphatic Congestion

When tissues become congested due to poor lymphatic drainage, cells experience accumulation of toxic acid waste and low oxygenation. Ear aches, sore throats, menstrual pain and headaches can all occur because of swelling in the lymph nodes and congestion of the lymphatic system. Besides using herbs that clear the lymphatic system, the techniques in the *Lymph-Moving Pain Relief* strategy will help with the lymphatic stagnation associated with pain.

Massage is one of these strategies that can relieve stagnant lymph, especially if you use an *Analgesic EO Blend* when you do the massage. The secret is to massage the painful areas six to eight times per day or more to keep the lymph flowing. Moderate physical activity such as walking or swimming helps increase lymphatic drainage.

Overacidity

Cells produce acid waste in the process of metabolism. If this acid waste isn't flushed properly from the system it leads to an over acid condition in the tissues. This reduces oxygenation and causes muscle tension and pain. Drinking enough water and breathing deeply will help reduce overacidity.

Drinking alkaline water or going on a short fast using lemon water can also help. Use the juice of four lemons in half a gallon of water, sweetened with a little real maple syrup. Don't eat anything for a couple of days and just drink this mixture whenever you are hungry. Often after two or three days of fasting like this, the body becomes more alkaline and many aches and pains simply disappear. To maintain a more alkaline system, read the suggestions under the *Alkalize the Body* strategy and the condition *Overacidity*.

Muscle Tension

Cramps and spasms are a frequent cause of pain. This may be due to stress, but it can also be due to repetitive movements or bad posture that stress the structural alignment of the body. For example, sitting at a computer and typing all day can cause chronic tension in the neck, shoulders, and upper back. This can lead to sore throats, headaches, and back pain.

Periodic stretching and better posture will often correct this type of pain. Chiropractic adjustments, massage therapy or other forms of body work can help a person have better structural alignment, thereby easing pain. See the *Good Posture* and *Bodywork* strategies.

Antispasmodic herbs can also help. Lobelia and kava kava are two great herbs for easing muscle tension to relieve pain. Muscle tension can also be eased by taking magnesium.

Chronic Inflammation

All of these causes of pain are linked with chronic inflammation. Try the *Anti-Inflammatory Pain Formula*, curcumin or turmeric, or omega-3 essential fatty acids. See *Inflammation* for more suggestions on how to reduce chronic inflammation.

Using Natural Analgesics

While you are working to identify the cause of your pain you can use natural remedies for pain relief instead of over-the-counter pain relievers or drugs. Herbs that contain salycilates act like natural aspirin and include willow bark, wintergreen, and meadowsweet. Corydalis is a fairly dependable pain reliever and is especially helpful when pain interferes with sleep. Two other herbs that are useful for symptomatic relief are Indian pipe and Jamaican dogwood. Many people also find CBD to be a dependable pain reliever, especially for chronic pain.

Strategies: Alkalize the Body, Aromatherapy, Bodywork, Deep Breathing, Emotional Healing Work, Enhance Nitric Oxide, Fasting, Good Posture, Healthy Fats, Hydration, Lymph-Moving Pain Relief, Poultice, and Sleep

Formulas: Stan Malstrom's Herbal Aspirin, Proanthocyanidins, Herbal Sleep Aid, Chinese Yang-Reducing, Liquid Lymph, **Topical Analgesic**, **Anti-Inflammatory Pain**, Antioxidant, **General Analgesic**, Christopher's Nervine, CBD Relaxing, **CBD Anti-inflammatory**, Nitric Oxide Boosting, Digestive Support, and CBD Joint

Essential Oil Blends: Analgesic EO

Herbs: Aloe vera, arnica, barley, **boswellia**, California poppy, cannabis, capsicum, **corydalis**, **dogwood (Jamaican)**, gastrodia, hops, Indian pipe, **kava kava**, ligusticum, **lobelia**, meadowsweet, noni, prickly ash, safflower, Saint John's wort, teasel, **turmeric**, valerian, wild lettuce, and **willow bark**

Supplements: CBD, chlorophyll, **curcumin**, L-phenylalaine, L-tryptophan, magnesium, **MSM**, and **omega-3 EFAs**

Essential Oils: Camphor, clove, eucalyptus, fir, frankincense, helichrysum, lavender, lemon, marjoram, **menthol**, spruce (hemlock), tansy (blue), and **wintergreen**

Palpitations
see *heart fibrillation/palpitations*

Pancreatitis

See also inflammation

Pancreatitis is an inflammation of the pancreas. Normally, the digestive enzymes produced by the pancreas do not become active until they reach the small intestine, where they begin digesting food. But if these enzymes become active inside the pancreas, they start "digesting" the pancreas itself, causing inflammation.

Acute pancreatitis occurs suddenly and lasts for a short period. It usually resolves itself with no medical treatment. It is often caused by gallstones or drinking too much alcohol, although it can be due to other causes. Remedies that reduce inflammation may be helpful.

Chronic pancreatitis does not resolve itself and results in a slow destruction of the pancreas. Either form can cause serious complications that can become life-threatening. Seek professional assistance.

Strategies: Hydration and Low-Glycemic Diet

Formulas: Digestive Support, Plant Enzyme, Probiotic, and Anti-Inflammatory Pain

Herbs: Amalaki, **bilberry leaf**, black walnut, dandelion, **goldenseal**, horsetail, **juniper**, **licorice**, and uva ursi

Supplements: Chlorophyll, silicon, and vitamin B-complex

Essential Oils: Helichrysum and juniper

Panic Attack   see *anxiety attacks*

Pap Smear, Abnormal

See also cervical dysplasia

An abnormal Pap smear is caused by cervical dysplasia. See that listing for more information. The following may be helpful in correcting an abnormal Pap smear. Mix lemon and clove oils in a carrier oil (such as olive oil) and apply topically to the abdomen. (See the *Aromatherapy* strategy.) Decongest the liver with liver-cleansing herbs.

Strategies: Compress or Fomentation

Formulas: Detoxifying and Chinese Wood-Decreasing

Programs: Chinese Balanced Cleansing

Essential Oils: Clove and lemon

Paralysis

See also nerve damage

Paralysis is a complete or partial loss of motor function usually involving loss of motion with or without loss of sensation in any part of the body. This is usually due to damage to the nervous system, especially the spinal cord.

Obviously, this is a condition that requires medical attention, but there are some remedies that may help nerves to heal. The extent of their ability to heal depends on the amount of damage.

Saint John's wort has been called the "arnica of the nervous system" because of its ability to stimulate nerve repair. It can be used internally (as an herb or homeopathic remedy) or topically (as an oil).

Good fats are essential for the nerves as nerves are 50 percent fat by dry weight. Magnesium and B-complex vitamins are also helpful for nutritionally supporting nerve function. Lobelia and capsicum applied topically over injured areas can stimulate healing, and improving circulation by using prickly ash internally may also be helpful.

Strategies: Eat Healthy and Healthy Fats

Formulas: Anti-Stress B-Complex and Herbal Potassium

Herbs: Capsicum, lobelia, muira puama, prickly ash, and **Saint John's wort**

Supplements: Magnesium, omega-3 EFAs, vitamin B-complex, and **vitamin B**$_{12}$

Essential Oils: Lavender

Paranoia   see *fear* and *anxiety disorders*

Parasites

See also giardia, parasites (tapeworm), parasites (nematodes, and worms)

When most of us think of parasites, hideous images come to mind, such as ten-foot-tape worms being coaxed out of human hosts—or starving children in developing countries with swollen bellies. But not all parasites are giant worms; many are microscopic single-cell organisms. Furthermore, parasites aren't limited to people living in developing countries. Many people in North American also have problems with parasites and don't realize it.

People can pick up parasites from food, water or pets, or through the skin or mucous membranes. Fortunately, where clean food and water are the norm, odds are very small that people will have a serious parasite problem. However, as more and more food is coming out of developing countries, parasite problems are on the rise.

Furthermore, if you have pets or animals with parasites, there is a high probability that you have them too. It's also easy to pick up parasites while traveling in foreign countries. So if you've experienced a change in your health after traveling, parasites may be the reason.

Diagnosing Parasitic Infections

Once parasites are in the body, they can be very hard to diagnose. A standard stool analysis may or may not reveal their presence, because a particular sample may not contain them. In fact, parasite problems are often so evasive to standard medical investigation that no one can accurately estimate how much of the population may be afflicted. Fortunately, stool tests that not only check with a microscope but also check for parasite antibodies have recently increased the reliability of diagnosis.

Parasites leave telltale signs, including chronic fatigue, anemia, an illness that won't go away, nervousness, teeth grinding, diarrhea, ulcers or digestive pain, nausea or diarrhea, extremes of appetite, weight loss or gain, itching (especially in the rectal area), aches and pains that move from place to place, chronic foul breath, furred tongue, liver jaundice, wide mood swings, fever, colitis, insomnia, and lowered immune response. Just because you have these symptoms doesn't mean that you have parasites, but if you do have a lot of these symptoms and other therapies you've tried aren't working, a parasite cleanse may be useful.

Strategies for Eliminating Parasites

The core of a parasite cleanse are antiparasitic herbs. Some of the best options are mugwort, wormwood, sweet annie, and black walnut. Ideally several antiparasitic herbs should be taken together as part of an *Antiparasitic Formula*. This should be taken along with herbs to help cleanse the colon, such as a good *General Detoxifying Formula*. In some cases, cascara sagrada or a *Stimulant Laxative Formula* may also be a helpful part of the cleanse.

Enzymes can be taken between meals to help destroy parasites. Protease enzyme supplements are particularly helpful.

One can also use foods that tend to be antiparasitic. One of the best is raw garlic. It has been used for worms (pinworms, roundworms, hookworms, tapeworms), giardia, amoebic dysentery, and yeast. A garlic enema is an effective way to get rid of worms. See the *Colon Hydrotherapy* strategy for instructions.

Other antiparasitic foods and herbs include cloves, pumpkin seeds, watermelon seeds, and horsetail, raw almonds (with skins), raw carrots, raw onions, raw papaya, figs, cucumbers, and lemon water. Food-based remedies can be especially helpful for parasites in children.

During the cleanse it is helpful to avoid simple sugars, starchy foods, alcohol, and caffeine. In fact, fasting on water for several days while taking the antiparasitic herbs will greatly intensify the effectiveness of the program as it starves the parasites.

Always drink plenty of water when doing any cleanse. Follow up a parasite cleanse with probiotics to help restore normal gut flora. See specific parasites in related conditions for more specific remedies.

Strategies: Blood Type Diet, Colon Hydrotherapy, Fasting, Friendly Flora, Gut-Healing Diet, and Hydration

Formulas: Antiparasitic, H. Pylori-Fighting, **Standardized Acetogenin**, **Stabilized Allicin**, Stimulant Laxative, Detoxifying, Digestive Support, and Probiotic

Programs: Parasite Cleansing

Herbs: Aloe vera, **andrographis**, bitter melon, **black walnut**, cascara sagrada, chaparral, clove, elecampane, **garlic**, goldenseal, haritaki, horsetail, **mugwort**, neem, oregano, pau d'arco, **pawpaw**, picrorhiza, purslane, quassia, **sweet annie**, and **wormwood**

Supplements: Protease

Essential Oils: Cinnamon, clove, fennel, lemon, neroli, oregano, and pine

Parasites (Nematodes, Worms)

See also parasites

Nematodes are tiny worms such a pinworms (*Enterobius vermicularis*), whipworms (*Trichuris trichiura*), and hookworms (*Ancylostoma duodenale* and *Necator americanus*). The most prevalent of these are pinworms, which are common in school-children. They are highly contagious and easily passed around the family.

Pinworm eggs can contaminate clothing, bed linens, and toilet seats. When the eggs are ingested, the worms hatch in the intestines and their eggs are passed from the rectum. Pinworms can also infect the vulva, uterus, and fallopian tubes in women.

Fortunately, pinworms are one of the easier parasites to detect because they cause rectal itching. If one examines the rectal area at night with a flashlight, the worms appear as white threads at the anal opening. Other symptoms include nervousness, inability to concentrate, lack of appetite, and unusual dark circles around the eyes.

Take precautions to prevent pinworms from spreading by washing bed linens, bed-clothes, and underwear of the entire family, having the infected child take daily morning showers to remove eggs deposited in the rectal region during the night; disinfecting toilet seats, bathtubs, sinks, and door handles daily; and being sure everybody washes their hands (and fingernails) before meals. Clean cat litter boxes daily.

Also, avoid a diet high in sugar and other junk food, which gives parasites more to feed on.

Whipworms and hookworms are less common but pose a more serious threat to human health. Whipworms inject a fluid that liquefies colon tissue so the worms can ingest it. This creates severe nutritional deficiencies and infections.

Hookworms bite and suck on the intestinal wall, causing bleeding and destroying tissue. This can be severe enough to cause death. Since they consume iron, they cause severe anemia, which can help in detecting them.

Natural therapies for nematodes include garlic enemas (see *Colon Hydrotherapy* strategy) or suppositories and *Antiparasitic Formulas*. The Parasite Cleansing Pack is a good program. You can enhance its effectiveness by taking protease enzyme supplements between meals. For serious parasite infections seek medical assistance. See *parasites* for more basic information on getting rid of parasites.

Strategies: Colon Hydrotherapy and Detoxification

Formulas: Antiparasitic, Stabilized Allicin, Standardized Acetogenin, Digestive Support, and Stimulant Laxative

Programs: Parasite Cleansing

Herbs: Black walnut, boswellia, butternut, cascara sagrada, chirata, false unicorn, garlic, horseradish, horsetail, papaya, pawpaw, **pumpkin seeds**, sage, **sweet annie**, thuja, thyme, vervain (blue), and **wormwood**

Supplements: Protease

Essential Oils: Bay leaf and chamomile (Roman)

Parasites (Tapeworm)

See also parasites

Other parasites may actually be more dangerous to one's health, but tapeworms (*Taenia saginata*, beef tapeworm and *T. solium*, pork tapeworm) are emotionally disturbing because of their size. Tapeworms require an intermediate host, so they are usually ingested by eating improperly cooked beef, pork, or fish.

Tapeworms are composed of three to four thousand segments per worm. New segments are formed near the head, and the ones on the end are cast off with egg packets. When passed, these segments look like grains of uncooked rice or cucumber seeds. This is one of the ways they can be diagnosed. Other symptoms of tapeworms include diarrhea or constipation—or alternating diarrhea and constipation. Some people lose weight with tapeworms, but it is more common for the host to be overweight and retaining water. Tapeworms raise blood sugar levels, cause anemia, and interfere with vitamin B_{12} uptake.

Natural therapies for tapeworms include *Antiparasitic Formulas* and protease enzyme supplements. Fasting on raw

pineapple has helped in destroying them. Raw fig juice and pumpkin seeds have also proven helpful. See *parasites* for more information.

Strategies: Detoxification

Formulas: Antiparasitic, **Standardized Acetogenin**, and Stimulant Laxative

Programs: Parasite Cleansing

Herbs: Aloe vera, **black walnut**, **pawpaw**, and wormwood

Supplements: Nanoparticle silver and protease

Parkinson's Disease

See also neurodegenerative diseases

Parkinson's disease is a chronic, progressive disease of the nervous system, usually occurring later in life. It involves the destruction of neurotransmitters that produce acetylcholine and dopamine and is marked by tremor and weakness in resting muscles and a gradual loss of muscle control. Seek appropriate medical assistance, because this disease is not easy to treat naturally once it has begun.

To prevent this disease, protect the brain by making sure your diet contains good fats and fat-soluble vitamins. Also make sure you get adequate amounts of antioxidant foods and nutrients and stay well hydrated. Avoid heavy metals and other environmental toxins.

Once the disease has started, natural remedies can be helpful in slowing its progress. *Antioxidant* and *Brain* and *Memory Tonic Formulas* may be helpful in protecting neurons from damage. Since the brain is 50 percent fat by dry weight, it is essential to use healthy fats in the diet and possibly supplement with omega-3 fatty acids or DHA (the most prominent fatty acid in the brain). *Antispasmodic Formulas* and nervine herbs like skullcap, valerian, and wood betony may help to ease tremors. Velvet bean is a natural source of l-DOPA, a precursor to dopamine that be helpful for some people. CBD can also be helpful for neurological disorders like Parkinson's.

Strategies: Eat Healthy, Gut-Healing Diet, Healthy Fats, Heavy Metal Cleanse, and Hydration

Formulas: Anti-Stress B-Complex, Oral Chelation, GLA Oil, **Brain and Memory Protection**, Herbal Sleep Aid, Watkin's Hair, Skin, and Nails, Brain Calming, Proanthocyanidins, and **Antioxidant**

Herbs: Coconut oil, evening primrose, ginkgo, hops, horsetail, licorice, milk thistle, passion flower, schisandra, skullcap, valerian, **velvet bean**, vervain (blue), and wood betony

Supplements: 7-keto, **alpha-lipoic acid**, **CBD**, Co-Q10, GABA, L-methionine, L-phenylalaine, **N-acetyl cysteine**, omega-3 DHA, **omega-3 EFAs**, omega-6 GLA, vitamin B-complex, **vitamin B_5**, vitamin C, and vitamin E

Peptic Ulcer see *ulcers*

Periods, Lack Of see *amenorrhea*

Peripheral Neuropathy

See also diabetes, neuralgia & neuritis, and mitochondrial dysfunction

Peripheral neuropathy is a disorder where the peripheral nerves that carry signals to and from the spinal cord to the rest of the body aren't working properly. It can involve damage to just one nerve or damage to the nerves in general.

Diabetes is the most common cause of peripheral neuropathy, but it can be caused by autoimmune conditions, chronic kidney disease, infections, nutritional deficiencies, poor blood flow, and low thyroid. Drugs and toxins can also damage nerves. In some cases, mechanical pressure may be the cause (as in carpal tunnel syndrome) or a physical injury may damage a nerve.

Symptoms of neuropathy include pain, numbness, tingling, or burning sensations. You may also start to lose feeling in your arms or legs. Nerve damage can also make it harder to control your muscles.

Damage to nerves can also affect internal organs. It can cause digestive problems and heart problems, for example. It can cause problems with the bladder and sweat glands. It can also affect reproductive function, causing erectile dysfunction in men or vaginal dryness in women.

In treating peripheral neuropathy, it is essential that you work with a medical doctor or other qualified health-care practitioner to help you determine and correct the cause. You may need to control your blood sugar, stop taking certain medications, or get bodywork to take pressure off nerves.

Natural remedies may be of help. Start by eating a whole food diet (preferably a low-glycemic one). Eat plenty of fresh fruits and vegetables. Avoid caffeine, sugar, and artificial sweeteners, particularly aspartame. Alpha-lipoic acid can be helpful when the neuropathy is due to blood sugar problems. In this case, it will also be helpful to take a *Blood Sugar Control Formula.*

Since nerves are composed of fat, eating healthy fats like omega-3 fatty acids or DHA will provide nutrition for the nerve cells. The fat-soluble vitamins, particularly D and E, can be very helpful in protecting the nerves from damage. B-complex vitamins, especially methylated B_{12} and B_9, are also helpful for nerve function and repair.

Sometimes using herbs which improve peripheral circulation will help too. These include prickly ash and capsicum.

Nerve tonic like skullcap and milky oat seed may also be helpful.

Strategies: Avoid Sugar, Eat Healthy, Healthy Fats, Hydration, and Stress Management

Formulas: Methyl B12 Vitamin, **Methylated B Vitamin**, and Blood Sugar Control

Herbs: Asparagus, capsicum, oat seed (milky), **prickly ash**, Saint John's wort, skullcap, and wood betony

Supplements: Alpha-lipoic acid, **krill oil**, **L-carnitine**, **omega-3 DHA**, omega-3 EFAs, vitamin B-complex, **vitamin B_1**, **vitamin B_{12}**, vitamin B_6, **vitamin B_9**, vitamin C, **vitamin D**, and **vitamin E**

Pernicious Anemia

See also anemia

Pernicious anemia is one form of megaloblastic anemia, and is marked by a progressive decrease in number and increase in size and hemoglobin content of red blood cells. Pernicious anemia is caused by an immune attack on the gastric parietal cells in the stomach that produce intrinsic factor. This causes a deficiency in B_{12}. The condition is characterized by paleness, weakness, and gastrointestinal and nervous disturbances. B_{12} shots may be needed, although B_{12} can also be taken sublingually in some cases.

Formulas: Christopher's Herbal Iron, **Methyl B12 Vitamin**, and **Methylated B Vitamin**

Herbs: Astragalus, licorice, and reishi

Supplements: Vitamin B-complex, **vitamin B_{12}**, vitamin B_9, and vitamin C

Perspiration, Deficient

When a person has a difficult time sweating, the skin does not detoxify the body properly and the body has a hard time cooling down. Sudorifics (also known as diaphoretics) are herbs used to induce perspiration. They are taken as a hot tea or infusion for this purpose. Sudorifics can also be used to encourage sweating to help throw off acute illnesses like colds and flu. Yarrow is one of the best sudorific herbs. It can be mixed with peppermint to make the tea palatable. Catnip is a good sudorific for children and can be mixed with elderflowers and/or peppermint.

Strategies: Sweat Bath

Formulas: Steven Horne's Children's Composition, **Ed Millet's Herbal Crisis**, and Herbal Composition

Herbs: Boneset, **capsicum**, catnip, **elder flowers**, ginger, lemon balm, peppermint, pleurisy, **vervain (blue)**, and **yarrow**

Perspiration, Excessive
Sweating

See also night sweating

When a person perspires too easily or suffers from night sweats, it is often a sign of an imbalance in the hypothalamus or adrenal glands. Sage is a good remedy for reducing excessive perspiration. It needs to be taken as a cold decoction or a capsule because a hot tea of sage increases perspiration. *Adaptogen Formulas* or herbs like atractylodes or lycium may also be helpful. Chlorophyll, while not reducing perspiration, can be helpful in reducing odor associated with perspiration.

> **Formulas: Chinese Qi and Blood Tonic, Chinese Fire-Increasing**, Chinese Water-Increasing, and Hot Flash
>
> **Herbs:** Atractylodes, lycium, **sage**, and **schisandra**
>
> **Supplements:** Chlorophyll
>
> **Essential Oils:** Cypress

Pertussis
Whooping Cough

See also cough (spastic)

Pertussis is a contagious bacterial infection, usually seen in children, marked by a spasmodic cough. It is also called whooping cough. It is one of the diseases children are inoculated against with the DPT shot, so outbreaks are now fairly rare. There are outbreaks from time-to-time, however, even in vaccinated children.

Herbs used traditionally to treat this condition include garlic, wild cherry, elecampane, thyme, and rosemary. Because the cough associated with this disease is often spastic, antispasmodic herbs like lobelia, khella, or blue vervain can also be helpful. You can also diffuse essential oils for the lungs into the room, especially those that have an antispasmodic effect. Inducing perspiration using the *Sweat Bath* strategy and perhaps clearing the colon with an enema (see *Colon Hydrotherapy* strategy) will also be helpful in promoting rapid recovery.

> **Strategies:** Colon Hydrotherapy and Sweat Bath
>
> **Formulas: Stabilized Allicin** and Antispasmodic
>
> **Herbs:** Black cohosh, **cherry**, elecampane, **garlic**, grindelia, khella, licorice, **lobelia**, marshmallow, oregano, pleurisy, **red clover**, rosemary, rosemary, skunk cabbage, thyme, and **vervain (blue)**
>
> **Supplements: Nanoparticle silver, vitamin A**, vitamin C, and **vitamin D**
>
> **Essential Oils:** Cypress, eucalyptus, helichrysum, oregano, pine, ravensara, rosemary, and thyme

Pet Supplements

Pets can benefit from herbs and nutritional supplements too. Here are some basic suggestions.

Many pet owners add liquid chlorophyll to the drinking water of their pets. Chlorophyll is found in green plants and is nature's blood cleanser for animals. It helps red blood cells take up oxygen and supports the immune system. It also aids digestion and deodorizes the body. Taken daily, it will help prevent halitosis, reduce body odors, and dispel gas.

Animals need good fats in their diet, so omega-3 fatty acids or flax seed oil can be a good supplement for your pet. Good fats will help maintain healthy skin and bones and protects cell membranes form oxidative damage. They also support the immune system, helping your pet resist inflammation and arthritis.

The *Mineral Rich Herbs Formula* was originally designed as an herbal supplement for pet health. Simply empty the capsules and mix the powder with the animal's food.

A good supplement for your pet's immune system is a mixture of goldenseal, echinacea, and garlic powders in equal parts. Just mix the powders with their food. This strengthens the immune system, promotes gastrointestinal health, and prevents parasites and infections.

One of the big problems pets often have is parasites. Pets can have both external and internal parasites, the most common being fleas, lice, ear mites, fly larvae, ticks, and giardia. Prevention is the best treatment. To avoid topical parasites, treat injuries properly. Regular grooming will reveal the occasional hitchhiker, especially ticks. Keeping a clean environment for your pet, provide fresh drinking water everyday, and give them clean food to help prevent internal parasites.

Artemesia, black walnut, and garlic have all been used for getting rid of amoebas, tapeworm, and other parasites of the respiratory, digestive, and intestinal system. *Antiparasitic Formulas* containing these herbs can be used for dogs and cats as well as people. Just mix the antiparasitic formula or herbs with the animal's food. If you have pets in your household, it is probably a good idea to give *Antiparasitic Formulas* not only to your pets but also to everyone in the family twice a year.

To repel fleas you can use add essential oils like lemongrass, citronella, geranium, or peppermint to the *Enzyme Spray Formula* and spray this on the pet's fur. The *Enzyme Spray Formula* is a handy product to have around for pets in general as it helps remove odors and stains.

Generally speaking, most dogs and cats will respond to the same remedies you use for human beings, but I recommend getting a book specifically about treating animals with herbs for more information on this topic.

Strategies: Friendly Flora, Healthy Fats, and Mineralization

Formulas: Pet Supplement, Stabilized Allicin, **Antiparasitic, Enzyme Spray**, and Colloidal Mineral

Herbs: Echinacea, flax seed oil, garlic, goldenseal, neem, and wormwood

Supplements: Chlorophyll, Co-Q10, collagen, **nanoparticle silver**, and **omega-3 EFAs**

Essential Oils: Lemongrass and peppermint

Peyronie's Disease

This disease is caused by scar tissue, called plaque, in the penis that causes it to be bent rather than straight when erect. It may make sex painful or contribute to erectile dysfunction. The condition often improves without treatment, so doctors often suggest waiting one to two years or longer before they try to correct it.

Remedies that aid circulation such as acetyl-l-carnitine and Co-Q10 have proven helpful for some men. The *Oral Chelation* and *Caster Oil Pack* strategies may also be helpful.

Strategies: Castor Oil Pack and Oral Chelation

Formulas: Oral Chelation and Nitric Oxide Boosting

Herbs: Gotu kola

Supplements: Bromelain, **Co-Q10**, L-arginine, **L-carnitine**, and vitamin E

Essential Oils: Ylang ylang

Phlebitis

See also varicose veins

Phlebitis is inflammation of a vein, usually in the legs. A *Vein Tonic Formula* containing butcher's broom and/or horse chestnut can be very helpful. It is also important to use fat-soluble vitamins like vitamin E. A decoction of oak bark or another astringent can be applied topically using the *Compress or Fomentation* strategy to reduce the inflammation.

Strategies: Compress or Fomentation

Formulas: Vein Tonic and Anti-Inflammatory Pain

Herbs: Butcher's broom, capsicum, **horse chestnut**, and white oak

Supplements: Lecithin and **vitamin E**

Essential Oils: Helichrysum, lavender, and lemon

Phobias

See also fear and anxiety disorders

A phobia is an excessive, unreasonable desire to avoid something because of fear that is not actually dangerous. When this fear is beyond control and interferes with daily life, the phobia becomes an anxiety disorder. Some form of counseling or therapy will probably be necessary to help overcome a phobia, but there are some herbs and supplements that may aid the process.

For starters, flower essences can be helpful for dealing with phobias and other fears. Mimulus is a basic flower essence for fears of specific things, while aspen is helpful for generalized fear. The *Fear-Reducing FE Blend* contains both.

As with other anxiety disorders, adaptogens, an *Adrenal Glandular Formula,* and/or the *Anti-Stress B-Complex Formula* may be helpful for feeding the nervous system and reducing levels of anxiety.

Strategies: Counseling or Therapy, Emotional Healing Work, and Flower Essence

Formulas: Adrenal Glandular, Chinese Fire-Increasing, Anti-Anxiety, and **Anti-Stress B-Complex**

Flower Essence Blends: Shock and Injury FE and **Fear-Reducing FE**

Herbs: Licorice and vervain (blue)

Supplements: Vitamin B-complex and vitamin C

Piles   **see** *hemorrhoids*

Pimples   **see** *acne*

Pin Worms   **see** *parasites (nematodes, worms)*

Pink Eye   **see** *conjunctivitis*

Pleurisy

Pleurisy is inflammation of the tissues that cover the lungs and line the thoracic cavity, creating painful and difficult breathing, cough, and collection of fluid or fibrous tissue in the thoracic cavity. The herb pleurisy root is a specific for this problem. Lobelia and various expectorant and decongestant herbs may also be helpful.

Formulas: Lung Moistening and Antioxidant

Herbs: Cherry, coltsfoot, fenugreek, **lobelia**, marshmallow, **pleurisy**, and yarrow

Supplements: MSM and vitamin C

Essential Oils: Thyme

PMS

See also dysmenorrhea, menstrual cramps, and menorrhagia

PMS is an abbreviation for premenstrual syndrome and is not a specific ailment. A *syndrome* is a collection of symptoms with multiple causes. Premenstrual Syndrome includes over one hundred and fifty signs and symptoms that women may experience during the latter half of their menstrual cycle.

Four major types of PMS were identified by Dr. Guy Abraham, MD, a research gynecologist and endocrinologist who also pioneered the use of nutrients for PMS. This model helps to break down this very complex problem, making it easier to identify possible nutrients, herbs, and therapies that may be helpful.

Here are the four major types. PMS type A involves high estrogen and low progesterone. PMS type D involves high progesterone and low estrogen. PMS type C involves food cravings and PMS type H involves bloating and swelling.

Two other minor PMS types have also been identified by some. The first is PMS type S, which involves skin problems associated with the menstrual cycle and the second is PMS type P which involves pain or cramping prior to the period. A woman may have a mixture of PMS symptoms, meaning her symptoms may be a blend of more than one type.

In working with PMS, start by simply adopting a healthier diet and lifestyle. Many women experience improvement by just taking magnesium and vitamin B_6. Getting more omega-3 essential fatty acids and less omega-6 essential fatty acids (see the *Healthy Fats* strategy) has also helped many women. Others have benefited from the GLA found in evening primrose oil.

If these basic remedies don't work for you, then read about the various PMS types that follow. Figure out which type or combination of types you are and try some of the more specific remedies. You can also review related conditions like *dysmenorrhea* (painful periods), *menorrhagia* (heavy menstrual bleeding), and *menstrual cramps* for other ideas on natural therapies to balance out the cycle.

Strategies: Avoid Xenoestrogens, Emotional Healing Work, Healthy Fats, Liver Detoxification, and Reduce Chemical Exposure

Formulas: Chinese Wood-Increasing, GLA Oil, Female Cycle, and **Female Tonic**

Herbs: Black cohosh, blue cohosh, **chaste tree**, and peony

Supplements: Magnesium, omega-3 EFAs, omega-6 GLA, vitamin B_6, and vitamin E

PMS Type A

See also PMS, anger (excessive), and methylation (under)

PMS type A is characterized by high levels of estrogen and low levels of progesterone. This is the most common PMS imbalance, affecting about 80 percent of women with PMS.

The *A* stands for *anxiety*, because one of the major symptoms with this hormonal imbalance is nervous tension or anxiety. Emotional sensitivity is also common with this PMS type, which may also involve mood swings and irritability. The moodiness and anger associated with this PMS type is what most PMS jokes center on.

Excessive levels of estrogen in relationship to progesterone cause an increase in levels of adrenaline, noradrenaline, and serotonin, while the levels of dopamine and phenylethylamine drop. This is what causes the feelings of irritability and nervousness. Too much estrogen also seems to interfere with vitamin B_6, which is instrumental in many important functions of the body, including maintaining normal blood sugar levels and stabilizing one's moods. Another problem that can happen with excessive estrogen is heavy menstrual bleeding.

This type of PMS often involves congestion in the liver, which helps keep hormones in balance by breaking them down when they are no longer needed. Overconsumption of sugar and other simple carbohydrates, foods fried in refined vegetable oils, excessive exposure to chemical additives, and consumption of alcohol may all contribute to this liver congestion. Eating more dark, leafy green vegetables and fresh berries and taking the *Chinese Wood-Decreasing Formula* may be helpful in easing this congestion.

Xenoestrogens, chemical compounds that mimic estrogen, may also tip the balance of estrogenic activity and progesterone. Read how to avoid these endocrine disruptors in the *Avoid Xenoestrogens* strategy. You can also help the liver eliminate excessive estrogens (natural or chemical) by eating more cruciferous vegetables (like broccoli, cauliflower, or cabbage) and/or taking indole-3 carbinol.

Two herbs that are particularly helpful for this PMS type are chaste tree and false unicorn. Chaste tree seems to help balance progesterone and estrogen naturally, while false unicorn seems to tip the hormonal balance toward progesterone. *The Female Cycle Formula* contains chaste tree. Progesterone creams could also be used during the latter half of the cycle to help balance the hormones.

See *PMS* for additional suggestions.

Strategies: Avoid Xenoestrogens, Healthy Fats, Liver Detoxification, and Stress Management

Formulas: Blood Purifier, **Chinese Wood-Decreasing**, Anti-Anxiety, Detoxifying, and **Female Cycle**

Essential Oil Blends: Menopause Support EO

Herbs: Angelica, black currant, chamomile, **chaste tree**, evening primrose, and **false unicorn**

Supplements: Indole-3-carbinol, **magnesium**, and **vitamin B_6**

Essential Oils: Chamomile (Roman), geranium, and lavender

PMS Type C

See also hypoglycemia and PMS

Blood sugar levels tend to fall naturally during the latter half of the menstrual cycle (between ovulation and the onset of menses), but in this type the reaction is more pronounced. The drop in blood sugar (a hypoglycemic reaction) results in food cravings, particularly for carbohydrates. Thus PMS type C is named for these cravings for excessive amounts of sugary sweets. Other symptoms that can occur with this type include weight gain, fatigue, headaches, dizziness, and heart palpitations, which may involve low levels of prostaglandin 1 (PGE1).

Magnesium levels are often low in type C. Chocolate is a good source of magnesium and the cravings for chocolate many women experience with PMS may be a sign of low blood sugar coupled with magnesium deficiency. Many women have found their cravings for chocolate subside when they increase their magnesium intake. Of course, there is nothing wrong with eating a little dark chocolate either.

Working with PMS type C requires increasing protein and good fats to stabilize blood sugar levels, while reducing the intake of simple carbohydrates. Vitamin B_6, zinc, and chromium are also helpful for this type as they help to balance serotonin levels as well as blood sugar and insulin. Licorice root may also be helpful for curbing sugar cravings. See *hypoglycemia* for more suggestions on balancing blood sugar.

Strategies: Avoid Sugar and Low-Glycemic Diet

Formulas: Algae and Chinese Yin-Increasing

Herbs: Cocoa, dandelion, evening primrose, **licorice**, and milk thistle

Supplements: Chromium, L-glutamine, magnesium, omega-3 EFAs, vitamin B-complex, vitamin B_6, and zinc

Essential Oils: Ylang ylang

PMS Type D

See also depression and PMS

PMS type D is caused by the opposite hormonal imbalance to PMS type A. In this case progesterone levels are too high in relationship to estrogen. In balance, progesterone has a calming effect on a woman, but when progesterone is in excess, it can act as a depressant to the brain. Thus, the *D* stands for *depression*. It can also stand for drama, which can also be seen in this type. The drama is characterized by alternating moods of depression, anxiety, and rage—coupled with confusion, forgetfulness, crying easily, and being accident-prone. High progesterone will also cause scanty menstruation.

Exercise is very important for PMS type D. At the very least talk a walk every day for twenty to thirty minutes. Foods rich in phytoestrogens can also be helpful, which include dark green leafy vegetables, whole grains, and beans. Black cohosh can be helpful for balancing this PMS type and can be used as a single tincture in doses of five to fifteen drops two or three times per day. The two *Female Tonic Formulas* which feature black cohosh as a primary ingredient can also be used. The *Chinese Qi-Regulating Formula*, which helps lift depression, may also be helpful. Magnesium and vitamin B_6 are also important supplements for this type.

Strategies: Aromatherapy

Formulas: Hot Flash, **Chinese Qi-Regulating**, and **Female Tonic**

Herbs: Black cohosh, cocoa, and Saint John's wort

Supplements: Magnesium, SAM-e, and **vitamin B_6**

Essential Oils: Bergamot, clary sage, lavender, and **rose**

PMS Type H

See also edema and PMS

Some women experience water retention during PMS, which is believed to be caused by too much aldosterone, a hormone produced by the adrenal glands. The *H* stands for *hyperhydration*, a term which represents the abdominal bloating and breast swelling and tenderness found in this type. There may also be high levels of estrogen and low levels of magnesium.

Reducing salt consumption and increasing potassium-rich foods such as bananas and other fresh fruits and vegetables will be helpful. The *Chinese Water-Decreasing Formula* or any other *Diuretic Formula* can be helpful for reducing the excess fluid.

Formulas: Chinese Water-Decreasing, Liquid Kidney, Liquid Lymph, and **Diuretic**

Herbs: Dandelion leaf, evening primrose, juniper, **nettle, and stinging leaf**

Supplements: Magnesium, potassium, vitamin B_6, and vitamin E

Essential Oils: Frankincense and lemon

PMS Type P

See also dysmenorrhea

P is for pain. Pain associated with menstruation is called dysmenorrhea. Try using the *Antispasmodic Formula* and/or magnesium supplements. Ginger can be used to enhance pelvic circulation when the pain is congestive. See *dysmenorrhea* for more options.

Formulas: Antispasmodic

Herbs: Ginger, **kava kava**, and lobelia

Supplements: Magnesium

PMS Type S

See also acne, adrenal fatigue, and skin problems

S is for *skin*. Some women get outbreaks of acne due to high levels of androgens, which are a side effect of stress. Chronic stress will eventually fatigue the adrenal glands. Exhausted adrenal glands are aggravated by animal fats and dairy products. Eat more green leafy vegetables, vegetable proteins, and fruit. A colon and liver cleanse would add vital energy to the body and clear the skin. A *Blood Purifier Formula* or the *Ayurvedic Skin Healing Formula* may help to clear the skin. Decrease nicotine, caffeine, sugar, and salt consumption.

Strategies: Avoid Caffeine, Avoid Sugar, and Detoxification

Formulas: Blood Purifier, Adrenal Glandular, **Ayurvedic Skin Healing**, and Liquid Lymph

Herbs: Black currant, **burdock**, **dandelion**, and **red clover**

Supplements: Vitamin B-complex and vitamin C

Pneumonia

Pneumonia is a disease of the lungs characterized by inflammation and fluid accumulation, usually caused by infection. Seek appropriate medical assistance, especially when pneumonia occurs in the elderly.

Pneumonia is usually caused by a viral or a bacterial infection, so antiviral or antibacterial remedies like garlic, either raw or in the *Stabilized Allicin Formula*, nanoparticle silver, and andrographis will help clear the infection.

However, it's more important to use herbs that decongest the lungs and expel the mucus and fluids. A good basic program is four capsules of *Jeannie Burgess' Allergy-Lung Formula* along with one tablet of *Stabilized Allicin Formula* every two to four hours until the lungs clear.

It's common for elderly people to develop pneumonia after the death of their spouse as grief adversely affects the lungs. The *Grief and Sadness FE Blend* or the *Lung-Supporting EO Blend* can be helpful when the disease is associated with the recent loss of loved ones.

Strategies: Colon Hydrotherapy

Formulas: Jeannie Burgess' Allergy-Lung, **Stabilized Allicin**, Chinese Metal-Decreasing, Ayurvedic Bronchial Decongestant, and Immune-Boosting

Essential Oil Blends: Lung-Supporting EO

Flower Essence Blends: Grief and Sadness FE

Herbs: Andrographis, **cherry**, **garlic**, licorice, lobelia, lomatium, olive, **osha**, pleurisy, quince (Bengal), usnea, and yarrow

Supplements: N-acetyl cysteine, **nanoparticle silver**, omega-3 EFAs, vitamin C, and zinc

Essential Oils: Lemon

Poison Ivy/Oak

See also dermatitis and rashes & hives

Certain plants cause a mild to severe contact allergic reaction when touched, such as poison ivy or poison oak. This is known as contact dermatitis. Symptoms of this allergic reaction may include mild to severe redness, rash, itching, burning, and/or oozing blisters.

When exposed to these plants, wash the skin immediately with plenty of soap and water as soon as possible after contact. One can then apply herbs topically to reduce swelling and inflammation. Jewelweed, which is not sold commercially but often grows near these plants in the Eastern United States, is one of the best remedies for poison ivy or oak.

Other possible remedies include plantain, uva ursi, yerba santa, grindelia (gumweed), and aloe vera. Almost any astringent herb will be helpful. Crush the fresh plants and apply them using the *Poultice* strategy or make an infusion or decoction and apply them using the *Compress or Fomentation* strategies.

Internally, vitamin C, and *Blood Purifier Formulas* containing burdock, yellow dock, or red clover may be helpful. If you are hypersensitive to these plants, try using homeopathic poison ivy (*Rhus tox*) to desensitize the body.

Strategies: Compress or Fomentation and Poultice

Formulas: Blood Purifier and Detoxifying

Herbs: Aloe vera, black walnut, burdock, collinsonia, ginseng (American), ginseng (Asian/Korean), **grindelia**, honeysuckle, lobelia, **plantain**, red clover, **uva ursi**, white oak, yellow dock, and yerba santa

Supplements: Vitamin A, vitamin C, and vitamin D

Essential Oils: Tea tree

Poisoning

See also food poisoning

There are numerous toxic substances that can accidentally be inhaled, ingested, or absorbed through the skin. Call a poison control center near you for help with any kind of acute poisoning.

Activated charcoal absorbs many toxins, and milk thistle helps protect the liver against many toxins. It's a good item to keep in your herbal first aid kit. For some toxins, lobelia or ipecac can be taken to induce vomiting. These and other remedies that may help, but always contact a poison control center for advice before treatment.

Formulas: Hepatoprotective and Detoxifying

Herbs: Lobelia and **milk thistle**

Supplements: Charcoal, chlorophyll, and vitamin C

Polycystic Ovarian Syndrome
PCOS

See also metabolic syndrome

Polycystic ovary syndrome is a hormonal imbalance that women can get during their childbearing years. It is usually related to metabolic syndrome and high insulin levels, which throw female hormones out of balance. It may involve cysts on the ovaries, but this is not always the case. It's primary symptoms are darkened skin or excess skin (skin tags) on the neck or in the armpits, mood changes, pain in the pelvic area, and weight gain. It may also cause acne and unwanted facial hair. The primary way to treat it is to get blood sugar under control (see *metabolic syndrome*).

Women with PCOS should also avoid xenoestrogens and sugar and consume healthy fats. Soy should be avoided. B-complex vitamins and formulas to aid liver detoxification may also be helpful.

Strategies: Avoid Sugar, Avoid Xenoestrogens, and Healthy Fats

Formulas: Blood Sugar Control, Detoxifying, and Liver Cleanse

Programs: Chinese Balanced Cleansing

Herbs: Chaste tree, cinnamon, and fenugreek

Supplements: Omega-3 EFAs

Polyps

A polyp is a projecting mass of swollen, overgrown, or tumorous tissue, usually found in the nasal cavity or intestine. They are benign (noncancerous) growths. Natural healers typically view polyps as a toxic condition in the body and use blood purifiers to clean up the system. Internally, consider using a *Blood Purifier* or *Detoxifying Formula* containing herbs like burdock, pau d'arco, and red clover. Also consider using the *Detoxification* strategy.

Bayberry is an astringent and can be used to shrink polyps. For nasal polyps make some of *Steven Horne's Sinus Snuff Powder* using and snuffing it up the nose once or twice daily.

Strategies: Detoxification

Formulas: Chinese Wood-Increasing, Blood Purifier, **Detoxifying**, and **Steven Horne's Sinus Snuff**

Herbs: Aloe vera, **bayberry**, burdock, **goldenseal**, pau d'arco, and red clover

Supplements: Vitamin A, vitamin B_9, vitamin C, and vitamin D

Postpartum Depression

See also depression

After a mother gives birth, she faces a lot of new challenges. There are new responsibilities and a loss of sleep from waking up to care for the newborn baby. Hormone levels are higher when a woman is pregnant and fall soon after childbirth. These are possible reasons that a mother may become depressed after giving birth. Many women experience a mild depression, the "baby blues," which typically resolves itself in a week or two, but other women experience clinical depression.

Symptoms of postpartum depression include feelings of sadness and loss of hope, feeling unable to care for the baby, crying a lot for no apparent reason, sleeping too much, or loss of interest in things the mother normally enjoys. This may also interfere with the mother's ability to bond with her baby.

Medical treatment for postpartum depression includes counseling and antidepressant medications. From a natural perspective, counseling can be very helpful in dealing with the stress or emotional issues surrounding being a mother, and things like surrounding yourself with people who care, getting some exercise, and making time for having some fun can also be helpful.

Black cohosh has been helpful for women with postpartum depression where they feel trapped or have a sensation of having a "dark cloud" over them. It can be used in drop doses as a tincture or as a flower essence. The *Chinese Qi-Regulating Formula* might also be a helpful. Mariposa flower essence can also be used to aid mother-infant bonding. If depression is severe, seek professional help.

Strategies: Emotional Healing Work and Flower Essence

Formulas: Female Tonic, **Chinese Qi-Regulating**, and Chinese Wood-Increasing

Herbs: Black cohosh, **blessed thistle**, and partridge berry

Supplements: Vitamin B_3

Essential Oils: Jasmine

Postpartum Weakness

The following may be safely used to help a woman gain strength after giving birth.

Strategies: Sitz Bath

Formulas: Antioxidant, **Mitochondria Energy**, Colloidal Mineral, Christopher's Herbal Iron, and **Whole Food Green Drink**

Supplements: Chlorophyll and vitamin C

Posttraumatic Stress Disorder   see *PTSD*

Preeclampsia
Toxemia

See also pregnancy

Formerly known as toxemia, preeclampsia is a disorder that occurs only during pregnancy and the period after delivery, known as the postpartum period. It typically occurs during the second and third trimesters and can last until six weeks after delivery. Occurring in about 5 percent of pregnancies, it is most common in first-time pregnancies.

Symptoms include an increase in blood pressure, leakage of albumin into the urine, edema, headaches, and changes in vision, although some women with this disorder experience few symptoms, making proper prenatal care essential to preventing or diagnosing preeclampsia. Appropriate medical attention should be sought for this potentially serious condition, which is the leading cause of maternal and infant death worldwide.

A healthy diet and supplement program during pregnancy will reduce the risk of preeclampsia. See *pregnancy* for suggestions.

If a woman develops preeclampsia, bed rest is typically recommended, and sometimes medication. Utah midwives have used alterative teas like red clover and burdock to aid recovery. Other possible remedies are listed below, but these should be used only in conjunction with proper medical care.

Strategies: Drawing Bath and Hydration

Formulas: Blood Purifier, **Detoxifying**, Antioxidant, Chinese Wood-Decreasing, and Hepatoprotective

Programs: Ivy Bridge's Cleansing and **Chinese Balanced Cleansing**

Herbs: Aloe vera, **burdock**, **milk thistle**, pau d'arco, and **red clover**

Supplements: Chlorophyll, MSM, and **vitamin C**

Pregnancy

See also labor & delivery and avoid during pregnancy

During pregnancy, a woman needs the nutrients necessary to form two extra pounds of uterine muscle, several pounds of amniotic fluid, and the placenta. She also experiences a 50 percent increase in blood volume, and her liver and kidney cells need to process the waste from two living beings—all in addition to forming the bones, muscles, skin, glands, nervous system and other vital organs of her developing child.

This means her body will require larger-than-normal amounts of protein, good fats, vitamins, and minerals—nutrients she isn't going to get from eating a diet of refined and processed foods. Here are some basic guidelines to follow.

Get Good Protein

Adequate intake of protein is essential to a healthy pregnancy. It is a good idea to use meat, eggs, and dairy products from pasture raised animals, preferably organic to avoid chemicals. For vegetarians or vegans, use a good protein powder.

A great meal replacement is the *Whole Food Green Drink Formula*. Try mixing it with pineapple juice. Many women have found it very helpful for extra nutrition during pregnancy. Another good meal replacement is the *Green Food Protein Powder* (listed under *Whole Food Protein*).

Eat Good Fats

Good fats are a must for pregnancy, as a developing child's brain and nervous system need essential fatty acids. Supplementing with omega-3 fatty acids has been shown to reduce the risk of developing preeclampsia, postpartum depression, and preterm labor. Deep-ocean fish (especially sardines), walnuts, flaxseeds, hemp seeds, avocados, coconut oil, and organic butter from grass-fed cows are also great sources of good fats for pregnancy (see the *Healthy Fats* strategy).

Use Supplements

Traditional cultures used special foods for pregnant women to ensure healthy babies. Supplements can do the same for modern pregnant women. Megadoses of vitamins and minerals aren't wise, but a good prenatal vitamin and mineral supplement can be beneficial. These contain essential nutrients for energy and basic health during pregnancy, such as 800 mg of folic acid (as 5MTHF or methylfolate), which is essential in the prevention of neural tube defects.

Herbs for Pregnancy

Many women have found herbs to be helpful during pregnancy, both in reducing problems like morning sickness and also in preparing the body for childbirth. Red raspberry is a traditional uterine tonic and is typically taken as a tea. The *Pregnancy Tea Formula* is easy to make and very helpful for most pregnant women. Prepare the tea by steeping three to four heaping tablespoons of this mixture in a quart of boiling water for about one hour. Drink a quart each day. An alternative is to use *Joan Patton's Herbal Minerals Formula*.

There are also herbs that should be avoided during pregnancy. They are listed under *pregnancy, remedies to avoid*.

Iron for Pregnancy

Iron levels often fall during pregnancy. Eating dark-green leafy vegetables, organic red meat, and the pregnancy tea mentioned above can keep iron levels normal during pregnancy. Consider supplementing with *Christopher's Herbal Iron Formula* or two to four capsules of yellow dock in addition to the pregnancy tea if iron levels fall. See *anemia* for more suggestions.

Emotional Support

Mental and emotional factors are also important during pregnancy. The baby picks up on the mother's emotions and mood. Keeping a positive attitude about life and minimizing stress during this time helps ensure a healthy pregnancy and a calmer baby after birth. The *Flower Essence* and *Stress Management* strategies are helpful here.

Strategies: Affirmation and Visualization, Bone Broth, Eat Healthy, Flower Essence, Healthy Fats, Mineralization, and Stress Management

Formulas: Watkin's Hair, Skin, and Nails, **Christopher's Herbal Iron**, **Prenatal Support**, **Colloidal Mineral**, Antioxidant, **Whole Food Green Drink**, Algae, **Methylated B Vitamin**, **Pregnancy Tea**, **Joan Patton's Herbal Minerals**, and **Whole Food Protein**

Herbs: Alfalfa, blessed thistle, dulse, kelp, **nettle, stinging**, **red raspberry**, and yellow dock

Supplements: **Calcium**, chlorophyll, iron, **magnesium**, **multiple vitamin and mineral**, **omega-3 EFAs**, and **vitamin B$_9$**

Essential Oils: Marjoram and myrrh

Pregnancy, Remedies to Avoid

During pregnancy, it is important to avoid taking any herb or supplement that might adversely affect the pregnancy. The most important herbs to avoid are those that have potential abortifacient properties. These include blue cohosh, pennyroyal, and cotton root, along with all strong antiparasitics, like anamu, wormwood, tansy, pawpaw, and thuja.

Herbs that have strong effects on a woman's hormonal system should also be avoided, such as black cohosh, partridge berry, and dong quai. Substances that raise estrogen levels should also be avoided, such as DHEA. I have highlighted all these remedies in the list below.

Since many of these substances are especially harmful during the first trimester, it is wise to avoid them when a woman is trying to conceive as well. Some herbs such as blue cohosh and black cohosh may be safe to use to help induce or aid labor after the due date.

Many of the other herbs and supplements on this list may be problematic in pregnancy, but have been used safely by some women to address specific health concerns. These remedies are the ones that are not highlighted. For example, stimulant laxatives and herbal cleansing programs are generally not recommended during pregnancy. If these herbs are a small part of an herbal formula they will likely be safe during pregnancy.

The following is a list of remedies to avoid during pregnancy. Only use these remedies during pregnancy under the guidance of a professional herbalist or naturopath (findanherbalist.com or americanherbalistsguild.com).

Again, the following is a list of remedies to *avoid* during pregnancy, not a list of remedies to use during pregnancy.

Formulas: **Antiparasitic**, **Standardized Acetogenin**, 5-HTP Adaptogen, Prebirth, Adaptogen-Immune, **Chrisopher's Menopause**, **Hot Flash**, Green Tea Polyphenols, Brain Calming, Metabolic Stimulant, **Female Tonic**, Anti-Snoring, Gut Immune, **DHEA with Herbs**, Heavy Metal Cleansing, and Women's Aphrodisiac

Programs: Parasite Cleansing

Herbs: Angelica, **arnica**, barberry, **black cohosh**, black walnut, blessed thistle, **blue cohosh**, borage, buchu, buckthorn, butternut, cascara sagrada, cat's claw, **chaparral**, **comfrey**, cordyceps, cramp bark, damiana, dong quai, elecampane, eleuthero, fenugreek, feverfew, gentian, goldenseal, guggul, horehound, hyssop, licorice, mistletoe, motherwort, myrrh, osha, **pawpaw**, rosemary, sage, saw palmetto, **thuja**, thyme, wood betony, and **wormwood**

Supplements: 5-HTP, 7-keto, **DHEA**, GABA, melatonin, and SAM-e

Essential Oils: Jasmine

Premature Ejaculation

See also erectile dysfunction

Men who experience problems with premature ejaculation may benefit from taking herbs to balance male reproductive hormones, such as maca, damiana, or ginseng. The *Chinese Water-Increasing* and *Fire-Increasing Formulas* may be helpful for some men. It's also wise to follow the *Avoid Xenoestrogens* strategy.

This problem is often due to stress and tension and the inability to relax. If this is the case, adaptogens and nervines along with the *Stress Management* strategy will be helpful. A strategy involving *Counseling or Therapy* may also be needed, as the problem is often an expression of relationship problems.

Strategies: Avoid Xenoestrogens, Counseling or Therapy, and Stress Management

Formulas: **Chinese Water-Increasing** and Chinese Fire-Increasing

Herbs: Damiana, ginseng (Asian/Korean), **maca**, noni root, and **schisandra**

Supplements: Zinc

Progesterone, Low

See also PMS Type A

With exposure to xenoestrogens and an excess burden on the liver, many women have too much estrogen and not enough progesterone. Good reproductive health requires a balance between these two hormones.

Herbs such as sarsaparilla and false unicorn can also be used to counteract excess estrogen by enhancing progesterone. These herbs have been used to help sustain pregnancy and prevent miscarriage and to relieve heavy menstrual bleeding and cramps. Chaste tree, taken regularly for several months, can also balance out estrogen and progesterone.

Strategies: Avoid Xenoestrogens and Healthy Fats

Formulas: Female Cycle, Chrisopher's Menopause, Adrenal Glandular, and General Glandular

Herbs: Blue cohosh, **chaste tree**, **false unicorn**, and wild yam

Supplements: Magnesium

Prolapsed Colon

A falling-down or sagging of the colon from its usual position is called a prolapsed colon. This condition often involves the transverse or horizontal portion of the colon. Lying on a slant board with one's feet elevated and massaging the colon can help. An inversion table can also be helpful.

Taking a *Fiber Blend* along with a *Stimulant Laxative Formula* or *Gentle Bowel Cleansing Formula* to keep the colon working properly may help to tone the colon. Yellow dock and bayberry are specific herbs that help to tone up the bowel tissues. Vitamin C and calcium can help to build structural integrity in tissues too.

If the abdomen lacks tone and the person tends to feel discouraged or depressed, the *Chinese Qi-Regulating Formula* may be helpful. It lifts the person's energy and helps tone up the internal organs.

Formulas: Intestinal Detoxification, Chinese Qi-Regulating, Gentle Bowel Cleansing, Fiber, and Stimulant Laxative

Herbs: Bayberry, red raspberry, solomon's seal, uva ursi, white oak, and **yellow dock**

Supplements: Calcium and vitamin C

Prolapsed Uterus

See also prolapsed colon

A falling-down or sagging of the uterus from its usual position is called a prolapsed uterus. It is more common after pregnancies. It may prevent conception and often puts pressure on the bladder, which may lead to incontinence.

Lying on a slant board with one's feet elevated or hanging on an inversion table while massaging the uterus can help. The *Good Posture* strategy (standing and sitting erect) is also helpful.

Red raspberry, white pond lily, and yellow dock may all be helpful in toning up the weakened tissues. The *Chinese Qi-Regulating Formula* also lifts up the body and helps with sagging internal organs. This condition may be associated with a prolapsed colon.

Strategies: Mineralization

Formulas: Chinese Qi-Regulating and UTI Prevention

Herbs: Astragalus, bayberry, black walnut, cranberry, dong quai, orange (bitter), **red raspberry**, uva ursi, white oak bark, **white pond lily**, and **yellow dock**

Supplements: Calcium, magnesium, and vitamin C

Prostate Problems   see *BPH* and *prostatitis*

Prostatitis

See also BPH

Prostatitis is inflammation of the prostate gland that causes painful urination, frequent trips to the men's room, misaim, and dribbling because the weak stream of urine is insufficient to fully open the flaps at the tip of the penis. It is sometimes due to infection but is more often due to other unknown causes.

One reason the prostate may become inflamed involves its proximity to both the bladder and the rectum. If the body is toxic, the irritants being eliminated from the colon and urinary passages may be irritating the prostate gland, causing it to swell.

If the problem is due to an acute or chronic infection, consider some herbs with natural antibacterial action, such as goldenseal or uva ursi. One can also use *Christopher's Prostate Formula* for this.

Omega-3 essential fatty acids can also reduce prostate inflammation. Eskimo men who have a fish-rich diet have significantly lower rates of prostatitis and prostate cancer than other men. Omega-3 fatty acids have also been shown to inhibit prostate cell growth and reduce prostate enlargement. They help decrease pain and fatigue, reduce nighttime urination, increase elimination (stream), and increase libido.

Zinc may also be beneficial at reducing inflammation and prostate swelling. Daily exercise to increase circulation is also beneficial for prostatitis because it increases circulation to the prostate and reduces swelling. As with all urinary problems, make sure you are adequately hydrated.

Strategies: Avoid Xenoestrogens, Detoxification, Eat Healthy, Exercise, Healthy Fats, and Hydration

Formulas: Chinese Water-Increasing, Anti-Inflammatory Pain, Antioxidant, **Chinese Water-Decreasing**, Antiparasitic, **Prostate**, and Probiotic

Herbs: Amalaki, barberry, buchu, couchgrass, **goldenseal**, **gravel root**, **hydrangea**, pumpkin seed, pygeum, saw palmetto, uva ursi, and **white sage**

Supplements: Bromelain, chondroitin, equol, nanoparticle silver, **omega-3 EFAs**, **quercetin**, and zinc

Protein Digestion, Poor

See also hiatal hernia and low stomach acid

The following help to improve protein digestion and metabolism. This is often due to a hiatal hernia or low stomach acid. People with the A blood type are prone to low stomach acid and often have a hard time digesting protein.

Formulas: Betaine HCl, **Chinese Earth-Increasing**, **Digestive Support**, and **Herbal Bitters**

Herbs: Ginseng (American) and orange (bitter)

Supplements: Pancreatin and **protease**

Psoriasis

See also eczema and leaky gut

Psoriasis differs from eczema because it involves rapid skin growth and appears to be an autoimmune disorder, like multiple sclerosis or lupus. Psoriasis primarily affects the skin, but in about 10 percent of the cases, the joints are also affected. Research suggests that psoriasis is triggered when certain T-cells reproduce very rapidly, which starts an inflammatory reaction that causes skin cells to multiply seven to twelve times faster than normal. In natural medicine this may be taking place because the skin is malnourished and weak or because of allergic reactions to food.

Because this hyperactivity of the immune system also creates a form of inflammation, psoriasis has symptoms similar to eczema. The skin is often itchy and dry and frequently cracking or blistering. Oils are needed to keep the skin moist. In particular, omega-3 essential fatty acids may be helpful.

Diet is important in the effective treatment of psoriasis. Using the *Gluten-Free Diet* strategy has also benefited some sufferers. Since food allergies are a contributing factor in psoriasis, it would also be a good idea to follow the *Eliminate Allergy-Causing Foods* strategy.

Incomplete protein digestion and bowel toxemia may be underlying factors in psoriasis. Digestive enzyme supplements, taken between meals, will help break down undigested protein and detoxify the colon. Psoriasis is often linked to leaky gut syndrome, so healing the gut can help.

Detoxifying the liver is also important. Products containing liver-protecting herbs like milk thistle and nutrients that enhance liver detoxification like N-acetyl-cysteine and detoxifying herbs like burdock and red clover can accomplish this. The *Detoxification* strategy may also be helpful.

Nutrients that have been reported helpful for psoriasis include vitamin A (in large doses of about 50,000 to 75,000 IU per day for a short time), vitamin E (400 to 800 IU per day), B-complex vitamins and vitamin B_6 in particular, vitamin C, zinc, and chromium.

Feverfew can be used both internally and topically to ease psoriasis. The polyphenols in green tea can also help to reduce irritation of the skin and ease psoriasis. Since acetogenins slow the metabolism of rapidly growing cells, one can mix the *Standardized Acetogenin Formula* into a fixed oil or a lotion made with pau d'arco and apply it topically to the skin, leaving it in place for four to eight hours.

This can be a tricky problem to overcome. You may wish to get help from a qualified herbalist or naturopath (findanherbalist.com or americanherbalistsguild.com).

Strategies: Detoxification, Eliminate Allergy-Causing Foods, and Healthy Fats

Formulas: Blood Purifier, Detoxifying, Liver Cleanse, GLA Oil, Hepatoprotective, **Green Tea Polyphenols**, Whole Food Green Drink, **Standardized Acetogenin**, Digestive Support, and Ayurvedic Skin Healing

Herbs: Aloe vera, amur cork, **burdock**, chamomile, chickweed, evening primrose oil, **feverfew**, flax, gotu kola, Indian madder, licorice, milk thistle, pau d'arco, **pawpaw**, psyllium, **red clover**, tea, and **turmeric**

Supplements: Chromium, MSM, N-acetyl cysteine, omega-3 DHA, omega-3 EFAs, omega-6 GLA, protease, **vitamin A**, vitamin B-complex, **vitamin B_6**, vitamin C, **vitamin D**, **vitamin E**, and zinc

Essential Oils: Cajeput, sandalwood, and thyme

PTSD

See also adrenal fatigue, stress, nervous exhaustion, anxiety disorders, and trauma

PTSD (posttraumatic stress disorder) used to be called "shell shock" or "battle fatigue." It was identified as a condition affecting soldiers who had undergone so much stress that they simply couldn't cope anymore. You don't have to have gone to war to suffer PTSD, however. Any extremely frightening, shocking, or dangerous situation that overwhelms a person's ability to cope can trigger someone into PTSD.

To be diagnosed with PTSD, one must experience four things for at least one month. First, they must be re-experiencing the traumatic situation. This can include flashbacks, bad dreams, and recurring frightening thoughts. They must also have at least one symptom of avoidance, where they are doing something to try to escape reminders of or feelings about the trauma. They must also show arousal and reactivity symptoms, which include things like being easily startled, angry outbursts, or difficulty sleeping. Finally, they must also have mood or cognitive symptoms such as distorted feelings of guilt or blame, loss of interest in enjoyable activities, and negative thoughts about themselves or life.

Children and teenagers may also develop PTSD, but their symptoms will differ. Children may be unable to talk, become excessively clingy with a parent or other adults, or struggle with bedwetting. Teenagers may develop disruptive, disrespectful, or destructive behaviors.

Not everyone who experiences a traumatic event will develop PTSD. Factors such as childhood abuse, long-term stress, or general feelings of helplessness will increase the likelihood that a traumatic event will result in PTSD. Having support from other people, feeling good about one's actions in the situation, and being able to act responsibly in the face of fear will reduce the chances of experiencing PTSD.

Medical therapy is typically medications like antidepressants and/or some form of talk therapy to help a person work through their fear and make sense of their memories. A person who has PTSD definitely needs some form of *Counseling or Therapy*. In addition to counseling, here are some natural strategies for recovery from PTSD.

Support the Adrenal Glands

PTSD often involves an extreme state of nervous exhaustion or adrenal fatigue. Hence, an *Adrenal Glandular Formula* or nourishing adaptogens like ashwagandha and holy basil may be helpful. See *adrenal fatigue* for more information.

Take CBD

Low levels of endocannabinoids have been found in people with PTSD. This suggests that the endocannabinoid system, which helps to rebalance the nervous system after a stressful event, may not be working properly. Also, people with PTSD often use cannabis (marijuana) recreationally, reporting it eases symptoms.

The problem with using marijuana, however, is that the THC it contains will decrease the number of cannabinoid receptors over time. CBD helps restore cannabinoid receptor functions and would work well especially if combined with nervine herbs to reduce feelings of stress. If a person with PTSD has been using THC-rich cannabis, CBD will also help counteract the negative effects of the THC.

Take Parasympathetic Nervines

In the stress response, the sympathetic nervous system activates. In PTSD, it appears this branch of the autonomic nervous system is hyperactive, while the parasympathetic branch, which helps a person relax, is inhibited. Nervine herbs like kava kava, motherwort, vervain, and skullcap help to activate the parasympathetic nervous system so the person can feel more relaxed. The *Anti-Anxiety Formula* may be helpful here. PTSD is considered an anxiety disorder so you may also want to read about *anxiety disorders* for more ideas.

Additional Suggestions

Moderate, nonstressful physical activities such as walking or swimming will be helpful, as will meditation, prayer, and spending time with trusted friends. The *Pleasure Prescription* is a good strategy for people with PTSD as well.

Flower essences may also be helpful. The *Shock and Injury FE Blend* can help deal with past as well as current trauma. Where the person with PTSD is using addictions to cope, the *Self-Responsibility FE Blend* will be helpful. You can also use the information under *addictions*.

Strategies: Counseling or Therapy, Emotional Healing Work, Flower Essence, Forgiveness, Hiatal Hernia Correction, Hydration, Low-Glycemic Diet, Meditation, Pleasure Prescription, and Sleep

Formulas: Adrenal Glandular, **Chinese Fire-Increasing**, Anti-Stress B-Complex, **Anti-Anxiety**, and Memory Enhancing

Flower Essence Blends: Shock and Injury FE and Self-Responsibility FE

Herbs: Ashwagandha, cannabis, eleuthero, **holy basil**, **kava kava**, motherwort, passion flower, schisandra, and **skullcap**

Supplements: CBD, GABA, lithium, **magnesium**, multiple vitamin and mineral, vitamin B-complex, and vitamin B_5

Essential Oils: Chamomile (Roman), frankincense, lavender, and ylang ylang

Puberty

See also acne, menstrual irregularity, mood swings, and sex drive (excessive)

It's no great secret that teenagers experience major hormonal changes. These changes affect not only a teen's body but also their thoughts and emotions, so it is important to talk with kids about these changes and help them through this critical time in their lives. The transition through puberty is going to be easier if children are being raised with a healthy lifestyle.

Excessive consumption of carbohydrates, especially refined sugar and white flour products, upsets hormonal balance and can contribute to teenager acne, mood swings, and other puberty related problems. It's also wise to encourage young children to avoid caffeinated sodas and especially the so-called energy drinks.

Nutritional supplements and herbs can help this transition period. A multiple vitamin and mineral is a good idea to ensure basic nutrients are present in the diet. Omega-3 fatty acids are also helpful, both for mental development and for healthy skin. *Mineral Tonic Formulas* may also be helpful for growing bones, teeth and tissues.

It's important to have teens eat a breakfast that contains protein. This has been shown to improve performance at school and keep blood sugar levels more stable. Try making a smoothie for your teens using a *Whole Food Protein*. If you can get them to drink it, try giving them the *Whole Food Green Drink Formula* mixed in pineapple or apple juice.

There are also some herbs that can be helpful. Red raspberry is a good female tonic and is safe for young women. It helps to tone the uterus and may help with periods. Chaste tree has a balancing effect on reproductive hormones and may be helpful for teenage acne and menstrual cramps in young women. See related conditions for more information on dealing with problems kids face during puberty.

Strategies: Avoid Caffeine, Avoid Sugar, Avoid Xenoestrogens, Exercise, Healthy Fats, Low-Glycemic Diet, and Mineralization

Formulas: Female Cycle, Blood Purifier, **Female Tonic**, Colloidal Mineral, **Whole Food Protein**, and Whole Food Green Drink

Herbs: Chaste tree and red raspberry

Supplements: Magnesium, multiple vitamin and mineral, **omega-3 EFAs**, and vitamin B$_6$

Puncture Wounds   **see** *tetanus* **and** *wounds & sores*

Pyorrhea   **see** *gingivitis*

Radiation

See also electromagnetic pollution

When the body is exposed to radiation, cellular DNA is damaged and a toxic condition is created in the body. X-rays, radon, microwave ovens, radar, and radiation treatments for cancer are among the ways the body can be exposed to radiation. There is also some concern over cell phone radiation, especially with the high cell phone use by young people. This is discussed in the *Reduce EMF Pollution* strategy.

One of the most important supplements to take when one has been or will be exposed to actual nuclear radiation is iodine, as it protects the thyroid against radioactive iodine. If you're into emergency preparedness, an iodine supplement, such as Lugol's solution or Iororal® is a good thing to keep with in your emergency supplies.

Radiation of all kinds, not just nuclear, has the potential to cause free radical damage, so antioxidants are helpful in reducing problems from radiation exposure. Algae and seaweeds have been shown to have protective effects against radiation.

If a person is undergoing radiation treatments for cancer, they should consider taking an *Algae Formula* and the *Chinese Qi and Blood Tonic* to reduce the damage these treatments can cause to healthy tissue. It's also a good idea to take these supplements if you work around any potential source of radiation or electromagnetic pollution. See *electromagnetic pollution* for more information.

Strategies: Eat Healthy and Reduce Chemical Exposure

Formulas: Gut Immune, **Algae**, Hypothyroid, Antioxidant, **Chinese Qi and Blood Tonic**, and Adaptogen

Herbs: Aloe vera, barley grass, blue-green algae, chaparral, chlorella, **codonopsis**, **dulse**, eleuthero, ginseng (American), ginseng (Asian/Korean), gynostemma, kelp, **reishi**, rhodiola, and **spirulina**

Supplements: Iodine, **sodium alginate**, vitamin A, and vitamin D

Rapid Heart Rate   **see** *tachycardia*

Rashes & Hives

See also itching and dermatitis

A rash is a skin eruption, which can be local or general. It is an inflammatory process (dermatitis) and may involve allergic reactions or toxicity. Symptoms include redness, swelling, itching, burning and sometimes blisters.

The *Drawing Bath* strategy is very helpful in easing rashes and hives. It can soothe the irritated skin and reduce itching. Any of the following could be used in the bath: chickweed (good for itching), comfrey (healing and soothing to the skin), marshmallow (soothing), or seaweeds like kelp (soothing and nourishing to the skin).

Also consider topical applications of herbs like aloe vera, chickweed, and burdock that soothe irritated skin. Internally, *Blood Purifier* or *Detoxifying Formulas*, containing herbs like burdock, Oregon grape, pau d'arco, and yellow dock, have been traditionally used to clear up skin conditions. A particularly good formula for skin problems is the *Ayurvedic Skin Healing Formula*.

CBD may have beneficial effects in calming down rashes and other skin eruptions. It can also reduce itching. It can be applied topically or taken internally. A lotion made with pau d'arco or a little rose or helichrysum essential oil, diluted in a fixed oil, can be applied topically to soothe the skin.

Strategies: Drawing Bath, Eliminate Salicylates, and Hydration

Formulas: Essiac Immune Tea, Chinese Yang-Reducing, **Enzyme Spray**, **Antihistamine**, Blood Purifier, Detoxifying, **Ayurvedic Skin Healing**, and **Chinese Wood-Decreasing**

Herbs: Aloe vera, baical skullcap, black walnut, **burdock**, chamomile, **chickweed**, dandelion, grindelia, marshmallow, mullein, **Oregon grape**, pau d'arco, polygala, turmeric, and **yellow dock**

Supplements: **CBD**, **clay (bentonite)**, clay (Redmond), manganese, **MSM**, vitamin A, and vitamin D

Essential Oils: Helichrysum, lemon, **rose**, and tea tree

Raynaud's Disease

Raynaud's disease is a vascular disorder marked by recurrent spasm of the capillaries (especially those of the fingers and toes upon exposure to cold), skin changes from white to blue to red in succession, and pain. Remedies that enhance peripheral circulation, such as capsicum, ginkgo, and prickly ash, can be helpful. Other potentially helpful remedies include turmeric, vitamin B_{12}, and magnesium.

Formulas: **Brain-Heart** and **Methyl B12 Vitamin**

Programs: Cardiovascular Nutritional

Herbs: **Astragalus**, butcher's broom, capsicum, ginger, **ginkgo**, hawthorn, lobelia, **prickly ash**, and **turmeric**

Supplements: Chlorophyll, Co-Q10, **magnesium**, vitamin B-complex, and **vitamin B_{12}**

Recuperation   see *convalescence*

Red/Itching Eyes   see *eyes (red/itching)*

Respiratory Congestion
see *congestion (lungs)*

Respiratory Infections
see *congestion (lungs)*, *infection (bacterial)*, *infection (viral)*, *pleurisy*, **and** *pneumonia*

Restless Dreams
See also adrenal fatigue

Restless and disturbing dreams are often one of the first indications that a person is under too much stress and in danger of developing enervation and adrenal burnout. Practice some of the skills listed under the *Stress Management* strategy

and take an some herbs or nutrients to help reduce the stress. The *Chinese Fire-Increasing Formula* is often very helpful. As a single herb, passion flower is very helpful in calming the mind. The flower essences of chaparral and Saint John's wort may be helpful for children (or adults) who have nightmares. It also helps to balance blood sugar using the *Low-Glycemic Diet* and to *Avoid Caffeine* strategies.

Strategies: Avoid Caffeine, Emotional Healing Work, Low-Glycemic Diet, and Stress Management

Formulas: **Adrenal Glandular**, **Chinese Fire-Increasing**, and **Anti-Stress B-Complex**

Herbs: Chamomile, lotus, and **passion flower**

Supplements: Amber (succinum) and GABA

Restless Leg
See also anemia

Restless leg syndrome is a condition where the legs itch, tickle, or burn, often at night. Moving them brings temporary relief, but the urge to move them returns seconds or minutes later. It can hinder sleep. Food allergies, mineral deficiencies, anemia, and stress could be underlying problems. Start by taking magnesium, B-complex vitamins, and some herbs to calm the nerves. If there are signs of anemia, build up the blood. Seek professional help to determine the underlying cause if symptoms persist.

Strategies: Mineralization and Stress Management

Formulas: Herbal Sleep Aid, GLA Oil, Methyl B12 Vitamin, **Methylated B Vitamin**, and Colloidal Mineral

Herbs: Kava kava, lobelia, Saint John's wort, and **skullcap**

Supplements: **Iron**, **magnesium**, **vitamin B-complex**, vitamin B_{12}, **vitamin B_9**, and vitamin E

Reversed Polarity
See also electromagnetic pollution

Reversed polarity is a problem encountered by people who do muscle testing. The energy fields of the body reverse so the "poles" are incorrect. This causes a person to test incorrectly. The *Chinese Qi and Blood Tonic* is very helpful in correcting this problem.

People with reversed polarity are attracted to negative influences and have weakened immune systems. Exposure to electromagnetic pollution (computers, microwave ovens, cell phones, etc.) is often the cause. If you work around computers and other electronic equipment or live near high-voltage power line or a power substation and feel frequently tired and drained, you may have reversed polarity. See the *Reduce Electromagnetic Exposure* strategy and the *electromagnetic pollution* condition for additional information.

Strategies: Hydration and Reduce EMF Exposure

Formulas: Chinese Qi and Blood Tonic, Jeannie Burgess' Thymus, **Chinese Qi-Regulating**, Algae, and Adaptogen

Herbs: Bee pollen, damiana, and spirulina

Reye's Syndrome

Reye's syndrome is a serious illness that occurs after a viral infection such as a cold, flu, or chicken pox. Research has linked the development of this disease to the use of aspirin and other salicylates to treat symptoms. It is important to know that natural sources of salycilates, such as willow bark, can also trigger Reye's syndrome. I do not recommend the use of herbal pain formulas containing salicylate-bearing herbs to treat symptoms of viral diseases.

In Reye's syndrome, abnormal accumulations of fat begin to develop in the liver and other organs of the body. Pressure in the brain also increases. Early diagnosis and treatment is essential, as death can occur rapidly. This disorder requires immediate medical attention. Supplements listed may be beneficial as adjuncts to medical treatment.

Formulas: Chinese Wind-Heat Evil, Gut Immune, and Antioxidant

Herbs: Cat's claw

Supplements: L-carnitine and lecithin

Rheumatic Fever

Rheumatic fever is an acute, often recurrent, disease found mainly in children and young adults. It is characterized by fever, inflammation, pain, and swelling in and around the joints. The inflammation also affects the surface and valves of the heart and may involve the formation of small nodules in the heart or other tissues. Appropriate medical assistance should be sought as this disease can damage the heart.

Garlic and Oregon grape are good remedies to help with infection. Co-Q10 and l-carnitine can help protect the heart. These should be used as adjuncts to medical treatment.

Formulas: Stabilized Allicin

Herbs: Garlic, **hawthorn**, **Oregon grape**, and passion flower

Supplements: Co-Q10, L-carnitine, and **nanoparticle silver**

Essential Oils: Peppermint

Rhinitis

See also allergies (respiratory)

Rhinitis is an inflammatory condition that affects the sensitive membranes of the nasal and sinus passages, the eyes, and the throat. In allergic rhinitis, the inflammation is caused by allergic reactions, but any irritation to the sensitive membranes of the upper respiratory passages and eyes can cause rhinitis. Whatever the cause, having congested nasal passages, a runny nose, itchy and watery eyes, and an irritated throat can make life miserable.

Here's what's happening: anytime the sensitive membranes in your upper respiratory tract are exposed to irritants, inflammation can occur. Tissues swell and mucus is secreted to try to flush the irritation away.

In most people, these symptoms include sneezing, wheezing, stuffiness, itchy and runny nose and throat, post-nasal drip, itchy and watery eyes, conjunctivitis, earaches, and insomnia. Many feel a reduced sense of taste or smell and even difficulty hearing. Others have a nasal voice, breathe noisily, or snore. Still others complain of frequent headaches and feeling chronically tired. Some people are more sensitive and will experience nasal and respiratory congestion, pain, and pressure in the face. In more severe cases, rhinitis can produce yellow or greenish discharge from the nose, a chronic cough that produces mucus, poor appetite, nausea, and sometimes a fever.

To deal with this problem, you need to identify, if possible, the source of the irritation. If the problem is an allergy, see *Allergies (Respiratory)*. In the case of non-allergic rhinitis, what we're discussing here, the irritation is usually chemical in nature. Avoid household cleaning products or other chemicals that cause respiratory irritation. People have found permanent relief just by switching to nontoxic household cleaning products.

Eyebright, nettles, and osha are herbs that can provide symptomatic relief for both allergic and non-allergic rhinitis. The *Herbal Eyewash Formula* is good for rhinitis when taken internally because of the eyebright in it. Vitamin C can break down the histamine involved in the immune reactions and reduce symptoms. You can also try using *Jeannie Burgess' Allergy-Lung Formula* to ease congestion and reduce reactions.

A very simple way to ease rhinitis is to drink lots of water and take a small amount of natural salt with it. The salt and water increase secretions of tears and mucus, which helps the body flush away irritants faster. By staying well hydrated, the body is able to keep irritants flushed away, which prevents the inflammatory reactions. It can also help to take an *Antioxidant Formula* along with the water.

For a long-term solution to rhinitis, use the *Detoxification* and *Eliminate Allergy-Causing Foods* strategies.

Strategies: Detoxification, Eliminate Allergy-Causing Foods, and Hydration

Formulas: Enzyme Spray, **Jeannie Burgess' Allergy-Lung**, Christopher's Sinus, **Antioxidant**, Anti-Inflammatory

Pain, Seasonal Cold and Flu, Steven Horne's Anti-Allergy, Herbal Eyewash, Digestive Support, and Chinese Metal-Decreasing

Herbs: Bibhitaki, burdock, butterbur, **eyebright**, holy basil, lycium, mangosteen, **nettle, stinging**, and osha

Supplements: **Quercetin** and **vitamin C**

Essential Oils: Lavender and ravensara

Ringing In Ears   see *tinnitus*

Ringworm   see *parasites (nematodes, worms)*

Rosacea

See also food allergies/intolerances, leaky gut, SIBO, and dysbiosis

Rosacea is a chronic inflammatory skin condition. It is very similar to facial acne, except that it typically appears after the age of thirty. Rosacea is usually restricted to the face but occasionally spreads to other parts of the body.

It is more commonly experienced by people with deficient amounts of hydrochloric acid and poor digestion and is directly linked to small intestinal bacterial overgrowth (SIBO), dysbiosis, and leaky gut. Red raspberry, chamomile, or feverfew can help when applied topically as a facial mask. Healthy fats, especially omega-3 fatty acids, and the fat-soluble vitamins A, D, and E may be helpful.

Strategies: Bone Broth, Eat Healthy, Eliminate Allergy-Causing Foods, Gut-Healing Diet, Healthy Fats, and Reduce Chemical Exposure

Formulas: **Betaine HCl**, Intestinal Soothing, and Digestive Support

Herbs: Alfalfa, aloe vera, **chamomile**, evening primrose, **feverfew, goldenseal**, hawthorn, and red raspberry

Supplements: Chlorophyll, **L-glutamine**, **omega-3 EFAs**, **vitamin A**, **vitamin D**, vitamin E, and **zinc**

Essential Oils: Tea tree

Runny Nose   see *congestion (sinus)*

Scabies

Scabies is caused by a mite (*Sarcoptes scabiei*) that burrows into the skin, causing itching. It is contagious and can spread quickly through close physical contact. Symptoms include itching, which is often severe and usually worse at night. There are also thin, irregular burrow tracks in the skin made up of tiny blisters or bumps. These typically occur in folds of the skin such as armpits, wrists, elbows, knees, between fingers, and so forth.

Since other conditions such as dermatitis or eczema are associated with itching and bumps on the skin, a medical diagnosis is required. If scabies is diagnosed, it is treated medically with medications that kill the mites and their eggs. It is also important to wash all clothes and linens in hot, soapy water and dry with high heat to help kill the mites.

To aid recovery, the *Standardized Acetogenin Formula*, lemon oil, tea tree oil, and/or thyme oil can be added to a shampoo or soap and used as a wash. They could also be added to a lotion and applied topically to the affected areas.

Formulas: **Standardized Acetogenin**

Herbs: Garlic, goldenseal, pau d'arco, and pawpaw

Supplements: Nanoparticle silver

Essential Oils: **Lemon**, lemongrass, **tea tree**, and **thyme**

Scars/Scar Tissue

A scar is a mark left in the skin by the healing of injured tissue. Scarring can be prevented by proper treatment of injuries. Remedies with a cicatrizant property help injuries heal without scarring. Examples include the essential oils of lavender, helichrysum, and tea tree or herbs like yarrow or calendula. To soften and aid the healing of existing scars, mix helichrysum essential oil with vitamin E and apply it to the scars. Helichrysum can also applied topically over areas of the body where there is internal scar tissue to help heal it.

Strategies: Bodywork and Compress or Fomentation

Herbs: Aloe vera, **calendula**, chamomile, and yarrow

Supplements: MSM and **vitamin E**

Essential Oils: Bergamot, chamomile (Roman), frankincense, **helichrysum**, jasmine, **lavender**, patchouli, red mandarin, rose, and tea tree

Schizophrenia

See also hypoglycemia, mental illness, trauma, and methylation (under)

Schizophrenia is a serious mental disorder characterized by loss of contact with reality and by noticeable deterioration in a person's ability to deal with ordinary life. Symptoms include hallucinations, delusions, dysfunctional ways of thinking, and agitated body movements. A person suffering from schizophrenia may have reduced feelings of pleasure, reduced emotional expression, difficulty beginning and sustaining activities, and a reduction in vocal expression with a flat tone of voice. They may also experience difficulty focusing or paying attention, making decisions, or utilizing new information.

Schizophrenia tends to run in families. No specific genetic markers for the disease have been discovered, so there may be environmental factors that trigger epigenetic changes. Possible triggering factors include viral infection, malnutrition during pregnancy, birth trauma, and social factors such as experiencing trauma or abuse in childhood. Symptoms usually start between ages sixteen and thirty, but sometimes begin in childhood.

It is generally believed that schizophrenia is due to changes in the brain and neurotransmitter function. There may be a higher level of dopamine in the brain for example. Medical treatments largely involve drugs that affect the balance of neurotransmitters, primarily antipsychotic medications, which are usually taken daily in pill or liquid form. This is usually coupled with counseling or other psychiatric therapy.

Along with using the *Counseling or Therapy* and *Emotional Healing Work* strategies, there are many natural things a person can do to help schizophrenia. Here are the basic strategies.

Adopt a Healthy Diet

Helping schizophrenia using a natural approach involves first adopting the *Healthy Diet* strategy. Many schizophrenia people have serious blood sugar imbalances. Research on the link between nutrition and mental ability has been around for a long time. Michael Lesser testified before the Senate Select Committee on Nutrition and Human Needs in the 1970s that 70 percent of all previously uncontrollable schizophrenics showed improvement when put on a diet to counter hypoglycemia. See *Avoid Sugar* and *Low-Glycemic Diet* strategies. It's also wise to avoid stimulants like caffeine. Licorice root and the *Algae Blend* can use used to help curb cravings for sugar and balance blood sugar levels. See *hypoglycemia* for more information on this problem.

Supplement the Diet

Dr. Lessor and my own experience is that schizophrenics also show improvement with vitamin supplements, particularly certain B vitamins. The *Anti-Stress B-Complex*, which also contains vitamin C is a good formula to try. Some people have also found extra niacin to be helpful.

Zinc and magnesium deficiencies are also common in people with schizophrenia. See *mental illness* for more suggestions on specific nutritional imbalances that could be involved.

Deal with Previous Trauma

As with other mental illnesses, trauma or abuse may be a factor in the development of schizophrenia and helping the person deal with these painful memories can be helpful. Flower essences may be helpful in this process. Bodywork, massage therapy, Rolfing, chiropractic, and other *Bodywork* strategies are often helpful in release trauma from the tissues. See *trauma* for more suggestions.

Don't Abruptly Discontinue Medications

If someone is on antipsychotic medications, they should not discontinue them abruptly. This can cause serious reactions in brain chemistry. If a person wishes to get off these medications, it's best to work on improving overall health and gradually back off the dose of medication under proper medical supervision.

Treat the Person with Respect

When dealing with someone who has schizophrena, remember that their beliefs or hallucinations seem very real to them. Reassure them that it is OK that they see things the way they do and be respectful, supportive, and kind. However, do not tolerate dangerous or inappropriate behavior. It is always best to work with qualified medical professionals when dealing with someone with schizophrenia.

Strategies: Avoid Caffeine, Avoid Sugar, Balance Methylation, Blood Type Diet, Bodywork, Counseling or Therapy, Emotional Healing Work, Flower Essence, and Low-Glycemic Diet

Formulas: **Anti-Stress B-Complex**, Brain Calming, Anti-Anxiety, **Methyl B12 Vitamin**, **Methylated B Vitamin**, Hypoglycemic, and Algae

Herbs: Evening primrose, licorice, and **skullcap**

Supplements: **CBD**, **GABA**, **L-glutamine**, **magnesium**, **omega-3 EFAs**, **vitamin B-complex**, **vitamin B$_{12}$**, **vitamin B$_3$**, **vitamin B$_9$**, **vitamin C**, **vitamin D**, and **zinc**

Sciatica

See also backache

Sciatica is a pain along the course of the sciatic nerve, making pain common in the lower back, buttocks, hips, and back of the thighs. This usually is isolated to one side of the body. It may involve pressure on the nerve from the hips being out of alignment. Chiropractic care and other *Bodywork* strategies can be very helpful, including the *Herbal Back Adjustment*.

In traditional Chinese medicine, the kidney energy (qi) builds the bones and structural misalignment may indicate poor kidney function. Hence, the *Hydration* strategy and a *Chinese Water-Increasing Formula* may be of help. A *Topical Analgesic Formula* or MSM may be used to help the pain.

Strategies: Bodywork, Good Posture, Herbal Back Adjustment, Hydration, and Lymph-Moving Pain Relief

Formulas: Herbal Calcium, **Chinese Water-Increasing**, Enzyme Spray, Analgesic Nerve, and Topical Analgesic

Herbs: Black cohosh, capsicum, corydalis, dogwood (Jamaican), lobelia, prickly ash, and **Saint John's wort**

Supplements: MSM

Essential Oils: Helichrysum and thyme

Scoliosis

This is a disorder where the spine is abnormally curved like an S. It may also be rotated. It can be very painful. It is due to a number of underlying causes, but the following remedies may help to strengthen the spine along with appropriate physical therapy and and the *Bodywork* strategy.

Strategies: Bodywork, Good Posture, and Herbal Back Adjustment

Formulas: Chinese Water-Increasing, Watkin's Hair, Skin, and Nails, Enzyme Spray, Colloidal Mineral, and Skeletal Support

Scratches
see *abrasions/scratches* **and** *wounds & sores*

Scrofula   **see** *tuberculosis*

Scurvy

Scurvy is a deficiency of vitamin C.

Herbs: Acerola fruit, lemon juice, and rose hips
Supplements: Vitamin C

Seasonal Affective Disorder

See also depression

Seasonal affective disorder (SAD) is a form of depression that occurs in the dark and dreary fall and winter months. It is believed to be due to a lack of exposure to natural sunlight. Full spectrum lighting is very helpful in preventing this condition, as is taking the sunshine vitamin, vitamin D_3. See *depression* for additional suggestions.

Strategies: Affirmation and Visualization, Healthy Fats, and Stress Management
Formulas: Chinese Qi-Regulating
Herbs: Lemon balm and Saint John's wort
Supplements: Omega-3 EFAs, **SAM-e**, vitamin B_5, and **vitamin D**

Seborrhea

Seborrhea is characterized by scaly patches of skin. It is caused by a disorder of the oil-producing glands. Good fats and fat-soluble vitamins may be helpful, as well as topical applications of aloe vera gel mixed with a few drops of lemon or tea tree oil.

Strategies: Aromatherapy and Healthy Fats
Formulas: GLA Oil and Skinny
Herbs: Aloe vera and burdock

Supplements: Omega-3 EFAs, **vitamin A**, and vitamin D
Essential Oils: Atlas cedarwood, **lemon**, and **tea tree**

Seizures

See also epilepsy

A seizure is a sudden convulsive attack. There is usually a clouding of consciousness involved. These are often a result of epilepsy. Seizures should be treated medically, but there are some herbs and nutrients that may be helpful as well.

GABA is a calming neurotransmitter in the brain that keeps the brain from over-firing. It may be helpful for some seizures. Passionflower and valerian affect GABA receptors. Scullcap, lobelia, blue vervain, and mistletoe are single herbs that have been historically used for seizures.

Animal research has shown CBD to have anti-convulsive effects. Double-blind studies have shown that CBD has helped some people with seizures, but not everyone. In a 2013 Stanford University study, a survey of ten children with intractable epilepsy that used a CBD-rich whole-plant hemp extract, the results were 11 percent became seizure-free, 42 percent reported a greater than 80 percent reduction and 32 percent reported a 25 to 60 percent reduction with better sleep, improved alertness, and better mood overall. The only adverse affect was drowsiness.

In 2013 two Colorado neurologists presented a survey of eleven patients using CBD rich oil with 75 percent reported a 98 to 100 percent decrease in seizures.

A high fat-diet (see *Ketogenic Diet* strategy) may be helpful in controlling seizures. It may also be helpful to supplement with omega-3 essential fatty acids, particularly DHA.

Strategies: Healthy Fats and Ketogenic Diet
Formulas: Brain Calming and Memory Enhancing
Flower Essence Blends: Shock and Injury FE
Herbs: Coconut, **coconut oil**, hyssop, **lobelia**, mistletoe, passion flower, polygala, **skullcap**, and valerian
Supplements: CBD, GABA, and **omega-3 DHA**
Essential Oils: Helichrysum

Senility
see *Alzheimer's*, *memory/brain function*, **and** *dementia*

Sepsis   **see** *blood poisoning*

Sex Drive, Excessive

See also trauma

If a person feels their sexual drive is excessive and wants to calm it down for some reason, there are a number of remedies that may be helpful. Chaste tree, for example, has been traditionally used to calm sexual desire, especially in males who are under a vow of chastity. Marjoram essential oils is also known to reduce sex drive. Excessive sexual desire can also be the result of sexual abuse during childhood, in which case counseling, *Flower Essence* or *Emotional Healing Work* strategy may be helpful.

Strategies: Counseling or Therapy, Emotional Healing Work, Fasting, and Flower Essence

Formulas: Female Cycle

Flower Essence Blends: Self-Responsibility FE

Herbs: Chaste tree, hops, oat seed (milky), and **white pond lily**

Essential Oils: Jasmine, **marjoram**, sandalwood, and ylang ylang

Sex Drive, Low

Frigidity

See also adrenal fatigue, cholesterol (low), endometriosis, estrogen (low), fibroids (uterine), hypothyroidism, erectile dysfunction, testosterone (low), vaginal dryness, and trauma

Health problems that interfere with sexual intimacy are not life-threatening, but they do interfere with the health of a marriage or relationship. When there is a lack of desire for intimacy in a relationship, the first thing to examine is the relationship itself.

Touch and intimacy are forms of nonverbal communication, and according to David Schnarch, author of *Passionate Marriage*, what is happening in the bedroom is communicating very clearly what is happening in the marriage. When there is no physical reason for loss of desire, honest communication and perhaps even counseling may be necessary.

There are, of course, physical things that can interfere with sexual desire as well. A person who is physically exhausted or sick is going to naturally lose their desire for intimacy, so maintaining overall health will help maintain normal sexual desire. Good general health also enhances physical attractiveness by promoting healthier skin and normal weight.

Here are some specific health issues that can interfere with sexual desire.

Manage Stress

The adrenal glands convert cholesterol into a hormone called pregnenolone, which is then converted into other hormones like cortisol and DHEA. DHEA is the precursor to the sex hormones estrogen and testosterone.

During times of stress, pregnenolone is used to create more cortisol, which can lower levels of DHEA and sex hormones. This can result in fatigue, emotional sensitivity, poor sleep, and the loss of interest in sex. When this is happening supplementing with a *DHEA with Herbs* or an *Adrenal Glandular Formula* may help. See *nervous exhaustion* and *adrenal fatigue* for other suggestions.

Raise Cholesterol if Low

It is worth noting that cholesterol is necessary for the production of sex hormones, which is why low cholesterol levels (below 175 mg/dl) can result in reduced sex drive and infertility. See *cholesterol (low)*.

Balance Hormones

Males: Testosterone is essential for a healthy male sex drive. Levels for males have fallen in recent decades. A combination of factors may be contributing to this, such as poor nutrition and exposure to endocrine disruptors like xenoestrogens. Besides loss of sexual drive, low testosterone may manifest as a loss of self-confidence, weight gain, mild depression, and erectile dysfunction. Low testosterone levels can easily be diagnosed through medical testing. See *testosterone (low)* for more information.

Females: Estrogen is essential for a healthy female sex drive. This can also be determined by medical testing. If low estrogen is a problem or there are other hormonal imbalances, a woman might find a *Female Aphrodisiac Formula* containing herbs like chaste tree and maca helpful. See *estrogen (low)* for more information.

Address Low Thyroid

Low thyroid hormones may cause loss of sexual desire as well. Symptoms of low thyroid hormones may include weight gain, dry and lackluster skin, hair thinning, fatigue, and depression. See *hypothyroidism* for suggestions on dealing with this.

Deal with Sexual or Emotional Abuse

If a person has experienced trauma with the opposite sex, it may interfere with normal sexual desires. For instance, if a person (female or male) was raped or sexually molested as a child it may be difficult for them to perceive sexual activity as a loving act. Likewise, if they have experienced emotional abuse in previous relationships, it may be difficult for them to feel completely safe with a partner.

These barriers to intimacy require patience, love and good communication between the partners to overcome them. The *Counseling or Therapy* strategy may be necessary to help heal from these issues, but there are some flower essences that can help. These include basil, crab apple, Easter lily, pink monkey flower, purple monkey flower, and sticky monkey flower.

Other Barriers to Intimacy

For some women vaginal dryness may interfere with the pleasure of intimacy. A natural lubricant can help. See *vaginal dryness* for more suggestions.

Uterine fibroids or endometriosis can make intimacy painful for women. It these are problems see the appropriate entry for suggestions about natural therapy. If intercourse is painful, seek medical help to determine the cause before determining an approach to treatment.

Strategies: Affirmation and Visualization, Counseling or Therapy, Emotional Healing Work, and Pleasure Prescription

Formulas: Chrisopher's Menopause, **Chinese Fire-Increasing**, Suma Adaptogen, **Male Performance**, **Women's Aphrodisiac**, Thyroid Glandular, Anti-Anxiety, Adrenal Glandular, **DHEA with Herbs**, **Testosterone**, and Adaptogen

Herbs: Black cohosh, **cocoa**, cordyceps, **damiana**, eleuthero, **epimedium**, ginseng (American), ginseng (Asian/Korean), gotu kola, kava kava, licorice, **maca**, muira puama, oat seed (milky), suma, vanilla, and yohimbe

Supplements: DHEA, **L-arginine**, omega-3 EFAs, and vitamin E

Essential Oils: Cinnamon, clary sage, clove, jasmine, neroli, patchouli, **rose**, **sandalwood**, and **ylang ylang**

Shame & Guilt

See also trauma

The concept of guilt is associated with committing a trespass or crime against another person. When I injure someone by harming them, stealing from them, or otherwise violating their inalienable rights, I am guilty. When we are guilty of a trespass against others, it is natural and healthy to experience shame. Shame allows us to recognize that we have done something wrong and change our behavior. To be without shame, or "shameless," is to be without conscience and to be capable of harming others without remorse.

Shame is not healthy, however, when that shame is a result of being abused. Many times abusers try to make their victims feel like they were deserving of the abuse. The person internalizes this sense of guilt and feels ashamed of being who they are, even when they are not actually harming others. This toxic shame and guilt is unhealthy and needs healing.

Toxic shame not only creates poor self-esteem, which causes a person to tolerate abuse; it can actually cause a person's immune system to weaken. Because they have a hard time standing up for themselves, they lack the "fight" neces-

sary to defend themselves and their body against harm. The *Counseling or Therapy* and *Flower Essence* strategies can be helpful in healing this toxic shame.

Strategies: Aromatherapy, Counseling or Therapy, Emotional Healing Work, and Flower Essence

Flower Essence Blends: Personal Boundaries FE, Grief and Sadness FE, and Shock and Injury FE

Essential Oils: Clary sage, jasmine, lime, **pine**, rose, and ylang ylang

Shingles

See also chicken pox

Shingles is an infection by the *herpes zoster* virus that causes chicken pox. It is theorized that by suppressing the fever in chicken pox, it inhibits the immune system from expelling the virus, which allows it to lie dormant until it flares up. Then, it causes acute inflammation and severe pain along the path of a specific nerve or nerves.

Antiviral herbs may be helpful, particularly the *Chinese Wind-Heat Evil Formula*. Saint John's wort can also be helpful, since it is anti-inflammatory and antiviral and also helps to ease nerve pain. Since flare-ups tend to occur when a person is under stress, the *Stress Management* strategy is also helpful.

Strategies: Stress Management

Formulas: Chinese Wind-Heat Evil, **Standardized Acetogenin**, and Colostrum-Immune Stimulator

Herbs: Astragalus, isatis, **lemon balm**, licorice, olive, **pawpaw**, **Saint John's wort**, and **yarrow**

Supplements: L-lysine and **vitamin A**

Essential Oils: Bergamot, eucalyptus, lemon, and tea tree

Shock (Medical)

Shock is characterized by an insufficient flow of blood throughout the body. This life-threatening medical condition typically accompanies severe injury or illness such as internal bleeding, heart conditions, severe allergic reactions, serious infections, burns, or spinal cord injuries. Medical shock is different from emotional or psychological shock, which occurs after a traumatic or frightening event. See *shock (emotional)* for information on dealing with emotional shock.

There are several different types of medical shock. Septic shock results from a bacterial infection releasing toxins in the blood. Anaphylactic shock is caused by allergic reactions to things like bee stings, medications or food. Cardiogenic shock can occur when the heart is damaged from a heart attack or congestive heart failure. Hypovolemic shock is caused by a severe loss of blood or other fluids, often from a serious injury. It can also be caused by severe anemia. Neurogenic shock happens when the spinal cord is injured.

Primary symptoms of shock include rapid and shallow breathing, rapid and weak pulse, cold and clammy skin, and weakness, dizziness or fainting. Other symptoms may include anxiety, confusion, sweating, chest pain, seizures and eyes that appear to stare.

All cases of medical shock require emergency medical assistance. Call 911 immediately. While waiting for emergency assistance, it may be helpful to cover the person with a blanket (if they feel cold). If there is no sign of spinal injury, you may wish to have them lie down and try to elevate their feet above the heart. If they are thirsty, let them sip some water to help them stay hydrated.

A small amount of capsicum powder or tincture on the tongue may be helpful too. In the absence of capsicum, other strong pungent or aromatic herbs might help. The *Shock and Injury FE Blend* is helpful taken under the tongue or applied to the pulse points on the wrists to aid shock. Allowing the person to smell pungent, vaporous or spicy essential oils or oil blends can also be helpful.

Strategies: Hydration

Essential Oil Blends: Analgesic EO

Flower Essence Blends: Shock and Injury FE

Herbs: Capsicum, ginger, and hawthorn

Essential Oils: Cinnamon, eucalyptus, lemongrass, peppermint, pine, tea tree, thyme, and wintergreen

Shortness of Breath   see *wheezing*

SIBO

Small Intestinal Bacterial Overgrowth

See also belching, gas & bloating, gastritis, hiatal hernia, ileocecal valve, leaky gut, low stomach acid, and dysbiosis

Intestinal microflora, also called friendly flora or probiotics, play a role in regulating the immune system and keeping the colon healthy. However, most of the bacteria in your intestines should be in your colon or large intestines, not your small intestines.

When abnormally large numbers of bacteria (even friendly bacteria) start growing in the small intestines, they actually cause problems with your health. SIBO (small intestinal bacterial overgrowth) is a condition where abnormally large numbers of bacteria are present in the small intestines.

These bacteria feed off sugars and starches in the diet (both refined sugars and natural sugars) and produce methane and hydrogen gas. They also inhibit the enzymes in the small intestines that break down starches into simple sugars for absorption. This can result in abdominal bloating, belching, and/or flatulence (intestinal gas), especially when you eat grains and other carbohydrates. The gases produced by these bacteria can also cause abdominal pain, intestinal cramping, and IBS with constipation and/or diarrhea. Gas pressure in the small intestines can push upward against the stomach, contributing to the development of a hiatal hernia and causing heartburn, acid reflux (GERD), and nausea.

SIBO increases a hormone called zonulin, causing an increase in small intestinal permeability (see *leaky gut syndrome*), which results in the intestines absorbing large molecules they shouldn't. The bacteria also like to gobble up essential nutrients like fats, iron, and vitamin B_{12}. The nutrient deficiencies from SIBO along with the absorption of large protein molecules can cause problems with the immune system and contribute to allergies, asthma, autoimmune disorders, and a general decline in health.

Recognizing SIBO

Experts in SIBO have estimated that about 35 to 50 percent of the general public have this problem. Unfortunately, it is not widely understood and, hence, is not properly diagnosed. Many people who have SIBO think they have a candida or yeast infection. However, while yeast overgrowth can occur with or without SIBO, candida is often overdiagnosed and SIBO is underdiagnosed.

If you have an autoimmune disorder, pain in multiple joints, chronic allergies, chronic skin conditions, chronic fatigue or depression, or general malaise (just don't feel good), you may have leaky gut. When you have symptoms of leaky gut coupled with chronic diarrhea or constipation, regular abdominal pain, IBS, bloating or belching after meals, GERD, and/or regular indigestion, you may have SIBO.

Other clues include having better bowel movements after taking antibiotics and bowel problems getting worse when taking probiotics or fiber. If bowel problems began after using opiates for pain, this is another clue that SIBO may be a factor in your health problems.

What Causes SIBO?

There are several major factors that contribute to the development of SIBO. The first is a lack of hydrochloric acid (HCl) in the stomach. HCl helps the body digest proteins, but it also helps to kill bacteria in the food we eat and prevents them from colonizing the small intestines.

A second factor is a lack of intestinal motility. In between meals, migrating motor complexes (MMCs) sweep down the intestines, helping to flush bacteria. These movements of the small intestine are responsible for what we call hunger pangs, the "rumblings" we feel in our gut when we haven't eaten in a while. These MMCs may be damaged by surgery, intestinal scarring, various diseases, intestinal infections, and certain drugs. Medications that can inhibit these intestinal movements include antibiotics, proton pump inhibitors, antacids, and opiates like morphine.

Stress can be a factor in both low hydrochloric acid and the lack of intestinal motility, as the sympathetic nervous system (responsible for the fight-or-flight response) inhibits both digestive secretion and intestinal motility. When we are relaxed, the parasympathetic nervous system is more active and digestion and intestinal motility are enhanced. Unfortunately, many people in our society are eating on the run and do not take time to relax, chew their food thoroughly, and enjoy their meals.

A final factor in SIBO is a malfunctioning ileocecal valve (see *ileocecal valve*). This valve lies between the small and large intestines and is designed to prevent back flow (that is, to keep material in the large intestine from migrating back into the small intestine). When this valve is not shutting properly, intestinal bacteria migrate from the colon into the small intestine, causing gas, bloating, and general weakness and malaise.

Strategies for SIBO

Here are seven strategies you can use to overcome SIBO. Many of these things are also done for leaky gut.

Step 1. Remove irritants

Dietary adjustments are essential to overcoming both SIBO and leaky gut. It is absolutely essential to eliminate all refined sugars from the diet and most starchy foods. At the least, one should eliminate grains containing gluten (wheat, rye, barley), but eliminating all grains may be required.

Dairy may also be problematic because the bacteria love to feast on lactose, the sugar in dairy. Goat-milk products and cultured dairy foods can be beneficial for some people, yet other people may have to eliminate all dairy foods. More information about diet for SIBO can be found under the *Gut-Healing Diet* strategy. A particularly helpful strategy may be to *Eliminate FODMAPs*, which are fermentable foods that feed bacterial overgrowth.

Step 2. Increase HCl and/or enzymes

There are two ways to increase stomach acid and enzymes. One is to take supplements like a *Betaine HCl Formula* and the other is to take herbs and nutrients that stimulate their production, such as an *Herbal Bitters Formula*. With SIBO it is normally necessary to do both. See *low stomach acid* for information on how to fix low stomach acid.

Step 3. Improve intestinal motility

With SIBO, it is also important to make certain that there is good intestinal motility between meals to flush the intestines and clear out bacteria. One way to do this is to allow adequate time between meals, by practicing intermittent fasting (see the *Fasting* strategy). Depending on the efficiency of your digestion, you need three to five hours between meals. Ideally, you should wait until you get stomach rumblings indicating your digestive tract is clear before eating the next meal.

If motility is slow take carminative herbs. Many people find that a cup of ginger tea is most helpful. It may also help to take 100 mg of 5-HTP twice daily as it helps the body produce the hormone that causes intestinal motility.

Step 4. Close the ileocecal valve

If there is severe gas and bloating, you probably need to work on the ileocecal valve. This is done by massaging the valve to reduce swelling and inflammation and get it to close properly. See *ileocecal valve* for more information.

Step 5. Reduce bacterial overgrowth

It is necessary to take herbs to reduce the number of bacteria in the small intestines. For starters, take an *Herbal Bitters Formula* mixed with antibacterial herbs like goldenseal. Enteric coated peppermint oil is also helpful; take one capsule with three meals each day for about twenty days. In clinical trials this was shown to cause a 25-50 percent reduction in small intestinal bacteria.

Cinnamon kills both lactic acid bacteria and yeast. It is much more active than peppermint. Use it when you are sensitive to taking probiotics. Take two capsules three times daily with meals.

Goldenseal may also be helpful. It not only reduces intestinal bacteria, it also tones up digestive membranes and reduces irritation. It also lowers blood sugar levels. Take two capsules three times daily with meals. As an alternative you can take one capsule of berberine twice daily.

Note: It is not necessary to take *all* of the above remedies. That would be overkill. Pick one or two only, depending on your circumstances and what's available to you. You may also wish to read the suggestions under *dysbiosis* too.

Step 6. Restore beneficial bacteria

People with SIBO often do not do well on probiotic supplements, especially if they contain prebiotics which feed the small intestinal bacteria as well as friendly flora.

Cultured vegetables are usually more valuable in treating SIBO. You can make your own cultured vegetables or you can purchase them from a health food store or some supermarkets. If you do take probiotics, make sure to complete the previous five steps and start slowly to see how you react to them. See the *Friendly Flora* strategy for more information.

Step 7. Repair gut integrity

Since SIBO always causes leaky gut, it is important to rebuild the integrity of the intestinal membranes. One of the best ways to do this is by using the *Bone Broth* strategy. Bone broth is high in glutamine and glycine, both of which are essential in healing the gut.

If you can't take the bone broth, you can use L-glutamine, which can also be used along with bone broth. L-glutamine is a major part of the *Gut-Healing Fiber*, but you won't be able to take this product until you've reduced the bacterial overgrowth as it also contains the prebiotic inulin.

Other remedies that help heal the gut include chamomile tea (one cup three times daily), deglycyrrhizinated licorice (two capsules three times daily) and colostrum powder, one teaspoon twice daily. The *Cat's Claw Combination* is also good for healing the gut.

Strategies: Avoid Sugar, Bone Broth, Eliminate FODMAPs, Fasting, Friendly Flora, Gut-Healing Diet, and Stress Management

Formulas: Betaine HCl, **Probiotic**, **H. Pylori-Fighting**, **Gut Immune**, Herbal Bitters, **Digestive Support**, Anti-Fungal, Stimulant Laxative, and **Gut-Healing Fiber**

Herbs: Cinnamon, garlic, **ginger**, **goldenseal**, nopal, and pau d'arco

Supplements: 5-HTP, **berberine**, **L-glutamine**, and melatonin

Essential Oils: Peppermint

Sickle Cell Anemia

See also anemia

Sickle cell anemia is a hereditary form of anemia that causes abnormally shaped red blood cells. Although natural remedies may not cure the condition, some can be helpful in easing symptoms. Chlorophyll and zinc have helped some people. Herbs that help to build the blood such as *Christopher's Herbal Iron Formula* may also be helpful.

Strategies: Mineralization

Formulas: Christopher's Herbal Iron and Chinese Wood-Increasing

Herbs: Alfalfa and nettle, stinging leaf

Supplements: Chlorophyll and zinc

Sinus Infection

See also congestion (sinus) and rhinitis

Although antibiotics are commonly recommended for sinus infections, they rarely have a positive effect. Chronic sinus infections are typically the result of problems in the digestive tract and may be related to food allergies, food sen-sitivities, intestinal dysbiosis, and/or leaky gut syndrome. Using the *Colon Cleansing* and *Eliminate Allergy-Causing Foods* strategies is often the best long-term solution.

Two effective herbs for sinus problems are fenugreek and thyme. These herbs are found in the *Sinus Formula* which can be used along with *Christopher's Sinus Formula*. Osha, Brigham tea, and horseradish can also help clear the sinuses.

Drink plenty of water and take a small pinch of salt with it. This helps increase mucus flow and helps the sinuses to drain properly.

For rapid relief, make a solution of sea salt and water, add a little xylitol to it, and use it as a nasal wash (neti pots are the perfect tool to use). You can also use liquid silver as a nasal spray. *Steven Horne's Sinus Snuff* can bring rapid relief, but this can be an uncomfortable therapy for some.

Putting some essential oils into a pot of water that has been brought to a boil and removed from the stove and then inhaling the steam can also help decongest the sinuses. The essential oils I like best for this are pine and eucalyptus.

Strategies: Aromatherapy, Avoid Sugar, Detoxification, Eliminate Allergy-Causing Foods, Eliminate Salicylates, Friendly Flora, Hydration, and Increase Dietary Fiber

Formulas: Antibacterial, **Christopher's Sinus**, **Sinus**, Topical Analgesic, Ed Millet's Herbal Crisis, **Steven Horne's Sinus Snuff**, Probiotic, Triphala, Chinese Earth-Increasing, and Chinese Metal-Decreasing

Essential Oil Blends: Lung-Supporting EO

Herbs: Andrographis, bayberry, echinacea, **fenugreek**, goldenseal, **horseradish**, lomatium, **osha**, **thyme**, and yerba santa

Supplements: Bromelain, **nanoparticle silver**, **vitamin A**, **vitamin C**, and xylitol

Essential Oils: Cajeput, **eucalyptus**, frankincense, helichrysum, **pine**, ravensara, rosemary, tea tree, and thyme

Sinus Problems
see *congestion (sinus)* **and** *rhinitis*

Situational Anxiety **see** *anxiety (situational)*

Sjögren's Syndrome
see *autoimmune disorders*

Skin (Infections)

See also infection (fungal), infection (bacterial), and infection (viral)

When there is an infection in the skin, you can apply a silver gel or an *Antibacterial Formula* directly to the affected areas using the *Compress or Fomentation* strategy. You can also dilute essential oils like rosemary, tea tree, and/or thyme with a fixed oil and apply this to affected areas.

Internally, *Blood Purifier* or *Detoxifying Formulas* containing burdock, red clover, and other alteratives have been used traditionally to help clear up skin infections. Gotu kola is also a good herb to take internally for fighting skin infections. If you know whether the infection is viral, fungal, or bacterial, you can look up additional remedies under those related conditions.

Strategies: Aromatherapy and Compress or Fomentation

Formulas: Antibacterial, Ayurvedic Skin Healing, Blood Purifier, and Detoxifying

Herbs: Burdock, chicory, **echinacea**, **goldenseal**, **gotu kola**, honeysuckle, **pau d'arco**, **red clover**, and yarrow

Supplements: Nanoparticle silver, **vitamin A**, vitamin C, and vitamin D

Essential Oils: Clary sage, clove, helichrysum, lemongrass, rosemary, **tea tree**, and thyme

Skin Problems

See also acne, hypothyroidism, and leaky gut

The skin is the largest sensory organ in the body. Loaded with nerves that allow us to sense heat, cold, texture, pressure, and pain, the skin allows us to "touch" the outside world. The fact that the skin is so connected with our nervous system is also revealed by how our skin communicates what is going on inside of us mentally and emotionally.

Through our skin we flush from excitement, we blush when we're embarrassed, we grow pale because of fear, and we sweat over the "small stuff" that sometimes makes us feel overwhelmed and nervous. It is why we say that a person who is confident is "comfortable in their own skin." This strong connection to our emotions suggests we shouldn't discount the importance of positive mental attitudes and emotional health in keeping the skin healthy.

Unhealed shame can be a big factor in skin diseases because how we look affects our self-esteem. Feeling ashamed of who we are, not wanting to be "seen," or feeling undesirable and unattractive can manifest in our skin. Likewise, skin conditions that arise from physical problems with our skin, can contribute to these emotional issues. The two go hand in hand and should always be worked on together.

Physically, the skin needs nutrition to be healthy, just like any other organ of the body. Skin conditions are not just "skin deep." They point to more deep-seated conditions like poor nutrition, toxicity of the liver, poor kidney function,

and problems with the mucous membranes of the gut. They can also point to imbalances in the glandular system.

Nutrients the skin needs include silica, calcium, trace minerals, good fats, fat-soluble vitamins like A, D, E and K, and vitamin C. Antioxidants protect the skin from damage from the sun and other environmental influences. Herbs helpful for topical application to the skin include seaweeds (dulse, kelp, etc.), rosemary, sage, and chamomile. Internally, horsetail, dulse, and gotu kola are helpful.

Traditionally *Blood Purifier* and *Detoxifying Formulas* have been used to clear up skin conditions. The *Sweat Bath* and *Drawing Bath* strategies are also great ways to detoxify the body and improve skin health.

When using products on your skin such as cosmetics, soaps, and beauty care products, remember that your skin absorbs things. Don't put chemicals on your skin that you don't want in your body.

Strategies: Aromatherapy, Counseling or Therapy, Drawing Bath, Eat Healthy, Healthy Fats, Mineralization, Poultice, and Sweat Bath

Formulas: Watkin's Hair, Skin, and Nails, Ayurvedic Skin Healing, Enzyme Spray, Thyroid Glandular, Chinese Wood-Decreasing, Blood Purifier, **Antioxidant**, Detoxifying, and Alterative-Immune

Essential Oil Blends: Relaxing and Soothing EO

Herbs: Aloe vera, bladderwrack, chamomile, chickweed, comfrey, **dulse**, elder flowers, **gotu kola**, horsetail, Irish moss, kelp, **rosemary**, and tea

Supplements: Calcium, **CBD**, collagen, multiple vitamin and mineral, **nanoparticle silver**, **omega-3 EFAs**, **silicon**, vitamin A, vitamin C, vitamin D, and vitamin E

Essential Oils: Chamomile (Roman), copaiba, helichrysum, rose, sandalwood, tansy (blue), tea tree, and ylang ylang

Skin, Dry/Flaky

See also fat metabolism (poor), gallbladder problems, Hashimoto's disease, and hypothyroidism

The skin is kept moist by the secretion of sebum, a waxy, oily substance secreted by the sebaceous glands in the skin. This substance holds moisture in the skin, helping to keep it soft and moist. Dry skin is typically due to a lack of this secretion. A lack of healthy fats in the diet, poor fat digestion and metabolism, and low thyroid function are all possible causes of dry and flaky skin.

If you have problems with dry skin, make sure you are eating healthy fats and avoiding processed fats like margarine, shortening, and refined vegetable oils. Make sure you are able to properly digest fats by taking lipase enzyme or a *Digestive Support Formula*. Also make sure your liver and gallbladder are secreting bile to emulsify and digest the fats. Herbs that aid fat metabolism by supporting the liver and promoting bile flow include burdock, turmeric and fringetree.

Most frequently, however, dry skin is a sign of poor thyroid function. If your dry skin is accompanied by feeling easily chilled and tired, you may have a thyroid problem. The thyroid hormone regulates the combustion of fats and is essential for soft, moist skin. An *Herbal Thyroid Formula* may help, but be sure to look up additional suggestions under *hypothyroidism* and *Hashimoto's disease*.

The essential oils listed below can aid dry skin when mixed with a lotion or fixed vegetable oil and applied topically. Baths with seaweeds in the water can also be helpful (see the *Drawing Bath* strategy).

Strategies: Aromatherapy, Drawing Bath, and Healthy Fats

Formulas: Chinese Yin-Increasing, GLA Oil, **Hypothyroid**, Thyroid Glandular, Adrenal Glandular, and Digestive Support

Herbs: Black currant, **burdock**, **coconut**, **flax**, fringe tree, Irish moss, kelp, and turmeric

Supplements: Krill oil, **lipase**, MSM, **omega-3 EFAs**, and omega-6 GLA

Essential Oils: Chamomile (Roman), **geranium**, **helichrysum**, jasmine, lavender, neroli, and peppermint

Skin, Oily

Oily skin can be a sign of problems with fat metabolism. Lipase enzyme supplements and herbs for the liver and gallbladder, like burdock, can help the body process fats more effectively.

The *Drawing Bath* strategy, using a fine clay like Redmond clay, can be used to pull excess oil from the skin. The clay can also be moistened and applied to the skin as a mask to draw out excess oils. Adding a drop or two of rosemary or rose essential oils to the mask will also be helpful.

Strategies: Detoxification and Drawing Bath

Formulas: Detoxifying and Blood Purifier

Herbs: Burdock and **rosemary**

Supplements: Clay (Redmond) and **lipase**

Essential Oils: Bergamot, cypress, frankincense, geranium, grapefruit (pink), lemon, lime, red mandarin, **rose**, tea tree, and ylang ylang

Sleep Apnea

See also excess weight

Sleep apnea occurs when the throat closes down completely, making it impossible to breathe while sleeping. This starves your tissues for oxygen, which can cause you to wake up after about a minute of not breathing, shift positions and go back to sleep. The problem is that you are not aware that you are waking up numerous times each night starved for oxygen.

Sleep apnea doesn't just interfere with your sleep; it is dangerous. Not only does it stress your heart and increase your risk of heart disease, but you also risk dying in your sleep from oxygen starvation. If you snore very loudly, get checked for sleep apnea. If you do have sleep apnea, medical help may be necessary to ensure you get enough oxygen for a sound night's sleep. To protect your heart, try taking Co-Q10 and four hawthorn capsules at bedtime.

Factors that can contribute to snoring and sleep apnea include excess weight, swollen lymph nodes, sinus congestion, or any inflammation of the mucous membranes. The *Anti-Snoring Formula* may help shrink swelling of inflamed mucous membranes, reduce sinus congestion and swollen lymph nodes, and otherwise help to open respiratory passages. Food and respiratory allergies may be a factor, so try following the *Eliminate Allergy-Causing Foods* strategy. High doses of vitamin C with bioflavonoids (2,000-3,000 mg per day) can help to counteract histamine reactions if allergies are a factor. Weight loss and colon cleansing are also helpful.

Strategies: Detoxification and Eliminate Allergy-Causing Foods

Formulas: Antihistamine, **Anti-Snoring**, and Liquid Lymph

Herbs: Hawthorn

Supplements: Alpha-lipoic acid, bioflavonoids, **Co-Q10**, **quercetin**, and **vitamin C**

Slivers

Slivers are tiny pieces of wood or other material embedded in the skin. A Drawing Salve can help draw slivers out of the skin. Pine gum and crushed leaves of lily of the valley are also good for this. Apply the remedy and cover with a bandage. Tea tree oil or silver gel can help prevent infection.

Strategies: Poultice

Formulas: Drawing Salve and Intestinal Soothing

Herbs: Pine gum

Supplements: Nanoparticle silver

Essential Oils: Tea tree

Smell, Loss Of

See also congestion (sinus)

A loss of the sense of smell is sometimes due to a zinc deficiency. It can also be due to sinus congestion and nasal polyps, in which case a *Sinus Formula* or *Steven Horne's Sinus Snuff Formula* may be helpful.

Formulas: Sinus and Steven Horne's Sinus Snuff

Herbs: Bayberry, fenugreek, goldenseal, and thyme

Supplements: Nanoparticle silver and **zinc**

Smoking   see *addictions (tobacco)*

Snakebite

Seek medical attention if bitten by a poisonous snake and only use these remedies while en route to the hospital. Astringent herbs have traditionally been applied topically to snakebites to promote healing and counteract the venom. One of the best astringent herbs for this purpose is plantain. Black cohosh and echinacea are also traditional snake bite remedies. They should be applied topically using the *Compress or Fomentation* or *Poultice* strategies, but may also be taken internally. Large doses of vitamin C internally (5,000 mg or more) may also be helpful.

Strategies: Compress or Fomentation and Poultice

Herbs: **Black cohosh**, **echinacea**, pau d'arco, and **plantain**

Supplements: Vitamin C

Sneezing   see *congestion (sinus)*

Snoring

See also food allergies/intolerances, allergies (respiratory), congestion (sinus), and sleep apnea

Snoring is caused by blockage in the respiratory passages that narrows the airways when sleeping. To clear this congestion, use the *Detoxification* and *Eliminate Allergy-Causing Foods* strategies. Try using the *Anti-Snoring* or *Sinus Formula* to clear the sinuses. The *Hydration* strategy helps too. If you snore a lot, get checked for sleep apnea.

Strategies: Detoxification, Eliminate Allergy-Causing Foods, and Hydration

Formulas: **Anti-Snoring**, **Jeannie Burgess' Allergy-Lung**, Seasonal Cold and Flu, Antihistamine, and **Sinus**

Herbs: **Fenugreek** and **thyme**

Supplements: Co-Q10 and MSM

Sore Gums   see *gingivitis*

Sore Throat

See also strep throat

Sore throat is a discomfort in the pharynx due to inflammation. A number of herbs can be used as infusions (teas) and a gargle for sore throats. You can also make the gargle by diluting a tincture or extract in water. Good herbs for gargles include capsicum (stings at first, then numbs the pain), bayberry (great for loosening mucus), goldenseal (fights infection and reduces inflammation), myrrh (antiseptic), and sage (antiseptic).

Silver can be used as a gargle too. Swallow the silver after gargling with it so that you get the benefits of it internally too. You can also use *Herbal Composition* or *Ed Millet's Herbal Crisis Formulas* diluted in warm water as gargles for sore throats.

Another approach is to apply a *Topical Analgesic Formula* to the throat and gently massage it. See the *Lymph-Moving Pain Relief* strategy. Lobelia and capsicum extracts mixed in equal parts also make a great topical massage for sore throats.

Sucking on slippery elm or licorice powder will ease irritation and dryness. Internally, the *Liquid Lymph Formula* or lymphatic herbs like red root and echinacea can be used to clear swollen lymph nodes, which also helps.

If the problem is a bacterial infection (such as strep throat), then garlic and echinacea are good remedies. They are taken internally, but garlic oil can also be massaged topically into the throat. See *strep throat* for details.

Strategies: Hydration and Lymph-Moving Pain Relief

Formulas: **Antibacterial**, **Chinese Yang-Reducing**, Stabilized Allicin, Anti-Inflammatory Pain, **Cold Lozenges**, Lymphatic Infection, Liquid Lymph, **Herbal Composition**, **Ed Millet's Herbal Crisis**, Steven Horne's Children's Composition, and Chinese Metal-Decreasing

Essential Oil Blends: Lung-Supporting EO

Herbs: Acacia (Indian), aloe vera, andrographis, balloon flower, **bayberry**, **capsicum**, collinsonia, **echinacea**, elder berries, forsythia, **garlic**, **goldenseal**, isatis, **licorice**, lobelia, lomatium, **myrrh**, osha, **red root**, sage, **slippery elm**, stillingia, trichosanthes, and usnea

Supplements: **Nanoparticle silver**, vanadium, vitamin A, vitamin C, and vitamin D

Essential Oils: Clary sage, eucalyptus, lemon, **menthol**, peppermint, sandalwood, tea tree, and thyme

Sore/Geographic Tongue

A tongue that is covered with bare red patches alternating with heavily coated areas is called a geographic tongue. Both a geographic tongue and a sore tongue can be a sign of a vitamin B_{12}, iron, folate, or niacin deficiency. They can also indicate digestive mucosal irritation. Bitter herbs, particularly yellow dock and dandelion, can be helpful for cooling down this digestive irritation. You can also mix some goldenseal or yellow dock with marshmallow root or aloe vera juice and take this fifteen to twenty minutes prior to meals. A *Digestive Support Formula* may also be helpful.

> **Strategies:** Eat Healthy, Friendly Flora, and Increase Dietary Fiber
>
> **Formulas: Herbal Bitters**, Plant Enzyme, Antioxidant, **Methyl B12 Vitamin**, **Methylated B Vitamin**, **Probiotic**, and Digestive Support
>
> **Herbs:** Aloe vera, dandelion, **goldenseal**, marshmallow, and **yellow dock**
>
> **Supplements:** Iron, vitamin B-complex, **vitamin B$_{12}$**, vitamin B$_3$, vitamin B$_6$, and **vitamin B$_9$**

Sores   see *wounds & sores*

Spasms   see *cramps & spasms*

Spastic Colon   see *colon (spastic)*

Spider Veins

See also cardiovascular disease

Spider veins can be an early warning sign of cardiovascular inflammation that can lead to cardiovascular disease. *Vein Tonic* and *Anti-Inflammatory Formulas* can be helpful. Co-Q10, vitamin C, and bioflavonoids will strengthen capillaries and help to reduce these unsightly veins. Spider veins can also indicate a copper deficiency. If this is the case, taking sodium copper chlorophyllin (liquid chlorophyll) may help. Using the *Compress or Fomentation* strategy to apply an extract of rose hips, butcher's broom, or bilberry will also help.

> **Strategies:** Compress or Fomentation, Eat Healthy, and Healthy Fats
>
> **Formulas:** Enzyme Spray, **Vein Tonic**, Oral Chelation, and Anti-Inflammatory Pain
>
> **Herbs:** Bilberry, **butcher's broom**, **horse chestnut**, and rose hips
>
> **Supplements:** Bioflavonoids, chlorophyll, **Co-Q10**, copper, omega-3 EFAs, and **vitamin C**

Spinal Disks
Herniated or Slipped Disks

See also backache

When the disks between the vertebrae are bulging, better posture, stretching exercises, and body work such as chiropractic care will help them realign. You can also use a slant-board or inversion table to take stress off the disks. Even when disks rupture or herniate, surgery is not usually the best option. It is better to try to help the disks heal and then work on improving posture and spinal flexibility.

One possible way to speed the healing of herniated disks is to apply a poultice over the area where the injured disk is. Use mucilaginous herbs along with goldenseal and yarrow. Change the poultice at least twice daily (see the *Poultice* strategy).

Many people have also reported that using the *Enzyme Spray Formula* topically on the back has eased pain and promoted healing. Supplements that help tissues heal can also be helpful.

> **Strategies:** Aromatherapy, Bodywork, Herbal Back Adjustment, Mineralization, Poultice, and Stress Management
>
> **Formulas: Enzyme Spray**, **Chinese Water-Increasing**, Herbal Arthritis, Anti-Inflammatory Pain, **Vulnerary**, and Colloidal Mineral
>
> **Herbs:** Boswellia, **goldenseal**, lobelia, **solomon's seal**, thyme, turmeric, and willow
>
> **Supplements: Bromelain**, chlorophyll, collagen, **MSM**, vitamin A, and vitamin D
>
> **Essential Oils:** Helichrysum

Spinal Meningitis   see *meningitis*

Sprains

A sprain is caused by a sudden or violent twisting of a joint that causes stretching or tearing of ligaments, resulting in swelling, pain, inflammation, bruising, and discoloration. Arnica is a wonderful remedy for sprains and can be applied topically as an oil or ointment and used internally as a homeopathic. Soaking the sprained joint in Epsom salts will help to reduce swelling. You can also make a soak or fomentation using decoctions of herbs like comfrey, willow, white oak bark, and/or plantain. Using a *Tissue Healing Formula* internally can also speed healing.

> **Strategies:** Compress or Fomentation and Epsom Salt Bath
>
> **Formulas: Enzyme Spray**, Vulnerary, Topical Analgesic, **CBD Topical Analgesic**, and Enzyme Spray
>
> **Essential Oil Blends: Topical Injury**
>
> **Flower Essence Blends:** Shock and Injury FE
>
> **Herbs:** Aloe vera, angelica, **arnica**, chickweed, **comfrey**, lobelia, marshmallow, pau d'arco, **plantain**, Saint John's wort, **solomon's seal**, **white oak**, and willow
>
> **Supplements:** L-lysine, MSM, and vitamin C
>
> **Essential Oils:** Camphor, helichrysum, jasmine, marjoram, and rose

Staph Infections

See also infection (bacterial)

Staphylococcus are a particular type of bacteria that can invade the body. Serious infections may require medical attention, but raw garlic, goldenseal, Oregon grape, wild indigo, and echinacea can be effective in fighting staph infections when taken internally and applied externally. You can also use an *Antibacterial* or *Immune Stimulant Formula*. Vitamins A, D, and C can also be helpful. If you take an antibiotic, be sure to supplement with probiotics afterwards.

Strategies: Friendly Flora

Formulas: Stabilized Allicin, Lymphatic Infection, **Immune-Boosting**, Antibacterial, and Probiotic

Herbs: Aloe vera, baptisia, **echinacea**, garlic, **goldenseal**, and Oregon grape

Supplements: Nanoparticle silver, vitamin A, vitamin C, and **vitamin D**

Essential Oils: Tea tree

Stiff Neck

See also cramps & spasms and whiplash

Pain, inflammation, and lack of mobility between the head and shoulders can be aided by massaging a *Topical Analgesic Formula* or lobelia extract into the neck and shoulders using the *Lymph-Moving Pain Relief* strategy. Chiropractic care or other applications of the *Bodywork* strategy can be helpful too. Blue vervain and kudzu are two helpful herbs for a stiff neck. Make sure to drink plenty of water too.

If the stiffness is due to an injury, black coshosh tincture, taken in doses of five to fifteen drops, may be helpful. See *whiplash* for other suggestions.

Stress and fatigue, especially from working too much at a computer or other desk job can contribute to this problem (see the *Good Posture* strategy). Take period breaks to stretch and relax.

Strategies: Bodywork, Detoxification, Good Posture, Hydration, Lymph-Moving Pain Relief, and Stress Management

Formulas: Topical Analgesic and Enzyme Spray

Herbs: Black cohosh, dogwood (Jamaican), **kava kava**, **kudzu**, lobelia, siler, **vervain (blue)**, and **wood betony**

Supplements: Magnesium and MSM

Stomachache   see *indigestion*

Strep Throat

See also sore throat

Strep throat is a sore throat that is caused by a particular type of infectious bacteria. It can have serious complications and medical attention should be sought. A type of strep, specifically group A beta hemolytic streptococcal infection can lead to rheumatic fever, a serious condition. Untreated strep will lead to rheumatic fever in about 3 percent of people. I recommend any child younger than twelve years old who tests positive for strep and is running a fever higher that 102 be treated with antibiotics.

There are some herbs that can be effective against strep. These include garlic (especially when raw), echinacea, usnea, and goldenseal. Try making a gargle using the *Antibacterial Formula, Herbal Crisis,* or *Herbal Composition Formulas* diluted in warm water. Also take an *Antibacterial Formula* internally and drink plenty of water. It also helps to follow some of the general procedures listed under *sore throat*.

Strategies: Hydration

Formulas: Stabilized Allicin, Immune-Boosting, Antibacterial, Lymphatic Infection, Ed Millet's Herbal Crisis, and **Herbal Composition**

Herbs: Andrographis, baptisia, **echinacea**, garlic, **goldenseal**, pine, **usnea**, and white sage

Supplements: Nanoparticle silver, vitamin A, vitamin C, and zinc

Essential Oils: Tea tree

Stress

See also nervousness and anxiety disorders

Stress is a physical, chemical or emotional factor that causes bodily or mental tension and is a contributing factor to disease. See the *Stress Management* strategy. Basic strategies for handling stress include the following.

When we're under stress, it's important to take good care of our health. Eating right, getting enough sleep, drinking enough water, and making time for ourselves becomes very important. Avoid caffeine and sugar when under stress, as they cause further depletion of the nerves. Drink plenty of pure water, as hydration also helps the body cope better with stress.

Nervines help the body relax, which can reduce anxiety and nervousness. They can also promote better sleep, which also helps a person cope with stress. The *Chinese Fire-Decreasing Formula* is a good nervine for people who tend to be prone to nervousness, hyperactivity, and stress.

Adaptogens and adaptogen formulas can reduce the output of stress hormones, thus lowering baseline stress levels. This increases energy, boosts immunity and helps a person cope better both physically and emotionally with stress.

Ashwagandha Complex and the *Chinese Fire-Increasing Formula* are two good formulas for coping with stress, especially when feeling burned out.

B-complex vitamins and vitamin C help with stress too. The *Anti-Stress B-Complex Formula* helps support a person who is under stress. It helps the person feel more relaxed and energized at the same time.

When nerves feel shot because of stress, borage, milky oat seed, skullcap, and magnesium can all be helpful remedies. Various essential oil blend can also help you relax when you're faced with a lot of stress, especially when used for massage or the *Epsom Salt Bath* strategy. It's also a good idea to use the *Pleasure Prescription* strategy.

Strategies: Avoid Caffeine, Avoid Sugar, Blood Type Diet, Emotional Healing Work, Epsom Salt Bath, Hydration, Meditation, Pleasure Prescription, Sleep, and Stress Management

Formulas: Adaptogen-Immune, Herbal Sleep Aid, Christopher's Nervine, **Anti-Stress B-Complex**, **Chinese Fire-Decreasing**, Jeannie Burgess' Stress, **Chinese Fire-Increasing**, Cortisol-Reducing, Electrolyte Drink, **Anti-Anxiety**, Adrenal Glandular, **Ashwagandha Complex**, **Colloidal Mineral**, Nitric Oxide Boosting, **CBD Relaxing**, and **Adaptogen**

Essential Oil Blends: Menopause Support EO, Balancing EO, Mood Lifting EO, Calming and Relaxing EO, and Relaxing and Soothing EO

Herbs: **Ashwagandha**, borage, **chamomile**, **eleuthero**, ginseng (American), ginseng (Asian/Korean), gotu kola, **holy basil**, Indian pipe, **kava kava**, licorice, maca, **motherwort**, **oat seed (milky)**, passion flower, **rhodiola**, Saint John's wort, **skullcap**, suma, valerian, and **vervain (blue)**

Supplements: 5-HTP, **magnesium**, **multiple vitamin and mineral**, potassium, **vitamin B-complex**, vitamin B_3, vitamin B_5, and **vitamin C**

Essential Oils: Atlas cedarwood, bay leaf, bergamot, chamomile (Roman), clary sage, copaiba, grapefruit (pink), lavender, lime, orange (sweet), ravensara, ravintsara, sandalwood, spearmint, spruce (blue), tansy (blue), and ylang ylang

Stretch Marks

Stretch marks are lines of scarred tissue that form on the surface of the skin when the skin is stressed from rapid growth. For instance, stretch marks are common from pregnancy or rapid weight gain. In pregnancy, they are commonly found on the belly, hips, and or thighs. Vitamin E and zinc can help prevent stretch marks. Massaging cocoa butter, coconut, olive, or peanut oil into the skin also helps. Adding some of the listed essential oils may prevent stretch marks or help them heal.

Herbs: **Cocoa butter**, coconut oil, and olive oil
Supplements: **Vitamin C**, vitamin E, and **zinc**
Essential Oils: Copaiba, grapefruit (pink), helichrysum, lavender, myrrh, and red mandarin

Strokes

See also blood clot prevention, hypertension, and thrombosis

A stroke causes temporary or permanent loss of blood flow to an artery of the brain and the part of the brain that artery feeds. It may be caused by an arterial rupture or a blood clot. The type and degree of damage depends on the size and location of the portion of the brain affected.

Appropriate medical attention should be sought immediately following a stroke. Capsicum and ginkgo can be administered while waiting for medical assistance. Lily of the valley was also a traditional remedy given to people who had suffered a stroke.

To reduce one's risk of stroke make sure to keep blood pressure managed, as high blood pressure increases the risk of stroke (see *hypertension*). The *Nitric Oxide Boosting Formula* is a good choice.

Magnesium, potassium, vitamin C, and omega-3 essential fatty acids can all reduce one's risk of stroke. Butcher's broom, horse chestnut, nattozimes, vitamin E, and *Vein Tonic Formulas* can all reduce the risk of blood clots that cause strokes. See *blood clot prevention* for additional information.

Strategies: Eat Healthy and Healthy Fats
Formulas: **Oral Chelation**, Colloidal Mineral, Anti-Stress B-Complex, Nattokinase Enzyme, **Nitric Oxide Boosting**, and Vein Tonic
Programs: Cardiovascular Nutritional
Herbs: **Butcher's broom**, **capsicum**, **ginkgo**, and horse chestnut
Supplements: Lecithin, magnesium, omega-3 EFAs, potassium, vitamin C, and vitamin E

Sty

See also eye infection

An inflamed swelling of a sebaceous gland at the margin of the eyelid is called a sty. Eyebright or chamomile, made into a tea and applied to the eyes using the *Compress or Fomentation* strategy, can be effective for treating a sty. You could also try an *Herbal Eye Wash Formula* used as a wash or a compress. Vitamins A and D help eye infections to heal more rapidly.

Strategies: Compress or Fomentation
Formulas: **Herbal Eyewash**

Herbs: Bayberry, **chamomile**, **eyebright**, goldenseal, and horsetail

Supplements: Vitamin A and **vitamin D**

Sugar Cravings

see *addictions (sugar/carbohydrates)* **and** *hypoglycemia*

Sunburn

See also burns & scalds

Varying degrees of damage to the skin due to overexposure to sunlight can be aided by applying aloe vera gel topically. It can be used by itself or with added lavender oil. Keep the burn moist by spraying purified water or the *Enzyme Spray Formula* on the skin. Large doses of vitamin C taken internally also speed recovery.

Strategies: Eat Healthy and Hydration

Formulas: Enzyme Spray

Herbs: Aloe vera, chamomile, and nopal

Supplements: Vitamin C

Essential Oils: Chamomile (Roman), **lavender**, and tea tree

Surgery (Preparation)

Prior to surgery, discontinue any herbs that may have a blood-thinning effect, including alfalfa, ginkgo, garlic, and willow. It may also be wise to discontinue taking vitamin E.

Hepatoprotective Formulas containing milk thistle, schisandra, and other remedies that aid the liver's ability to cope with chemicals can be taken prior to surgery to help the liver handle the drugs used in the hospital. *Christopher's Herbal Iron Formula, Colloidal Mineral Formulas* and a good multivitamin might also be helpful in making sure the body is adequately prepared for the surgery.

Since surgery is a stressful event, the *Stress Management* strategy can be practiced before-hand to keep stress hormones at a minimum. This will help the body be better prepared to handle the stress of surgery. It also helps to use the strategy *Affirmation and Visualization*, affirming or visualizing that all will go well during the procedure. Prayer has also been documented to improve outcomes during surgery, so have family and friends pray for you while in the hospital.

Strategies: Affirmation and Visualization, Mineralization, and Stress Management

Formulas: Vulnerary, **Watkin's Hair, Skin, and Nails, Colloidal Mineral**, and Christopher's Herbal Iron

Herbs: Butcher's broom, capsicum, **milk thistle**, and schisandra

Supplements: Multiple vitamin and mineral, vitamin B-complex, and **vitamin C**

Surgery (Recovery)

See also injuries

After surgery, the body needs support to complete the healing process. Vulnerary herbs, such as calendula, comfrey, marshmallow, oak bark, and plantain, can be used to stimulate tissue repair. You can obtain several of these herbs at once by using a *Vulnerary Formula* either topically or internally.

A number of nutrients also aid the healing process, including vitamin C, vitamin E, and zinc. These nutrients help prevent scarring. Taking 2,000 mg of MSM and 2,000 mg of vitamin C twice a day after surgery greatly speeds the healing process. Minerals also aid tissue repair when recovering from injury or surgery.

Arnica homeopathic can be taken several times a day to reduce inflammation and pain. The *Anti-Inflammatory Pain Formula* also reduces pain and speeds healing.

The liver has to detoxify any anesthetic drugs used during surgery, so using a *Blood Purifier* or *Detoxifying Formula* can aid this process. B-complex vitamins, milk thistle, N-acetylcysteine, and red clover are also helpful for post surgery detoxification.

Since antibiotics are used to prevent infection during and after surgery, it is very important to restore normal gut flora by using probiotic supplements and/or eating fermented foods following surgery.

Strategies: Affirmation and Visualization, Friendly Flora, Liver Detoxification, Mineralization, and Poultice

Formulas: Vulnerary, Proanthocyanidins, Algae, **Detoxifying**, Chinese Qi-Increasing, Watkin's Hair, Skin, and Nails, **Anti-Inflammatory Pain**, **Herbal Calcium**, Colloidal Mineral, CBD Topical Analgesic, Hemp Oil with Terpenes, and **Probiotic**

Herbs: Alfalfa, arnica homeopathic, burdock, **calendula**, **comfrey**, milk thistle, **plantain**, and red clover

Supplements: Bromelain, L-arginine, **MSM**, N-acetyl cysteine, omega-3 EFAs, vitamin B-complex, vitamin B_5, **vitamin C**, **vitamin E**, and **zinc**

Sweating   **see** *perspiration (excessive)*

Swelling   **see** *edema*

Swollen Lymph Glands

See also congestion (lymphatic) and tonsillitis

When the lymph glands or nodes are irritated they can cause swelling at the neck, throat, armpits, groin, and chest, where they are located. They can feel like hard bumps under the skin in these areas. Swollen lymph glands are usually present in respiratory congestion, earaches, sore throats, and breast swelling.

Use herbs that promote lymphatic drainage like cleavers, red clover, ocotillo, and red root. It is important to drink plenty of water and get some moderate exercise, as movement increases lymph flow.

A *Lymphatic Infection* or *Liquid Lymph Formula* can be helpful. If infection is present add echinacea or an *Antibacterial Formula*. Topically, lobelia extract or poke oil can be helpful.

Tea tree or thyme essential oils can be diluted in a carrier oil or a lotion and massaged into swollen glands. Garlic oil can also be massaged into swollen lymph nodes.

Strategies: Aromatherapy, Compress or Fomentation, Detoxification, Exercise, and Hydration

Formulas: Lymphatic Infection, Antibacterial, **Liquid Lymph**, **Lymph Cleansing**, and Alterative-Immune

Herbs: Baptisia, burdock, **cleavers**, dulse, **echinacea**, forsythia, fritillary, garlic, kelp, lobelia, **mullein**, Oregon grape, **red clover**, **red root**, and yarrow

Supplements: Vitamin A, vitamin D, and vitamin K

Essential Oils: Tea tree and thyme

Syndrome X   see *metabolic syndrome*

Syphilis

Syphilis is a sexually transmitted bacterial infection. It is best treated medically with antibiotics. Echinacea and goldenseal may be somewhat helpful, but antibiotics are generally needed. After taking antibiotics, be sure to replace friendly flora with probiotic supplements. The disease can be prevented by having sexual relations only within committed relationships or using condoms when having sex with partners who have not been tested for sexually transmitted diseases.

Strategies: Friendly Flora

Formulas: Probiotic

Herbs: Echinacea, **goldenseal**, and Oregon grape

Supplements: **Nanoparticle silver**

Essential Oils: Lemon and myrrh

Tachycardia
Rapid Heart Rate

See also Graves' disease

Tachycardia is a rapid beating of the heart. This may happen occasionally from physical exertion or stress, but when it is ongoing, it requires medical attention

Under proper medical supervision, it may be aided by natural remedies. Motherwort, lobelia, and mistletoe are the best single herbs I know for this problem. Motherwort is a dependable remedy in mild cases. Lobelia acts as a natural beta-blocker, which slows and strengthens the heartbeat. Magnesium can also help calm and strengthen the heart beat.

Strategies: Deep Breathing, Hiatal Hernia Correction, Mineralization, and Stress Management

Formulas: Chinese Yang-Reducing, Herbal Potassium, Colloidal Mineral, Anti-Anxiety, and Thyroid Calming

Herbs: Biota, bugleweed, cherry, hawthorn, lemon balm, **lobelia**, **mistletoe**, **motherwort**, and quince (Bengal)

Supplements: Calcium, **magnesium**, potassium, and vitamin B_5

Essential Oils: Lavender, rosemary, and ylang ylang

TBI   see *traumatic brain injury*

Teeth, Grinding

See also parasites and stress

The often-unconscious habit of gritting the teeth together during sleep or periods of stress is often due to a lack of trace minerals, calcium deficiency, parasites, or stress. Look under related conditions for information on how to treat these root causes. Mineral supplements and nervines may help relieve this condition.

Strategies: Mineralization and Stress Management

Formulas: Herbal Calcium, **Watkin's Hair, Skin, and Nails**, Anti-Stress B-Complex, Joan Patton's Herbal Minerals, and **Skeletal Support**

Programs: Parasite Cleansing

Herbs: Bacopa, **motherwort**, and **vervain (blue)**

Supplements: Calcium, **magnesium**, vitamin B_3, and vitamin B_5

Teeth, Loose

See also gingivitis

Teeth that are not properly rooted or firmly attached into the gums of the mouth and thus wiggle back and forth in their sockets may be aided by remedies that strengthen tissue integrity and reduce inflammation. This problem is usually the result of infection in the bone, which may require the abscessed teeth to be removed. However, there are herbs that can help fight the infection and possibly strengthen the bones. White oak bark tea can be used as a mouthwash. Brushing with an *Herbal Toothpowder Formula* can also be helpful.

Strategies: Eat Healthy and Mineralization

Formulas: Herbal Calcium, **Herbal Tooth Powder**, and Colloidal Mineral

Herbs: Black walnut and **white oak**

Supplements: Co-Q10 and **vitamin C**

Essential Oils: Lavender and lemon

Teething

In the process of developing the first set of teeth and having them push through the gums, infants often develop pain, irritability, fever, and earache. Rubbing clove oil diluted in olive oil can ease gum pain. Lobelia can also be rubbed on the gums. Other remedies taken internally can also ease teething pain. Chamomile tea is a traditional remedy for this.

Formulas: Children's Colic and Herbal Calcium

Herbs: Catnip, **chamomile**, lobelia, marshmallow, and passion flower

Supplements: Calcium

Essential Oils: Chamomile (Roman) and clove

Tendonitis

See also inflammation

Tendonitis is inflammation of a tendon and is often due to injury or overexertion. Remedies that reduce inflammation will speed recovery. Use a *Topical Analgesic Formula* to ease pain. See *inflammation* for more ideas.

Formulas: Topical Analgesic, Herbal Calcium, Vulnerary, and **Anti-Inflammatory Pain**

Herbs: Aloe vera, boswellia, licorice, **safflower**, **solomon's seal**, teasel, and willow

Supplements: MSM

Essential Oils: Wintergreen

Tension
see *cramps & spasms*, *stress*, and *anxiety disorders*

Testosterone, Low

See also cholesterol (low), erectile dysfunction, and sex drive (low)

Testosterone is the principal male hormone. It stimulates sperm production, libido, muscular strength, and the physical characteristics of the male. Low testosterone has become an increasingly common problem. Testosterone levels in men appear to have been falling steadily for the past two decades, although it may be that recognition of the problem has simply become more common.

Testosterone levels in men naturally decline with age. The extent to which low testosterone levels affect men varies, but for every ten years increase of age, the chance of having low testosterone increased 17 percent. Here are some strategies for increasing testosterone levels.

Symptoms of low testosterone may include reduced libido, erectile dysfunction, reduced energy and fatigue, depression, loss of muscle mass, decreased muscle mass and increased body fat, difficulties with concentration and memory, loss of muscular strength, and low bone mineral density or osteoporosis. Here are some strategies for increasing testosterone levels.

Avoid Xenoetrogens

Excess estrogens upset the balance between testosterone and estrogen in men, and xenoestrogens are a principal cause of this imbalance. So follow the strategy *Avoid Xenoestrogens* to promote better testosterone levels.

Men suffering from any kind of male reproductive problems should also be aware that too many phytoestrogens (estrogenic compounds found in plants) can cause imbalances in testosterone and estrogen levels. One of the principal culprits here is soy. Widely touted as a beneficial health food, according to the Weston Price Foundation, "numerous animals studies show that soy foods cause infertility in animals… Japanese housewives feed tofu to their husbands frequently when they want to reduce his virility." So use soy sparingly.

Men should also avoid consuming large amounts of licorice, as it enhances cortisol and decreases testosterone. Hops is another highly estrogenic herb. It contains very potent estrogens that can reduce male sex drive. Since most beer is made with hops, men who are concerned about their fertility or who are suffering from male reproductive health problems should avoid drinking beer made from hops. Finally, grapefruit interferes with estrogen breakdown and should also be consumed sparingly by men who wish to enhance their testosterone levels.

Check Drug Medications

Drugs can also adversely affect testosterone levels. Classes of medications that may interfere with male reproductive function include anti-inflammatories, antibiotics, antifungals, statins (cholesterol-lowering medications), antidepressants, calcium channel blockers, sleeping pills, and high blood pressure medications. Carefully read warning labels to discover if any medications you take may be affecting your reproductive health. If medications are causing your low testosterone, work with your natural health consultant to see about natural alternatives.

Eat a Healthy Diet

Diets that are high in refined carbohydrates and low in good fats and protein will also damage male reproductive health. High-carbohydrate diets stress the adrenal glands and pancreas, resulting in increased levels of insulin and reduced levels of DHEA, a building block for male hormones.

Make Sure You Have Enough Cholesterol

The current drive to lower cholesterol levels is increasing depression and reproductive health problems in men. DHEA and all reproductive hormones are made from cholesterol, so driving cholesterol levels too low will actually cause reproductive problems. If your cholesterol is low, organic meat, eggs, and dairy products will actually good for you, especially if they are from grass-fed animals. See *cholesterol (low)* for more information.

Exercise and Success

Men's testosterone fluctuates with how they feel about themselves and response to specific stimuli. For instance, winning in sports or seeing an attractive woman can increase testosterone levels, while being rejected by a woman or losing in competition will decrease them. Regular exercise helps you feel better about yourself and also increases testosterone production. Resistance training with weights is especially important for men as they grow older. It also helps for men to be pursuing and achieving worthwhile goals for themselves to boost their self-confidence and self esteem.

Avoid Fluoride

A compound which may be causing a drop in testosterone levels is fluoride. High doses of fluoride are known to suppress testosterone production, but a study published in *Environmental Research* in 2003 suggested that even low levels can reduce the amount of available testosterone. Most water supplies in the United States are now fluoridated. So to protect testosterone levels, avoid fluoridated water and fluoridated toothpastes, mouthwashes, and dental treatments. You can help the body detoxify from fluoride by taking iodine supplements or seaweeds.

Use Herbs and Supplements

There are many herbs that have either been used traditionally or have some research backing their ability to increase testosterone. The *Male DHEA with Herbs Formula*

is one option. However, it may be a good idea to get your DHEA levels tested before using DHEA supplements. The other is to use a *Testosterone Formula* containing a variety of testosterone enhancing herbs and nutrients.

Strategies: Avoid Sugar, Avoid Xenoestrogens, Exercise, Healthy Fats, and Low-Glycemic Diet

Formulas: Male Performance, **DHEA with Herbs**, and **Testosterone**

Herbs: Cinnamon, cordyceps, damiana, eleuthero, epimedium, ginseng (American), **ginseng (Asian/Korean)**, **maca**, **muira puama**, and pine pollen

Supplements: DHEA, omega-3 EFAs, and zinc

Essential Oils: Cinnamon

Tetanus
Lockjaw

See also wounds & sores

Tetanus is an acute infectious disease characterized by tonic spasm of voluntary muscles, especially those of the jaw. It is caused by a toxin from a specific bacteria, which is usually introduced through a wound. Medical advice is to obtain a tetanus shot for any deep puncture wounds; however, if wounds are properly cleansed and topical antiseptics, such as a nanoparticle silver gel along with a disinfectant essential oil like tea tree, are applied the risk of tetanus is very slight. If tetanus does develop, medical attention should be sought immediately.

Strategies: Compress or Fomentation

Herbs: Lobelia

Supplements: Nanoparticle silver

Essential Oils: Cajeput, **tea tree**, and thyme

Thrombosis

See also blood clot prevention

A blood clot within a blood vessel is called thrombosis. The formation of these clots is dangerous because if they break loose, they can lodge in the heart or brain, causing a heart attack or stroke. Medical doctors often prescribe blood thinners to avoid thrombosis, but there are natural remedies that can help too.

Start by keeping your blood pressure down and staying properly hydrated, as this also helps prevent thrombosis. Nattokinase is a natural enzyme that reduces the risk of blood clots. Butcher's broom, horse chestnut, garlic, and ginkgo all help to prevent blood clots from forming in the circulatory system. Vitamin E is also helpful. Be cautious using natural blood thinners with people who are on blood-thinning medication. See *blood clots (prevention of)* for additional information.

Strategies: Hydration

Formulas: Heart Health, Vein Tonic, and **Nattokinase Enzyme**

Herbs: Alfalfa, **butcher's broom**, garlic, ginkgo, guggul, and horse chestnut

Supplements: Colostrum and **vitamin E**

Essential Oils: Lemon

Thrush

See also infection (fungal)

Thrush is a candida or yeast infection of the mouth marked by white patches in the oral cavity. It typically occurs in infants and children. For rapid relief, mix up the *Antifungal EO Blend*. Give one drop of this mixture twice daily. You can also combine these essential oils about forty to one (40:1) with Silver Shield. Also give the child probiotics.

Strategies: Friendly Flora

Formulas: **Probiotic** and Chinese Wind-Heat Evil

Essential Oil Blends: **Antifungal EO**

Herbs: Licorice and pau d'arco

Supplements: **Nanoparticle silver**

Essential Oils: Cajeput, **lavender**, lemon, marjoram, myrrh, rose, tea tree, and thyme

Thyroid, High   see *hyperthyroid*

Thyroid, Low   see *hypothyroidism*

Tick

See also lyme disease

A tick is a small blood-sucking insect whose bite can carry diseases such as Lyme or Rocky Mountain spotted fever. The current recommendation for removing ticks is to use fine-tipped tweezers to grasp the tick as close to the skin's surface as possible. You then pull upward with a steady, even pressure, being careful not to twist or jerk the tick. The goal is to remove the tick without breaking off the mouth parts. If they do break off, remove them with tweezers.

Ticks should not be crushed when removed. They should also be put in alcohol, flushed down the toilet, or disposed of in a sealed plastic bag. If you suspect infection you can put the tick in a plastic bag in the freezer so it can be checked later if necessary.

After removing the tick, thoroughly clean the bite area and your hands with soap and water. Apply andrographis to the tick bite if you have it. You can also apply rubbing alcohol, silver gel, or tea tree oil to disinfect the area.

Raw garlic rubbed on the skin is a natural tick repellant, but it can be a people repellant too. Several essential oils might help repel ticks; these include geranium, lemongrass, and eucalyptus.

If you develop a bull's eye rash or fever after being bitten by a tick, see a doctor immediately. Antibiotics can be very helpful in treating tick-borne illness if used early on.

Herbs: **Andrographis**, garlic, and pawpaw

Supplements: **Nanoparticle silver** and vitamin C

Essential Oils: Eucalyptus, **geranium**, lemon, lemongrass, and **tea tree**

Tickle in Throat

See also cough (dry)

An annoying sensation in the pharynx that feels like a tickle can often be relieved by sucking on licorice or slippery elm powder. It can also be a sign you aren't drinking enough water.

Strategies: Hydration

Herbs: **Licorice**, marshmallow, and **slippery elm**

Tics

See also twitching and tremors

A tic is a spasmodic muscular contraction. The movement may appear voluntary or purposeful but is involuntary. These are often due to deficiencies of mineral electrolytes like magnesium, potassium, and calcium. Antispasmodic herbs like lobelia and blue vervain may be helpful for tics.

Strategies: Epsom Salt Bath

Formulas: **Herbal Potassium**, Mitochondria Energy, Brain Calming, and Methyl B12 Vitamin

Herbs: Lobelia, **vervain (blue)**, and wood betony

Supplements: Calcium, **magnesium**, potassium, vitamin B-complex, and vitamin B_{12}

Tinnitus
Ringing in the Ears

See also earache

Tinnitus refers to a sound in the ears when no outside sound is present. Tinnitus can sound like ringing, hissing, roaring, pulsing, whooshing, chirping, humming, whistling, or clicking. One-third of all adults experience tinnitus at some time in their lives.

Signs you might have problems with tinnitus include dizziness, ringing in the ears, and difficulty hearing, such as trouble following conversations or having to ask people to repeat themselves. If you have symptoms like these, you should have your hearing evaluated by a certified audiologist.

Tinnitus may be caused by ear infections, circulatory problems, or nerve damage. It can also be caused by chronic tension in the muscles holding the bones of the middle ear. These muscles tense to reduce vibration when we hear loud noises, and like any other muscle, can fatigue from chronic tension. Exposure to loud noises makes them tense, which is why it is important to protect your ears from excessively load noises.

Lobelia extract warmed to body temperature to use as eardrops may be helpful in treating tinnitus, as it will help to relax these tiny muscles. Ginkgo biloba, the *Oral Chelation Formula,* and other remedies that aid circulation may be helpful when the problem is due to circulatory problems.

Some people have found using the *Antispasmodic Ear Formula* in the ears is helpful. Saint Johns wort may be helpful when the problem is due to nerve damage. Herbalist Matthew Wood reports successfully using drop doses of bergamot or beebalm for this problem.

If the problem is temporary and related to an infection, see *earache.*

Strategies: Eliminate Salicylates and Oral Chelation

Formulas: Chinese Yin-Increasing, Chinese Water-Increasing, Oral Chelation, **Antispasmodic Ear**, Stabilized Allicin, Chinese Yang-Reducing, **Brain-Heart**, and Methyl B12 Vitamin

Herbs: Aloe vera, **bee balm**, black cohosh, cordyceps, dodder, dogwood (Asian), drynaria, garlic, **ginkgo**, gotu kola, hawthorn, kudzu, **lobelia**, mistletoe, **Saint John's wort**, and wood betony

Supplements: Potassium, vitamin B-complex, vitamin B_{12}, and zinc

Essential Oils: Lemon

TMJ

See also tension

TMJ stands for *temporomandibular joint* or the point at which the lower jaw meets the temple region of the skull. Those who suffer from TMJ experience headaches and radiating pain from this region. Mechanical work by a massage therapist or chiropractor is often helpful. Magnesium or antispasmodic herbs to relax muscle tension may also be helpful, both taken internally and applied topically. The flower essence of snapdragon can be helpful for people who hold tension in their jaw.

Strategies: Bodywork and Stress Management

Formulas: Chinese Yang-Reducing and Enzyme Spray

Herbs: Kava kava and lobelia

Supplements: Glucosamine and **magnesium**

Tonsillitis
Adenoids

See also congestion (lymphatic)

When there is inflammation and swelling of the tonsils or lymph nodes located at the back of the throat (also known as adenoids), they can obstruct the nasal and ear passages, resulting in mouth breathing, snoring, and nasal discharge. If chronically inflamed, they can become a site of infection.

Traditionally the tonsils were removed when they became infected because they were thought to have no function. Now we understand that they are actually part of the lymphtic-immune system and removing them actually lowers the immune system.

Some herbs that can be helpful for tonsillitis include echinacea, garlic, red root, and wild indigo. I have found the combination of red root and echinacea particularly helpful. Since the tonsils are part of the lymphatic system, remedies for clearing the lymph system will also be helpful (see *congestion, lymphatic*).

Gargling with silver every two hours will also be helpful. Essential oils can be diluted in a carrier oil and massaged into the throat.

If the tonsils are severely infected medical attention should be sought.

Strategies: Detoxification and Eliminate Allergy-Causing Foods

Formulas: Lymph Cleansing, Stabilized Allicin, Liquid Lymph, **Lymphatic Infection**, Chinese Yang-Reducing, and **Antibacterial**

Herbs: Andrographis, baptisia, capsicum, **echinacea**, gardenia, garlic, goldenseal, oregano, **red root**, slippery elm, vervain (blue), and white oak

Supplements: Nanoparticle silver, vitamin A, and vitamin C

Essential Oils: Bergamot, **lemon**, oregano, tea tree, and **thyme**

Tooth Extraction

See also surgery (recovery)

After a tooth has been removed by pulling or surgery, herbs like goldenseal, oak bark, or plantain can be used topically to ease pain and promote more rapid healing. Crushed plantain leaves or a compress with plantain tincture can help pull material from the gums that wasn't properly removed in the extraction. I've also found the *Anti-Inflammatory Pain Formula* very helpful in reducing pain and speeding healing.

Strategies: Compress or Fomentation and Lymph-Moving Pain Relief

Formulas: Stan Malstrom's Herbal Aspirin and **Anti-Inflammatory Pain**

Herbs: Goldenseal, **plantain**, valerian, and **white oak**

Supplements: MSM and vitamin C

Tooth Grinding   see *teeth (grinding)*

Toothache

Pain in or around a tooth often as a result of a cavity or gum disease can be eased by diluting a little clove oil in a fixed oil and applying it to the gums. You can also slice a piece of garlic, coat it with olive oil, and put it in between the cheek and the gum to fight the infection, relieve pain, and ease the swelling of dental abscesses until a dentist can repair the tooth. You can also apply a silver gel around the tooth every couple of hours and take liquid nanoparticle silver internally at the same time. Some of the best herbs for easing the pain are Jamaican dogwood, kava-kava, and lobelia. All of these are temporary measures to use while seeking dental assistance.

Formulas: Topical Analgesic

Herbs: Achyranthes, chamomile, clove, dogwood (Jamaican), drynaria, **garlic**, ginger, kava kava, lobelia, **spilanthes**, and thyme

Supplements: Nanoparticle silver

Essential Oils: Clove and tea tree

Tourette's Syndrome

See also tics

Tourette's syndrome is a neurological disorder involving repetitive involuntary movements and vocalizations known as tics. Symptoms can include simple tics like eye blinking or darting, head jerking, lip or nose twitching, shoulder shrugging, or grunting. It may also involve more severe tics such as obscene gestures, swearing, and repeating words or phrases.

The cause of tourette's syndrome is unknown, but it is believed there is a hereditary aspect. It may respond to some types of *Counseling or Therapy* that work on behavior modification. Adopting the *Eat Healthy, Reduce Chemical Exposure* and *Liver Detoxification* strategies may help.

A study at Germany's Medical School of Hanover reported in 1998 that 82 percent of tourette's syndrome patients reported a "reduction or complete remission of motor or vocal tics and amelioration of premonitory urges and OCD symptoms" with cannabis use. This effect appears to be mainly due to THC-rich cannabis, but CBD might be helpful too.

Strategies: Counseling or Therapy, Eat Healthy, Liver Detoxification, and Reduce Chemical Exposure

Formulas: Methyl B12 Vitamin

Herbs: Cannabis, chamomile, passion flower, and vervain (blue)

Supplements: CBD, **magnesium**, vitamin B-complex, vitamin B_{12}, and vitamin D

Toxic Blood   see *blood poisoning*

Trauma

See also depression, insomnia, mental illness, anxiety disorders, and PTSD

Trauma is anything which triggers the body's fight-flight-or-freeze response. Trauma comes in many forms and can be both physical and emotional. Accidents, surgery, and physical assaults can be traumatizing on a physical level. Abandonment, abuse, neglect, ridicule, and belittling are emotionally traumatizing.

Unresolved trauma is an underlying cause of many health problems. The trauma may be experienced in childhood or later in life. Consider the need to work on healing trauma in people who have a long history of ill health and multiple health problems.

Problems caused by unresolved trauma include mental health issues such as depression, post-traumatic stress disorder, anxiety disorders, and feelings of tension and stress. Physical health problems can include constipation, loss of sex drive, digestive upset, and headaches. Trauma may weaken the immune system, laying the groundwork for immune-related diseases like frequent infections, autoimmune diseases, and cancer. It also affects nerve and glandular function.

Understanding Trauma

When people are traumatized, the higher brain shuts down and the amygdala takes over, creating an involuntary response to fight, flee, or freeze. In the fight response, people get angry and try to fight back against what is hurting or threatening them. Flight involves running away from what is hurting or threatening the person. When a person perceives themselves unable to fight or flee, as often happens in childhood abuse, they freeze. In this state, the body remains highly charged, ready to fight or flee, but does not move.

Just as the response to trauma is automatic, so are the responses that allow healing to occur. When the trauma passes and a person feels safe, they instinctively try to discharge the tension in their body, allowing the nervous system to return to normal. Animals in the wild do this automatically.

In human beings, this discharging process may involve the following:

Anger: shouting, yelling, kicking, punching, stomping feet

Grief: crying, moaning, wailing, sighing, screaming

Fear and anxiety: shaking, trembling, breathing rapidly, pacing, wringing the hands, running

Laughter: talking about the event or the problem until one starts to find humor in it and begins to laugh

People are conditioned to interrupt the trauma recovery process. They are told not to get angry, not to be sad, not to be afraid, or not to laugh so loud. This is usually done through criticism or punishment, comforting the person with the intent to make them stop expressing their feelings, or showing disapproval for the discharging behavior.

When a person's attempts to discharge emotional tension and trauma are repeatedly interrupted, a cycle of trauma is created within them. Every time they encounter a situation that reminds them of the original traumatic event, the same intense emotions they felt during that initial event are triggered. They may experience a sense of helplessness, rage, fear, sadness, or other intense emotions.

Left unresolved, these cycles of trauma grow stronger over time. Dr. Peter A. Levine calls this a *trauma vortex* and has written several good books on this process. I recommend reading *In an Unspoken Voice* as a start.

Signs of Unresolved Trauma

There are two major signs that a person's unresolved trauma is being triggered. First, the person's thoughts and words may become negative and incoherent, tending to spiral downwards. Second, the person may think and speak in absolute terms: "Everybody does this," "Nobody does that," "This always happens to me," and "That never happens to me."

Strategies for Healing Trauma

The *Counseling or Therapy* strategy may be helpful for resolving trauma, but counselors are often too head-based. The *Emotional Healing Work* strategy is designed to help a person discharge the emotional tension from their nervous system. Often a person being willing to listen with patience and kindness and allowing the person to just express their emotions freely is all that is needed.

Flower essences can be a helpful part of working through trauma. Black-eyed Susan and golden ear drops are two flower essences I've used to help people get in touch with suppressed memories of trauma. Arnica flower essence, which is found in the *Shock and Injury FE Blend*, helps people heal from past trauma. Pine, found in the *Personal Boundaries FE Blend*, helps people get over toxic shame from abuse. I've also used echinacea flower essence along myrrh and frankincense

essential oils to rebuild self-esteem damaged by trauma or abuse. See the *Flower Essences* and *Aromatherapy* strategies.

Herbs and supplements can be used alongside these therapies to support recovery. The *Anti-Stress B-Complex Formula* can be used as a general support for the nervous system. Nervines and adaptogens like ashwagandha, holy basil, and skullcap can help calm the nerves and aid the process of healing. More suggestions for remedies that can help traumatized people to heal can be found under *PTSD* and *Anxiety Disorders*.

Strategies: Affirmation and Visualization, Aromatherapy, Bodywork, Counseling or Therapy, Flower Essence, Healthy Fats, and Meditation

Formulas: **Adrenal Glandular**, **Anti-Stress B-Complex**, Chinese Fire-Increasing, Chinese Fire-Decreasing, Jeannie Burgess' Stress, Anti-Anxiety, Adaptogen-Immune, Ashwagandha Complex, and **Adaptogen**

Flower Essence Blends: Personal Boundaries FE, **Shock and Injury FE**, and Self-Responsibility FE

Herbs: **Ashwagandha**, holy basil, kava kava, passion flower, and **skullcap**

Supplements: Magnesium and **vitamin B-complex**

Essential Oils: Frankincense, myrrh, and **pine**

Traumatic Brain Injury
TBI, Concussions

See also injuries

Your brain is sort of like Jell-O in consistency. It's made of soft, fatty tissue that floats inside your skull surrounded by cerebrospinal fluid. The skull and the fluid inside it cushion the brain to reduce the risk of damage. However, if your head is hit hard enough or is shaken about violently, the brain can be physically damaged by the trauma. Damage like this is called a traumatic brain injury (TBI).

The most common and mildest form of TBIs are concussions. The word *concussion* comes from the Latin *concutere*, which means "to shake violently." The word shows the nature of the injury, which occurs from the jarring movement of the brain inside the skull.

Obviously, serious TBIs, such as those which occur in motorcycle and automobile accidents, should receive immediate medical attention. However, concussions from other causes like falls, bicycle, and skateboard accidents, and injuries incurred while playing sports should not be ignored and these often fail to receive the attention they deserve.

Symptoms of Concussion

A concussion is sort of like a bruise in your brain. The damage causes an inflammatory process, and the localized inflammation and swelling causes that portion of the brain to cease to function correctly, resulting in a loss of cognitive ability or motor control. The most extreme example of this is getting knocked out, which is commonly depicted in movies.

Most head injuries don't make you pass out. They can simply cause you to feel confused, dazed, clumsy, or dizzy. This is what is depicted in the cartoon images by the stars spinning around the head of a cartoon character who has had a concussion.

Concussions can also cause nausea, vomiting, headache, blurred vision, or sensitivity to lights or sounds. There may also be cognitive changes after a concussion such as a loss of memory, difficulty putting thoughts into words, or poor concentration. Concussions can even cause changes in behavior or personality such as depression, outbursts of anger, irritability, or anxiety.

These symptoms of a concussion can last for hours, days, weeks, or even longer. And, they may not be recognized as being linked with the concussion.

Concussions and Chronic Brain Disorders

Normally the brain heals just fine from this type of injury, although the process typically takes about two weeks, as the brain appears to heal more slowly than many other tissues. The primary treatment doctors recommend for concussions is rest. You need to avoid anything that would further jar and injure your brain, which means you need to avoid excessive activity for a while.

Resting after a concussion is very important because the evidence suggests that when multiple physical injuries to the brain occur, it can set up a chronic inflammatory cascade. This can definitely happen from repeated sports injuries or falls or from severe abuse, such as where a small child is repeatedly shaken and/or struck in the head in a violent manner.

Unresolved chronic inflammation in any tissue, including the brain, lays the foundation for more serious chronic and degenerative conditions to develop. There is evidence that chronic brain inflammation may be involved in anxiety, depression, drug and alcohol abuse, mental illness, ADHD, and suicide. We also know that chronic inflammation is involved in neurological disorders like Alzheimer's and Parkinson's. There is even evidence that cancer develops in areas of chronic inflammation, being a type of injury that never fully healed.

So if you or someone close to you has an injury to the head, fall, or suffers from any violent jarring of the head, it's a good idea to carefully monitor them for signs of con-

cussion. If you see any of these signs, you should seek medical advice and the person with the concussion should take it easy, avoiding all jarring activities for a couple of weeks. It may also be helpful to take some of the supplements listed below to help the brain heal faster.

Strategies: Eat Healthy, Healthy Fats, Lymph-Moving Pain Relief, and Sleep

Formulas: Enzyme Spray, Brain and Memory Protection, and Digestive Support

Herbs: Ginkgo, rosemary, **Saint John's wort**, **turmeric**, and yarrow

Supplements: **Alpha-lipoic acid**, CBD, **curcumin**, huperzine A, **omega-3 DHA**, and omega-3 EFAs

Essential Oils: Copaiba

Tremors

See also adrenal fatigue, twitching, and tics

A tremor is an involuntary quivering of a muscle. This can be due to severe depletion of muscle energy or nervous system problems. It often indicates low levels of potassium or magnesium and may also be a sign of exhausted adrenals. Besides these minerals, B-complex vitamins, and herbs like skullcap and wood betony may be helpful.

Formulas: **Mitochondria Energy**, **Fibromyalgia**, Chinese Fire-Increasing, Adrenal Glandular, **Herbal Potassium**, and Methyl B12 Vitamin

Herbs: Ginkgo, siler, **skullcap**, vervain (blue), and **wood betony**

Supplements: **Magnesium**, **potassium**, vitamin B_1, and vitamin B_{12}

Triglycerides, High

Triglycerides are blood fats composed of three fatty acids linked together. They travel with cholesterol in the bloodstream and are used to produce energy. When triglycerides are high, there may be problems with digestion, adrenal function, or the hypothalamus. Contrary to popular belief, eating healthy fats is not necessarily what elevates triglycerides. Excess consumption of alcohol, sugar, starches, and other simple carbohydrates is the primary reason triglycerides are elevated, because the excess calories are converted into fats. So adopting the *Low-Glycemic Diet* strategy is your first step to lowering triglycerides.

The *Cholesterol-Regulating Formula* may help with the metabolism of excess triglycerides. The *Mushroom Immune Formula* can also be helpful in balancing triglycerides and cholesterol.

Strategies: Avoid Sugar, Enhance Nitric Oxide, Increase Dietary Fiber, and Low-Glycemic Diet

Formulas: Whole Food Green Drink, Digestive Support, Adrenal Glandular, Anti-Stress B-Complex, Garcinia Fat-Burning, **Blood Sugar Control**, **Cholesterol-Regulating**, and **Mushroom Immune**

Herbs: Garcinia, goldenseal, **guggul**, gymnema, gynostemma, licorice, **orange (bergamot)**, red yeast rice, reishi, shitake, spirulina, and turmeric

Supplements: Alpha-lipoic acid, **berberine**, equol, lipase, omega-3 DHA, **omega-3 EFAs**, and omega-6 CLA

Triglycerides, Low

See also fatty liver disease

Low triglycerides may be due to a lack of dietary fats, fatty congestion in the liver, or digestive problems. If you're on a low-fat diet, see the *Healthy Fats* strategy to add them to your diet. Cholagogue herbs like dandelion, barberry, and turmeric, and lipase enzymes can help your body break down fats better. L-carnitine, burdock and chickweed can help the body metabolize fats more efficiently.

Strategies: Healthy Fats

Formulas: Adrenal Glandular, Digestive Support, Skinny, and **Chinese Wood-Decreasing**

Herbs: Barberry, burdock, chickweed, **dandelion root**, fringe tree, gentian, and turmeric

Supplements: L-carnitine, **lipase**, and **omega-3 EFAs**

Tuberculosis
Consumption, Scrofula

An infectious disease caused by a bacterial infection, tuberculosis used to be called consumption. Scrofula is a particular variety of tuberculosis, involving lymph nodes, especially in the neck.

Tuberculosis was once very common but the discovery of antibiotics has caused this condition to become very rare. Unfortunately, antibiotic-resistant strains have developed; so it is making a comeback. Herbs that have historically been used for tuberculosis are listed below. Supporting the immune system with nutrients like vitamins A, C, and D$_3$ can also be helpful.

Formulas: **Stabilized Allicin**, Chinese Metal-Increasing, and Immune-Boosting

Herbs: Astragalus, cherry, **elecampane**, **garlic**, goldenseal, he shou wu, **lobelia**, **lomatium**, mangosteen, mullein, olive, red clover, Saint John's wort, and **usnea**

Supplements: N-acetyl cysteine, **nanoparticle silver**, **vitamin A**, **vitamin C**, and **vitamin D**

Essential Oils: Bergamot, lemon, oregano, rose, tea tree, and thyme

Tumors   see *cancer* and *fatty tumors/deposits*

Twitching

See also tics and tremors

A twitch is a quick spasmodic contraction of a muscle. When repeated in rapid succession this is twitching. Minerals like calcium, magnesium, and potassium and antispasmodic herbs may be helpful for twitching.

Formulas: **Herbal Potassium** and Skeletal Support

Herbs: Dogwood (Jamaican), hops, **lobelia**, valerian, and wood betony

Supplements: Calcium, **magnesium**, and **potassium**

Typhoid

Typhoid is a severe contagious disease marked by high fever, stupor alternating with delirium, intense headache, diarrhea, intestinal inflammation, and a dark red rash. It is medically treated with antibiotics. Supporting the immune system with vitamins A, C, and D$_3$, as well as echinacea, would be helpful supportive therapies. Silver may also be helpful.

Formulas: Immune-Boosting

Herbs: Coptis, **echinacea**, and goldenseal

Supplements: **Nanoparticle silver**, **vitamin A**, **vitamin C**, and **vitamin D**

Essential Oils: Cinnamon and lemon

Ulcerations (External)

See also wounds & sores

An open sore or break in the skin, often containing pus, can often be healed by topical application of herbs like goldenseal, myrrh, propolis, or tea tree oil using the *Compress or Fomentation* or *Poultice* strategy. Internally, remedies to enhance circulation and immune function may be helpful. Vitamin C and zinc helps tissues to heal more rapidly.

Strategies: Compress or Fomentation and Poultice

Formulas: **Ayurvedic Skin Healing** and **Oral Chelation**

Herbs: Aloe vera, astragalus, bayberry, calendula, coptis, echinacea, **goldenseal**, grindelia, marshmallow, **myrrh**, Saint John's wort, and slippery elm

Supplements: **Propolis**, **vitamin C**, and **zinc**

Essential Oils: Myrrh and **tea tree**

Ulcerative Colitis
see *inflammatory bowel disorders*

Ulcers

There are two major kinds of ulcers, gastric or peptic ulcers (found in the stomach) and duodenal ulcers (found in the first part of the small intestine). In both kinds of ulcers, the lining and the tissue underneath it have been damaged and eroded by the digestive acids. In essence, the hydrochloric acid used in digestion starts to digest the body's own tissues. This leaves an open wound inside of the stomach or duodenum and causes irritation and swelling in the surrounding tissues.

Even though some peptic ulcers are asymptomatic, they are most often experienced as abdominal pain or discomfort about forty-five minutes to an hour after eating or during the night. The pain feels like cramping, gnawing, burning, aching, or is described as "heartburn." Relief occurs when the stomach acids are neutralized by antacids or by vomiting or drinking water. Other symptoms can be headaches, low back pain, choking sensations, itching, and nausea.

Contributing factors can be as diverse as food allergies, a poor diet that is too low in fiber, stress, medications and over-the-counter drugs such as aspirin and other pain relievers, cigarette smoking, alcohol consumption, and infections. The bacteria *Helicobacter pylori* (*H. pylori*) is believed to be responsible for causing many ulcers and is reported to be found in 95 percent of patients with ulcers.

If an ulcer is suspected and symptoms cannot be controlled by natural means, it is important to seek medical help to find out exactly what the problem is. Complications of peptic ulcers can be serious and may need hospitalization.

To deal with peptic ulcers in a natural way, one must first identify and reduce the factors that may have contributed to causing the ulcer. Once the causative factors have been eliminated, the next step is to heal and protect the tissues with proper supplementation and continued lifestyle changes. Here are the strategies.

Eliminate irritants. Restrict the use of sugar, which increases stomach acid. Restrict salt, as it irritates stomach and intestinal tissues. Eliminate dairy products. Food allergies can cause stomach bleeding, so eliminate suspected foods. Aspirin, alcohol, coffee, and tea increase stomach acidity and can interfere with healing.

Take fiber. A high-fiber diet is important because fiber slows the movement of food and acidic fluid from the stomach to the intestines and will reduce the frequency of recurrence. Aloe vera and slippery elm are two helpful fiber supplements. Bananas and banana chips have also been proved to help. Fresh cabbage juice has been proved to accelerate the healing of peptic ulcers.

Take licorice root. Licorice root soothes inflamed and injured mucous membranes in the digestive tract. It is the most highly recommended of all single herbs for the treatment of peptic ulcers. Licorice root taken one-half hour before meals has been known to be very effective in the healing of ulcers.

Take supplements to fight H. Pylori. Remedies that inhibit the *H. pylori* bacteria may be helpful in fighting ulcers. These include cloves, pau d'arco, and licorice. All are found in the *H. Pylori-Fighting Herbal Formula*. Myrrh and goldenseal are also antimicrobial and have been helpful for some people with ulcers.

Use a natural antacid. It may be necessary to use a *Natural Antiacid Formula* or a calcium supplement to calm down acid production in the stomach while the ulcer heals. This is one case where a prescription for an acid blocker may be useful to give the ulcer time to heal.

Additional suggestions. Drinking adequate amounts of water is very helpful. See the *Hydration* strategy. Supplements that may help peptic ulcers include vitamin C, but it needs to be buffered so as to not irritate the ulcer. Vitamin A, zinc, and bioflavonoids may also be helpful.

Believe it or not, some people have healed ulcers using capsicum, which acts as a styptic. I don't personally recommend this, but you can take a little capsicum with the fiber and licorice to buffer its burning effects.

Strategies: Eat Healthy, Hydration, and Increase Dietary Fiber

Formulas: Intestinal Soothing, Vulnerary, **H. Pylori-Fighting**, and Natural Antacid

Herbs: Alfalfa, **aloe vera**, amalaki, astragalus, bayberry, bitter melon, calendula, capsicum, cat's claw, chaga, chamomile, chirata, cyperus, elecampane, forsythia, ginger, goldenseal, gotu kola, **licorice**, lobelia, myrrh, quince (Bengal), **slippery elm**, and stillingia

Supplements: Bioflavonoids, **L-glutamine**, **vitamin A**, **vitamin C buffered**, and **zinc**

Essential Oils: Frankincense, myrrh, peppermint, and rose

Underweight

See also Graves' disease, hiatal hernia, and wasting

The inability to gain muscle weight is often due to a stress-induced hiatal hernia. It can also be due to other digestive problems like malabsorption and occasionally to glandular imbalances like hyperthyroidism.

Using the *Hiatal Hernia Correction* strategy will often result in improved muscle tone and healthy weight gain. The *Digestive Support Formula* or the *Plant Enzyme Supplement* may improve digestion and assimilation of nutrients. The *Chinese Earth-Increasing Formula* is often helpful as well. See related conditions for more suggestions.

Strategies: Hiatal Hernia Correction and Stress Management

Formulas: Chinese Metal-Increasing, Betaine HCl, **Chinese Earth-Increasing**, **Plant Enzyme**, Chinese Qi and Blood Tonic, Whole Food Protein, **Digestive Support**, and Testosterone

Herbs: Astragalus, barley, ginseng (American), licorice, **saw palmetto**, and spirulina

Supplements: Protease

Urethritis

See also urination (burning/painful) and urinary tract infections

Inflammation of the urethra or tube that carries urine from the bladder to the outside of the body is called urethritis. Remedies that soothe inflammation in the urinary passages are helpful, such as corn silk, marshmallow, and pipsissewa. If an herbal *Diuretic* or *Urinary Support Formula* is used, look for one that is high in these soothing urinary remedies. Drinking more water helps dilute irritants in the urine, which also soothes irritation and promotes healing.

Strategies: Hydration

Formulas: Chinese Water-Decreasing, Diuretic, **Urinary Support**, and Liquid Lymph

Herbs: Barberry, buchu, **corn silk**, couchgrass, damiana, gravel root, horsetail, hydrangea, **marshmallow**, **pipsissewa**, spilanthes, and uva ursi

Uric Acid Retention

See also gout

The inability of the body to eliminate uric acid results in painful uric acid crystal formation in the joints of the body, which can weaken bones and joints and increase the risk of calcium deposits and kidney stones. When uric acid retention is a problem decrease proteins containing purines and eat more vegetables (especially dark green, leafy vegetables), drink more water, and use herbs that help to neutralize the acid. Some of the best herbs to reduce uric acid levels are nettles, celery seed, and black cherries.

While most people know that eating foods high in purine raise uric acid levels, what many don't know is that fructose is a bigger culprit! In fact the consumption of fructose from table sugar, high-fructose corn syrup, and fruits high in fruc-

tose is one of the primary causes of not only elevated uric acid, but also metabolic syndrome and high blood pressure.

Strategies: Eat Healthy and Hydration

Formulas: **Herbal Arthritis** and **Chinese Water-Increasing**

Herbs: Alfalfa, barley, **celery seed**, devil's claw, **nettle, stinging leaf**, **safflower**, and yucca

Supplements: **Alpha-lipoic acid** and vitamin B-complex

Essential Oils: Pine

Urinary Tract Infections
UTI

See also bladder infection

You can get infections in any part of the urinary system, but most infections involve the urethra and bladder. If the infection spreads to the kidneys, it's much more serious. Women are more prone to them than men. Symptoms of UTIs include: a strong, persistent urge to urinate, burning sensations when urinating, frequent urination with only small amounts of urine, and urine that is cloudy or strong smelling.

Cranberry is helpful for preventing UTIs, but is not very effective at treating them once they are active. If you are prone to UTIs, try taking cranberry or the *UTI Prevention Formula* and drinking more water.

Some of my favorite remedies for active UTIs include uva ursi (taken as a tea), pipsissewa (for frequent small urination), any herb with berberine (such as goldenseal or coptis), and goldenrod. Kava kava is helpful if there is pain when urinating. The *Urinary Immune Formula* taken along with some berberine or the *Antibacterial Formula* may be helpful.

Strategies: Blood Type Diet and Hydration

Formulas: **UTI Prevention**, **Antibacterial**, Chinese Water-Decreasing, Diuretic, **Urinary Immune**, and Nitric Oxide Boosting

Herbs: Agrimony, amur cork, asparagus, bee balm, bilberry, buchu, **coptis**, couchgrass, **cranberry**, **goldenrod**, **goldenseal**, juniper, kava kava, mangosteen, **pipsissewa**, usnea, **uva ursi**, and yerba santa

Supplements: Nanoparticle silver

Essential Oils: Atlas cedarwood, bergamot, fennel, juniper, and lemon

Urination, Burning/Painful

See also interstitial cystitis

Painful urination is a sign of inflammation and/or infection. Avoid stimulating diuretics like juniper and buchu. Drink plenty of water to dilute irritants in the urine and take soothing non-irritating diuretics. Some of my favorites are corn silk, kava kava, and pipsissewa. If there is infection uva ursi can be helpful.

Strategies: Hydration

Formulas: Urinary Support, Liquid Kidney, **Prostate**, UTI Prevention, Diuretic, and Chinese Water-Decreasing

Herbs: Corn silk, **couchgrass**, goldenseal, kava kava, **lobelia**, **marshmallow**, nopal, **pipsissewa**, and uva ursi

Supplements: Nanoparticle silver

Urination, Frequent

See also adrenal fatigue, prolapsed uterus, BPH, stress, urinary tract infections, and prostatitis

This may be a sign of a urinary tract infection (see *urinary tract infections*). It can also be a sign the person isn't drinking enough water. When a person doesn't drink enough water, the body concentrates the irritants it's trying to eliminate through the urinary system making the urine more irritating to the bladder. This can result in the frequent urge to urinate. Unfortunately, this often leads someone to drink less water, which actually makes the problem worse. (See the *Hydration* strategy.)

To reduce irritation to the bladder, you can use soothing herbs like corn silk, marshmallow, schisandra, and pipsissewa. These can calm down the bladder and reduce trips to the bathroom, but must be taken with plenty of water.

When a person has a dry mouth and constant thirst, then drinks water and has to go to the bathroom frequently, this is a sign of yin deficiency in TCM. (It can also be an early warning indication for diabetes.) The *Chinese Yin-Increasing Formula* will help the body hold onto moisture better, reducing both thirst and the frequent urge to urinate, as well as helping to balance blood sugar.

Frequent nighttime urination is often a sign of stress and adrenal fatigue. Schisandra or the *Chinese Fire-Increasing Formula* may be helpful.

This can also be a sign of prostate problems in men, especially if it's difficult to start the flow of urine. In women, it can be a symptom of a prolapsed uterus. See these related conditions for information on deal with them.

Strategies: Hydration

Formulas: Chinese Water-Increasing, Antioxidant, **Chinese Yin-Increasing**, Chinese Fire-Increasing, and Prostate

Herbs: Corn silk, dogwood (Asian), eucommia, jambul, lotus, **marshmallow**, nettle, stinging, **pipsissewa**, **schisandra**, and uva ursi

Urine, Scant

See also edema, BPH, and prostatitis

When urine production is scant, the kidneys need stimulation and support. In men, this can be a sign of prostate problems. Diuretic herbs, like those found in the *Diuretic Formulas*, can increase output of urine. Make sure you are drinking adequate amounts of water. If the problem persists you should seek medical attention.

Strategies: Hydration

Formulas: Diuretic, **Chinese Water-Decreasing**, Urinary Support, UTI Prevention, Liquid Kidney, Liquid Lymph, and Prostate

Herbs: Buchu, butcher's broom, cleavers, dandelion leaf, **juniper**, pipsissewa, and uva ursi

Uterine Fibroids   **see** *fibroids (uterine)*

Vaccine Side Effects

See also mercury poisoning and aluminum toxicity

The basic principle of vaccination is scientifically sound in that the body creates antibodies to tag bacteria and viruses for destruction. Once exposed to a microbe, the body memorizes the configuration of that infective agent and is prepared to respond rapidly to repeated exposure. A vaccine presents a dead or weakened organism to the body to cause it to develop these antibodies.

Vaccines are a controversial topic, especially in natural health circles. As with any medical treatment, vaccines are not without potential side effects, and it is important to weight risks versus benefits before accepting treatment. I suggest that readers do their own research and make their own determination about what is best for themselves and their children.

These options could include following the full recommended immunization schedule, creating a modified schedule with fewer immunizations, or opting for no vaccines at all. It is not my intention here to convince readers to follow any particular course of vaccination, as I believe in informed freedom of choice in all matter pertaining to health care. I do, however, wish to make a few suggestions about vaccination and immunity.

Vaccines and the Immune System

First, vaccines do not confer immunity directly. Instead, they challenge the immune system, which has to respond to the vaccine by mounting a healthy immune response. Therefore, the real hero in preventing contagious disease is ultimately the immune system. A healthy immune system is the best way to not only reduce your risk of infection, but also to reduce your risk of allergic reactions, autoimmune diseases, and even cancer.

A healthy immune system requires good nutrition, a healthy intestinal biome, and the ability to handle stress effectively. Many people give these issues little or no thought.

I personally believe it is not wise to vaccinate people whose immune system may be compromised in any way. Don't get vaccines when you're already sick, weak, or malnourished. It's also not a good idea to get too many vaccines in a short period of time as this can overwhelm the immune system and increase the risk of adverse reactions.

If You Choose to Vaccinate

If you do choose to vaccinate or are compelled to because of your work, you can reduce the risk of adverse effects by boosting the immune system prior to the vaccination. This can be done with a *Mushroom Immune* or *Immune-Boosting Formula*. One could also take vitamin extra A and D along with vitamin C and zinc to boost the immune system prior to the vaccination. These remedies put the immune system on alert, which improves the body's ability to react properly to the challenge.

Because vaccines contain toxic chemicals (which are used to weaken or kill the infectious organisms), it's also wise to do some gentle detoxification following a vaccination. This can be done by taking a *Blood Purifier* or *Detoxifying Formula* containing herbs like red clover, dandelion, burdock, pau d'arco, and milk thistle. A tea made from red clover and dandelion is a good detoxifier for children.

Some vaccines still contain mercury compounds, particularly flu shots (see *mercury poisoning*). If you do get a vaccine with mercury, you may also want to do a *Heavy Metal Cleanse*. Many vaccines now contain aluminum compounds. See *aluminum toxicity* for suggestions on detoxifying aluminum.

Handling Vaccine Reactions

If a child or adult gets feverish or irritable within twenty-four hours of a vaccine, you can administer the same types of herbs or nutrients you'd use to help the body fight an natural infection or fever. These remedies include as yarrow, elderberry, chamomile, and feverfew. I've given *Steven Horne's Children's Composition Formula* to infants who are crying and fussing after a vaccine with good results. If it's a viral vaccine, you can also use the *Chinese Wind-Heat Evil Formula*.

You should alert your physician if you have a bad reaction to a vaccine. He may not do anything, or say it is unrelated to the vaccine, but you want a record that you reported the problem in case there are problems down the road.

Important Note: None of the above applies to the new COVID-19 vaccines, as they are not vaccines in the traditional sense. They don't present you with a weakened virus but rather inject you with RNA that enters your cells and replicates itself in a similar manner to a virus. This is a new technology and more of a genetic therapy than a vaccine. Its safety is yet to be determined. So I'm also unsure if boosting the immune system or detoxifying after receiving it will be of any help.

Choosing Not to Vaccinate

The main proof that vaccines are effective is the historical decline in infectious disease. However, evidence suggests that improved sanitation was what caused this worldwide reduction in contagious diseases, because diseases for which vaccines weren't developed also declined. Furthermore many diseases for which vaccines were developed were declining before the vaccines were introduced.

Before you assume that any vaccine is safe, you should ask the doctor if you can read the label. You may also find this information online. Look at the ingredients and the list of potential side effects and decide if you believe the potential benefits are worth the risk.

If you decide not to vaccinate be prepared to defend your position with government authorities and other people. Make sure you have done your research and are clear about your position. Some states make it more difficult to refuse vaccines than others, but there are ways to defend your rights.

If you don't vaccinate, be sure to take steps to create a healthy immune system. Eat a healthy diet, exercise, manage stress, get adequate sleep, and otherwise take good care of your health. I chose not to vaccinate my children or receive any more vaccines myself. I fortify my immune system during cold and flu season with extra vitamins, A, C, and D_3 in particular, and minerals like zinc. I also take immune-boosting herbs.

Strategies: Drawing Bath, Friendly Flora, Healthy Fats, Heavy Metal Cleanse, Liver Detoxification, and Sweat Bath

Formulas: Blood Purifier, **Antispasmodic Ear**, **Detoxifying**, Liquid Lymph, **Chinese Wind-Heat Evil**, Antioxidant, **Heavy Metal Cleansing**, Children's Elderberry Cold and Flu, Elderberry Cold and Flu, **Steven Horne's Children's Composition**, Immune-Boosting, and **Mushroom Immune**

Programs: Chinese Balanced Cleansing

Herbs: Baptisia, chamomile, echinacea, **elder flower**, feverfew, lobelia, mullein, Oregon grape, thuja, and yarrow

Supplements: L-glutamine, **omega-3 EFAs**, **vitamin A**, **vitamin C**, **vitamin D**, and **zinc**

Vaginal Discharge   **see** *leucorrhea*

Vaginal Dryness

See also estrogen (low)

During menopause, levels of estrogen are reduced. One of the effects of these lower estrogen levels can be vaginal dryness. It can also occur at other times in a woman's life for a variety of reasons, including childbirth and breastfeeding, radiation and chemotherapy, antiestrogen medications, or following the surgical removal of the ovaries. It is also an effect in Sjogren's syndrome, an autoimmune disorder, and may be a side effect of excessive douching.

Assessing the cause of the vaginal dryness is important. Some women with severely low estrogen might need to use an estrogen cream. In most cases, improving nutrition, increasing sleep, and decreasing stress can help with hormonal balance and vaginal dryness. Moistening remedies like shatavari, marshmallow, and linden taken as a tea are helpful in increasing mucus membrane moisture. Any kind of chronic burning, itching, discomfort, or pain should be checked by a doctor to determine the cause before embarking on a course of treatment.

If vaginal dryness is interfering with sexual relations, here are some tips. Vaginal lubrication increases during sexual arousal, so it is important to spend adequate time in sexual foreplay before intercourse to allow time for arousal and lubrication to occur. A water-based lubricant can also be applied prior to sexual activity. Some women have found that nanoparticle silver gel works as a nice lubricant.

Formulas: Hot Flash, Chrisopher's Menopause, GLA Oil, and Female Tonic

Herbs: Hops, linden, **marshmallow**, and white pond lily

Supplements: Omega-3 EFAs and vitamin E

Essential Oils: Geranium and tea tree

Vaginitis

See also leucorrhea

Inflammation of the vagina is known as vaginitis. It arises from a variety of causes primarily bacterial or yeast infections, though infection with the sexually transmitted parasite trichomoniasis isn't uncommon. Vaginitis can also be caused by irritation from douches and sprays.

About 50 percent of vaginitis is caused by excessive growth of certain vaginal bacteria. Bacterial vaginitis is characterized by an off-white vaginal discharge (especially after vaginal intercourse) with an unpleasant smell. Discharge occurs without significant irritation, pain, or redness, although mild itching can sometimes occur. Most cases of mild bacterial vaginitis can be remedied by the use of lactobacillus probiotics vaginally using the *Douche* strategy.

In more severe cases a Povidone iodine solution (betadine) one ounce in a quart of water used as a douche daily for seven days can remedy most infections. Follow with a probiotic douche. Make it by dissolving a couple of capsules of probiotic powders or one tablespoon of plain yoghurt with live cultures into one cup warm purified water. Use this as a douche two times a day for seven days to replace friendly bacteria.

Vaginitis caused by candida or yeast overgrowth causes vulval itching, soreness, and irritation, with pain or discomfort during sexual intercourse or urination and vaginal discharge, which is usually odorless. Take pau d'arco, other anti-fungal herbs, or a *Yeast Cleansing Formula* internally. Douche with something to knock down the yeast. For mild candida infections, simply use two teaspoons of apple cider vinegar mixed in one cup warm water or pau d'arco tea for two days. For severe candida infections mix one tablespoon of boric acid powder USP in one quart of warm water. Used as a douche one or two times per day for seven days, it is generally very effective. You should follow these douches with the probiotic douche described above.

Silver has also also been used as a douche. Some women have also used essential oils for douches, but these must be diluted as follows. Use only oils that are safe to use neat (undiluted) on the skin, such as lavender, cajeput, or tea tree oil. Mix one drop of essential oil with five to ten drops of a natural soap like Dr. Bronner's Supermild Baby Soap. Mix this in a pint of water and use as a douche. See the *Aromatherapy* strategy for instructions on using essential oils. As before, follow this with the probiotic douche.

Strategies: Douche, Eat Healthy, Friendly Flora, Sitz Bath, and Stress Management

Formulas: Probiotic and **Anti-Fungal**

Programs: Yeast Cleansing

Herbs: Aloe vera, amur cork, barberry, bayberry, garlic, **kava kava**, Oregon grape, pau d'arco, red raspberry, and usnea

Supplements: Nanoparticle silver

Essential Oils: Bergamot, cajeput, eucalyptus, lavender, rosemary, and tea tree

Varicose Veins
Peripheral Vascular Disease

See also hemorrhoids

Externally visible, prominent veins are called varicose veins. They are common on the legs and are a sign of poor circulation and venous valve collapse. They are not just a cosmetic problem; they may be painful and indicate a lack of tone in the blood vessels. They can also be a sign of congestion in the liver. Eat lots of fresh fruits and vegetables (especially berries) for their antioxidant value. These foods also contain vitamin C, which helps to tone veins.

Herbs like butcher's broom, ginkgo, and horse chestnut, which help to tone up varicose veins and improve venous circulation, can be taken internally or applied topically. The *Vein Tonic Formula* is a good blend of these. You can also use white oak bark, bayberry, or yarrow topically, using the *Compress or Fomentation* strategy, to help veins to shrink more rapidly.

You can also apply essential oils, diluted in a carrier oil, topically. Lemon, lemongrass, and rosemary are good options. See the *Aromatherapy* strategy for instructions on using essential oils.

Strategies: Compress or Fomentation, Eat Healthy, Increase Dietary Fiber, and Oral Chelation

Formulas: Oral Chelation, **Vein Tonic**, Antioxidant, and Nattokinase Enzyme

Programs: Cardiovascular Nutritional

Herbs: Aloe vera, bayberry, **bilberry**, **butcher's broom**, capsicum, ginkgo, **horse chestnut**, milk thistle, **white oak**, and yarrow

Supplements: Bioflavonoids, copper, and **vitamin C**

Essential Oils: Bergamot, copaiba, cypress, geranium, lemon, lemongrass, neroli, peppermint, and rosemary

Vertigo   see *dizziness*

Viral Infection   see *infection (viral)*

Vitiligo

See also autoimmune disorders and Hashimoto's disease

Vitiligo is a skin condition where there are white patches of skin surrounded by a dark border. It occurs when melanocytes, the cells responsible for producing pigment, or skin color, die or are unable to function properly. While the exact cause is unknown, it is thought to be autoimmune in nature. Treatment with ultra violet B (UVB) light, either from the sun or a special UVB lamp, combined with high doses of B_{12} and folate, is a good basic therapy. In a study of one hundred people with vitiligo, B_{12}, folate, and UVB together stopped depigmentation in 65 percent of people, caused 52 percent of people to develop new pigment, and totally cured 6 percent of the people involved in the study.

There is a strong link with vitiligo and Hashimoto's thyroidiitis. Screen people with vitiligo for thyroid peroxidase and thyroglobulin antibodies to see if this is a problem. If so, follow the recommendations for *Hashimotos's thyroiditis*.

Formulas: GLA Oil, Watkin's Hair, Skin, and Nails, General Glandular, **Methyl B12 Vitamin**, and **Methylated B Vitamin**

Herbs: Evening primrose

Supplements: Vitamin B-complex, **vitamin B_{12}**, **vitamin B_9**, vitamin C, vitamin D, and zinc

Vomiting   see *nausea & vomiting*

Warts

A wart is a horny projection on the skin usually caused by a virus. Remedies may be taken internally and applied topically.

Raw garlic has also been applied topically to get rid of warts. A banana peel taped over the wart has also been an effective wart remedy. The *Chinese Wind-Heat Evil Formula* can also be taken internally.

A *Drawing Salve Formula* can be applied topically to help get rid of warts. Mixing the *Standardized Acetogenin Formula* with a healing salve can make a good ointment for warts. Cover with a bandage and change twice daily.

One can also use the *Compress or Fomentation* or *Poultice* strategies on warts using herbs like bloodroot or celandine. These herbs are somewhat caustic, so this should be done with the supervision of a skilled herbalist or naturopath (findanherbalist.com or americanherbalistsguild.com).

Strategies: Compress or Fomentation and Poultice

Formulas: Standardized Acetogenin, **Chinese Wind-Heat Evil**, and **Drawing Salve**

Herbs: Aloe vera, **celandine**, and **garlic**

Supplements: Vitamin C

Essential Oils: Cinnamon, clove, tea tree, and thyme

Wasting

See also underweight

Wasting is a condition where a person begins to lose muscle mass and general body weight. In most cases it is caused by not consuming adequate calories and nutrients to sustain body weight. Voluntary weight loss and eating disorders will cause this, but are not considered wasting. It can also occur due to infections or chronic illness. Tuberculosis, cancer, AIDS, and chronic diarrhea, for example, can all cause wasting. Elderly people sometimes experience wasting due to a loss of appetite and digestive function.

Therapy for wasting depends on what is causing it. General approaches include eating foods rich in protein and good fats such as nut butters, eggs, cheese, and high quality animal foods. The *Digestive Support Formula* and/or the *Betaine HCL Formula* may be necessary to aid the breakdown of these foods. For children, mix about one-fourth of a capsule of the *Plant Enzyme Formula* with food before feeding it to the child.

The *Chinese Earth-Increasing Formula* can improve appetite and help counteract wasting. When the wasting involve cancer treatments like chemotherapy and radiation, the *Chinese Qi and Blood Tonic* may be helpful.

Herbalists have sometimes used marshmallow or slippery elm as nourishing gruel (eaten like porridge) to rebuild health in people who are wasting. The *Whole Food Green Drink Formula* is also a good food for people who are experiencing wasting.

Strategies: Eat Enzyme-Rich Foods, Gluten-Free Diet, and Stress Management

Formulas: Chinese Earth-Increasing, Plant Enzyme, **Digestive Support**, **Chinese Qi and Blood Tonic**, Whole Food Green Drink, Algae, and Betaine HCl

Herbs: Ashwagandha, **astragalus**, barley grass & juice, **cocoa**, ginseng (American), marshmallow, saw palmetto, **slippery elm**, and spirulina

Supplements: Multiple vitamin and mineral

Water Retention   see *edema*

Weak Knees

Excess weight and a lack of physical activity can weaken the knees. There may also be problems with connective tissue, nerves, or posture. Get help to determine the cause, but the following may be helpful.

Strategies: Bodywork and Good Posture

Formulas: Chinese Water-Increasing, **Joint Healing Nutrients**, and Colloidal Mineral

Supplements: Collagen

Weight (Under)
see *underweight* **and** *wasting*

Weight, Excess   see *excess weight*

Wheezing
Shortness of Breath

See also COPD

Wheezing can occur from constriction of the respiratory passages or by a loss of elasticity to the respiratory membranes. The following may help wheezing and shortness of breath.

Formulas: Chinese Metal-Increasing, Christopher's Sinus, and Chinese Metal-Decreasing

Herbs: Apricot, **cordyceps**, ginkgo, horsetail, **lobelia**, and **mullein**

Essential Oils: Anise

Whiplash

Whiplash is an injury to the neck caused by auto accidents or any sudden distortion of the neck. Black cohosh is a good remedy for whiplash. Other antispasmodic herbs like lobelia or vervain may also be helpful, either taken internally or applied topically. Magnesium oil or homeopathic arnica can also be applied topically. Find a chiropractor or other therapist following the *Bodywork* strategy will be helpful.

Strategies: Bodywork

Formulas: Enzyme Spray

Herbs: Arnica homeopathic, **black cohosh**, lobelia, **skunk cabbage**, **vervain (blue)**, and wood betony

Supplements: Magnesium

Essential Oils: Frankincense, geranium, and lavender

Whooping Cough   see *pertussis*

Worms   see *parasites (nematodes, worms)*

Worry   see *fear*

Wounds & Sores

See also abrasions/scratches, cuts, and injuries

There are many herbs that can help wounds and sores to heal more rapidly. Many of these herbs also prevent infection. You can also use the *Compress or Fomentation* or *Poultice* strategies using herbs like calendula, goldenseal, comfrey, and yarrow. Essential oils, such as tea tree or thyme, can also be applied to inhibit infection and promote healing. The *Lymph-Moving Pain Relief* strategies work very well in helping various types of wounds and sores to heal faster.

Strategies: Aromatherapy, Compress or Fomentation, Lymph-Moving Pain Relief, and Poultice

Formulas: Vulnerary, **Healing Salve**, Drawing Salve, **Enzyme Spray**, CBD Topical Analgesic, and Hemp Oil with Terpenes

Essential Oil Blends: Disinfectant EO and Topical Injury

Herbs: Aloe vera, baptisia, bayberry, black walnut, **calendula**, capsicum, chamomile, chickweed, comfrey, cyperus, devil's claw, **echinacea**, goldenseal, grindelia, he shou wu, horsetail, lady's mantle, marshmallow, pau d'arco, purslane, sage, Saint John's wort, slippery elm, thyme, white oak, **yarrow**, and yellow dock

Supplements: MSM, **nanoparticle silver**, **vitamin C**, and **zinc**

Essential Oils: Bergamot, cajeput, chamomile (Roman), clary sage, clove, copaiba, eucalyptus, geranium, helichrysum, jasmine, lemon, ravensara, rose, and **tea tree**

Wrinkles

See also skin problems

The development of wrinkles in the skin is a natural part of the aging process. As skin ages, it starts to lose its ability to hold on to moisture and is slower to heal. With age, skin cells renew themselves more slowly, which causes the skin's inner layer to thin. These factors cause the skin to lose its flexibility and elasticity.

The type of wrinkles we tend to form is based on our general mood. People who are always frowning develop different kinds of wrinkles than people who smile a lot. So as we age our face also reveals our general character. So learning how to deal with our emotions and manage our stress will also help us avoid unattractive wrinkles.

Excessive wrinkling of the skin can be caused by a variety of factors. Smoking curbs the skin's production of collagen, which reduces the skins elasticity and contributes to development of wrinkles. Dehydration also increases wrinkling, so anything that contributes to loss of moisture in the body will contribute to the development of wrinkles. Oxidative stress from factors like excessive sun exposure will also cause premature wrinkles.

Of course, good nutrition and proper hydration are helpful for keeping the skin looking youthful and healthy. Good fats like omega-3 fatty acids and fat-soluble vitamins are especially important, as is vitamin C, which aids in the production of collagen. Topical application of an astringent, like witch hazel, can help to tone the skin and reduce wrinkles.

Strategies: Eat Healthy, Healthy Fats, Hydration, Mineralization, and Stress Management

Formulas: GLA Oil, Watkin's Hair, Skin, and Nails, **Enzyme Spray**, and Colloidal Mineral

Herbs: Horsetail

Supplements: Co-Q10, **collagen**, krill oil, **nanoparticle silver**, **omega-3 EFAs**, vitamin A, vitamin C, and vitamin D

Essential Oils: Lemon, patchouli, and rose

Yeast Infections   **see** *infection (fungal)*

Remedies

Formulas, Herbs, Nutrients, Essential Oils, and Flower Essences

This section contains all the remedies referenced in the book. After determining which remedies might be beneficial for your healing strategy, you can read about what it is and how it is used and might benefit you.

These remedies include formulas or blends (combinations of multiple ingredients) as well as single supplements (herbs, essential oils, vitamins, minerals, enzymes, fatty acids, amino acids, and other nutrients). The type of remedy (herb, phytochemical, nutrient, etc.) is listed in italics to the right of the supplement name. Single supplements also list their herbal energetic category or aromatic category along with the type of supplement.

It is important to note the type of supplement because there are several herbs with an essential oil that has the same name. So make sure you're looking at the right entry. Herbs and essential oils will also list the Latin name for that remedy under the common name.

Each remedy has a short description highlighting what it is and its primary actions and uses. Single herbs and nutrients also list the formulas or blends in which they are key ingredients. Formulas where they are a minor ingredient are not included. Where applicable, strategies for suggested uses are listed and can be found in the "Strategies" section.

Here are the additional sections a remedy may have and what they mean.

Warnings: Any situations where the remedy should not be used or other cautions about using it are listed here.

Usage: Any specific directions to use the remedy will be listed here; otherwise, follow the manufacturer's usage. We have not included dosages for most single herbs because the potency of products varies, which is why you should rely on label recommendations. Label recommendations are usually conservative, which means it is usually safe to double the dose in many cases. It's always best to start slowly, however, and work up gradually.

Energetics: The energetics of the remedy—that is, how it affects the biological terrain of the body (the six tissue states). This is explained in the introduction.

Used For: This is a list of major health problems for which the remedy is used. The conditions the remedy is particularly helpful for are listed in bold. Look under the *Conditions Section* to learn more about a condition.

Properties: These are the properties (or actions) the remedy has. A glossary of these terms is in the *Properties Section*.

Affects: The body systems, organs, tissues, hormones, neurotransmitters, or Chinese elements that the remedy affects. Look under the *System Section* to learn more about a system.

Ingredients: Formulas and blends include a list of ingredients that you can use to identify a given product for use. Only the ingredients that are important for the primary purpose are listed. So, a specific commercial product may have additional ingredients and still work.

In some cases, there are several similar formulas that you can use. When this is the case an additional name is given along with any specific characteristics, ingredients and usage information that make that variant unique.

The names of these formulas have been created for this book and are not the names of commercial products. Most of the formulas and blends listed have readily available commercial counterparts. We suggest that you do your own research to find commercial formulas that contain ingredients similar to the ones listed. Visit stevenhorne.com for help.

Where a suitable commercial formula might be hard to find we've also included a few do-it-yourself formulas. These give you the parts so you can make it yourself. Directions for making all of these formulas can be found in the book *Modern Herbal Dispensatory* by Thomas Easley and Steven Horne.

5-HTP   *Phytochemical*

A direct precursor to the neurotransmitter serotonin, 5-hydroxytryptophan is the intermediate metabolite of the amino acid l-tryptophan. While a tryptophan deficiency isn't common, stress, insulin resistance, vitamin B_6 deficiency, and a magnesium deficiency all inhibit the body's ability to convert tryptophan to 5-HTP and then serotonin. Numerous studies have shown 5-HTP to be as or more effective than many prescription antidepressants.

Studies have also shown 5-HTP to be an effective remedy for insomnia. When using 5-HTP to aid sleep, turn the lights down low or otherwise darken the room before bedtime as 5-HTP is first converted to serotonin and then when it is dark, the pineal gland converts the serotonin to melatonin, the hormone that induces sleep.

Warnings: Avoid during pregnancy. 5-HTP should not be taken with an SSRI unless under the supervision of a health professional.

Usage: For depression, headaches, fibromyalgia and obesity start with 50 mg, three times a day with meals and increase to 100–200 mg, three times a day for 2 weeks if necessary. For insomnia take 100–300 mg before bedtime.

Used For: Addictions (sugar/carbohydrates), **appetite (deficient)**, **appetite (excessive)**, **depression**, down syndrome, excess weight, fibromyalgia, headache, **insomnia**, mental illness, SIBO, and stress

Properties: Antidepressant, appetite suppressant, and soporific

5-HTP Adaptogen Formula

See also *Antidepressant Formula*

A blend of 5-HTP mixed with adaptogenic herbs can help with stress and insomnia. See *5-HTP* for additional information.

Warnings: If taking a prescription SSRI, consult a healthcare practitioner before taking this product. Pregnant or nursing women should seek the advice of a healthcare practitioner before using this supplement. Avoid use with ADHD since high dopamine levels are associated with hyperactivity.

Used For: Addictions (sugar/carbohydrates), appetite (deficient), appetite (excessive), depression, excess weight, and **insomnia**

Affects: Brain depression, hypothalamus, pineal, and **serotonin**

Take 1 capsule three times daily with a meal for depression. Or as a sleep aid, take 3 capsules with an evening meal about thirty to sixty minutes before bedtime. Take no more than 3 capsules per day in total.

Ingredients: 5-HTP, eleuthero root, ashwagandha root, and suma bark

7-Keto   *Hormone*

This supplement stimulates the conversion of T4, the inactive form of the thyroid hormone, to T3, the active form. This increases the metabolic rate and causes the body to burn fat at an accelerated rate. It may be helpful when there are symptoms of hypothyroid, but thyroid hormones are at normal levels. Clinical trials have also shown this supplement to enhance the immune system, increase energy, and enhance memory. 7-keto

does not convert into the sex steroids, testosterone and estrogen, as does DHEA, so it may provide some of the same benefits as DHEA but without the hormonal side effects.

Warnings: Avoid during pregnancy. Consult a health-care professional when thyroid problems are present. Use of 7-keto consumes T4 reserves in the blood, and long-term use may affect thyroid function. Should not be used by people with low levels of T4. Prolonged use may cause some symptoms of hypothyroid.

Usage: As an aid to weight loss, take 1–2 capsules (75–150 mg) daily with a meal.

Used For: Excess weight, hypothyroidism, lupus, and Parkinson's disease

Properties: Antiobesic and immune stimulant

Acacia   *Mucilant Herb*

Acacia greggii

A source of mucilaginous fiber, used as a bulk laxative. It feeds the friendly flora, soothes digestive irritation and tones leaky gut. It can be applied topically for gum or skin inflammation.

Look for *acacia* in *Gut-Healing Fiber Formula*

Energetics: Cooling and moistening

Used For: Cholesterol (high), constipation (adults), excess weight, gingivitis, and leaky gut

Properties: Emulsifier and mucilant

Acacia (Indian)   *Astringent Herb*

Acacia catechu

Native to India, Myanmar (Burma), Sri Lanka, and East Africa, this tree is cultivated for its lumber. It is used like other astringents to stop bleeding or dry up excessive secretions.

Look for *acacia (Indian)* in *Ayurvedic Skin Healing Formula*

Warnings: Do not take for more than 2-3 weeks at a time or if suffering from kidney inflammation. Black catechu is subject to legal restrictions in some countries.

Energetics: Constricting and drying

Used For: Bleeding (external), bleeding (internal), congestion, diarrhea, eczema, hemorrhoids, and sore throat

Properties: Astringent

Açaí   *Sour Herb*

Euterpe oleracea

Açaí berries are loaded with antioxidants that help to protect cells from damage that may lead to chronic diseases, such as heart disease, diabetes, and cancer. The *Journal of*

Agriculture and Food Chemistry published a 2008 study showing that the açaí berry has more antioxidants than blackberries, blueberries, strawberries, and raspberries. A 2006 study by the American Chemical Society showed that açaí mimics the anti-inflammatory effects of prescription medications, such as the COX-1 and COX-2 inhibitors.

Look for *açaí* in *Antioxidant Formula*

Energetics: Cooling and nourishing

Used For: Cancer prevention, cardiovascular disease, **free radical damage**, and overacidity

Properties: Anti-inflammatory, antioxidant, and nutritive

Acerola
Sour Herb

Malpighia emarginata

A cherry like fruit from a shrub native to Central America, northern South America, Mexico, and the Caribbean. It is a rich source of vitamin C.

Used For: Colds and scurvy

Properties: Food and nutritive

Achyranthes
Bitter & Sour Herb

Achyranthes bidentata

Used in Chinese herbalism to invigorate blood flow and ease menstrual pain. It enters the liver and kidney meridians.

Look for *achyranthes* in *Chinese Water-Increasing Formula*

Warnings: Do not take if pregnant or if experiencing diarrhea or heavy menstruation.

Energetics: Neutral, drying, and relaxing

Used For: Backache, bleeding (external), canker sores, dysmenorrhea, gingivitis, kidney stones, menstruation (scant), nosebleeds, and toothache

Properties: Analgesic, antispasmodic, and diuretic

Adaptogen Formula

These are adaptogen formulas. Adaptogens help to reduce stress reactions and help the body cope with stressful situations. They tend to balance the immune system and normalize hormones.

Used For: Addictions (drugs), addictions (sugar/carbohydrates), **adrenal fatigue**, altitude sickness, **anxiety disorders**, autoimmune disorders, **cancer treatment side effects**, confusion, convalescence, **electromagnetic pollution**, environmental pollution, **exercise (performance)**, exercise (recovery), fibromyalgia, hypertension, hypotension, irritability, lyme disease, metabolic syndrome, mood swings, **nervous exhaustion**, **nervous-**

ness, radiation, reversed polarity, sex drive (low), **stress**, and **trauma**

Balanced Adaptogen

A blend of stimulating and nourishing adaptagens. Take 2 capsules once or twice daily.

Ingredients: Eleuthero root extract, schisandra fruit extract, astragalus root extract, ashwagandha root extract, gynostemma leaf extract, and rhodiola root extract

Regular Adaptogen

An slightly stimulating adaptogen formula for daily use. Do not take at bedtime or if you have bipolar disorder. Take 50-70 drops two or three times daily.

Ingredients: Eleuthero, oat seed (milky), schisandra, rhodiola, and american ginseng

Relaxing Adaptogen

An adpatogen formula with relaxing nervine action. Take 50-70 drops two or three times daily.

Ingredients: Ashwagandha root, linden flower & leaf, oat seed (milky), reishi mushroom, and schisandra berry

Adaptogen-Immune Formula

See also *Suma Adaptogen Formula*

These are blends of adaptogenic and immune enhancing herbs. They help with fatigue, immune weakness, and symptoms of aging brought on by excessive stress.

Warnings: Pregnant or lactating women should consult their healthcare professional prior to taking this supplement.

Used For: ADD/ADHD, Addison's disease, **aging**, AIDS, anxiety disorders, autoimmune disorders, cancer treatment side effects, cloudy thinking, exercise (performance), **fatigue**, fear, Hashimoto's disease, stress, and trauma

Affects: Adrenal depression

Immune Adapt

Take 2 capsules with a meal two to three times daily for stress or for immune weakness brought on by stress.

Ingredients: Korean ginseng root extract, rhodiola root extract, eleuthero root, gynostemma whole plant extract, ashwagandha root, schisandra fruit, suma bark, and reishi mycelium

David Winston's Immune Adapt

Take 2 capsules once daily or 60-100 drops four times daily.

Ingredients: Codonopsis root, eleuthero root, reishi, schisandra berry, astragalus root, atractylodes root, and ligustrum berry

Adrenal Glandular Formula

See also *Adaptogen-Immune Formula, Chinese Fire-Increasing Formula,* and *Suma Adaptogen Formula*

A formula containing adrenal substance may help strengthen weak adrenal glands. Additional herbs and nutrients support the production of thyroid hormones. A formula like this is particularly helpful for people whose adrenal glands are depleted from long term stress or chronic inflammation, including autoimmune disorders. It can also be helpful in overcoming addictions.

This product is ideally used for a short period of time (two to three months) to rebuild severely depleted adrenals, but can be taken for six to twelve months under supervision from a qualified natural health practitioner. Following the use of an adrenal glandular, the *Chinese Fire-Increasing Formula* or one of the adaptogen formulas (*Adaptogen-Immune* or *Suma Adaptogen Formula*) may be used for longer term care.

Used For: **ADD/ADHD**, **addictions (coffee, caffeine)**, **addictions (drugs)**, **addictions (sugar/carbohydrates)**, **Addison's disease**, **adrenal fatigue**, **alcoholism**, allergies (respiratory), **anxiety attacks**, **anxiety disorders**, **asthma**, **autoimmune disorders**, body building, **cholesterol (low)**, **concentration (poor)**, **confusion**, depression, **eczema**, **emotional sensitivity**, **endurance**, **fatigue**, **fear**, Graves' disease, hair loss/thinning, Hashimoto's disease, **hot flashes**, **hypochondria**, **hypotension**, hypothyroidism, hysteria, insomnia, **jet lag**, **lupus**, lyme disease, **menopause**, **mental illness**, mood swings, **narcolepsy**, nervous exhaustion, **nervousness**, night sweating, **nightmares**, **OCD**, **phobias**, PMS Type S, progesterone (low), **PTSD**, **restless dreams**, sex drive (low), skin (dry/flaky), stress, **trauma**, tremors, triglycerides (high), and triglycerides (low)

Affects: **Adrenal cortex**, **adrenal depression**, low cortisol, low DHEA, **nerve depression (exhaustion)**, and thyroid irritation

To strengthen under active adrenal function take 1 capsule one to two times daily.

Ingredients: Vitamin C, vitamin B$_5$, magnesium, zinc, adrenal substance, borage seed oil, licorice root, and schisandra fruit

Agrimony   *Astringent, Sour, & Mildly Sweet Herb*

Agrimonia eupatoria

Agrimony has an almost-paradoxical action. On one hand, it is an astringent, so it helps stop bleeding in wounds and diarrhea. On the other hand, it relieves tension in the nervous system. Its indication as a flower remedy is a good guide to its herbal use—it helps people who mask their pain behind a facade of cheerfulness. I find it very helpful for peo-ple who have a tense pulse and appear friendly and cheerful but are actually very tense and stressed. It is a great urinary tract remedy and helps urinary tract infections, cystitis, and incontinence. It also helps "constricted liver qi," a condition from Chinese herbalism that is commonly seen in many Americans. This involves an inner resistance, anger, or frustration that constricts blood flow to the liver and creates a tense, wiry pulse. It relaxes blood flow to the liver and helps a person relax and go with the flow of life.

Energetics: Drying and relaxing

Used For: Anger (excessive), bleeding (internal), blood in urine, diarrhea, incontinence, interstitial cystitis, and urinary tract infections

Properties: Anti-inflammatory, astringent, hemostatic, and vulnerary

Alfalfa   *Mildly Bitter & Salty Herb*

Medicago sativa

Alfalfa has been called the king of herbs, and it has been used since the ancient times. Roots can grow thirty to sixty feet deep to pick up minerals and water other plants can't reach. This makes alfalfa a rich source of vitamins, minerals, trace minerals, and other nutrients. Its trace mineral content is probably what makes it valuable for the pituitary, since trace mineral deficiencies often affect this gland. It acts as a mild alterative and blood purifier. Alfalfa and peppermint make a good tea for digestive troubles.

Look for *alfalfa* in *General Glandular, Herbal Arthritis, Herbal Calcium, Herbal Potassium, Joan Patton's Herbal Minerals, Pet Supplement,* and *Pregnancy Tea Formulas*

Warnings: Alfalfa is contraindicated in lupus.

Energetics: Moistening and nourishing

Used For: Anemia, aneurysm, arthritis, arthritis (rheumatoid), birth defect prevention, calcium deficiency, convalescence, cystic fibrosis, dental health, endometriosis, gout, hemochromatosis, indigestion, jaundice (adults), morning sickness, nursing, osteoporosis, overacidity, **pregnancy**, rosacea, sickle cell anemia, surgery (recovery), thrombosis, ulcers, and uric acid retention

Properties: Alterative, antiarthritic, **anticarious**, **anticoagulant**, antilipemic, **aperitive**, digestive tonic, **galactagogue**, **mineralizer**, nutritive, stimulant (appetite), and stomachic

Algae Blend

Algae supplies protein, carbohydrates, carotenoids, amino acids and trace minerals. Their high amino acid content make them helpful for reducing sugar cravings (especially when taken with licorice root) and stabilizing neurotransmitter function. The blend can enhance memory, concentration and learning, as well as stabilize mood. It can be taken as a natural energy booster when feeling tired or sluggish.

Used For: ADD/ADHD, **addictions (sugar/carbohydrates)**, aluminum toxicity, anemia, appetite (excessive), bipolar mood disorder, cadmium toxicity, confusion, convalescence, **debility**, electromagnetic pollution, exercise (performance), failure to thrive, fatigue, **hypoglycemia**, mania, **memory/brain function**, mercury poisoning, metabolic syndrome, mood swings, **PMS Type C**, pregnancy, **radiation**, reversed polarity, schizophrenia, surgery (recovery), and wasting

Affects: Brain, brain irritation, nails, **pancreatic irritation**, and pituitary (anterior)

Take 2-4 capsules one to three times daily. Add 1 capsule of licorice with each dose to stabilize blood sugar levels.

Ingredients: Blue-green algae, spirulina, and chlorella

Alisma   *Sweet Herb*

Alisma plantago-aquatica

Used as a cooling diuretic in Chinese herbalism, alisma is a fast-acting diuretic that enters the kidney and bladder meridians.

Energetics: Cooling and drying

Used For: Diarrhea, dizziness, edema, and nausea & vomiting

Properties: Antibacterial, diuretic, hypertensive, and hypoglycemic

Aloe Vera   *Mucilant & Mildly Sour Herb*

Aloe vera

Aloe vera juice and gel are made from the inner pulp of the aloe vera leaf. Aloe is extremely soothing to irritated skin and mucous membranes, burns and other damaged tissues. Whole-leaf aloe vera juice also builds the immune system to help fight arthritis, AIDS, cancer, and other degenerative diseases.

Aloe vera gel may be applied full strength topically for burns and skin irritations. Apply liberally and keep the skin moist for best results. Aloe vera works best when fresh. It's easy to keep an aloe plant in the home for treating burns.

The green part of the leaf is a strong purgative, but it is filtered out in the juice and gel. This is why the leaf, which contains anthraquinone glycosides, is a stimulant laxative.

Look for *aloe vera* in *Ivy Bridge's Cleansing* and *Vein Tonic Formulas*

Warnings: Some herbalists suggest that children, the elderly, and pregnant women should not drink whole aloe vera juice. However, this may apply only to the green leaf portion (which is strongly cathartic) or to aloe vera concentrates. The diluted juice is a mild, harmless remedy.

Usage: Apply gel liberally for topical applications. Cut leaves in half to apply gel from the fresh plant. Drink 1–3 ounces of aloe vera juice once or twice daily.

Energetics: Cooling and moistening

Used For: Abrasions/scratches, **acid indigestion**, acne, AIDS, **arthritis (rheumatoid)**, autoimmune disorders, blood in stool, **burns & scalds**, cancer, **cancer treatment side effects**, **celiac disease**, **colitis**, constipation (adults), convalescence, corns, cough (dry), **cradle cap**, dandruff, **denture sores**, **dermatitis**, **diaper rash**, **duodenal ulcers**, dyspepsia, eczema, food allergies/intolerances, food poisoning, **gastritis**, hepatitis, hysteria, ileocecal valve, indigestion, infection (viral), inflammation, **inflammatory bowel disorders**, irritability, **itching**, leaky gut, leukemia, lupus, menopause, nausea & vomiting, pain, parasites, parasites (tapeworm), poison ivy/oak, polyps, preeclampsia, psoriasis, radiation, rashes & hives, rosacea, scars/scar tissue, **seborrhea**, skin problems, sore throat, sore/geographic tongue, sprains, staph infections, **sunburn**, tendonitis, tinnitus, ulcerations (external), **ulcers**, vaginitis, varicose veins, warts, and wounds & sores

Properties: Anti-inflammatory, antiarthritic, aperient, **balsamic**, **emollient**, laxative, laxative (bulk), moistening, **mucilant**, **soothing**, tonic, vermifuge, and **vulnerary**

Alpha Linolenic Acid   **see** *omega-3 ALA*

Alpha-Lipoic Acid   *Nutrient*

Alpha-lipoic acid (ALA) is a vitamin-like enzyme cofactor or a coenzyme. It is chemically similar to a vitamin, and like vitamin C and E is part of the body's first line of defense against free radical damage. ALA is both water- and fat-soluble and is capable of extending the life of other antioxidants in the body like vitamin E, vitamin C, and glutathione, while at the same time directly preventing oxidative damage. While ALA is naturally made by the body, we still need to get most of it from our diet or supplements, especially as we age or during disease processes.

ALA is hepatoprotective and is currently being studied in the treatment of liver cirrhosis and fatty liver. It also aids liver detoxification and helps remove toxins like heavy metals, organophosphates, latex, and pesticides from the body. In addition ALA is an effective treatment for peripheral neuropathy associated with insulin resistance and, while research isn't conclusive, might actually help overcome insulin resistance as well. ALA crosses both cell membranes and the blood-brain barrier, protecting the entire body from oxidative damage.

Usage: Take 600–1800 mg daily with meals. For R-lipoic acid, the active component of ALA, 200–400 mg daily.

Used For: Addictions (sugar/carbohydrates), aging, Alzheimer's, arsenic poisoning, burning feet/hands, cadmium toxicity, cancer treatment side effects, cardiovascular disease, chemical exposure, **dementia**, **diabetes**, **diabetic retinopathy**, down syndrome, environmental pollution, **free radical damage**, **gangrene**, glaucoma, **heavy metal poisoning**, **hypertension**, hypoglycemia, inflammation, **lead poisoning**, **mental illness**, **mercury poisoning**, **metabolic syndrome**, **mitochondrial dysfunction**, neurodegenerative diseases, **Parkinson's disease**, **peripheral neuropathy**, sleep apnea, **traumatic brain injury**, triglycerides (high), and **uric acid retention**

Properties: Antidiabetic, **antioxidant**, detoxifying, and hypolipidemic

Alterative-Immune Formula

See also *Essiac Immune Tea Formula*

These are blood purifying formulas which also contain herbs traditionally used to fight cancer. They are used as part of a comprehensive natural program for cancer and not as stand-alone remedies. They can also be used to clear up other problems where alterative or blood purifying herbs are indicated.

Used For: Abscesses, boils, **cancer**, **congestion (lymphatic)**, lymphoma, skin problems, and swollen lymph glands

Ingredients: Burdock root, poke, red clover, and stillingia

Use 10–40 drops internally 2–3 times daily.

Ingredients: Burdock root, red clover flower, stillingia, poke, and prickly ash

Amalaki   *Astringent, Bitter, Pungent, & Sour Herb*

Phyllanthus emblica

One of the three fruits in triphala, this fruit has a balancing energy like schisandra because it contains multiple tastes—sour, astringent, sweet, pungent and bitter. It is used to heal ulcers and reduce intestinal inflammation and is one of the most frequently used herbs in Ayurvedic herbalism.

Look for *amalaki* in *Triphala Formula*

Energetics: Cooling, mildly constricting, and mildly drying

Used For: Asthma, colitis, colon (spastic), constipation (adults), cough, diabetes, dizziness, dyspepsia, gastritis, gingivitis, gout, hemorrhoids, inflammatory bowel disorders, leucorrhea, pancreatitis, prostatitis, and ulcers

Properties: Alterative, anti-inflammatory, antibacterial, anticancer, antidiabetic, antioxidant, aperient, astringent, febrifuge, and hepatoprotective

Amber (Succinum)   *Mineral*

Amber is the fossilized resin of trees in the pine family. It is used in Chinese herbalism for the heart, liver and bladder meridians. It decreases fear and helps the mind be calm. It opens awareness and mental perception. In essential oil-like liquid form, it makes a grounding perfume oil that can be applied to the forehead to wake up the mind and increase perception and rational thought processes.

Energetics: Mildly warming, mildly drying, and relaxing

Used For: Fear, heart fibrillation/palpitations, insomnia, and restless dreams

Properties: Relaxant

Amur Cork (Phellodendron)   *Bitter Herb*

Phellodendron amurense

A cooling detoxifier, the bark of this tree contains berberine, which has antimicrobial properties. It is used in Chinese herbalism for inflammation and swelling (damp heat).

Look for *amur cork* in *Cortisol-Reducing* and *Myelin Sheath Formulas*

Energetics: Cooling

Used For: Abscesses, arthritis, boils, eczema, inflammation, jaundice (adults), psoriasis, urinary tract infections, and vaginitis

Properties: Anti-inflammatory, **antibacterial**, and cholagogue

Amylase   *Enzyme*

Amylase is a starch digesting enzyme. There are various forms of it. It helps break down starches in foods into sugars for absorption.

Used For: Digestion (poor) and gas & bloating

Properties: Digestant

Analgesic EO Blend

See also *Topical Analgesic Formula*

These essential oil blends have analgesic and anti-inflammatory effects, making them useful for aches and pains in the muscles and joints.

See the strategy *Aromatherapy* for suggested uses.

Warnings: Do not use internally.

Used For: Anger (excessive), **arthritis**, backache, bites & stings, concentration (poor), confusion, exercise (recovery), fatigue, **headache**, **headache (cluster)**, **pain**, and shock (medical)

Affects: Joints, muscles, **nerve irritation (pain)**, and **structural depression**

Topical Analgesic Essential Oils

My favorite topical analgesic. Use topically to ease aches and pains. Apply to temples for migraines. Inhale to ease respiratory congestion and promote mental alterness.

Ingredients: Menthol EO, eucalyptus EO, camphor EO, wintergreen EO, lavender EO, and clove EO

Topical Soothing Blend

A topical analgesic that may helps with infection. Apply topically as needed.

Ingredients: Wintergreen EO, camphor EO, rosemary EO, cajeput EO, clove EO, and helichrysum EO

Analgesic Nerve Formula

See also *Anti-Inflammatory Pain Formula, General Analgesic Formula,* and *Stan Malstrom's Herbal Aspirin Formula*

Pain, inflammation, and stress are often connected. Inflammation causes pain, pain causes tension, and tension causes more pain. This formula can help to break this vicious cycle. It contains herbs that reduce inflammation, ease pain, relax muscle spasms, and reduce tension and stress.

Used For: **Arthritis**, arthritis (rheumatoid), **Bell's palsy**, burning feet/hands, cramps (menstrual), dislocation, **headache**, **headache (tension)**, **inflammation**, injuries, **lupus**, multiple sclerosis, **neuralgia & neuritis**, and sciatica

Affects: Joints, nerve irritation (pain), **prostaglandins**, structural constriction, and structural irritation

Take 2 capsules three times daily or as needed.

Ingredients: Willow bark, hops flower, valerian root, wood betony aerial parts, devil's claw root, and black cohosh root & rhizome

Andrographis   *Bitter Herb*

Andrographis paniculata

Widely used in Ayurvedic herbalism, andrographis extracts have been shown to mildly inhibit *Staphylococcus aurea, Psudomonas aeruginosa, Proteus vulgaris, Shigella dysenteriae,* and *Escherichia coli.* Extracts have also been shown to inhibit lipid peroxidation and inflammation. In a clinical study, patients treated with andrographis for three months were two times less likely to catch colds than the placebo group. It is also a major remedy for Lyme infection.

Look for *andrographis* in *Anti-Inflammatory Pain* and *Seasonal Cold* and *Flu Formulas*

Warnings: Do not use during pregnancy or while nursing.

Energetics: Cooling and drying

Used For: Colds, **diarrhea**, earache, **flu**, **giardia**, **hepatitis**, infection (viral), **lyme disease**, **malaria**, **mononucleosis**, **parasites**, **pneumonia**, sinus infection, sore throat, **strep throat**, **tick**, and **tonsillitis**

Properties: Anti-inflammatory, antibacterial, cholagogue, febrifuge, and immune stimulant

Anemarrhena   *Bitter Herb*

Anemarrhena asphodeloides

A cooling Chinese remedy used to reduce fever, heat, and irritability. It affects the lung, stomach, and liver merididans.

Look for *anemarrhena* in *Chinese Metal-Increasing Formula*

Energetics: Cooling and moistening

Used For: Cough, diabetes, fainting, fever, and irritability

Properties: Antibacterial, febrifuge, and hypoglycemic

Angelica   *Aromatic & Mildly Sweet Herb*

Angelica archangelica

Angelica is a warming, aromatic tonic for a cold, stiff, weakened body and digestive system. It also helps respiratory congestion. Angelica is an important female remedy that helps to regulate menses and balance hormones, as it is related to dong quai and has similar actions. It can also be applied topically.

Look for *angelica* in *Headache, Herbal Bitters,* and *Prebirth Formulas*

Warnings: Not for use during pregnancy or while nursing. Also contraindicated in heavy menstrual bleeding.

Energetics: Warming and drying

Used For: Anemia, anorexia, belching, bruises, colds with fever, colic (adults), **congestion (lungs)**, cough (dry), **cramps (menstrual)**, dysmenorrhea, dyspepsia, flu, **gas & bloating**, low stomach acid, menstrual irregularity, PMS Type A, and sprains

Properties: Decongestant, digestive tonic, and stomachic

Anger-Reducing FE Blend

A flower essence for people who have issues with anger. It is helpful for those who feel irritated, impatient and easily lose their temper. It helps a person be more receptive to other people's points of view and work for cooperation rather than competition. It promotes forgiveness, tolerance, and acceptance of others, as well as open and loving communication. People who have issues with venting their anger on others are more prone to liver disease and heart problems.

See the strategy *Flower Essence* for suggested uses.

Used For: Anger (excessive), cardiovascular disease, cirrhosis of the liver, hepatitis, and irritability

Take 3-10 drops under the tongue as need. See *Flower Essence* strategy for additional suggestions.

Ingredients: Calendula FE, snapdragon FE, impatiens FE, vine FE, holly FE, and pretty face FE

Anise   *Aromatic Herb*

Pimpinella anisum

Anise is a soothing aromatic with properties similar to fennel. Tea, tincture, or oil can be used to settle the stomach and expel gas. It is useful for colic in infants and helps promote lactation. It is a mucolytic agent and helps to thin and expel mucus from the lungs. It is a common ingredient in formulas for indigestion, but is not a key herb in these formulas.

Look for *anise* in *Herbal Bitters Formula*

Warnings: Avoid during pregnancy.

Energetics: Warming and drying

Used For: Colic (children), **congestion (bronchial)**, **gas & bloating**, **nausea & vomiting**, and nursing

Properties: Carminative and galactagogue

Anise EO   *Sweet Essential Oil*

Pimpinella anisum

Anise EO has a clean, sweet, licorice-like odor. It's fragrance is warming and uplifting and is helpful for people who tend to be introverted, withdrawn, and melancholic.

See the strategy *Aromatherapy* for suggested uses.

Warnings: Probably safe for internal use but should be diluted 20:1 for internal use. Occasionally causes allergic reactions topically.

Used For: Anxiety (situational), asthma, circulation (poor), colic (children), congestion, cough, digestion (poor), **gas & bloating**, nursing, and wheezing

Properties: Analgesic, anti-inflammatory, antibacterial, antidepressant, antiepileptic, antifungal, antioxidant, antiparasitic, antirheumatic, antiseptic, antispasmodic, **carminative**, expectorant, galactagogue, insecticide, sedative, and stomachic

Anti-Anxiety Formula

Take this to reduce anxiety and nervousness. Use it to improve mood without creating drowsiness. It contains a standardized, patented extract of *Sceletium tortuosum*, a plant from South Africa that was traditionally chewed to ease anxiety, depression and stress. It also contains L-theanine, an amino acid found in green tea. It has some effects on GABA and serotonin, causing relaxing and anxiety-reducing effects.

Used For: Anxiety (situational), **anxiety attacks**, **anxiety disorders**, emotional sensitivity, fear, Graves' disease, hypochondria, hysteria, irritability, **mental illness**, **nervous exhaustion**, **nervousness**, OCD, phobias, PMS Type A, **PTSD**, schizophrenia, sex drive (low), **stress**, tachycardia, and trauma

Affects: Adrenal irritation, **brain irritation**, and sympathetic-dominant ANS

Take 1 capsule as needed up to 3-4 capsules per day.

Ingredients: Vitamin B_1, magnesium, zinc, and zembrin® plant extract

Anti-Fungal Formula

See also *Yeast Cleansing Program*

These formulas are used to fight fungal infections such as *Candida albicans*.

Warnings: If bloating or gas gets too uncomfortable (due to candida kill off), reduce the amount taken.

Used For: Athlete's foot, **infection (fungal)**, jock itch, leaky gut, leucorrhea, SIBO, and **vaginitis**

Affects: Digestive stagnation, intestinal stagnation, large intestines (colon), and **vagina**

Ed's Herbal Antifungal Formula

An good anti-fungal tincture. 1 dropper two to four times daily in water or juice.

Ingredients: Usnea, oregano leaf & flower, spilanthes whole plant, and pau d'arco

Anti-Fungal with Caprylic Acid

Capryllic acid is a medium-chain saturated fatty acid from coconut oil that helps the immune system regulate gut bacteria. Take 2 capsules twice daiily.

Ingredients: Caprylic acid, elecampane root, and black walnut hulls

Antifungal Formula

A blend of herbs and nutrients that reduce yeast overgrowth and harmful bacteria in the GI tract, plus boost the immune system. Take 1 capsule two to three times daily with plenty of water.

Ingredients: Zinc, selenium, caprylic acid, pau d'arco bark, garlic bulb, and oregano (mexico) leaf

Candida Clearing Blend

A strong antifungal blend, avoid with liver problems. Use as directed on the label.

Ingredients: Pau d'arco, chaparral, and purple loosestrife

Anti-Inflammatory Pain Formula

See also *Analgesic Nerve Formula*, *General Analgesic Formula*, and *Stan Malstrom's Herbal Aspirin Formula*

This formula is a great alternative to NSAIDs for easing aches and pains. It contains herbs that act as natural COX-2 inhibitors. It not only reduces pain and inflammation following injuries or surgery but also promotes tissue repair and healing.

Warnings: Thins the blood and probably should be avoided if taking blood thinners.

Used For: Afterbirth pain, **allergies (respiratory)**, appendicitis, arthritis, backache, bunions, bursitis, **dislocation**, enteritis, gingivitis, Hashimoto's disease, headache, **inflammation**, **inflammatory bowel disorders**, **injuries**, interstitial cystitis, laryngitis, lupus, mastitis, meningitis, nephritis, **neuralgia & neuritis**, **oral surgery**, **pain**, pancreatitis, phlebitis, prostatitis, rhinitis, sore throat, spider veins, spinal disks, **surgery (recovery)**, **tendonitis**, and **tooth extraction**

Affects: **General irritation**, gums, joints, **nerve irritation (pain)**, **prostaglandins**, spinal discs, **structural irritation**, and substance P

For acute pain, take 2 capsules every two hours to a maximum of 10 capsules per day. For chronic pain and inflammation, take 2 capsules two to four times daily. Drink a lot of water.

Ingredients: Andrographis whole plant extract, boswellia gum extract, mangosteen pericarp extract, turmeric root extract, and white willow bark extract

Anti-Snoring Formula

See also *Sinus Formula*

A natural sinus decongestant that can be taken to help open the respiratory passages and inhibit snoring.

Warnings: Do not use during pregnancy.

Used For: Congestion (sinus), headache (sinus), **sleep apnea**, and **snoring**

Affects: Respiratory stagnation

Take 1-3 capsules daily 30 minutes before bedtime for snoring. For sinus problems take 1-2 capsules two to three times daily.

Ingredients: Co-Q10, orange (bitter) fruit, and bromelain

Anti-Stress B-Complex Formula

This supplement helps calm nervous and high-strung individuals. It feeds the nerves and adrenal glands, making it a good supplement for anyone who feels depleted from nervous stress. It does not cause drowsiness and can increase energy while maintaining a sense of calm.

Used For: ADD/ADHD, **addictions (drugs)**, **addictions (tobacco)**, **adrenal fatigue**, **alcoholism**, angina, anorexia, **anxiety (situational)**, anxiety attacks, **anxiety disorders**, Bell's palsy, bipolar mood disorder, burning feet/hands, cloudy thinking, confusion, **copper toxicity**, Cushing's disease, dandruff, depression, eczema, **emotional sensitivity**, **fear**, **fingernail biting**, hypochondria, insomnia, irritability, **mania**, **memory/brain function**, **mental illness**, mitochondrial dysfunction, mitral valve, narcolepsy, **nerve damage**, **nervous exhaustion**, **nervousness**, **numbness**, **paralysis**, Parkinson's disease, **phobias**, PTSD, **restless dreams**, **schizophrenia**, **stress**, strokes, teeth (grinding), **trauma**, and triglycerides (high)

Affects: **Adrenal irritation**, **adrenal medulla**, central nervous system, pineal, and stressed fire

Use 1 tablet three times a day.

Ingredients: Vitamin C, vitamin B_1, vitamin B_2, vitamin B_3, vitamin B_6, vitamin B_9, vitamin B_{12}, biotin, vitamin B_5, schisandra fruit, hops flower extract, passion flower flower extract, and valerian root extract

Antibacterial Formula

The blend of goldenseal and echinacea is a basic formula for fighting bacterial infections. It is helpful in the later stages of a cold (when mucus turns yellow or green), but not as helpful in the early stages (when mucus is clear or white). It can be used with garlic to treat respiratory infections and may also be helpful for urinary infections. It can be applied topically for skin infections or diluted with water and used as a mouthwash or gargle.

Warnings: See warnings for the herbs echinacea purpurea and goldenseal.

Used For: Antibiotic resistance, **food poisoning**, gangrene, giardia, gonorrhea, **impetigo**, **infection (bacterial)**, leucorrhea, **mastitis**, **sinus infection**, **skin (infections)**, **sore throat**, staph infections, **strep throat**, swollen lymph glands, **tonsillitis**, and **urinary tract infections**

Affects: **Subacute disease stage**

Use 1-2 capsules or 1/2 teaspoon of the extract three times daily with meals. For children, use 1/8-1/4 teaspoon every two to four hours.

Ingredients: Echinacea aerial parts & root, echinacea root, and goldenseal root extract

Antidepressant Formula

See also *5-HTP Adaptogen Formula* and *Chinese Qi-Regulating Formula*

These are blends of herbs that may be helpful in improving ones mood when depressed due to grief, anxiety, or stressful situations. By themselves, they are not sufficient remedies for severe depression. (See *depression*.)

Warnings: When taking antidepressant medications seek professional advise about using these formulas.

David Winston's Mood Elevating Formula

A good choice for gloomy, sad feelings. Use as directed on the label.

Ingredients: Saint John's wort flower, lemon balm, mimosa bark, black cohosh, and night-blooming cereus stem

Bright Mood

Helpful for depression associated with stress. Use as directed on the label.

Ingredients: Rhodiola, lemon balm, passion flower, and damiana

Antifungal EO Blend

I got this formula from Carl Robinson, who created it to help with thrush in infants. It works well for adults as well as children, both topically and internally.

Used For: Athlete's foot, colic (children), dysbiosis, infection (fungal), **jock itch**, and **thrush**

Affects: Digestive depression and digestive stagnation

Take 1-2 drops twice daily for 3-4 days or up to a maximum of 7 days. For children dilute the oils in 40 drops of olive oil and only give 1 drop twice daily. For topical use dilute with only 20 drops of olive oil.

30 drops Olive oil
4 drops Cajeput EO
3 drops Lavender EO
2 drops Thyme EO
1 drop Lemon EO

Antihistamine Formula

See also *Steven Horne's Anti-Allergy Formula*

These formulas act as natural antihistamines. They help to stabilize the white blood cells involved in allergic reactions, making them less likely to rupture and release more histamine. They are helpful for respiratory allergies (hay fever) as well as food allergies and leaky gut syndrome. They can also help reduce allergic reactions in the skin in eczema and dermatitis taken internally or applied topically.

Used For: ADD/ADHD, **allergies (respiratory)**, bites & stings, congestion (bronchial), congestion (sinus), **dermatitis**, **eczema**, eyes (red/itching), **food allergies/intolerances**, headache (migraine), **itching**, **rashes & hives**, sleep apnea, and snoring

Affects: Bronchi, eustachian tubes, and sinuses

This blend has a drying effect on mucous membranes. Take 2 capsules with a meal twice daily.

Ingredients: Stinging nettle leaf, quercetin, bitter orange fruit, and bromelain

Antioxidant Eye Formula

See also *Antioxidant Formula*

This formula helps protect the eyes from damage due to oxidative stress. It can help diminish the effects of macular degeneration and may help to prevent damage to the eyes from diabetes. It can also help when eyes are irritated from environmental pollutants.

Used For: Cataracts, **diabetic retinopathy**, **eye health**, **eyes, bloodshot**, **glaucoma**, **macular degeneration**, and night blindness

Affects: Sight

Use 2 capsules one time daily.

Ingredients: Vitamin A, vitamin C, zinc, selenium, copper, lutein, zeaxanthin, carotenoid blend, bilberry fruit, N-acetyl cysteine, and taurine

Antioxidant Formula

See also *Antioxidant Eye Formula* and *Proanthocyanidins Formula*

Antioxidant formulas prevent and reduce free radical damage and reduce inflammation, the primary causes of aging and degenerative diseases. These formulas can also help reduce inflammation and fever, protect the liver from chemical damage, aid in the treatment or prevention of cancer, calm autoimmune responses, and reduce allergic reactions. They may also have protective effect on the brain and nervous system.

Warnings: High doses of antioxidants may cause a healing crisis, as it causes their body to detoxify. In these cases, some colon and lymphatic cleansing may be needed.

Used For: **Age spots**, **aging**, AIDS, **allergies (respiratory)**, Alzheimer's, anorexia, arteriosclerosis, arthritis (rheumatoid), **autoimmune disorders**, bruises, **burning feet/hands**, **cancer**, **cancer prevention**, cancer treatment side effects, capillary weakness, cardiovascular disease, carpal tunnel, cataracts, debility, dementia, diabetic retinopathy, **easily bruised**, electromagnetic pollution, emphysema, environmental pollution, Epstein-Barr virus, exercise (performance), eyes (red/itching), **fever**, fibromyalgia, **free radical damage**, **glaucoma**, **inflammation**, injuries, lupus, **macular degeneration**, memory/brain function, meningitis, mental illness, multiple sclerosis, myasthenia gravis, **nephritis**, **neuralgia & neuritis**, neurodegenerative diseases, night blindness, oral surgery, **overacidity**, pain, **Parkinson's disease**, pleurisy, postpartum weakness, preeclampsia, pregnancy, prostatitis, radiation, Reye's syndrome, **rhinitis**, **skin problems**, sore/geographic tongue, urination (frequent), vaccine side effects, and varicose veins

Affects: Arteries, capillaries, **circulatory irritation**, **general irritation**, gums, hepatic irritation, liver, respiratory irritation, and veins

Antioxidant Nutrient Blend

A capsule formula that has liver-protecting benefits. Take 1 capsule twice daily.

Ingredients: Turmeric root, milk thistle seed, lycopene, and alpha-lipoic acid

Antioxidant Mangosteen and Berry Drink

A liquid juice drink featuring the antioxidant rich fruits. Drink 1 ounce one or two times daily. Mix with lemonade made with fresh lemon juice and maple syrup for a cooling drink on hot summer days.

Ingredients: Mangosteen fruit & pericarp, Grape fruit & skin extracts, blueberry fruit, red raspberry fruit, lycium fruit extract, açaí berry, pomegranate fruit, sea buckthorn fruit, Grape seed extract, green tea leaf extract, and apple fruit extract

High ORAC Blend

An antioxidant formula in a capsule. Take 1–2 capsules once or twice daily.

Ingredients: Green tea leaf, mangosteen pericarp, turmeric root extract, açaí berry, quercetin, resveratrol, and selenium

Antiparasitic Formula

See also *Parasite Cleansing Program*

These formulas are used to aid in the expulsion of worms and other parasites. It's often a good idea to take a *Stimulant Laxative Formula* or cascara sagrada when doing a parasite cleanse, especially if the bowels are sluggish.

Warnings: Not recommended for pregnancy or when nursing or for children under the age of twelve. Drink plenty of water when on a cleanse of any kind.

Used For: Fingernail biting, infection (fungal), **malaria**, **parasites**, **parasites (nematodes, worms)**, **parasites (tapeworm)**, **pet supplements**, and prostatitis

Affects: Digestive stagnation, intestinal stagnation, and prostate

David Christopher's Antiparasitic Formula

A very strong liquid parasite cleanse in a glycerine base. One teaspoon morning and night for 3 days.

Ingredients: Wormwood leaf, wormseed seed, and male fern leaf

Antiparasitic Artemesia Blend

This formula contains two species of artemesias (mugwort and wormwood), which are good for worms. The Sweet Annie in this formula is helpful for malaria. Use 2 capsules three times per day.

Ingredients: Elecampane root, mugwort aerial parts, clove flower, garlic bulb, and sweet wormwood aerial parts

Antiparasitic Formula with Pumpkin Seed

A gentler antiparasitic formula that can also help the male prostate. A good antiparasitic formula for pets, especially in combination with black walnut. Use 2 capsules three times per day.

Ingredients: Pumpkin seed, black walnut hulls, and cascara sagrada bark

Ed Smith's Antiparasitic Formula

A liquid parasite cleanse that also acts as a digestive tonic. One dropper 3–4 times per day in water or juice.

Ingredients: Black walnut hulls, wormwood, quassia, and clove

Male Fern-Black Walnut Formula

Another strong antiparasitic formula.

Ingredients: Black walnut hulls, male fern, and pumpkin seed

Antispasmodic Ear Formula

This is a very unusual combination of herbs with broad applications. It has been used for nervous disorders (particularly muscle spasms, anxiety, and stress) and as ear drops for chronic ear problems. It can also be used to reduce inflammation and irritation in tissues.

Warnings: Hypoglycemics should use with caution.

Used For: **Deafness**, **dizziness**, **earache**, hearing loss, **Ménière's disease**, **tinnitus**, and **vaccine side effects**

Affects: Central nervous system, **general constriction**, **hearing**, and nerve constriction (tension)

For ear problems, warm the liquid to body temperature and then use 5–10 drops in the ear. For nervous system issues take 1/2 to 1 teaspoon with a glass of water three times a day. As a mouthwash, gargle with 1 teaspoon in water.

Ingredients: Black cohosh root, chickweed aerial parts, passion flower aerial parts, and valerian root

Antispasmodic Formula

An antispasmodic formula is helpful for any condition involving muscle spasms or cramping. These remedies correct the tissue condition known as *constriction*.

Warnings: Not advisable in cases of low blood pressure.

Used For: **Asthma**, **cramps (leg)**, **cramps (menstrual)**, cramps & spasms, **dysmenorrhea**, epilepsy, headache, hysteria, irritable bowel, nervous exhaustion, pertussis, and **PMS Type P**

Affects: Bronchi, **central nervous system**, **general constriction**, intestinal constriction, **muscles**, **nerve constriction (tension)**, respiratory constriction, and **structural constriction**

Menstrual Cramp Formula

Aimed primarily at easing menstrual cramps. Use 2 capsules with a meal two or three times daily, or for severe cramping, take 2 capsules every hour for up to six hours.

Ingredients: Cramp bark bark, black cohosh root, lobelia aerial parts, and wild yam root

Jethro Kloss' Antispasmodic Formula

A traditional antispasmodic formula for topical or internal use. Very helpful for asthma. Take 20–40 drops as needed.

Ingredients: Black cohosh root, skullcap flowering tops, skunk cabbage root, and lobelia flower & seed

Topical Antispasmodic Formula

A great formula to use with the Herbal Back Adjustment Therapy. Apply topically or use as directed on the label.

Ingredients: Black cohosh, blue vervain, cayenne pepper, and indian tobacco

Apricot   *Bitter Herb*

Prunus armeniaca

Apricot seeds are used in Chinese herbalism for problems in the lung and large intestine meridians. In Western medicine, an extract from the kernels known as laetrile has been used as a controversial cancer treatment.

Warnings: Apricot seeds are mildly toxic as they contain prussic acid and should only be used in small amounts.

Energetics: Cooling and moistening

Used For: Asthma, cancer, constipation (adults), cough (damp), and wheezing

Properties: Antitussive, expectorant, laxative (gentle), and moistening

Arjuna   *Astringent & Bitter Herb*

Terminalia arjuna

Valued as a remedy for the heart and poor circulation in Ayurvedic herbalism, arjuna is used as a treatment for angina, congestive heart failure, heart problems related to smoking,

and elevated blood pressure. It is used in a very similar manner to hawthorn and works well when combined with it.

Energetics: Cooling and mildly relaxing

Used For: **Angina**, **arrhythmia**, arteriosclerosis, **cardiovascular disease**, **congestive heart failure**, **heart weakness**, and **hypertension**

Properties: Antiarrhythmic, **cardiac**, hypotensive, and vasodilator

Arnica   *Acrid Herb*

Arnica montana

Arnica is used to reduce swelling, bruising, and pain from injury and trauma. It is most often used as a homeopathic preparation both internally and topically to treat swelling, bruises, and injuries. It is a good idea to keep homeopathic arnica (both tablets and topical cream) in your first aid kit.

Arnica tincture, taken internally, acts as a cardiac tonic and improves the supply of blood through the coronary vessels but should be taken only under professional supervision as it is highly toxic. It should be highly diluted when used internally—just a few drops diluted in water.

Look for *arnica* in *CBD Topical Analgesic* and *Topical Injury Formulas*

Warnings: Gastric irritation may develop with internal use of the herb. High doses taken internally can cause intoxication, dizziness, tremors, tachycardia, arrhythmia, and collapse. Arnica tincture should not be used during pregnancy or nursing. Homeopathic preparations do not cause these problems and are completely safe, but both the herb and the homeopathic preparations should not be applied to broken skin.

Usage: Use homeopathic preparations as directed on the label.

Energetics: Warming and drying

Used For: Angina, backache, **bruises**, bunions, congestive heart failure, **injuries**, ligaments (torn/injuried), numbness, pain, **sprains**, surgery (recovery), and **whiplash**

Properties: Analgesic, anticoagulant, vasodilator, and vulnerary

Artichoke   *Strongly Bitter Herb*

Cynara scolymus

This is the leaf of the globe artichoke that is eaten as a vegetable. It contains cynarine, which has liver-protective capabilities. Artichoke also contains silymarin, the active constituent of milk thistle. The leaves are used as a digestive bitter for a sluggish liver and poor digestion.

Look for *artichoke* in *Cholesterol-Regulating Formula*

Energetics: Cooling and drying

Used For: Appetite (deficient), **cholesterol (high)**, **fat metabolism (poor)**, **gallbladder problems**, indigestion, jaundice (adults), and **low stomach acid**

Properties: Alterative, **anticholesteremic**, antilipemic, **cholagogue**, digestive tonic, and hypolipidemic

Asafetida   *Aromatic Herb*

Ferula assafoetida

A perennial plant used in Ayurvedic herbalism for digestive problems. It is also used as a condiment in Indian curries.

Warnings: Not recommended for use by children.

Energetics: Mildly warming, relaxing, and drying

Used For: Asthma, bronchitis, cough, gas & bloating, indigestion, and indigestion

Properties: Carminative, condiment, and hypotensive

Ashwagandha

Bitter, Mildly Pungent, & Mildly Sweet Herb

Withania somnifera

An important herb from Ayurvedic herbalism, ashwagandha is a nervine and adrenal tonic that helps anxiety, depression, exhaustion and poor muscle tone. It is adaptogenic and reduces the effects of stress, while promoting energy and vitality. It is used as a supporting herb for recovery from debilitating diseases, and is effective for treating sexual dysfunction caused by stress. It is also an effective anti-inflammatory that can relieve symptoms associated with arthritis pain. ashwagandha is also helpful for boosting the conversion of T4 (the thyroid storage hormone) to T3 (the active thyroid hormone).

Look for *ashwagandha* in *5-HTP Adaptogen, Adaptogen, Adaptogen-Immune, Ashwagandha Complex, Herbal Arthritis, Hypothyroid, Sleep Support,* and *Testosterone Formulas*

Warnings: Use cautiously during pregnancy.

Usage: Take before bedtime to aid sleep. Take two or three times per day to reduce stress. Follow directions on product label for dose.

Energetics: Mildly warming

Used For: ADD/ADHD, **addictions (coffee, caffeine)**, **addictions (drugs)**, **adrenal fatigue**, **ALS**, **anxiety disorders**, arthritis (rheumatoid), **autoimmune disorders**, **bipolar mood disorder**, **bulimia**, cancer treatment side effects, **convalescence**, **depression**, **down syndrome**, **emotional sensitivity**, endurance, Epstein-Barr virus, erectile dysfunction, **fatigue**, **fibromyalgia**, **Hashimoto's disease**, **hot flashes**, **hypothyroidism**, **jet lag**, memory/brain function, **multiple sclerosis**, **narcolepsy**, nervous

exhaustion, **nervousness**, **OCD**, osteoporosis, **PTSD**, **stress**, **trauma**, and wasting

Properties: **Adaptogen**, anti-inflammatory, antidepressant, nervine, and **thyrotropic**

Ashwagandha Complex Formula

See also *Adaptogen-Immune Formula* and *Suma Adaptogen Formula*

Use this formula to help enhance mood, mental alertness, and energy. It may also be helpful for modulating autoimmune reactions. It can be used as nervine and adrenal tonic to help anxiety, depression, exhaustion, and poor muscle tone.

Warnings: Use caution taking it in the evening; it contains stimulating herbs that can contribute to insomnia

Used For: Addictions (coffee, caffeine), addictions (drugs), ALS, anxiety disorders, **autoimmune disorders**, **cloudy thinking**, convalescence, **depression**, excess weight, **fatigue**, Hashimoto's disease, hypothyroidism, **memory/brain function**, OCD, **stress**, and trauma

Affects: Adrenal irritation, **brain depression**, high cortisol, **nerve depression (exhaustion)**, thyroid depression, and weakened fire

Take 1 or 2 capsules once or twice daily.

Ingredients: Ashwagandha root extract, bacopa leaf extract, schisandra fruit, and rhodiola root extract

Asparagus   *Salty & Mildly Sweet Herb*

Asparagus officinalis

Asparagus acts as a kidney tonic, flushing acid waste from the system. The root of a different species is used in Chinese herbalism, see *Asparagus (Chinese)*.

Look for *asparagus* in *Liquid Kidney* and *Urinary Support Formulas*

Warnings: The root should not be used when there is kidney disease.

Used For: Appetite (deficient), backache, breast lumps, cancer, colds, congestion (lungs), congestive heart failure, debility, diarrhea, edema, erectile dysfunction, heart fibrillation/palpitations, kidney stones, nephritis, night sweating, peripheral neuropathy, and urinary tract infections

Properties: Food, kidney tonic, low glycemic, and lung tonic

Asparagus, Chinese
Mildly Bitter & Sweet Herb

Asparagus cochinchinesis

Also known as tien-men-tung, Chinese asparagus root is a tonic to the lung and kidney meridians. It nourishes the yin, moistens dryness, clears heat from the lungs, and helps to control coughing.

Look for *asparagus (Chinese)* in *Dry Cough Syrup Formula*

Energetics: Cooling, nourishing, and drying

Used For: Cancer, constipation (adults), cough, and hepatitis

Properties: Anti-inflammatory, antibacterial, antiseptic, antitussive, aperient, and diuretic

Astragalus   *Sweet Herb*

Astragalus membranaceus

Astragalus is an adaptogenic and tonic herb used in Chinese herbalism to boost energy and strengthen immunity. Research suggests that the polysaccharides and saponins in astragalus may be helpful to those with heart disease, improving heart function and providing relief from symptoms. Astragalus appears to restore immune and adrenal function in people whose immune systems have been weakened by chemotherapy or chronic illness. It has antibacterial and antiviral properties, making it useful as a topical treatment for healing wounds. It can be helpful both in preventing and treating common colds and respiratory infections.

Look for *astragalus* in *Adaptogen, Adaptogen-Immune, Children's Elderberry Cold* and *Flu, Chinese Earth-Increasing, Chinese Metal-Increasing, Chinese Qi* and *Blood Tonic, Chinese Water-Decreasing, Colostrum-Immune Stimulator, Dry Cough Syrup, Gut Immune,* and *Suma Adaptogen Formulas*

Usage: Astragalus can be taken in capsules or extracts but can also be cooked into rice or soups.

Energetics: Mildly warming and moistening

Used For: Arthritis (rheumatoid), asthma, **autism**, autoimmune disorders, bronchitis, **cancer**, cancer prevention, **cancer treatment side effects**, colds, **colds (antiviral)**, congestive heart failure, **convalescence**, COPD, cough (dry), diabetes, digestion (poor), flu, **Hashimoto's disease**, heart fibrillation/palpitations, heart weakness, hepatitis, hypertension, **infection (viral)**, **infection prevention**, **lupus**, mononucleosis, multiple sclerosis, nephritis, night sweating, overacidity, pernicious anemia, prolapsed uterus, **Raynaud's disease**, shingles, tuberculosis, ulcerations (external), ulcers, underweight, and **wasting**

Properties: Adaptogen, anti-inflammatory, antioxidant, antisudorific, antiviral, cardiac, diuretic, hypotensive, immune modulator, immune stimulant, tonic, and vasodilator

Atlas Cedarwood EO
Camphorous, Sweet, & Woody Essential Oil

Cedrus atlantica

This is a camphoric oil, with a sweet, woody undertone. It is energizing and promotes a grounded strength and dignity. It can strengthen a person's resistance to stress, reducing anxiety and tension, while promoting a calm, conscious mind. It can help a person stand up to difficult circumstances with strength and serenity.

See the strategy *Aromatherapy* for suggested uses.

Warnings: Do not use internally. Nontoxic and nonirritating for topical use. Avoid during pregnancy.

Used For: Anxiety (situational), bronchitis, cellulite, cough, seborrhea, stress, and urinary tract infections

Properties: Antiseptic, astringent, diuretic, expectorant, insecticide, and sedative

Atractylodes
Aromatic, Mildly Bitter, & Sweet Herb

Atractylodes ovata

This Chinese herb is used in digestive and urinary combinations. It may also be helpful for treating fungal and bacterial infections.

Look for *atractylodes* in *Chinese Earth-Increasing Formula*

Warnings: Contraindicated with high fever, excessive sweating, severe inflammation or dehydration.

Energetics: Warming and drying

Used For: Diarrhea, digestion (poor), and perspiration (excessive)

Properties: Anti-inflammatory, carminative, digestive tonic, and diuretic

Attention-Focus Formula

The herbs and nutrients in these formulas help balance activity in the brain's neurotransmitter system. They can help hyperactivity and ADD. They also help protect the brain from toxic chemicals. For best results, take with DHA or omega-3 essential fatty acids.

Warnings: Consult a healthcare provider before giving these products to children under three years.

Used For: ADD/ADHD, Alzheimer's, **cloudy thinking, concentration (poor)**, confusion, epilepsy, and memory/brain function

Affects: Acetylcholine, brain, brain irritation, and gaba

Michael Tierra's Calming Formula

An herbal formula for calming the brain. Take 2 tablets twice daily.

Ingredients: Gotu kola leaf extract, Saint John's wort aerial parts extract, passion flower aerial parts extract, jujube seed, lemon balm aerial parts extract, chamomile flower extract, hawthorn berry extract, and jujube fruit extract

Brain Calming Blend with DMAE

An encapsulated version for teens and adults. Adults or children over age twelve, take 2 capsules twice daily with meals, or as needed.

Ingredients: L-glutamine, DMAE, lemon balm leaf, and ginkgo leaf extract

Attention Enhancing Nutrients

A powdered version for young children. Children age 6–12: take 1/2 teaspoon of the powder in 1–1/2 ounces of water twice daily. Children age 3–6: take 1/4 teaspoon of the powder in 1 ounce of water twice daily. Mix well and drink immediately.

Ingredients: Vitamin B_1, vitamin B_2, vitamin B_3, vitamin B_6, vitamin B_9, vitamin B_{12}, vitamin B_5, DMAE, lemon balm leaf extract, bacopa leaf extract, and ginkgo leaf extract

Ayurvedic Bronchial Decongestant Formula

See also *Jeannie Burgess' Allergy-Lung Formula*

An Ayurvedic herbal formula that acts as an expectorant and decongestant, helping to dilate the bronchial passages for easier breathing. Besides being helpful for bronchitis, it may also be helpful for coughs, colds, indigestion and asthma.

Used For: Allergies (respiratory), asthma, **bronchitis**, **congestion (bronchial)**, congestion (lungs), cough (damp), and pneumonia

Affects: **Bronchi**, respiratory atrophy, and respiratory constriction

Use 2 capsules three times daily.

Ingredients: Malabar nut leaf extract, licorice root extract, mullein leaf & stem, asian bayberry bark extract, greater galandgal rhizome extract, indian elecampane root extract, picrorhiza root extract, and himalayan fir leaf

Ayurvedic Skin Healing Formula

See also *Blood Purifier Formula*

An Ayurvedic formula for chronic skin conditions and dermatitis. It acts as an alterative or blood purifier and nourishes the skin.

Used For: **Acne**, **boils**, carbuncles, **dermatitis**, **eczema**, PMS Type S, psoriasis, **rashes & hives**, skin (infections), **skin problems**, and **ulcerations (external)**

Affects: General stagnation, hepatic stagnation, **skin**, structural irritation, and structural stagnation

Use 2 capsules three times daily.

Ingredients: Dandelion root, catechu bark extract, Chinese smilax root, neem bark extract, picrorhiza root, indian sarsaparilla root, amla fruit, belleric myrobalan fruit, chebulic myrobalan fruit, and turmeric root

Bacillus coagulans   *Probiotic*

Bacillus coagulans

A lactic acid-producing probiotic that forms spores, making it shelf-stable. Helps to control unfriendly microbes in the GI tract and repopulate the intestinal biome with health microbes.

Used For: Convalescence, food poisoning, gas & bloating, infection prevention, and irritable bowel

Properties: Antifungal

Bacopa   *Mildly Bitter Herb*

Bacopa monnieri

Used in India to treat nervous disorders such as anxiety, mental illness, seizures and poor memory, bacopa has become a popular herb for aiding brain function in Western herbalism. In a recent clinical trial of ninety-eight healthy people over age fifty-five, Bacopa significantly improved memory acquisition and retention.

Look for *bacopa* in *Ashwagandha Complex* and *Memory Enhancing Formulas*

Warnings: Do not use for hyperthyroidism.

Energetics: Cooling

Used For: ADD/ADHD, aging, Alzheimer's, anxiety disorders, **cloudy thinking**, **concentration (poor)**, confusion, **dementia**, **memory/brain function**, mental illness, OCD, and teeth (grinding)

Properties: Anti-inflammatory, antioxidant, **cerebral tonic**, mucilant, and nervine

Baical Skullcap   *Bitter Herb*

Scutellaria baicalensis

A Chinese medicinal herb related to the Western herb skullcap. It is used to remove heat and moisture from the body and to prevent spontaneous abortion. It is also used for inflammatory conditions like asthma, hay fever, eczema, and rashes.

Energetics: Cooling and drying

Used For: Allergies (respiratory), eczema, edema, fever, miscarriage prevention, and rashes & hives

Properties: Anti-inflammatory, antiabortive, antiallergenic, antifungal, diuretic, and febrifuge

Balancing EO Formula

Use this blend to promote calm awareness and centeredness. It can also enhance feelings of self-esteem and empower you to stand up for yourself. It can aid meditation and reduce emotional tension.

See the strategy *Aromatherapy* for suggested uses.

Warnings: Not for use during pregnancy. Not for internal use.

Used For: Fatigue, fear, headache (tension), and stress

Affects: Central nervous system

Ingredients: Spruce leaf EO, ho leaf EO, blue tansy EO, frankincense EO, and roman chamomile EO

Balloon Flower   *Acrid & Bitter Herb*

Platycodon grandiflorum

This Chinese herb helps decongest the lungs when there is an excess of mucus. It is typically combined with other herbs and is believed to direct their action toward the lungs.

Look for *balloon flower* in *Chinese Metal-Increasing, Damp Cough Syrup,* and *Dry Cough Syrup Formulas*

Warnings: Do not use when there is blood in the expectoration.

Energetics: Drying, mildly relaxing, and neutral

Used For: Congestion, cough (damp), and sore throat

Properties: Expectorant

Bamboo   *Sweet Herb*

Bambusa vulgaris

Bamboo shavings are used in Chinese herbalism for the lung and stomach meridians. The sap is used for reducing irritation and expelling phlegm.

Look for *bamboo* in *Chinese Metal-Decreasing* and *Chinese Qi-Regulating Formulas*

Energetics: Cooling

Used For: Fever and nausea & vomiting

Properties: Antibacterial and febrifuge

Baptisia (Wild Indigo)

Stimulant Bitter Herb

Baptisia tinctoria

A very valuable remedy for serious infections causing toxicity and blood poisoning, wild indigo is indicated in conditions where there is foul discharge and an odor reminiscent of decaying meat. It works very well for these conditions when combined with echinacea and other anti-infective herbs.

Warnings: This herb should be used with caution. It is potentially toxic and is a strong purgative and emetic in larger doses. It is best used as part of a formula.

Energetics: Cooling and drying

Used For: Adenitis, AIDS, appendicitis, **blood poisoning**, boils, cervical dysplasia, gangrene, gonorrhea, **infection (bacterial)**, **leukemia**, mastitis, mononucleosis, staph infections, strep throat, swollen lymph glands, tonsillitis, vaccine side effects, and wounds & sores

Properties: Emetic and lymphatic

Barberry   *Stimulant Bitter Herb*

Berberis spp.

One of the best bitter liver tonics, barberry contains the antiseptic berberine for fighting bacterial infections. It also has antifungal properties. It has been shown to triple bile production for an hour and a half. This herb can also be helpful for multiple personality disorder either as an herb or a homeopathic.

Look for *barberry* in *Liver Cleanse Formula*

Warnings: Not for use during pregnancy or when emaciated.

Energetics: Cooling and drying

Used For: Antibiotic side effects, **bladder infection**, cancer, cholesterol (high), conjunctivitis, dissociative identity disorder, dysbiosis, **fat cravings**, **fat metabolism (poor)**, **gallbladder problems**, **gallstones**, **gas & bloating**, headache (cluster), infection (bacterial), **infection (fungal)**, mental illness, prostatitis, triglycerides (low), urethritis, and vaginitis

Properties: Alterative, antiseptic, aperient, and **cholagogue**

Barley   *Salty & Sweet Herb*

Hordeum vulgare

Barley grass is an excellent source of many essential vitamins and minerals and is high in amino acids, chlorophyll, and enzymes. Barley is also an ancient and widely cultivated grain known for its strengthening, nourishing, and soothing properties. A porridge of barley grain is recommended for people recovering from illness and soothing intestinal inflammation. Barley cereal has also been used for poultices.

Warnings: Barley grass can dry mother's milk; do not use when lactating. People with gluten intolerance or allergies should avoid barley as a grain, but can still take barley grass.

Energetics: Neutral, moistening, and nourishing

Used For: AIDS, appetite (excessive), convalescence, eczema, **electromagnetic pollution**, exercise (recovery), food allergies/intolerances, free radical damage, gout, pain, radiation, underweight, uric acid retention, and wasting

Properties: Anti-inflammatory, antioxidant, appetite suppressant, detoxifying, food, galactagogue, mineralizer, nutritive, tonic, and vulnerary

Bay Leaf EO (Bay Laurel)

Fresh & Sweet Essential Oil

Laurus nobilis

Also known as bay laurel, this essential oil has a fresh, sweet, and camphorous smell. A garland of laurel leaves was used to honor victory among the Romans and men of distinction were crowned with a wreath of laurel with its berries in the Middle Age—hence the phrase, "Earning one's laurels."

The oil has bactericidal and fungicidal properties. It can be helpful topically for skin infections and inhaled for respiratory infections.

It is a nerve tonic for people who doubt themselves. It is believed to inspire creativity in artists, promoting confidence, insight and courage. It's a good oil for those who lack self-esteem or doubt their intellectual abilities.

See the strategy *Aromatherapy* for suggested uses.

Warnings: Do not use internally. Dilute for topical application.

Used For: Abscesses, acne, appetite (deficient), boils, congestion, depression, fever, gas & bloating, infection (fungal), inflammation, malaria, parasites (nematodes, worms), and stress

Properties: Anesthetic, anti-inflammatory, antibacterial, anticancer, antifungal, antimicrobial, antirheumatic, antiseptic, bactericidal, carminative, diaphoretic, digestive tonic, diuretic, expectorant, mucolytic, sedative, and tonic

Bayberry   *Mildly Aromatic & Astringent Herb*

Myrica cerifera

A powerful astringent with a mild aromatic (stimulant) action, bayberry is good for toning the GI tract, arresting diarrhea, and removing mucus. It loosens mucus from the sinuses and throat.

Look for *bayberry* in *Ed Millet's Herbal Crisis, Herbal Composition, Herbal Eyewash, Herbal Tooth Powder, Lymph Cleansing,* and *Steven Horne's Sinus Snuff Formulas*

Warnings: In large doses bayberry is emetic (induces vomiting). Bayberry should not be given internally to children under age two. For older children and people over sixty-five, start with a low-strength preparation and increase strength if necessary. Use with caution internally during pregnancy. Topical application is completely safe.

Energetics: Mildly warming, drying, and constricting

Used For: Bites & stings, bleeding (external), bleeding (internal), **blood in stool**, blood in urine, cancer treatment side effects, congestion (sinus), **cough (damp)**, cuts, **diarrhea**, endometriosis, floaters, gingivitis, injuries, labor & delivery, menorrhagia, nosebleeds, **polyps**, **prolapsed colon**, prolapsed uterus, sinus infection, smell (loss of), **sore throat**, sty, ulcerations (external), ulcers, vaginitis, varicose veins, and wounds & sores

Properties: **Astringent**, **coagulant**, expectorant, **hemostatic**, insecticide, mucolytic, **styptic**, vermifuge, and vulnerary

Bee Balm (Bergamot)

Aromatic & Mildly Pungent Herb

Monarda didyma

Bergamot or beebalm is in the mint family and is a warming aromatic remedy similar to oregano. It can helpful in cases of dysbiosis and is helpful for yeast infections.

Energetics: Mildly warming and mildly relaxing

Used For: **Dysbiosis**, infection (fungal), leaky gut, leaky gut, **Ménière's disease**, **tinnitus**, and urinary tract infections

Properties: Antifungal, antimicrobial, and relaxant

Bee Pollen   *Sweet Herb*

Bee pollen contains every known nutrient in trace amounts. It is highly energizing and therefore used to increase energy, stamina, and endurance. It supports the glands and aids the immune system. Bee pollen has been used to overcome allergies to pollen. In overcoming allergies, it is best to get bee pollen from local beekeepers and start with a small amount (just a few grains). Gradually increase the dose over a period of several weeks to develop a tolerance to pollen and improve immune function.

Look for *bee pollen* in *Vandergriff's Energy Booster Formula*

Warnings: A few allergic attacks have been reported from use of bee pollen. Symptoms of allergy include itching, dizziness, and difficulty swallowing.

Usage: Take 1–2 capsules or 1/2 to 1 teaspoon once or twice daily. If you have allergies, be sure to start with a small amount (a few grains).

Energetics: Neutral and nourishing

Used For: ADD/ADHD, addictions (sugar/carbohydrates), aging, **allergies (respiratory)**, anger (excessive), bulimia, concentration (poor), convalescence, **debility**, **electromagnetic pollution**, endurance, excess weight, exercise (recovery), **fatigue**, **hypoglycemia**, jet lag, mercury poisoning, and **reversed polarity**

Properties: Adrenal tonic, corrects polarity, food, glandular, nutritive, stimulant (appetite), and stimulant (metabolic)

Beet   *Sweet Herb*

Beta vulgaris

Beet root's high iron content helps build the blood and restore color to the skin. It contains betaine HCl which helps produce hydrochloric acid for digestion. Beet is high in antioxidants, which eliminate free radicals. Nitrates in beets help enhance nitric oxide levels, which helps control high blood pressure and aid recovery from exercise.

Look for *beet* in *Christopher's Herbal Iron, Hypoglycemic, Liver Cleanse,* and *Nitric Oxide Boosting Formulas*

Usage: The best way to derive these benefits is to eat beets as a vegetable.

Energetics: Neutral, moistening, and nourishing

Used For: Anemia, exercise (recovery), **hypertension**, and hypoglycemia

Properties: Antioxidant, **blood building**, food, hepatic, hypotensive, nutritive, and tonic

Berberine   *Phytochemical*

Berberine is an alkaloid found in many herbs traditionally used for fighting infection and improving the health of the gastrointestinal tract. It is a bright-yellow color, which means some of the plants containing it have also been used as yellow dyes.

Berberine has shown some benefits in the treatment of insulin-resistant (type 2) diabetes. It helps to reduce blood glucose levels and appears to reduce insulin resistance. It has been shown to help lower triglycerides and cholesterol, working by a different method than statins, so it lacks the dangerous side effects associated with these drugs.

Berberine has antimicrobial activity against many types of bacteria, viruses, and fungi. it helps balance the microbiome in the gastrointestinal (GI) tract. See *dysbiosis* for more information.

Studies also suggest that berberine may be helpful for heart problems. A study published in the *American Journal of Cardiology* in 2002 showed that patients being treated medically for congestive heart failure showed greater improvement when berberine was added to their program in comparison to a placebo. Exercise capacity improved, heart function

improved and mortality was reduced. Berberine also appears to help lower blood pressure.

While the research isn't robust, Berberine might also have antidepressant activity, increasing norepinephrine and serotonin levels while lowering dopamine. It may also have protective effects against Alzheimer's disease.

Warnings: It is not recommended for infants or children under two, and should not be given to children in general (use herbs containing berberine, like Oregon grape, instead). It should also be avoided while pregnant or nursing. It may also be contraindicated with low blood pressure. People taking prescription medications should use berberine with caution as it can alter the way drugs are metabolized in the liver. Berberine in high doses can cause diarrhea.

Usage: Take 300 to 500 mg three times daily.

Used For: **Alzheimer's**, **antibiotic resistance**, bladder infection, cancer, cardiovascular disease, **cholera**, cholesterol (high), congestive heart failure, depression, **diabetes**, **dysbiosis**, **excess weight**, food allergies/intolerances, giardia, hypertension, **infection (bacterial)**, **infection (fungal)**, irritable bowel, **metabolic syndrome**, **SIBO**, and **triglycerides (high)**

Properties: **Antibacterial**, **antidiabetic**, **antifungal**, antilipemic, **antimicrobial**, antiobesic, cholagogue, and hepatic

Bergamot EO *Fresh, Fruity, & Sweet Essential Oil*

Citrus x bergamia

A floral, slightly citrus-smelling oil, bergamot tends to be balancing to the nerves. It is relaxing and uplifting at the same time. It can help with anxiety and depression, especially when these are associated with low self-esteem and excessive self-judgment. It helps overcome core beliefs that one is bad or just not good enough.

Bergamot is a valuable antiseptic and anti-inflammatory. It aids urinary conditions like cystitis. It also aids respiratory problems like bronchitis when inhaled. Combined with tea tree oil and a carrier oil, it is useful for skin infections and erruptions. In douches and baths, bergamot has proved helpful in gonococcal infections and urinary infections. It also makes a refreshing bath during late pregnancy. It acts as a carminative on the digestive system, making it useful for relieving colic, flatulence and indigestion.

The oil soothes anger and frustration by decreasing the activity of the sympathetic nervous system. It helps with self-confidence and exhaustion from physical or psychological illnesses. An effective antidepressant, it uplifts and refreshes the spirit, evokes joy, aids self-confidence, and warms the heart. It also helps overcome emotions like bitterness, fear, grief, helplessness, and loneliness.

See the strategy *Aromatherapy* for suggested uses.

Warnings: Do not use internally without the supervision of a professionally trained aromatherapy practitioner. Avoid exposure to the sun after using bergamot in a massage or bath. Oil may oxidize over time, so discard old oil.

Used For: Chicken pox, cold sores, colic (adults), eczema, fear, herpes, leucorrhea, menopause, mood swings, nervous exhaustion, nervousness, PMS Type D, scars/scar tissue, shingles, skin (oily), stress, tonsillitis, tuberculosis, urinary tract infections, vaginitis, varicose veins, and wounds & sores

Properties: Analgesic, anti-inflammatory, antidepressant, antiseptic, antiviral, carminative, cicatrizant, deodorant, digestive tonic, febrifuge, sedative, stimulant (appetite), stomachic, tonic, vermifuge, and vulnerary

Beta-Glucans   *Phytochemical*

Beta-glucans are polysaccharides, found in many medicinal mushrooms, that stimulate the immune system. They active macrophages, T cells, natural killer cells, and cytokines.

Warnings: Do not use with autoimmune disorders.

Used For: Cancer and **infection prevention**

Properties: Immune stimulant

Betaine HCl Formula

Betaine hydrochloric acid adds hydrochloric acid (HCl) production to the stomach. HCl assists protein digestion, kills orally ingested pathogens, prevents bacterial and fungal overgrowths in the small intestines, and is essential for bile and pancreatic enzyme release. HCl is required for the absorption of folic acid, ascorbic acid, beta-carotene, iron, calcium, magnesium, and zinc. Many studies have shown that HCL production declines with age, and impaired HCl production and secretion is seen in a variety of conditions. In this formula, it is combined with pepsin, a protein digesting enzyme in the stomach, which assists in breaking proteins down into amino acids for absorption.

Warnings: Do not take if stomach ulcers are present. Discontinue if stomach irritation occurs. It is not a good idea to constantly take HCL, as this reduces the need for the body to make it for itself. Use digestive bitters to stimulate the body's own production of HCl.

Used For: Acid indigestion, aging, anemia, appetite (deficient), asthma, autoimmune disorders, belching, cancer, celiac disease, cholesterol (low), colitis, cystic fibrosis, **digestion (poor)**, **dysbiosis**, dyspepsia, eczema, **food**

allergies/intolerances, **gas & bloating**, **gastritis**, **gout**, Graves' disease, **hair (graying)**, **hair loss/thinning**, **Hashimoto's disease**, hepatitis, hypothyroidism, **indigestion**, **infection (fungal)**, irritable bowel, **leaky gut**, **low stomach acid**, **lupus**, methylation (under), **osteoporosis**, **overalkalinity**, **protein digestion**, **rosacea**, **SIBO**, underweight, and wasting

Affects: Stomach

Take 1-2 capsules with meals as an aid to digestion of proteins.

Ingredients: Betaine hydrochloric acid (hcl) and pepsin

Bibhitaki
Astringent, Bitter, Pungent, & Sweet Herb
Terminalia bellerica

This is an antispasmodic herb that is pungent and warming. It is an expectorant and decongestant and used to treat asthma, bronchial problems, and allergies. It has a balancing action because it contains all five of the Chinese tastes.

Look for *bibhitaki* in *Triphala Formula*

Energetics: Warming

Used For: Allergies (respiratory), asthma, bronchitis, and rhinitis

Properties: Antiallergenic, antispasmodic, decongestant, and expectorant

Bilberry   *Sour Herb*
Vaccinum spp.

Bilberry has been shown to improve night vision and help heal eye irritations. It protects collagen structures in the eyes, thereby preventing and treating macular degeneration and retinopathy. It is also used to tone blood vessels and improve circulation. Scientific studies suggest that this antioxidant-rich berry can protect against diseases of the circulatory system. Blueberries are a cousin of bilberry and can be used interchangeably. Blueberries and bilberries can improve atherosclerosis and varicose veins. The leaves of bilberries and blueberries may be helpful in reducing blood sugar in diabetes.

Look for *bilberry* in *Antioxidant Formula*

Warnings: Fruits are completely safe; long-term use of leaves can cause gastric irritation and kidney damage.

Energetics: Cooling, mildly drying, and nourishing

Used For: Bruises, capillary weakness, **cataracts**, diabetes, diabetic retinopathy, easily bruised, **eye health**, eyes, bloodshot, free radical damage, glaucoma, hemorrhoids, macular degeneration, night blindness, nosebleeds, **pancreatitis**, spider veins, urinary tract infections, and **varicose veins**

Properties: Antidiabetic, antioxidant, diuretic, food, nutritive, opthalmicum, tonic, and vascular tonic

Bile Salt *Nutrient*

Bile salt comes from the bile of animals. It supplements the bile produced in the liver for digestion fats. Taking bile salts can be helpful for people who have had their gallbladder removed or who have sluggish gallbladder function.

Used For: Fat cravings, **fat metabolism (poor)**, and **gallbladder problems**

Properties: Digestant

Bioflavonoids *Phytochemical*

Bioflavonoids are a class of plant secondary metabolites known for their antioxidant activity. Until the 1950s, flavonoids were referred to as Vitamin P, probably due to their beneficial effect on the permeability of vascular capillaries.

High amounts of bioflavonoids are found in the rind of green citrus fruits, rose hips, and black currants. They have been used in alternative medicine as an aid to enhance the action of vitamin C, to support blood circulation, treat allergies, viruses, arthritis and other inflammatory conditions, and as an antioxidant.

Usage: Bioflavonoids are often added to vitamin C and multivitamin formulas. Follow manufacturer's recommendations.

Used For: Anal fistula/fissure, aneurysm, bleeding (internal), blood in urine, bruises, **capillary weakness**, diabetic retinopathy, **easily bruised**, hemorrhoids, nosebleeds, sleep apnea, spider veins, ulcers, and **varicose veins**

Properties: Vascular tonic

Biota *Pungent & Sweet Herb*

Platycladus orientalis

The dried seeds of the oriental arborvitae are used in Chinese herbalism as a superior tonic. They affect the heart, liver, and kidney meridians. They calm the heart, quiet the emotions, and moisten the intestines to improve bowel movements.

I came up with an interesting theory about this herb and its effect on blood sugar. I read a report where John Christopher told a man who had edema to use juniper berries. He later told Christopher the juniper berries hadn't worked for the edema, but had helped his blood sugar. Christopher looked at the berries he had been taking and said they were cedar berries, not juniper berries.

Since some species of juniper are called cedars in Utah, this lead to a species of juniper berries being used in blood sugar

formulas. However, since all juniper berries are diuretic, this didn't make sense to me. I felt it must be a different plant the man had used.

I decided it was probably arborvitae and tested the green "berries" (technically cones) in making blood sugar formulas. This is different than the mature seeds used in Chinese herbalism. They seemed to work quite well, and the formula I made using them as a key ingredient even helped some children with type 1 diabetes. I think this warrants further investigation.

Look for *biota* in *Chinese Fire-Increasing Formula*

Energetics: Mildly warming and moistening

Used For: Constipation (adults), **diabetes**, heart fibrillation/palpitations, insomnia, and tachycardia

Properties: Antidiabetic, calmative, hypoglycemic, moistening, and relaxant

Biotin **see** *vitamin B₇*

Bitter Melon *Bitter Herb*

Momordica charantia

Bitter melon has long been used in Ayurvedic herbalism to treat type 2 diabetes. It is helpful for protecting the pancreas, while improving insulin resistance and lowering blood lipids. Compounds in the plant inhibit *H. pylori*, which is useful in cases of gastric ulcers. Leaf extracts have demonstrated anticancer and antitumor activity as well as antiviral activity against HIV and herpes simplex. It may be helpful for parasites and intestinal worms and stomach pain or colic accompanied with constipation.

Look for *bitter melon* in *Blood Sugar Control Formula*

Warnings: May cause diarrhea, stomach ache and bloating. Should not be taken with other diabetes medications without professional supervision.

Energetics: Cooling and drying

Used For: AIDS, cancer, **diabetes**, herpes, kidney stones, **metabolic syndrome**, parasites, and ulcers

Properties: Anthelmintic, antibacterial, anticancer, **antidiabetic**, antioxidant, and antiviral

Black Cohosh *Acrid Herb*

Cimicifuga racemosa

Black cohosh is typically used for its estrogenic effects, but it's role as a source of natural estrogens is questionable. It does help to regulate hormones during menopause, however. Black cohosh is also antispasmodic and mildly analgesic. It is a good remedy for venomous bites and stings. Black cohosh can help lower blood pressure and cholesterol, reduce mucus production, and enhance circulation by lowering blood pressure. It helps improve dark, gloomy depression and relives dark, twisted emotional congestion.

Look for *black cohosh* in *Antidepressant, Antispasmodic, Antispasmodic Ear, Christopher's Nervine, Female Tonic, Heart Health, Hot Flash, Prebirth,* and *Prostate Formulas*

Warnings: In large doses black cohosh can cause headaches, dizziness, irritation of the central nervous system, nausea, and vomiting. If headache or dizziness occurs, reduce dose or discontinue use. Most formulas do not contain enough to cause any of these side effects.

It is contraindicated during early pregnancy and when trying to get pregnant because it stimulates uterine contractions. It can be used (especially as part of a formula) during the last weeks of pregnancy or during labor.

Usage: Black cohosh is best used in tincture form or as part of a formula because it is easier to regulate the dose. For many people, one capsule is a large dose. Follow directions on the product label.

Energetics: Cooling, relaxing, and drying

Used For: Angina, arrhythmia, **bites & stings**, breasts (swelling/tenderness), chest pain, cough (spastic), **cramps (menstrual)**, cramps & spasms, **depression**, diphtheria, dizziness, **dysmenorrhea**, **estrogen (low)**, frozen shoulder, **headache**, **headache (tension)**, **hot flashes**, **hypertension**, **hysteria**, **labor & delivery**, measles, **menopause**, menstrual irregularity, menstruation (scant), neuralgia & neuritis, night sweating, **osteoporosis**, **ovarian pain**, pertussis, PMS, **PMS Type D**, **postpartum depression**, sciatica, sex drive (low), **snakebite**, stiff neck, tinnitus, and **whiplash**

Properties: Analgesic, antiarrhythmic, antiarthritic, **antidepressant**, antidote, antirheumatic, **antispasmodic**, **antitoxic**, **antivenomous**, aphrodisiac, **bronchial dilator**, **cephalalgic**, emmenagogue, **estrogenic**, expectorant, female tonic, glandular, **hypotensive**, **insecticide**, nervine, parturient, **phytoestrogen**, and relaxant

Black Currant   *Herb*

Ribes nigrum

Black currant oil is a good source of GLA (gamma-linolenic acid). It contains 16 to 18 percent GLA (more than evening primrose oil) plus two essential fatty acids—linoleic and alpha-linolenic. Oils containing GLA have been used to aid temperature regulation, cell construction, energy, low immune response, and inflammation. They also help to relieve some PMS symptoms. GLA is frequently deficient in people with eczema, atherosclerosis, and diabetes mellitus. The oil may help the myelin sheath on nerve cells.

Look for *black currant* in *GLA Oil Formula*

Usage: As a nutritional supplement use 1–3 capsules per day.

Used For: ADD/ADHD, allergies (respiratory), angina, arteriosclerosis, arthritis, asthma, breast lumps, breasts (swelling/tenderness), cystic fibrosis, down syndrome, eczema, epilepsy, excess weight, fat cravings, fear, fibrosis, lupus, multiple sclerosis, PMS Type A, PMS Type S, and skin (dry/flaky)

Properties: Analgesic, anti-inflammatory, anticholesteremic, immune modulator, and nutritive

Black Haw   *Astringent Herb*

Viburnum prunifolium

Black haw is used to relieve painful menstruation and low back pain. It is similar in action to cramp bark, though not as strong. Decoctions are useful for menstrual cramps and headaches. It may be added to remedies for high blood pressure.

Warnings: Contraindicated during pregnancy, except in cases of threatened miscarriage or in the last five weeks. Large doses can be hypotensive.

Energetics: Neutral, drying, relaxing, and

Used For: Cramps (menstrual), cramps & spasms, dysmenorrhea, and **miscarriage prevention**

Properties: Analgesic, antiabortive, and **antispasmodic**

Black Pepper   *Pungent Herb*

Piper nigrum

Pepper is the world's most traded spice and has been used since ancient times for culinary and medicinal purposes. It stimulates digestion and intestinal mobility to ease gas and bloating.

Warnings: Large doses can cause gastrointestinal irritation in some people.

Energetics: Warming and mildly drying

Used For: Appetite (deficient) and gas & bloating

Properties: Antiseptic, aperitive, **carminative**, catalyst, and stimulant (circulatory)

Black Walnut   *Mildly Fragrant Bitter Herb*

Juglans nigra

Black walnut hulls are a remedy for hypothyroid, parasites, and infections, The dried hulls have some medicinal value, but a tincture made from the green hulls is much stronger. It is a good parasite cleanser for children and pets. It can be applied topically or taken internally. It also builds tooth enamel when used as a tooth powder mixed with white oak bark.

Look for *black walnut* in *Anti-Fungal, Antiparasitic, Drawing Salve, General Glandular, Healing Salve, Herbal Tooth Powder,* and *Lymphatic Infection Formulas*

Warnings: Avoid during pregnancy.

Energetics: Mildly warming, drying, and mildly constricting

Used For: Antibiotic side effects, appetite (excessive), **athlete's foot**, autism, boils, cholesterol (low), **cold sores**, colon (atonic), cradle cap, **dandruff**, **dental health**, depression, **diverticulitis**, eczema, Epstein-Barr virus, **fibromyalgia**, **food allergies/intolerances**, giardia, **gingivitis**, goiter, Hashimoto's disease, **herpes**, **hypothyroidism**, **impetigo**, infection (fungal), inflammatory bowel disorders, irritable bowel, **leaky gut**, lice, lupus, lyme disease, pancreatitis, **parasites**, **parasites (nematodes, worms)**, **parasites (tapeworm)**, poison ivy/oak, prolapsed uterus, rashes & hives, teeth (loose), and wounds & sores

Properties: Antiamebic, **anticarious**, antifungal, **antiparasitic**, antiseptic, antiviral, astringent, **dentifrice**, **immune modulator**, insecticide, laxative (gentle), **thyrotropic**, and vermifuge

Blackberry *Astringent Herb*

Rubus fruticosus

This plant's berries are found in jams, jellies, and pies and are a good source of antioxidants. However, the root bark is one of the best remedies for watery diarrhea. It can also be used topically as an astringent for injuries.

Energetics: Drying and constricting

Used For: Bites & stings, cancer treatment side effects, and **diarrhea**

Properties: **Antidiarrheal**, antifungal, antiseptic, and astringent

Bladderwrack *Salty Herb*

Fucus vesiculosus

Bladderwrack contains iodine, which stimulates digestion and metabolism. It also contains and alginic acid, which helps remove heavy metals and eases acid indigestion, and fucoidan, a type of fiber that helps lower cholesterol and glucose levels, while removing toxic waste from the body. Fucoidan is known to have a variety of antitumor and anti-angiogenic properties. Bladderwrack helps reduce inflammation and pain in joints caused by rheumatoid arthritis.

Look for *bladderwrack* in *Hypothyroid Formula*

Warnings: Not for use with hyperthyroidism or Grave's disease. Use cautiously with Hashimoto's thyroiditis and during pregnancy.

Energetics: Cooling, moistening, and nourishing

Used For: Arthritis (rheumatoid), excess weight, **fatty tumors/deposits**, goiter, hypothyroidism, and skin problems

Properties: Anti-inflammatory, anticholesteremic, antirheumatic, detoxifying, mucilant, nutritive, and thyrotropic

Blessed Thistle *Bitter Herb*

Cnicus benedictus

Blessed thistle is a bitter herb with high mineral content. It is used to strengthen the liver and digestive system with properties similar to milk thistle. It is also taken with marshmallow by nursing mothers to enrich and increase breast milk.

Look for *blessed thistle* in *Chrisopher's Menopause, Female Tonic,* and *Steven Horne's Anti-Allergy Formulas*

Warnings: Avoid during pregnancy.

Energetics: Cooling and drying

Used For: Acid indigestion, allergies (respiratory), anorexia, appetite (deficient), calcium deposits, circulation (brain), gas & bloating, hiccups, indigestion, memory/brain function, **menstrual irregularity**, nausea & vomiting, **nursing**, **postpartum depression**, and pregnancy

Properties: Alterative, cephalic, cholagogue, digestive tonic, emmenagogue, female tonic, **galactagogue**, **hepatic**, hepatoprotective, nervine, stomachic, and tonic

Blood Pressure Reducing Formula

See also *Nitric Oxide Boosting Formula*

These formulas help reduce blood pressure by reducing arterial inflammation and helping to dilate peripheral blood vessels. Blood pressure is a complex problem, read the about the condition *hypertension* for more information.

Used For: Blood clot prevention, cardiovascular disease, and **hypertension**

Affects: Arteries and **circulatory constriction**

Cardiac Relaxing Formula

Contains mistletoe and linden, two excellent herbs for relaxing arterial tension. Use 30–60 drops three times daily.

Ingredients: Hawthorn berry, hawthorn leaf, hawthorn flower, linden flower, motherwort flowering tops, olive leaf, and mistletoe

Blood Pressure Reducing Formula

Enhances nitric oxide and reduces inflammation. Take 1 capsule with a meal three times daily.

Ingredients: L-arginine, olive leaf extract, Grape seed extract, coleus root extract, hawthorn berry extract, and goldenrod aerial parts

Cardiovascular L-Arginine Formula

Enhances nitric oxide and helps reduce cardiovascular inflammation. Empty the contents of one packet into eight to ten ounces of cold water, shake and drink. Use one packet per day.

Ingredients: Grape skin extract, vitamin D, pomegranate fruit, vitamin K, L-arginine, N-acetyl cysteine, L-carnitine, and resveratrol

Blood Purifier Formula

See also *Detoxifying Formula* and *Liver Cleanse Formula*

Blood purifiers, also known as alteratives, are generally bitter and or salty herbs that help clear up morbid conditions in the body. They are generally helpful for skin eruptive diseases, sluggish liver function, lymphatic stagnation, and toxic accumulations. These formulas combine several blood purifiers together.

Warnings: Use with caution with inflammatory bowel disorders. Avoid cleansing when pregnant or nursing.

Used For: **Abscesses**, **acne**, addictions (drugs), adenitis, autoimmune disorders, blood poisoning, chicken pox, cystic breast disease, dermatitis, eczema, impetigo, itching, jaundice (adults), measles, myasthenia gravis, PMS Type A, **PMS Type S**, poison ivy/oak, polyps, preeclampsia, psoriasis, puberty, rashes & hives, skin (infections), skin (oily), skin problems, and vaccine side effects

Affects: Hepatic stagnation, skin, and **structural stagnation**

Christopher's Blood Purifier

Traditional adult blood purifier. Use 2 capsules with two meals.

Ingredients: Burdock root, pau d'arco bark, red clover flowering tops, dandelion root, sarsaparilla root, yellow dock root, buckthorn bark, cascara sagrada bark, Oregon grape root & rhizome, and prickly ash bark

Blood Purifier Extract with Red Clover

Liquid blood purifier, can be used for children. Use 1/2–1 teaspoon two to three times daily.

Ingredients: Red clover flower, burdock root, and pau d'arco bark

Blood Sugar Control Formula

Use these formulas to help reduce high blood sugar. They are helpful for diabetes, metabolic syndrome, and reducing sugar cravings. Reducing high blood sugar can help reduce inflammation and the risk of chronic and degenerative disease. It can also help control blood fats (triglycerides) and cholesterol.

Warnings: Avoid with hypoglycemia. These are not replacements for diabetes medication. Do not stop taking medication without advice of a medical doctor. Type 1 diabetics usually need to remain on insulin. Check blood sugar levels frequently when taking herbs and supplements for diabetes so that dosages of medications can be adjusted as the situation improves.

Used For: Addictions (sugar/carbohydrates), cloudy thinking, **diabetes**, **metabolic syndrome**, peripheral neuropathy, **polycystic ovarian syndrome**, and **triglycerides (high)**

Affects: **Pancreatic depression** and small intestines

Ayurvedic Blood Sugar Balancing Formula

This blood sugar formula from India may be helpful for type 1 as well as type 2 diabetes. Use 1–2 capsules three times daily.

Ingredients: Gymnema leaf & leaf extract, bitter melon fruit extract, andrographis herb extract, jambolan seed extract, jambul seed, and fenugreek seed extract

Pancreas Blood Sugar Formula

A traditional herbal blend. Use 2 capsules three times daily.

Ingredients: Nopal leaf, burdock root, eleuthero root, and goldenseal root & rhizome

Blood Sugar Regulating Formula

Uses both Ayurvedic and Western herbs along with chromium and vanadium to regulate blood sugar. Use 1 capsule three times daily.

Ingredients: Vanadium, cinnamon bark extract, fenugreek seed, bitter melon fruit, gymnema leaf extract, nopal leaf, banaba leaf, and chromium

Blood Sugar Energy Drink

This drink packet provides an energy boost while helping to regulate blood pressure. A good product to use in place of coffee for breakfast. Mix one packet with four to six ounces of hot water.

Ingredients: Yerba maté, nopal fruit, cinnamon bark extract, and banaba leaf extract

Cinnamon-Nopal Blood Sugar Control

A formula I helped to create that also regulates gut flora. Use 2 capsules two to four times daily.

Ingredients: Cassia cinnamon bark, nopal leaf, and fenugreek seed

Blue Cohosh (Squaw or Papoose Root) *Acrid Herb*

Caulophyllum thalictroides

Blue cohosh root is used to help induce labor and support contractions during labor. Today, herbalists use the herb in small doses to induce delayed labor. This also works for inducing delayed menstruation. Taken during labor, blue cohosh strengthens contractions and eases the pain of childbirth. Its tonic action actually stimulates and relaxes the uterus at the same time, making it helpful for relieving painful menstrual symptoms such as cramps and breast pain. It can also be used to help ovarian pain.

Look for *blue cohosh* in *Prebirth Formula*

Warnings: Contraindicated during early pregnancy and when trying to get pregnant because it stimulates uterine contractions. It should also be avoided with heavy menstrual bleeding. It can be used by women after their due date to induce labor, but professional supervision is advised. Blue cohosh can be mildly toxic in large doses.

Energetics: Cooling, drying, and relaxing

Used For: Amenorrhea, arthritis (rheumatoid), cramps (menstrual), dysmenorrhea, epilepsy, hysteria, labor & delivery, menorrhagia, menstruation (scant), PMS, and progesterone (low)

Properties: Abortifacient, anti-inflammatory, antiepileptic, antirheumatic, **antispasmodic**, contraceptive, diuretic, **emmenagogue**, **oxytocic**, **parturient**, and uterine tonic

Blue Flag *Bitter Herb*

Iris versicolor

This powerful liver-cleansing herb is best used in small doses or as part of a combination. It is considered helpful for chronic skin diseases and gallbladder problems involving a lack of bile flow. It helps with hypoglycemia associated with migraines, sugar cravings and red-colored skin.

Warnings: The fresh root is too strong for internal use and can be toxic. Only the dried herb should be used. Large doses of the dried herb can cause nausea, vomiting, intestinal pain, and diarrhea. Not for use during pregnancy or lactation.

Energetics: Cooling and drying

Used For: Acne, eczema, and gallbladder problems

Properties: Cholagogue, emetic, and lymphatic

Blue-Green Algae

Mildly Salty & Sweet Herb

Aphanizomenon flos-aquae

This algae comes from Klamath Lake in Oregon. It contains chlorophyll, protein and amino acids, neuropeptides, fatty-acids, B vitamins, and beta-carotene. There is some research suggesting it may be helpful for reducing allergic reactions, boosting immune activity, balancing brain function in ADHD, normalizing blood sugar levels, and reducing levels of heavy metals like arsenic.

Look for *blue-green algae* in *Algae Formula*

Energetics: Nourishing, neutral, and balancing

Used For: ADD/ADHD, allergies (respiratory), appetite (excessive), convalescence, electromagnetic pollution, heavy metal poisoning, **hypoglycemia**, mania, metabolic syndrome, and radiation

Properties: Antiallergenic, antidiabetic, appetite suppressant, food, immune stimulant, and low glycemic

Boneset *Aromatic & Bitter Herb*

Eupatorium perfoliatum

An aromatic and bitter herb traditionally used for colds, fevers and flu. Taken as a warm tea it helps to promote perspiration and acts as an emetic. Taken as a cold tea, it acts as a tonic. Combined with mint, it helps to relieve vomiting and bloating. Combined with ginger and anise it aids coughs. It is very helpful for flu accompanied by aches in the muscles.

Look for *boneset* in *Jeannie Burgess' Allergy-Lung Formula*

Warnings: Use cautiously during pregnancy. Long term use is not recommended.

Energetics: Cooling, drying, and mildly relaxing

Used For: Colds, **fever**, **flu**, lyme disease, and perspiration (deficient)

Properties: Analgesic, diaphoretic, and emetic

Borage *Oily Herb*

Borago officinalis

Borage seed oil is high in polyunsaturated fatty acids and is used for inflammation, skin conditions and arthritis. Borage herb is a mood-elevating remedy that boosts adrenal function and lifts sadness and depression. Used as a flower essence, it promotes cheerful courage when facing adversity.

Look for *borage* in *Adrenal Glandular* and *GLA Oil Formulas*

Warnings: None for the oil, but the herb itself contains pyrrolizidine alkaloids and should be used with caution. Avoid while pregnant.

Energetics: Cooling, moistening, and nourishing

Used For: Adrenal fatigue, anorexia, arthritis, convalescence, eczema, fever, hangover, and stress

Properties: Adrenal tonic, anti-inflammatory, **antidepressant**, cell proliferant, decongestant, and expectorant

Boron   *Mineral*

Boron is an essential trace mineral that seems to affect the way the body handles other minerals such as calcium, magnesium, and phosphorus. It is necessary for bone development and may help to increase estrogen levels in post-menopausal women. It can also be helpful for relieving painful periods. It may also have antioxidant effects.

Boric acid, a common form of boron, can kill yeast that causes vaginal infections. It is has been used topically to treat vaginal yeast infections.

Used For: Arthritis, broken bones, dysmenorrhea, menopause, and **osteoporosis**

Properties: Nutritive

Boswellia   *Aromatic & Bitter Herb*

Boswellia serrata

Boswellia resin has been used in traditional Ayurvedic herbalism as a remedy for arthritis, pulmonary diseases, ringworm and diarrhea. The active constituent in boswellia is boswellic acid, which appears to have anti-inflammatory and anti-arthritic actions.

Look for *boswellia* in *Anti-Inflammatory Pain, CBD Joint, General Analgesic,* and *Herbal Arthritis Formulas*

Energetics: Cooling and mildly drying

Used For: **Arthritis**, arthritis (rheumatoid), bursitis, cancer, carpal tunnel, cartilage damage, diarrhea, dislocation, **inflammation**, **inflammatory bowel disorders**, **pain**, parasites (nematodes, worms), spinal disks, and tendonitis

Properties: Analgesic, **anti-inflammatory, antiarthritic**, and expectorant

Brain and Memory Protection Formula

See also *Brain Tonic*

Use this formula to support the brain cells involved in memory and learning that utilize the neurotransmitter acetylcholine. Huperzine A is a key ingredient in this formula that helps prevent the break down of acetylcholine. See more information under *Huperzine A*.

Used For: Aging, **Alzheimer's**, circulation (brain), cloudy thinking, **dementia**, **memory/brain function**, mental illness, **Parkinson's disease**, and traumatic brain injury

Affects: Acetylcholine, brain, brain atrophy, and central nervous system

Take 2 capsules with a meal twice daily.

Ingredients: Phosphatidylserine, phosphatidylcholine, ginkgo leaf, alpha-lipoic acid, and huperzine A

Brain Calming Formula

See also *Attention-Focus Formula*

This formula combines GABA with herbs and nutrients that may aid it's production. GABA acts as a calming neurotransmitter in the brain inhibiting overactivity of nerve cells. Many people with anxiety, insomnia, epilepsy, and other brain disorders do not manufacture sufficient levels of GABA. See more information under *GABA*.

Warnings: Do not exceed directed amount; do not combine with prescription drugs or use with pregnancy or nursing.

Used For: ADD/ADHD, **addictions (coffee, caffeine)**, **anxiety disorders**, autism, concentration (poor), epilepsy, **insomnia**, OCD, Parkinson's disease, schizophrenia, **seizures**, and tics

Affects: Brain, **brain irritation**, central nervous system, and **gaba**

Use 1-2 capsules per day. Take one capsule prior to bedtime to promote sleep. If you wake up and can't go back to sleep because of excessive thoughts, take a second capsule.

Ingredients: GABA, L-glutamine, passion flower aerial parts, taurine, and spirulina

Brain-Heart Formula

The combination of ginkgo and hawthorn is very popular in Europe. It improves blood circulation and enzyme metabolism throughout the body and supports the utilization of oxygen to the heart. It is a gentle and safe remedy, but works best with extended use as the improvements are gradual.

Used For: Alzheimer's, **angina**, cardiac arrest, cardiovascular disease, **circulation (brain)**, **circulation (poor)**, cold hands/feet, concentration (poor), dizziness, fainting, **heart valves**, heart weakness, memory/brain function, Ménière's disease, **numbness**, **Raynaud's disease**, and **tinnitus**

Affects: Brain, hearing, and **heart**

Take 1-2 capsules two to three times daily with a meal.

Ingredients: Hawthorn berry and ginkgo leaf & leaf extract

Broken and Hardened Hearts FE Blend

This is a flower essence blend I formulated for people who are unable to face the grief and pain of their losses, who have a tendency to harden their hearts against love. They are afraid of intimacy and warmth because they fear the pain they will feel if they lose it.

People who need this remedy have closed their hearts because of unresolved wounds from childhood and previous relationships. They have difficulty trusting others or being vulnerable in a relationship.

This remedy helps a person face their suppressed pain and grief, open their heart, and find healing. It helps them learn to open up to the connection of love and feel warmth and pleasure again. It increases empathy, compassion, and trust in relationships by helping a person find the healthy vulnerability that love requires.

See the strategy *Flower Essence* for suggested uses.

Used For: Cardiac arrest, cardiovascular disease, cirrhosis of the liver, COPD, **grief & sadness**, heart fibrillation/palpitations, and heart weakness

Affects: Circulatory atrophy, circulatory constriction, heart, and lungs

Ingredients: California wild rose FE, baby blue eyes FE, yerba santa FE, star tulip FE, evening primrose FE, pink monkeyflower FE, and golden ear drops FE

Bromelain
Enzyme

Bromelain is a proteolytic (protein-digesting) enzyme from the pineapple plant. It reduces inflammation by inhibiting the formation of bradykinin and COX2 enzymes. It also inhibits platelet aggregation, preventing blood clot formation. Bromelain has been studied extensively and has been shown to be an effective treatment for musculoskeletal injuries as well as speeding post-operative recovery. It also helps potentiate some antibiotics, increasing their effectiveness.

Usage: 300 mg taken four times a day with food or on an empty stomach. Don't take bromelain if you are allergic to pineapples or bees. If you are prone to heart palpitations, limit dosage to 400 mg daily.

Used For: **Allergies (respiratory)**, angina, arthritis (rheumatoid), **autoimmune disorders**, backache, congestion (sinus), diarrhea, digestion (poor), dysmenorrhea, inflammation, inflammatory bowel disorders, injuries, Peyronie's disease, prostatitis, sinus infection, **spinal disks**, and **surgery (recovery)**

Properties: Antithrombotic

Broomrape
Salty & Sweet Herb

Cistanche salsa

Broomrape is a superior tonic in Chinese herbalism. It is nutritious and not harsh-acting. It enters the kidney and large intestine meridians and has tonifying and laxative qualities. It helps moisten the intestines and has slight blood-pressure-reducing effect. It also tonifies the kidney yang.

Look for *broomrape* in *Chinese Fire-Increasing* and *Chinese Water-Increasing Formulas*

Energetics: Warming and moistening

Used For: Backache, constipation (adults), erectile dysfunction, and infertility

Properties: Aperient and hypotensive

Buchu
Pungent Herb

Barosma betulina

A strong diuretic native to Africa, buchu is used primarily for problems with the urinary tract. It can also be helpful for the prostate.

Look for *buchu* in *UTI Prevention Formula*

Warnings: Avoid during pregnancy. Contraindicated with dryness. Not recommended for children under two years of age. Not to be used with acute inflammation of the urinary tract.

Energetics: Warming and drying

Used For: **Edema**, incontinence, kidney infection, prostatitis, urethritis, urinary tract infections, and **urine (scant)**

Properties: Antiseptic, carminative, and **diuretic**

Buckthorn
Bitter Herb

Rhamnus frangula

A bitter laxative with properties similar to cascara sagrada but not as harsh, buckthorn is most often used to relieve constipation.

Look for *buckthorn* in *Stimulant Laxative Formula*

Warnings: Avoid during pregnancy or by persons who are weak. Avoid prolonged use.

Energetics: Cooling and drying

Used For: Colon (atonic), **constipation (adults)**, and gallbladder problems

Properties: Anthelmintic and **laxative**

Bugleweed
Bitter Herb

Lycopus virginicus

Bugleweed inhibits iodine metabolism and helps to reduce an overactive thyroid. It is used with lemon balm and motherwort for Graves' disease. It also influences the lungs and heart and can be beneficial for a rapid or irregular heartbeat, especially when it coincides with sleep difficulties.

Look for *bugleweed* in *Heart Health* and *Thyroid Calming Formulas*

Warnings: Bugleweed should not be used in cases of underactive thyroid (hypothyroidism). Do not take during pregnancy or with excessive menstrual bleeding.

Energetics: Cooling and drying

Used For: Anxiety disorders, **Graves' disease**, heart fibrillation/palpitations, and tachycardia

Properties: **Antithyrotropic** and cardiac

Bupleurum   *Bitter Herb*

Bupleurum chinense

A bitter and aromatic Chinese herb, bupleurum is an ingredient in many Chinese formulas for liver, blood and skin conditions. Bupleurum contains saikosides, which strengthen liver function while protecting the liver from toxins. It has an anti-inflammatory effect and can reduce the risk of liver cancer in people with cirrhosis. Tradition says it helps release anger and sadness stored in the liver.

Look for *bupleurum* in *Chinese Metal-Decreasing, Chinese Wind-Heat Evil,* and *Chinese Wood-Decreasing Formulas*

Energetics: Cooling and drying

Used For: **Anger (excessive)**, depression, fever, gas & bloating, grief & sadness, **hepatitis**, indigestion, and inflammation

Properties: Alterative, anti-inflammatory, antidepressant, carminative, **hepatic**, and hepatoprotective

Burdock   *Mildly Bitter & Sweet Herb*

Arctium lappa

Burdock root is a nourishing alterative used for skin diseases, issues with fat metabolism, cancer, and lymphatic congestion. A strong decoction can be used in baths for itching. Burdock helps to stabilize mast cells, which reduces allergic reactions. The leaves can be used as a poultice.

Look for *burdock* in *Alterative-Immune, Blood Purifier, Blood Sugar Control, Chinese Balanced Cleansing, Christopher's Herbal Iron, Christopher's Sinus, Detoxifying, Drawing Salve, Essiac Immune Tea, Herbal Bitters, Lymph Cleansing,* and *Steven Horne's Anti-Allergy Formulas*

Warnings: Use with caution during pregnancy.

Energetics: Cooling, moistening, and nourishing

Used For: Abscesses, **acne**, allergies (respiratory), arthritis, boils, breasts (swelling/tenderness), bunions, bursitis, **cancer**, **cartilage damage**, cellulite, chicken pox, con-

stipation (adults), cysts, **dermatitis**, **eczema**, fat cravings, fat metabolism (poor), **fatty liver disease**, fatty tumors/deposits, food allergies/intolerances, gallbladder problems, gout, hypoglycemia, itching, leukemia, measles, mumps, **PMS Type S**, poison ivy/oak, polyps, **preeclampsia**, **psoriasis**, **rashes & hives**, rhinitis, seborrhea, **skin (dry/flaky)**, **skin (infections)**, **skin (oily)**, surgery (recovery), swollen lymph glands, and triglycerides (low)

Properties: **Alterative**, **antiallergenic**, **anticancer**, antimutagenic, **antipruritic**, aperient, cholagogue, detoxifying, diuretic, food, hepatic, hypoglycemic, lipotropic, lymphatic, **mast cell stabilizer**, and stomachic

Butcher's Broom   *Mildly Bitter Herb*

Ruscus aculeatus

Butcher's broom is a tonic for the vascular system, helping to prevent blood clots and to tone arteries and veins. It works well in combination with vitamin E and horse chestnut.

Look for *butcher's broom* in *Vein Tonic Formula*

Warnings: May be contraindicated in cases of high blood pressure.

Energetics: Cooling, drying, and mildly constricting

Used For: Anal fistula/fissure, aneurysm, **blood clot prevention**, bruises, cancer treatment side effects, **capillary weakness**, **easily bruised**, hemorrhoids, jaundice (adults), **phlebitis**, Raynaud's disease, **spider veins**, **strokes**, surgery (preparation), **thrombosis**, urine (scant), and **varicose veins**

Properties: **Anticoagulant**, **antithrombotic**, cardiac, deobstruent, and **vascular tonic**

Butterbur   *Stimulant Bitter Herb*

Petasites hybridus

This herb was tested on hay fever (allergic rhinitis) symptoms and found to be as effective as many OTC and prescription drugs. Butterbur has also been shown to reduce the frequency, intensity and duration of migraines. It is also a useful remedy for cramps and asthma.

Warnings: The plant contains pyrrolizidine alkaloids (which can be toxic to the liver), but extracts are available with these alkaloids removed.

Energetics: Cooling, drying, and relaxing

Used For: Allergies (respiratory), asthma, cramps (menstrual), **headache (migraine)**, and rhinitis

Properties: Analgesic, antiallergenic, antitussive, and expectorant

Butternut
Bitter Herb

Juglans cinerea

Butternut bark is a milder alternative to cascara sagrada and buckthorn. The unripe nut is used to kill intestinal worms.

Warnings: Avoid during pregnancy and lactation.

Energetics: Cooling and drying

Used For: Colon (atonic), constipation (adults), parasites (nematodes, and worms)

Properties: Laxative and **vermifuge**

Cajeput EO
Sweet & Woody Essential Oil

Melaleuca leucadendron

Cajeput EO is related to tea tree and has a eucalyptus-like and camphorous odor. It is very warming and stimulating. It has antiseptic and disinfectant properties and can be applied topically to injuries to prevent infection and ease healing. It helps relieve itchy skin in eczema and psoriasis and is also helpful for insect bites. It can be used in massage to relieve back pain and muscle stiffness.

See the strategy *Aromatherapy* for suggested uses.

Warnings: Do not use internally without the supervision of a professionally trained aromatherapy practitioner. Can be irritating to the skin so it is best to dilute it before application.

Used For: Abrasions/scratches, bites & stings, circulation (poor), colic (children), congestion, congestion (lymphatic), cough, digestion (poor), eczema, fever, flu, gas & bloating, gout, **infection (bacterial)**, infection prevention, jock itch, neuralgia & neuritis, psoriasis, sinus infection, tetanus, thrush, vaginitis, and wounds & sores

Properties: Analgesic, anti-inflammatory, antibacterial, antifungal, antimicrobial, antiparasitic, **antiseptic**, antispasmodic, antiviral, carminative, disinfectant, and expectorant

Calamus (Sweet Flag)
Pungent Herb

Acorus calamus

Calamus has been used in Ayurvedic herbalism as a tonic for the brain and nervous system. It has been used in both Ayurveda and Western herbalism as an aid for indigestion and intestinal gas.

Energetics: Warming, drying, and relaxing

Used For: Colic (adults), gas & bloating, and indigestion

Properties: Antispasmodic, aphrodisiac, carminative, diaphoretic, stimulant (appetite), and tonic

Calcium
Mineral

Calcium is the most abundant mineral in the body and is important for healthy bones and teeth, muscular contractions, nerve function, and many other body processes. Calcium intake in Paleolithic people and among healthy populations in the world today averages between 1,500 and 2,500 mg daily. Compare that to the average American female's intake of around 500 mg daily.

Calcium cannot be properly utilized without adequate stomach acid. Even if with good digestion, your body still cannot process more than about 400 mg at a time, so the dosage should be spread out throughout the day. Calcium also requires magnesium, boron, vitamin D, vitamin K_2 and trace minerals for proper utilization. Women with PMS, leg cramps associated with pregnancy, pre-eclampsia, and people with low bone density should supplement with calcium or increase dietary intake.

Usage: 400–800 mg daily. Always take calcium with equal amounts of magnesium, and preferably with other trace minerals.

Used For: Acid indigestion, allergies (respiratory), arrhythmia, Bell's palsy, broken bones, cadmium toxicity, calcium deficiency, dyspepsia, emotional sensitivity, gastritis, hearing loss, heart fibrillation/palpitations, hypertension, insomnia, mental illness, mitochondrial dysfunction, narcolepsy, osteoporosis, **overacidity**, **pregnancy**, prolapsed colon, prolapsed uterus, skin problems, tachycardia, teeth (grinding), teething, tics, and twitching

Properties: Alkalinizer and antiarrhythmic

Calendula (Marigold)
Astringent Herb

Calendula officinalis

Calendula is used topically, either as an herb or homeopathic remedy, for cuts, burns, and other injuries. It speeds wound healing and soothes irritated tissues.

Look for *calendula* in *Ear Drop, Healing Salve,* and *Topical Injury Formulas*

Warnings: Avoid taking internally during pregnancy. Topical use is completely safe.

Energetics: Cooling, drying, and constricting

Used For: Abrasions/scratches, anal fistula/fissure, athlete's foot, bites & stings, **bleeding (external), blisters**, breasts (swelling/tenderness), celiac disease, conjunctivitis, cradle cap, **cuts**, depression, **diaper rash**, gingivitis, **inflammatory bowel disorders, injuries, leaky gut**, leucorrhea, ligaments (torn/injuried), menorrhagia, **scars/scar tissue, surgery (recovery)**, ulcerations (external), ulcers, and **wounds & sores**

Properties: Astringent, hemostatic, styptic, and vulnerary

California Poppy　　　*Bitter Herb*

Eschscholzia californica

California poppy is in the same family as opium poppy and has mild sedative and analgesic properties but is not narcotic. It helps to normalize nervous system function to ease nervous tension, anxiety, insomnia and pain (internal and external). It has an affinity for GABA receptors in the brain, calming the mind without depressing the central nervous system.

Look for *California poppy* in *Herbal Sleep Aid Formula*

Energetics: Cooling and relaxing

Used For: Addictions (drugs), anxiety disorders, headache (tension), heart fibrillation/palpitations, **insomnia, nervousness**, and pain

Properties: Analgesic, **sedative**, and **soporific**

Calming and Relaxing EO Blend

This is a soothing and relaxing blend of essential oils that is helpful for calming anxiety, stress, and emotional sensitivity. It may also aid sleep and ease tension headaches.

See the strategy *Aromatherapy* for suggested uses.

Warnings: Phototoxic—avoid sun exposure after topical application. Use with caution during pregnancy.

Used For: Anxiety attacks, emotional sensitivity, headache, headache (tension), insomnia, and stress

Affects: Central nervous system

Ingredients: Lavender EO, orange EO, atlas cedarwood EO, and ylang ylang EO

Camphor EO　　　*Fresh & Woody Essential Oil*

Cinnamomum camphora

The oil from *Cinnamonum camphora* is called camphor. There are several types, but the white camphor oil is typically used topically to relieve pain and inhaled to ease congestion. Camphor is a local anesthetic, numbing the nerve endings where it is applied. Inhaled it is stimulating and invigorating and helps open congested air passages.

See the strategy *Aromatherapy* for suggested uses.

Warnings: Do not use internally.

Energetics: Warming and relaxing

Used For: Arthritis, backache, bronchitis, **congestion (bronchial)**, **congestion (sinus)**, dislocation, **pain**, and sprains

Properties: Anti-inflammatory, antiseptic, and expectorant

Cannabis (Hemp, Marijuana)

Aromatic, Oily, & Sweet Herb

Cannabis sativa

There are two basic varieties of cannabis. One is known as hemp (the industrial, non-psychoactive variety) and the other marijuana (the psychoactive variety).

Hemp has been a valuable resource for the whole of Western civilization. Hemp fibers have been used to make paper, clothing, rope and sails. In fact, until 1883, 75—90 percent of all paper was made from hemp fiber, including Bibles, maps, books, newspapers, and money. Early American clothing was often made from hemp, too.

Hemp seeds are also highly nutritious and a great plant source of omega-3 fatty acids and protein. Hemp oil is a better source of essential fatty acids than flax seed oil.

Both hemp and marijuana contain phytocannabinoids, compounds that interact with a newly discovered body system, which was named after the cannabis plant. It's called the endocannabinoid system (ECS) and it helps to regulate homeostasis. Both plants have medicinal properties, and can be used to ease pain, reduce inflammation, and possibly help with neurological disorders and cancer.

About one hundred different phytocannabinoids have been identified in cannabis, but the primary ones are THC and CBD. Phytocannabinoids have also been found in other herbs such as echinacea and kava kava as well as in chocolate and truffles.

Personally, I believe recreational marijuana is problematic because growers have been deliberately creating strains of cannabis with higher levels of THC, the psychoactive cannabinoid responsible for the high produced by the drug. Marijuana grown in the 1970s had only about 1–3 percent THC, whereas today's varieties range from 5–30 percent. Both THC and CBD are made from the same precursor chemical, which means that breeding higher levels of THC reduce the level of CBD in cannabis.

Because THC binds to ECS receptors, it causes the body to produce fewer endocannabinoids, thus down-regulating your ECS. Since your ECS kicks in to help you cope with pain and stress, using THC regularly makes you less able to deal with pain and stress naturally.

The use of THC-rich cannabis is especially risky for teenagers, whose ECS system is still developing as they learn to adapt and cope with the normal stresses of life. Heavy use of THC-rich cannabis in young people has been shown to decrease IQ and increase the risk of mental illness, including schizophrenia. The down-regulation of the ECS is also what makes a person dependent and causes withdrawal symptoms when a person discontinues the use of marijuana.

Fortunately, high-CBD hemp does not have the drawbacks of marijuana and actually helps to counter the negative aspects of THC. Hemp can now be legally grown in the United States. The THC content of legal hemp must be under 0.3 percent. See the entry on CBD for more information on using this non-psychoactive compound from cannabis. The uses listed here are for high-CBD, low-THC cannabis.

Look for *cannabis* in *CBD Anti-inflammatory, CBD Brain, CBD Joint, CBD Relaxing, CBD Topical Analgesic, Hemp Oil with Terpenes,* and *Sleep Support Formulas*

Used For: ALS, cancer, **cancer treatment side effects**, **epilepsy**, fibromyalgia, headache (migraine), Huntington's disease, inflammation, insomnia, multiple sclerosis, **neurodegenerative diseases**, pain, PTSD, and **Tourette's**

Properties: Analgesic, anti-inflammatory, **antiepileptic**, antinausa, antispasmodic, **euphoretic**, and **immune modulator**

Caprylic Acid
Fatty Acid

A medium-chain saturated fatty acid that helps the body fight fungal and bacterial infections. It is naturally found in coconut oil (8 percent), palm kernel (4 percent) and butter (1–2 percent).

Capsicum (Cayenne)
Pungent Herb

Capsicum annuum

Capsicum is a major stimulant for the circulatory system. It increases circulation to every area of the body it comes in contact with, internally or externally. Capsicum also strengthens the heartbeat. Because adequate blood supply is necessary for all tissues to heal, capsicum has earned a reputation in the West as a kind of "cure-all." The capsaicin in capsicum blocks pain receptors, giving it an analgesic effect.

Look for *capsicum* in *Antispasmodic, Circulatory, Fire Cider, Flu* and *Vomiting, Heart Health, Herbal Composition, Paavo Airola's Cold,* and *Stan Malstrom's Herbal Aspirin Formulas*

Warnings: Due to its irritating nature some people have a hard time taking capsicum. Large doses can be irritating to the stomach and cause painful bowel eliminations. Although capsicum stops bleeding and has been used to heal ulcers, this herb can cause pain when used for these purposes; hence, it should be used with caution. It is best to start with extremely small doses to build up tolerance. Capsicum causes burning sensations in sensitive areas, such as genitals, sinuses, etc. It is not recommended for people with hemorrhoids or anal fissures.

Energetics: Warming and drying

Used For: Aneurysm, arteriosclerosis, arthritis, bleeding (external), bleeding (internal), blood clot prevention, blood in stool, burning feet/hands, **cardiac arrest**, cardiovascular disease, chest pain, chills, **circulation (poor)**, **cold hands/feet**, colds, cuts, dysmenorrhea, fainting, fatigue, fever, flu, **frostbite prevention**, gangrene, headache, headache (cluster), heart fibrillation/palpitations, heart weakness, hypertension, hypotension, indigestion, labor & delivery, laryngitis, menorrhagia, miscarriage prevention, **nosebleeds**, numbness, pain, paralysis, peripheral neuropathy, **perspiration (deficient)**, phlebitis, Raynaud's disease, sciatica, **shock (medical)**, **sore throat**, **strokes**, surgery (preparation), tonsillitis, ulcers, varicose veins, and wounds & sores

Properties: Analgesic, **anesthetic**, antiarthritic, anticoagulant, antithrombotic, aperient, cardiac, carminative, **catalyst**, **coagulant**, condiment, counterirritant, dacryagogue, **diaphoretic**, **hemostatic**, hypertensive, **hypotensive**, panacea, rubefacient, sialogogue, **stimulant (circulatory)**, stimulant (metabolic), stomachic, **styptic**, and vulnerary

Cardamom
Aromatic Herb

Elettaria cardamomum

An aromatic spice, cardamon acts as a carminative and digestive aid. It has a reputation as an aphrodisiac and has been used in India for respiratory and kidney ailments.

Look for *cardamom* in *Herbal Bitters Formula*

Energetics: Warming and mildly drying

Used For: Anorexia, gas & bloating, halitosis, and indigestion

Properties: Aperitive, **carminative**, condiment, and digestive tonic

Cardiovascular Antioxidant Formula

This blend of high-ORAC antioxidants helps to prevent cholesterol from oxidizing, as well as reduce total cholesterol and LDL cholesterol. Cholesterol does not adhere to the arterial lining unless it has been oxidized. So by preventing oxidization this decreases arterial inflammation and the risk and heart disease.

Used For: Cardiovascular disease and **cholesterol (high)**

Affects: Arteries, circulatory atrophy, circulatory stagnation, and heart

Take 2 capsules with your evening meal.

Ingredients: Orange (bergamot) fruit extract, turmeric root & rhizome extract, tea leaf, mangosteen pericarp extract, and olive leaf extract

Cardiovascular Nutritional Program

See also *Oral Chelation Formula*

This is a complete nutritional program for the cardiovascular system. It can be used like the oral chelation program to improve blood flow, aid heart health and prevent cardiovascular disease. It can be used for a wide variety of circulatory problems. It has many of the same potential benefits as the *Oral Chelation Formula* and *Oral Chelation* strategy.

Used For: **Aging**, **arteriosclerosis**, blood clot prevention, **cholesterol (high)**, circulation (brain), circulation (poor), cold hands/feet, erectile dysfunction, hypertension, hypotension, macular degeneration, Raynaud's disease, strokes, and varicose veins

Affects: Arteries, circulatory constriction, and circulatory irritation
Take 1 packet daily.

Ingredients: Vitamin A, vitamin C, vitamin d3, vitamin B_1, vitamin B_2, vitamin B_3, vitamin B_6, folate, biotin, vitamin B_{12}, vitamin B_5, choline, calcium, phosphorus, iodine, magnesium, zinc, selenium, copper, manganese, chromium, potassium, orange (bergamot) fruit extract, and fish oil

Cascara Sagrada   *Bitter Herb*

Rhamnus purshiana

A bitter purgative, cascara sagrada increases bile flow and stimulates peristalsis of the colon. The name "cascara sagrada" means holy or sacred bark. It is known for its effectiveness in relieving constipation and colon cleansing.

Look for *cascara sagrada* in *Antiparasitic, Detoxifying, Intestinal Detoxification, Skinny,* and *Stimulant Laxative Formulas*

Warnings: Avoid during pregnancy or for weak persons. Avoid prolonged use. If a person appears dependent on this or other stimulant laxatives or if cramps or griping become a problem, use nervines or magnesium to counteract bowel spasms. In case of diarrhea caused by excessive use, use charcoal or mucilaginous herbs. Long term use will darken the tissue color of the bowel and create laxative dependency.

Energetics: Cooling and drying
Used For: Colon (atonic), **constipation (adults)**, gallbladder problems, parasites, parasites (nematodes, and worms)
Properties: Cholagogue and **laxative**

Cat's Claw (Uña de Gato)

Bitter & Mildly Astringent Herb
Uncaria spp.

Cat's claw is one of the very best remedies for normalizing function of the gastrointestinal tract. It is helpful for inflammation of the bowel and intestines and can also address inflammation of the joints and muscles. Cats claw seems to have antiviral and anti-mutagenic properties, making it a good complimentary treatment for a variety of degenerative diseases and helping to strengthen the immune system against the effects of chemotherapy.

Look for *cat's claw* in *Gut Immune Formula*

Warnings: Avoid during pregnancy.
Energetics: Cooling and mildly constricting
Used For: Arthritis, **arthritis (rheumatoid)**, **cancer**, cancer treatment side effects, cartilage damage, colitis, **diverticulitis**, **dysbiosis**, **Epstein-Barr virus**, fibromyalgia, **food allergies/intolerances**, gastritis, herpes, **inflammatory bowel disorders**, **irritable bowel**, **leaky gut**, **lyme disease**, Reye's syndrome, and ulcers
Properties: Anti-inflammatory, anticancer, antimutagenic, and antioxidant

Catnip   *Aromatic & Mildly Bitter Herb*

Nepeta cataria

A mild aromatic herb which is soothing and settling to the stomach and nerves, catnip is helpful for colds, chills, congestion, sore throat and indigestion. It is excellent for colic in infants when combined with fennel. Catnip tea is often used in enemas to bring down fevers or reduce respiratory congestion. It helps produce perspiration without increasing body heat. Catnip can also be used for nervousness or stress and at bedtime as a sleep aid. Catnip is excellent for children and babies it is mild and extremely safe.

Look for *catnip* in *Children's Colic* and *Stimulant Laxative Formulas*

Warnings: Extremely large doses can cause vomiting. Avoid during pregnancy.
Energetics: Cooling and drying
Used For: **Acid indigestion**, addictions (tobacco), anorexia, belching, colds, **colic (children)**, **colitis**, **colon (spastic)**, **croup**, **dyspepsia**, fever, flu, gas & bloating, hiatal hernia, hiccups, indigestion, inflammatory bowel disorders, insomnia, **irritable bowel**, measles, mumps, perspiration (deficient), and teething

Properties: Analgesic, **antacid**, antispasmodic, carminative, diaphoretic, **nervine**, **sedative**, stimulant (metabolic), and stomachic

CBD (Cannabinol) *Phytochemical*

CBD is a nonpsychoactive cannabinoid found in the cannabis plant. It doesn't directly bind to cannabinoid receptors like THC (the other major cannabinoid in cannabis) does. Instead it attaches to the receptors and makes them more sensitive to the body's own endocannabinoids. So not only does it not have the brain-altering properties of THC, and actually reduces the psychoactive effects of THC. So it can be taken to aid withdrawal symptoms for someone discontinuing the use of marijuana.

Also unlike THC, CBD does not build tolerance, nor do there appear to be any withdrawal symptoms when discontinuing it. So CBD has many potential health benefits without the problems associated with THC. CBD is anti-inflammatory, anticonvulsant, reduces anxiety, eases depression, and helps to ease pain and relax muscles.

Anyone who is concerned about the dangers of marijuana and therefore concerned about the fact that CBD comes from the cannabis plant, needs to understand that CBD itself and cannabis that is high in CBD and low in THC (which the federally mandated 0.3 percent for legal hemp is) cannot make you high and is completely safe for medicinal use.

One drawback of CBD products is that having a small amount of THC in them will actually help them be more effective medicinally, but it also means you could test positive on a drug test. So if you are concerned about this, make sure you get CBD products that are THC-free.

Used For: ADD/ADHD, addictions, **addictions (drugs)**, **ALS**, Alzheimer's, anorexia, anxiety attacks, **anxiety disorders**, **arthritis**, **arthritis (rheumatoid)**, asthma, **autism**, **autoimmune disorders**, **cancer**, **cancer treatment side effects**, depression, dermatitis, diabetes, **dislocation**, **eczema**, emotional sensitivity, **epilepsy**, **fibromyalgia**, glaucoma, Graves' disease, **headache**, **headache (migraine)**, hepatitis, Huntington's disease, **inflammation**, inflammatory bowel disorders, **itching**, lupus, **multiple sclerosis**, **nerve damage**, **neurodegenerative diseases**, **pain**, **Parkinson's disease**, PTSD, **rashes & hives**, **schizophrenia**, **seizures**, **skin problems**, Tourette's, and traumatic brain injury

Properties: Analgesic, **anti-inflammatory**, anticancer, antidepressant, **antiepileptic**, antinausa, antioxidant, antispasmodic, and **anxiolytic**

CBD Anti-inflammatory Formula

Use this formula to reduce inflammation and ease pain. It can be taken internally or applied topically.

Used For: Arthritis, backache, **dislocation**, **inflammation**, inflammatory bowel disorders, injuries, and **pain**

Affects: CB2 receptors, **nerve irritation (pain)**, prostaglandins, and **structural irritation**

Ingredients: Cannabis whole plant extract, CBD, cannabis seed oil, copaiba EO, turmeric rhizome oil, and holy basil aerial parts oil

CBD Brain Formula

This blend combines CBD with remedies that enhance the brain function and calm the mind.

Used For: Anxiety disorders and neurodegenerative diseases

30 drops once daily

Ingredients: Hemp whole plant extract, cinnamon bark oil, kanna extract, clove EO flower oil, rosemary EO leaf oil, and lemongrass EO

CBD Joint Formula

See also *Herbal Arthritis Formula* and *Joint Healing Nutrients Formula*

This blend combines CBD with herbs that enhance circulation, reduce inflammation and ease pain.

Used For: Arthritis, bursitis, and pain

Take 20-30 drops once or twice daily.

Ingredients: Hemp aerial parts extract, CBD, boswellia resin extract, turmeric root extract, clove EO, and frankincense EO

CBD Relaxing Formula

See also *Herbal Sleep Aid Formula* and *Sleep Aid*

Use this formula to help promote relaxation and better sleep.

Used For: Insomnia, irritability, pain, and **stress**

Affects: CB1 receptors, **central nervous system**, and sympathetic-dominant ANS

Ingredients: Cannabis seed oil, cannabis aerial parts extract, lavender EO, lemongrass EO, hops cone oil, rosemary EO, and magnolia flower oil

CBD Topical Analgesic Formula

See also *Analgesic EO Blend* and *Topical Analgesic Formula*

This is a topical cream which helps to ease inflammation and pain. It can also help promote healing of minor injuries.

Used For: Abrasions/scratches, **arthritis**, **backache**, bruises, bursitis, dislocation, exercise (recovery), headache, **inflammation**, injuries, **sprains**, surgery (recovery), and wounds & sores

Affects: **CB2 receptors**, **nerve irritation (pain)**, **prostaglandins**, skin, **spinal discs**, **structural irritation**, and **substance P**

Apply topically as needed.

Ingredients: Methyl salicylate, eucalyptus EO, menthol, camphor EO, hemp (cbd extract), and arnica extract

Celandine   *Bitter Herb*

Chelidonium majus

A bitter herb with strong affinity for the liver and gallbladder, celandine is usually used in combination with other herbs. The juice of celandine has traditionally been used for warts, corns and ringworm.

Warnings: Contraindicated with emaciation or weak digestion. Not for long term use. Not for use during pregnancy.

Energetics: Cooling and drying

Used For: Corns, gallbladder problems, gallstones, headache (cluster), and **warts**

Properties: Cholagogue

Celery   *Aromatic Herb*

Apium graveolens

The seeds of celery help the kidneys to dispose of urine and other unwanted waste products. They to disinfect the bladder and urinary tubules. Celery stalks are also good remedy for urinary problems and for alkalizing the body.

Look for *celery* in *Herbal Arthritis* and *Kidney Stone Formulas*

Warnings: Use seeds cautiously during pregnancy and while lactating

Energetics: Warming and drying

Used For: Arthritis, **arthritis (rheumatoid)**, gout, interstitial cystitis, and **uric acid retention**

Properties: Antirheumatic, condiment, diuretic, food, and low glycemic

Chaga   *Mildly Bitter & Sweet Herb*

Inonotus obliquus

A medicinal mushroom that grows on birch trees in Northern Europe, Asia, and Canada used for cancer and immune deficiency. An extract was approved as an anticancer drug in Russia in 1955.

Look for *chaga* in *Mushroom Immune Formula*

Energetics: Cooling, balancing, and nourishing

Used For: AIDS, cancer, cholesterol (high), gastritis, hypertension, and ulcers

Properties: Anticancer, antioxidant, antiviral, and immune modulator

Chamomile (Roman, German)

Aromatic & Mildly Bitter Herb

Chamomilla recutita

Chamomile has properties similar to catnip and peppermint. It calms the nerves and settles the stomach. It also helps to expel gas. This is an excellent nervine agent, especially for children. Use it homeopathically or make it into a tea and sweeten for colic, hyperactivity, teething, fussiness, fever or irritability in infants and children.

Chamomile is useful for colds and flu in children when combined with elderflower, peppermint and/or yarrow. It contains an anti-inflammatory volatile oil similar to the oil in yarrow. Use it in combination with other nervines and anti-inflammatory agents for pain, swelling and infection. It can be applied topically to help heal injuries and is helpful for quitting smoking when used with lobelia.

Due to its anti-inflammatory properties and its effects on the digestive and nervous systems, chamomile is a common ingredient in herbal formulas.

Look for *chamomile* in *Herbal Bitters, Herbal Sleep Aid, Intestinal Soothing, Irritable Bowel Fiber, Jeannie Burgess' Stress,* and *Paavo Airola's Cold Formulas*

Warnings: There is a rare chance of an allergic reaction to chamomile.

Energetics: Cooling and relaxing

Used For: Acid indigestion, acne, ADD/ADHD, addictions (drugs), addictions (tobacco), alcoholism, anger (excessive), anorexia, anxiety (situational), anxiety disorders, appetite (deficient), cancer treatment side effects, celiac disease, colds, colic (adults), colic (children), colitis, colon (spastic), **conjunctivitis**, corns, Cushing's disease, cystic breast disease, **denture sores**, dermatitis, digestion (poor), diverticulitis, dyspepsia, **emotional sensitivity**, **eyes (red/itching)**, **eyes, bloodshot**, fear, fever, **floaters**,

gas & bloating, hysteria, ileocecal valve, **indigestion**, **inflammation**, **inflammatory bowel disorders**, **insomnia**, **irritability**, irritable bowel, labor & delivery, leaky gut, menopause, nervousness, PMS Type A, psoriasis, rashes & hives, restless dreams, **rosacea**, scars/scar tissue, skin problems, **stress**, **sty**, sunburn, **teething**, toothache, Tourette's, ulcers, vaccine side effects, and wounds & sores

Properties: Analgesic, **anti-inflammatory**, antiphlogistic, antiseptic, antismoking, antispasmodic, **antiviral**, **calmative**, **carminative**, diaphoretic, **digestive tonic**, febrifuge, **nervine**, opthalmicum, relaxant, sedative, **stimulant (appetite)**, **stomachic**, vermifuge, and vulneraries

Chamomile, Roman EO

Fresh, Fruity, & Sweet Essential Oil

Anthemis nobilis

Chamomile EO is a sweet, floral oil that has a calming effect on the nerves. It is particularly helpful for people who are peevish or irritable, as it helps to promote a calm, sunny disposition. It is a very good essential oil for easing stress and irritability in children, but is also good for anyone who is constantly complaining about little, insignificant things.

Chamomile has anti-inflammatory and antispasmodic effects. It helps with irregular periods and PMS, especially when used in a bath or as a massage oil. To ease gall-bladder problems, sore throats, abdominal pain, and colic in children it can be applied topically in a warm, moist compress. As an inhalant, it helps with emotional anxiety and tension associated with asthma, hay fever, and other allergies. Roman chamomile is used when someone feels grumpy, morose, discontented or impatient, short-tempered, self-involved, overly sensitive or rarely satisfied. It is a remedy for children who are feeling impatient, disagreeable or tense. The oil is beneficial for teething pain, colic or flatulence as the underlying cause for emotional distresses. It has mildly sedating properties, a calming but not a depressing effect.

See the strategy *Aromatherapy* for suggested uses.

Warnings: Do not use internally without the supervision of a professionally trained aromatherapy practitioner. When applying topically, always use in a carrier oil as it may cause contact dermatitis. It should not be used where there is prolonged exposure to direct sunlight. Contraindicated in chronic anxiety and narcolepsy.

Used For: Abscesses, acne, ADD/ADHD, adrenal fatigue, anger (excessive), anxiety (situational), Cushing's disease, dermatitis, dysmenorrhea, eczema, emotional sensitivity, fear, fever, gas & bloating, hysteria, inflammation, insect repellant, insomnia, **irritability**, menopause, nervousness, neuralgia & neuritis, parasites (nematodes, worms), PMS Type A, PTSD, scars/scar tissue, skin (dry/flaky),

skin problems, stress, sunburn, teething, and wounds & sores

Properties: Adrenal tonic, analgesic, anti-inflammatory, antiphlogistic, antiseptic, antispasmodic, bactericidal, carminative, cholagogue, cicatrizant, digestive tonic, emmenagogue, febrifuge, hepatic, parasympatholytic, sedative, stomachic, sympatholytic, and vulnerary

Chaparral   *Fragrant Bitter Herb*

Larrea tridentata

A bitter, acrid herb, chaparral has long been used as a cancer remedy and blood purifier. It contains an antioxidant substance known as NDGA. Chaparral cleanses and tones the liver, blood and lymphatics. It is helpful for drug withdrawal.

Look for *chaparral* in *Anti-Fungal* and *Drawing Salve Formulas*

Warnings: Potentially hepatotoxic, although the evidence is circumstantial. It may be due to taking the plant in capsules instead of its traditional form as a tea. Nevertheless, it is contraindicated in liver disease and when pregnant. It has a strong action on the kidneys and should be taken with ample amounts of water to protect the kidneys.

Energetics: Cooling and drying

Used For: Acne, **cancer**, congestion (lymphatic), heavy metal poisoning, infection (bacterial), infection (fungal), infection (viral), parasites, and radiation

Properties: Alterative, anthelmintic, antibacterial, **anticancer**, **antioxidant**, antiparasitic, antiseptic, and **cytotoxic**

Charcoal   *Non-Nutrient*

Charcoal absorbs irritants and many poisonous substances. Applied to wounds it draws out pus and infection. Taken internally, it lowers cholesterol, reduces gas and bloating and eases diarrhea. As a poultice it is helpful for venomous insect bites, especially brown recluse spider bites.

Warnings: Charcoal can interfere with assimilation of medicines and nutrients. Do not take with prescription medications. Do not take for more than a few days at a time. Large doses may cause constipation.

Usage: For poisoning, hospitals normally administer between 50–100 grams, but smaller doses like 1,000 milligrams (1 gram) taken at the first sign of intestinal distress works well. Repeat after two hours if needed, up to a maximum of 10 capsules per day. For severe diarrhea, combine with psyllium seed capsules or bulk slippery elm. For treating poisoning, contact the Poison Control Center and follow their recommendations. First-aid application may require 30 to 200 capsules, depending on quantity and toxicity of the material ingested. and Charcoal can also be applied as a poultice to spider bites. It is even effective with brown recluse bites. Change poultice the every hour for maximum benefit.

Used For: **Belching**, **bites & stings**, blood poisoning, cancer treatment side effects, **chemical exposure**, **cholera**, cholesterol (high), **diarrhea**, **food poisoning**, **gas & bloating**, **giardia**, **jaundice (adults)**, **jaundice (infants)**, motion sickness, and **poisoning**

Properties: **Adsorbent**, **antidiarrheal**, **antidote**, **antitoxic**, antivenomous, and drawing

Chaste Tree   *Bitter & Pungent Herb*

Vitex agnus-castus

Chaste tree berries help to regulate hormones, making them useful for menstrual irregularity, PMS and menopause. They reduce sex drive in men and were used by Monks under vows of celibacy (which is where the plant gets its common name). It is a good remedy to balance reproductive hormones in teenagers suffering from acne. It is a slow acting remedy and should be taken for three to six months to see optimal results.

Look for *chaste tree* in *DHEA with Herbs* and *Female Cycle Formulas*

Warnings: Although a traditional remedy to prevent miscarriages, it has the potential to cause miscarriages in some women. It might reduce the effectiveness of hormonal birth control.

Energetics: Drying and cooling

Used For: **Acne**, **birth control side effects**, **breast lumps**, **breasts (swelling/tenderness)**, cramps (menstrual), dysmenorrhea, **estrogen dominance**, **fibroids (uterine)**, **hot flashes**, lupus, **menopause**, **menorrhagia**, **menstrual irregularity**, **nocturnal emission**, **ovarian pain**, **PMS**, **PMS Type A**, polycystic ovarian syndrome, **progesterone (low)**, **puberty**, and **sex drive (excessive)**

Properties: **Anaphrodisiac** and female tonic

Cherry   *Sour Herb*

Prunus spp.

The bark of some species of cherries, especially wild cherries, has a long history of use as a cough remedy (which may explain why so many cough remedies are cherry-flavored). It is a cooling remedy that expels phlegm and soothes and dries out mucous membranes. It may also help normalize histamine reactions in allergies. In Chinese herbalism, it is indicated when there is "heart fire blazing," consisting of mental restlessness, agitation, insomnia, rapid pulse, and a yellow-coated tongue with a red tip.

Look for *cherry* in *Dry Cough Syrup Formula*

Warnings: Wild cherry is slight toxic so it should not be used in large amounts or for long periods of time. Contains hydrocyanic acid which, in high doses, may cause spasms and difficulty breathing. Medicinal doses have never proved harmful. Avoid during pregnancy.

Energetics: Cooling and drying

Used For: Allergies (respiratory), asthma, bronchitis, congestion (bronchial), COPD, cough, **cough (damp)**, heart fibrillation/palpitations, irritability, nervousness, **pertussis**, **pleurisy**, **pneumonia**, tachycardia, and tuberculosis

Properties: Astringent and **expectorant**

Chia   *Oily & Sweet Herb*

Salvia hispanica

Chia seeds are a nutrient rich food containing good fats, protein and mucilaginous fiber. Consumed as a food they can help to balance blood sugar, aid weight management and reduce chronic inflammation.

Energetics: Nourishing, moistening, and mildly cooling

Used For: Excess weight, inflammation, and metabolic syndrome

Properties: Antioxidant, mucilant, and nutritive

Chickweed   *Salty Herb*

Stellaria racemosamedia

Chickweed is a mucilaginous herb thought to break down fats and fatty tumors in the body. It acts as a mild appetite suppressant and weight loss aid when taken one hour before mealtimes. It can be used in poultices for skin irritations and the tea can be used as an eyewash for soothing irritated eyes. Applied topically, it is helpful for relieving itchy skin.

Look for *chickweed* in *Antispasmodic Ear*, *Fat-Absorbing Fiber*, *Garcinia Fat-Burning*, and *Healing Salve Formulas*

Energetics: Cooling and balancing

Used For: Acne, appetite (excessive), arthritis (rheumatoid), boils, **cellulite**, chicken pox, cholesterol (low), cysts, diaper rash, **eczema**, **excess weight**, eyes (red/itching), fat cravings, fat metabolism (poor), **fatty liver disease**, **fatty tumors/deposits**, gout, hemorrhoids, **itching**, psoriasis, **rashes & hives**, skin problems, sprains, triglycerides (low), and wounds & sores

Properties: Alterative, antiobesic, **antipruritic**, emollient, **emulsifier**, expectorant, laxative (bulk), **lipotropic**, mineralizer, mucilant, and nutritive

Chicory   *Bitter & Sweet Herb*

Cichorium intybus

Chicory is related to dandelion and has similar uses. It contains inulin, which feeds the friendly flora of the digestive tract. It is a bitter tonic for the digestive system and liver. The roasted roots are also used as a coffee substitute.

Energetics: Cooling, drying, and nourishing

Used For: Anemia, arthritis, asthma, cataracts, dysbiosis, eyes (red/itching), fever, gallstones, gout, headache (cluster), infertility, mastitis, and skin (infections)

Properties: Aperient, digestant, food, and hepatoprotective

Children's Colic Formula

Catnip and fennel are a traditional remedy to help infants with colic. The blend calms the nerves and can be helpful for cold and flu symptoms. A mild and safe remedy for children, it is also helpful for adults.

Used For: Acid indigestion, belching, **colic (children)**, dyspepsia, **gas & bloating**, indigestion, irritability, and teething

Affects: Digestive depression, **digestive irritation**, and **stomach**

To help ease colic, diarrhea, teething and fussiness in infants use 3-10 drops straight or diluted in water for tea. For indigestion, nervousness, insomnia in older children, take 1/2 teaspoon or more as needed. For the same conditions in adults use 1 teaspoon three times daily or as needed.

Ingredients: Catnip leaf extract and fennel seed oil

Children's Elderberry Cold and Flu Formula

See also *Steven Horne's Children's Composition Formula*

A chewable product with immune-boosting nutrients for children, this can be helpful for warding off colds and flu, especially during the cold winter months, or boosting children's immune systems when they are sick.

Used For: Colds (antiviral), flu, infection (viral), **infection prevention**, and vaccine side effects

Affects: Acute disease stage

Chew up 2 as needed.

Ingredients: Elder berry, astragalus root, echinacea root, reishi, maitake, vitamin C, vitamin D, and zinc

Chinese Balanced Cleansing Program

See also *Ivy Bridge's Cleansing Program*

This is a general cleansing and detoxification program developed by a Chinese herbalist that helps balance the whole body. It stimulates bowel elimination, but more importantly helps to cleanse the liver and the tissues. Using the cleanse should produce two or three bowel movements daily. If stools become too loose, reduce the number of packets being used. It can be helpful to add fiber to this cleanse. Take 1 teaspoon of a *Fiber Blend* in a large glass of water or juice in the morning. Be sure to drink plenty of water when cleansing.

Warnings: Avoided in cases of irritable or inflammatory bowel conditions. Do not use if diarrhea, loose stools, or abdominal pain are present or develop. Not for prolonged use.

Used For: Cervical dysplasia, **chemical exposure**, cholesterol (high), **constipation (adults)**, dysbiosis, eczema, environmental pollution, **halitosis**, headache (migraine), **leaky gut**, pap smear (abnormal), polycystic ovarian syndrome, **preeclampsia**, and vaccine side effects

Affects: Digestive stagnation, hepatic stagnation, **intestinal stagnation**, and liver

Take the contents of 1 packet 15 minutes before meals up to three times daily for 10 days. Drink one glass (8 ounces) of pure water with the capsules, followed by another glass of water.

Ingredients: Chinese Wood Decreasing, special cellular cleansing formula, stan malstrom's lower bowel formula, psyllium hulls, burdock root, and concentrated black walnut

Chinese Earth-Decreasing Formula

Xiao Dao

See also *Christopher's Carminative Formula*

This Chinese herbal formula reduces excessive earth energy. It decongests the stomach and gastrointestinal tract, helping to relieve acute indigestion. It can ease nausea, expel excess gas, restore appetite, and ease sensations of fullness after eating. It can also be used when there is a general sluggish, heavy feeling in the body or a tendency to sugar cravings and weight problems. It is also helpful for people who have indigestion because they are overly pensive, absorbed in their own activities.

Used For: Appetite (deficient), **belching**, congestion, diarrhea, digestion (poor), **dyspepsia**, **gas & bloating**, **halitosis**, ileocecal valve, **indigestion**, and nausea & vomiting

Affects: Digestive depression, **digestive stagnation**, intestinal depression, pancreas head, **stomach**, and **stressed earth**

To strengthen digestion and relieve problems with gas, take 4 capsules o with a meal two times daily. For acute indigestion, take 4 capsules at the first sign of indigestion. There is also a TCM concentrate of this formula where the dose is 1 capsule instead of four.

Ingredients: Chinese giant hyssop tops, Chinese hawthorn fruit, hoelen sclerotium, magnolia bark, rice seed sprout, gastrodia rhizome, and bai-zhu atractylodes rhizome

Chinese Earth-Increasing Formula

Wen Zhong

This formula boosts the earth element by tonifying the spleen chi. It improves the digestion and metabolism of proteins, minerals and other nutrients to enhance muscle tone, improve physical development, enhance energy and increase appetite for healthy foods. It is helpful for elderly people who are losing weight, people who are losing weight because of prolonged illness, and people who are skinny and can't gain muscle mass. Emotionally, a lack of earth element energy will lead to chronic worries and fears, a sense of hopelessness, lack of control over one's own life and sluggish thought processes.

Used For: Anorexia, **bulimia**, convalescence, cramps & spasms, debility, diarrhea, **digestion (poor)**, fear, food allergies/intolerances, gas & bloating, heart fibrillation/palpitations, hemorrhoids, hernias, hiatal hernia, ileocecal valve, indigestion, **muscle tone**, **protein digestion**, sinus infection, **underweight**, and **wasting**
Affects: Digestive atrophy, digestive constriction, general atrophy, **intestinal atrophy**, **spleen**, stomach, and **weakened earth**

To improve chronic digestive system weakness take 3 capsules three times daily. There is also a TCM concentrate of this formula where the dose is one capsule instead of three.

Ingredients: Asian ginseng root, astragalus root, bai-zhu atractylodes rhizome, hoelen sclerotium, Chinese yam rhizome, sacred lotus seed, licorice (Chinese) root, lesser galangal, and sichuan pepper seed

Chinese Fire-Decreasing Formula

An Shen

See also *Anti-Anxiety Formula* and *Anti-Stress B-Complex Formula*

This traditional Chinese formula reduces excessive fire energy. The traditional Chinese name, An Shen, means "pacify the spirit." It is used for conditions associated with a high strung and tense personality. People who talk rapidly and are constantly busy, having a difficult time relaxing, may find this formula helpful. Other indications include absentmindedness, dizziness, pains in the chest due to stress, emotional instability and excessive perspiration. It can ease feelings of fear and insecurity and reduce conditions involving over acidity, such as urinary tract irritation and mouth sores.

Used For: Angina, **anxiety disorders**, Bell's palsy, canker sores, dizziness, emotional sensitivity, fear, **Graves' disease**, headache (tension), heart fibrillation/palpitations, hypertension, insomnia, irritability, mental illness, **stress**, and trauma
Affects: Acute disease stage, central nervous system, general constriction, **stressed fire**, **sympathetic-dominant ANS**, and thyroid irritation

To help nervous problems the suggested dose is 4 capsules once or twice daily. There is also a TCM concentrate of this formula where the dose is 1 capsule once or twice daily.

Ingredients: Oyster shell, silk tree bark, haliotus shell, hoelen sclerotium with hostwood root, asian ginseng root, jujube seed, and polygala root

Chinese Fire-Increasing Formula

Yang Xin

See also *Adrenal Glandular Formula*

This Chinese herbal formula nourishes deficient fire energy. It is a tonic for the heart, nerves and glands, particularly the adrenal glands, which become exhausted under constant stress. A key indication that a person could benefit from this formula is fatigue during the day coupled with disturbed and restless sleep patterns at night. Disturbing dreams are often an early warning sign that one is approaching "burnout." As the problem becomes more severe, a person wakes up frequently at night or suffers from night sweats.

This state of chronic stress may also involve sensations of pressure or pain on the left side of the chest, loss of sexual desire, nervous exhaustion, trembling, and burning sensations in the palms of the hands, the souls of the feet or over the heart area. The fire-weakened person has muddled thoughts, mental confusion, hypersensitive emotions and a loss of short-term memory. Frequently, the person suffering from this burnout has dark circles under their eyes and a quivering tongue.

Used For: Addictions (coffee, caffeine), addictions (drugs), addictions (sugar/carbohydrates), **adrenal fatigue**, anemia, **angina**, anorexia, anxiety disorders, chest pain, **cloudy thinking**, **concentration (poor)**, **confusion**, dehydration, depression, diabetes, **emotional sensitivity**, erectile dysfunction, **fatigue**, **fear**, **Graves' disease**, **heart weakness**, hot flashes, **hysteria**, **insomnia**, jet lag, memory/brain function, **mental illness**, **mood swings**, **nervous exhaustion**, **nervousness**, **night sweating**, **nightmares**, OCD, **perspiration (excessive)**, phobias, premature ejaculation, **PTSD**, **restless dreams**, **sex drive (low)**, **stress**, trauma, tremors, and urination (frequent)

Affects: **Adrenal depression**, brain, **central nervous system**, heart, hepatic stagnation, **nerve depression (exhaustion)**, **thyroid irritation**, and **weakened fire**

For those who are "burned-out" and need to strengthen the heart, nerves and glands take 3-4 capsules two or three times daily. It is also available in a TCM concentrate where the dose is 1 capsule two to three times daily. It can also be taken when a person wakes up at night and can't seem to go back to sleep.

Ingredients: Schisandra fruit, oriental arborvitae seed, broomrape stem, dodder seed, lycium fruit, ophiopogon, amber (succinum), hoelen sclerotium, sacred lotus seed, and asian ginseng root

Chinese Metal-Decreasing Formula

Xuan Fei

See also *Jeannie Burgess' Allergy-Lung Formula*

This Chinese formula reduces acute respiratory congestion. Its traditional name, Xuan Fei, means "ventilate the lungs," referring to its ability to open up the respiratory passages and get rid of mucus congestion. It dilates the bronchi, decongests and expels phlegm, and enhances immune activity.

Xuan Fei can be helpful for a wide variety of respiratory conditions. Emotionally, the formula can be helpful for grief, sadness and dogmatic, defensive people. It can also be helpful for a wide variety of problems not directly associated with the lungs, but related to lymphatic congestion.

Warnings: Pregnant or lactating women should consult their healthcare provider or a professional herbalist prior to taking because of the stimulants it contains.

Used For: Allergies (respiratory), **asthma**, breasts (swelling/tenderness), bronchitis, colds, **congestion (bronchial)**, congestion (lymphatic), **cough (damp)**, earache, edema, **grief & sadness**, headache (sinus), lymphoma, pneumonia, rhinitis, sinus infection, sore throat, and wheezing

Affects: Bronchi, lungs, respiratory constriction, **respiratory stagnation**, and **stressed metal**

For respiratory congestion take 1 capsule of the TCM concentrate every four hours. For an acute asthma attack, take 1 capsule every 15 minutes with two glasses of water until the attack subsides.

Ingredients: Typhonium rhizome, bamboo sap, bupleurum root, fritillary bulb, hoelen sclerotium, perilla leaf, platycodon root, apricot seed, and coltsfoot flowering tops

Chinese Metal-Increasing Formula

Fu Lei

This traditional Chinese formula enhances deficient metal energy. It enhances the function of the mucous membranes lining the lungs and the colon to improve immune response. It is useful for people who suffer from chronic infections of the lungs, dry cough, tightness in the chest, shortness of breath, and general weakness. It can also be helpful for chronic lung diseases.

The deficiency of metal energy can also be associated with deep-seated grief and sadness that can make a person aloof, cold and withdrawn. This formula can help to resolve this deep-seated grief. People who are unnaturally thin, suffer from weak muscles and energy loss or who are pale with flushed cheeks may also find this formula helpful.

Used For: **Addictions (tobacco)**, asthma, bronchitis, convalescence, **COPD**, **cough (dry)**, dizziness, **emphysema**, grief & sadness, infection prevention, muscle tone, overacidity, tuberculosis, underweight, and **wheezing**

Affects: Bronchi, **lungs**, **respiratory atrophy**, respiratory depression, and **weakened metal**

For respiratory weakness to take 3 capsules two to four times daily. It is also available in a TCM concentrate where the dose is 1 capsule two to four times daily.

Ingredients: Astragalus root, tartarian aster root, large-leaf gentian root, platycodon root, anemarrhena rhizome, tangerine (Mandarin) green fruit rind, tangerine (Mandarin) mature fruit rind, and typhonium rhizome

Chinese Qi and Blood Tonic Formula

Sheng Mai

The formula is for when the body seems overall run-down. It is a blood and qi tonic in Chinese medicine, which means it overcomes anemia and weakness. It strengthens immunity and resistance to negative environmental influences, including electromagnetic radiation. It corrects reversed polarity in muscle testing. It is an excellent formula to fortify the body when fighting cancer. It helps the body resist the harmful effects of chemotherapy and radiation.

Warnings: This formula is not for acute illnesses, high fever or severe inflammation.

Used For: **Anorexia**, **cancer**, cancer prevention, **cancer treatment side effects**, chills, **cold hands/feet**, **convalescence**, **debility**, dizziness, **electromagnetic pollution**, endurance, **Epstein-Barr virus**, **fatigue**, infection prevention, memory/brain function, **menstruation (scant)**, **perspiration (excessive)**, **radiation**, **reversed polarity**, underweight, and **wasting**

Affects: **Blood**, brain depression, central nervous system, **chi**, **chronic disease stage**, degenerative disease stage, **general atrophy**, low cortisol, and **thymus**

For recovery from long-term fatigue, illness and general weakness, use 3 capsules three times daily. It is also available as a TCM concentrate where the dose is 1 capsule instead of three.

Ingredients: Astragalus root, asian ginseng root, ganoderma mushroom, barrenwort leaf, eucommia bark, lycium fruit, rehmannia root tuber, achyranthes root, bai-zhu atractylodes rhizome, hoelen sclerotium, and ligustrum fruit

Chinese Qi-Increasing Formula

See also *Vandergriff's Energy Booster Formula*

This is an energy tonic that nourishes both blood and chi according to the principles of traditional Chinese medicine. Instead of providing a boost of instant energy followed by a crash, it gradually builds energy reserves in the body and aids the body's ability to adapt to stress. It helps increase metabolism and reduce appetite, which may be helpful for weight loss. It can be used to help wean off of caffeine, refined sugar and other stimulants. It also helps overcome anemia and supports a healthy immune system.

Warnings: Excessive or long term use could cause nervousness or insomnia. It is not a substitute for adequate sleep and rest.

Used For: Addictions (coffee, caffeine), addictions (drugs), addictions (sugar/carbohydrates), **appetite (excessive)**, debility, excess weight, exercise (performance), **fatigue**, and surgery (recovery)

Affects: **Chi**, chronic disease stage, and nerve depression (exhaustion)

As an energy tonic, take 1 capsule once or twice daily. For appetite reduction take 2 capsules in between breakfast and lunch.

Ingredients: Eleuthero root, cassia twig, Chinese peony root without bark, asian ginseng root, Chinese mint leaf, forsythia fruit, and gardenia fruit

Chinese Qi-Regulating Formula

Jie Yu

See also *Antidepressant Formula*

This formula is used to relieve sagging energy (qi or chi). It is helpful for sadness, depression, fatigue, insomnia and anxiety. Unlike modern Western approaches to depression which focus on the neurotransmitter serotonin, this traditional Chinese formula works in a holistic manner to relieve depression and sadness by balancing liver, digestive, intestinal and nervous functions. It is useful not only for depression, but for condigions involving lymphatic congestion and sluggishness of the liver.

Many people have been able to get off antidepressant drugs with this formula, taking the formula along with their medication, until they begin to feel better. They then gradually reduce the dose of their medication. Never discontinue antidepressant medications abruptly as this can cause major emotional imbalances, including the risk of violent behavior and suicide. Ideally, this process should be done under professional supervision over a period of many months.

Warnings: This is not a replacement for prescription medications. Consult a doctor before discontinuing antidepressants.

Used For: Anxiety (situational), backache, **bipolar mood disorder**, congestion (lymphatic), **depression**, dizziness, emotional sensitivity, fatigue, insomnia, menopause, mental illness, nervousness, **PMS Type D**, **postpartum depression**, **prolapsed colon**, **prolapsed uterus**, **reversed polarity**, and **seasonal affective disorder**

Affects: Brain, **brain depression**, chi, dopamine, liver, and weakened wood

For depression and nervous problems, recommended dose is 4 capsules twice daily. For digestive upset and liver problems use 2-3 capsules three times daily. The formula is also available as a TCM concentrate where 1 capsule replaces 4 capsules of the regular formula.

Ingredients: Perilla leaf, cyperus rhizome, typhonium rhizome, orange (bitter) young fruit, bamboo sap, bupleurum root, and hoelen

Chinese Water-Decreasing Formula

Qu Shi

See also *Diuretic Formula*

This traditional Chinese formula reduces excess water energy. It acts as a diuretic and it works with other body systems and processes that flush excess fluid from the tissues.

The emotional issues associated with excess water energy include fear and a "wishy-washy" personality. It can improve these emotional issues by redistributing and eliminating excess moisture.

Warnings: Avoid in conditions of dryness or fluid deficiency.

Used For: Backache, breasts (swelling/tenderness), congestion (lymphatic), dizziness, **edema**, fear, kidney stones, **PMS Type H**, **prostatitis**, urethritis, urinary tract infections, urination (burning/painful), and **urine (scant)**

Affects: Bladder, kidneys, lymphatics, spinal discs, **stressed water**, and **urinary stagnation**

To build the kidneys and eliminate excess moisture from the body take 4 capsules three times daily. A TCM concentrate is also available where 1 capsule replaces 4 capsules of the regular formula.

Ingredients: Hoelen sclerotium, siler root, flowering quince fruit, white mulberry root bark, astragalus root, asian plantain seed, and asian water plantain rhizome

Chinese Water-Increasing Formula

Jian Gui

This Chinese formula enhances water energy. It strengthens the organs associated with water in the body, the kidneys and bladder. It also aids muscular skeletal function which is connected with the water element and kidney qi in TCM. It helps the kidneys function more efficiently to remove acid waste, thus helping to keep the system alkaline. It can help with a variety of back, muscle, bone and joint problems.

Fear is the emotion associated with the kidneys, and this formula can also be helpful for a person who is fearful and timid and lacks backbone. It rejuvenates and strengthens the bones (especially the spine), kidneys, connective tissues, and sexual organs. This leads to a healthier urogenital system and more energy and sexual vitality.

Used For: Arthritis, **backache**, bladder infection, blood in urine, BPH, calcium deposits, dizziness, erectile dysfunction, **fear**, **gout**, **hair (graying)**, **incontinence**, infertility, **interstitial cystitis**, kidney infection, **kidney weakness/ failure**, **nocturnal emission**, **osteoporosis**, **overacidity**, overalkalinity, perspiration (excessive), **premature ejaculation**, **prostatitis**, **sciatica**, **scoliosis**, **spinal disks**, tinnitus, **uric acid retention**, **urination (frequent)**, and **weak knees**

Affects: Bladder, bones, hair, **kidneys**, prostate, **spinal discs**, **urinary atrophy**, and **weakened water**

To strengthen weak bones and kidneys take 3 capsules two or three times daily. It is also available as a TCM concentrate where the dose is 1 capsule two to three times daily.

Ingredients: Eucommia bark, broomrape stem, achyranthes root, sichuan teasel root, drynaria rhizome, hoelen sclerotium, and morinda root

Chinese Wind-Heat Evil Formula

Kang Weng

This formula was developed by Dr. Wenwei Xie of Beijing, China for use against the herpes simplex virus. Testing in the United States confirmed its effectiveness against the virus, but no useful drugs were found in any of the herbs and research was abandoned.

The formula is used for cold sores, canker sores and herpes infections. Its Chinese indications are weak chi (or vital energy) with external heat. Hence, it is useful for viral disorders in which the immune system is weak, but external heat (sores, fever, etc.) is present. Dr. Xie thought it might also benefit AIDS patients.

Used For: Adenitis, **AIDS**, **Bell's palsy**, **canker sores**, cervical dysplasia, **chicken pox**, **cold sores**, dizziness, **Epstein-Barr virus**, hepatitis, **herpes**, **infection (viral)**, **measles**, Ménière's disease, meningitis, **mononucleosis**, **Reye's syndrome**, **shingles**, thrush, **vaccine side effects**, and **warts**

Affects: Chi, **chronic disease stage**, and excess yang

Use 4 capsules two times a day for mild cases, 4 capsules three times daily for moderate cases and 4 capsules four times daily for severe cases.It is available as a TCM concentrate where 1 capsule replaces four of the regular formula. It is also available as a liquid, where the dose is 1/2 to 1 teaspoon.

Ingredients: Indigo (assam) leaf & root, dandelion root, purslane tops, thlaspi whole plant, bupleurum root, baical skullcap root, typhonium rhizome, and cinnamon twig

Chinese Wood-Decreasing Formula

Tiao He

See also *Detoxifying Formula* and *Liver Cleanse Formula*

The Chinese name for this formula, Tiao He, means "mediate harmony" because the wood element in Chinese medicine helps all the systems of the body work harmoniously together. Anytime a person has a lot of vague health problems where it's difficult to determine what the source of the problem is, this formula may be helpful. It will help to cleanse the liver, nourish the blood, improve digestive function and promote elimination.

This formula can also help temper feelings of excess anger and irritability. It is helpful for someone who loses their temper easily.

Used For: Age spots, **anger (excessive)**, chemical exposure, dysmenorrhea, dyspepsia, **estrogen dominance**, fat cravings, fat metabolism (poor), food allergies/intolerances, **gallbladder problems**, gallstones, **hangover**, **headache (migraine)**, hemochromatosis, **hepatitis**, **hypochondria**, hypoglycemia, **insomnia**, **irritability**, leaky gut, **mood swings**, **morning sickness**, nightmares, pap smear (abnormal), **PMS Type A**, preeclampsia, **rashes & hives**, skin problems, and **triglycerides (low)**

Affects: Blood, digestive atrophy, gallbladder, **hepatic irritation**, hepatic stagnation, **liver**, ovaries, and **stressed wood**

Use 4 capsules two times daily or 1 capsule one to two times daily of the TCM concentrate.

Ingredients: Bupleurum root, Chinese peony root, typhonium rhizome, cassia twig, dong quai root, hoelen sclerotium w/hostwood root, and scute root

Chinese Wood-Increasing Formula

Bu Xue

Bu Xue, the traditional Chinese name, means "build the blood." It helps increase blood volume and flow, combating anemia, scanty menstruation and fatigue. It is very helpful for pale, anemic women who experience heavy menstrual bleeding.

It also works to remove congested fat in the liver and lower cholesterol. It has an immune-balancing action, making it potentially useful in autoimmune disorders, particularly myasthenia gravis and systemic lupus erythematosus. It is also a good formula for people who have hypochondriac feelings or suppressed anger.

Warnings: Use with caution where colitis is present.

Used For: Alcoholism, **anemia**, appetite (excessive), cholesterol (high), cirrhosis of the liver, **cold hands/feet**, convalescence, depression, dizziness, dysmenorrhea, exercise (performance), fatigue, hepatitis, hypertension, **hypochondria**, hypoglycemia, itching, jaundice (adults), leukemia, lupus, **menorrhagia**, **menstrual irregularity**, mood swings, morning sickness, myasthenia gravis, nausea & vomiting, **PMS**, polyps, postpartum depression, and sickle cell anemia

Affects: **Blood**, brain depression, **hepatic atrophy**, **hepatic depression**, **liver**, sight, skin, and **weakened wood**

To build the liver and the blood take 3 capsules three times daily. The formula is also available as a TCM concentrate where the dose is 1 capsule twice daily.

Ingredients: Chinese peony root without bark, dong quai root, ganoderma mushroom fruiting body, lycium fruit, asiatic dogwood fruit without seeds, bupleurum root, Chinese salvia root & rhizome, ligustrum fruit, ligusticum rhizome, and rehmannia root

Chinese Yang-Reducing Formula

Qing Re

This Chinese formula reduces inflammation or evil heat. It does this by supporting mechanisms that help to detoxify the blood, fight infection, promote tissue healing and reduce the inflammation. Anytime you see swollen, red or painful tissue, it can be helpful. Also consider using it anytime you see someone with a bright red tongue and a rapid heart rate.

Warnings: Not for cold conditions. Thins the blood, should probably be avoided if taking blood thinners.

Used For: Arthritis, autoimmune disorders, blood poisoning, **burning feet/hands**, bursitis, chicken pox, chills, colds, **colds with fever**, dizziness, **earache**, **endometriosis**, **fever**, flu, gingivitis, Graves' disease, **Hashimoto's disease**, headache, **inflammation**, inflammatory bowel disorders, nephritis, pain, rashes & hives, **sore throat**, tachycardia, tinnitus, TMJ, and tonsillitis

Affects: Excess yang, general irritation, **gums**, intestinal irritation, and sight

Use 4 capsules of the regular formula two times daily or take 4 capsules every two hours for severe acute conditions. Taking 1 capsule of the concentrate is equivalent to 4 capsules of the regular formula.

Ingredients: Japanese honeysuckle flower bud, forsythia fruit, ligusticum rhizome, chrysanthemum flower, gardenia fruit, schizonepeta flower, scute root, phellodendron stem bark, and coptis rhizome

Chinese Yin-Increasing Formula

Bu Yin

This formula is indicated in conditions of excessive dryness coupled with thirst. The symptoms are dry skin, mouth, cough and eyes and burning sensations in the hands and feet. This is accompanied by constant thirst and frequent urination. These may be indications of metabolic syndrome or the early stages of diabetes.

In traditional Chinese philosophy yin is associated with moisture and coolness. This formula increases the ability of the cells to hydrate. It also helps balance blood sugar. It can ease constipation and tissue irritation (inflammation) caused by dehydration.

Used For: Addictions (sugar/carbohydrates), **burning feet/ hands**, constipation (adults), cough (dry), **dehydration**, hot flashes, **metabolic syndrome**, **night sweating**, numbness, PMS Type C, **skin (dry/flaky)**, tinnitus, and **urination (frequent)**

Affects: Adrenal medulla, deficient yin, **intestinal atrophy**, and pancreatic irritation

Use 3 capsules three times daily of the regular formula or 1 capsule once or twice daily for the TCM concentrate.

Ingredients: Eucommia bark, glehnia root, rehmannia root tuber, kudzu root, ophiopogon root tuber, trichosanthes root, achyranthes rhizome, and anemarrhena rhizome

Chirata   *Bitter Herb*

Swertia chirata

A member of the gentian family, known for it's bitter digestive herbs, chirata or chirayata is used to increase appetite, relieve acid indigestion and nausea and expel intestinal parasites. It is also helpful for respiratory congestion.

Energetics: Cooling and drying

Used For: Acid indigestion, asthma, bronchitis, cough (damp), debility, fever, nausea & vomiting, parasites (nematodes, worms), and ulcers

Properties: Alterative, anti-inflammatory, antibacterial, antifungal, antiviral, CNS depressant, febrifuge, hepatoprotective, hypoglycemic, laxative (gentle), sedative, and vermifuge

Chlorella   *Sweet Herb*

Chlorella sp.

Chlorella is a single-celled green algae that grows in fresh water. It has high contents of chlorophyll, vitamins and minerals and amino acids. A hot infusion has been shown to increase interferon production. Chlorella also stimulates the production of macrophages in the body that can reduce tumors.

Look for *chlorella* in *Algae Formula*

Energetics: Neutral, balancing, and nourishing

Used For: Cadmium toxicity, cancer prevention, convalescence, debility, **electromagnetic pollution**, heavy metal poisoning, hypoglycemia, mania, memory/brain function, and radiation

Chlorophyll   *Phytochemical*

Chlorophyll is the molecule that makes leaves green and captures the sun's energy during photosynthesis. Chlorophyll has an affinity for human blood, where it prevents the clumping of red blood cells and increases the oxygen-carrying capacity of the blood. It can help to detoxify the blood and accelerate wound healing by increasing oxygen uptake. It is also used for reducing colostomy odor, bad breath, and constipation. Chlorophyll also seems to nutritionally build the blood when taken regularly. Intravenously, chlorophyll is used for treating chronic relapsing pancreatitis.

Natural chlorophyll from green leafy vegetables is a good source of magnesium, a mineral many people are deficient in. Natural chlorophyll is sometimes sold in gel capsules and has a beneficial action on the bowel. Liquid chlorophyll is sodium copper chlorophyllin, which means that the magnesium at the center of the chlorophyll molecule has been displaced by copper and sodium. Copper and zinc are antagonists, so people with high levels of copper and low levels of zinc should not use liquid chlorophyll.

Chlorophyll contains components that are activated by light and can cause mild photosensitization when taken internally. Certain carotenoids such as beta-carotene and canthaxanthin seem to prevent or lessen the photosensitivity that results from taking chlorophyll.

Warnings: Sodium copper chlorophyllin contains copper. People low in zinc and high in copper should avoid it.

Usage: Add a small amount of liquid chlorophyll to water and drink, or follow the directions on the bottle.

Used For: Anemia, **body odor**, cancer, cancer prevention, cold sores, diaper rash, emphysema, fatigue, **foot odor**, free radical damage, gout, **halitosis**, heart fibrillation/palpitations, hemochromatosis, labor & delivery, nursing, **overacidity**, pain, pancreatitis, perspiration (excessive), **pet supplements**, poisoning, postpartum weakness, preeclampsia, pregnancy, Raynaud's disease, rosacea, sickle cell anemia, spider veins, and spinal disks

Properties: Alkalinizer, anticoagulant, antiemetic, antimutagenic, blood building, carminative, and **deodorant**

Cholesterol-Regulating Formula

These formula contains a number of supplements that have some clinical evidence that they can reduce cholesterol levels. They may also help liver and gallbladder function and aid in peripheral circulation.

Used For: Cardiovascular disease, **cholesterol (high)**, circulation (poor), gallbladder problems, gallstones, and **triglycerides (high)**

Affects: Arteries and heart

Take 1 capsule three times daily.

Ingredients: Phytosterols, resveratrol, and artichoke leaf

Choline
Nutrient

Choline was only acknowledged as a required nutrient by the Institute of Medicine in 1998. Your body makes some, but you need to get it from your diet. It's not a vitamin, but is often included with vitamin supplements, especially vitamin B supplements. Choline is important for liver function, muscles, nerves and metabolism.

It plays a role along with folate in converting homocysteine to methionine. Elevated levels of homocysteine a sign of poor methylation and are linked to an increased risk of heart disease.

Choline is required to produce acetylcholine, the neurotransmitter involved in memory and muscle movement.

Used For: Cardiovascular disease, **fatty liver disease**, memory/ brain function, and **methylation (under)**

Properties: Nutritive

Chondroitin
Nutrient

Chondroitin is a long chain of repeating sugars found naturally in the joints and connective tissues of healthy people and animals. Chondroitin is available from animal sources such as the gristle near the joints, but is not often consumed. This sulfate is important to healthy joints and when taken as a supplement, studies show that it may treat the inflammation and pain of osteoarthritis. Chondroitin helps produce both new cartilage and enhances synovial fluid viscosity. It interferes with enzymes that destroy cartilage molecules as well as those that prevent nutrients from reaching the cartilage. These actions are especially important to those with osteoarthritis who are often suffering because their cartilage is unable to rebuild or protect itself.

Chondroitin is also beneficial to those with psoriasis and inflammatory bowel disorders. It is found naturally in bone broths, a staple of many cultures and a super food in its own right. The improvements in joint function from chondroitin are not permanent, so continued supplementation is warranted for those who see results.

Usage: 1,200–2,000 mg taken once daily.

Used For: **Arthritis**, inflammatory bowel disorders, and prostatitis

Properties: Antiarthritic

Chrisopher's Menopause Formula

See also *Female Tonic Formula* and *Menopause Support*

Created by the famous herbalist John Christopher, the herbal formula helps to balance female hormones, especially during menopause. It may also help other female issues.

Warnings: Avoid during pregnancy or lactation.

Used For: Estrogen (low), hot flashes, infertility, **menopause**, mood swings, osteoporosis, progesterone (low), sex drive (low), and vaginal dryness

Affects: Ovaries

Work up gradually to about 2 capsules three times daily.

Ingredients: Dong quai root, blessed thistle aerial parts, sarsaparilla root extract, black cohosh root & rhizome extract, partridge berry whole plant, and false unicorn root

Christopher's Carminative Formula

See also *Chinese Earth-Decreasing Formula*

This a Western formula is for indigestion, gas, belching, bloating and other acute digestive disturbances. It supplements digestive enzymes with papaya and contains carminatives and antispasmodics to expel gas and relieve intestinal cramping.

Used For: Acid indigestion, anorexia, appetite (deficient), **belching**, digestion (poor), dyspepsia, **gas & bloating**, halitosis, indigestion, lactose intolerance, and morning sickness

Affects: Digestive depression, pancreas head, **stomach**, and stressed earth

Use 2 capsules after meals as a digestive aid or 2-4 capsules as needed to relieve gas, bloating and indigestion.

Ingredients: Papaya fruit concentrate, ginger rhizome, peppermint leaf, fennel seed, and spearmint leaf & flower

Christopher's Gallbladder Formula

This is a Western formula for the gallbladder and gastrointestinal system. It stimulates bile flow and digestive secretions. It also contains antispasmodics to relax cramping in the digestive system.

Used For: Cholesterol (high), constipation (adults), fat cravings, fat metabolism (poor), **gallbladder problems**, gallstones, indigestion, and jaundice (adults)

Affects: Digestive irritation, **gallbladder**, hepatic constriction, and hepatic stagnation

Use 2 capsules with meals as an aid to liver congestion, jaundice, sluggish gall bladder production or frequent bloating or stuffiness in the abdomen.

Ingredients: Oregon grape root & rhizome, cramp bark bark, fennel seed, and wild yam root

Christopher's Herbal Iron Formula

This formula contains herbs that are rich in iron and iron cofactors. While it contains only a fraction of the iron found in traditional iron supplements, it is better at building up iron levels in the blood because it contains whole foods and herbs that contain synergistic ingredients to rebuild iron levels. This is important because iron is especially difficult to absorb from isolated iron supplements.

Used For: Anemia, fatigue, **hemochromatosis**, **menorrhagia**, pernicious anemia, postpartum weakness, **pregnancy**, **sickle cell anemia**, and surgery (preparation)

Affects: Blood and liver

Take 2 capsules three times daily with meals. It works better when taken 1 capsule of yellow dock twice daily.

Ingredients: Beet root, yellow dock root, burdock root, nettle, and stinging leaf

Christopher's Nervine Formula

See also *Jeannie Burgess' Stress Formula*

Use this formula to aid in relaxation, reduce stress and inflammation. It is a natural sedative and has mild pain-reducing qualities.

Used For: Alcoholism, headache (tension), pain, and stress

Affects: Central nervous system

Take 2 capsules two to three times daily with meals for nervous stress and other nervous disorders.

Ingredients: Black cohosh root, valerian root, passion flower aerial parts, hops flower, and wood betony aerial parts

Christopher's Sinus Formula

See also *Sinus Formula*

Use this formula to dry up excessive sinus flow, improve digestion and expel excess phlegm. It helps to detoxify the body to remove the underlying causes of sinus problems.

Used For: Allergies (respiratory), **congestion (sinus)**, rhinitis, **sinus infection**, and wheezing

Affects: Mucous membranes, respiratory stagnation, and **sinuses**

Use 2 capsules three to four times daily. It works better if you also take 1-2 capsules of the Sinus Blend with it.

Ingredients: Burdock root, goldenseal root & rhizome, horehound leaf & flower, and orange (bitter) fruit extract

Chromium *Mineral*

Chromium is a trace mineral that helps to improve sensitivity to insulin. Adequate intake is essential for maintenance of normal blood sugar levels. Not only does it help with type 2 diabetes, it also helps type 1 diabetics improve the action of insulin. It is indicated for people with pre-diabetes and women with Poly Cystic Ovarian Syndrome (PCOS). A couple of small studies have shown that chromium is helpful for people with hypoglycemia.

Usage: Take about 500 to 1,000 mcg with a meal (preferably lunch).

Used For: Addictions (sugar/carbohydrates), alcoholism, anger (excessive), arteriosclerosis, bedwetting, cardiovascular disease, confusion, **diabetes**, erectile dysfunction, hypertension, hypoglycemia, mental illness, **metabolic syndrome**, narcolepsy, **PMS Type C**, and psoriasis

Properties: Antidiabetic, hypolipidemic, and immune modulator

Chrysanthemum *Bitter & Sweet Herb*

Chrysanthemum spp.

Used primarily as an ornamental plant in the West, chrysanthemum is a popular medicinal herb in China. Besides being consumed as a beverage, it is used to soothe irritated eyes, reduce fevers and lower high blood pressure.

Look for *chrysanthemum* in *Chinese Yang-Reducing Formula*

Energetics: Cooling, relaxing, and mildly drying

Used For: Colds with fever, conjunctivitis, dizziness, eyes (red/itching), headache, and infection (viral)

Properties: Anti-inflammatory, antibacterial, antiviral, detoxifying, and hypotensive

Cilantro/Coriander *Aromatic Herb*

Coriandrum sativum

A widely popular culinary herb, cilantro is used by herbalists to detoxify the body and help remove heavy metals. The research on its ability to bind heavy metals is mixed, but it may be helpful, especially when combined with other herbs and nutrients. Coriander seeds come from the cilantro plant and are used as a carminative and digestive aid.

Look for *cilantro/coriander* in *Heavy Metal Cleansing Formula*

Energetics: Cooling and drying

Used For: Gas & bloating, heavy metal poisoning, **mercury poisoning**, and multiple sclerosis

Properties: Carminative, condiment, and food

Cinnamon (Cassia)

Astringent & Pungent Herb

Cinnamomum spp.

A spicy aromatic herb used in Chinese herbalism as a warming stimulant, cinnamon is useful as a digestive and circulatory stimulant. Modern research has shown that cinnamon can help to reduce blood sugar levels. Cinnamon also has astringent properties and can help control heavy menstrual flows and postpartum bleeding.

Look for *cinnamon* in *Analgesic EO, Blood Sugar Control, CBD Brain, Chinese Qi-Increasing, Chinese Wood-Decreasing,* and *Sugar Craving Reducer Formulas*

Warnings: Taking over two grams of cinnamon bark a day can cause gastrointestinal irritation. Avoid during pregnancy, except as a seasoning. Avoid spices like cinnamon while breast feeding.

Energetics: Warming, drying, and constricting

Used For: Alzheimer's, anorexia, **bleeding (external)**, **bleeding (internal)**, bronchitis, chills, circulation (poor), colds, **diabetes**, **diarrhea**, **dysbiosis**, fatigue, flu, gas & bloating, hypoglycemia, **menorrhagia**, **metabolic syndrome**, nausea & vomiting, polycystic ovarian syndrome, SIBO, and testosterone (low)

Properties: Analgesic, **antidiabetic**, antiseptic, antithrombotic, **astringent**, carminative, condiment, hemostatic, and **stimulant (metabolic)**

Cinnamon EO   *Spicy Essential Oil*

Cinnamomun aromaticum

A spicy, pungent oil that is very warming and stimulating, cinnamon is helpful for people who feel devitalized and weak. They may be suffering from depression due to extreme fatigue. It helps awaken the fire in a person, motivating them to get up and start doing something about their life. It can also help to arouse passion and sensuality in men.

Cinnamon essential oil is very warming. It stimulates digestion and circulation. It is helpful for easing digestive upset such as colitis, diarrhea, nausea and vomiting. The smell has a testosterone-enhancing action, which makes it useful for inhaling to stimulate contractions during childbirth or increase sexual desire in men and women. It is also antiseptic and antiparasitic, so it can be used topically to destroy harmful organisms. It has a calming effect on the nerves, but helps improve energy while overcoming feelings of depression and anxiety. Apply diluted oil topically or smell.

See the strategy *Aromatherapy* for suggested uses.

Warnings: Do not use internally without the supervision of a professionally trained aromatherapy practitioner. It must be highly diluted to avoid irritating skin or mucous membranes. Dilute to greater than 100:1.

Used For: Anorexia, antibiotic resistance, chills, circulation (poor), colds (antiviral), colitis, congestion, **dental health**, depression, diarrhea, erectile dysfunction, fatigue, flu, gingivitis, infection (bacterial), lice, metabolic syndrome, nausea & vomiting, parasites, sex drive (low), shock (medical), testosterone (low), typhoid, and warts

Properties: Antimicrobial, antiparasitic, **antiseptic**, aphrodisiac, cardiac, carminative, emmenagogue, glandular, hemostatic, insecticide, parturient, preservative, stimulant (metabolic), stomachic, and vermifuge

Circulatory Formula

These formulas are typically used for high blood pressure. The parsley helps counteract some of the garlic odor and it acts as a mild diuretic to stimulate kidney function. They can also be used for general circulatory disorders, including cold hands and feet, arteriosclerosis and cholesterol problems. They can also be used for fighting acute viral infections.

Warnings: Capsicum and garlic may cause some digestive upset. Do not use where gastric ulcers are present.

Used For: Arteriosclerosis, chills, **circulation (poor)**, cold hands/feet, **hypertension**, hypotension, and infection (viral)

Affects: Arteries, **circulatory depression**, general depression, and heart

Circulatory Stimulant Formula

Use 1–2 capsules three to four times daily for circulatory problems. For infection use 2–4 capsules every two to four hours with plenty of water.

Ingredients: Capsicum fruit, garlic bulb, and parsley leaf

Christopher's Circulatory Formula

Use 1–2 capsules three times daily.

Ingredients: Garlic bulb, capsicum fruit, parsley leaf, and ginger rhizome

Clary Sage EO

Herbaceous, Musky, & Sharp Essential Oil

Salvia sclarea

Clary sage EO is a floral and herbaceous oil that has a euphoric or uplifting effect. It is balancing to the nerves, so it helps both anxiety and depression. And while it has an energizing and uplifting effect, it also helps people stay grounded. It calms the mind reducing tension and stress while helping to overcome fatigue and increase energy. It also enhances estrogen in women, so it can be helpful for women who are suffering from depression due to low estrogen.

Clary sage helps with uterine problems such as PMS, regulating scanty periods and easing cramps in the lower back area. It encourages labor by helping the mother to relax and also eases postnatal depression. It promotes estrogen secretion by acting with the pituitary. It inhibits prolactin, so it tends to dry up breast milk. Clary sage can be used for asthma to relax spasms of the bronchial tubes and ease emotional tension found in asthma sufferers. Its effects on the central nervous system make it a good choice for impotency, mid-life crisis, frigidity, and as an aphrodisiac. It can be used topically to reduce excessive sebum production in oily hair and skin.

Emotionally, it regenerates energy and inspires both mind and spirit. It is used for nervousness, weakness, fear, paranoia and depression. It brings a long-lasting inner tranquility and helps to remedy melancholy. It diverts one from negative thoughts and helps guide energies.

See the strategy *Aromatherapy* for suggested uses.

Warnings: Do not use internally without the supervision of a professionally trained aromatherapy practitioner. Nontoxic and nonirritating for topical use. Avoid during pregnancy. Contraindicated in states of high anxiety. Women with breast cysts, uterine fibroids and estrogen-dependent cancers should probably avoid this oil as it contains a rare ketone compound called sclareol that mimics estrogen. Large amounts can be stupefying, especially when combined with alcohol or hypnotic drugs.

Used For: Alzheimer's, amenorrhea, anxiety (situational), bipolar mood disorder, breast milk (surplus), breasts (undersized), bronchitis, cholesterol (high), convalescence, **cramps (menstrual)**, cramps & spasms, digestion (poor), dysmenorrhea, eczema, **estrogen (low)**, gas & bloating, hot flashes, irritability, mania, menopause, menstrual irregularity, menstruation (scant), nervous exhaustion, night sweating, PMS Type D, sex drive (low), shame & guilt, skin (infections), sore throat, stress, and wounds & sores

Properties: Antibacterial, antidepressant, antigalactagogue, antiseptic, antispasmodic, antiviral, aphrodisiac, deodorant, emmenagogue, estrogenic, hypotensive, nervine, parturient, sedative, and tonic

Clay, Bentonite   *Non-Nutrient*

A natural clay from volcanic ash suspended in water. When taken internally, the clay attracts irritating substances and binds them for removal from the body. It can help remove viruses, mold, pesticides, herbicides and heavy met-

als from the body. It can absorb some heavy metals and may help shrink diverticula.

Usage: As an aid to colon cleansing use 1 tablespoon with a glass of water one or two times daily. Use one-half of a bottle of liquid bentonite in a bath to help with rashes, psoriasis, eczema, and to detoxify the skin.

Used For: Acne, chicken pox, diarrhea, diverticulitis, food allergies/intolerances, food poisoning, heavy metal poisoning, itching, lead poisoning, mercury poisoning, and **rashes & hives**

Properties: Adsorbent, antidiarrheal, antitoxic, and detoxifying

Clay, Redmond   *Non-Nutrient*

A fine clay, like this clay from Redmond, Utah, can be used for drawing baths, poultices or other topical applications for a wide variety of conditions. It pulls both toxins and excess oil out of the skin. See the *Drawing Bath* and *Poultice* strategies for information on how to use it.

Usage: Use one cup in a bath. Mix with water to form a paste to apply topically as a poultice.

Used For: Acne, chicken pox, **heavy metal poisoning**, **itching**, measles, **mercury poisoning**, rashes & hives, and **skin (oily)**

Properties: Adsorbent, antitoxic, drawing, and soothing

Cleavers (Bedstraw)   *Salty Herb*

Galium aparine

Cleavers, also known as bedstraw, are used to promote urination and stimulate the lymphatic system. They are a gentle kidney and lymphatic remedy, suitable for children. They have also been used externally as a poultice for cancerous growths, inflammation and as a decoction for sunburn and freckles.

Look for *cleavers* in *Liquid Lymph* and *Lymph Cleansing Formulas*

Energetics: Cooling and drying

Used For: Adenitis, bladder (irritable), breasts (swelling/tenderness), congestion, congestion (lymphatic), edema, interstitial cystitis, kidney weakness/failure, leukemia, **nephritis**, **swollen lymph glands**, and urine (scant)

Properties: Diuretic, kidney tonic, and lymphatic

Clove   *Pungent Herb*

Eugenia carophyllata

A spicy aromatic often used in combination with other herbs, cloves are valuable in liniments, gargles and digestive formulas. Powdered cloves have been used to expel parasites. It also helps with colds and other viral diseases.

Look for *clove* in *Analgesic EO, Antiparasitic, H. Pylori-Fighting,* and *Herbal Composition Formulas*

Warnings: Clove can be irritating in large quantities. Clove oil should not be used internally without professional supervision. Use with caution during pregnancy.

Energetics: Warming and drying

Used For: Bronchitis, colds, denture sores, diarrhea, gas & bloating, gingivitis, indigestion, mumps, nausea & vomiting, parasites, and toothache

Properties: Analgesic, anesthetic, antiseptic, carminative, condiment, counterirritant, stimulant (circulatory), and **vermifuge**

Clove EO   *Sweet & Woody Essential Oil*

Eugenia carophyllata

The strong, pungent, slightly woody and sweet odor of clove EO is highly stimulating to the nervous system, although topically it numbs the nerves. It is a very invigorating fragrance, promoting a strong, self-assured and energetic state of being. It helps people to stand up for themselves, breaking people from patterns of tolerating abuse.

Clove essential oil is an excellent antiseptic because of its high eugenol content. It is useful in the prevention of viral diseases. It is an antiparasitic, helps to stimulate digestion, restores appetite and relieves flatulence. It has a mild anesthetic effect and is commonly used for toothaches. It triggers the release of anti-inflammatory substances and inhibits the prostaglandins type 2 which are well-known mediators of inflammatory processes. It can be diluted with a fixed oil and applied topically for pain. It is used by dentists to numb the gums prior to giving shots.

Emotionally it lifts depression and is useful when feeling weak and lethargic. It has a positive, stimulating effect on the mind. Although traditionally used for teething infants, it's better to use chamomile, as clove can be too irritating. You can also mix clove with carrier oil and apply topically over the abdominal area to help make a parasite cleanse more effective.

See the strategy *Aromatherapy* for suggested uses.

Warnings: Do not use internally without the supervision of a professionally trained aromatherapy practitioner. Do not use unless highly diluted (100:1) as it can be highly irritating to skin and mucus membranes.

Used For: Addictions (tobacco), arthritis (rheumatoid), belching, bronchitis, cervical dysplasia, colds (decongestant), corns, cough (damp), denture sores, diarrhea, digestion (poor), gas & bloating, **gingivitis**, halitosis, hernias, hiccups, hypotension, indigestion, infection (fungal), insect repellant, labor & delivery, laryngitis, leucorrhea, memory/brain function, mumps, nausea & vomiting, pain, pap smear (abnormal), parasites, sex drive (low), skin (infections), teething, **toothache**, warts, and wounds & sores

Properties: Analgesic, anesthetic, anti-inflammatory, antibacterial, anticancer, antiepileptic, antifungal, antimicrobial, antioxidant, antiparasitic, antiseptic, antispasmodic, antiviral, aphrodisiac, carminative, disinfectant, expectorant, stimulant (metabolic), stomachic, and vermifuge

Co-Q10   *Nutrient*

Co-Q10 stands for co-enzyme Q10. It assists the mitochondria, our sub-cellular power plants, in producing energy by facilitating the production of ATP, the basic energy molecule in the cell. By helping our cells to produce energy, Co-Q10 also helps them to live longer, be healthier and to reproduce properly.

Most of the research on Co-Q10 has focused on the heart, because of how hard the heart works and its high energy requirements. Co-Q10 has been found to strengthen the heart in people who have suffered heart disease and to protect it from further damage. Other studies have documented its ability to raise or lower blood pressure. Co-Q10 also has antioxidant functions.

Although Co-Q10 is found in many foods, the levels in our bodies tend decline with age. Furthermore, statin drugs deplete Co-Q10. This includes the natural alternative to statins, red yeast rice. The beta blockers propranolol and metoprolol, phenothiazines, and tricyclic antidepressants also lower Co-Q10 levels. Anyone these drugs or supplements should also take Co-Q10.

Besides helping the heart and circulation, Co-Q10 can help heal bleeding gums, potentially reduce the side effects of chemotherapy, and reduce allergic reactions. In a well-designed study conducted in 2003, Co-Q10 supplementation reduced the need for dialysis and significantly improved creatine clearance and kidney function in those with renal failure.

Usage: 60–300 mg daily.

Used For: Adrenal fatigue, aging, AIDS, allergies (respiratory), Alzheimer's, **angina, arteriosclerosis,** asthma, autism, cancer, cancer treatment side effects, cardiac arrest, cardiovascular disease, cholesterol (high), **congestive heart failure,** convalescence, debility, diabetes, down syndrome, emphysema, fatigue, food allergies/intolerances, free radical damage, **gingivitis,** glaucoma, Graves' disease, hair loss/thinning, Hashimoto's disease, **headache (migraine),** heart fibrillation/palpitations, **heart weakness,** Huntington's disease, **hypertension,** incontinence, inflammation, jet lag, kidney weakness/failure, **mitochondrial dysfunction,**

mitral valve, muscle tone, muscular dystrophy, narcolepsy, neurodegenerative diseases, Parkinson's disease, pet supplements, **Peyronie's disease**, Raynaud's disease, rheumatic fever, **sleep apnea**, snoring, **spider veins**, teeth (loose), and wrinkles

Properties: Anti-inflammatory, antiaging, antiallergenic, **antioxidant**, **cardiac**, **hypotensive**, and tonic

Cocoa
Bitter & Oily Herb

Theobroma cacao

Everyone is familiar with cocoa or chocolate, but few people are aware that it has a long tradition as a medicinal plant. The Latin name, *Theobroma*, means "food of the gods," which is how the ancient Aztecs viewed chocolate. When it was first introduced to Europeans, it was viewed as a tonic, restorative, and virtual cure-all.

Modern research shows cocoa has many positive health benefits. For starters, it is one of the strongest antioxidant foods. It also has a number of feel good chemicals, which is why many people get cravings for it. One of these is phenylethylamine which affects neurotransmitters like dopamine, oxytocin and endorphins, and produces a feeling similar to falling in love. This is probably why chocolates are such a popular present for Valentine's Day.

Because of its mild oxytocic effect a midwife friend of mine used to keep chocolate bars in her medical kit. If the placenta failed to deliver, she would have the woman eat the chocolate and it would stimulate the uterine contractions that delivered the placenta.

Another compound in chocolate is anandamide, which is an endogenous cannabinoid. Anandamide plays a role in the regulation of appetite, pleasure, pain regulation, sleep and numerous other body processes.

Chocolate contains a modest amount of caffeine, but most of its stimulating effect comes from theobromine. Theobromine produces a milder, more gentle stimulant effect that is also longer lasting. It also acts as a mild antidepressant, which is another reason people self-medicate with chocolate when they feel down. Furthermore, unlike coffee which tends to elevate blood pressure and produce insomnia, cocoa helps to lower blood sugar and can actually aid sleep.

Cocoa is also quite nutritious. It has a healthy fat called cocoa butter, which can be applied topically for stretch marks and makes a good addition to lotions and salves. It also has significant amounts of magnesium, potassium, zinc, and manganese. A three-ounce piece of dark chocolate supplies about 58 percent of the RDA for magnesium, which may be why some women crave it when they're experiencing PMS, as magnesium deficiency is common in PMS. A three-ounce piece of chocolate also provides 100 percent of the RDA for manganese, which appears to play a critical role in women's reproductive health.

The biggest problem with chocolate is the large amount of sugar added to it, so for medicinal uses stick to dark chocolate (70 percent cocoa or more) or cocoa powder. Cocoa is an underutilized herb in herbal formulas, too, and could be used as a medicinal ingredient for many purposes, not just a flavoring agent.

Used For: Addictions (coffee, caffeine), afterbirth pain, cardiovascular disease, debility, depression, fatigue, free radical damage, insomnia, **nervous exhaustion**, **PMS Type C**, PMS Type D, **sex drive (low)**, **stretch marks**, and **wasting**

Properties: Antidepressant, **antioxidant**, aphrodisiac, food, hypertensive, oxytocic, and **stimulant (metabolic)**

Coconut
Oily Herb

Cocos nucifera

Coconut oil is a very helpful supplement for the nervous system. It contains medium chain saturated fats that aid the heart, brain and immune system. Many people have found that taking coconut oil daily has helped with neurodegenerative diseases such as Alzheimer's disease. It can also help to boost the thyroid and aid weight loss. The caprylic acid in coconut oil helps fight yeast infections and improve the intestinal microbiome. Coconut oil is also a good carrier oil to use to apply essential oils topically for dry or irritated skin or to take essential oils internally. Add one or two drops of the essential oil to a tablespoon of melted coconut oil.

Usage: Take 1–3 tablespoons one to three times daily.

Energetics: Cooling, moistening, and nourishing

Used For: **Alzheimer's**, dementia, dysbiosis, **epilepsy**, excess weight, hypothyroidism, infection (fungal), **metabolic syndrome**, multiple sclerosis, **neurodegenerative diseases**, Parkinson's disease, seizures, **seizures**, **skin (dry/flaky)**, and stretch marks

Properties: Antiepileptic, antifungal, **emollient**, food, immune modulator, and low glycemic

Codonopsis
Sweet Herb

Codonopsis pilosula

Used as an expectorant and a tonic, codonopsis increases vital energy. It can replace ginseng as a milder and safer general tonic for both men and women. It dilates peripheral blood vessels and inhibits adrenal cortex activity (to lower cortisol), thereby lowering blood pressure and improving immune function. Used in Fu Zheng therapies to prevent side effects from chemotherapy or radiation, it also increases hemoglobin levels and red blood cells, stimulates appetite and strengthens the immune system.

Look for *codonopsis* in *Adaptogen-Immune Formula*

Energetics: Moistening, nourishing, and mildly warming

Used For: Addison's disease, appetite (deficient), autism, **auto-immune disorders**, cancer, cancer treatment side effects, **convalescence**, diarrhea, **fatigue**, multiple sclerosis, and **radiation**

Properties: Adaptogen, lung tonic, and **tonic**

Coffee   *Stimulant Bitter Herb*

Coffea spp.

Coffee is widely used as a stimulant to reduce drowsiness and aid energy. Coffee contains xanthones and acts as an antioxidant. It has been used for relieving migraine headaches. Coffee enemas have been used for detoxification of the liver.

Green (unroasted) coffee beans have become popular as a supplement for weight loss. They contain higher amounts of chlorogenic acid which has a blood sugar reducing effect and is antibacterial.

Look for *coffee* in *Metabolic Stimulant Formula*

Warnings: Overuse of coffee can contribute to high blood pressure, anxiety, insomnia, and other health issues. Generally speaking it's not wise for most people to drink more than one, or perhaps two, cups a day.

Used For: Appetite (excessive), edema, excess weight, fatigue, headache (migraine), and heart weakness

Properties: Antioxidant, digestant, **stimulant (metabolic)**, and sympathomimetic

Cold Lozenges Formula

Suck on these lozenges to aid recovery from colds and irritated throats. They can also be used as a zinc supplement.

Used For: Colds, **laryngitis**, and **sore throat**

Affects: Acute disease stage

Take 1 lozenge each hour or as needed. Allow lozenge to dissolve slowly in the mouth. Do not use more than 6 lozenges in a 24-hour period.

Ingredients: Vitamin C and zinc

Coleus   *Aromatic & Bitter Herb*

Coleus forskohlii

Coleus is used in India for digestive problems, but research showing it increases cAMP levels, which results in an increase in energy production throughout the body, has led to its use in a variety of cardiac problems. It is used for congestive heart failure, poor coronary blood flow and glaucoma (topical use). When used with hawthorn it can help reduce high blood pressure. Coleus's basic cardiovascular action is to lower blood pressure while simultaneously increasing the contractility of the heart.

Look for *coleus* in *Blood Pressure Reducing* and *Hypothyroid Formulas*

Warnings: Don't take if you have hyperthyroidism or low blood pressure. May interact with cardiac medications.

Energetics: Cooling

Used For: Asthma, bronchitis, congestive heart failure, gas & bloating, glaucoma, **hypertension**, hypothyroidism, and insomnia

Properties: Anti-inflammatory, antispasmodic, cardiac, carminative, and hypotensive

Collagen   *Nutrient*

Collagen is used to build cartilage, tendons, heart muscle tissue, skin and lean muscle mass. It can be used for weight loss or for helping to repair damaged tissues. It also helps the skin to be healthier.

Usage: For joint support and general health take about 15–20 grams with a meal one to three times a day. For weight management, take it on an empty stomach with a glass of water just before bedtime.

Used For: Abrasions/scratches, AIDS, **arthritis**, arthritis (rheumatoid), backache, **bedwetting**, **body building**, broken bones, **cartilage damage**, **excess weight**, fingernails (weak/brittle), **injuries**, **leaky gut**, **ligaments (torn/injuried)**, pet supplements, skin problems, spinal disks, weak knees, and **wrinkles**

Properties: Nutritive and vulnerary

Collinsonia   *Mildly Bitter & Sour Herb*

Collinsonia canadensis

Collinsonia is an excellent astringent for rectal problems such as anal fistulae and hemorrhoids. It can be taken orally and applied topically. It is also useful for sore throats and laryngitis, being a specific remedy for speakers and singers who develop throat irritation. It can also be used on skin for poison oak and ivy and as a topical application for injuries.

Energetics: Cooling and constricting

Used For: Anal fistula/fissure, **BPH**, **hemorrhoids**, injuries, **laryngitis**, poison ivy/oak, and sore throat

Properties: Astringent and vascular tonic

Colloidal Mineral Formula

Minerals play critical roles in every part of our body, but they are especially needed for healthy bones, teeth and other structural systems of the body. Minerals are also catalysts for all biochemical processes and enzyme systems. Colloidal minerals are derived from mineral rich deposits from ancient sea beds. Mineral rich water from springs that come from these beds have long been sought out as places of healing. Since most people don't get enough trace minerals in their diet due to refined and processed foods and poor agricultural practices, many people find that using a colloidal mineral formula increases their over-all health.

Used For: ALS, amenorrhea, anorexia, appetite (excessive), **arthritis**, **bipolar mood disorder**, birth defect prevention, **broken bones**, convalescence, cystic fibrosis, debility, **dental health**, diarrhea, eczema, endurance, exercise (recovery), **fingernail biting**, **fingernails (weak/brittle)**, gingivitis, **hair (graying)**, hair loss/thinning, hearing loss, **infertility**, injuries, menorrhagia, mental illness, multiple sclerosis, myasthenia gravis, oral surgery, osteoporosis, **overacidity**, pet supplements, postpartum weakness, **pregnancy**, puberty, restless leg, scoliosis, spinal disks, **stress**, strokes, **surgery (preparation)**, surgery (recovery), tachycardia, teeth (loose), weak knees, and wrinkles

Affects: Bones, **general relaxation**, muscles, **structural atrophy**, structural relaxation, and **teeth**

Chinese Mineral Qi Adaptogen Formula

Provides colloidal minerals in a base of Chinese herbs that help to balance the entire body (all five of the Chinese elements). Has adaptogenic properties and supplies extra potassium. Take 1 ounce one or two times daily. Mixing with juice will help disguise the taste.

Ingredients: Potassium, trace minerals, lycium fruit, schisandra fruit extract, gynostemma plant extract, licorice root extract, reishi mushroom, astragalus root extract, eleuthero root, and ginkgo leaf

Colloidal Minerals

Basic colloidal mineral supplement. Take 1 tablespoon twice daily with meals.

Ingredients: Trace minerals

Colostrum   *Nutrient*

When a baby is born, the first milk produced by the mammary glands is called colostrum. It contains immune-boosting factors that help build the infant's resistance to disease. Colostrum is made from bovine colostrum and is used to help balance the immune system. It helps to normalize the gut flora and heal leaky gut, a root cause of many ailments. Because it doesn't over stimulate the immune system, it is very suitable for autoimmune disorders.

Colostrum contains naturally occurring IGF-1, which stimulates cell growth and repair. It contains dipeptides that stimulate the production of glutathione an important intracellular antioxidant. It helps lower blood pressure and prevent blood clots. It contains leptin, which helps reduce appetite.

It is very essential to get high quality colostrum. True colostrum comes from the first twelve hours after birth. Many manufacturers use milk that is taken between twenty-four to seventy-two hours after birth, which contains some colostrum, but is not as potent. They may also skim the fat off the colostrum, which reduces its potency.

Usage: Take 1500 milligrams twice daily.

Used For: Allergies (respiratory), Alzheimer's, antibiotic side effects, **autoimmune disorders**, **cancer**, debility, dysbiosis, excess weight, exercise (performance), fibromyalgia, food allergies/intolerances, hypertension, interstitial cystitis, **leaky gut**, lupus, and thrombosis

Properties: Antiaging, hypotensive, and immune modulator

Colostrum-Immune Stimulator Formula

Use whenever the immune system needs to be stimulated to fight infection or for helping with natural cancer therapy.

Warnings: Contraindicated with autoimmune disorders.

Used For: Allergies (respiratory), cancer, convalescence, infection prevention, and shingles

Take 1 capsule three times daily, preferably on an empty stomach with a large glass of water.

Ingredients: Colostrum, astragalus root, maitake, and shitake

Coltsfoot   *Stimulant Bitter & Sweet Herb*

Tussilago farfara

Coltsfoot is a great remedy for debilitated individuals with chronic respiratory conditions. It is indicated for asthma and emphysema, as the active constituents can decrease the time for bronchial cilia to recover after damage from smoking. Extracts of the plant have been shown to increase immune resistance. The University of Michigan Health System states that coltsfoot has been found to be just as effective as some allopathic antihistamine medicines in alleviating symptoms, without producing side effects such as drowsiness.

Warnings: Do not use during pregnancy and lactation. May be toxic in higher doses. Use only as directed and for no longer than six weeks a year.

Energetics: Cooling and moistening

Used For: Asthma, COPD, **cough**, cough (spastic), **emphysema**, and pleurisy

Properties: Antihistamine, **antitussive**, and expectorant

Comfrey   *Mucilant & Mildly Astringent Herb*

Symphytum officinale

Comfrey is a mucilaginous herb with a slight astringent quality. it also contains allantoin, a substance with stimulates cell growth. It has been used for generations to aid in the healing of injuries. In modern herbalism it is primarily used topically because of concerns over liver toxicity. I personally believe that comfrey leaf tea can be safely taken by people who don't have liver problems for two to four weeks without a problem.

Apply comfrey or comfrey products topically to help injured tissues heal. Use internally to speed the healing of broken bones and other injuries.

Look for *comfrey* in *Healing Salve Formula*

Warnings: Completely safe for topical use. It contains pyrrolizidine alkaloids, which are believed to cause liver problems. Many people have used comfrey internally with no reported ill effects and it is probably safe to use internally for short periods. It should be avoided during pregnancy, where cancer or tumors are present, and where there is a history of liver problems.

Energetics: Cooling, moistening, and mildly constricting

Used For: Abrasions/scratches, **blisters**, breasts (swelling/tenderness), **broken bones**, bruises, **injuries**, itching, **ligaments (torn/injuried)**, skin problems, **sprains**, **surgery (recovery)**, and wounds & sores

Properties: Cell proliferant, cicatrizant, **emollient**, mucilant, and **vulnerary**

Conjugated Linolenic Acid   **see** *omega-6 CLA*

Copaiba EO

Balsamic, Sweet, & Woody Essential Oil

Copaifera reticulata, officinalis, coriacea, and langsdorffiii

Copaiba is a resin from a South American tree. An essential oil can be distilled from the resin. The oil contains B- caryophyllene, a terpene that acts as a phytocannabinoid on CB_2 receptors, which modulates immune reactions. It can be combined with CBD for relieving inflammation. The resin has been used historically as an antiseptic and expectorant. The essential oil has neuroprotective effects and may have hepatoprotective effects. It may help with dental infections and root canals.

See the strategy *Aromatherapy* for suggested uses.

Warnings: Use internally as part of a formula.

Used For: Acne, anxiety (situational), arthritis, bites & stings, **cramps & spasms**, digestion (poor), **dislocation**, **fibromyalgia**, headache, infection prevention, skin problems, stress, stretch marks, traumatic brain injury, varicose veins, and wounds & sores

Properties: Analgesic, anti-inflammatory, antibacterial, antifungal, antiseptic, disinfectant, expectorant, hepatoprotective, and relaxant

Copper   *Mineral*

Copper is an essential mineral required for hemoglobin production, the absorption and use of iron, energy metabolism, the development and repair of bone and connective tissue, the formation of myelin sheath, adrenal hormone production, thyroid hormone production, immunity, and the pigmentation of hair and skin. The lack of accuracy in determining a copper deficiency with a single blood test combined with the potential toxicity of copper supplementation has resulted in many people not being properly treated for this deficiency.

A deficiency of copper causes fatigue, anemia, low level of neutrophils and leukocytes, the impairment of nerve and muscle function, under activity of adrenal and thyroid gland function, reproductive difficulties, premature graying of the hair, brittle bones, premature aging of the skin, and varicose veins. Copper is found in liver, oysters, nuts, seeds, whole grains, and cocoa. Deficiency can occur with poor diet and malabsorption.

Usage: Consumption of copper rich foods is best. For supplementation please consult a qualified practitioner. Normal supplementation is with 1–5 mg daily if, and only if, you have signs of a copper deficiency. Toxicity if the form of liver damage, renal failure and death has occurred with doses higher than 10 mg daily.

Used For: Appetite (deficient), arthritis, burning feet/hands, cadmium toxicity, calcium deficiency, **hair (graying)**, osteoporosis, spider veins, and varicose veins

Coptis   *Bitter Herb*

Coptis chinensis

Coptis is one of the infection-fighting herbs that contain berberine. It's a good alternative to the endangered goldenseal for fighting infections. Like all berberine containing plants it's a mild cholagogue and alterative.

Warnings: Use with caution during pregnancy.

Energetics: Cooling, drying, and mildly constricting

Used For: Belching, blood in stool, blood in urine, carbuncles, colitis, dermatitis, eczema, halitosis, infection (bacterial), inflammatory bowel disorders, nosebleeds, typhoid, ulcerations (external), and **urinary tract infections**

Properties: Alterative, antibacterial, antiviral, astringent, and cholagogue

Cordyceps   *Sweet Herb*

Cordyceps spp.

Cordyceps entered Western medicine after the Chinese government demonstrated its efficacy at the Olympic games in Beijing, where the Chinese athletes set new world records in nearly every competition they entered. The spectacular performance of the athletes stimulated a burst of pharmacological and clinical research into its health benefits. It is an adaptogen and general health tonic. It benefits the lungs, kidneys, glands and cardiovascular system.

Because it tonifies both the yin and yang, the Chinese consider this a very safe substance that can be taken over long periods of time. It modulates the immune system, so it can be helpful for boosting the immune system or calming it down.

Look for *cordyceps* in *Immune-Boosting, Mushroom Immune,* and *Testosterone Formulas*

Warnings: People using immune-suppressing drugs, anticoagulant drugs, or bronchodilators should consult their healthcare practitioners before using this product. Pregnant or lactating women should avoid using this product.

Energetics: Mildly warming, balancing, and nourishing

Used For: Addison's disease, adrenal fatigue, **aging**, altitude sickness, **asthma**, autoimmune disorders, **body building, bronchitis, cancer**, cancer prevention, **cancer treatment side effects**, cardiovascular disease, **convalescence, COPD**, cough, cough (damp), cough (dry), COVID-19, cystic fibrosis, **debility**, diabetes, diphtheria, dizziness, electromagnetic pollution, **emphysema**, endurance, erectile dysfunction, **exercise (performance), exercise (recovery)**, fatigue, hepatitis, hypertension, **infection prevention**, infertility, lupus, memory/brain function, menopause, **mood swings, nephritis, nervous exhaustion**, overacidity, sex drive (low), testosterone (low), tinnitus, and **wheezing**

Properties: Adaptogen, anti-inflammatory, anticancer, anticholesteremic, antifungal, antioxidant, antiviral, aphrodisiac, bronchial dilator, glandular, hepatoprotective, immune modulator, kidney tonic, **lung tonic**, and **tonic**

Corn Silk   *Mucilant Herb*

Zea mays

A mild, soothing diuretic agent, corn silk is useful for kidney inflammation and relieving discomfort associated with urinary tract conditions such as inflamed bladder and painful urination.

Look for *corn silk* in *Urinary Support Formula*

Energetics: Cooling and mildly drying

Used For: Bladder (irritable), bladder (ulcerated), cysts, diaper rash, edema, incontinence, **interstitial cystitis, nephritis, urethritis, urination (burning/painful)**, and **urination (frequent)**

Properties: Diuretic, mucilant, and **soothing**

Cortisol-Reducing Formula

Use this formula to reduce the output of stress hormones, including cortisol, from the adrenals. Cortisol reduces inflammation but too much cortisol also leads to a breakdown of lean muscle tissue and an accumulation of fat. This formula can help boost metabolism and may aid to weight loss when weight problems are related to stress.

Warnings: Avoid when the adrenals are underactive or exhausted or when there is a lot of chronic inflammation present, as is usually the case in autoimmune disorders.

Used For: Cushing's disease, excess weight, and stress

Affects: High cortisol

Use 1 capsule with a meal three times daily.

Ingredients: Vitamin C, chromium, magnolia bark extract, amur cork bark extract, holy basil leaf extract, green tea leaf extract, banaba leaf extract, L-threonine, DHEA, and vanadium

Corydalis   *Bitter Herb*

Corydalis yanhusuo

Corydalis is a natural pain reliever that contains an alkaloid called THP, which acts similar on endorphin receptors like opium poppy. However it is much milder in its effect and also has warming properties to move stagnant blood. It is a good remedy for pain associated with rheumatism, arthritis or menstruation. It can also be used as an aid for sleep, especially when sleep is disturbed by pain. I've also found it helpful in weaning people off of opioid pain killers. I have them start using corydalis and slowly back off the dose of their pain medication.

Warnings: Avoid during pregnancy.

Energetics: Warming and relaxing

Used For: Addictions (drugs), backache, cancer treatment side effects, **insomnia, pain**, and sciatica

Properties: Analgesic, narcotic, **sedative**, and soporific

Couchgrass *Sweet Herb*

Agropyrum repens

A cooling and soothing urinary remedy for inflammation in the urinary tract, prostatitis, and irritable bladder.

Energetics: Cooling and moistening

Used For: Arthritis (rheumatoid), bladder (irritable), cough (damp), digestion (poor), diverticulitis, gout, incontinence, kidney stones, prostatitis, urethritis, urinary tract infections, and **urination (burning/painful)**

Properties: Anti-inflammatory, cephalalgic, emetic, and mucilant

Cramp Bark *Astringent Herb*

Viburnum opulus

As its name implies, cramp bark is used to relax muscle spasms. It is commonly used for women as a uterine tonic since it both relaxes and tones the uterus. It has been used to ease menstrual cramps and prevent miscarriage, but may also be helpful for angina, backache, and other problems involving tension.

Look for *cramp bark* in *Antispasmodic, Christopher's Gallbladder,* and *Female Tonic Formulas*

Warnings: Avoid during pregnancy. Don't take with low blood pressure.

Energetics: Relaxing

Used For: **Angina**, backache, cramps (leg), **cramps (menstrual)**, **cramps & spasms**, **dysmenorrhea**, **hiccups**, irritable bowel, and **miscarriage prevention**

Properties: Antiabortive and antispasmodic

Cranberry *Sour Herb*

Vaccinium macrocarpon

Cranberries contain antioxidants that mitigate the damaging effects of free radicals in the body. They also contain hippuric acid, which is an antibacterial agent. For this reason they are commonly used to prevent urinary tract infections, although they can be used to help prevent other infections. They are high in vitamin C content and were used to prevent scurvy in sailors. Even commercially prepared cranberry juice cocktails have medicinal benefits, although they work better without the added sugar.

Look for *cranberry* in *UTI Prevention Formula*

Energetics: Cooling and mildly drying

Used For: Bladder infection, incontinence, kidney infection, prolapsed uterus, and **urinary tract infections**

Properties: Antibacterial, antioxidant, and nutritive

Curcumin *Phytochemical*

Curcumin is a pigment from the Indian spice, turmeric, which gives curry its yellow color. It's also a powerful anti-inflammatory agent. It inhibits activity of the transcription factor NF-kB, a pro-inflammatory messenger. Clinical research suggests it can be a valuable remedy in treating rheumatoid arthritis, osteoarthritis, and other inflammatory conditions.

Curcumin also has hepatoprotective properties and aids liver detoxification. It increases glutathione levels and glutathione-S-transferase activity, which gives it antioxidant properties. It acts as a free radical scavenger, inhibiting peroxidation of lipids (fats) and protecting nervous tissue from toxins like lead and other heavy metals. The research suggests that curcumin's antioxidant action may help to prevent certain cancers, Alzheimer's disease, and cardiovascular conditions.

Several studies have shown that curcumin has a positive effect on the brain and nervous system. It has been found to help protect the brain in injury and to reduce the risk of stroke. In one animal study, curcumin was shown to protect against toxicity and impairment of mental ability caused by an amyloid-protein infusion. Another study found that curcumin shrank the size of plaques and reduced neurite dystrophy in an Alzheimer mouse model.

In one study, curcumin induced apoptosis (cell death) in cancer cells without cytotoxic effects on healthy cells. In an animal study, curcumin inhibited the growth of cancer cells in the stomach, liver, and colon as well as oral cancers.

Usage: Take one capsule twice daily. Curcumin is more easily absorbed when taken with fats.

Used For: Alzheimer's, **arthritis**, **arthritis (rheumatoid)**, autoimmune disorders, **bursitis**, cancer prevention, cardiovascular disease, depression, **dislocation**, **down syndrome**, gallbladder problems, gallstones, inflammation, **pain**, and **traumatic brain injury**

Properties: Anti-inflammatory, **antiarthritic**, antioxidant, antioxidant, cholagogue, and hepatoprotective

Cyperus *Mildly Bitter, Pungent, & Sweet Herb*

Cyperus rotundus

The tuberous roots and rhizomes of this fast growing weed are used in Ayurvedic and Chinese herbalism. The enters the lung and spleen (digestive) meridians and is used for digestive problems. It regulates qi and moves stagnant water and mucus.

Look for *cyperus* in *Chinese Qi-Regulating Formula*

Energetics: Relaxing, drying, and neutral

Used For: Amenorrhea, asthma, bites & stings, diarrhea, dysmenorrhea, dyspepsia, excess weight, hypertension, ulcers, and wounds & sores

Properties: Antifungal, carminative, diuretic, emmenagogue, febrifuge, hypotensive, mucilant, and stomachic

Cypress EO   *Fresh & Woody Essential Oil*

Cupressus sempervirens

A sweet balsamic fragrance, with a refreshing or vaporous quality, cypress EO strengths the nervous system when one feels burdened or overwhelmed. It is helpful for those who have lost touch with their own center and need to find calmness and strength in life. It can be helpful during times of transition in one's life, such as moving, changing jobs or the ending of close relationships. Topically, it is helpful for oily skin and excessive perspiration.

See the strategy *Aromatherapy* for suggested uses.

Warnings: Do not use internally. Topically it is nonirritating and nonsensitizing and may be used neat (undiluted).

Used For: Acne, bronchitis, dysmenorrhea, hemorrhoids, hot flashes, perspiration (excessive), pertussis, skin (oily), and varicose veins

Properties: Antiseptic, deodorant, diuretic, hemostatic, hepatic, styptic, and tonic

Damiana   *Aromatic & Mildly Bitter Herb*

Turnera spp.

Damiana is most commonly used to increase libido, but it is really a tonic for stress and low energy. In other words, it works best when low sex drive is due to fatigue and stress. It also has antidepressant effects.

Look for *damiana* in *Antidepressant, DHEA with Herbs, Male Performance,* and *Women's Aphrodisiac Formulas*

Warnings: Use with caution during pregnancy.

Energetics: Warming, mildly drying, and mildly relaxing

Used For: Addictions (tobacco), **anxiety disorders**, bipolar mood disorder, BPH, **depression, erectile dysfunction, fatigue, hot flashes, infertility**, interstitial cystitis, narcolepsy, **nervous exhaustion**, premature ejaculation, reversed polarity, **sex drive (low)**, testosterone (low), and urethritis

Properties: Antidepressant, aperient, **aphrodisiac**, cardiac, diuretic, euphoretic, glandular, nervine, and stimulant (metabolic)

Damp Cough Syrup Formula

See also *Dry Cough Syrup Formula* and *Steven Horne's Horehound Cough Formula*

These formulas help loosen and expel mucus. They are used to clear congestion in the lungs and are helpful where there is excess mucus production and drainage.

Used For: Colds (decongestant), congestion (lungs), and **cough (damp)**

Traditional Cherry Bark Syrup

Take 1 tablespoon every two hours, as needed.

Ingredients: Yerba santa, osha, elecampane root & flower, grindelia flower bud, black cherry bark, and horehound leaf

Children's Cough Syrup

Use as directed on the label.

Ingredients: Yerba santa, elecampane flower & root, grindelia flower bud, balloon flower, and horehound leaf

Dandelion   *Bitter Herb*

Taraxacum officinale

This common weed in lawns and gardens has a beneficial effect on the digestive system, the urinary system and the pancreas. The root is primarily used to stimulate bile flow and aid the liver, while the leaf is more often employed as a diuretic to aid kidney function. It has a beneficial effect on the microflora of the gut and helps stimulate digestive secretions.

Look for *dandelion* in *Ayurvedic Skin Healing, Blood Purifier, Chinese Wind-Heat Evil, Detoxifying, Diuretic, Hepatoprotective, Herbal Bitters, Hypoglycemic, Lactase Enzyme, Lipase Enzyme, Liver Cleanse, Nattokinase Enzyme, Pet Supplement,* and *Urinary Support Formulas*

Warnings: Contraindicated for conditions involving fluid deficiency or dryness.

Energetics: Cooling and drying

Used For: Acne, anger (excessive), appetite (deficient), blood poisoning, **cirrhosis of the liver, digestion (poor)**, dysbiosis, **eczema, edema**, fat cravings, fat metabolism (poor), **gallbladder problems**, gout, hepatitis, **indigestion, jaundice (adults)**, kidney weakness/failure, low stomach acid, metabolic syndrome, nephritis, overacidity, pancreatitis, PMS Type C, PMS Type H, **PMS Type S**, rashes & hives, sore/geographic tongue, **triglycerides (low)**, and urine (scant)

Properties: Alterative, antacid, **cholagogue, digestive tonic, diuretic**, food, hepatic, hepatoprotective, lipotropic, stimulant (appetite), and **stomachic**

Detoxifying Formula

See also *Blood Purifier Formula* and *Chinese Wood-Decreasing Formula*

These formulas strengthens all eliminative organs to help the body expel toxins of all sorts. Use them as part of a periodic cleanse to remove the effects of environmental pollution. They are also good to take if you have been exposed to chemicals on a regular basis, such as painting, manufacturing, lab work, farm chemicals.

Warnings: Individuals with colon problems (especially spastic or colitis) should use this formula carefully as it will increase bile flow and may further irritate the colon.

Used For: **Abscesses**, **acne**, addictions (drugs), blood poisoning, body odor, **boils**, breast lumps, cancer, cancer treatment side effects, cervical dysplasia, chemical exposure, chicken pox, **cysts**, **eczema**, **environmental pollution**, fibroids (uterine), fibromyalgia, irritability, itching, pap smear (abnormal), parasites, PMS Type A, poison ivy/oak, poisoning, polycystic ovarian syndrome, **polyps**, **preeclampsia**, psoriasis, rashes & hives, skin (infections), skin (oily), skin problems, **surgery (recovery)**, and **vaccine side effects**

Affects: Digestive stagnation, gallbladder, **general stagnation**, **hepatic stagnation**, **intestinal stagnation**, **liver**, mitochondria, skin, stressed wood, and structural stagnation

Special Cellular Cleansing Formula

My favorite traditional cleansing formula, helps the colon, kidneys, liver, and lymphatics. Use 1–2 capsules two or three times daily with plenty of water.

Ingredients: Gentian root, cascara sagrada bark, black walnut hulls, yellow dock root, dandelion root, Oregon grape rhizome & root, and goldenseal root extract

Environmental Detoxifying Formula

A newer formula for general detoxification from environmental pollutants, aids gut microbiome. Take 2–3 capsules once or twice daily with plenty of water.

Ingredients: Burdock root, dandelion root, pepsin, red clover flower, yellow dock root, sarsaparilla root extract, Bacillus coagulans, echinacea root extract, and milk thistle seed extract

Devil's Claw   *Bitter Herb*

Harpagophytum procumbens

Used by indigenous people for thousands of years to treat pain, stomach disorders and fever, Devil's claw is used as an anti-inflammatory in modern herbalism for treating problems like arthritis and low back pain. It Increases mobility in the joints and is a common ingredient in formulas for inflammation and arthritis.

Look for *devil's claw* in *Herbal Arthritis Formula*

Warnings: Contraindicated in gastric and duodenal ulcers.

Energetics: Cooling and drying

Used For: Acid indigestion, allergies (respiratory), **arthritis**, **arthritis (rheumatoid)**, backache, bursitis, fever, fibrosis, food allergies/intolerances, gout, indigestion, **inflammation**, neuralgia & neuritis, uric acid retention, and wounds & sores

Properties: Analgesic, **anti-inflammatory**, **antiarthritic**, and digestive tonic

DHEA   *Hormone*

The adrenal glands produce numerous hormones, but the most abundant hormone they produce is DHEA (dehydroepiandrosterone). DHEA is a building block for the sex hormones, including androgens (male hormones such as testosterone) and estrogens. DHEA levels tend to drop as we age.

DHEA is also an antagonist to cortisol, a stress hormone that also reduces inflammation. Stress reduces DHEA production and low levels are often found in people with cancer, autoimmune diseases and chronic inflammation. However, taking DHEA will not necessarily help these conditions.

DHEA has been shown to improve immune function. For instance, DHEA supplements have been helpful for some people with lupus, an autoimmune condition.

DHEA is probably most helpful if you have low levels of testosterone or estrogen. However, if you're going to take DHEA, it's probably wise to get your levels tested first to see if you're actually low in it. Otherwise, small doses are best because getting too much of a particular hormone can be just as bad as getting too little.

Warnings: Because DHEA is a naturally occurring hormone, long-term supplementation may alter the body's ability to produce sufficient amounts of it on its own. DHEA is best used for short-term treatment hormone imbalance. Excessive levels of DHEA can cause acne and hormonal imbalances like those found in teenagers. It's best to get your hormones tested to determine if you actually need DHEA before taking it for any length of time. DHEA should not be taken by children, teenagers, pregnant women or nursing mothers. It should be avoided by people with reproductive cancers, such as prostate or uterine cancer. High levels of DHEA have been reported to cause symptoms of hypothyroidism, heart palpitations and arrhythmia.

Usage: 5–15 mg daily for women, 10–30 mg daily for men.

Used For: Aging, AIDS, cramps (menstrual), diabetes, emotional sensitivity, erectile dysfunction, estrogen (low), lupus, menopause, menstrual irregularity, osteoporosis, sex drive (low), and **testosterone (low)**

Properties: Estrogenic, glandular, and testosterone-enhancing

DHEA with Herbs Formula

DHEA is the precursor to estrogen and testosterone. Levels tend to drop as we age. (See *DHEA* for more information.) These formulas combine DHEA with herbs traditionally used to support male or female reproductive health.

Warnings: Avoid during pregnancy. See warnings under DHEA

Used For: AIDS, Alzheimer's, **erectile dysfunction**, **estrogen (low)**, **lupus**, **sex drive (low)**, and **testosterone (low)**

Affects: Adrenal cortex, high progesterone, low cortisol, **low DHEA**, **low estrogen**, **low testosterone**, and **testes**

Women's DHEA with Herbs

This blend contains 25 mg. of DHEA in a base of herbs designed to help balance female hormones. Take 1 capsule daily with a meal.

Ingredients: DHEA, wild yam root, false unicorn root, and chaste tree berry extract

Men's DHEA with Herbs

This blend contains 25 mg. of DHEA in a base of herbs designed to support the production of testosterone aid common male reproductive problems. Take 1 capsule daily with a meal.

Ingredients: DHEA, sarsaparilla root, damiana leaf, and ginseng (Asian/Korean) root extract

Digestive Settling EO Blend

Use this essential oil blend to help settle the stomach. It can help reduce gas, bloating, indigestion, and nausea. It can also be helpful for motion sickness.

See the strategy *Aromatherapy* for suggested uses.

Used For: Gas & bloating, indigestion, motion sickness, and nausea & vomiting

Affects: Digestive depression, digestive stagnation, and stomach

Ingredients: Ginger EO, anise EO, peppermint EO, lemongrass EO, and fennel seed

Digestive Support Formula

See also *Plant Enzyme Formula*

The body makes substances like hydrochloric acid (HCl), pancreatic enzymes and bile salts to break down food. Digestive function may decline with age or be compromised by chronic disease. People with autoimmune diseases often tend to be low in enzymes, too. In these situations people do not release enough digestive secretions to properly break down their food. This formula contains these digestive secretions along with additional enzymes to help people break down their food better.

Enzyme supplements can also aid immunity. They may be helpful as part of a holistic approach to cancer if taken between meals or in the early hours of the morning (between midnight and 3 AM) on an empty stomach.

Warnings: Do not take if stomach ulcers are present. It may cause stomach irritation in some persons. Always take with food. I recommend that this product not be used continually, except in the case of people over 50 with chronically-poor digestion, as supplementing these digestive secretions will tend to atrophy the body's ability to produce them. Use to help rebuild a person while supplementing their diet with herbs and nutrients that rebuild the digestive organs. For regular long-term use take a Plant Enzyme Formula as it does not duplicate the body's natural digestive secretions.

Used For: Acid indigestion, **aging**, allergies (respiratory), ALS, anorexia, **appetite (deficient)**, **autoimmune disorders**, **belching**, bulimia, **cancer**, cancer treatment side effects, celiac disease, cloudy thinking, congestion, convalescence, COPD, cystic breast disease, **cystic fibrosis**, dandruff, debility, **digestion (poor)**, dysbiosis, dyspepsia, eczema, endurance, Epstein-Barr virus, excess weight, fat cravings, fat metabolism (poor), fatty liver disease, fibroids (uterine), **fibromyalgia**, fibrosis, fingernails (weak/brittle), **food allergies/intolerances**, gallbladder problems, gallstones, **gas & bloating, gastritis**, gastritis, **hair loss/thinning, halitosis, hiatal hernia**, hypoglycemia, **ileocecal valve, indigestion**, infection (bacterial), infection (fungal), inflammatory bowel disorders, **irritable bowel, leaky gut**, low stomach acid, **lymphoma**, menopause, multiple sclerosis, myasthenia gravis, overacidity, **overalkalinity**, pain, pancreatitis, parasites, parasites (nematodes, worms), **protein digestion**, psoriasis, rhinitis, rosacea, **SIBO**, skin (dry/flaky), sore/geographic tongue, traumatic brain injury, triglycerides (high), triglycerides (low), **underweight**, and **wasting**

Affects: Digestive depression, gallbladder, **pancreas head**, small intestines, **stomach**, and weakened earth

Take 1-2 capsules during or after meals as an aid to digestion.

Ingredients: Betaine hydrochloric acid (hcl), alpha amylase, pepsin, bromelain, papain, bile salt, pancreatin, and lipase

Disinfectant EO Blend

This blend of essential oils is antiseptic and antifungal. It is helpful for preventing the spread of infection or aiding recovery from colds, flu, coughs, and bronchitis.

See the strategy *Aromatherapy* for suggested uses.

Warnings: Not for internal use. Use with caution with asthma, pregnancy and children under the age of eight. Phototoxic—avoid sun exposure after topical application.

Used For: Blood poisoning, bronchitis, **carbuncles**, colds (antiviral), colds (decongestant), cough (damp), flu, infection (bacterial), infection (viral), **infection prevention**, injuries, and wounds & sores

Affects: Lungs and sinuses

Ingredients: Clove EO, eucalyptus EO, cinnamon bark EO, lemon EO, pine EO, wild rosemary EO, and thyme EO

Diuretic Formula

See also *Chinese Water-Decreasing Formula*

These formulas help increase urine output in cases of edema or kidney problems.

Warnings: These formulas are stimulating diuretics and should be avoided when the kidneys are inflamed. They also contains herbs that should be used with caution in the early stages of pregnancy.

Used For: Bedwetting, bladder infection, **edema**, interstitial cystitis, kidney stones, **PMS Type H**, urethritis, urinary tract infections, urination (burning/painful), and **urine (scant)**

Affects: Bladder, **kidneys**, stressed water, **urinary depression**, and urinary stagnation

Christopher's Diuretic Blend

This blend contains goldenseal, making it more useful for UTIs. 1–2 capsules three times daily with plenty of water. Combine with goldenseal or berberine for UTIs.

Ingredients: Juniper berry, parsley leaf, uva ursi leaf, and goldenseal root extract

Herbal Diuretic Formula

A slightly stronger diuretic, less suitable for UTIs, but better for edema. 1–2 capsules three times daily with plenty of water.

Ingredients: Juniper berry, parsley leaf, uva ursi leaf, and dandelion root

Docosahexaenoic Acid   **see** *omega-3 DHA*

Dodder   *Pungent & Sweet Herb*

Cuscuta chinensis

Dodder enters the liver and kidney meridians. It supplements the kidney energy and aids male reproductive problems like impotency, infertility and nocturnal emissions. It stimulates the uterus in women and helps prevent miscarriage. It has a tonic effect on the heart and helps to lower blood pressure. It also helps decrease the size of the spleen.

Look for *dodder* in *Chinese Fire-Increasing Formula*

Energetics: Warming and balancing

Used For: Diarrhea, dizziness, erectile dysfunction, infertility, nocturnal emission, and tinnitus

Properties: Antidiarrheal, cardiac, and hypertensive

Dogwood, Asian   *Mildly Bitter & Sour Herb*

Cornus officinalis

The fruits of Asian dogwood enter the liver and kidney meridians and have a tonifying effect on the kidney. It aids the kidney qi and promotes normal urination.

Look for *dogwood (Asian)* in *Chinese Wood-Increasing Formula*

Energetics: Mildly warming and mildly drying

Used For: Hearing loss, tinnitus, and urination (frequent)

Properties: Antibacterial, antihistamine, and diuretic

Dogwood, Jamaican   *Acrid & Bitter Herb*

Piscidia erythrina

A mild narcotic and anodyne herb, Jamaican dogwood is a relatively potent sedative known as a remedy for migraine headaches, neuralgia, and the treatment of insomnia caused by pain, nervous tension and stress. The bark is anti-inflammatory and antispasmodic and can be used for painful menstrual periods. It is used in combination with other herbs to treat the musculoskeletal pain of arthritis and rheumatism.

Warnings: Use with caution with hypotension and with children or pregnant women. May amplify the effects of sedative medications.

Energetics: Cooling and relaxing

Used For: Arthritis, **backache**, cough (spastic), **cramps & spasms**, **dysmenorrhea**, **headache**, **headache (migraine)**, neuralgia & neuritis, **pain**, sciatica, stiff neck, toothache, and twitching

Properties: Analgesic, antispasmodic, narcotic, sedative, and soporific

Dong Quai
Aromatic & Sweet Herb

Angelica sinensis

Dong quai has been used extensively in the Orient for improving the general health of women. Millions of Chinese women take it regularly throughout their childbearing years. It is a blood tonic and helps to rebuild the blood from the monthly blood loss women experience during their childbearing years. It also eases pain and congestion associated with periods. It also stimulates circulation in the abdomen and aids digestive function.

Look for *dong quai* in *Chinese Wood-Decreasing, Chinese Wood-Increasing, Chrisopher's Menopause, Female Tonic, Hot Flash, Intestinal Soothing,* and *Prebirth Formulas*

Warnings: Avoid during pregnancy, while menstruating or with excessive menstrual flow.

Energetics: Warming, moistening, and nourishing

Used For: Amenorrhea, anemia, breasts (swelling/tenderness), circulation (poor), cramps (menstrual), dysmenorrhea, fibroids (uterine), headache (migraine), infertility, labor & delivery, menopause, menstrual irregularity, and prolapsed uterus

Properties: Anticoagulant, antispasmodic, **blood building**, deobstruent, diuretic, emmenagogue, female tonic, glandular, phytoestrogen, and uterine

Drawing Salve

Drawing salves are used to disinfect wounds and pull pus and infection out of the skin. They may also be helpful for slivers. Stronger versions of drawing salves are called escharotics and are used to remove moles, warts, and skin cancers. The *Escharotic Formula* and *Black Salve* are examples of escharotics. To make an simple escharatic ointment, mix the contents of one capsule of a standardized extract of acetogenins from Paw Paw enough Healing Salve to form a paste.

Apply eschortics only to the tissue you wish to remove and discontinue use once the morbid tissue is gone. Carefully observe the warnings below. Follow this up with a *Healing Salve* or a poultice of healing herbs. Discontinue application if excessive redness or irritation occur. Ideally these products should be used only under the direction of a skilled herbalist who is familiar with this therapy (findanherbalist.com or americanherbalistsguild.com).

Warnings: A mild black salve is not likely to cause skin irritation or redness, but if it does, discontinue use. Escharotics will typically cause redness around the wart, mole, or skin cancer. If the irritation becomes excessive, discontinue use.

Using escharotics to remove morbid tissue can leave scars, so be cautious about using them on the face or neck. Once the offending material is drawn to the surface, discontinue their use and use and apply a Healing Salve or poultice with astringent and mucilant herbs to promote healing. Carefully follow directions for any product you use.

Used For: Abscesses, acne, **boils**, **cysts**, infection (bacterial), **slivers**, **warts**, and wounds & sores

Black Salve

A mild, non-irritating drawing salve. Apply a thick layer over the desired area and cover with a bandage.

Ingredients: Chaparral leaf, red clover, pine gum resin, plantain, and poke

Escharotic Formula

A potent escharotic paste for professional use only. Apply a small amount to the wart, mole, etc. with a toothpick. Do not apply to surrounding skin. Cover with a bandage. When a ring appears around the affected area, discontinue use.

Ingredients: Black walnut, burdock, and white oak bark

Traditional Black Salve

These are key ingredients for traditional black salves. Apply as directed on the label of the product you buy and follow the above warnings.

Bloodroot *Sanguinaria canadensis*

Zinc *chloride*

Chaparral *Larrea tridentata*

Dry Cough Syrup Formula

See also *Damp Cough Syrup Formula*

These formulas help moisten the lung tissue when there is a lack of mucus production. They help to clear irritants from the lungs and ease chronic coughing.

Used For: Congestion, congestion (lungs), COPD, **cough (dry)**, and emphysema

Loquat Lung Formula

A good formula for dry, irritated lungs. Take 1 tablespoon every two hours.

Ingredients: Loquat leaf, fritillary bulb, black cherry bark, and balloon flower

David Winston's Cold-Dry Formula

Relieves dry cough when the lungs are cold (underactive). 50–60 drops three times daily.

Ingredients: Astragalus root, prince seng root, asparagus (Chinese) root, licorice root, and spikenard root

David Winston's Hot-Dry Formula

Relieves dry cough when the lungs are hot (irritated). 60–80 drops in juice or water three to four times per day.

Ingredients: Horehound, balloon flower, red clover, elecampane root, and ophiopogon

Drynaria *Bitter Herb*

Drynaria fortunei

The dried rhizome of this herb from Chinese herbalism supports the kidney and heart meridians. It helps heal broken bones, strengthens tendons and helps heal pain in the knees.

Look for *drynaria* in *Chinese Water-Increasing Formula*

Energetics: Mildly warming and nourishing

Used For: Broken bones, diarrhea, kidney weakness/failure, tinnitus, and toothache

Properties: Analgesic and kidney tonic

Dulse *Salty and Mucilant Herb*

Palmaria palmata

Dulse is a nourishing food containing numerous trace minerals as well as iodine to support the thyroid. Liquid dulse is a great way to get iodine and five to ten drops make a great mineral supplement for kids. It can be used in baths and other topical preparations to promote healthy skin as well.

Look for *dulse* in *Herbal Potassium* and *Watkin's Hair, Skin, and Nails Formulas*

Warnings: Not recommended for hyperactive thyroid.

Energetics: Cooling, moistening, and nourishing

Used For: **Aluminum toxicity**, cholesterol (low), depression, **dermatitis**, eczema, excess weight, fatigue, fatty tumors/deposits, **goiter**, hair loss/thinning, Hashimoto's disease, **hypothyroidism**, itching, pregnancy, **radiation**, **skin problems**, and swollen lymph glands

Properties: Emollient, glandular, mineralizer, mucilant, nutritive, and thyrotropic

Ear Drop Formula

Wen Zhong

See also *Antispasmodic Ear Formula*

These are blends designed to be warmed to body temperature and used in the ear for earaches.

Used For: Earache and hearing loss

David Winston's Ear Drops

Ingredients: Mullein flower, Saint John's wort flower, garlic bulb, and tea tree EO

Traditional Ear Drop Formula

Ingredients: Mullein flower, Saint John's wort flower & leaf, and garlic oil

Herbal Ed's Ear Drops

Ingredients: Calendula flower, Saint John's wort flowering tops, mullein flower, and garlic bulb

Echinacea *Mildly Acrid & Bitter Herb*

Echinacea spp.

Echinacea is a popular herb for boosting the immune system. It helps the body fight both bacterial and viral infections, although I don't find it that effective a remedy for colds or flu after you catch one. It can be used for prevention during cold and flu season.

It's very effective for infections where there is pus and redness. It inhibits the spread of infection. It was also traditionally used as a remedy for snakebites, insect bites and bee stings.

Look for *echinacea* in *Antibacterial, Children's Elderberry Cold and Flu, Elderberry Cold and Flu, Gut Immune, Immune-Boosting, Lymph Cleansing, Lymphatic Infection,* and *Suma Adaptogen Formulas*

Warnings: Avoid when there are autoimmune disorders where the immune system is over active (i.e. M.S. Lupus, Hodgkins). In excessive amounts it can cause excessive salivation and a scratchy, tingling sensation in the throat.

Usage: For maximum effectiveness, a blend of echinacea needs to be taken in large, frequently repeated doses. A low dose for adults is 15–20 drops (1 ml), but most herbalists suggest 45–90 drops (3–5 ml) three times daily. When fighting infection take every two hours.

Energetics: Cooling and drying

Used For: Abscesses, acne, **adenitis**, anal fistula/fissure, **antibiotic resistance**, antibiotic resistance, appendicitis, **bites & stings**, **blood poisoning**, **boils**, **bronchitis**, cancer, **cancer treatment side effects**, canker sores, **carbuncles**, **cervical dysplasia**, cholera, colds, colds (antiviral), **congestion (lymphatic)**, croup, **diphtheria**, earache, eczema, Epstein-Barr virus, fever, flu, food poisoning, **gangrene**, giardia, gingivitis, gonorrhea, headache (sinus), **impetigo**, **infection (bacterial)**, infection (viral), **infection prevention**, **kidney infection**, lyme disease, malaria, **mastitis**, meningitis, mercury poisoning, **mononucleosis**, **mumps**, nephritis, pet supplements, sinus infection, **skin (infections)**, **snakebite**, **sore throat**, **staph infections**, **strep throat**, **swollen lymph glands**, **syphilis**, **tonsillitis**, **typhoid**, ulcerations (external), vaccine side effects, and **wounds & sores**

Properties: Alterative, analgesic, anti-inflammatory, antiallergenic, **antibacterial**, antiseptic, antitoxic, antivenomous, **antiviral**, detoxifying, febrifuge, **immune stimulant**, lymphatic, and vulnerary

Ed Millet's Herbal Crisis Formula

See also *Fire Cider Formula* and *Herbal Composition Formula*

Herbal Crisis is a modified version of Samuel Thomson's Composition Powder, originally created by Edward Milo Millet. It is a very effective formula for knocking out colds and flu quickly. Directions for this make-it-yourself formula can be found in the book *Modern Herbal Dispensatory*.

Used For: **Colds**, congestion (sinus), cough (damp), fever, **flu**, **perspiration (deficient)**, sinus infection, **sore throat**, and strep throat

Affects: Digestive depression, **intestinal relaxation**, intestinal stagnation, **mucous membranes**, **respiratory depression**, **respiratory stagnation**, sinuses, and sweat glands

Take 1/2 teaspoon at the first sign of acute illness with plenty of water. Fast and continue to take 1/2 teaspoon every hour with water until the symptoms subside. You can also dilute it with water and use it as a gargle for sore throats. It can also be added to an enema solution for clearing the colon of mucus.

> *4 parts* Bayberry root bark
> *2 parts* White pine bark
> *1 part* Goldenseal root
> *1 part* Lobelia
> *1 part* Ginger root
> *1/2 part* Clove bud
> *1/2 part* Capsicum

Eicosapentaenoic Acid   see *omega-3 EPA*

Elder   *Sour Herb*

Sambucus canadensis

Elder is a very versatile herb. Elderberries are a popular antiviral remedy and useful for colds and flu. The flowers are cooling and anti-inflammatory. They also have antiviral properties and act as a febrifuge for colds and flu. They are traditionally combined with peppermint. The flowers are also used in skin lotions. The leaves may be applied topically to injuries and the bark is a laxative, but rarely used in modern herbalism due to potential toxicity.

Look for *elder* in *Children's Elderberry Cold* and *Flu*, *Elderberry Cold* and *Flu*, *Immune-Boosting*, *Myelin Sheath*, and *Steven Horne's Children's Composition Formulas*

Warnings: Stems, bark and root can be toxic. No known warnings for flowers and berries.

Energetics: Cooling and drying

Used For: AIDS, cataracts, cervical dysplasia, **colds**, **colds (antiviral)**, cough (damp), Epstein-Barr virus, **fever**, **flu**, hepatitis, **infection (viral)**, **infection prevention**, mononucleosis, **perspiration (deficient)**, skin problems, sore throat, and **vaccine side effects**

Properties: Anti-inflammatory, anticatarrhal, **antiviral**, decongestant, diaphoretic, **febrifuge**, food, nutritive, and virostatic

Elderberry Cold and Flu Formula

See also *Steven Horne's Children's Composition Formula*

This formula helps support the body in fighting off colds, flu and other forms of contagious disease, particularly those with a viral base. It boosts the immune system, improves lymphatic drainage and prevents the spread of infection. It's a great product for both children and adults to take during the cold and flu season to stay healthy. It can also be taken to speed recovery.

Used For: **Colds (antiviral)**, fever, **flu**, **infection (viral)**, **infection prevention**, and vaccine side effects

Affects: Acute disease stage

Take 2 capsules three times daily, plus 2 capsules before going to bed. You can also take 1 capsule two or three times a day to boost the immune system during cold and flu season.

Ingredients: Vitamin d3, elder berry extract, echinacea aerial parts, and olive leaf extract

Elecampane

Acrid, Aromatic, & Mildly Bitter Herb

Inula helenium

Elecampane is an outstanding remedy for clearing phlegm and mucus from the lungs, urinary system and digestive system. Elecampane is specific for chronic irritation and infection of the respiratory system. It contains inulin which feeds friendly bacteria in the colon.

Look for *elecampane* in *Anti-Fungal, Antiparasitic, Damp Cough Syrup, Dry Cough Syrup, H. Pylori-Fighting,* and *Herbal Tooth Powder Formulas*

Warnings: Avoid during pregnancy.

Energetics: Warming and drying

Used For: Asthma, bronchitis, congestion, congestion (bronchial), **congestion (lungs)**, cough, dental health, parasites, pertussis, **tuberculosis**, and ulcers

Properties: Antiseptic, diaphoretic, **expectorant**, and pulmonary

Electrolyte Drink Powder

This formula helps replenish electrolytes (calcium, magnesium, sodium and potassium) after exercise. It can be consumed before, during and after strenuous physical activity or used as a beverage anytime during the day to replenish energy. It is also helpful for loss of electrolytes following a bout of diarrhea or intense sweating. It also supports bone and muscle health.

Used For: Dehydration, diarrhea, **exercise (performance)**, **exercise (recovery)**, giardia, night sweating, and stress

Affects: Muscles

Empty the contents of one packet into 14-16 ounces of cold water, mix and drink.

Ingredients: Vitamin C, vitamin E, vitamin B_1, vitamin B_2, vitamin B_3, vitamin B_6, vitamin B_{12}, pantothenic acid, calcium, magnesium, potassium, glucosamine, inulin, d-ribose, L-carnitine, glycine, and taurine

Eleuthero (Siberian Ginseng) *Sweet Herb*

Eleutherococcus senticosus

This herb was the first plant identified as an adaptogen by Russian scientists. It not only helps the body cope better with stress, it increases stamina and endurance, stimulates the brain to improve concentration and stimulates male hormone production. Soviet researchers found eleuthero improved athletic performance, aided cosmonauts in preventing space sickness, caused secretaries to make fewer mistakes and helped workers have fewer sick days. In other words, it enhances endurance, immunity, brain function and general good health. Eleuthero aids adrenal function and improves the body's ability to resist disease.

Look for *eleuthero* in *5-HTP Adaptogen, Adaptogen, Adaptogen-Immune, Blood Sugar Control, Chinese Qi-Increasing, Jeannie Burgess' Thymus, Seasonal Cold* and *Flu, Suma Adaptogen, Vandergriff's Energy Booster,* and *Women's Aphrodisiac Formulas*

Warnings: Avoid during pregnancy. Not recommended for acute diseases, high fever, severe inflammations, hyperactivity or extreme, nervous anxiety.

Energetics: Mildly warming and balancing

Used For: Addictions (coffee, caffeine), **addictions (drugs)**, addictions (sugar/carbohydrates), Addison's disease, altitude sickness, **body building**, bulimia, cancer, **cancer** treatment side effects, **Cushing's disease**, depression, dizziness, emotional sensitivity, **endurance**, Epstein-Barr virus, erectile dysfunction, **exercise (performance)**, **exercise (recovery)**, **fatigue**, fear, Graves' disease, hair loss/thinning, Hashimoto's disease, headache (tension), heart fibrillation/palpitations, heart weakness, hot flashes, hypertension, hypoglycemia, infection prevention, infertility, insomnia, **jet lag**, mercury poisoning, **mood swings**, narcolepsy, **nervousness**, **OCD**, PTSD, radiation, sex drive (low), **stress**, and testosterone (low)

Properties: **Adaptogen**, antiadrenergic, antirheumatic, aphrodisiac, hypotensive, immune modulator, serotonergic, sympatholytic, and tonic

Enzyme Spray Formula

While this formula was originally designed to break down odors without harming fabrics and to help remove stains, a number of people discovered it was also therapeutic for a wide variety of conditions. It can be sprayed topically on the body to reduce pain and inflammation for a wide variety of injuries and ailments.

For sunburn, apply aloe vera gel to the burned areas and keep moist with this spray. For back and muscle pain, apply lobelia and capsicum extracts topically, follow up with essential oils with topical analgesic properties and then spray on the enzymes to activate healing.

For general skin care try applying a silver gel to the face and other areas of the skin that need attention after showering or bathing. Follow this up with this enzyme spray.

This formula has proved helpful in repairing damaged disks in the spine. Applying a goldenseal tincture to the areas where the damaged disks are, along with and following up with this spray can be very helpful.

The product also makes an excellent deodorizer, spot remover, and cleaner. The enzymes it contains break down stains and odors. You can also use it as a natural deodorant. It works better if you add essential oils to it.

Used For: Abrasions/scratches, acne, **age spots**, arthritis, **backache**, **bites & stings**, **body odor**, boils, **breast lumps**, broken bones, bruises, **burns & scalds**, cartilage damage, corns, **cystic breast disease**, **cysts**, dandruff, **denture sores**, dermatitis, diaper rash, eczema, fleas, **foot odor**, gingivitis, inflammation, **injuries**, **itching**, **pet supplements**, **rashes & hives**, rhinitis, sciatica, scoliosis, **skin problems**, spider veins, **spinal disks**, **sprains**, sprains, stiff neck, **sunburn**, TMJ, traumatic brain injury, whiplash, **wounds & sores**, and **wrinkles**

Affects: Breasts, nails, **skin**, **spinal discs**, and structural depression

Spray on the skin over injured areas of the body.

Ingredients: Oxidoreductases, transferases, lyases, hudroloses, isomerases, and ligases

Epimedium (Horny Goat Weed)

Pungent Herb

Epimedium grandiflorum

Epimedium contains Icariin, which acts on the PDE-5 enzyme, which breaks down cyclic guanosine monophosphate (cGMP). cGMP is necessary for an erection in men because it triggers the release of nitric oxide, which dilates genital blood vessels. Many men over forty have a cGMP deficiency due to excessive PDE-5 activity, resulting in nitric oxide deficiency and erectile dysfunction. Icariin inhibits PDE-5, thereby allowing nitric oxide release sufficient to maintain an erection. It also stimulates the production of osteoblasts, specialized cells involved in building bone mass. The flavonoids in horny goat weed are believed to stimulate the nerves, improving the sensation of touch.

Look for *epimedium* in *Male Performance* and *Testosterone Formulas*

Warnings: High doses of horny goat weed may result in breathing trouble, dizziness, vomiting or thirst and dry mouth.

Energetics: Warming, drying, and mildly relaxing

Used For: Arthritis, endurance, **erectile dysfunction**, fatigue, infertility, **sex drive (low)**, and testosterone (low)

Properties: Aphrodisiac and vasodilator

Equol   *Nutrient*

Equol is a substance produced from the isoflavone daidzein. The richest sources of daidzein are soy beans, fava beans and kudzu. Certain strains of intestinal bacteria transform daidzein into equol. Only about 25–30 percent of people in Western countries appear to be able to make this conversion as opposed to 50–60 percent of people from Asian countries like Japan, Korea and China.

Equol binds to dihydrotestosterone (DHT) a metabolite of testosterone that stimulates prostate growth. Excess DHT is believed to cause benign prostatic hyperplasia (BPH) as men grow older. Most drugs for BPH work by blocking the enzyme that converts testosterone to DHT. Unfortunately, this enzyme is also involved in numerous other body processes, so side effects are numerous. Equol simply prevents DHT from binding to the prostate. In addition to binding to DHT, equol also binds and acts as an agonist to the estrogen receptor beta, which down-regulates the androgen receptors

that DHT binds to, which further reduces the tendency of prostate cells to proliferate.

In addition to aiding BPH, research suggests that may be useful for menopausal symptoms and the prevention of estrogen-dependent cancers such as prostate cancer and breast cancer. One study suggested in may prevent breast cancer cells from proliferating.

Equol may be helpful for reducing BPH in men when taken regularly for three to six months, although some men may notice benefits within four to six weeks.

Warnings: Consult with a physician before taking Equol supplements with prescription prostate medications.

Used For: BPH, cancer prevention, hot flashes, menopause, prostatitis, and triglycerides (high)

Properties: Anti-inflammatory, anticancer, antioxidant, and vasodilator

Essiac Immune Tea Formula

See also *Alterative-Immune Formula*

This is a Native American formula for cancer that was given to Rene Caisse of Canada, a nurse who used it to help many people with cancer. She prepared it in a fresh liquid form and called it Essiac Tea (Essiac is Caisse spelled backward). Essiac is a blood purifier so it may also be helpful for eruptive skin diseases.

Warnings: Cancer is a serious illness. Do not rely on one herbal formula as your sole treatment. Consult a qualified practitioner and develop a complete health program.

Used For: Acne, **cancer**, cancer treatment side effects, congestion (lymphatic), **leukemia**, measles, and rashes & hives

Affects: Hypoactive immune activity, liver, lymphatics, spleen, and thymus

Take 2–4 capsules at bedtime or 2 capsules three times daily. It is best used in liquid form. Use 2 capsules in four ounces of hot water to make tea, or take capsules with warm water.

Ingredients: Burdock root extract, sheep sorrel aerial parts extract, slippery elm bark extract, and turkey rhubarb root extract

Eucalyptus EO   *Fresh & Woody Essential Oil*

Eucalyptus globulus

Eucalyptus EO has a refreshing, camphoric odor. It is opening, cleansing and refreshing, helping a person feel like they can breathe freely in life. It helps a person let go of negativity and the problems of the past and approach life with a renewed sense of hope, optimism and vigor. If you feel stifled or stuck in life the smell of eucalyptus can help you feel free and alive again.

Eucalyptus essential oil is best known for its expectorant properties. It reduces the swelling of mucous membranes and loosens phlegm to make breathing easier, while increasing oxygen supply to the body's cells. It can help with airborne staphylococci bacteria and is stimulating to the immune system. These properties make it very useful for colds and flu as well as sinus problems and throat infections. Eucalyptus is also helpful for pain of a cold cramping nature like muscle pain and neuralgia.

Emotionally, eucalyptus restores vitality and positive outlook and assists concentration. It dispels stagnant feelings that can keep one bound to a limiting environment. Relieving a sense of emotional suffocation, it helps one to achieve freedom and reduce fear and excessive caution.

See the strategy *Aromatherapy* for suggested uses.

Warnings: Do not use internally. Dilute for topical application.

Used For: Acne, arthritis, asthma, blisters, body odor, bronchitis, cloudy thinking, **colds (decongestant)**, concentration (poor), **congestion**, **congestion (lungs)**, congestion (sinus), COPD, **cough**, **cough (damp)**, croup, **diphtheria**, earache, fear, fleas, grief & sadness, herpes, infection (bacterial), infection prevention, **lice**, pain, pertussis, shingles, shock (medical), **sinus infection**, sore throat, tick, vaginitis, and wounds & sores

Properties: Analgesic, anti-inflammatory, antibacterial, antifungal, antirheumatic, **antiseptic**, antispasmodic, antiviral, balsamic, cicatrizant, decongestant, deodorant, diuretic, **expectorant**, febrifuge, hypoglycemic, nervine, rubefacient, vermifuge, and vulnerary

Eucommia *Mildly Acrid & Sweet Herb*
Eucommia ulmoides

Eucommia is a Chinese herb used to strengthen the liver and kidneys. It has a calming effect on the nerves and is indicated where there is weakness in the muscles of the back or lower extremities. It can also help with frequent urination and impotence.

Look for *eucommia* in *Chinese Qi* and *Blood Tonic*, *Chinese Water-Increasing*, and *Chinese Yin-Increasing Formulas*

Energetics: Cooling, moistening, and relaxing

Used For: Backache, erectile dysfunction, hypertension, kidney weakness/failure, and urination (frequent)

Properties: Kidney tonic and nervine

Evening Primrose *Oily Herb*
Oenothera biennis

Evening primrose oil is a source of gamma-linoleic acid (GLA), an important essential fatty acid that helps the immune system. See omega-3 GLA for more information.

Look for *evening primrose* in *GLA Oil Formula*

Usage: As a nutritional supplement use 1–2 capsules daily.

Energetics: Neutral, moistening, and nourishing

Used For: Alcoholism, arthritis, breast lumps, breasts (swelling/tenderness), cardiovascular disease, cystic breast disease, cystic fibrosis, dandruff, down syndrome, eczema, epilepsy, fat cravings, fibrosis, leucorrhea, menopause, menstrual irregularity, multiple sclerosis, neuralgia & neuritis, Parkinson's disease, PMS Type A, PMS Type C, PMS Type H, psoriasis, rosacea, schizophrenia, and vitiligo

Properties: Analgesic, anti-inflammatory, antiarthritic, anticholesteremic, anticoagulant, immune modulator, and nutritive

Eyebright *Astringent Herb*
Euphrasia officinalis

Eyebright is commonly used to treat eye infections and strengthen the eyes. Although it is often taken internally for these conditions, it works best when used as an eyewash. The best use of eyebright internally, however, is as an internal remedy for upper respiratory congestion involving acute irritation of the sinuses and eyes with thin, watery mucus and itching eyes and ears, such as rhinitis or the early stages of a cold. A tincture made from the fresh plant will open the Eustachian tubes in children, allowing the inner ear to drain and thus preventing earaches.

Look for *eyebright* in *Antihistamine*, *Herbal Eyewash*, and *Steven Horne's Anti-Allergy Formulas*

Warnings: Eyebright tinctures used as eye drops can cause increased eye pressure, redness, watering and swelling. When using it topically, use the tea.

Energetics: Cooling, drying, and mildly constricting

Used For: Allergies (respiratory), cataracts, colds (decongestant), conjunctivitis, **earache**, eye health, eyes (red/itching), eyes, bloodshot, **floaters**, glaucoma, nosebleeds, **rhinitis**, and **sty**

Properties: Anti-inflammatory, **antiallergenic**, anticatarrhal, astringent, expectorant, and **opthalmicum**

False Unicorn (Helonias)   *Bitter Herb*

Chamaelirium luteum

False unicorn appears to have a progesterone-enhancing effect. It is used as a female tonic to balance excess estrogen and has been used to help prevent miscarriage.

Look for *false unicorn* in *DHEA with Herbs* and *Prebirth Formulas*

Warnings: Not recommended with emaciation or inflammation.

Energetics: Cooling and moistening

Used For: Amenorrhea, **cystic breast disease**, dysmenorrhea, **endometriosis**, erectile dysfunction, **estrogen dominance**, fibroids (uterine), infertility, leucorrhea, lice, menopause, menorrhagia, **menstrual irregularity**, **miscarriage prevention**, morning sickness, nocturnal emission, **ovarian pain**, parasites (nematodes, worms), **PMS Type A**, and **progesterone (low)**

Properties: **Antiabortive**, diuretic, emmenagogue, **female tonic**, kidney tonic, and uterine tonic

Fat-Absorbing Fiber Formula

See also *Fiber Blend*

Helps to slow the absorption of fats in the intestines, reducing appetite and helping balance blood sugar. It also absorbs the cholesterol in bile, helping to reduce cholesterol levels. Being a fiber supplement it also helps cleanse the colon and balance gut microflora.

Warnings: May cause constipation without adequate hydration. Mucilants like psyllium and guar gum absorb a large amount of water.

Used For: **Cholesterol (high)**, excess weight, and fatty liver disease

Affects: Digestive atrophy, gallbladder, and small intestines

Take 4 capsules three times daily, drinking one glass of water before taking them with another glass of water.

Ingredients: Guar gum, psyllium hulls, and chickweed leaf extract

Fear-Reducing FE Blend

This is a blend of flower essences I formulated to help people to move through their fears and take the actions needed to overcome them. It is also useful for people who are overly dependent on the advice of others or the opinions of experts. It helps people to trust their own inner light and judgment. As they learn to make decisions for themselves and take action, they build greater self-confidence and self-esteem.

See the strategy *Flower Essence* for suggested uses.

Used For: Anxiety disorders, **apathy**, **bedwetting**, emotional sensitivity, **fear**, and **phobias**

Ingredients: Mountain pride FE, aspen FE, scleranthus FE, mimulus FE, cerato FE, blackberry FE, and red clover FE

Female Cycle Formula

See also *Female Tonic Formula*

This formula helps regulate excessive estrogen levels in the body. It may ease severe menstrual cramping or reduce excessive hormones in teenagers. It can be helpful for teenage acne caused by hormones. The formula may also help women who have been on birth control pills and are experiencing irregular cycles after discontinuing those pills.

Warnings: Chaste tree may reduce sexual desire, primarily in men. Women who are trying to get pregnant should avoid this formula (see wild yam). Avoid using while taking birth control pills or other female hormone replacement drugs. Very high doses could cause nausea, vomiting, and mild headache.

Used For: **Acne**, birth control side effects, **cramps (menstrual)**, dysmenorrhea, estrogen dominance, menopause, **menstrual irregularity**, nocturnal emission, **ovarian pain**, PMS, **PMS Type A**, **progesterone (low)**, **puberty**, and **sex drive (excessive)**

Affects: High estrogen, low progesterone, and pituitary (anterior)

Take 1-2 capsules with a meal twice daily.

Ingredients: Wild yam root extract and chaste tree berry extract

Female Tonic Formula

See also *Female Cycle Formula*

These formulas can help balance female hormones to normalize monthly cycles and help with the transition through menopause. They all help tone the uterus and have mild analgesic properties for menstrual pain. They may also aid liver and urinary function.

Warnings: Avoid during pregnancy or when trying to become pregnant or nursing.

Used For: Acne, amenorrhea, birth control side effects, breasts (swelling/tenderness), cramps (menstrual), **dysmenorrhea**, endometriosis, fibroids (uterine), hot flashes, infertility, menopause, nephritis, **PMS**, **PMS Type D**, postpartum depression, **puberty**, and vaginal dryness

Affects: High progesterone, **ovaries**, and uterus

Stan Malstrom's Female Balancing Formula

Contains black cohosh and dong quai, which support estrogen. Has mild analgesic and uterine toning properties.

Good formula for long term use. Typical dose is 1–2 capsules three times daily. Start with small dose (1–2 capsules a day) and work up to find best dose.

Ingredients: Red raspberry leaf, blessed thistle aerial parts, dong quai root, meadowsweet leaf, and black cohosh root & rhizome extract

Christopher's Female Tonic Formula

This blend does not contain black cohosh, but does have false unicorn, making it more progesterone enhancing. Good for PMS Type D. Typical dose is 1–2 capsules three times daily.

Ingredients: Goldenseal root, uva ursi leaf, cramp bark bark, blessed thistle aerial parts, and false unicorn root

Female Balancing Formula

Very similar action to Stan Malstrom's formula but stronger in action. Good for PMS Type A. Typical dose is 1–2 capsules three times daily. Start with small dose (1–2 capsules a day) and work up to find best dose.

Ingredients: Red raspberry leaf, dong quai root, black cohosh root, blessed thistle aerial parts, and meadowsweet leaf

Fennel   *Aromatic & Sweet Herb*

Foeniculum vulgare

Fennel is a wonderful carminative, commonly used in combination with catnip for colic. Catnip and fennel is an excellent remedy for colic, indigestion and diarrhea in infants and young children, as well as adults. Fennel, like most carminatives, stimulates digestion and reduces intestinal gas. It also helps to sweeten and increase breast milk.

Look for *fennel* in *Children's Colic, Christopher's Carminative, Christopher's Gallbladder, Herbal Bitters, Hypoglycemic, Irritable Bowel Fiber, Lactase Enzyme, Liver Cleanse,* and *Stimulant Laxative Formulas*

Warnings: Use with caution during pregnancy.

Energetics: Warming and drying

Used For: Belching, colic (children), dyspepsia, gas & bloating, indigestion, and lactose intolerance

Properties: Carminative, condiment, food, and galactagogue

Fennel EO   *Sweet Essential Oil*

Foeniculum vulgare

A sweet smelling oil with an earthy quality fennel is a good oil for those who are overly intellectual and/or constantly busy and need to become more grounded. Fennel is antispasmodic and carminative, making it a good remedy for gas, bloating, and stomach cramps. It also helps clear edema and lymphatic congestion.

See the strategy *Aromatherapy* for suggested uses.

Warnings: Dilute at least 20:1 for internal use. For example, use one drop in a tablespoon of honey. Do not use internally with children or pregnant women. Nontoxic and nonirritating for topical use. Avoid using with epilepsy.

Used For: Anxiety (situational), bites & stings, colic (adults), congestion (lungs), congestion (lymphatic), cough, diarrhea, digestion (poor), earache, **gas & bloating,** gout, **indigestion,** menopause, nursing, parasites, and urinary tract infections

Properties: Analgesic, antifungal, antiparasitic, antiseptic, **antispasmodic, carminative,** diuretic, emmenagogue, expectorant, galactagogue, and stomachic

Fenugreek   *Aromatic & Sweet Herb*

Trigonella foenum-graecum

Fenugreek encourages weight gain and is helpful for strengthening the body during convalescence. It helps to balance blood sugar and therefore may be helpful for diabetes. Fenugreek also helps to enrich breast milk in nursing mothers. It is a soothing remedy for ulcers, burns, abscesses and other injuries. Used with thyme it helps decongest the sinuses.

Look for *fenugreek* in *Blood Sugar Control, Jeannie Burgess' Allergy-Lung, Lung Moistening, Sinus, Vein Tonic,* and *Vulnerary Formulas*

Warnings: Avoid during pregnancy.

Energetics: Warming and drying

Used For: Congestion, **congestion (sinus),** cough (dry), **croup,** cystic fibrosis, diabetes, dyspepsia, emphysema, **headache (sinus),** metabolic syndrome, **nursing,** pleurisy, polycystic ovarian syndrome, **sinus infection,** smell (loss of), and **snoring**

Properties: Antidiabetic, condiment, decongestant, galactagogue, and hypolipidemic

Feverfew   *Bitter Herb*

Tanacetum parthenium

Feverfew is a very popular natural remedy for migraine headaches. It doesn't work very well once the migraine has started, but taken regularly it helps to prevent migraines and lessen their severity. It has anti-inflammatory properties and its name comes from its traditional use as a remedy for fevers. It is applied topically to aid rosacea and psoriasis.

Look for *feverfew* in *Headache* and *Jeannie Burgess' Stress Formulas*

Warnings: Avoid during pregnancy. If mouth soreness or ulcerations develop, reduce dosage or discontinue use. It does not work on migraine headaches caused by weakness or deficiency (i.e., anemia).

Energetics: Cooling and drying

Used For: Allergies (respiratory), **fever**, **headache (migraine)**, inflammation, **psoriasis**, **rosacea**, and vaccine side effects

Properties: Analgesic, anthelmintic, anti-inflammatory, antibacterial, **anticephalalgic**, carminative, diuretic, emmenagogue, **febrifuge**, insecticide, nervine, stomachic, and vermifuge

Fiber Blend

See also *Irritable Bowel Fiber Formula*

A blend of various plant fibers can be beneficial for colon health. Fiber absorbs toxins in the colon, reduces cholesterol, slows absorption of nutrients that balances blood sugar and reduces hunger, and helps feed friendly bacteria. Best times to take fiber are on an empty stomach, such as first thing in the morning, at least half an hour before meals.

Fiber can be taken in water or juice, but citrus juices are not recommended. Try apple or grape juice. Drink quickly after stirring fiber into the liquid. It gels and becomes undrinkable. Drink six to eight glasses of water per day when taking a fiber supplement.

If you have a dry stool, try mixing the fiber blend with equal parts freshly ground flax, hemp, or chia seeds. This helps moisten and lubricate the bowels. If you have a lot of colon problems you can also mix a fiber blend with equal parts *triphalia*, which tones and improves colon health.

Warnings: May cause constipation without adequate hydration. Long-term use can weaken digestion unless you also take some ginger, capsicum or other aromatic stomachic herbs occasionally. When taking fiber, start with a small amount and slowly increase it as your body adapts to it.

Used For: Cancer treatment side effects, chemical exposure, cholera, **cholesterol (high)**, colon (atonic), **constipation (adults)**, **diarrhea**, fatty liver disease, fibromyalgia, heavy metal poisoning, **hemorrhoids**, inflammatory bowel disorders, and prolapsed colon

Affects: Gallbladder, intestinal atrophy, large intestines (colon), rectum, and small intestines

Three Fiber Blend

This is a blend of three fibers. It is less harsh than the *Psyllium Hulls Fiber Blend* and is also good for lowering cholesterol Take 1/2 teaspoon to 1 tablespoon and mix in a small glass of water or juice.

Ingredients: Psyllium hulls, apple pectin, and oat bran

Cholesterol Lowering Fiber Blend

This blend was designed primarily to lower cholesterol. It is the gentlest of the three formulas and most suitable for people with irritable bowels. Add 1 tablespoon to 8 ounces of liquid, stir, and drink immediately.

Ingredients: Psyllium hulls, apple fiber, gum arabic, flax seed, guar gum, and oat bran

Psyllium Hulls Fiber Blend

This formula is mostly psyllium. It's the strongest of the fiber supplements and useful for atonic colons. Take 1/2 teaspoon to 1 tablespoon and mix in a small glass of water or juice.

Ingredients: Psyllium seed & husk and licorice root

Fibromyalgia Formula

Both chronic fatigue syndrome and fibromyalgia seem to be caused when the body fails to produce ATP (adenosine triphosphate). ATP is generally formed from the energy in foods. When foods are broken down, the vitamins, minerals and coenzymes provide electrical charges to carry out enzymatic reactions. Once this step occurs, ATP is made and energy is released.

Malic acid is a fruit acid mostly found in apples and it plays an important role in ATP production in low oxygen conditions. When malic acid is combined with magnesium, it provides fuel that generates energy to operate the body. (See *magnesium* for more information.)

Used For: **Cramps & spasms**, Epstein-Barr virus, **fibromyalgia**, and **tremors**

Affects: General constriction, hyperactive immune activity, **muscles**, nerve constriction (tension), and **structural constriction**

Take 2 capsules twice per day, with meals.

Ingredients: Magnesium and malic acid

Fir EO   *Fresh & Woody Essential Oil*

Abies alba

Fir EO is applied topically to ease muscle or joint pain. It can be inhaled to reduce mucus in the respiratory passages, but is contraindicated with asthma and whooping cough. Emotionally, it eases anxiety and stress, aids clairity of mind and spirit and produces a sense of strength and protection. It is both grounding and uplifting, promoting a greater sense of inner wholeness.

See the strategy *Aromatherapy* for suggested uses.

Warnings: Do not use internally. Topically it is nonirritating and nonsensitizing and may be used neat (undiluted).

Used For: Arthritis, bronchitis, circulation (poor), cough, fatigue, fever, fever, and pain

Properties: Analgesic, anti-inflammatory, anticancer, antimicrobial, antioxidant, antirheumatic, antiseptic, antispasmodic, deodorant, disinfectant, expectorant, rubefacient, and stimulant (circulatory)

Fire Cider Formula

This is a great cold and flu remedy originally developed by Rosemary Gladstar. There are companies that sell various versions of it. You can also make-it-yourself. Directions can be found in the book *Modern Herbal Dispensatory*.

Used For: Colds, flu, and infection (viral)

Affects: Circulatory depression, lungs, **respiratory depression**, **respiratory stagnation**, sinuses, and sweat glands

Take 1/2 to 1 teaspoon with warm water at the first sign of colds or flu. Continue taking every one to two hours with lots of water until you feel better.

1/2 cup Horseradish root
1 medium Onion
1/2 cup Ginger root
1/4 cup Garlic
2 Jalepeno peppers
1 whole Lemon zest & juice
2 tablespoons Rosemary

Flax *Oily Herb*

Linum usitatissimum

Freshly ground flax seed is amazingly healing to an inflamed gut. It is a stool softener and bulk laxative for chronic constipation. Flax lignans are phytoestrogens and may be helpful in preventing estrogen-dependent cancers. Flax seed oil is a vegetarian source of omega-3 and omega-6 fatty acids. The oil is also a good supplement for pets.

Look for *flax* in *Fiber, Gut-Healing Fiber, Irritable Bowel Fiber, Phytoestrogen Breast,* and *Whole Food Green Drink Formulas*

Warnings: Flax sees oxidize very rapidly after being ground. Fresh flax seeds are best. Keep oil refrigerated.

Usage: As a nutritional supplement, take 1–2 soft gels of flax seed oil three times daily with meals. Use oil for salads or other food, but not for cooking.

Energetics: Cooling, moistening, and nourishing

Used For: Cholesterol (high), **constipation (adults)**, **constipation (children)**, cough (dry), eczema, estrogen (low),

failure to thrive, pet supplements, psoriasis, and **skin (dry/flaky)**

Properties: Food, **laxative (bulk)**, **moistening**, nutritive, and phytoestrogen

Flu and Vomiting Formula

See also *Children's Colic Formula*

Use this to help settle the stomach and fight infection when you have the flu. It can also be helpful for colds.

Warnings: Capsicum and ginger may be irritating to sensitive stomachs.

Used For: Colds, **flu**, indigestion, motion sickness, and **nausea & vomiting**

Affects: Digestive stagnation, pancreas head, and stomach

Use 2-4 capsules every hour to help settle the stomach during acute flu, nausea, vomiting. For colds, use 2 capsules every two hours with a large glass of water until you start to feel better.

Ingredients: Ginger rhizome, capsicum fruit, goldenseal root extract, and licorice root

Folic Acid **see** *vitamin B*$_9$

Forsythia *Bitter Herb*

Forsythia suspensa

The fruit of forsythia is a cooling remedy used in Chinese herbalism for inflammatory diseases and high fevers.

Look for *forsythia* in *Chinese Yang-Reducing Formula*

Energetics: Cooling

Used For: Abscesses, chills, fever, headache, sore throat, swollen lymph glands, and ulcers

Properties: Anti-inflammatory, antibacterial, antiviral, detoxifying, detoxifying, and diuretic

Frankincense EO

Balsamic, Spicy, Sweet, & Woody Essential Oil
Boswellia carteri

This oil has a turpentine-like odor that is refreshing and uplifting. It eases feelings of stress and muscle tension, helping someone to relax and breathe freely. It has been traditionally used to help purify a person's environment, driving away negative or dark feelings. It helps people with poor self-esteem to feel less vulnerable. It helps reduce mental chatter, calm the mind, cut ties with the past and become more present and focused. For these reasons it has been considered a valuable aid to prayer and meditation.

Frankincense essential oil is effective for respiratory problems. It eases stress and strengthens the immune system.

Frankincense has been applied topically to help shrink tumors or lumps, especially in the breasts. It has also been massaged over the ovaries to ease ovarian inflammation and pain during menses. It acts as a uterine tonic.

Emotionally it slows down breathing and produces feelings of calm. Possessing an elevating and soothing effect on the mind, frankincense allows the consciousness to expand. It works well with anxious and obsessive states linked to worrying about the past and is a strong support tool for agitation, worry, or conditions where the mind is distracted and overwhelmed by a multitude of thoughts.

See the strategy *Aromatherapy* for suggested uses.

Warnings: Do not use internally. Topically it is nonirritating and nonsensitizing and may be used neat (undiluted).

Used For: Aging, aneurysm, anxiety disorders, apathy, arthritis, asthma, autism, bipolar mood disorder, **breast lumps**, breasts (swelling/tenderness), cancer, cirrhosis of the liver, confusion, COPD, cystic breast disease, dementia, depression, **eczema**, electromagnetic pollution, **fear**, fibroids (uterine), grief & sadness, hepatitis, **infection prevention**, inflammation, irritability, laryngitis, menorrhagia, nightmares, ovarian pain, pain, PMS Type H, PTSD, scars/scar tissue, sinus infection, skin (oily), trauma, ulcers, and whiplash

Properties: Antimicrobial, antiseptic, carminative, cicatrizant, disinfectant, diuretic, emmenagogue, expectorant, immune stimulant, preservative, sedative, uterine, uterine tonic, and vulnerary

Fringe Tree   *Bitter Herb*

Chionanthus virginicus

A bitter tonic with blood purifying, laxative and mild diuretic actions, fringetree is my favorite gallbladder remedy. It stimulates bile flow and helps relieve intestinal gas, bloating and a stuffy feeling under the right rib cage. It is one of the best herbs for gallstones, especially when combined with other liver/gallbladder herbs like wild yam, turmeric, dandelion, barberry and milk thistle.

Warnings: Do not use with bile duct obstruction or pregnancy.

Energetics: Cooling and drying

Used For: Appetite (deficient), cholesterol (high), **fat cravings**, **fat metabolism (poor)**, **gallbladder problems**, **gallstones**, jaundice (adults), skin (dry/flaky), and triglycerides (low)

Properties: Anticholesteremic and **cholagogue**

Fritillary   *Sweet and Mildly Bitter Herb*

Fritillaria thumbergii

Fritillary bulbs are used in Chinese herbalism for dry conditions of the lungs, swollen lymph glands and abscesses. They have a cough suppressing action and are especially helpful for dry cough.

Look for *fritillary* in *Chinese Metal-Decreasing* and *Dry Cough Syrup Formulas*

Warnings: Raw, unprocessed herb is toxic and should not be taken internally.

Energetics: Cooling, moistening, and nourishing

Used For: Abscesses, **cough (dry)**, and swollen lymph glands

Properties: Antitussive, decongestant, expectorant, lymphatic, and mucilant

GABA   *Amino Acid*

GABA (Gamma-Amino Butyric Acid) is an amino acid that acts as a major calming neurotransmitter in the brain. It is an inhibitory neurotransmitter, which means it inhibits overactivity of nerve cells in the brain. GABA plays a critical role in normalizing the nervous system. Proper levels of this amino acid in the brain contribute to motor control and vision and calm the mind, reducing anxiety, fear, hyperactivity, and stress-related sleep disorders. Many people with anxiety, insomnia, epilepsy, and other brain disorders do not manufacture sufficient levels of GABA.

Research has shown that GABA increases the production of alpha brain waves (a state often achieved by meditation, characterized by being relaxed with greater mental focus and mental alertness) and reduces beta waves (associated with nervousness, scattered thoughts, and hyperactivity). GABA also increases mental clarity, while reducing the effects of stress. Valium, Xanax, and other benzodiazepene drugs mimic or bind to GABA receptors and have a calming effect but are addicting, while GABA is not.

Warnings: Avoid during pregnancy.

Usage: 50–200 mg, three times a day.

Used For: **ADD/ADHD**, **addictions (drugs)**, **anxiety attacks**, **anxiety disorders**, concentration (poor), **epilepsy**, fear, **insomnia**, mental illness, Parkinson's disease, PTSD, restless dreams, **schizophrenia**, and **seizures**

Properties: **Anxiolytic**, calmative, gaba-enhancing, and soporific

Galangal   *Pungent Herb*

Alpinia galanga

Both greater and lesser galangal are used in Chinese herbalism to disperse cold, relieve pain, and strengthen digestion.

Energetics: Warming

Used For: Diarrhea, indigestion, and nausea & vomiting
Properties: Analgesic and stomachic

Gamma Linolenic Acid   see *omega-6 GLA*

Garcinia (Brindleberry)   *Sour Herb*

Garcinia cambogia

Animal research suggests that this herb can control the appetite by activating fatty acid oxidation in the liver due to an ingredient called hydroxycitric acid. Based on this research the herb is used in formulas to control appetite, aid weight loss and stabilize blood sugar. Unfortunately, very little research has been done demonstrating garcinia has the ability to promote weight loss in human beings. However, garcinia has also been shown to reduce LDL cholesterol and triglycerides and promote HDL cholesterol.

Look for *garcinia* in *Garcinia Fat-Burning Formula*

Energetics: Cooling

Used For: Appetite (excessive), cholesterol (high), excess weight, fatty tumors/deposits, hypoglycemia, and triglycerides (high)

Properties: Anticholesteremic and appetite suppressant

Garcinia Fat-Burning Formula

This formula aids weight loss. It helps to control appetite and aid the body in burning fat. This formula may help to prevent the formation of arterial plaque and be of some benefit in cardiovascular disease and fatty congestion of the liver.

Used For: Appetite (excessive), cardiovascular disease, cholesterol (high), **excess weight**, fatty tumors/deposits, and triglycerides (high)

Affects: Heart

Take 2 capsules 30 minutes before a meal three times daily.

Ingredients: Chromium, garcinia fruit rind extract, chickweed aerial parts, and L-carnitine

Gardenia   *Bitter Herb*

Gardenia jasminoidis

A cooling remedy used in Chinese herbalism for reducing high fever which produces insomnia and delirium. It has been called the happiness herb because it relieves irritability.

Look for *gardenia* in *Chinese Yang-Reducing Formula*

Energetics: Cooling and drying

Used For: Blood in urine, canker sores, copper toxicity, **fever**, insomnia, irritability, jaundice (adults), mastitis, nosebleeds, and tonsillitis

Properties: Anti-inflammatory, antibacterial, antifungal, cholagogue, febrifuge, and hypotensive

Garlic   *Pungent Herb*

Allium sativum

Garlic has been called nature's penicillin. It is a strong aromatic herb with powerful antibiotic, antifungal, and antiviral action. It acts as an expectorant to expel phlegm from the lungs and as a circulatory tonic to lower high blood pressure and prevent arteriosclerosis. It is also helpful for parasites.

For hypertension (high blood pressure) and/or high cholesterol, it must be taken daily for at least three to six months. For fighting infections, freshly crushed garlic is the best, with the *Stabilized Allicin Formula* being the second best form. Garlic oil is also useful for infections.

Garlic extracted in a vegetable oil can be rubbed on the chest and back to relieve lung congestion. The warm oil can also be dropped into the ears and/or rubbed on the ears and sides of the neck to help relieve earaches.

Garlic is useful in enemas for reducing fevers, relieving respiratory congestion, earaches, infection and worms. For a garlic enema, blend one chopped clove in one pint of warm water or use six to eight capsules and steep as tea for three to five minutes. Strain before using.

Look for *garlic* in *Antiparasitic, Circulatory, Ear Drop, Fire Cider, Heart Health,* and *Stabilized Allicin Formulas*

Warnings: Not for feeble, emaciated or wasting conditions. Gastric irritation is possible; eat or take with food to lessen this effect.

Energetics: Warming and drying

Used For: AIDS, altitude sickness, antibiotic resistance, antibiotic side effects, arsenic poisoning, arteriosclerosis, athlete's foot, blood clot prevention, blood poisoning, bronchitis, cancer, chills, cholera, cholesterol (high), circulation (poor), cold hands/feet, colds, colds (antiviral), colds (decongestant), colds with fever, congestion, **congestion (lungs)**, congestion (lymphatic), corns, **cough, cough (damp)**, diabetes, diarrhea, **diphtheria**, dyspepsia, **earache**, emphysema, fever, flu, food poisoning, **gangrene**, gas & bloating, gonorrhea, **hypertension**, hypotension, **infection (bacterial)**, infection (fungal), **infection (viral)**, infection prevention, **insect repellant**, interstitial cystitis, itchy ears, jock itch, lead poisoning, leucorrhea, lupus, lyme disease, mercury poisoning, mumps, mumps, overalkalinity, **parasites**, parasites (nematodes, worms), **pertussis**, pet supplements, **pneumonia, rheumatic fever**, scabies, SIBO, **sore throat**, staph infections, strep throat, swollen lymph glands, thrombosis, tick, tinnitus, tonsillitis, **toothache**, **tuberculosis**, vaginitis, and **warts**

Properties: **Anthelmintic**, antiamebic, **antibacterial**, anticholesteremic, anticoagulant, antidiabetic, antifungal, antilipemic, antimicrobial, **antiparasitic**, **antiseptic**, antithrombotic, antiviral, aphrodisiac, cardiac, carminative, cholagogue, condiment, dacryagogue, **decongestant**, **diaphoretic**, **expectorant**, febrifuge, food, hypertensive, hypolipidemic, **hypotensive**, lung tonic, lymphatic, pectoral, preservative, pulmonary, **stimulant (circulatory)**, stimulant (metabolic), stomachic, vasodilator, and **vermifuge**

Gastrodia   *Sweet Herb*

Gastrodia elata

Gastrodia rhizome is a sweet herb that enters the liver meridian in Chinese herbalism. It helps control pain and invigorate the meridians. It can ease headache, convulsions, and pain.

Energetics: Relaxing, mildly warming, and drying

Used For: Dizziness, epilepsy, and pain

Properties: Analgesic, antiepileptic, antispasmodic, and cholagogue

General Analgesic Formula

See also *Analgesic Nerve Formula* and *Stan Malstrom's Herbal Aspirin Formula*

A natural pain relief formula for reducing inflammation and easing minor aches and pains.

Used For: Arthritis, headache, inflammation, injuries, and **pain**

Affects: Joints, muscles, and nerve irritation (pain)

Take two capsules twice daily for arthritis and other chronic aches and pains. For acute injuries or acute pain take 2-5 capsules.

Ingredients: Hops cone extract, turmeric root extract, willow bark extract, boswellia gum extract, mangosteen pericarp, phellodendron bark, dl-plenylalanine, and andrographis whole plant

General Glandular Formula

This is a general glandular supplement containing herbs for each gland in a base of vitamins and minerals. This formula is useful as an overall glandular tonic.

Used For: Acne, ADD/ADHD, hot flashes, **infertility**, labor & delivery, myasthenia gravis, progesterone (low), and vitiligo

Affects: Pituitary (anterior)

Take 1-2 capsules three times daily.

Ingredients: Vitamin A, vitamin C, vitamin E, pantothenic acid, zinc, manganese, potassium, licorice root, alfalfa aerial parts, black walnut hulls, thyme leaf, eleuthero root, kelp leaf & stem, and schisandra fruit

Gentian   *Strongly Bitter Herb*

Gentiana lutea

This intensely bitter herb is commonly used to stimulate digestive system function. It is often combined with other bitters and carminatives for this purpose. It is best taken in liquid form prior to meals.

Look for *gentian* in *Chinese Metal-Increasing*, *Detoxifying*, and *Lipase Enzyme Formulas*

Warnings: Do not use during pregnancy or acute GI inflammation.

Energetics: Cooling and drying

Used For: **Acid indigestion**, anemia, **anorexia**, **appetite (deficient)**, belching, bulimia, cystic breast disease, cysts, **digestion (poor)**, endometriosis, fat cravings, gallbladder problems, **gas & bloating**, **indigestion**, **low stomach acid**, and triglycerides (low)

Properties: Alterative, antacid, anthelmintic, antiseptic, aperitive, **digestive tonic**, and **stimulant (appetite)**

Gentle Bowel Cleansing Formula

See also *Triphala Formula*

This is an effective alternative to herbal stimulant laxatives. It helps to hydrate the colon and improve bowel tone to promote natural elimination. It can be used to wean someone off of stimulant laxatives and restore normal tone to the colon. The key ingredient is magnesium hydroxide, a salt of magnesium that attracts water to the bowel. This helps hydrate the stool and make it easier to pass. It also contains a blend of three herbs used in Ayurvedic medicine called triphala. (See *triphala* for more information.)

It is a safe bowel formula for people who are suffering from inflammatory diseases. It is also safe for pregnancy. Take the formula with plenty of water. It also works well with marshmallow, slippery elm, or other soft fibers for irritable and inflammatory bowel disorders.

Used For: **Anal fistula/fissure**, celiac disease, **colitis**, **colon (atonic)**, **colon (spastic)**, **constipation (adults)**, **constipation (children)**, diverticulitis, hemorrhoids, inflammatory bowel disorders, **irritable bowel**, **leaky gut**, and **prolapsed colon**

Affects: Intestinal atrophy, intestinal depression, **large intestines (colon)**, and **small intestines**

A safe long-term dose (for maintenance of normal bowel function) is 2 capsules once or twice daily. People who have serious constipation problems or have become dependent on stimulant laxatives for normal bowel function will need to start with a higher dose, about 6-9 capsules daily. This could be 2-3 capsules three times daily or 3-4 capsules twice daily (morning and evening are best). As bowel function improves, the dose can be reduced.

Ingredients: Magnesium, triphala, and yellow dock root

Geranium EO

Floral, Fresh, & Sweet Essential Oil

Pelagonium graveolens

Geranium EO has a stimulating effect on the adrenal cortex and a regulatory effect on the hormonal system. It helps with PMS and menopausal problems such as depression, lack of vaginal secretion and heavy periods. It may even be helpful with infertility. As a lymphatic stimulant it helps relieve congestion, fluid retention and swollen extremities. Geranium also reduces inflammation, relaxes nerves and calms feelings of anxiety. With both analgesic and antispasmodic properties, it is useful for nerve, eye, and joint pain.

Emotionally, geranium works for chronic and acute anxiety where there is stress due to feeling overworked. It is ideal for workaholics and those with perfectionist attitudes. Ideal for someone who has forgotten imagination, intuition and sensory experience, it reconnects one to a feeling for life.

See the strategy *Aromatherapy* for suggested uses.

Warnings: Do not use internally. Don't use with oily skin conditions. Avoid with anxiety, high stress levels, and estrogen dominant PMS Type A.

Used For: Adrenal fatigue, AIDS, amenorrhea, anorexia, apathy, breasts (swelling/tenderness), cancer, capillary weakness, confusion, congestion (lymphatic), dermatitis, diarrhea, dysmenorrhea, eczema, edema, **estrogen (low)**, fatty liver disease, fatty tumors/deposits, gallbladder problems, gastritis, hot flashes, impetigo, infertility, inflammation, **insect repellant**, jaundice (adults), kidney stones, menopause, menorrhagia, mood swings, nosebleeds, PMS Type A, **skin (dry/flaky)**, skin (oily), **tick**, vaginal dryness, varicose veins, whiplash, and wounds & sores

Properties: Analgesic, anti-inflammatory, antidepressant, antiseptic, antiviral, anxiolytic, astringent, cicatrizant, decongestant, deodorant, diuretic, hemostatic, relaxant, stimulant (metabolic), styptic, tonic, uterine tonic, vermifuge, and vulnerary

Ginger   *Pungent Herb*

Zingiber officinale

A pungent aromatic, ginger is used to relieve nausea, vomiting and motion sickness. Take capsules or extract before traveling to prevent motion sickness. Taken with or after meals it stimulates digestive secretions. Research indicates that ginger root also enhances immune function, promotes the secretion of bile and gastric fluids and increases blood circulation by inhibiting platelet aggregation. It may also reduce pain and inflammation associated with arthritis and ulcerative colitis. It is very helpful for treating colds and chills.

Look for *ginger* in *Christopher's Carminative, Circulatory, Ed Millet's Herbal Crisis, Fire Cider, Flu* and *Vomiting, Herbal Arthritis, Herbal Composition,* and *Stimulant Laxative Formulas*

Warnings: Use with caution during pregnancy, but no adverse effects have been reported by women using ginger for morning sickness.

Energetics: Warming and drying

Used For: Altitude sickness, amenorrhea, burning feet/hands, cancer treatment side effects, chills, **circulation (poor)**, **cold hands/feet**, colds, congestion (lungs), cough (damp), diarrhea, diverticulitis, **dizziness, dysmenorrhea**, dyspepsia, fever, **flu**, food allergies/intolerances, **gas & bloating**, headache (migraine), indigestion, lactose intolerance, **morning sickness, motion sickness, nausea & vomiting**, perspiration (deficient), **PMS Type P**, Raynaud's disease, shock (medical), **SIBO**, toothache, and ulcers

Properties: Analgesic, antacid, **antiemetic**, antihistamine, antinausa, antioxidant, aperient, aperitive, **carminative**, catalyst, condiment, counterirritant, **diaphoretic**, digestive tonic, hypotensive, nervine, sialogogue, **stimulant (circulatory)**, stimulant (metabolic), and **stomachic**

Ginkgo   *Mildly Bitter & Mildly Sour Herb*

Ginkgo biloba

Extensive research has been conducted in Europe using concentrated extracts of the flavonoids in this herb. This is one herb that is best used as a standardized extract. Ginkgo is commonly used to enhance memory and brain function. It improves blood flow to the brain and acts as an antioxidant to protect brain cells from damage. It also improves peripheral circulation and may be beneficial in diabetic retinopathy, tinnitus, vertigo, and dizziness. Best results are obtained when the herb is used consistently for two to three months. Ginkgo is an excellent remedy to take to slow the aging process and protect the nervous and cardiovascular systems.

Look for *ginkgo* in *Brain* and *Memory Protection, Brain-Heart, Memory Enhancing,* and *Vein Tonic Formulas*

Warnings: Use with caution when taking blood thinners. Some authors advise caution during pregnancy, but the herb appears safe. Consult a professional herbalist (findanherbalist.com) for advice.

Energetics: Mildly cooling and balancing

Used For: Age spots, aging, **altitude sickness**, **Alzheimer's**, angina, arteriosclerosis, autism, **blood clot prevention**, **cardiovascular disease**, **circulation (brain)**, circulation (poor), cloudy thinking, cold hands/feet, concentration (poor), confusion, **dementia**, depression, diabetic retinopathy, **dizziness**, down syndrome, easily bruised, erectile dysfunction, free radical damage, glaucoma, headache (migraine), **hearing loss**, heart valves, heart weakness, **hypertension**, irritability, **macular degeneration**, **memory/brain function**, Ménière's disease, mental illness, multiple sclerosis, narcolepsy, numbness, Parkinson's disease, **Raynaud's disease**, **strokes**, thrombosis, **tinnitus**, traumatic brain injury, tremors, varicose veins, and wheezing

Properties: Anti-inflammatory, **antiaging**, antiallergenic, **anticoagulant**, antioxidant, antithrombotic, **cephalalgic**, **cerebral tonic**, hypotensive, serotonergic, tonic, vascular tonic, and **vasodilator**

Ginseng, American   *Sweet Herb*

Panax quinquefolius

American ginseng is used as a tonic for strengthening the overall system, improving stamina and resistance to disease. It helps counteract the effects of aging and improves overall health when taken in very small doses. American ginseng is less stimulating than Asian (Korean) ginseng. It helps regulate blood sugar, improves digestion, helps the body cope better with stress, and strengthens adrenal and general glandular function.

Look for *ginseng (American)* in *Adaptogen Formula*

Warnings: Should not be taken by persons with high blood pressure, fevers, acute inflammation, and acute diseases like colds and flu. Large doses can cause insomnia and nervous over stimulation.

Usage: American ginseng works best in small doses—15-30 drops of the tincture or 1 capsule daily.

Energetics: Cooling and moistening

Used For: Addictions (coffee, caffeine), **aging**, ALS, body building, cancer, cardiovascular disease, cloudy thinking, debility, depression, diabetes, digestion (poor), **endurance**, erectile dysfunction, excess weight, exercise (performance), fatigue, fear, hypertension, **hypotension**, **infertility**, metabolic syndrome, poison ivy/oak, protein digestion, radiation, sex drive (low), stress, testosterone (low), underweight, and wasting

Properties: Adaptogen, adrenal tonic, androgenic, antidiabetic, antioxidant, aphrodisiac, cardiac, cholinergic, hypertensive, immune stimulant, nervine, panacea, **spleen chi tonic**, stimulant (metabolic), and **tonic**

Ginseng, Asian/Korean   *Sweet Herb*

Panax ginseng

Ginseng is one of the most highly prized herbs in the world. Asian or Korean ginseng has been shown to increase energy, help fight fatigue and increase physical stamina and agility. It may even enhance the body's ability to recover from physical injuries. Small doses of ginseng are used to slow aging, reduce stress, balance mood and enhance a person's general health. Ginseng may lower the risk of cancer and build up a weakened immune system. Asian ginseng is more warming than American ginseng and is well-suited to older men and women who tend to be cold, pale and easily fatigued. Red ginseng, which is steamed before drying, is more warming in energy, while white ginseng, which is just peeled and dried, is more neutral in energy.

Look for *ginseng (Asian/Korean)* in *Adaptogen-Immune, Chinese Earth-Increasing, Chinese Fire-Decreasing, Chinese Qi* and *Blood Tonic, Chinese Qi-Increasing, DHEA with Herbs, Myelin Sheath,* and *Testosterone Formulas*

Warnings: Contraindicated in acute diseases, high fevers or inflammation.

Energetics: Warming and moistening

Used For: Addictions (coffee, caffeine), addictions (drugs), **aging**, ALS, body building, cancer, cardiovascular disease, debility, depression, diabetes, dysmenorrhea, **endurance**, erectile dysfunction, exercise (performance), fatigue, hypertension, hypotension, infertility, jet lag, metabolic syndrome, poison ivy/oak, premature ejaculation, radiation, sex drive (low), stress, and **testosterone (low)**

Properties: Adaptogen, **androgenic**, antiaging, antioxidant, **aphrodisiac**, blood building, cardiac, cholinergic, hypertensive, immune stimulant, nervine, panacea, stimulant (metabolic), sympathomimetic, and tonic

GLA Oil Blend

The three oils in this blend are all high in the omega-6 essential fatty acids, linoleic acid and gamma-linolenic acid (GLA). These oils are used in the creation of eicosanoids that play essential roles in maintaining normal blood pressure and body weight, and in reducing platelet aggregation and inflammation. (See *omega-3 GLA* for more information.)

Warnings: In the presence of high insulin levels and a lack of omega-3 essential fatty acids, however, GLA is converted into eicosanoids that are pro-inflammatory and have opposing effects to the benefits listed above. So it is also important to obtain adequate omega-3 in the diet and to avoid refined carbohydrates for maximum effects.

Used For: Age spots, appetite (excessive), bipolar mood disorder, burning feet/hands, cradle cap, dandruff, dermatitis, down syndrome, eczema, endometriosis, epilepsy, fat cravings, food allergies/intolerances, leucorrhea, lupus, memory/brain function, **menopause**, menstrual irregularity, multiple sclerosis, nerve damage, neuralgia & neuritis, Parkinson's disease, **PMS**, psoriasis, restless leg, seborrhea, skin (dry/flaky), vaginal dryness, vitiligo, and wrinkles

Affects: Central nervous system, general atrophy, intestinal atrophy, nails, and prostaglandins

Normal dose is 1 capsule three times daily with food.

Ingredients: Evening primrose oil, black currant oil, borage oil, and gamma linolenic acid (gla)

Glucosamine *Nutrient*

Glucosamine is an amino acid/sugar substance used by the body to produce connective tissues. The supplement is derived from crab shells. Research done on glucosamine showed that glucosamine sulfate brings relief from joint tenderness, swelling, and pain. In tests, people who took at least one gram a day of glucosamine salts, chondroitin sulfates, or glucosamine sulfate found a dramatic relief from the pain of osteoarthritis. Not only did they have less pain, but the studies showed that the connective tissues gained the ability of self-healing. Even after the patients stopped taking these supplements, the relief continued for another six to twelve weeks. In several clinical trials where glucosamine sulfate was compared to NSAIDs, long-term reductions in pain were greater in patients receiving glucosamine sulfate.

Warnings: May irritate ulcers if not taken with food. Do not take if you have an allergy to shellfish.

Usage: 500–1,000 mg three times daily.

Used For: Arthritis, arthritis (rheumatoid), backache, inflammation, overalkalinity, and TMJ

Properties: Anti-inflammatory, **antiarthritic**, tonic, and vulnerary

Goldenrod *Bitter & Pungent Herb*

Solidago canadensis

A useful diuretic for urinary tract problems, obstructions, kidney stones and inflammation, goldenrod is very soothing and healing. It is also helpful for hay fever and allergies to cats. It can be helpful for upper respiratory infections and yeast infections like thrush.

Look for *goldenrod* in *Blood Pressure Reducing, Liquid Kidney,* and *Steven Horne's Anti-Allergy Formulas*

Warnings: Not for use with edema from kidney failure.

Energetics: Warming and drying

Used For: Allergies (respiratory), **edema**, food allergies/intolerances, kidney stones, **kidney weakness/failure**, and **urinary tract infections**

Properties: Anti-inflammatory, antiseptic, **diuretic**, and **kidney tonic**

Goldenseal *Bitter & Mildly Astringent Herb*

Hydrastis canadensis

Goldenseal is a natural antibiotic and immune stimulant with diuretic and antibiotic properties, making it useful in urinary and digestive tract infections. It is particularly helpful for sub acute inflammation of the respiratory, digestive or urinary mucous membranes. It lowers blood sugar and stimulates digestion. It is a specific remedy for amoebic dysentery (giardia). Topically, it heals injuries. It has been used as a wash for sore red eyes and as a topical application for canker sores. Goldenseal has been over harvested and other herbs should be used as substitutes where possible. Coptis root, Oregon grape, and barberry all contain berberine alkaloids and have similar antimicrobial properties.

Look for *goldenseal* in *Antibacterial, Antihistamine, Blood Sugar Control, Christopher's Sinus, Ed Millet's Herbal Crisis, Female Tonic, Flu* and *Vomiting, Herbal Eyewash, Herbal Tooth Powder, Lymphatic Infection, Prostate, Steven Horne's Sinus Snuff, Stimulant Laxative, Urinary Immune,* and *Vulnerary Formulas*

Warnings: Goldenseal is safe when used at recommended dosages and times, but should not to be used as a single herb for long periods (over four weeks). It can cause malabsorption of vitamin B, resulting in fatigue and listlessness, when used for long periods. It is contraindicated for hypoglycemics because it lowers blood sugar levels. Hypoglycemics can use Oregon grape, coptis, or myrrh gum instead of goldenseal. It should be used under professional supervision during pregnancy.

Energetics: Cooling, drying, and mildly constricting

Used For: Abrasions/scratches, **acid indigestion**, aneurysm, **anorexia**, **antibiotic resistance**, **appendicitis**, **bladder (ulcerated)**, **canker sores**, chicken pox, **cholera**, cirrhosis of the liver, congestion (sinus), **conjunctivitis**, cuts, diabetes, **diarrhea**, digestion (poor), **dysbiosis**, dyspepsia, **eyes (red/itching)**, floaters, food allergies/intolerances, **food poisoning**, gangrene, **gastritis**, **giardia**, gingivitis, gonorrhea, **headache (sinus)**, hemorrhoids, impetigo, **infection (bacterial)**, inflammation, itching, **kidney infection**, low stomach acid, measles, meningitis, metabolic syndrome, morning sickness, nephritis, **oral surgery**, **pancreatitis**, parasites, pet supplements, **polyps**, **prostatitis**, **rosacea**, scabies, **SIBO**, sinus infection, **skin (infections)**, smell (loss of), **sore throat**, **sore/geographic tongue**, **spinal disks**, **staph infections**, **strep throat**, sty, **syphilis**, tonsillitis, **tooth extraction**, triglycerides (high), tuberculosis, typhoid, **ulcerations (external)**, ulcers, **urinary tract infections**, urination (burning/painful), and wounds & sores

Properties: Alterative, **antacid**, antiamebic, **antibacterial**, anticatarrhal, antidiabetic, antimicrobial, antiparasitic, antipruritic, antiseptic, antiviral, **aperitive**, astringent, cholagogue, detergent, digestive tonic, emmenagogue, hemostatic, **hypoglycemic**, immune stimulant, nervine, opthalmicum, oxytocic, **stimulant (appetite)**, and stomachic

Gotu Kola   *Bitter & Sweet Herb*

Centella asiatica

Gotu kola has a reputation for improving memory and brain function. It also has a positive effect on the adrenals, giving it adaptogenic effects. It is used in India for skin diseases and wasting diseases such as leprosy.

Look for *gotu kola* in *Attention-Focus, Memory Enhancing, Prostate,* and *Vandergriff's Energy Booster Formulas*

Warnings: Overdose may cause dizziness. Use caution with blood thinning medications. It appears safe during pregnancy and lactation, but some sources suggest caution. Consult with a professional herbalist for advice.

Energetics: Cooling and balancing

Used For: **Abrasions/scratches**, aging, Alzheimer's, **circulation (brain)**, cloudy thinking, **concentration (poor)**, confusion, dementia, depression, dermatitis, dizziness, eczema, epilepsy, fatigue, Hashimoto's disease, inflammation, jaundice (adults), leprosy, **memory/brain function**, meningitis, myasthenia gravis, narcolepsy, **Peyronie's disease**, psoriasis, sex drive (low), **skin (infections)**, **skin problems**, stress, tinnitus, and ulcers

Properties: Adaptogen, alterative, anti-inflammatory, anti-aging, antibacterial, antiepileptic, aphrodisiac, cephalic, **cerebral tonic**, hypotensive, insecticide, nervine, and vulnerary

Grape   *Sour & Sweet Herb*

Vitis vinifera

Grapes have long been used for healing. The famous herbalist, Juliette de Bairacli Levy, recommended the grape cure "when the human body has become sick almost beyond reasonable hope of recovery." It consists of living off of fresh, unsprayed grapes (and a few leaves and tendrils). Other famous healers have also used a diet of grapes as a cure for many chronic ailments. They are highly alkalizing and help to remove acid waste from the body. Grape seeds contain the antioxidant compounds oligomeric procyanidins (OPCs) and grape skins are also loaded with antioxidants. The leaves are edible and act as a mild diuretic.

Look for *Grape* in *Antioxidant, Blood Pressure Reducing,* and *Proanthocyanidins Formulas*

Energetics: Cooling, moistening, and nourishing

Used For: Arthritis, cancer prevention, convalescence, debility, free radical damage, gout, and inflammation

Properties: Alkalinizer, anti-inflammatory, antioxidant, diuretic, food, and nutritive

Grapefruit, Pink EO

Fresh & Sweet Essential Oil

Citrus paradisi

Pink grapefruit EO has a sweet, citrus aroma that is both cooling and relaxing. It reduces muscle tension and is helpful for easing depression, stress, and nervous exhaustion. It is particularly helpful for the wintertime blues, when people feel depressed and lethargic in the dark months of winter. It helps to promote feelings of self-worth, self-esteem, and euphoria. It also helps people who tend to eat for comfort when they are under stress.

Pink grapefruit is beneficial for an overheated liver and a sluggish lymphatic system. It acts as a blood purifier, helping the body to eliminate toxins, which makes it useful in drug withdrawal. Its diuretic properties and ability to help break down fats make it useful for treating water retention and cellulite. It can also help to prevent and reverse arteriosclerosis and hypertension. Having a stimulating effect on the digestive system, it helps with abdominal distention, constipation and nausea. Grapefruit oil helps with rheumatic pain of a hot nature when the joints feel warm and swollen, mixed with a burning sensation. Topically it is good for oily skin, acne and stretch marks.

Emotionally, pink grapefruit helps with feelings of tension, frustration, irritability and moodiness. It is an uplifting antidepressive agent and helps with nervous exhaustion. It helps reverse obesity in those who, under pressure and tension, resort to comfort eating to deal with emotions, because it eases the hunger for immediate satisfaction or the desperate need to be full. It also helps those who have high expectations of life, other people, and themselves, and feel let down when their expectations have not been met. When people react with anger, blame, and self-criticism, often followed by feelings of guilt and depression, grapefruit oil helps clear the emotional congestion with its cleansing, clarifying and refreshing effects.

See the strategy *Aromatherapy* for suggested uses.

Warnings: Dilute for topical use. Can be phototoxic when applied topically, so avoid direct exposure to sunlight after use.

Used For: Addictions (drugs), anorexia, appetite (excessive), arteriosclerosis, arthritis (rheumatoid), cellulite, confusion, congestion (lymphatic), digestion (poor), dyspepsia, edema, estrogen (low), excess weight, herpes, hot flashes, hypertension, irritability, mood swings, nausea & vomiting, nervous exhaustion, skin (oily), stress, and stretch marks

Properties: Alterative, analgesic, antibacterial, antidepressant, antidepressant, antioxidant, antiseptic, appetite suppressant, decongestant, detoxifying, disinfectant, diuretic, estrogenic, and nervine

Gravel Root   *Aromatic & Bitter Herb*

Eupatorium purpureum

Gravel root is a diuretic that helps to remove urinary stones and flush the urinary passages. It is also used for kidney infections, prostatitis, pelvic inflammatory disease, gout, and diabetes.

Warnings: Contains pyrrolizidine alkaloids. Avoid long-term use or while pregnant or nursing.

Energetics: Cooling and drying

Used For: Arthritis (rheumatoid), calcium deposits, **gout**, interstitial cystitis, **kidney stones**, **prostatitis**, and urethritis

Properties: Antilithic, antiurolithic, diuretic, and lithotriptic

Green Tea Polyphenols Formula

This is a decaffeinated, standardized green tea extract that has concentrated amounts of polyphenols, which are known to be two hundred times stronger than vitamin E in neutralizing free radicals. It helps normalize vascular blood clotting and total cholesterol levels as well as having antimicrobial properties.

Warnings: Not recommended for children under six or pregnant or nursing women.

Used For: Aging, Alzheimer's, anorexia, arteriosclerosis, autism, bedwetting, blood in stool, cancer, free radical damage, inflammation, and **psoriasis**

Take 1 capsule three times daily with a meal; three capsules have the polyphenol content of ten cups of liquid green tea.

Ingredients: Green tea standardized extract

Grief and Sadness FE Blend

This is a blend of flower essences I formulated to help people with the grieving process. It is helpful for people who are going through breakups, divorce, or death of loved ones or pets. It is helpful for people who are suffering losses of any kind in their lives. It is also a useful remedy for people who feel victimized by life, who complain a lot and blame others for their problems and lack of success. It helps people find the strength to let go of what they have lost, release the past, find spiritual comfort, and have hope and confidence to face the future.

People who are unable to complete a grieving process often develop respiratory problems, such as chronic coughs, frequent respiratory infections, or even pneumonia. If a person is experiencing respiratory problems after death, divorce or other major loses, this remedy can be helpful in their healing.

See the strategy *Flower Essence* for suggested uses.

Used For: Congestion (lungs), **depression**, **grief & sadness**, pneumonia, and shame & guilt

Affects: Heart and lungs

Ingredients: Self-heal FE, love-lies-bleeding FE, chicory FE, bleeding heart FE, chrysanthemum FE, borage FE, and yellow star tulip FE

Grindelia (Gumweed)

Aromatic & Astringent Herb

Grindelia camporum

This resinous expectorant and decongestant is very good at breaking up hardened mucus in the respiratory tract. It eases breathing in bronchitis and asthma. It has antispasmodic action that opens the smaller passages in the lungs and can make breathing easier. Combined with plantain it pulls thick mucus out of the lungs. It has also been applied topically as a salve to heal skin afflictions like poison ivy and rashes. It is also helpful topically for insect bites.

Look for *grindelia* in *Damp Cough Syrup Formula*

Warnings: Can be toxic in large doses. Not for long term use or for use by people suffering from kidney or heart disease.

Energetics: Warming, drying, and constricting

Used For: **Asthma**, **bites & stings**, bronchitis, congestion (bronchial), congestion (lungs), cuts, dermatitis, eczema, **emphysema**, **itching**, pertussis, **poison ivy/oak**, rashes & hives, ulcerations (external), and wounds & sores

Properties: Antiseptic, astringent, decongestant, **decongestant**, **expectorant**, and pulmonary

Guar gum   *Mucilant Herb*

Cyamopsis tetregonoloba

A high-fiber plant in Ayurvedic herbalism that is used as a bulk laxative similar to psyllium.

Look for *guar gum* in *Fat-Absorbing Fiber, Gut-Healing Fiber,* and *Natural Antacid Formulas*

Used For: Cholesterol (high) and constipation (adults)

Properties: Laxative (bulk) and mucilant

Guarana   *Stimulant Bitter Herb*

Paullinia cupana

Guarana is a stimulant containing a form of caffeine and is often used as a substitute for coffee or kola drinks.

Look for *guarana* in *Metabolic Stimulant Formula*

Warnings: Avoid taking guarana if combined with ephedrine, or if you have high blood pressure, heart disease, or sensitivity to caffeine. May cause irregular heartbeat, anxiety, jitteriness, and insomnia in susceptible persons.

Energetics: Warming and drying

Used For: Fatigue

Properties: Diuretic, **stimulant (metabolic)**, sympathomimetic, and vasoconstrictor

Guggul   *Astringent, Bitter, & Pungent Herb*

Commiphora mukul

Research has shown that guggul may be able to lower both cholesterol and triglycerides. It also inhibits platelet aggregation and can help prevent and possibly reverse arterial plaque. It mildly stimulates the thyroid and may be helpful for weight loss.

Look for *guggul* in *Heart Health, Herbal Arthritis, Hypothyroid,* and *Metabolic Stimulant Formulas*

Warnings: Because it thins the blood, it should not be used in persons who bleed easily or during pregnancy. Also avoid with hyperthyroid disorders.

Energetics: Warming and drying

Used For: Arteriosclerosis, **cholesterol (high)**, circulation (poor), **excess weight, fatty tumors/deposits**, hypertension, thrombosis, and **triglycerides (high)**

Properties: Anti-inflammatory, antibacterial, anticholesteremic, **anticoagulant**, antilipemic, antirheumatic, hepatic, and hypolipidemic

Gut Immune Formula

This formula contains several immune enhancing herbs and helps to regulate the immune system in the intestinal tract. It helps to tone and strengthen the intestinal membranes.

Warnings: Contraindicated with autoimmune disorders. Cat's claw has contraceptive effects and should be avoided by women who are pregnant or who are trying to conceive.

Used For: AIDS, arthritis, bursitis, **cancer**, cancer treatment side effects, cartilage damage, **diverticulitis, dysbiosis, Epstein-Barr virus**, food allergies/intolerances, herpes, **leaky gut, lyme disease**, radiation, Reye's syndrome, and **SIBO**

Affects: Immune system, large intestines (colon), and **small intestines**

Take 1 capsule one to three times daily.

Ingredients: Cat's claw bark, astragalus root, and echinacea root

Gut-Healing Fiber Formula

See also *Fiber Blend*

This fiber formula contains psyllium, inulin, and L-glutamine. Inulin feeds friendly intestinal flora and glutamine helps heal leaky gut. It also contains other ingredients to soothe and heal the mucous membrane linings. It also aids in heavy metal detoxification. People with small intestinal bacterial overgrowth may experience gas and bloating taking this formula.

Used For: Chemical exposure, **colitis**, environmental pollution, food allergies/intolerances, **heavy metal poisoning, leaky gut, mercury poisoning**, and **SIBO**

Affects: Intestinal atrophy and intestinal relaxation

Mix 1 pack in 9 ounces of water and drink immediately. Use once or twice daily between meals on an empty stomach.

Ingredients: Psyllium hulls, inulin, L-glutamine, flax seed, acacia gum, and guar gum

Gymnema   *Bitter Herb*

Gymnema sylvestre

Ayurvedic practitioners have used gymnema to treat type 2 diabetes for at least two thousand years. When placed on the tongue, gymnema makes it impossible to taste sugar. It is believed that it not only blocks sweet receptors on the tongue, it also slows absorption of sugar in the digestive tract. Dozens of peer-reviewed studies now support the use of gymnema as a treatment for high blood sugar.

Look for *gymnema* in *Blood Sugar Control Formula*

Warnings: Gymnema is generally regarded as safe and associated with few side effects or drug interactions.

Energetics: Cooling and drying

Used For: **Diabetes**, excess weight, and triglycerides (high)

Properties: Antidiabetic, astringent, diuretic, refrigerant, and stomachic

Gynostemma   *Mildly Bitter & Sweet Herb*

Gynostemma pentaphyllum

This calming adapatogen contains triterpenoid saponins like those found in the ginseng family. It enhances the immune system and can be helpful in counteracting the effects of radiation and chemotherapy. It enhances levels of superoxide dismutase an important free radical scavenger. It tones the cardiovascular system, reducing platelet aggregation and lowering cholesterol and triglycerides.

Look for *gynostemma* in *Adaptogen, Adaptogen-Immune,* and *Colloidal Mineral Formulas*

Warnings: Can cause gastric upset when taken on an empty stomach. High doses may cause rash, fatigue, dizziness and palpitations.

Energetics: Mildly relaxing, neutral, and balancing

Used For: Angina, **cancer treatment side effects**, cardiovascular disease, cholesterol (high), headache (tension), hypotension, insomnia, radiation, and triglycerides (high)

Properties: Adaptogen, anticholesteremic, antioxidant, cardiac, expectorant, hepatoprotective, immune modulator, and nervine

H. Pylori-Fighting Formula

See also *Gut Immune Formula*

Studies have suggested that the bacteria *Helicobater pylori* is involved in the formation of ulcers. This combination combines several herbs tested to be effective against *H. pylori* with digestive stimulants and antiulcer herbs. It is helpful for ulcers but can also correct dysbiosis of the intestinal tract to promote a better microbiome.

Used For: Belching, celiac disease, **diarrhea**, **duodenal ulcers**, dysbiosis, gastritis, leaky gut, parasites, **SIBO**, and **ulcers**

Affects: Digestive irritation, immune system, **mucous membranes**, and stomach

To combat ulcers take 2 capsules four times daily with plenty of water. For altering the intestinal flora take 1-2 capsules three times daily.

Ingredients: Dgle (deglycyrrhizinated licorice root extract), clove flower extract, indian elecampane root extract, pau d'arco bark extract, and capsicum fruit

Haritaki

Astringent, Bitter, Salty, Sour, & Sweet Herb

Terminalla chebula

Haritaki, also known as chebulic is one of the three herbs in the widely used Ayurvedic combination triphala. It has a balanced energy, containing all five flavors in Ayurvedic herbalism (bitter, sour, astringent, salty, and sweet). It has a balancing effect on intestinal function as it is both laxative and astringent. It is used to ease chronic constipation, remove parasites, and reduce nervousness.

Look for *haritaki* in *Triphala Formula*

Energetics: Warming, relaxing, and moistening

Used For: Allergies (respiratory), anxiety attacks, asthma, constipation (adults), constipation (children), nervousness, and parasites

Properties: Alterative, anti-inflammatory, antimicrobial, antioxidant, antiparasitic, antispasmodic, hepatoprotective, hypoglycemic, laxative (gentle), moistening, and nervine

Hawthorn   *Sour & Sweet Herb*

Crataegus spp.

Hawthorn berries are an excellent herbal food for building up the heart muscle. Studies around the world have confirmed that hawthorn berries improve the tone of the cardiac muscle, improve oxygen uptake by the heart, improve circulation in the heart, energize the heart cells and dilate blood vessels in the extremities to reduce strain on the heart. The flowers and leaves are also used as cardiac tonics, and a blend of all three may be the most effective. Hawthorn needs to be taken on a regular basis for best results. Hawthorn berries are also used to reduce stress and improve digestion.

Look for *hawthorn* in *Blood Pressure Reducing, Brain-Heart, Chinese Earth-Decreasing, Cholesterol-Regulating, Heart Health, Hypoglycemic,* and *Skinny Formulas*

Warnings: Hawthorn should not be used with digitalis (a heart drug). Dangerous side effects may occur when used together unless the dosage is carefully monitored and adjusted by a qualified physician.

Energetics: Cooling and moistening

Used For: Age spots, aneurysm, **angina**, arrhythmia, **arteriosclerosis**, capillary weakness, **cardiac arrest, cardiovascular disease**, circulation (poor), cold hands/feet, **congestive heart failure**, dizziness, easily bruised, Graves' disease, **heart fibrillation/palpitations, heart valves, heart weakness, hypertension**, hypotension, memory/brain function, mitral valve, numbness, Raynaud's disease, **rheumatic fever**, rosacea, shock (medical), **sleep apnea**, tachycardia, and tinnitus

Properties: Antiarrhythmic, antilipemic, antioxidant, antiseptic, **cardiac**, food, food, hypertensive, hypotensive, sympatholytic, and **vasodilator**

He Shou Wu *Mildly Bitter & Sweet Herb*

Polygonum multiflorum

This herb is considered an anti-aging tonic and is believed to help prevent (and possibly reverse) the graying of hair when taken regularly. It helps to balance blood sugar levels and increases glycogen reserves in the liver. It helps build up the thyroid and reduces cholesterol.

Look for *he shou wu* in *Hypothyroid Formula*

Warnings: Not for persons with diarrhea, weak digestion and heavy mucus congestion.

Energetics: Neutral, moistening, and nourishing

Used For: Angina, dizziness, erectile dysfunction, **hair (graying)**, hair loss/thinning, **Hashimoto's disease**, hypoglycemia, hypothyroidism, infertility, numbness, tuberculosis, and wounds & sores

Properties: Antiaging, anticholesteremic, blood building, glandular, kidney tonic, thyrotropic, and tonic

Headache Formula

See also *Analgesic Nerve Formula* and *Stan Malstrom's Herbal Aspirin Formula*

These are formulas designed to ease headaches. They provide symptomatic relief but one always needs to identify and address the underlying cause for lasting relief.

Used For: Headache (migraine) and headache (tension)

Periwinkle Headache Formula

The periwinkle in this formula makes it helpful for vasoconstrictive migraines where the head feels like it's being squeezed. One dropper two to four times per day between meals.

Ingredients: Feverfew leaf & flower, meadowsweet leaf & flower, and periwinkle flowering tops

Headache Formula with Chinese Herbs

A blend of Western and Chinese herbs for easing headaches, especially migraines. One tablet three times daily between meals.

Ingredients: Schizonepeta aerial parts, notopterygium root, green tea leaf, angelica root, cyperus rhizome, white willow bark, and feverfew leaf

Healing Salve

These salves soften and soothe irritated, rough, chafed or chapped skin. They promotes healing of damaged tissue and are useful for all minor injuries to the skin as well as damaged, dry, rough, or chapped skin and lips. They can be mixed with powdered white oak bark or another astringent to apply topically for hemorrhoids.

Warnings: Not recommended for deep wounds or cuts.

Used For: Abrasions/scratches, **abscesses**, anal fistula/fissure, blisters, cuts, **diaper rash**, **hemorrhoids**, injuries, and **wounds & sores**

Affects: Rectum, **skin**, structural atrophy, and structural irritation

Ed Smith's Healing Salve

Ingredients: Comfrey root, Saint John's wort flowers & buds, calendula flower, chickweed, mullein leaf, and plantain

Golden Healing Salve

Apply topically as needed.

Ingredients: Black walnut hulls, comfrey root, goldenseal root, myrrh gum, white oak bark, and yarrow flower

Heart Health Formula

These formulas are for strengthening the heart and the entire circulatory system. Specific ingredients make different formulas more useful for specific conditions as indicated.

Used For: Angina, **arrhythmia**, **arteriosclerosis**, cardiac arrest, cardiovascular disease, circulation (poor), **congestive heart failure**, edema, **heart weakness**, hypertension, hypotension, mitral valve, and thrombosis

Affects: Circulatory atrophy, circulatory depression, and **heart**

David Winston's Heart Formula

The addition of night blooming cereus makes this formula more useful for problems with heart valves. Take 40-60 drops three times daily in water or juice.

Ingredients: Hawthorn berry, night-blooming cereus stem, and motherwort leaf

Arjuna & Hawthorn Formula

This is a general heart tonic for strengthening a weak heart. 2 tablets twice daily.

Ingredients: Hawthorn leaf & flower, guggul, and arjuna bark

Stan Malstrom's Heart Formula

A basic heart and circulatory formula. Take 1–2 capsules three times daily.

Ingredients: Hawthorn berry, capsicum fruit, and garlic bulb

Heart Support Formula

The lily of the valley in this formula makes it especially helpful for congestive heart failure. Use as directed on the label.

Ingredients: Black cohosh, bugleweed, hawthorn, and lily of the valley

Heavy Metal Cleansing Formula

These formulas aid the body in detoxifying and expelling mercury and other heavy metals. They help the liver bind and eliminate these toxins. They are good products to take after removal of amalgam fillings or if you suspect you have been exposed to other heavy metals like lead or cadmium.

Warnings: Avoid during pregnancy. Do not exceed the recommended dosage as this can create too rapid of a detoxification process. If headache, nausea, or diarrhea develops, reduce dosage. It's a good idea to take extra fiber (three to four capsules of algin are recommended) in order to bind heavy metals in the gut. Drawing baths using clay and Epsom salts may also aid the detoxification process.

Used For: ADD/ADHD, **aluminum toxicity**, Alzheimer's, **autism**, autoimmune disorders, **cadmium toxicity**, chemical exposure, **heavy metal poisoning**, **lead poisoning**, mental illness, **mercury poisoning**, **multiple sclerosis**, and **vaccine side effects**

Affects: Hepatic stagnation, immune system, and liver

Metal Cleansing

A gentler heavy metal cleansing formula. Take 1 capsule twice daily with plenty of water.

Ingredients: Vitamin B$_6$, cilantro/coriander leaf, sodium alginate, N-acetyl cysteine, L-methionine, and alpha-lipoic acid

Metal Detox

A more comprehensive cleansing formula. Take 1 capsule in between meals two or three times daily.

Ingredients: Zinc, selenium, chlorella, broccoli, N-acetyl cysteine, L-methionine, and alpha linolenic acid *see omega-3 ALA*

Helichrysum EO

Fresh, Herbaceous, & Sweet Essential Oil

Helichrysum italicum

Helichrysum EO, also known as immortelle or everlasting, has been a preferred remedy for chronic ailments of the skin and lymphatic system. It is an essential oil that helps with respiratory complaints and allergic conditions that involve nasal catarrh, sneezing, and itchy skin rashes. For earaches, it can be diluted in a carrier oil and dropped into the ear to reduce inflammation and fight infection.

Topically it speeds cellular growth, eases eczema and dermatitis, and assists in wound healing of all types. It reduces inflammation, helps heal old scar tissue and stretch marks, and loosens adhesions after injuries. It has anticoagulant actions making it useful for any severe bruising that results in clotted blood.

Emotionally, helichrysum alleviates the tension that arises from issues involving excessive effort and overcontrol. Easing long-standing frustrations and helping a person break through negative "stuck" emotions, it is highly effective on stubborn, negative attitudes. These may be blockages in expressing anger and despair or even in admitting the depth of one's emotional wounds. Though secretly despairing, they cannot bear to see others admit vulnerability and may feel rage when they do so. Helichrysum can loosen the hardest of attitudes, restoring compassion for self and others. It also increases dream activity and awareness to stimulate the right side of the brain.

See the strategy *Aromatherapy* for suggested uses.

Warnings: Do not use internally without the supervision of a professionally trained aromatherapy practitioner. Nontoxic and nonirritating for topical use.

Used For: Abrasions/scratches, alcoholism, allergies (respiratory), aneurysm, anger (excessive), arthritis, asthma, bronchitis, bruises, cholesterol (high), cirrhosis of the liver, colds (antiviral), colitis, confusion, **congestion (lymphatic)**, cramps & spasms, **cuts**, cysts, deafness, depression, dermatitis, digestion (poor), diphtheria, dislocation, earache, **eczema**, fibroids (uterine), gallbladder problems, gingivitis, grief & sadness, headache, headache (migraine), **hearing loss**, **hepatitis**, herpes, infection (viral), inflammation, injuries, mood swings, **nerve damage**, pain, pancreatitis, pertussis, phlebitis, rashes & hives, **scars/scar tissue**, sciatica, seizures, sinus infection, **skin (dry/flaky)**, skin (infections), skin problems, spinal disks, sprains, stretch marks, and wounds & sores

Properties: Analgesic, anti-inflammatory, antiallergenic, antibacterial, anticatarrhal, anticoagulant, antifungal, antimicrobial, antioxidant, antispasmodic, antiviral, **cicatrizant**, expectorant, hepatic, mucolytic, and **vulnerary**

Hemp Oil with Terpenes Formula

This formula uses hemp-seed oil with terpenes to create a similar effect to CBD but without the presence of any phytocannabinoids which could cause legal problems in some states. It helps to build the endocannabinoid receptors and may be helpful for reducing inflammation and pain.

Used For: Abrasions/scratches, arthritis, autoimmune disorders, broken bones, bruises, bursitis, **inflammation**, injuries, surgery (recovery), and wounds & sores

Affects: CB1 receptors and immune system

Use one dropper once daily.

Ingredients: Hemp seed oil, turmeric root extract, and peppermint EO

Hepatoprotective Formula

See also *Liver Cleanse Formula*

These formulas aid liver detoxification and protect the liver from environmental poisons. They are very helpful for people who work around chemicals on a regular basis, which includes painters, auto mechanics, dry cleaners, carpet and house cleaners, beauticians, and health professionals. Both can be used safely for long periods of time, but drink plenty of water when taking them.

Warnings: Cleansing is generally contraindicated during pregnancy and nursing, but these formulas are probably safe for pregnant women and nursing mothers.

Used For: Addictions (drugs), **alcoholism**, **cancer prevention**, **chemical exposure**, **cirrhosis of the liver**, **environmental pollution**, **fatty liver disease**, fibromyalgia, gallbladder problems, gallstones, **hangover**, heavy metal poisoning, **hepatitis**, insomnia, irritable bowel, **jaundice (adults)**, leaky gut, menstrual irregularity, mercury poisoning, nightmares, **poisoning**, preeclampsia, and psoriasis

Affects: General stagnation, hepatic atrophy, hepatic depression, hepatic irritation, **hepatic stagnation**, immune system, and liver

Liver Protecting Nutrients with Milk Thistle

Primarily hepatoprotective, this is a less expensive option for people who wish to protect themselves from chemicals. Take 1-2 tablets twice daily.

Ingredients: Vitamin A, vitamin C, choline, N-acetyl cysteine, inositol, milk thistle seed extract, and dandelion root

Liver Detox Program

In addition to its detoxifying and hepatoprotective effects, this formula also supports a healthy intestinal flora. Take the contents of 1 packet (which contains 2 tablets and 4 capsules) before a meal, ideally breakfast, once daily.

Ingredients: Vitamin A, vitamin C, choline, Bacillus coagulans, berberine root, N-acetyl cysteine, milk thistle seed extract, dandelion root, and turmeric rhizome

Herbal Arthritis Formula

These are herbal formulas for arthritis. They all work on underlying aspects of the disease providing gentle detoxification, anti-inflammatory, and analgesic effects along with herbs to aid joint healing. Do not expect instant results as these formulas takes effect gradually over a period of about one to two weeks.

Used For: Arthritis, **arthritis (rheumatoid)**, bunions, **bursitis**, calcium deposits, cartilage damage, gout, inflammation, lupus, neuralgia & neuritis, spinal disks, and **uric acid retention**

Affects: Bones, **joints**, and **structural stagnation**

Paavo Airola's Arthritis Formula

A traditional blend of Western herbs for arthritis. Can be helpful for arthritis in pets. This blend combines well the *Herbal Calcium* and *Watkin's Hair, Skin, and Nails Formula* for healing joints in osteoarthritis. Take 2 capsules three times daily. This formula has also been used with pets. Mix 1–2 capsule with their food.

Ingredients: Alfalfa aerial parts, horsetail stem & strobilus, celery seed, hydrangea root extract, yucca root extract, white willow bark, burdock root, sarsaparilla root, and bromelain

David Winston's Arthritis Formula

This formula eases inflammation in both joints and muscles. Take 40-60 drops three or four times daily.

Ingredients: Sarsaparilla rhizome, turmeric rhizome, devil's claw tuber, ginger rhizome, sichuan teasel root, and willow bark

Ayurvedic Arthritis Formula

An arthritic formula from India. Take 2 capsules with a meal three times daily.

Ingredients: Ashwagandha root, guggul gum extract, sarsaparilla (chinese) root, boswellia gum, skunkvine leaf extract, and celery seed

Herbal Bitters Formula

The taste of something bitter in the mouth has an effect on the nervous system that stimulates appetite and digestion. Traditionally, bitters have been made as alcohol beverages, aperitifs, and liqueurs. Various blends of bitter herbs have traditionally been used as tonics to improve digestive function, ease acid indigestion, reduce gas and bloating, and improve liver detoxification.

Used For: Acid indigestion, **anorexia**, **appetite (deficient)**, belching, **bulimia**, cancer treatment side effects, congestion, **digestion (poor)**, dysbiosis, **dyspepsia**, food allergies/intolerances, gas & bloating, **gastritis**, **headache**

(migraine), **indigestion**, **low stomach acid**, overacidity, **protein digestion**, SIBO, and **sore/geographic tongue**

Affects: **Digestive stagnation**, **gallbladder**, hepatic stagnation, **intestinal stagnation**, **pancreas head**, and **small intestines**

Bitter Digestive Tonic

This formula was overly sweetened. However, the sweetness makes it more suitable for children. Adding a little goldenseal to it will make it more bitter and improve its effectiveness for adults. Adults should take one teaspoon fifteen to thirty minutes before meals. For children over six, use 1/2 teaspoon fifteen minutes before meals.

Ingredients: Cardamom seed, dandelion root, orange (sweet) peel, and gentian root

Basic Digestive Bitters

A good basic bitters formula. Take 1/2–1 teaspoonful about fifteen to thirty minutes prior to meals with a glass of water.

Ingredients: Dandelion leaf & root, burdock root, orange (sweet) peel, fennel seed, yellow dock root, angelica root, ginger root, and gentian root

Chamomile Bitters

Take 1/2–1 teaspoonful about fifteen to thirty minutes prior to meals with a glass of water.

Ingredients: Dandelion root & leaf, chamomile flower, burdock root, yellow dock root, and ginger root

Balanced Bitters

A make-it-yourself formula from *Modern Herbal Dispensatory*. Take 1/2–1 teaspoonful about fifteen to thirty minutes prior to meals with a glass of water.

Ingredients: Dandelion root, orange peel, angelica, cardamom, and anise

Herbal Calcium Formula

See also *Joan Patton's Herbal Minerals Formula*

This formula consists primarily of vulnerary (tissue-healing) mucilants. It does not contain a large amount of calcium but does help bones and injured tissues to heal. It contains many trace elements that help the body utilize calcium and other major minerals better. It would also help enrich breast milk and make an excellent tonic for pregnant women in combination with red raspberry.

Used For: Arthritis, backache, **broken bones**, calcium deficiency, calcium deposits, dental health, **dislocation**, fingernail biting, fingernails (weak/brittle), hernias, **ligaments (torn/injuried)**, menopause, multiple sclerosis,

nursing, sciatica, **surgery (recovery)**, teeth (grinding), teeth (loose), teething, and tendonitis

Affects: Bones, general atrophy, general relaxation, structural atrophy, and teeth

For injuries take 2-4 capsules three to six times daily with a large glass of water. This formula can also be used externally as a poultice for swelling and injuries.

Ingredients: Alfalfa aerial parts, horsetail stem & strobilus, oat straw extract, and plantain leaf

Herbal Composition Formula

See also *Ed Millet's Herbal Crisis Formula*

Herbal composition is a traditional formula that has been used successfully for over two hundred years for colds, flu, sore throats, coughs, congestion, and other acute ailments. Developed by the pioneer herbalist Samuel Thomson, it was originally called composition or composition powder. Thomson claimed said the formula was used to "scour the bowels and remove the canker [mucus and/or toxins]." He used it as a tea, along with lobelia and capsicum, as part of a system of eliminating infectious diseases.

Herbal Composition helps reduce mucus congestion in the system. It breaks up congested mucus and helps the body expel it. It also helps to promote perspiration and stimulates circulation. It is a very useful formula for colds, flu, fevers, sore throats and other acute ailments. Directions for this make-it-yourself formula can be found in *Modern Herbal Dispensatory*.

Used For: Colds, fever, flu, perspiration (deficient), **sore throat**, and **strep throat**

Affects: Digestive depression, immune system, intestinal stagnation, mucous membranes, and **respiratory stagnation**

Make the tea at the very first sign of a cold or flu and sip it frequently until you feel better.

4 parts Bayberry root bark

2 parts Pine bark

1 part Ginger root

1/2 part Clove

1/2 part Capsicum

Herbal Eyewash Formula

An herbal eye wash can help with poor vision, cataracts, eye infections, such as pink eye and other eye problems. This is a do-it-yourself formula made by blending equal parts eyebright, goldenseal, bayberry and red raspberry.

To make the eyewash, use one-half to one teaspoon teaspoon of the above mixture per cup of purified, boiling water.

Distilled water is ideal for making this preparation. Allow the herbs to steep for five to ten minutes and strain thoroughly through a fine cloth or coffee filter. You don't want any of the herb powders getting into your eyes.

Store extra tea in the refrigerator and make a fresh batch every three to four days. You can help preserve the tea and make the eyewash more sanitary by adding one teaspoon of liquid silver to each cup.

Use an eyewash cup to wash the eyes or put drops of the tea into the eyes. You can also soak cotton balls with the tea and use them as a compress over the eyes. Christopher claimed that used daily the eyewash would improve eyesight and even aid cataracts and glaucoma. I've heard stories of people successfully using it for these purposes but it typically takes anywhere from a couple of weeks to a couple of months to see results. I've personally used it for eye infections but never had the patience to use it daily to try to improve my own eyesight.

The formula can be taken internally. It has a strong affinity for the respiratory system and mucous membranes. It contains herbs that may relieve itchy, red eyes, itchy nose with watery sinus drainage, swollen Eustachian tubes that can cause frequent ear infections, and itchy ears.

Used For: Allergies (respiratory), cataracts, **conjunctivitis**, eye health, **eyes (red/itching)**, glaucoma, rhinitis, and **sty**

Affects: Sight

Ingredients: Eyebright, goldenseal, bayberry, and red raspberry

Herbal Potassium Formula

A natural potassium supplement benefits the kidneys and helps to maintain fluid and electrolyte balance. This formula is naturally high in sodium as well as potassium and contains many herbs beneficial to the thyroid.

Used For: Cramps (leg), cramps (menstrual), cramps & spasms, dehydration, diarrhea, edema, giardia, heart fibrillation/palpitations, lyme disease, Ménière's disease, overacidity, paralysis, tachycardia, **tics**, **tremors**, and **twitching**

Affects: Aldosterone, hypothalamus, **kidneys**, parotids (salivary glands), **pituitary (posterior)**, structural constriction, and urinary atrophy

Take 2 capsules with a meal three times daily.

Ingredients: Potassium, kelp leaf & stem, alfalfa aerial parts, and dulse fronds

Herbal Sleep Aid Formula

See also *Sleep Aid*

These formulas contain relaxing nervine herbs that can aid sleep. They can also be helpful for nervousness, anxiety, and health conditions arising from stress.

Warnings: See cautions for valerian.

Used For: ADD/ADHD, alcoholism, **insomnia**, jet lag, pain, Parkinson's disease, restless leg, and stress

Affects: Brain and **sympathetic-dominant ANS**

Sleep Soundly Formula

A great herbal formula to relax the body to aid sleep. Take 1–2 capsules about one hour before bedtime.

Ingredients: California poppy whole plant, valerian root, passion flower, chamomile flower, and oat seed (milky)

Traditional Sleep Formula

Take 2–4 capsules about one hour before bedtime. You can also take 1–2 capsules along with 1 capsule kava kava if you have a lot of muscle tension. Take 2 capsules three times daily for stress.

Ingredients: Valerian root, passion flower aerial parts, and hops flower

David Winston's Sleep Formula

A very good sleep formula in tincture form. Take 30–60 drops one hour prior to bedtime.

Ingredients: Skullcap flowering tops, hops strobile, passion flower herb, California poppy whole plant, and valerian root

Herbal Tooth Powder Formula

These formulas are simple to make yourself. Just mix the herbal powders together in a container. Put a small amount of powder into the palm of your hand. Dip a wet toothbrush into the powder and brush your teeth with it. Leaving the powder on for a few minutes before rinsing helps strengthen the gums.

Used For: Dental health, **gingivitis**, and **teeth (loose)**

Affects: Gums, structural relaxation, and **teeth**

Thomas Easley's Tooth Powder

This is a more antimicrobial tooth powder.

2 parts White oak bark

2 parts Elecampane

1 part Thyme

1 part Myrrh

Steven Horne's Tooth Powder

This version is more astringent for toning gums and teeth.

2 parts White oak bark

2 parts Black walnut hulls

1 part Bayberry root bark

1 part Goldenseal root

Hoelen   *Sweet Herb*

Poria cocos

This white fungus grows on trees, usually pine. The part used is the sclerotium, which is a compact mass of hardened fungal mycelium containing the food reserves. It resembles a coconut. It is a relaxing nervine, a nourishing diuretic that drains fluid from the tissues, and a tonic for weak digestion. It is used as a fortifying agent in Chinese formulas.

Look for *hoelen* in *Chinese Earth-Decreasing, Chinese Earth-Increasing, Chinese Fire-Decreasing, Chinese Metal-Decreasing,* and *Chinese Water-Decreasing Formulas*

Energetics: Neutral, nourishing, and drying

Used For: Anxiety (situational), appetite (deficient), edema, heart fibrillation/palpitations, insomnia, and nervousness

Properties: Antibacterial, diuretic, lymphatic, nutritive, and relaxant

Holy Basil   *Aromatic & Sweet Herb*

Ocimum sanctum

Used in Ayurvedic herbalism, holy basil is considered an adaptogen and general tonic in modern herbalism. It protects the heart from stress, lowers blood pressure and cholesterol levels, and stabilizes blood sugar levels. It reduces feelings of stress and down regulates excessive immune responses in conditions like hay fever (allergic rhinitis) and asthma. At the same time it enhances cerebral circulation, memory, concentration, and mental acuity.

Look for *holy basil* in *Cortisol-Reducing* and *Hypothyroid Formulas*

Energetics: Cooling and drying

Used For: Allergies (respiratory), anxiety disorders, asthma, bipolar mood disorder, cardiovascular disease, colds, concentration (poor), **Cushing's disease**, diabetes, inflammation, **memory/brain function**, PTSD, rhinitis, **stress**, and trauma

Properties: Adaptogen, antibacterial, antiviral, carminative, hypotensive, and immune modulator

Honeysuckle   *Sweet Herb*

Lonicera japonica

Honeysuckle flowers were traditionally used in Chinese herbalism to treat fevers, inflammation, diarrhea and skin infections. Modern herbalists use honeysuckle for its anti-inflammatory, antibacterial and calming properties. It can be used to treat skin rashes such as poison oak, cuts, and abrasions on the skin. Honeysuckle has antibiotic properties, making it helpful for treating infections caused by streptococcal bacteria. Helpful for other types of inflammation and infection, including upper respiratory tract infections and asthma. It is combined with chrysanthemum flowers to treat colds. May also be used as a massage oil to relax the muscles and calm the nerves.

Look for *honeysuckle* in *Chinese Yang-Reducing Formula*

Energetics: Cooling

Used For: Abrasions/scratches, asthma, carbuncles, colds with fever, cuts, diarrhea, fever, poison ivy/oak, and skin (infections)

Properties: Anti-inflammatory, antibacterial, antispasmodic, antiviral, diuretic, and **febrifuge**

Hops   *Aromatic & Bitter Herb*

Humulus lupulus

This herb is a powerful nervine and sleep aid, and can be combined with other carminatives for settling a nervous, acidic stomach. It is also estrogenic and has been used to increase sex drive in women and reduce it in men. Hops is indicated for a hot digestive system and/or irritated nervous system. It works best on hot, damp people who are often overweight, red-faced with fiery personalities, poor digestion, and insomnia.

Look for *hops* in *Analgesic Nerve, CBD Relaxing, General Analgesic, Herbal Sleep Aid, Hypothyroid, Jeannie Burgess' Stress,* and *Sleep Support Formulas*

Warnings: Contraindicated in clinical depression, estrogen dominance, or with allergies to hops. Not the best choice as a nervine for young children, but all right as part of a formula. Use with caution during pregnancy because of its estrogenic effects. Men with low testosterone should avoid hops, too.

Energetics: Cooling, relaxing, and mildly drying

Used For: Addictions (drugs), **alcoholism**, anxiety disorders, colic (adults), cramps (leg), cramps & spasms, Cushing's disease, epilepsy, estrogen (low), Graves' disease, headache (tension), **insomnia**, pain, Parkinson's disease, sex drive (excessive), twitching, and **vaginal dryness**

Properties: Analgesic, **anaphrodisiac**, antacid, anthelmintic, antiepileptic, antispasmodic, carminative, cholagogue,

CNS depressant, diaphoretic, diuretic, **estrogenic**, febrifuge, gaba-enhancing, narcotic, **nervine**, **phytoestrogen**, **sedative**, **soporific**, **sympatholytic**, tonic, tranquilizer, and vermifuge

Horehound   *Bitter Herb*

Marrubium vulgare

Horehound has traditionally been used to make cough drops or cough syrup. You can still find horehound drops in some stores. It is an excellent remedy for increasing the secretion of thinner mucus to break up congestion. It also stimulates digestion and has a mild cardiac effect.

Look for *horehound* in *Christopher's Sinus, Dry Cough Syrup,* and *Steven Horne's Horehound Cough Formulas*

Warnings: Use with caution during pregnancy.

Energetics: Cooling and drying

Used For: Appetite (deficient), **bronchitis**, **congestion (lungs)**, **cough**, **cough (damp)**, digestion (poor), and fever

Properties: Antiarrhythmic, cardiac, **decongestant**, and **expectorant**

Horse Chestnut
Mildly Astringent & Bitter Herb

Aesculus hippocastanum

Horse chestnut is a specific a tonic to the vascular system. It improves the tone of veins making it helpful for varicose veins, bruises, and hemorrhoids. It can be taken internally or applied topically.

Look for *horse chestnut* in *Vein Tonic Formula*

Warnings: There is some toxicity to the horse chestnut plant, but extracts of the seeds are safe when used as directed. Avoid with children, during pregnancy, and with nursing mothers. Use cautiously when taking blood thinning medications.

Energetics: Cooling, drying, and mildly constricting

Used For: Anal fistula/fissure, **aneurysm**, bruises, cancer treatment side effects, capillary weakness, **hemorrhoids**, **phlebitis**, **spider veins**, strokes, thrombosis, and **varicose veins**

Properties: Astringent and **vascular tonic**

Horseradish   *Pungent Herb*

Armoracia rusticana

Horseradish is a very good remedy for people who have a hard time digesting and metabolizing protein. Eaten with meat it helps stimulate both the digestion and metabolism of protein. It can be used for colds, flu, and other acute ailments and may be helpful for allergies, hay fever, and congestion in the lungs.

Look for *horseradish* in *Antihistamine, Fire Cider,* and *Jeannie Burgess' Allergy-Lung Formulas*

Warnings: Large amounts can cause gastrointestinal upset.

Energetics: Warming and drying

Used For: Allergies (respiratory), bronchitis, colds, congestion (lungs), **congestion (sinus)**, cough, cough (damp), digestion (poor), parasites (nematodes, worms), and **sinus infection**

Properties: Anticatarrhal, carminative, condiment, **decongestant**, **expectorant**, and stimulant (metabolic)

Horsetail   *Mildly Astringent & Mildly Salty Herb*

Equisetum arvense

Horsetail is rich in the mineral silica, which is used with calcium in bones, nails, hair, and the skin. Silica adds elasticity to tissues, making them strong but not brittle. It is astringent and is useful for internal bleeding, such as blood in the urine. It has a mild diuretic effect as well.

Look for *horsetail* in *Herbal Arthritis, Herbal Calcium, Joan Patton's Herbal Minerals, Skeletal Support, Watkin's Hair, Skin,* and *and Nails Formulas*

Warnings: Excessive consumption may lead to thiamin deficiencies. Powdered herb not recommended for children, but tea is okay.

Energetics: Cooling, drying, and mildly constricting

Used For: **Aluminum toxicity**, anal fistula/fissure, arthritis, bladder (ulcerated), bleeding (internal), **blood in urine**, broken bones, bruises, calcium deficiency, COPD, **dental health**, edema, **emphysema**, fingernail biting, **fingernails (weak/brittle)**, **hair loss/thinning**, hemorrhoids, **incontinence**, **interstitial cystitis**, multiple sclerosis, nephritis, nerve damage, nosebleeds, **osteoporosis**, pancreatitis, parasites, parasites (nematodes, worms), Parkinson's disease, skin problems, sty, urethritis, wheezing, wounds & sores, and wrinkles

Properties: **Astringent**, diuretic, hemostatic, **kidney tonic**, **mineralizer**, parasympatholytic, styptic, vermifuge, and vulnerary

Hot Flash Formula

See also *Female Tonic Formula* and *Menopause Support*

This formula is used to reduce or alleviate the hot flashes and other menopausal symptoms. The black cohosh found in it is a standardized extract of the rhizome containing 2.5 percent triterpene glycosides. The ingredients are also time-released so that they are introduced into the system gradually offering a full ten hours of benefits.

Warnings: Pregnant or lactating women should consult their healthcare providers before using this product.

Used For: Estrogen (low), **hot flashes**, **menopause**, **night sweating**, perspiration (excessive), PMS Type D, and vaginal dryness

Take 1 tablet in the morning and 1 at bed time.

Ingredients: Dong quai root and black cohosh root & rhizome extract

Huperzine A *Phytochemical*

This is a compound found in Chinese club moss, an herb which has a traditional history of use for treating memory loss, dementia, and mental illness in Chinese herbalism. Modern research found this compound which inhibits the enzyme acetylcholinesterase, which breaks down acetylcholine, the neurotransmitter involved in memory. Research suggests that huperzine-A may be helpful in Alzheimer's disease. In one US study where twenty-nine Alzheimer's patients were given huperzine-A, more than half seemed to show improvement. Research in China suggests that 60 percent of people with Alzheimer's disease show significant cognitive improvement when given huperzine-A. Other research suggests this alkaloid from the Chinese club moss may help protect brain cells from certain types of toxic chemicals. It can also be helpful for dementia and for improving memory function in general.

Used For: **Alzheimer's**, **dementia**, and traumatic brain injury
Properties: Cephalic and cerebral tonic

Hyacinth *Astringent Herb*

Dolichos lablab

The root of hyracinth bean used in Chinese herbalism to arrest discharge. The flowers and bean pods are also used. The bean capsule is used for diarrhea and vomiting. The flowers are used for bleeding, diarrhea and vaginal discharge.

Energetics: Drying and constricting
Used For: Bleeding (internal), diarrhea, earache, hemorrhoids, leucorrhea, and nausea & vomiting
Properties: Antiemetic, astringent, and styptic

Hydrangea *Bitter Herb*

Hydrangea

Used as a diuretic and a calcium solvent, hydrangea is used to help rid the body of kidney stones and calcium deposits. It can also be helpful for bladder pain, back pain, and arthritis.

Look for *hydrangea* in *Kidney Stone Formula*

Warnings: Not recommended in cases of fluid deficiency, wasting, or dryness. Overdose can cause vertigo and stuffiness of the chest. Not recommended for long term use.

Energetics: Cooling and mildly drying
Used For: Autoimmune disorders, bladder (ulcerated), **calcium deposits**, cystic breast disease, interstitial cystitis, **kidney stones**, **prostatitis**, and urethritis
Properties: Analgesic, **antilithic**, **antiurolithic**, diuretic, **lithotriptic**, and sialogogue

Hypoglycemic Formula

These formulas are used to stabilize blood sugar in people who are fasting or who have hypoglycemia. They may also help to reduce sugar cravings.

Used For: Alcoholism, anorexia, bedwetting, confusion, dizziness, fainting, **hypoglycemia**, mental illness, mood swings, and schizophrenia
Affects: Pancreatic irritation

Paavo Airola's Hypoglycemic Formula

A formula for stabilizing blood sugar in people with hypoglycemia. Take 2 capsules with meals

Ingredients: Licorice root, safflower flower, and dandelion root

Fasting Blood Sugar Formula

An aid to boosting low blood sugar while fasting. Use 2 capsules five times daily while fasting.

Ingredients: Licorice root, beet root, fennel seed, and hawthorn berry

Hypothyroid Formula

See also *Target Mineral Thyroid Formula* and *Thyroid Glandular Formula*

These are traditional herbal formulas for low thyroid. They may contain seaweeds that supply iodine and small amounts of thyroid hormone precursors. They may also contain herbs to help strengthen and build the thyroid gland. Seaweeds are less effective with Hashimoto's diease, which is an autoimmune condition and not caused by a lack of iodine.

Warnings: Contraindicated in cases of Graves' disease and other hyperthyroid/overactive thyroid conditions.
Used For: ADD/ADHD, epilepsy, excess weight, fatigue, fatty tumors/deposits, fibrosis, **goiter**, hair loss/thinning, Hashimoto's disease, **hypothyroidism**, radiation, and **skin (dry/flaky)**

Affects: Parathyroid, **thyroid depression**, **thyroxin**, and **tri-iodothyronine**

Thyroid Boosting Formula

This formula combines thyroid-building herbs with seaweed for iodine. Take 2 capsules in the morning and 1 capsule in the evening.

Ingredients: Coleus root, ashwagandha root, schisandra, mermaid's bladder, and bladderwrack

Christopher's Thyroid Formula

This is generally the stronger formula and more effective for most people. Take 2 capsules one to three times daily.

Ingredients: Irish moss and kelp leaf & stem

Stan Malstrom's Thyroid Formula

The hops in this formula acts to calm the nerves, since many individuals with thyroid problems have nervous stress as well. To aid thyroid function take 2 capsules one to three times daily.

Ingredients: Kelp leaf & stem, Irish moss whole plant, and hops flower

Thyroid Building Formula

Instead of supplying iodine from seaweed, this formula focuses on rebuilding the thyroid gland. Take 2 tablets twice daily.

Ingredients: Guggul, ashwagandha root, holy basil leaf, he shou wu, and coleus root

Hyssop   *Aromatic & Mildly Bitter Herb*

Hyssopus officinalis

A traditional remedy that is considered a cure-all for respiratory ailments. It helps clear thick and congested phlegm from the lungs to restore free breathing. Having antiseptic properties that are helpful in the treatment of cuts and abrasions, it can also be used to provide immediate relief from insect bites.

Warnings: The essential oil of hyssop is toxic. Avoid during pregnancy.

Energetics: Warming and drying

Used For: Asthma, colds, cough (damp), flu, and seizures

Properties: Antiseptic, antiviral, carminative, decongestant, emmenagogue, and expectorant

Immune-Boosting Formula

These formulas are general immune stimulators. By boosting white blood cell count and enhancing antibody and white blood cell activity, they can enhance the body's natural ability to destroy viruses, bacteria, fungus, and even cancer cells. They can be helpful for problems as simple as warding off a cold in the early stages or as difficult as dealing with serious infections such as pneumonia. They can even be helpful when dealing with immune disorders such as AIDS and cancer.

Warnings: Contraindicated when there are autoimmune disorders. Not recommended for long-term use.

Used For: AIDS, antibiotic resistance, antibiotic side effects, **cancer**, **cancer treatment side effects**, colds, colds (antiviral), Epstein-Barr virus, flu, **infection (bacterial)**, **infection (viral)**, **infection prevention**, **leukemia**, **meningitis**, **mononucleosis**, pneumonia, **staph infections**, **strep throat**, tuberculosis, typhoid, and vaccine side effects

Affects: **Chronic disease stage**, degenerative disease stage, **hypoactive immune activity**, immune system, lungs, and spleen

Immune-Boosting Herbs with Beta-Glucans

This is a powerful immune stimulant that can be used for immune deficiency or fighting infection. It is also used in natural therapy for cancer. Use it to strengthen a weakened immune system by taking 1 capsule between meals two or three times daily. For cancer or fighting acute bacterial infections larger doses are needed. Use 1–2 capsules every two hours for a total of 6–10 capsules per day.

Ingredients: Beta-glucans, arbinogalactan, colostrum, cordyceps mycelium, reishi mycelium, and maitake mushroom

Immune-Boosting Herbs and Vitamins

A drink pack containing immune-boosting herbs and vitamins. A better choice for fighting off or preventing acute infections. Empty the contents of one packet into fourteen to sixteen ounces of cold water, mix and drink. Take one to three times daily.

Ingredients: Zinc, elder berry, echinacea root, vitamin C, and vitamin D

Indian Madder   *Acrid, Bitter, & Sweet Herb*

Rubia cordifolia

Used to create a brilliant red dye the herb has been used in Ayurveda as a purifier of the blood, increasing hemoglobin in red blood cells and improving circulation. It is also used as a urinary remedy and contains a compound, ruberythic acid, which helps dissolve kidney stones. It enters the liver meridian and is used in Chinese herbalism primarily for controlling bleeding and stagnant blood.

Energetics: Cooling, constricting, and drying

Used For: Acne, bleeding (external), dysmenorrhea, kidney stones, and psoriasis

Properties: Alterative, anti-inflammatory, antibacterial, blood building, hemostatic, hepatoprotective, lithotriptic, and styptic

Indian Pipe (Ghost Pipe)

Slightly Sweet Herb

Monotropa uniflora

Used primarily to help ease pain, Indian pipe doesn't actually numb pain. Instead, it has the ability to take your pain and puts it beside you, whether physical or emotional. You remain aware of the pain but you no longer care about it. It can also be helpful for panic attacks from emotional pain and bad trips from LSD.

Warnings: Consumption of large doses can bring deep sleep and ultra vivid dreams.

Energetics: Relaxing and cooling

Used For: Addictions (drugs), pain, and stress

Properties: Antispasmodic, nervine, and sedative

Indole-3-Carbinol   *Nutrient*

Indole-3-carbinol is a constituent of cruciferous vegetables of the *Brassica* genus including broccoli, cabbage and Brussels sprouts. In fact one head of cabbage contains approximately 1,200 milligrams of indole-3-carbinol. Researchers think that indole-3-carbinol is one of several compounds responsible for the reduced risk of cancer in people that have diets high in fruits and vegetables.

Indole-3-carbinol helps with both phase 1 and phase 2 detoxification in the liver. It helps to break down excess estrogen compounds, including xenoestrogens, which may contribute to breast, prostate, and uterine cancers. This also makes it useful for PMS symptoms brought on by estrogen dominance.

Usage: Take 200–400 mg daily.

Used For: BPH, **breast lumps**, cancer, **cancer prevention**, cervical dysplasia, **cystic breast disease**, **endometriosis**, **estrogen dominance**, **fibroids (uterine)**, fibromyalgia, lupus, and PMS Type A

Properties: Anticancer and detoxifying

Internal Bleeding Formula

This formula contains herbs that reduce heavy menstrual bleeding through a variety of mechanisms. It helps balance hormones, as well as slow blood flow. The herbs in this formula can also arrest bleeding in the gastrointestinal tract in cases of ulceration or hemorrhoids.

Used For: Bleeding (internal), **blood in stool**, blood in urine, estrogen dominance, **fibroids (uterine)**, **menorrhagia**, and nosebleeds

Affects: Blood, circulatory relaxation, and intestinal relaxation

To reduce heavy menstrual bleeding and uterine fibroids take 2–3 capsules with a meal three times daily. For best results, this formula should be taken over a period of several months. For a more immediate effect while bleeding is actually in progress, it can be taken in larger amounts for short periods of time, such as 2-3 capsules every two hours for a period of several days. Take 1-2 capsules of yarrow with it for an even stronger effect.

Ingredients: Lady's mantle aerial parts, shepherd's purse aerial parts, yarrow aerial parts, leaf & flower, black haw root, nettle, stinging leaf, sarsaparilla root, chaste tree fruit, and false unicorn root

Intestinal Detoxification Formula

This formula contains many substances that absorb various types of toxins and irritants. It also contains enzymes and HCl to break down food, along with fiber and cascara to aid bowel movements.

Warnings: May cause constipation without proper hydration.

Used For: Constipation (adults), diverticulitis, gas & bloating, heavy metal poisoning, and **prolapsed colon**

Affects: Intestinal stagnation and large intestines (colon)

Take 1-2 capsules two to three times daily with a large glass of water. Best taken 20-30 minutes before breakfast and at bedtime. Drink 6-8 glasses of water per day when taking this formula for best results.

Ingredients: Betaine hydrochloric acid (hcl), bile extract, pancreatin, pepsin, psyllium hulls, sodium alginate, cascara sagrada bark, sodium copper chlorophyllin, and clay (bentonite)

Intestinal Soothing Formula

See also *Irritable Bowel Fiber Formula*

These formulas are helpful for problems involving intestinal inflammation, including Crohn's disease, colitis, Celiac's disease and ulcers. They have also proved beneficial for IBS (irritable bowel syndrome), leaky gut syndrome, diverticulitis, hemorrhoids, and anal fistula. Drink six to eight glasses of water daily when taking these formulas.

Used For: Acid indigestion, anal fistula/fissure, **blood in stool**, blood in stool, cancer treatment side effects, **celiac disease**, **colitis**, colon (spastic), diarrhea, **diverticulitis**, duodenal ulcers, **enteritis**, **gastritis**, **ileocecal valve**, **inflammatory bowel disorders**, **irritable bowel**, leaky gut, rosacea, slivers, and ulcers

Affects: Appendix, general atrophy, **intestinal irritation**, **large intestines (colon)**, mucous membranes, and **small intestines**

Christopher's Colitis Formula

This formula is more antispasmodic and anti-inflammatory for easing gut pain. Take 2-3 capsules three times daily.

Ingredients: Slippery elm bark, marshmallow root, dong quai root, wild yam root, and lobelia aerial parts

Jeannie Burgess's Intestinal Soothing Formula

This formula is more soothing and healing for Inflammatory bowel disorders. It was designed to work along with *Jeanne Burgess's Nervine Formula* for intestinal problems. Take 2–3 capsules three times daily.

Ingredients: Slippery elm bark, chamomile flower, plantain leaf, and marshmallow root extract

Iodine   *Mineral*

Iodine is an essential trace mineral in humans and is necessary for the production of thyroid hormones. It is also important for breast, uterus and prostate health as well as adrenal and immune function.

Iodine supplementation is greatly promoted in the natural world. However studies clearly show that cultures with high iodine intake have a greater risk of autoimmune thyroid disease. While the research isn't definitive, this could be explained by a concomitant deficiency of selenium.

The widespread contamination of food and water supplies with the toxin perchlorate, as well as the ingestion of compounds that displace iodine like chlorine and fluoride may very well warrant supplementation with iodine. Supplementation with iodine should only be undertaken with adequate selenium status and only if autoimmune thyroid disease isn't present. Iodine supplementation is normally in the form of potassium iodide and iodine combined. Potassium iodide is taken in large doses

Warnings: Avoid with autoimmune thyroid disease or selenium deficiency.

Usage: Take 200–5,000 mcg daily. Higher doses, 25–50 mg (25,000–50,000 mcg), have been used to help detoxify halogens (fluoride or bromide) and boost low iodine levels. These higher doses should only be undertaken with the guidance of a qualified practitioner who can monitor their effects. and If one is exposed to radiation (such as a dirty bomb, reactor meltdown, or nuclear fallout), potassium iodide should be taken daily until the danger

is passed. Recommendations are as follows—adults: 130 mg, teenagers and children (13–18 years): 65 mg, young childre (1 month–3 years): 32 mg, and babies: 16 mg. So, it is wise to store potassium iodide as part of emergency preparedness supplies.

Used For: Arsenic poisoning, cancer prevention, **cholesterol (low)**, cystic breast disease, fatty liver disease, **fatty tumors/deposits**, fibroids (uterine), fibromyalgia, goiter, hair loss/thinning, Hashimoto's disease, heavy metal poisoning, **hypothyroidism**, lead poisoning, **leucorrhea**, and **radiation**

Irish Moss   *Salty Herb*
Chondrus crispus

A seaweed rich in iodine and trace minerals and a source of bromine, protein, amino acids and manganese, Irish moss soothes dry and irritated tissues. It is helpful for chronic, dry lung conditions, and sore throat. It soothes dry, irritated membranes and arrests diarrhea, but it may also act as a mild laxative in conditions involving dry, hard stools. Contains a mucilage (carrageenan), which is widely used as a stabilizer in dairy products and cosmetics.

Look for *Irish moss* in *Hypothyroid* and *Target Mineral Thyroid Formulas*

Energetics: Cooling, moistening, and nourishing

Used For: Convalescence, cough (dry), diarrhea, eczema, excess weight, fatty tumors/deposits, goiter, interstitial cystitis, itching, skin (dry/flaky), and skin problems

Properties: Anti-inflammatory, **emollient**, laxative (bulk), mucilant, nutritive, and thyrotropic

Iron   *Mineral*

Iron is an essential trace mineral, vital for the production of red blood cells and the synthesis of neurotransmitters including dopamine, norepinephrine and serotonin. The absorption of iron from food depends not only on the source of iron but also on the digestive health of the person.

Symptoms of an iron deficiency if mild, might go unnoticed. See *anemia* for more information. Iron deficiency is easily diagnosed with blood work, so get tested to see if you actually need more iron, because taking too much iron can cause organ damage. I personally prefer food sources like red meat and black strap molasses and/or herbal supplements (alfalfa, nettles, and yellow dock) to supply iron.

Usage: Take 10–50 mg daily with confirmed iron deficiency.

Used For: Acid indigestion, anemia, anxiety disorders, burning feet/hands, depression, **fatigue**, hair loss/thinning, headache (cluster), heart fibrillation/palpitations, irritability,

menorrhagia, muscle tone, pregnancy, **restless leg**, and sore/geographic tongue

Properties: Blood building and nutritive

Irritable Bowel Fiber Formula

See also *Fat-Absorbing Fiber Formula, Fiber Blend,* and *Intestinal Soothing Formula*

This is a soft fiber formula suitable for use with inflammatory conditions in the intestinal tract such as Chron's disease, celiac disease, colitis, spastic colon, and leaky gut syndrome. It feeds the friendly bacteria in the colon, reduces inflammation, and absorbs toxins, while acting as a very gentle bulk laxative.

Used For: Anal fistula/fissure, blood in stool, celiac disease, **colitis**, **colon (spastic)**, constipation (adults), diarrhea, **diverticulitis**, enteritis, hemorrhoids, **inflammatory bowel disorders**, and leaky gut

Affects: Circulatory irritation, intestinal atrophy, large intestines (colon), and **rectum**

Mix 1 scoop in water or juice and take before meals 2-4 times daily. Take with plenty of water.

Ingredients: Apple pectin, slippery elm bark, chamomile flower, flax seed, fennel seed, marshmallow root, peppermint leaf, and cat's claw bark

Isatis   *Bitter Herb*

Isatis tinctoria

Isatis is a potent antiviral, but is so cooling that if taken for extended periods it can make a person feel like they have an ice cube in their stomach and cause uncontrolled shivering. For this reason it is normally taken only for short periods or combined with ginger. It is used for infections involving fever and inflammation.

Warnings: Isatis is contraindicated for cold, chronic conditions and is not recommended for long-term use.

Energetics: Cooling

Used For: Blood poisoning, cervical dysplasia, fever, flu, herpes, lyme disease, **measles**, **meningitis**, mononucleosis, shingles, and sore throat

Properties: Antiviral and **refrigerant**

Ivy Bridge's Cleansing Program

See also *Chinese Balanced Cleansing Program*

This is convenient daily cleansing program based on a cleansing program called Ivy's recipe. The original cleanse is discussed in the *Detoxification* therapy. It is used for cleansing the colon and liver and for general detoxification.

Warnings: For occasional use only. May aggravate spastic or irritable bowel conditions. See also warnings for cascara sagrada and hydrated bentonite.

Used For: Allergies (respiratory), **chemical exposure**, **constipation (adults)**, excess weight, food allergies/intolerances, heavy metal poisoning, leaky gut, and preeclampsia

Affects: Intestinal depression, **intestinal stagnation**, **large intestines (colon)**, and liver

Ivy Bridge's Cleanse

This version contains a *Stimulant Laxative Formula* and is a stronger cleanse. Take the contents of one cleanse packet fifteen to thirty minutes before breakfast and fifteen to thirty minutes before dinner. Mix the cleanse packet in 8 ounces of juice or water. Shake, blend, or stir vigorously and drink immediately. Directly following this it is recommended to drink an additional glass of water. Drink plenty of water throughout the day.

Ingredients: Stan malstrom's lower bowel formula, environmental detoxifying formula, psyllium hulls, aloe vera whole plant, sodium copper chlorophyllin, and clay (bentonite)

Ivy Bridge's Gentle Cleanse

This version contains the *Gentle Laxative Formula* and is better for people with sensitive colons. Same directions as above.

Ingredients: Gentle bowel cleansing blend, environmental detoxifying formula, psyllium hulls, aloe vera whole leaf, sodium copper chlorophyllin, and clay (bentonite)

Jambul

Mildly Astringent, Bitter, Sour, & Sweet Herb

Syzygium cumini

Most commonly used to treat type 2 diabetes, Jambul helps to maintain blood sugar levels. The seeds regulate the conversion of starch into sugar, checking the production of glucose. A powder made from the fruit reduces sugar in the urine and abates thirst. It is also helpful for bile insufficiency, gallbladder troubles, and hepatitis.

Energetics: Cooling and constricting

Used For: Diabetes, diarrhea, dyspepsia, gallbladder problems, and urination (frequent)

Properties: Antidiabetic, antidiarrheal, and astringent

Jasmine EO   *Floral & Sweet Essential Oil*

Jasminum officinale

Jasmine EO has an exquisite floral scent that is sensual and luxuriant. It is an exotic aphrodisiac with a powerful fragrance and only small quantities are needed. It has beneficial effects on the reproductive system and can be used to relieve uterine pain, childbirth pain, and to strengthen contractions during childbirth. It is also used to create a sensual, romantic mood. Jasmine is beneficial for respiratory problems and is useful for inflammatory conditions of the skin. A powerful mood enhancer, jasmine helps overcome feelings of anxiety, bitterness, burnout, dejection, depression, guilt, indifference, jealousy, negativity, and repression. It brings feelings of confidence, creativity, happiness, intuition, peace, and self-awareness.

See the strategy *Aromatherapy* for suggested uses.

Warnings: Do not use internally. Do a patch test first before using on skin. Avoid in cases of epilepsy. Keep away from eyes. Not to be used on babies. Do not use during the first trimester of pregnancy.

Used For: Afterbirth pain, apathy, arthritis, colds (antiviral), cough (damp), **cramps (menstrual)**, depression, dermatitis, eczema, emotional sensitivity, fatigue, fear, fever, flu, headache (tension), hypochondria, hysteria, insomnia, labor & delivery, laryngitis, mood swings, postpartum depression, scars/scar tissue, sex drive (excessive), sex drive (low), shame & guilt, skin (dry/flaky), sprains, and wounds & sores

Properties: Analgesic, antibacterial, antidepressant, antifungal, antimicrobial, antiseptic, antispasmodic, aphrodisiac, calmative, expectorant, febrifuge, galactagogue, glandular, parturient, parturient, perfume, relaxant, **sedative**, and uterine

Jeannie Burgess' Allergy-Lung Formula

See also *Chinese Metal-Decreasing Formula* and *Damp Cough Syrup Formula*

One of the best all-round formulas for most types of respiratory problems involving excess mucus. It works well combined with garlic for lung infections. It can also be helpful for food and respiratory allergies. It doesn't work well with dry coughs, however.

Used For: Allergies (respiratory), **asthma**, **bronchitis**, **colds**, **colds (decongestant)**, **congestion**, **congestion (bronchial)**, **congestion (lungs)**, congestion (sinus), COPD, **cough**, **cough (damp)**, earache, **eyes (red/itching)**, food allergies/intolerances, grief & sadness, headache (sinus), **pneumonia**, **rhinitis**, and **snoring**

Affects: Acute disease stage, **bronchi**, digestive depression, **lungs**, mucous membranes, respiratory irritation, respiratory stagnation, sinuses, smell, and stressed metal

For chronic conditions take 2 capsules three times daily with meals. For acute problems take 2-4 capsules every two

to four hours. For the liquid version use 1/2-1 teaspoon every two to four hours.

Ingredients: Boneset aerial parts, fenugreek seed, horseradish root, and mullein leaf

Jeannie Burgess' Stress Formula

See also *Chinese Fire-Decreasing Formula* and *Stress Reduction*

This is a general nervine formulas for stress and tension. It is mild and suitable for children as well as adults. It is also helpful for inflammatory bowel disorders when combined with an *Intestinal Soothing Formula*.

Used For: ADD/ADHD, anorexia, anxiety (situational), anxiety attacks, colitis, croup, **inflammatory bowel disorders**, nervous exhaustion, **nervousness**, stress, and trauma

Affects: Adrenal medulla, **central nervous system**, digestive constriction, general constriction, stressed fire, structural constriction, and **sympathetic-dominant ANS**

To reduce stress and muscle tension, take 2-4 capsules or use 15-60 drops of the liquid every two to four hours. To aid sleep, take about one hour before bedtime.

Ingredients: Passion flower aerial parts, feverfew aerial parts, hops flower, and chamomile flower

Jeannie Burgess' Thymus Formula

This formula helps strengthen the thymus gland, which helps to regulate the immune system.

Used For: Cancer prevention, convalescence, infection (viral), infection prevention, and reversed polarity

Affects: Immune system and **thymus**

To help improve a weakened immune system or help prevent disease, take 2 capsules with each meal. In acute situations take 2 capsules every two hours.

Ingredients: Vitamin A, wheat grass, red clover flower, and eleuthero root

Joan Patton's Herbal Minerals Formula

See also *Herbal Calcium Formula*, *Pregnancy Tea Formula*, and *Skeletal Support Formula*

This is a great formula to help support pregnant woman and developing children and adults who aren't getting enough trace minerals. It has helped keep growing kids stay healthy and aided problems with teeth and bones.

Based on the *Pregnancy Tea Formula*, this blend was created originally by the midwife that helped deliver my children, Joan Patten. I've made some changes to the formula over the years. She gave it to all her pregnant women to reduce complications. I've also had parents claim it helped their kids stay healthy and also helped correct problems with teeth and bones, including help teeth straighten (when taken with fish liver oil to supply vitamins A and D).

Directions for a slightly different make-it-yourself version can be found in *Modern Herbal Dispensatory*.

Used For: Arthritis, **birth defect prevention**, **broken bones**, calcium deposits, **dental health**, food allergies/intolerances, **labor & delivery**, ligaments (torn/injuried), miscarriage prevention, nursing, **pregnancy**, and teeth (grinding)

Affects: Bones, **structural atrophy**, structural relaxation, and **teeth**

Take 1/4-1 teaspoon one to three times daily.

8 parts Nettle

4 parts Alfalfa

2 parts Red raspberry leaf

2 parts Oat straw

1 part Horsetail

1 part Peppermint leaf

Joint Healing Nutrients Formula

See also *Herbal Arthritis Formula*

This formula encourages joint health by helping to lubricate the joints, increasing shock absorption in the joints, improving flexibility, and promoting tissue and cartilage repair.

Used For: Arthritis, arthritis (rheumatoid), backache, **cartilage damage**, exercise (recovery), injuries, lupus, and **weak knees**

Affects: Bones, **joints**, structural atrophy, and structural irritation

Take 2 tablets two times daily with a meal.

Ingredients: Glucosamine, MSM, chondroitin, and hyaluronic acid

Jujube   *Sweet and Mildly Sour Herb*

Ziziphus spp.

Jujube dates are a nourishing herb used in Chinese herbalism to calm the nervous system, improve stamina, and aid recovery from illness.

Look for *jujube* in *Attention-Focus Formula*

Energetics: Cooling, mildly relaxing, and nourishing

Used For: ADD/ADHD and fatigue

Properties: Sedative

Juniper (Cedar)

Aromatic & Mildly Astringent Herb

Juniperus spp.

Juniper berry strongly stimulates kidney function and has antiseptic properties. It is commonly used for edema and other urinary problems. It also stimulates digestion. One species of juniper (*J. monosperma*), commonly known as cedar berries, has been used in formulas to reduce blood sugar.

Look for *juniper* in *Diuretic, Liquid Kidney,* and *Prostate Formulas*

Warnings: The volatile oils in juniper can be irritating to the kidneys and the nervous system with long-term use. Not recommended when kidneys are inflamed or in cases of nephritis and nephrosis. Avoid during pregnancy.

Energetics: Warming and drying

Used For: Bladder infection, cystic fibrosis, **edema**, incontinence, kidney stones, metabolic syndrome, **pancreatitis**, PMS Type H, urinary tract infections, and **urine (scant)**

Properties: Antifungal, antiseptic, astringent, carminative, diaphoretic, **diuretic**, fumigant, lipotropic, preservative, stimulant (metabolic), stomachic, and vermifuge

Juniper EO

Balsamic, Fresh, Sweet, & Woody Essential Oil

Juniperus communis

Juniper EO has a woody, fresh, pine-like fragrance with a fresh, warm energy. It is antiseptic and diuretic. Juniper is good for cold, damp conditions and has a purifying energy. It is used for spiritual purification, driving out negative influences. It also helps people who are too absorbed in their own thoughts, worries, and bad memories. Can be used topically to reduce swelling and skin infection.

See the strategy *Aromatherapy* for suggested uses.

Warnings: Do not use internally without the supervision of a professionally trained aromatherapy practitioner. Nontoxic and nonirritating for topical use, but should probably be diluted. Avoid during pregnancy or with kidney disease.

Used For: Acne, arthritis, congestion (lymphatic), digestion (poor), eczema, edema, kidney stones, pancreatitis, and urinary tract infections

Properties: Analgesic, antioxidant, antirheumatic, antiseptic, antispasmodic, carminative, detoxifying, diuretic, rubefacient, stomachic, tonic, and vulnerary

Kanna   *Sweet and Mildly Bitter Herb*

Sceletium tortuosum

A plant from South Africa, kanna was valued by Dutch settlers and tribesman in South Africa. It has been used to elevate mood, relieve anxiety, regulate sleep, and quench thirst and hunger. A small dose helps ease anxious feelings associated with stress. It acts as an inhibitor of serotonin reuptake, which also makes it helpful for depression.

Subjectively, kanna is said to help people experience more distance towards situations that provoke emotional responses. In some people it makes them more reserved in social situations, in others it can make them more social and talkative.

It promotes a sense of euphoria and self-confidence and can also give a a an energy boost. It may also improve the ability to think clearly.

In a higher dose it becomes sedative and promotes relaxation and may impair mental concentration. It also suppresses appetite. Some people find it helps reduce the desire for tobacco (nicotine).

Zembrin® is a proprietary extract of kanna that is used commercially to provide these benefits.

Look for *kanna* in *Anti-Anxiety* and *CBD Brain Formulas*

Used For: Addictions (tobacco), **anxiety (situational)**, depression, and insomnia

Properties: Analgesic, antidepressant, **anxiolytic**, appetite suppressant, and sedative

Kava Kava   *Acrid Herb*

Piper methysticum

Kava kava has long been used to treat stress, anxiety. and insomnia. It is used in Polynesian religious ceremonies to reduce anxiety and relax muscles while maintaining a mentally alert state. It also elevates mood. Kava is a diuretic and is also useful for urinary tract infections. It has a mild analgesic quality and is helpful for insomnia due to muscle tension or pain.

Warnings: Large daily doses taken over many years may cause liver problems and skin eruptions. Do not drive or operate heavy machinery under the influence of large doses of kava kava as it can impair motor function. If you have liver health problems or drink alcohol regularly you should avoid kava kava.

Energetics: Relaxing, drying, and mildly warming

Used For: Addictions, addictions (drugs), adrenal fatigue, alcoholism, **anxiety (situational)**, **anxiety attacks**, **anxiety disorders**, arthritis (rheumatoid), backache, bladder (irritable), cancer treatment side effects, cramps (leg), **cramps & spasms**, Cushing's disease, depression, dysmenorrhea,

emotional **sensitivity**, fibromyalgia, gas & bloating, glaucoma, gout, headache, **headache (tension)**, **insomnia**, **interstitial cystitis**, kidney infection, **kidney stones**, laryngitis, leucorrhea, nervous exhaustion, **nervousness**, OCD, **pain**, **PMS Type P**, **PTSD**, restless leg, sex drive (low), **stiff neck**, **stress**, TMJ, toothache, trauma, urinary tract infections, urination (burning/painful), and **vaginitis**

Properties: **Analgesic**, **anesthetic**, anticholinergic, antidepressant, antiseptic, **antispasmodic**, **anxiolytic**, aphrodisiac, diuretic, **euphoretic**, gaba-enhancing, **relaxant**, **sedative**, serotonergic, and **soporific**

Kelp   *Salty Herb*

Laminaria spp.

A large, fast-growing seaweed or brown algae rich in iodine, minerals, trace minerals, vitamins, and chlorophyll, kelp is sometimes considered a super-food because of the many nutrients it contains. Like other seaweeds, it contains sodium alginate, which has proven to be effective at protecting the body from radiation.

Look for *kelp* in *Herbal Potassium, Hypothyroid, Pet Supplement, Target Mineral Thyroid,* and *Thyroid Glandular Formulas*

Warnings: Avoid with hyperthyroid disorders. Use cautiously in Hashimoto's thyroiditis and selenium deficiencies.

Usage: To boost the thyroid take 3,000 to 6,000 mg daily. That would be about six to twelve 500 mg capsules per day. Kelp powder can be sprinkled on foods; it has a mild salty flavor.

Energetics: Cooling, moistening, and nourishing

Used For: Acne, birth defect prevention, calcium deficiency, cancer, cardiovascular disease, cholesterol (low), cysts, dandruff, **dehydration**, down syndrome, eczema, excess weight, fatigue, **fatty tumors/deposits**, **fingernails (weak/brittle)**, **goiter**, hair loss/thinning, **hypothyroidism**, itching, lead poisoning, pregnancy, radiation, skin (dry/flaky), skin problems, and swollen lymph glands

Properties: Antacid, condiment, emollient, mineralizer, mucilant, nutritive, stimulant (metabolic), and **thyrotropic**

Khella   *Mildly Acrid, Aromatic, & Bitter Herb*

Ammi visnaga

Khella is a vasodilator and calcium channel blocker used to treat cardiovascular problems. Its antispasmodic properties make it helpful for asthma and cramps. It may also be helpful for dissolving stones in the gallbladder and kidneys. It is antispasmodic and has been used for asthma in a similar manner to lobelia.

Warnings: Do not use during pregnancy.

Energetics: Warming and relaxing

Used For: Angina, arrhythmia, **asthma**, bronchitis, congestion (bronchial), congestive heart failure, COPD, **cough (spastic)**, **cramps (menstrual)**, gallstones, hair loss/thinning, headache (tension), hypertension, kidney stones, and pertussis

Properties: Antiarrhythmic, antispasmodic, bronchial dilator, cardiac, hypotensive, and **vasodilator**

Kidney Stone Formula

A kidney stone formula combines diuretics with herbs that help to dissolve calcium deposits and kidney stones. See Kidney Stones for more information.

Used For: Calcium deposits and **kidney stones**

Ingredients: Stone breaker herb, celery seed, parsley leaf, and hydrangea root

Krill Oil   *Nutrient*

Krill oil is derived from the shrimp-like crustacean, krill, and contains significant amounts of the omega-3 fatty acids eicosapentaenoic acid (EPA) and docosahexaenoic acid (DHA). It also contains significant amounts of omega-9 fatty acids and relatively small amounts of omega-6 fatty acids. It also contains phosphatidylcholine, vitamin A, vitamin E (alpha-tocopherol), and astaxanthin.

Warnings: Use with caution when taking blood thinners.

Usage: Take 1 capsule one to two times daily.

Used For: ADD/ADHD, **calcium deposits**, **cardiovascular disease**, dementia, dental health, fat cravings, inflammation, Ménière's disease, osteoporosis, **peripheral neuropathy**, **skin (dry/flaky)**, and wrinkles

Properties: Anti-inflammatory and nutritive

Kudzu   *Mildly Astringent & Sweet Herb*

Pueraria lobata

Kudzu has a history of use in Chinese herbalism for counteracting the effects of alcohol. Extracts of the flower are used for treating alcoholism and relieving hangover. The roots are used for neutralizing poisons and viral infections. The roots are also used to treat venous problems and the headache, dizziness, and numbness caused by high blood pressure. It helps tone up the intestines in leaky gut syndrome.

Look for *kudzu* in *Chinese Yin-Increasing* and *Phytoestrogen Breast Formulas*

Energetics: Cooling and constricting

Used For: Alcoholism, diarrhea, fibromyalgia, **hangover**, headache, hypertension, inflammatory bowel disorders, **leaky gut**, **stiff neck**, and tinnitus

Properties: Astringent, mucilant, and tonic

Kutki (Picrorhiza)   *Bitter Herb*

Picrorhiza kurroa

Over harvesting of this important plant from Ayurvedic herbalism has threatened it with near extinction. It aids the digestive system and liver, possessing hepatoprotective activity and there are some studies suggesting it may be beneficial for viral hepatitis. It may also have a protective effect on the kidneys. In Chinese herbalism, it is said to enter the liver, large intestine, and stomach meridians and is used to dispel heat and remove dampness.

Look for *kutki* in *Ayurvedic Skin Healing Formula*

Warnings: Due to its endangered status, avoid using where possible.

Energetics: Cooling and drying

Used For: Asthma, dyspepsia, hepatitis, jaundice (adults), and nausea & vomiting

Properties: Anti-inflammatory, antioxidant, cytotoxic, hepatoprotective, and immune modulator

L-Arginine   *Amino Acid*

L-arginine is a semi-essential amino acid. It is essential in protein production, wound healing, fertility, and the production of the chemical messenger nitric oxide, which dilates blood vessels.

Supplementation with L-arginine can be beneficial in reducing high blood pressure and relieving angina. It also improves tolerance to exercise.

The drug sildenafil citrate affects nitric oxide by blocking an enzyme that breaks down nitric oxide. It was originally developed as a medication for high blood pressure, but was found to be more helpful in erectile dysfunction. L-arginine supplements, which help the body make more nitric oxide, have also proved beneficial in erectile dysfunction. A study of fifty men with erectile dysfunction showed that the group taking five grams of L-arginine per day had improvement over those on the placebo. L-arginine must be taken daily to have this affect.

By increasing blood flow to the brain, L-arginine can help vasoconstrictive migraines. L-arginine may also improve recovery time after surgery, prevent wasting in AIDS patients, prevent pre-eclampsia, improve senile dementia, and help in recovery from recurring interstitial cystitis.

Usage: Take 3–15 grams daily.

Used For: AIDS, altitude sickness, **angina**, **arteriosclerosis**, **cardiovascular disease**, **congestive heart failure**, dementia, **erectile dysfunction**, **exercise (recovery)**, headache (migraine), headache (tension), **hypertension**, infertility, interstitial cystitis, Peyronie's disease, **sex drive (low)**, and surgery (recovery)

Properties: Hypotensive

L-Carnitine
Amino Acid

Carnitine is primarily derived from animal proteins, especially red meat. Although it is not an essential amino acid, supplementation with L-carnitine can have a number of beneficial actions on health. One of the most important functions of carnitine is that it moves fatty acids into the mitochondria of the cell so they can be converted to energy. Carnitine is helpful for the heart and has been shown to be deficient in the hearts of patients who have died from myocardial infarctions.

Used For: ADD/ADHD, angina, cataracts, cellulite, **cholesterol (low)**, **congestive heart failure**, diabetes, down syndrome, **excess weight**, fatigue, **fatty liver disease**, free radical damage, Graves' disease, heart fibrillation/palpitations, heart weakness, infertility, mitral valve, **peripheral neuropathy**, **Peyronie's disease**, Reye's syndrome, rheumatic fever, and triglycerides (low)

Properties: Nutritive

L-Citrulline
Amino Acid

L-citrulline is a non-essential amino acid that is changed by the kidneys into L-arginine, which enhances nitric oxide. It works with L-arginine to help improve blood flow.

Used For: Erectile dysfunction and hypertension

Properties: Hypotensive

L-Cysteine
Amino Acid

A sulfur-containing, non-essential amino acid found in poultry, yogurt, egg yolks, red peppers, garlic, onions, and broccoli. It is a building block for the antioxidant glutathione and is also a component of N-acetyl L-cysteine. It is also part of the glucose tolerance factor. It helps to eliminate excess copper, which has been linked to behavioral problems. It aids skin texture and flexibility. L-cysteine has the ability to break up mucus.

Used For: Addictions, congestion (bronchial), congestion (lungs), and mental illness

Properties: Antioxidant, detoxifying, expectorant, and mucolytic

L-Glutamine
Amino Acid

Glutamine is not an essential amino acid, but it plays a critical role in many of the body's functions nonetheless. It is converted into glutamic acid and, with the help of Vitamin B_6, gamma-aminobutryic acid (GABA)—two critical neurotransmitters in the brain. Glutamic acid is involved in mental activity and learning and GABA is a calming neurotransmitter. Glutamine improves the glucose supply to the brain and has been found to help reduce cravings for sugar and alcohol. L-glutamine helps repair the intestinal tract in leaky gut syndrome and other inflammatory bowel disorders. It is one of the amino acids needed to make the antioxidant glutathione, which helps the body detoxify heavy metals and recycle other antioxidants.

Usage: Take 1–5 grams taken three times daily. L-glutamine is found naturally in meat and bone broth and contributes greatly to the gut healing properties of bone broth.

Used For: **ADD/ADHD**, **addictions**, **addictions (drugs)**, **addictions (sugar/carbohydrates)**, **alcoholism**, anemia, anger (excessive), appetite (excessive), **autism**, birth control side effects, **blood in stool**, cloudy thinking, **colitis**, depression, dizziness, earache, **excess weight**, fat metabolism (poor), fatigue, gout, hypoglycemia, **itchy ears**, **leaky gut**, menopause, motion sickness, narcolepsy, **PMS Type C**, **rosacea**, **schizophrenia**, **SIBO**, **ulcers**, and vaccine side effects

Properties: Nutritive and vulneraries

L-Glycine
Amino Acid

A non essential amino acid found in fish, meat, beans and dairy products. It is a component of collagen, glutathione and the glucose tolerance factor.

L-Histadine
Amino Acid

An essential amino acid found in meat and dairy products. It aids the production of hydrochloric acid and is used in inflammatory immune reactions in the form of a neurotransmitter called histamine. It is also used in the detoxification of heavy metals.

L-Leucine
Amino Acid

Promotes the healing of bones, skin and muscles. It should be used in combination with L-valine and L-isoleucine.

L-Lysine
Amino Acid

Lysine is an essential amino acid found in meats and dairy but is deficient in most grains. Insufficient intake causes poor appetite, weight loss, and anemia. Lysine helps the immune system manufacture antibodies and has been used for viral infections such as mononucleosis, herpes, and shingles. It also helps ensure adequate absorption of calcium and the formation of collagen for bone, cartilage, and connective tissue. It is necessary for all amino acid assimilation and assists in the storage of fats.

Usage: Take 500–3,000 mg daily.

Used For: Canker sores, **cold sores**, failure to thrive, **herpes**, infection (viral), mononucleosis, shingles, and sprains

Properties: Antiherpetic, antiviral, and nutritive

L-Methionine   *Amino Acid*

An essential, sulfur-based amino acid found in beef, chicken, pork, soybeans, eggs, cottage cheese, liver, sardines, and yogurt. It is used to synthesize the amino acids cystine and cysteine. It protects against free radicals and aids heavy metal detoxification in the liver. It is used to make SAM-e and helps to build the bones. It may also help to reduce tremors in Parkinson's disease. Supplementation is usually not necessary, but it is sometimes used as an ingredient in formulas.

Used For: Heavy metal poisoning, mercury poisoning, and Parkinson's disease

Properties: Antioxidant, detoxifying, and nutritive

L-Phenylanaine   *Amino Acid*

An essential amino acid found in soybeans, cottage cheese, fish, meat, poultry, almonds, brazil nuts, and pecans. It is used to synthesize tyrosine, which is used to create the neurotransmitters dopamine, norepinephrine, and epinephrine. By upregulating these neurotransmitters, it may be helpful for depression. It also stimulates production of cholyscystokinin and thus induces satiety, which helps regulate appetite. It may also have benefits in helping to relieve chronic pain.

Warnings: Avoid when pregnant or nursing. Those with schizophrenia should also avoid taking phenylalanine as it may cause tardive dyskinesia, a disorder characterized by involuntary and repetitive movements. Avoid taking if the birth defect phenylketonuria (PKU) is present.

Used For: Appetite (excessive), depression, excess weight, pain, and Parkinson's disease

Properties: Antidepressant and appetite suppressant

L-Proline   *Amino Acid*

A nonessential amino acid found in dairy foods that is used as part of the protein collagen.

L-Taurine   *Amino Acid*

A nonessential amino acid found in eggs, fish, meats, and dairy products. It is one of the most abundant amino acids in the body and is used in the central nervous system. It conjugates with bile salts to maintain solubility of fats and cholesterol.

Usage: Take 500–2,000 mg per day.

L-Theanine   *Amino Acid*

This is an amino acid found in tea that has a relaxing effect on the body. It can reduce anxiety and promote better sleep.

Usage: Use between 100–300 mg as needed.

Used For: Anxiety (situational), anxiety disorders, congestion (sinus), hypertension, **insomnia**, and memory/brain function

Properties: Anxiolytic, cerebral tonic, hypotensive, **relaxant**, and **soporific**

L-Threonine   *Amino Acid*

An essential fatty acid found in dairy, beef, poultry, eggs, beans, nuts, and seeds. It helps digestive and intestinal function and aids in the liver's ability to metabolize fats. It is deficient in grains. It is also involved in the immune system.

Used For: Addictions (drugs), anxiety disorders, depression, and fatty liver disease

Properties: Nutritive

L-Tryptophan   *Amino Acid*

An essential amino acid found in turkey, chicken, beef, brown rice, nuts, fish, milk, eggs, cheese, fruit, and vegetables. It is the precursor to both serotonin and melatonin, which aid mood and sleep. It is used to create pincolinic acid, which helps with absorption and transportation of zinc. A lack of tryptophan causes carbohydrate cravings. Due to a contaminated batch of L-tryptophan, it was taken off the market as a supplement in the 1980s, but a form of it known as 5-HTP can be obtained as a supplement for mood, sleep, and carbohydrate cravings.

Used For: Addictions (sugar/carbohydrates), depression, excess weight, fibromyalgia, headache (migraine), insomnia, and pain

Properties: Nutritive

L-Tyrosine   *Amino Acid*

A nonessential amino acid found in almonds, avocados, bananas, dairy products, lima beans, pumpkin seeds, and sesame seeds. It can be synthesized from phenylalanine. It's need for both thyroid hormones and the catecholomines—dopamine, epinephrine and norepinephrine. People with Blood Type O who are vegetarians or do not eat red meat may find it helpful in stabilizing their mood.

Usage: Take 500–1,000 mg daily.

Used For: Cloudy thinking, hypothyroidism, and **mania**

Properties: Nutritive

Lactase Enzyme Formula

Contains enzymes that help digest milk and dairy products. It is used specifically for lactose intolerance and dairy allergies.

Used For: Food allergies/intolerances, gas & bloating, and **lactose intolerance**

Take 1-2 capsules to aid in digestion of milk, ice cream and other dairy foods.

Ingredients: Lactase, protease, lipase, dandelion root, and fennel seed

Lady's Mantle   *Astringent Herb*

Alchemilla vulgaris

Lady's mantle is used as a tonic for the uterus and as a remedy for vaginal discharge and heavy menstrual bleeding, internally or externally. It is a styptic and can also be used for other types of bleeding. It helps to heal ruptured membranes, such as the eardrum, and has a diuretic effect to ease edema.

Look for *lady's mantle* in *Internal Bleeding Formula*

Warnings: Avoid during pregnancy.

Energetics: Drying and constricting

Used For: Bleeding (external), bleeding (internal), diarrhea, leucorrhea, menorrhagia, and wounds & sores

Properties: Antidiarrheal, astringent, styptic, uterine, **uterine tonic**, and vulnerary

Lavender EO

Floral, Herbaceous, Sweet, & Woody Essential Oil

Lavandula angustifolia

The sweet, floral, and slightly herbaceous aroma of lavender EO has a powerful balancing effect on the nervous system. It can act as a sedative, helping to relax the body and promote sleep, or it can produce a refreshing, uplifting feeling when one is depressed or discouraged. It has been called the mother of essential oils, suggesting that it helps to nurture the person's soul. It helps to bring a relaxed, spiritual focus into practical, day-to-day affairs. When you are feeling wound-up, tense, nervous and stressed this is one of the best essential oils for helping you to relax, unwind and get the rest you need.

Add six drops to hot bath water to calm irritable children, and place one drop on the temple for headache relief. For enervation, nervous exhaustion, anxiety, excess stress, and even cancer, lavender oil baths with Epsom salts (two cups per tub) are very beneficial. Lavender baths can also help fight fungal infections in children and adults.

Use the undiluted essential oil topically as an antiseptic, mild sedative and painkiller, particularly on insect bites, stings and small (cooled) burns. Lavender oil can be blended for use as a relaxing and anti-inflammatory massage oil. Combined with chamomile, it can be massaged into the chest for asthmatic and bronchial spasm.

Other uses for lavender oil include these: add a few drops of oil to a little water, aloe vera gel, or colloidal silver for sunburn or scalds; massage diluted oil into the temples and nape of the neck for tension headaches or at the first hint of a migraine; dilute ten drops oil in twenty-five milliliters carrier oil for sunstroke (note: this is not an effective sun block); and add a few drops of the oil to a chamomile-based cream for eczema. Dilute in water and apply rinse to hair for lice.

See the strategy *Aromatherapy* for suggested uses.

Warnings: Dilute 20:1 for internal use. Nontoxic and non-irritating for topical use. Skin to which lavender oil or salves/lotions containing lavender has been applied should not be exposed to sunlight, because lavender is photo-reactive and will bleach and blotch the skin. Not recommended in cases of clinical depression.

Used For: Abrasions/scratches, acne, addictions (drugs), afterbirth pain, allergies (respiratory), anger (excessive), anxiety (situational), anxiety disorders, apathy, appetite (excessive), autism, bites & stings, body odor, **burns & scalds**, cancer, cardiovascular disease, carpal tunnel, chicken pox, colic (children), confusion, congestion (lymphatic), convalescence, cough (spastic), cramps (leg), cramps & spasms, Cushing's disease, cuts, dandruff, diaper rash, dysbiosis, dysmenorrhea, earache, eczema, edema, epilepsy, fainting, fear, fever, gangrene, hair loss/thinning, headache, headache (tension), herpes, hot flashes, hypotension, hysteria, impetigo, indigestion, **infection (fungal)**, insect repellant, **insomnia**, **irritability**, itching, jock itch, mania, menopause, nausea & vomiting, nervous exhaustion, nervousness, neuralgia & neuritis, pain, paralysis, phlebitis, PMS Type A, PMS Type D, PTSD, rhinitis, **scars/scar tissue**, skin (dry/flaky), stress, stretch marks, **sunburn**, tachycardia, teeth (loose), **thrush**, vaginitis, and whiplash

Properties: Analgesic, anti-inflammatory, antibacterial, anticoagulant, **antifungal**, antihistamine, antimicrobial, antimutagenic, antiseptic, antispasmodic, antitoxic, calmative, cholagogue, cicatrizant, CNS depressant, narcotic, nervine, parasympatholytic, perfume, **relaxant**, **sedative**, stimulant (circulatory), sympatholytic, and tonic

Lecithin   *Nutrient*

Used with cholesterol in cell membranes, lecithin helps emulsify fats in the body and may help with high cholesterol levels. It works well with ginkgo, garlic, hawthorn, and capsicum for circulatory problems. It may also aid brain function.

Usage: Use 1–3 capsules with meals.

Used For: Fibroids (uterine), Hashimoto's disease, myasthenia gravis, neuralgia & neuritis, phlebitis, Reye's syndrome, and strokes

Properties: Antioxidant and emulsifier

Lemon   *Sour Herb*

Citrus limon

Lemon juice has many wonderful medicinal properties. It is used to help fight colds and flu. It has cooling effect on the body and helps with calcium deposits, gallstones and kidney stones. Lemon is used as a flavoring in many herbal teas and remedies.

As a preventative remedy for liver and urinary problems, many people have found that the juice of a half lemon in water taken each morning upon arising is very beneficial. To cleanse the system, lemon can be taken as part of a fast using lemon water (sweetened with a small amount of pure maple syrup, preferably grade B). The juice of four lemons dissolved in a gallon of distilled water and consumed over the course of a day while fasting has been known to help dissolve kidney stones.

The lemon peel can be used as an immune tonic. It helps to strengthen the capillaries and weak tissues (similar to rose hips).

Energetics: Cooling

Used For: Calcium deposits, capillary weakness, colds, flu, gallstones, gout, **gout**, infection (viral), jaundice (adults), **kidney stones**, and scurvy

Properties: Antilithic, antiparasitic, antiscorbutic, antiseptic, condiment, **febrifuge**, food, lithotriptic, nutritive, and **refrigerant**

Lemon EO   *Fresh & Fruity Essential Oil*

Citrus limon

With its fresh, sweet citrus smell, lemon EO is a very uplifting and invigorating fragrance. It can help to overcome mental fatigue, clear the mind and aid decision-making. It eases fears and insecurities, promoting feelings of confidence and a radiant, warm and sparkling presence. It can be helpful for calming and centering children (or adults) who have ADHD.

Lemon essential oil is a disinfectant (topical) and immune booster. It also helps to move lymph and lift mood. When using the essential oil internally or externally dilute five to ten drops in a half pint of warm water. Mix with Epsom salts before adding to bath water to prevent the oil from floating on the surface and irritating the skin.

See the strategy *Aromatherapy* for suggested uses.

Warnings: May be used internally, but shouldn't be used regularly as overuse of lemon oil internally may cause nausea. Externally, lemon oil may cause dermal irritation. Lemon oil is phototoxic, so avoid using on skin and then exposing to the sun.

Used For: Abscesses, acid indigestion, ADD/ADHD, addictions (tobacco), aging, Alzheimer's, anemia, anxiety disorders, apathy, appetite (deficient), arthritis, arthritis (rheumatoid), asthma, bipolar mood disorder, bites & stings, boils, breasts (swelling/tenderness), canker sores, capillary weakness, cardiovascular disease, cellulite, cervical dysplasia, cholesterol (high), colds (antiviral), confusion, congestion (lymphatic), constipation (adults), cough (dry), cramps & spasms, depression, dermatitis, diarrhea, digestion (poor), eczema, edema, excess weight, fatigue, fear, fever, fleas, flu, gallstones, gas & bloating, gingivitis, gonorrhea, gout, grief & sadness, halitosis, headache, herpes, hot flashes, hypertension, hypotension, infection (bacterial), **infection (viral)**, **infection prevention**, insect repellant, jaundice (adults), kidney stones, malaria, mania, mood swings, nausea & vomiting, pain, pap smear (abnormal), parasites, phlebitis, PMS Type H, pneumonia, rashes & hives, **scabies, seborrhea**, shingles, skin (oily), sore throat, syphilis, teeth (loose), thrombosis, thrush, tick, tinnitus, **tonsillitis**, tuberculosis, typhoid, urinary tract infections, varicose veins, wounds & sores, and wrinkles

Properties: Antimicrobial, antirheumatic, antiseptic, astringent, bactericidal, carminative, cicatrizant, condiment, deodorant, diaphoretic, diuretic, febrifuge, food, hemostatic, hypotensive, insecticide, rubefacient, stomachic, sympathomimetic, tonic, and vermifuge

Lemon Balm

Aromatic & Mildly Astringent Herb

Melissa officinalis

An aromatic with a mild astringent action and lemony scent, lemon balm is useful for many acute ailments such as colds, digestive upset and flu. It is used in combination with bugleweed to calm an overactive thyroid. It is helpful for nervousness that affects the heart and digestion. The antiviral properties of lemon balm make it useful for herpes, cold sores, chicken pox and shingles. It also has a positive effect on the brain, helping to ease sadness and depression, enhance sleep and aid memory and concentration.

Look for *lemon balm* in *Antidepressant, Attention-Focus, Sleep Support,* and *Thyroid Calming Formulas*

Energetics: Cooling and mildly relaxing

Used For: **ADD/ADHD**, anxiety disorders, **autism**, chicken pox, cold sores, colic (children), **depression**, fever, flu,

Graves' disease, **grief & sadness**, heart fibrillation/palpitations, **herpes**, hysteria, indigestion, **infection (viral)**, insomnia, mania, memory/brain function, **nausea & vomiting**, perspiration (deficient), **seasonal affective disorder**, **shingles**, and tachycardia

Properties: **Antidepressant**, antiherpetic, antiseptic, antisudorific, antithrombotic, **antithyrotropic**, antiviral, carminative, diaphoretic, and nervine

Lemongrass EO *Sharp & Fresh Essential Oil*

Cymbopogon citratus

As its name suggests, lemongrass EO has a citrus fragrance coupled with a grassy or herbaceous quality. It is very refreshing, energizing and uplifting. It promotes concentration, clear thinking and may help people who are sluggish in the morning, acting like a morning shower to wake up their body and mind.

Lemongrass is a citrusy, uplifting fragrance. Is is antiseptic and helpful for urinary tract infections. It can also help to settle the stomach and ease stomach pain. It has analgesic properties and is said to remove lactic acid buildup from tired muscles. It is good for oily hair, acne, skin infections and scabes. Emotionally, lemongrass is soothing and calming, easing stress and nervous exhaustion.

See the strategy *Aromatherapy* for suggested uses.

Warnings: Do not use internally without the supervision of a professionally trained aromatherapy practitioner. Do not use internally for more than seven to ten days at a time. Undiluted lemongrass oil can be irritating to the skin.

Used For: Acne, bites & stings, bladder infection, congestion (lymphatic), digestion (poor), edema, fever, **fleas**, foot odor, **infection (viral)**, infection prevention, **insect repellant**, **pet supplements**, scabies, shock (medical), skin (infections), tick, and varicose veins

Properties: Analgesic, antidepressant, antimicrobial, antiseptic, astringent, bactericidal, carminative, deodorant, febrifuge, galactagogue, insecticide, lymphatic, nervine, refrigerant, and tonic

Licorice *Sweet Herb*

Glycyrrhiza glabra

Licorice root helps to stabilize blood sugar levels and is useful in treating both hypoglycemia and diabetes. It improves stamina and endurance, increasing energy without being stimulating. Licorice has anti-inflammatory properties and can be used to reduce inflammation and heal ulcerations. The herb also eases dry cough and sore throats when used as a tea or syrup.

Look for *licorice* in *Adrenal Glandular, Ayurvedic Bronchial Decongestant, Colloidal Mineral, Dry Cough Syrup, Fiber,* *Flu* and *Vomiting, General Glandular, H. Pylori-Fighting, Hypoglycemic, Skinny,* and *Vandergriff's Energy Booster Formulas*

Warnings: Although licorice is a safe herb, some cautions are necessary when taking large doses for long periods of time. Licorice should be avoided in cases of high blood pressure or when taking digitalis. It causes retention of water and sodium and excretion of potassium, which can cause edema (water retention), high blood pressure, heart palpitations, or a slowing of the heartbeat. Vertigo (dizziness) and headaches are early symptoms of overuse of licorice. Taking a potassium supplement with licorice can help counteract some of these effects. These effects are much more likely in individuals using licorice extracts or licorice derived drugs than in taking whole licorice root. Deglycyrrhizinated licorice is free of adverse effects.

Use larger doses in pregnancy only under the supervision of a qualified herbalist (herbiverse.com) or practitioner. Small quantities, or licorice as part of a formula are okay during pregnancy.

Energetics: Cooling and moistening

Used For: **Acid indigestion**, ADD/ADHD, addictions (coffee, caffeine), addictions (drugs), **addictions (sugar/carbohydrates)**, **Addison's disease**, alcoholism, allergies (respiratory), anorexia, arthritis, asthma, **autoimmune disorders**, bedwetting, **bronchitis**, cirrhosis of the liver, colitis, congestion (bronchial), constipation (children), **COPD**, **cough (dry)**, **dehydration**, **dizziness**, **duodenal ulcers**, eczema, **emphysema**, endurance, Epstein-Barr virus, **estrogen (low)**, excess weight, **fainting**, **fatigue**, fear, fibromyalgia, fibrosis, **gastritis**, Graves' disease, halitosis, hangover, Hashimoto's disease, hot flashes, **hypoglycemia**, **hypotension**, hypothyroidism, inflammation, inflammatory bowel disorders, **interstitial cystitis**, irritable bowel, **jet lag**, **laryngitis**, leaky gut, lupus, mental illness, metabolic syndrome, **mood swings**, muscular dystrophy, myasthenia gravis, **pancreatitis**, Parkinson's disease, pernicious anemia, pertussis, phobias, **PMS Type C**, pneumonia, psoriasis, schizophrenia, sex drive (low), shingles, **sore throat**, stress, tendonitis, thrush, **tickle in throat**, triglycerides (high), **ulcers**, and underweight

Properties: Adaptogen, **adrenal tonic**, **adrenergic**, **anti-inflammatory**, antiherpetic, antilipemic, **antitussive**, antiviral, aperient, aphrodisiac, bronchial dilator, **catalyst**, emollient, estrogenic, expectorant, **hypertensive**, **immune modulator**, lung tonic, **moistening**, mucilant, nutritive, **parasympatholytic**, phytoestrogen, refrigerant, sialogogue, stimulant (appetite), stimulant (metabolic), sweetener, **sympathomimetic**, vasoconstrictor, and vulneraries

Ligusticum
Pungent Herb

Ligusticum wallichii

Ligusticum is a Chinese remedy that enters the liver, gallbladder, and pericardium meridians. It promotes the flow of qi and blood and helps relieve pain and muscle spasm.

Look for *ligusticum* in *Chinese Yang-Reducing Formula*

Energetics: Warming, relaxing, and balancing

Used For: Amenorrhea, cramps & spasms, headache, menstrual irregularity, and pain

Properties: Analgesic, antibacterial, antifungal, antispasmodic, hypotensive, tranquilizer, and vasodilator

Ligustrum
Bitter & Sweet Herb

Ligustrum lucidum

The fruit of the privet plant, which is grown as a hedge in many parts of the world, is used in Chinese herbalism for yin deficient heat or false heat. These are inflammatory conditions caused by a lack of cooling (antioxidant) compounds in the body. It nourishes the yin (moistening the tissues) and supports liver and kidney health.

It is part of the Fu Zheng therapy in China, where it is combined with herbs like astragalus and ganoderma to help reduce side effects of chemotherapy and radiation treatments. It supports the health of the liver and is used to aid eye health in diminished vision or spots in the eyes.

Energetics: Moistening and mildly cooling

Used For: Constipation (adults), dizziness, heart fibrillation/palpitations, and insomnia

Properties: Cardiac, hepatic, and immune modulator

Lime EO
Fruity & Sharp Essential Oil

Citrus aurantifolia

Possessing a fresh, fruity, citrus-type fragrance, lime EO has a calmin-ethereal effect. It is relaxing, yet uplifting at the same time. It helps with anxiety and depression, especially when associated with low self-esteem and excessive self-judgment. It helps overcome the core belief that one is bad or just not good enough. It is also energizing to someone who is tired, especially mentally tired. It is antimicrobial and a digestive tonic. Applied topically, it stimulates lymphatic flow. It is helpful for oily skin.

See the strategy *Aromatherapy* for suggested uses.

Warnings: Do not use internally without the supervision of a professionally trained aromatherapy practitioner. Lime non-toxic and nonirritating topically, but may cause photosensitivity, so avoid direct sunlight after application.

Used For: Anxiety (situational), appetite (deficient), cloudy thinking, depression, fatigue, fever, indigestion, shame & guilt, skin (oily), and stress

Properties: Anti-inflammatory, antiseptic, antispasmodic, antiviral, astringent, bactericidal, disinfectant, febrifuge, hemostatic, insecticide, and tonic

Linden
Sweet Herb

Tilia sp.

Linden is a soothing nervine that relaxes tension and reduces blood pressure. It can also be helpful for headaches. It a very pleasant-tasting herbal teas and is a valuable but underused remedy.

Look for *linden* in *Adaptogen* and *Blood Pressure Reducing Formulas*

Energetics: Cooling, drying, and relaxing

Used For: Anger (excessive), anxiety (situational), autism, bipolar mood disorder, dizziness, headache, headache (migraine), heart fibrillation/palpitations, **hypertension**, insomnia, itching, neuralgia & neuritis, and vaginal dryness

Properties: Antispasmodic, hypotensive, **nervine**, **relaxant**, and **vasodilator**

Linoleic Acid
see *omega-6 LA*

Lipase
Enzyme

Lipase is an enzyme produced by the pancreas to help breakdown fats. Supplementing with lipase, normally in combination with protease and amylase, is useful for anyone who is having problems with poor fat metabolism such as indigestion after eating fats and people with celiac disease, Crohn's disease, or gall bladder problems. It is very helpful after a person has had their gallbladder surgically removed to help the body break down fats more effectively.

Used For: Acne, celiac disease, cholesterol (low), dermatitis, digestion (poor), **fat cravings**, **fat metabolism (poor)**, fatty liver disease, fatty tumors/deposits, **gallbladder problems**, gallstones, **skin (dry/flaky)**, **skin (oily)**, triglycerides (high), and **triglycerides (low)**

Lipase Enzyme Formula

This enzyme helps break down fats in the digestive system. It is useful for anyone who is having problems with poor fat metabolism such as indigestion after eating fats, dry skin or gall bladder problems. It is very helpful after a person has had their gallbladder surgically removed to help the body break down fats more effectively.

Used For: **Fat cravings**, **fat metabolism (poor)**, **fatty liver disease**, and **gallbladder problems**

Affects: **Gallbladder** and small intestines

Lipase Enzyme Blend

Take 1-2 capsules before consuming foods high in fat.

Ingredients: Lipase, amylase, cellulase, protease, dandelion root, and gentian root

Liquid Kidney Formula

See also *Chinese Water-Decreasing Formula*, *Diuretic Formula*, and *Liquid Lymph Formula*

This is a diuretic formula that enhances the kidneys' ability to filter acid from tissues. This formula is best suited for conditions where urinary function is underactive and there is fluid accumulation in the tissues. Its kidney tonic herbs make it especially nourishing for sluggish kidneys. It works well with the *Liquid Lymph Formula*.

Warnings: Use with caution with kidney inflammation.

Used For: Adenitis, angina, bedwetting, bladder (irritable), bladder (ulcerated), **breasts (swelling/tenderness)**, congestive heart failure, **edema**, gout, **interstitial cystitis**, PMS Type H, urination (burning/painful), and urine (scant)

Affects: **Bladder**, kidneys, lymphatics, urinary depression, and urinary irritation

Take approximately 15-20 drops or 1/4 teaspoon in water twice daily.

Ingredients: Asparagus tops, plantain leaf, juniper berry, and goldenrod aerial parts

Liquid Lymph Formula

See also *Lymph Cleansing Formula*

This formula helps stimulate lymphatic drainage and clear toxins from tissue spaces. To clear fluid and reduce edema and swollen lymph nodes mix between a half to a full teaspoon each of this formula and *Liquid Kidney Formula* in a quart of water and sip the water frequently throughout the day.

Used For: Abrasions/scratches, abscesses, **adenitis**, appendicitis, bladder (irritable), bladder (ulcerated), body odor, boils, breast lumps, **breasts (swelling/tenderness)**, **congestion**, **congestion (lymphatic)**, congestive heart failure, **cystic breast disease**, cysts, earache, **edema**, Epstein-Barr virus, **kidney infection**, lymphoma, **mastitis**, mumps, oral surgery, pain, PMS Type H, PMS Type S, sleep apnea, sore throat, **swollen lymph glands**, tonsillitis, urethritis, urine (scant), and vaccine side effects

Affects: Appendix, breasts, capillaries, eustachian tubes, immune system, kidneys, **lymphatics**, subacute disease stage, and tonsils

Use approximately 15-20 drops or 1/4 teaspoon, in water twice daily.

Ingredients: Cleavers aerial parts, red clover flower extract, stillingia root, and prickly ash bark

Lithium   *Mineral*

Lithium is on the periodic table of elements and is a naturally occurring trace mineral in water supplies of many places in the world. Lithium was originally a component of 7Up. It was found to benefit bipolar disorder in the late 1800s, and has been studied in depth since 1949. Research from animal models shows that it likely works by reducing arachidonic acid and increasing DHA in the brain, reducing the inflammatory cascade at the root of many diseases including depression, bipolar disorder and anxiety. Lithium can also reduce the inflammatory processes in ALS and is the only known effective drug for slowing ALS. It's currently being researched for dementia and Alzheimer's disease. In places where lithium is high in the water (2 mg per liter on average) there are reductions in suicide, homicide, and drug use. Lithium also helps to regulate circadian rhythm and improve sleep. Some researchers are now pushing for a RDA of 1–2 mg a day of lithium. Lithium orotate is available as a supplement, providing 5 mg of elemental lithium per 120 mg capsule of lithium orotate.

Warnings: High doses of lithium (from any source including orotate) can cause thirst, frequent urination, hand tremors, nausea, and vomiting, hypothyroidism, kidney, and heart damage. Do not exceed 15 mg of lithium without professional advice, and don't take at all if you have kidney disease. The first few days of taking lithium you can feel sluggish and sleepy. These effects normally wear off, and are minimized by taking lithium before bed.

Usage: A typical dose is one 100–150 mg tablet of lithium orotate three times daily; taking 100 mg of lithium orotate supples 5 mg of lithium.

Used For: ADD/ADHD, anxiety attacks, anxiety disorders, **bipolar mood disorder**, bulimia, depression, headache (migraine), insomnia, and PTSD

Properties: Antidepressant, anxiolytic, and nutritive

Liver Cleanse Formula

See also *Detoxifying Formula* and *Hepatoprotective Formula*

These are general liver and digestive formulas. They can help improve liver detoxification to remove chemicals from the body. Liver cleansers are also used for skin eruptive diseases and a general feeling of malaise.

Used For: Alcoholism, anger (excessive), appetite (deficient), food allergies/intolerances, gallbladder problems, gallstones, hangover, hepatitis, jaundice (adults), mononucleosis, morning sickness, polycystic ovarian syndrome, and psoriasis

Affects: Digestive stagnation, gallbladder, hepatic stagnation, and **liver**

Jeannie Burgess' Liver Formula

A gentle liver cleansing formula. Take 2–4 capsules with each meal and before bed.

Ingredients: Dandelion root, barberry root bark, fennel seed, beet root, and horseradish root

Paavo Airola's Liver Cleanse

A more comprehensive liver cleansing formula. Take 1–2 capsules two to three times per day.

Ingredients: Beet root, dandelion root, parsley leaf, yellow dock root, birch, white leaf, blessed thistle aerial parts, angelica root, gentian root, and goldenrod aerial parts

Lobelia   *Acrid Herb*

Lobelia inflata

Lobelia is a powerful antispasmodic herb. It dilates the bronchial passages to ease asthma attacks and relaxes spasms to ease pain caused by muscle tension. Take five to ten drops every two to five minutes until relief is obtained. It can also be applied topically to insect bites and stings or to ease muscle spasms.

Lobelia contains lobeline, which binds to the same receptors in the nervous system as nicotine, but inhibits rather than stimulates them. For this reason, lobelia has been prescribed to help people quit smoking.

Look for *lobelia* in *Antispasmodic* and *Ed Millet's Herbal Crisis Formulas*

Warnings: The FDA considers lobelia to be poisonous, and many sources claim it will cause convulsions, coma and death. These are potential effects of its principal alkaloid lobeline, but there is no record of the whole herb causing these problems in anyone because lobelia is an emetic and makes you throw up if you take too much. Lobelia can produce severe symptoms (nausea, profuse sweating, vomiting, and deep relaxation), but these symptoms typically pass quickly and the person feels better afterward. However, because of these effects, lobelia is not recommended for weak, debilitated persons or persons who are deeply relaxed. Also, lobelia is not recommended for long-term use and should be used cautiously during pregnancy. To avoid unpleasant effects such as nausea and vomiting, use small, repeated doses, instead of large infrequent doses, or use it as part of a formula.

Energetics: Mildly warming, mildly drying, and relaxing

Used For: Addictions (drugs), **addictions (tobacco)**, adenitis, afterbirth pain, allergies (respiratory), **angina**, **anxiety attacks**, anxiety disorders, arrhythmia, **asthma**, backache, bites & stings, blood poisoning, bronchitis, **cardiac arrest**, **chest pain**, chicken pox, colds, colds (decongestant), **colic (adults)**, colic (children), colon (spastic), **congestion**, **congestion (bronchial)**, congestion (lymphatic), **COPD**, **cough**, **cough (spastic)**, cramps (leg), **cramps & spasms**, **croup**, deafness, diphtheria, dislocation, **dysmenorrhea**, **earache**, emphysema, epilepsy, fever, fibromyalgia, **food poisoning**, **glaucoma**, Hashimoto's disease, **headache**, headache (migraine), headache (tension), hearing loss, **hiatal hernia**, **hiccups**, hypertension, insomnia, irritable bowel, kidney stones, labor & delivery, laryngitis, **lead poisoning**, mastitis, mercury poisoning, miscarriage prevention, mumps, **pain**, paralysis, **pertussis**, **pleurisy**, PMS Type P, pneumonia, poison ivy/oak, **poisoning**, Raynaud's disease, restless leg, sciatica, **seizures**, sore throat, spinal disks, sprains, stiff neck, swollen lymph glands, **tachycardia**, teething, tetanus, tics, **tinnitus**, TMJ, toothache, **tuberculosis**, **twitching**, ulcers, **urination (burning/painful)**, vaccine side effects, **wheezing**, and whiplash

Properties: Analgesic, antiabortive, antiadrenergic, antiarrhythmic, anticephalalgic, anticholinergic, **antidote**, **antiepileptic**, **antismoking**, **antispasmodic**, antitoxic, **antitussive**, **antivenomous**, anxiolytic, **bronchial dilator**, catalyst, decongestant, **deobstruent**, diaphoretic, **emetic**, expectorant, **hypotensive**, lymphatic, **nauseant**, nervine, panacea, **relaxant**, sedative, stimulant (metabolic), and **vasodilator**

Lomatium   *Mildly Aromatic & Sweet Herb*

Lomatium dissectum

An herb with powerful antiviral and antiseptic actions, lomatium is useful for a wide variety of viral conditions. It is also beneficial for respiratory problems. Applied topically it can ease pain and promote healing of wounds, sprains, cuts and other injuries.

Warnings: Do not use during pregnancy. Discontinue if rash develops.

Energetics: Cooling

Used For: Acne, AIDS, allergies (respiratory), chicken pox, congestion (lungs), **Epstein-Barr virus**, lyme disease, mononucleosis, pneumonia, sinus infection, sore throat, and **tuberculosis**

Properties: Antiseptic and **antiviral**

Loquat   *Sour & Sweet Herb*

Eriobotrya japonica

The fruits are used as a remedy for dry coughs with irritation in the lungs. They make a good ingredient in a cough syrup. A tea from the cooling leaves can ease thirst in the heat of summer.

Look for *loquat* in *Dry Cough Syrup Formula*

Energetics: Cooling, moistening, and nourishing

Used For: Bronchitis and cough (dry)

Properties: Anti-inflammatory, expectorant, and **refrigerant**

Lotus   *Mildly Astringent & Sweet Herb*

Nelumbo nucifera

The lotus plant is considered a sacred herb in the Orient. The seeds are used for the liver, kidney and heart meridians. They are said to dispel toxic heat from the heart and strengthen the kidneys. They aid deficiency of the spleen.

The stems have similar uses. They are used for the heart and kidney meridians. They calm frequent urination and have an antiviral effect.

Energetics: Mildly constricting, cooling, and moistening

Used For: Diarrhea, leucorrhea, nocturnal emission, restless dreams, and urination (frequent)

Properties: Antiviral, astringent, relaxant, and spleen chi tonic

Lung Moistening Formula

See also *Dry Cough Syrup Formula*

This is one of the few formulas that is moistening to the lung tissue, rather than drying. It helps where there is a deficient production of mucus, resulting in a dry cough.

Used For: Allergies (respiratory), angina, **asthma**, bronchitis, cough, **cough (dry)**, **emphysema**, laryngitis, **nursing**, and **pleurisy**

Affects: Intestinal atrophy, **lungs**, respiratory atrophy, and respiratory stagnation

For soothing irritated respiratory passages, dry cough or tickle in throat, take 2 capsules every hour with large glass of water.

For chronic lung conditions, take 2 capsules two to three times daily. Taking this formula with mullein or licorice root can enhance its effectiveness.

Ingredients: Fenugreek seed and marshmallow root

Lung-Supporting EO Blend

Use this essential oil blend to help relieve respiratory congestion and fight respiratory infections. Dilute with massage oil and apply to temples, forehead, chest and back for sinus problems, bronchitis, pneumonia, and asthma. It can also be massaged on the throat for sore throats.

See the strategy *Aromatherapy* for suggested uses.

Warnings: May aggravate asthma, try a small amount first before using.

Used For: Asthma, **bronchitis**, congestion (bronchial), **congestion (sinus)**, croup, grief & sadness, pneumonia, sinus infection, and sore throat

Affects: Immune system, **respiratory depression**, and respiratory stagnation

Ingredients: Eucalyptus EO, cypress EO, fir needle EO, ravensara EO, and tea tree EO

Lutein   *Phytochemical*

Lutein is a carotenoid that helps protect the macula lutea from oxidative damage. It may also help to improve vision, prevent age-related macular degeneration, cataracts, and also has a protective effect against breast cancer. Foods like broccoli, spinach, and kale are the best sources of lutein. It is a yellow pigment that is also found in egg yolks and animal fats.

Usage: Take 20–40 mg daily.

Used For: **Cataracts**, **eye health**, free radical damage, glaucoma, and **macular degeneration**

Properties: Antioxidant

Lycium (Gogi, Wolfberry)   *Sour Herb*

Lycium chinense

Lycium berries, also known as wolfberries or gogi berries have become very popular due to their antioxidant and anti-inflammatory effects. They are one of the richest sources of vitamin C and contain many other vitamins and nutrients. The berries are used in China as a blood, liver, and eye tonic and are also believed to extend human longevity. They are used for cooling hot, irritated tissues.

Look for *lycium* in *Chinese Fire-Increasing*, *Chinese Wood-Increasing*, and *Colloidal Mineral Formulas*

Energetics: Cooling and moistening

Used For: Cough (dry), environmental pollution, eye health, fever, **free radical damage**, hepatitis, overacidity, perspiration (excessive), and rhinitis

Properties: Antiscorbutic, febrifuge, food, hepatoprotective, nutritive, refrigerant, and tonic

Lycopene   *Phytochemical*

Lycopene is a bright-red carotenoid found in fruits and vegetables like tomatoes, red bell peppers and watermelon.

Preliminary research on lycopene has shown an inverse correlation between the consumption of lycopene rich foods and cancer risk. While lycopene is a carotenoid, it isn't converted to vitamin A, but acts as a strong antioxidant instead. Its strong antioxidant properties are what is theorized to reduce cancer risk as well as to help prevent cardiovascular disease by inhibiting the oxidation of low-density lipoproteins.

Lycopene supplements have been shown to increase blood levels of lycopene in the same manner as food lycopene consumption. Cooked tomato products like tomato paste are the best food source of lycopene.

Usage: 30 mg daily.

Used For: Cancer prevention, cardiovascular disease, and free radical damage

Lymph Cleansing Formula

See also *Liquid Lymph Formula*

This formula improves lymphatic drainage, shrinks swollen lymph nodes, supports the immune system in fighting chronic infections, and acts as an alterative. It is useful for problems involving lymphatic congestion and may help Hodgkin's disease.

Used For: Breasts (swelling/tenderness), **congestion (lymphatic)**, cystic breast disease, edema, **leukemia**, **lymphoma**, **mumps**, **swollen lymph glands**, and **tonsillitis**

Affects: Appendix, **general stagnation**, immune system, **lymphatics**, subacute disease stage, and **tonsils**

Lymphatic Tonic

A potent lymph cleanser in capsule formula. Take 2 capsules two to three times daily.

Ingredients: Mullein leaf, bayberry root bark, cleavers aerial parts, plantain leaf, echinacea root, yarrow aerial parts, red root root, and lobelia aerial parts

David Winston's Lymph

A potent lymph tonic and cleanser. Take 40-60 drops three times daily.

Ingredients: Burdock root, echinacea root, figwort, red clover flower, red root, and violet

Lymphatic Infection Formula

See also *Antibacterial Formula*

These formulas target low-grade infections that affect the lymph glands, resulting in swollen lymph nodes and inflammation. They may help the tonsils, bronchial passages, ear infections, and breast tissue

Used For: Abscesses, **adenitis**, **blood poisoning**, **congestion (lymphatic)**, **cystic breast disease**, earache, Epstein-Barr virus, **giardia**, impetigo, infection (bacterial), mastitis, sore throat, staph infections, strep throat, swollen lymph glands, and **tonsillitis**

Affects: Bronchi, general stagnation, hearing, immune system, **lymphatics**, **subacute disease stage**, and **tonsils**

Stan Malstrom's Lymphatic Infection Formula

A traditional lymph gland formula for shrinking swollen lymph nodes. Use 2 capsules three times daily or every two hours for swollen lymph nodes.

Ingredients: Parthenium root, goldenseal root & rhizome, and yarrow aerial parts

Lymphatic Immune

An lymphatic formula with potent infection-fighting properties. Take 30-40 drops three to four times daily with water.

Ingredients: Echinacea root, indigo, true, prickly ash, red root, stillingia, and thuja

Christopher's Infection Fighter

A lymph gland formula with stronger infection fighting properties. Use 2 capsules three times daily or every two hours for serious infection.

Ingredients: Black walnut hips, echinacea aerial parts, plantain leaf, and goldenseal root extract

Maca   *Sweet Herb*

Lepidium meyenii

A rejuvenating tonic for reproductive health in both men and women. Studies have shown that maca can be helpful for erectile dysfunction in men and increasing sexual desire in women. Maca has adaptogenic and tonic properties.

Look for *maca* in *Testosterone* and *Women's Aphrodisiac Formulas*

Warnings: May be contraindicated with acute inflammation.

Energetics: Warming and nourishing

Used For: Adrenal fatigue, Epstein-Barr virus, erectile dysfunction, **fatigue**, hair loss/thinning, **infertility**, **premature ejaculation**, **sex drive (low)**, stress, and **testosterone (low)**

Properties: Adaptogen, antiaging, **aphrodisiac**, stimulant (metabolic), testosterone-enhancing, and tonic

Magnesium   *Mineral*

A study published in the *Journal of the American College of Nutrition* and sponsored by the National Institutes of Health found that 68 percent of Americans are magnesium-deficient. In my own clinical work I find magnesium deficiency is much more common than calcium deficiency.

Magnesium is used in over three hundred enzymatic reactions in the body. It acts as a catalyst in the utilization of carbohydrates, fats, protein, calcium, phosphorus, and possibly potassium. It helps produce energy inside cells.

Magnesium works hand in hand with calcium to maintain muscle tone. Calcium ions make muscles contract, while magnesium ions help muscles relax. Magnesium helps relieve muscle spasms, colic, and spastic bowel conditions. It also helps prevent heart attacks. Tense muscles, anxiety, nervous twitching, colon cramps, hypersensitivity to noises, and calcium deposits are all symptoms of magnesium deficiency.

A magnesium deficiency interferes with vitamin D utilization as well as contributes to many of the listed health issues. Alcohol, diuretics, birth control pills, antibiotics, steroids, acid reflux medication, and fluoride deplete the body's supply of magnesium.

Usage: Take 100–400 mg two or three times daily. Most people need between 400 and 1,000 mg daily.

Used For: Acid indigestion, **ADD/ADHD**, Addison's disease, **adrenal fatigue**, **afterbirth pain**, **alcoholism**, Alzheimer's, anal fistula/fissure, aneurysm, angina, **anxiety (situational)**, anxiety attacks, **anxiety disorders**, **arrhythmia**, arthritis, **asthma**, **autism**, **backache**, **bedwetting**, **Bell's palsy**, **bipolar mood disorder**, birth control side effects, breasts (swelling/tenderness), broken bones, bulimia, bursitis, **calcium deficiency**, **calcium deposits**, cancer treatment side effects, cardiac arrest, **cardiovascular disease**, carpal tunnel, **celiac disease**, chest pain, **colic (children)**, **colon (spastic)**, concentration (poor), confusion, **congestive heart failure**, constipation (adults), **constipation (children)**, COPD, **cramps (leg)**, **cramps (menstrual)**, **cramps & spasms**, Cushing's disease, cystic breast disease, dehydration, **dementia**, **depression**, **diabetes**, digestion (poor), **dysmenorrhea**, dyspepsia, **emotional sensitivity**, **epilepsy**, Epstein-Barr virus, **erectile dysfunction**, fatigue, **fibromyalgia**, floaters, gallstones, **glaucoma**, gout, **Graves' disease**, **headache**, **headache (cluster)**, **headache (migraine)**, **headache (tension)**, **hearing loss**, **heart fibrillation/palpitations**, **heart valves**, **heart weakness**, **hiccups**, **hypertension**, **insomnia**, irritability, irritable bowel, **kidney stones**, **labor & delivery**, leaky gut, memory/brain function, **mental illness**, **metabolic syndrome**, **miscarriage prevention**, **mitochondrial dysfunction**, **mitral valve**, **myasthenia gravis**, narcolepsy, nephritis, nerve damage, **nervous exhaustion**, **nervousness**, **OCD**, osteoporosis, ovarian pain, **overacidity**, pain, **paralysis**, PMS, **PMS Type A**, **PMS Type C**, **PMS Type D**, **PMS Type H**, **PMS Type P**, **pregnancy**, progesterone (low),

prolapsed uterus, **PTSD**, **puberty**, **Raynaud's disease**, **restless leg**, **schizophrenia**, **stiff neck**, **stress**, strokes, **tachycardia**, **teeth (grinding)**, **tics**, **TMJ**, **Tourette's**, trauma, **tremors**, **twitching**, and **whiplash**

Properties: **Alkalinizer**, **antiarrhythmic**, antiepileptic, **antilithic**, **antispasmodic**, antiurolithic, anxiolytic, aperient, dopamine-enhancing, **hypotensive**, laxative (gentle), lithotriptic, and **vasodilator**

Magnolia

Aromatic, Mildly Bitter, & Pungent Herb

Magnolia officinalis

Used in Chinese herbalism to reduce dampness and inflammation in the digestive tract and lungs. It promotes downward peristalsis in the GI tract, helping to relieve nausea, hiccups, and the sensation of a lump in one's throat.

Look for *magnolia* in *Chinese Earth-Decreasing* and *Cortisol-Reducing Formulas*

Warnings: Not for use by infants and young children or pregnant women. The herb may cause dizziness and low blood pressure.

Energetics: Warming, drying, and mildly relaxing

Used For: Asthma, cough (damp), hiccups, and nausea & vomiting

Properties: Antibacterial, antifungal, antiseptic, antispasmodic, aperient, expectorant, and stomachic

Maitake   *Sweet Herb*

Grifola frondosa

A powerful immune enhancing mushroom, maitake is used to regulate the immune system. The beta-glucans in maitake mushrooms activate and increase production of immune system cells such as macrophages, T cells, natural killer cells, and neutrophils. These cells help the immune system to fight illness more quickly and efficiently. Maitake may help decrease insulin resistance, thereby increasing insulin sensitivity. It can also help to decrease blood pressure levels, lower total cholesterol levels, and help maintain weight, thereby promoting heart health.

Look for *maitake* in *Children's Elderberry Cold* and *Flu*, *Colostrum-Immune Stimulator,* and *Immune-Boosting Formulas*

Energetics: Drying and nourishing

Used For: Addison's disease, allergies (respiratory), **cancer**, cancer prevention, cancer treatment side effects, cholesterol (high), diabetes, hypertension, **infection (viral)**, and infection prevention

Properties: Anticancer, anticholesteremic, antifungal, antiviral, diuretic, hepatoprotective, hypotensive, immune stimulant, and tonic

Male Performance Formula

See also *Testosterone Formula*

These are combinations of herbs and nutrients that enhance male energy, sexual activity and vitality. They improve blood flow and may be helpful for hypertension and exercise recovery as well as sexual performance.

Warnings: Consult a doctor if you have a known medical condition, in particular those affecting blood pressure, hormone sensitivity, heart, liver, or kidney. Consult a doctor if taking any medication, in particular those affecting blood pressure, heart conditions, diabetes, depression, or erectile dysfunction. Discontinue use if adverse reactions occur. Not recommended for hot constitutions or teenagers.

Used For: Circulation (poor), **erectile dysfunction**, exercise (recovery), hypertension, infertility, **sex drive (low)**, and testosterone (low)

Affects: Circulatory constriction, low testosterone, and **testes**

Male Action

Primarily aids erectile dysfunction. Take 2–6 capsules one hour prior to sexual activity to enhance performance. As a general supplement to improve male performance, take 2 capsules nightly before bed.

Ingredients: DHEA, damiana leaf, muira puama stem, epimedium leaf extract, maca root extract, yohimbe root bark, and L-arginine

Libido-Circulation Formula

Ingredients focused on improving blood flow. Take four capsules daily as needed.

Ingredients: L-citruline, velvet bean extract, pumpkin seed oil, L-theanine, capsicum, ginseng (Asian/Korean) root extract, and Co-Q10

Libido Formula

Focused on boosting testosterone. Take four capsules daily as needed.

Ingredients: Ashwagandha standardized extract, maca root, epimedium standardized extract, muira puama, ginseng (Asian/Korean) standardized extract, and cayenne pepper

Manganese   *Mineral*

Manganese plays a role in carbohydrate and protein metabolism. It helps transport oxygen into the cells. It aids connective tissue health and joint fluid production. It is also important in vitamin B$_1$ utilization. It is important for nerve function and may play a role in abdominal muscle tone. Red raspberry leaf has a very high amount of manganese, which may contribute to its uterine toning and antinausea effects

Used For: Anemia, cadmium toxicity, cholesterol (low), dizziness, fingernails (weak/brittle), hair (graying), hearing loss, hernias, metabolic syndrome, mitochondrial dysfunction, nausea & vomiting, osteoporosis, and rashes & hives

Properties: Antiemetic, nutritive, and uterine tonic

Mangosteen   *Sour Herb*

Garcinia mangostana

Mangosteen fruit is rich in antioxidant polyphenols. In terms of their antioxidant potency, polyphenols are ten times stronger than vitamin C and one hundred times stronger than vitamin E and carotenoids. This gives the body a big boost in fighting free radicals and keeping the immune system strong.

Mangosteen rind contains high levels of xanthones. These highly studied constituents promote intestinal, respiratory and immune system health. Two of the most beneficial xanthones in mangosteen are alpha-manostin and gamma-mangostin. These compounds have been shown to be antibiotic, antiviral, and anti-inflammatory. They have histamine-blocking actions and may help protect arteries from damage.

Look for *mangosteen* in *Anti-Inflammatory Pain, Antioxidant,* and *Metabolic Stimulant Formulas*

Energetics: Cooling

Used For: **Allergies (respiratory)**, **cancer**, cancer prevention, cancer treatment side effects, cardiovascular disease, easily bruised, **free radical damage**, **inflammation**, overacidity, rhinitis, tuberculosis, and urinary tract infections

Properties: **Anti-inflammatory**, **antiaging**, **antiallergenic**, **antioxidant**, antiviral, and febrifuge

Marjoram EO

Herbaceous & Woody Essential Oil

Origanum majorana

Possessing a spicy, camphoric, and woody odor, marjoram EO is a muscle relaxant that has a calming effect on the body. It is regarded as an anaphrodisiac, meaning that it diminishes the desire for sexual contact. It can ease obsession and emotional craving, promoting a more self-contained and self-nurturing personality. If you need to be celibate and alone for a while, this is a good oil to use.

Marjoram can be used in massages and baths for insomnia, PMS, scanty or painful periods. A compress can be used for vasoconstrictive migraines, rheumatic pains, sprained or strained muscles, bruises, and sore throat.

Emotionally, marjoram brings a sense of peace, calmness, balance, and self-assurance. It reduces stress and anxiety and eases grief, hostility, anger, and irritability. It promotes courage and confidence in those with a weak will.

See the strategy *Aromatherapy* for suggested uses.

Warnings: Do not use internally. May cause skin irritation in some people. Avoid sun exposure after topical use. Avoid using if pregnant. Do not use with low blood pressure. Use only for short periods (seven to ten days).

Used For: Arthritis, arthritis (rheumatoid), asthma, bronchitis, bruises, carpal tunnel, colds (antiviral), colic (children), concentration (poor), **cramps (leg)**, **cramps & spasms**, diphtheria, dislocation, grief & sadness, headache (migraine), heart fibrillation/palpitations, heart valves, hypertension, hypochondria, insomnia, irritability, menstruation (scant), neuralgia & neuritis, pain, pregnancy, **sex drive (excessive)**, sprains, and thrush

Properties: Analgesic, **anaphrodisiac**, antibacterial, antiseptic, antispasmodic, antiviral, bactericidal, carminative, diaphoretic, digestant, diuretic, emmenagogue, expectorant, hypotensive, nervine, sedative, stomachic, vasodilator, and vulnerary

Marshmallow   *Mucilant Herb*

Althea officinalis

A mucilaginous herb which aids the bowels, mucous membranes, lungs, and kidneys, marshmallow is also a mild, nourishing food. It soothes inflamed and irritated tissues and reduces swelling. Marshmallow is used in combination with other kidney herbs to soothe burning urination, inflamed kidneys and ease the passing of kidney stones. It can also ease respiratory congestion and dry cough. It enriches breast milk in nursing mothers.

Look for *marshmallow* in *Intestinal Soothing, Lung Moistening, Pepsin Intestinal,* and *Vulnerary Formulas*

Warnings: Very mild and safe remedy for children, infants, and elderly persons. There are no known toxic effects of marshmallow, but if any diarrhea occurs from its use, cut back or discontinue use.

Energetics: Cooling and moistening

Used For: Allergies (respiratory), asthma, bedwetting, **bladder (irritable)**, bladder (ulcerated), blood in urine, **bronchitis**, burns & scalds, cancer treatment side effects, **celiac disease**, cholera, **colitis**, congestion, convalescence, cough, **cough (dry)**, cystic fibrosis, diarrhea, digestion (poor), **diverticulitis**, emphysema, eyes (red/itching), failure to thrive, **gastritis**, hemorrhoids, ileocecal valve, inflammation, **inflammatory bowel disorders**, injuries, **interstitial cystitis**, irritable bowel, kidney stones, laryngitis, nephritis, **nursing**, pertusis, pleurisy, rashes &

hives, sore/geographic tongue, sprains, teething, tickle in throat, ulcerations (external), **urethritis**, **urination (burning/painful)**, **urination (frequent)**, **vaginal dryness**, wasting, and wounds & sores

Properties: Absorbent, antacid, balsamic, diuretic, emollient, expectorant, **galactagogue**, low glycemic, mineralizer, moistening, **mucilant**, nutritive, **soothing**, and vulnerary

Meadowsweet   *Astringent & Bitter Herb*

Filipendula ulmaria

Meadowsweet contains salycin, the natural form of aspirin, making it useful for reducing pain and inflammation. It also settles the stomach and acts as a natural antacid. It also contains silica, which aids skin, joints, and connective tissues.

Look for *meadowsweet* in *Female Tonic* and *Headache Formulas*

Warnings: Because of its natural aspirin content, some herbalists feel it should not be given to small children suffering with fevers from colds, flu or chicken pox. It can cause nausea or vomiting in large doses.

Energetics: Cooling and drying

Used For: **Acid indigestion**, arthritis, arthritis (rheumatoid), **gastritis**, and pain

Properties: Analgesic, **antacid**, **anti-inflammatory**, and stomachic

Melatonin   *Hormone*

Melatonin is a hormone that is primarily produced in the pineal gland to induce sleep. Serotonin is converted to melatonin when it gets dark. In addition to regulating sleep, melatonin is a free radicals scavenger and helps to regulate the immune system. Melatonin also seems to directly interact with GABA receptors, inducing relaxation and combating anxiety in people with low natural production.

Melatonin helps to establish normal sleeping and waking rhythms in people who do shift work or are suffering from jet lag. It can also be helpful for occasional insomnia. Because melatonin is a naturally occurring hormone, long-term supplementation may alter the body's ability to produce sufficient amounts of it on its own.

Warnings: Not recommended for use by children, adolescents, pregnant or lactating women.

Usage: 1–9 mg, one hour before bed.

Used For: Aging, **down syndrome**, **insomnia**, **jet lag**, and SIBO

Properties: Antioxidant, anxiolytic, gaba-enhancing, immune modulator, and **soporific**

Memory Enhancing Formula

See also *Brain* and *Memory Protection Formula* and *Brain-Heart Formula*

Use this formula to improve memory and cognitive ability, especially when this loss of mental ability is associated with aging. It contains a special form of magnesium, magnesium L-threonate, which readily crosses the blood-brain barrier and helps form new synapses in the brain nerves. Research shows this form of magnesium improves memory and general cognitive function.

Warnings: May cause sleepiness, drowsiness, or headaches, especially if one is severely magnesium deficient. This is a temporary effect and should pass as one's levels of magnesium improve. Discontinue if symptoms last more than a week.

Used For: Aging, **Alzheimer's**, **cloudy thinking**, **dementia**, mania, **memory/brain function**, PTSD, and seizures

Affects: Acetylcholine, **brain**, and **brain atrophy**

Take three capsules at night before bed and three capsules in the morning before breakfast. Since this product may cause drowsiness, you may wish to start with only the nighttime doses.

Ingredients: Gotu kola aerial parts, bacopa leaf extract, ginkgo leaf, and magnesium

Menopause Support EO Blend

Use this essential oil blend to help with women's hormones and nervous system. It helps the body relax and eases tension and menstrual cramping associated with periods. It also helps women going through menopause with problems like hot flashes and night sweats.

See the strategy *Aromatherapy* for suggested uses.

Warnings: Not for use during pregnancy or with estrogen-dependent cancers. Not for internal use.

Used For: Hot flashes, infertility, **menopause**, night sweating, PMS Type A, and stress

Affects: Low estrogen

Ingredients: Clary sage EO, ho leaf EO, ylang ylang EO, and chamomile EO

Menopause Support Program

See also *Female Tonic Formula*

This package contains several products that help with menopausal symptoms. It can help reduce mood changes, hot flashes, and other symptoms of menopause.

Used For: Hot flashes, **menopause**, and **osteoporosis**

Take the contents of 1 packet in the morning and in the evening, for three weeks.

Ingredients: Anti-stress b-complex formula, chrisopher's menopause formula, female cycle formula, gla oil blend, and skeletal support formula

Menthol EO   *Minty & Sharp Essential Oil*

Menthol is a compound found in oils like peppermint. It can be extracted or synthesized. It is used topically as an analgesic and can be helpful for pain, inflammation, and indigestion. It also helps ease coughing.

See the strategy *Aromatherapy* for suggested uses.

Warnings: Do not use internally without the supervision of a professionally trained aromatherapy practitioner.

Used For: Arthritis, asthma, **bronchitis**, colds, congestion (bronchial), congestion (lungs), flu, inflammation, itching, **pain**, and **sore throat**

Properties: Analgesic and carminative

Metabolic Stimulant Formula

These products boost metabolism, increasing thermogenesis and metabolic fat burn and reducing appetite. They are used to aid weight loss, but they can also be used to balance the nervous system in people who have a parasympathetic-dominant autonomic nervous system. This is identified primarily by chronically small pupils. People who are parasympathetic-dominant are considered ADHD and have difficulty concentrating, rapid digestion and colon transit time, hypersensitivity to small noises and irritations, and may actually feel more relaxed when taking stimulants. Relaxing nervines will actually make them feel agitated.

Warnings: Not recommended for pregnant or nursing mothers or children under the age of twelve.

Formulas that contain caffeine should be avoided by people suffering from anxiety, nervous exhaustion and adrenal burnout.

Used For: ADD/ADHD, appetite (excessive), cellulite, excess weight, and fatigue

Caffeine-Free Metabolism Booster

A caffeine-free metabolism booster with bitter orange and guggul lipids. Recommended dose is 2 capsules two to three times daily.

Ingredients: Green tea leaf extract, orange (bitter) fruit extract, guggul, and chickweed aerial parts

Guarana Metabolism Booster

Uses caffeine-bearing herbs like yerba mate and guarana, along with stimulants like capsicum and bitter orange extract. Recommended dose is 2 capsules two to three times daily.

Ingredients: Green tea leaf, guarana seed, orange (bitter) fruit extract, guggul, yerba maté leaf extract, and chickweed aerial parts

Metabolic Booster with Caffeinated Herbs

A metabolism booster with four caffeinated herbs. For the first three days take 1 capsule with breakfast and another with lunch. After three days increase to 2 capsules.

Ingredients: Coffee bean, green tea leaf, guarana seed extract, and yerba maté leaf extract

Metabolic Booster without Caffeine

Contains decaffeinated green coffee bean and rhodiola. Take 2 capsules twice daily, preferably at breakfast and lunch.

Ingredients: East indian globe thistle flower extract, mangosteen fruit & pericarp, rhodiola root extract, coffee bean, and green tea leaf

Methyl B12 Vitamin Formula

Many people are deficient in B_{12} which plays a role in numerous body functions. Methylated B_{12} is the easiest form of B_{12} to assimilate. It is a very important supplement for people on vegan diets as vitamin B_{12} is very difficult to obtain without animal foods. It is also valuable as a methyl donor for people with poor methylation.

Used For: Adrenal fatigue, Alzheimer's, **anemia**, autism, **burning feet/hands**, canker sores, depression, dizziness, down syndrome, **epilepsy**, **fatigue**, heart fibrillation/palpitations, hemochromatosis, memory/brain function, **methylation (under)**, multiple sclerosis, nervousness, **neuralgia & neuritis**, numbness, **peripheral neuropathy**, **pernicious anemia**, **Raynaud's disease**, restless leg, **schizophrenia**, **sore/geographic tongue**, tics, tinnitus, **Tourette's**, tremors, and **vitiligo**

Affects: Blood, immune system, and mitochondria

Take 17-18 drops once daily under the tongue. Hold for thirty seconds before swallowing. May be taken twice daily for energy.

Ingredients: Vitamin B_1, vitamin B_2, vitamin B_3, vitamin B_6, and vitamin B_{12}

Methylated B Vitamin Formula

This formula contains highly active forms of vitamin B_{12} and folic acid—methylcobalamin and methylfolate. These vitamins aid in the production of the amino acid methionine.

This formula can assist methylation one of the six phase-two liver detoxification pathways. Problems with methylation can contribute to mental health issues like depression, aggression, and schizophrenia. Folate tends to balance over-methylation, but under-methylation can also contribute to mental health issues. If this formula makes symptoms worse, try SAM-e.

Used For: Adrenal fatigue, anemia, angina, autism, **birth defect prevention**, **canker sores**, cataracts, cholesterol (low), deafness, depression, dizziness, down syndrome, hemochromatosis, macular degeneration, memory/brain function, **mental illness**, **methylation (under)**, **numbness**, **peripheral neuropathy**, **pernicious anemia**, **pregnancy**, **restless leg**, **schizophrenia**, **sore/geographic tongue**, and **vitiligo**

Affects: Liver and mitochondria

Recommended dose is one capsule twice daily.

Ingredients: Vitamin B_9 and vitamin B_{12}

Milk Thistle *Bitter Herb*

Silybum marianum

The silymarin complex of flavinoids contained in milk thistle can protect the liver from various chemicals and toxins, such as carbon tetrachloride and the toxic effects of aminita (death cap) mushrooms. They also have an antioxidant effect and are very helpful for people who regularly work around chemicals. Milk thistle stimulates bile, may help in the healing of liver diseases like hepatitis, and works as a mild laxative in some people.

Look for *milk thistle* in *Antioxidant* and *Hepatoprotective Formulas*

Energetics: Moistening and cooling

Used For: Acne, addictions (drugs), aging, AIDS, **alcoholism**, birth control side effects, **cancer prevention**, **chemical exposure**, cholesterol (high), **cirrhosis of the liver**, constipation (adults), dermatitis, dysmenorrhea, **environmental pollution**, fat cravings, **fatty liver disease**, food poisoning, gallbladder problems, gallstones, **hangover**, Hashimoto's disease, **heavy metal poisoning**, **hepatitis**, **jaundice (adults)**, menstrual irregularity, **mercury poisoning**, nightmares, **nursing**, Parkinson's disease, PMS Type C, **poisoning**, **preeclampsia**, psoriasis, **surgery (preparation)**, surgery (recovery), and varicose veins

Properties: Alterative, anti-inflammatory, **anticholesteremic**, antidiabetic, antioxidant, **cholagogue**, emmenagogue, **galactagogue**, **hepatic**, **hepatoprotective**, immune stimulant, and tonic

Mimosa

Sweet Herb

Albizia julibrissin

Also known as albizia, mimosa has been used in Chinese herbalism to calm the spirit, relieve constriction and pain, invigorate the blood, heal bone fractures, and treat bad temper, depression, insomnia, irritability, and poor memory due to suppressed emotions. Mimosa is a good remedy for anxiety and depression. It is mildly uplifting and yet grounding. The bark slowly lifts one's energy and mood upward and softens the heart that has been hardened by stress and pain. The flowers can create a feeling of mild euphoria and giddiness. I find mimosa flowers and rose petals to be a great combination for healing a grieving or hardened heart.

Look for *mimosa* in *Antidepressant* and *Chinese Fire-Decreasing Formulas*

Warnings: Avoid while pregnant or nursing. Mimosa gum may interact with amoxicillin preventing the body from absorbing this antibiotic.

Energetics: Cooling, moistening, and mildly relaxing

Used For: Anxiety disorders, **apathy**, autism, **depression**, **grief & sadness**, insomnia, **irritability**, and **mood swings**

Properties: Antidepressant, calmative, euphoretic, relaxant, and vulnerary

Mistletoe

Bitter Herb

Viscum album

In small doses, mistletoe is helpful for hypertension (without fluid retention). In large doses mistletoe induces hypertension. Mistletoe is a powerful nervine and may help relieve vasoconstrictive headaches, petit mal seizures, and tinnitus. It is oxytocic and has been used during labor to strengthen and normalize uterine contractions.

Warnings: Mistletoe is not a contraceptive, but it may act as an abortifacient, so pregnant women should not take it. There have been some reports of ingestion of mistletoe leading to adverse reaction and even death in animals and small children. Upon further investigation, it was determined in these cases that the substance ingested was probably another species of mistletoe that is not used medicinally. Adults need not fear poisoning unless large amounts are ingested.

One other caution: mistletoe contains tyramine. When mixed with a prescription medicine that has a monoamineoxidase inhibitor, a person may experience a sudden drop in blood pressure. So it should not be taken with prescription blood pressure medications. This is an herb that may require the supervision of a skilled herbalist

(findanherbalist.com or americanherbalistsguild.com) or naturopath.

Energetics: Relaxing

Used For: Arrhythmia, dizziness, Graves' disease, headache (tension), **hypertension**, seizures, **tachycardia**, and tinnitus

Properties: Cardiac, **hypotensive**, nervine, and sedative

Mitochondria Energy Formula

Inside each cell of the body there are tiny energy-producing factories called mitochondria. Using a chemical process known as the Krebs cycle, the mitochondria utilize fuel (fats and carbohydrates) and oxygen to create an energy storage molecule called adenosine triphosphate (ATP). It powers the life processes within each cell. Without ATP, cells cannot function.

When the cells produce energy efficiently, they are inherently healthier. This, of course, makes the whole body function better. Increased cellular energy not only improves energy levels for better physical and mental performance but also speeds the healing of damaged tissues, enhances resistance to infections, and helps the body overcome chronic and degenerative diseases.

This formula is a blend of nutrients that support mitochondrial function. Mitochondrial dysfunction may be involved in aging and chronic illness and debility. Improving energy production in the mitochoncria may increase energy and stamina and aid athletic performance.

Used For: Addictions (coffee, caffeine), addictions (sugar/carbohydrates), aging, AIDS, convalescence, exercise (performance), **fatigue**, **fibromyalgia**, **mitochondrial dysfunction**, nervous exhaustion, neurodegenerative diseases, overalkalinity, **postpartum weakness**, tics, and **tremors**

Affects: General depression and **mitochondria**

Take 1 capsule twice daily.

Ingredients: Vitamin E, vitamin B_1, vitamin B_2, vitamin B_3, vitamin B_5, magnesium, zinc, manganese, L-carnitine, Co-Q10, and alpha-lipoic acid

Mood Lifting EO Blend

This blend of citrus oils and spices is uplifting and mood elevating. It can ease depression and sadness, as well as tension and stress. The blend may also be good for indigestion, bloating and gas. Citrus oils often have a calming effect on people with ADHD.

See the strategy *Aromatherapy* for suggested uses.

Warnings: Phototoxic—avoid sun exposure after topical application.

Used For: ADD/ADHD, apathy, appetite (excessive), depression, grief & sadness, headache (tension), and stress

Affects: Brain, central nervous system, dopamine, and serotonin

Ingredients: Pink grapefruit EO, orange EO, lemon EO, peppermint EO, and bergamot EO

Motherwort   *Mildly Aromatic & Bitter Herb*
Leonurus cardiaca

As its name implies, motherwort is often used as a remedy for calming stress in mothers. It relieves anxiety, reduces high blood pressure, and eases strain on the heart. It is especially helpful for tachycardia and heart palpitations. It is valuable for many female problems and for reducing some of the symptoms of hyperactive thyroid.

Look for *motherwort* in *Blood Pressure Reducing*, *Heart Health*, and *Thyroid Calming Formulas*

Warnings: Avoid during pregnancy and menstruation with excessive bleeding.

Energetics: Cooling, drying, and relaxing

Used For: Amenorrhea, angina, anxiety (situational), anxiety attacks, anxiety disorders, **arrhythmia**, cramps (menstrual), depression, **Graves' disease**, **heart fibrillation/palpitations**, hot flashes, **hypertension**, insomnia, menstruation (scant), **nervousness**, PTSD, **stress**, **tachycardia**, and **teeth (grinding)**

Properties: **Antiarrhythmic**, antispasmodic, antithyrotropic, calmative, cardiac, emmenagogue, female tonic, hypotensive, **nervine**, sedative, and vasodilator

MSM   *Nutrient*

Methylsulfonylmethane (MSM) is an organic sulfur compound found in vegetables, fruit, meat and dairy products. It is a crystalline derivative of DMSO, the first naturally derived NSAID discovered after aspirin. It is a potent anti-inflammatory and analgesic that aids healing.

Sulfur is crucial in the process of maintaining a vital healthy body and mind. It is part of the cellular structure and necessary for effecting repairs in the body. It promotes the health of hair, skin, nails, joints, and the immune system.

Usage: 1–3 grams two times daily. To promote collagen production, take with vitamin C.

Used For: Acne, allergies (respiratory), arsenic poisoning, **arthritis**, **arthritis (rheumatoid)**, asthma, **backache**, **bladder (irritable)**, **bladder (ulcerated)**, **blood in stool**, blood poisoning, body building, broken bones, bronchi-

tis, **bruises**, **bunions**, **burns & scalds**, **bursitis**, cancer treatment side effects, carpal tunnel, **cartilage damage**, celiac disease, cholesterol (low), cirrhosis of the liver, confusion, congestion (bronchial), copper toxicity, cystic fibrosis, dermatitis, diabetes, **dislocation**, Epstein-Barr virus, fibromyalgia, food allergies/intolerances, gangrene, hypothyroidism, **inflammation**, inflammatory bowel disorders, injuries, **interstitial cystitis**, itching, **ligaments (torn/injuried)**, lupus, memory/brain function, overalkalinity, **pain**, pleurisy, preeclampsia, psoriasis, **rashes & hives**, **scars/scar tissue**, **sciatica**, skin (dry/flaky), snoring, **spinal disks**, sprains, stiff neck, **surgery (recovery)**, **tendonitis**, tooth extraction, and **wounds & sores**

Properties: Analgesic, anti-inflammatory, **antiarthritic**, lipotropic, and vulnerary

Mugwort   *Fragrant bitter Herb*
Artemesia vulgaris

Used in low doses to improve appetite and digestive function. In larger doses, it is used as an antiparasitic remedy. It induces menstruation and acts as a uterine stimulant.

Look for *mugwort* in *Antiparasitic Formula*

Warnings: Avoid during pregnancy or when trying to become pregnant. Only use for short periods and preferably as part of a formula, under the supervision of a professional herbalist.

Energetics: Warming and drying

Used For: Parasites

Properties: **Antiparasitic**, digestive tonic, emmenagogue, and stimulant (appetite)

Muira Puama   *Bitter & Sweet Herb*
Ptychopetalum olacoides

Muira puama is a tonic that can help with impotency and performance anxiety in men as well as lack of desire in women. It was used by natives of the Amazon rain forest to promote sexual energy and arousal. It has a relaxing effect and has also been used as a remedy for neuromuscular pain and cramps, rheumatism and poor circulation. It has been used for depression, nervous exhaustion and some mild cases of paralysis.

Look for *muira puama* in *Male Performance Formula*

Warnings: Do not use during pregnancy.

Energetics: Warming and relaxing

Used For: Cramps (menstrual), depression, **erectile dysfunction**, fatigue, hair loss/thinning, nervous exhaustion, paralysis, sex drive (low), and **testosterone (low)**

Properties: Androgenic, antirheumatic, aphrodisiac, nervine, nervine, testosterone-enhancing, and tonic

Mulberry *Bitter, Pungent, Sour, & Sweet Herb*

Morus alba

The leaves, young twigs, fruits, and root bark of the white mulberry are used in Chinese herbalism. The different parts have different energetics and properties. The root bark is used for lung problems. It is sweet, warming and mildly toxic and is used is an expectorant, diuretic, and mild sedative for asthma and cough. The fruits are used for the liver, heart, and kidney meridians. They nourish the blood and help vision. The twigs are slightly pungent and enter the liver meridian. They promote meridian flow. The leaves are bitter and aid the liver and lung meridians. They soothe and cleanse the liver and are helpful for headaches.

Look for *mulberry* in *Chinese Water-Decreasing Formula*

Energetics: Drying, relaxing, and warming

Used For: Asthma, cough (damp), edema, and headache

Properties: Analgesic, blood building, diuretic, expectorant, food, hypotensive, and sedative

Mullein *Salty Herb*

Verbascum thapsus

Mullein leaves are most commonly used for respiratory complaints. They have a soothing, hydrating effect on the lungs and contain saponins that loosen mucus. It is often used for chronic lung problems such as asthma and COPD but is also helpful for colds and coughs, particularly dry coughs. Mullein flowers are used to make ear drops to soothe earache.

Look for *mullein* in *Ayurvedic Bronchial Decongestant, Ear Drop, Jeannie Burgess' Allergy-Lung, Lymph Cleansing,* and *Vulnerary Formulas*

Warnings: Mullein seeds contain the poisonous substance rotenone. The leaf and flowers are generally regarded as safe.

Energetics: Moistening and cooling

Used For: Allergies (respiratory), asthma, backache, **Bell's palsy**, **breasts (swelling/tenderness)**, **broken bones**, bronchitis, congestion, **congestion (bronchial)**, congestion (lungs), congestion (lymphatic), **COPD**, cough, **cough (dry)**, COVID-19, croup, cystic fibrosis, dislocation, **earache**, **emphysema**, Epstein-Barr virus, fibrosis, injuries, interstitial cystitis, lymphoma, mastitis, mumps, rashes & hives, **swollen lymph glands**, tuberculosis, vaccine side effects, and **wheezing**

Properties: Emollient, expectorant, lung tonic, lymphatic, mineralizer, mucilant, pulmonary, vermifuge, and vulnerary

Multiple Vitamin and Mineral *Nutrient*

A multiple vitamin and minerals supplement (multi) may be helpful to maintain health and healing. It is especially important during pregnancy or periods of excessive stress.

When looking for a multi ignore claims of being "whole food." Vitamins are produced by bacterial or yeast fermentation and are technically synthetic. The form of the vitamins and minerals in the supplement is more important. You may need to experiment a little to find the best multi for you.

Used For: ADD/ADHD, addictions, adrenal fatigue, aging, **anorexia**, appetite (deficient), appetite (excessive), **birth defect prevention**, body building, bulimia, burning feet/hands, cancer treatment side effects, canker sores, cartilage damage, cervical dysplasia, confusion, convalescence, endurance, exercise (performance), fatigue, **infertility**, lyme disease, **nervous exhaustion**, **pregnancy**, PTSD, puberty, skin problems, **stress**, **surgery (preparation)**, and wasting

Properties: Immune modulator, nutritive, and vulneraries

Mushroom Immune Formula

See also *Alterative-Immune Formula* and *Immune-Boosting Formula*

Medicinal mushrooms have many healing properties but are especially for the immune system. The mushrooms in this blend stimulate the immune system to help the body fight infections and cancer. They are also adaptogenic, antioxidant, and anti-inflammatory, which means they promote overall health. They may also help to protect the liver from environmental toxins, reduce blood pressure and cholesterol, and have calming effects on the nerves.

Many of these fungi contain polysaccharides called 1, 3 beta-glucans, which have been studied for their role in enhancing immunity, improving insulin resistance, and lowering cholesterol. Beta-glucans are not directly antiviral or cytotoxic to cancer cells, but they are effective in stimulating natural killer cell (NK cell) activity. In fact, medicinal mushrooms can increase NK cell activity by as much as 400 percent and can stimulate production of tumor necrosis factor alpha (TNF-a) and other substances used by NK cells to initiate programmed cell death and destroy cancerous and viral-infected cells. The resulting localized cytokine concentration draws macrophages, cytotoxic T cells, and more NK cells to the area, thereby mobilizing the immune system.

In addition to beta glucans, the polysaccharide fraction of tonic mushrooms includes resistant starch, essential sugars, and other constituents. Resistant starch, which makes up about 15 percent dry weight of many fungi, is an excellent prebiotic for promoting beneficial bacteria in the large intestine.

Essential sugars, or glyconutrients, make up about 10 percent dry weight of many fungi. These sugars have a stimulating effect on white blood cells and the formation of antibodies. They help the immune system recognize pathogens and cancer cells and communicate these discoveries to the rest of the immune system so it can perform its job more effectively.

Warnings: Avoid in autoimmune disorders.

Used For: Autism, **cancer**, cancer prevention, **cancer treatment side effects**, cholesterol (high), **convalescence**, **flu**, herpes, hypertension, **infection (viral)**, **infection prevention**, mononucleosis, **triglycerides (high)**, and **vaccine side effects**

Affects: Breasts, chronic disease stage, **hypoactive immune activity**, and immune system

Mix 1 scoop (3 g) into food or beverages one to three times daily.

Ingredients: Cordyceps mushroom, reishi mushroom, turkey tail mushroom, chaga mushroom, shitake mushroom, and agaricus mushroom

Myelin Sheath Formula

This formula was created by Alan Tillotson, who tested it and found it helped to help nourish and rebuild the myelin sheath in people who have multiple sclerosis. It is also helpful for reducing inflammation.

Used For: Inflammation and **multiple sclerosis**

Take two tablets twice daily.

Ingredients: Elder berry, ginseng (Asian/Korean), tienchi ginseng, amur cork bark, guggul, boswellia, ashwagandha root, turmeric, and lion's mane

Myrrh *Aromatic & Bitter Herb*

Commiphora spp.

An aromatic and bitter resin with antiseptic and disinfectant qualities, myrrh combines well with goldenseal, echinacea, and other herbs for fighting infection. It is especially helpful when used as a gargle, mouthwash, or liniment. Myrrh helps heal wounds and extracts can be blended with aloe vera gel to form a soothing barrier. It is also a bitter tonic for digestion.

Look for *myrrh* in *Herbal Tooth Powder Formula*

Warnings: Avoid taking internally while pregnant.

Energetics: Warming and drying

Used For: Adenitis, amenorrhea, athlete's foot, canker sores, cholesterol (high), **dental health**, diarrhea, eczema, **gingivitis**, infection (bacterial), infection prevention, inflammation, oral surgery, **sore throat**, **ulcerations (external)**, and ulcers

Properties: **Antibacterial**, **antiseptic**, carminative, digestive tonic, and disinfectant

Myrrh EO *Balsamic & Spicy Essential Oil*

Commiphora spp.

Myrrh EO is a warm and spicy fragrance with a balsamic note. It is deeply calming to the nervous system, and promotes a sense of grounded awareness, which is why it has been traditionally used to aid meditation.

Myrrh was traditionally used for embalming and the essential oil prevents infection, clears toxins, and promotes tissue repair. It acts as an expectorant in any condition involving excessive thick mucus. Traditionally, it has been used for mouth, gum, and throat infections. Myrrh promotes menstruation and helps relieve painful periods. Topically, myrrh is used for chronic wounds and ulcers. It can be used for wounds that are slow to heal and for weepy eczema and athlete's foot. It works to heal deep cracks on the heels and hands. Emotionally, myrrh is valuable for those that feel stuck emotionally or spiritually and want to move forward in their lives. It is calming to the nervous system and instills a deep sense of mental tranquility. It is a principal oil for those who overthink things, worry, and have mental distractions. The sense of peace it imparts helps to ease sorrow and grief. Myrrh helps with a connection of inner self so that dreams can be brought to reality.

It helps people who are prone to worry or over think things, as well as those who are easily distracted. People who are stuck in their lives, unable to decide a proper course of action, or those who feel restless and stuck will find myrrh useful in helping them to determine a course of action in life and move forward.

See the strategy *Aromatherapy* for suggested uses.

Warnings: Do not use internally without the supervision of a professionally trained aromatherapy practitioner. Nontoxic and nonirritating for topical use. It is a uterine stimulant and not for use with pregnancy.

Used For: Amenorrhea, antibiotic resistance, appetite (deficient), athlete's foot, autism, bronchitis, cancer, canker sores, cholesterol (high), cirrhosis of the liver, colds (antiviral), cough, dental health, diarrhea, dysmenorrhea, eczema, electromagnetic pollution, fear, gas & bloating, **gingivitis**, grief & sadness, **halitosis**, hepatitis, herpes, hypothyroidism, impetigo, **infection (bacterial)**, infection prevention, inflammation, leprosy, nightmares, oral surgery, pregnancy, stretch marks, syphilis, thrush, trauma, ulcerations (external), and ulcers

Properties: Abortifacient, anti-inflammatory, anticatarrhal, antimicrobial, antiphlogistic, **antiseptic**, antiviral, astringent, balsamic, carminative, cicatrizant, disinfectant, emmenagogue, expectorant, perfume, preservative, sedative, stomachic, tonic, uterine, and vulnerary

N-Acetyl Cysteine   *Nutrient*

N-acetylcysteine (NAC) is a stabilized form of cysteine, a sulfur-containing amino acid found in high protein foods. NAC is produced naturally in the body and is also obtained from the diet. It is a precursor to glutathione, which is the body's most important cellular antioxidant and detoxifier. Supplementing with NAC boosts glutathione levels in the liver, in plasma and in the bronchioles of the lungs.

Glutathione acts as a powerful antioxidant in cells that detoxifies chemicals into less harmful compounds. Taking vitamins B_6, B_9, and B_{12} along with NAC helps recycle glutathione in the body so that it can continue acting as an antioxidant.

NAC is helpful for those suffering from many chronic respiratory problems, including smoker's cough. It is a natural expectorant that helps thin mucus and loosen phlegm and bronchial secretions in the lungs. Double-blind research has found that dosages of 1,200 milligrams per day prevents influenza infection and reduces symptoms and the duration of existing influenza infections. It is being studied in the treatment of cystic fibrosis.

NAC also detoxifies and removes heavy metals like lead, mercury, and arsenic from the body. NAC has been used in hospitals for treating patients with acetaminophen toxicity (found in Tylenol) and for treating other causes of liver failure and septic shock. It is often recommended as a liver support for those taking chemotherapy drugs and those suffering from alcohol poisoning.

Warnings: It is important to supplement zinc and other trace minerals with NAC, as NAC increases the excretion minerals when taken over an extended period.

Usage: Take 600–1,200 mg three times daily.

Used For: Addictions (coffee, caffeine), aging, AIDS, **Alzheimer's**, anger (excessive), asthma, autism, Bell's palsy, bronchitis, cancer, cancer treatment side effects, cataracts, **chemical exposure**, cirrhosis of the liver, congestion, **congestion (bronchial)**, **COPD**, **cystic fibrosis**, **dementia**, **emphysema**, environmental pollution, exercise (performance), glaucoma, **hangover**, **heavy metal poisoning**, **hepatitis**, hypertension, hypothyroidism, inflammation, **lead poisoning**, **mercury poisoning**, mitochondrial dysfunction, multiple sclerosis, **Parkinson's disease**, **pneumonia**, psoriasis, surgery (recovery), and **tuberculosis**

Properties: Antioxidant, detoxifying, hepatic, and **mucolytic**

Nanoparticle Silver (Colloidal Silver)   *Mineral*

An alternative to antibiotics that has been around for a long time is pure silver. It has long been known that silver has an antimicrobial action. Pioneers, for example, learned that they could keep water from going bad by putting a few silver coins in the bottom of the water barrel. Nobility in ancient Europe were less prone to infection than the general population because they ate and drank using silverware. Royalty became known as "blue-blood" due to the fact that ingestion of high amounts of silver causes argyria, a condition characterized by a blue/gray discoloration of the skin and inflammation of the inner eyelids. A solution of just 100 parts per million (ppm) of colloidal silver taken daily is enough to cause argyria.

Fortunately there are some new forms of colloidal silver that use a nanoparticle technology. They don't accumulate in the body and work at lower potencies. My favorite silver products use the aquasol technology, but there are other brands with nanoparticle silver too. Any form of silver only works as an antimicrobial when it comes in contact with pathogens. Therefore, it is most effective when applied topically or used to treat gastrointestinal infections. In high doses—two to four ounces of a ten to twenty parts per million (10-20 ppm) silver daily for one week—nanoparticle silver can help resolve antibiotic-resistant infections.

Usage: Use as a mouthwash, nasal spray or apply topically to injuries as directed on the bottle. For internal use, follow the manufacturer's recommendations. Only use colloidal silver to fight an active infection. Do not take daily.

Used For: Abrasions/scratches, **acne**, **anal fistula/fissure**, **antibiotic resistance**, **blood poisoning**, bronchitis, carbuncles, cholera, **conjunctivitis**, cradle cap, cuts, **denture sores**, **diarrhea**, **diphtheria**, **earache**, fever, **food poisoning**, **gangrene**, **gingivitis**, **herpes**, infection prevention, interstitial cystitis, **leprosy**, **leucorrhea**, parasites (tapeworm), **pertussis**, **pet supplements**, **pneumonia**, prostatitis, **rheumatic fever**, scabies, **sinus infection**, **skin (infections)**, **skin problems**, slivers, smell (loss of), **sore throat**, **staph infections**, **strep throat**, **syphilis**, **tetanus**, **thrush**, **tick**, **tonsillitis**, **toothache**, **tuberculosis**, **typhoid**, urinary tract infections, urination (burning/painful), vaginitis, **wounds & sores**, and **wrinkles**

Properties: Antimalarial

Nattokinase Enzyme Formula

Nattokinase is a protease (protein-digesting) enzyme formed during the soybean fermentation process that produces natto. Research has shown that nattokinase helps dissolve fibrin in the blood. Fibrin thickens the blood and contributes to the formation of blood clots, which can cause heart attack, stroke, and other clotting disorders. It is a natural alternative to blood thinners.

Warnings: Do not take with blood thinning medications, when bleeding disorders are present or if you are allergic to Aspergillus.

Used For: Blood clot prevention, cardiovascular disease, strokes, **thrombosis**, and varicose veins

Affects: Blood and veins

To aid circulatory health take 1 capsule between meals twice daily on an empty stomach.

Ingredients: Enzyme blend from asperigillus orzae and a. melleus, dandelion leaf, and resveratrol root

Natural Antacid Formula

See also *Children's Colic Formula*

This natural alternative to antacids helps neutralize excess acid, soothe the stomach, improve digestion and prevent stomach acid from backwashing into the esophagus. It soothes burning sensations in the stomach and lessens acidic tastes in the throat and mouth. For suggestions for long-term relief see the condition *acid indigestion*.

Warnings: If symptoms persist, consult a competent healthcare provider. Digestive problems may be a sign of more serious health concerns.

Used For: Acid indigestion, dyspepsia, and ulcers

Affects: Stomach

Use for quick temporary relief by taking 2 tablets when experiencing digestive difficulty.

Ingredients: Calcium, alginic acid from brown seaweed, papaya fruit, guar gum, slippery elm bark, and licorice root

Neem   *Aromatic & Astringent Herb*

Azadirachta indica

Neem is one of the most popular anti-infective herbs in India. It has broad activity against both bacteria and fungi. It can be used in a mouthwash or tea for gingivitis and bleeding gums. It's particularly useful topically for bacterial and fungal infections. Neem oil is also a natural insecticide for the garden.

Look for *neem* in *Ayurvedic Skin Healing Formula*

Warnings: Not for young children, the elderly or the weak.

Energetics: Constricting and warming

Used For: Antibiotic side effects, cancer, **dental health**, **gingivitis**, infection (bacterial), infection (fungal), insect repellant, parasites, and pet supplements

Properties: Anti-inflammatory, antiamebic, antibacterial, antifungal, antiherpetic, **antiparasitic**, contraceptive, dentifrice, and insecticide

Neroli EO   *Floral, Fresh, & Sweet Essential Oil*

Citrus x aurantium amara

Neroli EO is extracted from the flowers of the bitter orange tree and has a soft, delicate aroma. Traditionally, it is associated with marriage and purity. It helps to relax the nerves and can be used in massages or baths for stress, depression, anxiety, shock, and insomnia. It can be inhaled for headaches, neuralgia, heart palpitations or vertigo. It has an affinity for the circulatory system and can be used in a massage oil for broken capillaries, constricted circulation, and varicose veins. It can be massaged on the abdomen for digestive problems and parasites. It can also be used in a soak for nail fungus and athlete's foot.

Emotionally, neroli helps a person to have positive, confident feelings and to believe in him or herself. It can help overcome moodiness and nervous exhaustion, irritability, grief, and fear, as well as inspire feelings of hope and joy. Neroli may also help to overcome amnesia, phobias, panic, hysteria, and withdrawal.

See the strategy *Aromatherapy* for suggested uses.

Warnings: Do not use internally. Nontoxic and nonirritating for topical use.

Used For: Angina, anxiety (situational), athlete's foot, body odor, bronchitis, circulation (poor), depression, dyspepsia, fear, gas & bloating, headache, heart fibrillation/palpitations, hysteria, infection (fungal), insomnia, mood swings, neuralgia & neuritis, parasites, sex drive (low), skin (dry/flaky), and varicose veins

Properties: Antibacterial, antidepressant, antiseptic, antispasmodic, anxiolytic, bactericidal, carminative, cicatrizant, deodorant, digestive tonic, nervine, perfume, stimulant (metabolic), and vulnerary

Nettle, Stinging   *Salty Herb*

Urtica dioica

The leaves, roots, and seeds of stinging nettles are useful in herbal herbalism. The leaves are a nourishing herbal food, rich in iron, calcium, magnesium, protein, and other nutrients. Nettles help to build healthy blood, bones, joints and skin. As a blood-nourishing source of iron, nettle leaves are an excellent remedy for anemia, low blood pressure, and general weakness. They expel uric acid and help with rheumatism and gout. They have anti-inflammatory and anti-allergenic properties, making them useful for respiratory allergies, asthma, and skin eruptive diseases. A blend of nettle leaf, red raspberry, and alfalfa makes a great tea for pregnancy.

Nettle seeds can slow, halt or even partially reverse progressive renal failure. They also act as an adrenal tonic.

The root is a urinary and prostate remedy. Studies have show the root to improved benign prostate hypertrophy (BPH) symptoms in 81 percent of men taking the herb compared with 16 percent improvement in the placebo group.

Look for *nettle, stinging* in *Antihistamine, Joan Patton's Herbal Minerals, Pregnancy Tea, Steven Horne's Anti-Allergy,* and *Thyroid Glandular Formulas*

Warnings: While the live plant can cause contact dermatitis, the dried plant does not and is safe to use both topically and internally. Taken over a period of months, nettle may be moderately hypertensive in some people.

Energetics: Neutral and nourishing

Used For: **Allergies (respiratory)**, **anemia**, arthritis, arthritis (rheumatoid), birth defect prevention, **BPH**, calcium deficiency, dermatitis, eczema, **edema**, erectile dysfunction, food allergies/intolerances, **gout**, hair loss/thinning, hemochromatosis, hypotension, **hypothyroidism**, kidney weakness/failure, **kidney weakness/failure**, menorrhagia, nursing, osteoporosis, **overalkalinity**, **PMS Type H**, **pregnancy**, **rhinitis**, sickle cell anemia, **uric acid retention**, and urination (frequent)

Properties: Anti-inflammatory, **antiallergenic**, antihistamine, diuretic, galactagogue, **hypertensive**, **kidney tonic**, low glycemic, mast cell stabilizer, mineralizer, **thyrotropic**, and tonic

Niacin   see *vitamin B₃*

Night-Blooming Cereus   *Sweet Herb*

Selenicereus grandiflorus

This species of cactus is used for all types of cardiopulmonary disorders, including angina, tachycardia, palpitations, and valvular disease. It has an effect like digitalis, but milder. It stimulates the action of the heart and has been used to aid recovery from heart attacks and combines well with hawthorn and motherwort for this purpose. Cactus and mimosa are favored by some herbalists for people suffering from emotional heartbreak.

Look for *night-blooming cereus* in *Heart Health Formula*

Warnings: Recommended for professional use only.

Energetics: Cooling

Used For: **Arrhythmia**, cardiovascular disease, congestive heart failure, grief & sadness, heart fibrillation/palpitations, **heart valves**, heart weakness, and **mitral valve**

Properties: Antiarrhythmic, **cardiac**, diuretic, relaxant, and sedative

Nitric Oxide Boosting Formula

See also *Cardiovascular L-Arginine Formula*

Nitric oxide is a signaling molecule in the cardiovascular system. (See the strategy *Enhance Nitric Oxide* for more information.) This formula enhances nitric oxide in both pathways of nitric oxide synthesis, the L-arginine pathway and the nitrate pathway. It also contains vitamins and minerals to enhance circulation. It is helpful for hypertension and erectile dysfunction, but can also aid many other conditions by improving blood flow.

Used For: Altitude sickness, **angina**, **arteriosclerosis**, arthritis, asthma, **cardiovascular disease**, chemical exposure, **chest pain**, circulation (brain), **circulation (poor)**, cold hands/feet, congestive heart failure, COPD, dementia, depression, diabetes, **erectile dysfunction**, **exercise (performance)**, exercise (recovery), glaucoma, **heart weakness**, **hypertension**, infection (bacterial), inflammation, insomnia, kidney weakness/failure, mercury poisoning, metabolic syndrome, pain, Peyronie's disease, stress, **strokes**, and urinary tract infections

Affects: **Arteries**, **circulatory atrophy**, **circulatory constriction**, **heart**, immune system, and sight

Mix one pack into 8 ounces of water and drink one or two times daily. Consume before exercise to enhance stamina or after to ease muscle soreness and aid recovery.

Ingredients: Vitamin C, vitamin D, thiamine, vitamin B_6, folate, vitamin B_{12}, magnesium, red beet root, and L-arginine

Noni (Morinda)   *Sour Herb*

Morinda citrifolia

Noni juice is used as an antioxidant and anti-inflammatory agent. The root is used in Chinese herbalism to tonify the kidney and fortify the yang energy. Deficiency of kidney yang is connected to symptoms like impotence, male or female infertility, premature ejaculation, frequent urination, urinary incontinence, irregular menstruation, and a sore back. The kidney energy is also thought to strengthen the bones. Energetics are for the fruit.

Warnings: Noni root is contraindicated with damp-heat (conditions of excess fluid and inflammation) or heat from yin deficiency (heat with fatigue). It is also contraindicated in people who have a difficult time urinating. No warnings for the juice.

Energetics: Warming and drying

Used For: Arthritis, arthritis (rheumatoid), cancer, cancer treatment side effects, diabetes, easily bruised, erectile dysfunction, hair loss/thinning, incontinence, inflammation, kidney weakness/failure, nervous exhaustion, overacidity, pain, and premature ejaculation

Properties: Analgesic, anti-inflammatory, anticoagulant, antidiabetic, cell proliferant, hypolipidemic, kidney tonic, and vulnerary

Nopal   *Mucilant Herb*

Opuntia spp.

Nopal is helpful for type 2 diabetes and has a very low glycemic index. Single doses have reportedly decreased blood sugar by 17–46 percent in clinical trials. It contains potent antioxidants, reduces inflammation, and helps promote healthy gut flora. It is also helpful for relieving hangover. Topically, fresh noni pulp can be applied for burns and other skin irritations in the same way aloe vera is used.

Look for *nopal* in *Blood Sugar Control Formula*

Energetics: Cooling and moistening

Used For: Burns & scalds, dehydration, **diabetes**, dysbiosis, hangover, hypertension, metabolic syndrome, SIBO, sunburn, and urination (burning/painful)

Properties: Analgesic, anti-inflammatory, **antidiabetic**, food, **hypoglycemic**, low glycemic, and mucilant

Oat   *Sweet Herb*

Avena sativa

The milky (unripe) seeds of the oat grain are used as a remedy for a depleted nervous system. Milky oat seed works best on people with mental and physical exhaustion, who are irritable and lack focus. They may also experience heart palpitations and loss of libido. Milky oat seed can also be used to aid recovery from drug addiction.

Oat seed and straw are used in formulas for female hormones. Like horsetail, oat straw is rich in silica. It is used as a mineralizer and a mild nervine. Oat bran is used as a bulk laxative and an agent to help lower cholesterol. Oatmeal can be used as a soothing poultice for itchy skin and minor skin irritations.

Look for *oat* in *Adaptogen, Fiber, Herbal Calcium, Joan Patton's Herbal Minerals,* and *Women's Aphrodisiac Formulas*

Energetics: Neutral, moistening, and nourishing

Used For: Addictions (drugs), addictions (tobacco), adrenal fatigue, anxiety disorders, apathy, depression, **emotional sensitivity**, fatigue, grief & sadness, hypochondria, insomnia, mental illness, **narcolepsy**, **nervous exhaustion**, **nervousness**, osteoporosis, peripheral neuropathy, sex drive (excessive), sex drive (low), and **stress**

Properties: Food, laxative (bulk), mineralizer, nervine, and nutritive

Olive   *Mildly Bitter Herb*

Olea europaea

Olive oil is nutritious and helps to lower cholesterol. It is often used in herbal salves and ointments. Olive oil is often used with lemon juice as a natural therapy for gallstones.

The leaf of the olive tree is used, along with other herbs, to treat high blood pressure and angina. Olive leaf is also widely recommended as a broad-spectrum antiviral and antibacterial agent, but its antimicrobial effects are mild. Energetics are for the leaf, not the oil.

Look for *olive* in *Antifungal EO, Blood Pressure Reducing,* and *Elderberry Cold* and *Flu Formulas*

Energetics: Cooling, drying, and mildly relaxing

Used For: Arteriosclerosis, chicken pox, colds (antiviral), Epstein-Barr virus, gastritis, hepatitis, hypertension, infection (fungal), infection (viral), **nervous exhaustion**, pneumonia, shingles, stretch marks, and tuberculosis

Properties: Antibacterial, antidiabetic, antifungal, antioxidant, antiviral, astringent, diuretic, food, **hypoglycemic**, hypotensive, and **vasodilator**

Omega-3 ALA (Alpha Linolenic Acid)

Fatty Acid

This is the plant-based form of omega-3 essential fatty acids. It is found in high amounts in flax seeds, flax seed oil, and hemp seeds. It is converted into eicosapentaenoic acid (EPA), and then into docosahexaenoic acid (DHA) in a healthy body. See omega-3 essential fatty acids for properties and uses of this family of fatty acids.

Omega-3 DHA (Docosahexaenoic Acid)   *Fatty Acid*

DHA is an essential fatty acid, and the most abundant fatty acid in the brain. It is essential for myelin sheath repair and the development, growth and maintenance of the brain. It may be helpful for the nerves, eyes, and cardiovascular system. In combination with EPA, DHA is a systemic anti-inflammatory and is also beneficial for the prevention and reversal of many diseases. It is especially important for the development of the brain in children.

Usage: Take 1 capsule of about 250 mg daily or take as part of an omega-3 supplement.

Used For: **ADD/ADHD**, Alzheimer's, arthritis, autism, bipolar mood disorder, cholesterol (high), circulation (poor), colitis, **concentration (poor)**, **dementia**, depression, diabetes, eye health, failure to thrive, fibromyalgia, gout, Huntington's disease, **memory/brain function**, **mental illness**, mercury poisoning, mood swings, **multiple sclerosis**, nerve damage, neuralgia & neuritis, **neurodegenerative diseases**, Parkinson's disease, **peripheral neuropathy**, psoriasis, **seizures**, **traumatic brain injury**, and triglycerides (high)

Properties: Anti-inflammatory, anticholesteremic, nutritive, and tonic

Omega-3 EFAs *Fatty Acid*

There are three basic forms of omega-3 fatty acids, alpha linolenic acid (ALA), eicosapentaenoic acid (EPA), and docosahexaenoic acid (DHA). You can look at the description of each for more information. The body uses these fatty acids in cell membranes and to make chemical messengers to mediate inflammation, immunity, and nerve functions. Most Americans are getting too many omega-6 fatty acids and not enough omega-3 fatty acids. This leads to the production of inflammatory prostaglandins, oxidative damage, and significantly raises the risk of heart disease. It can also cause problems with the brain and nerves.

American diets typically contain a 20:1–30:1 ratio of omega-6 to omega-3 essential fatty acid (EFA). The ratio should be about 6:1–7:1. To improve your ratio, reduce consumption of high omega-6 vegetable oils including: soybean, canola, cottonseed, corn, peanut, safflower, and sunflower oil, while at the same time increasing omega-3 by eating fatty fish or other omega-3-rich foods and/ or using an omega-3 supplement.

Omega-3 fatty acids EPA and DHA are used in the treatment of many chronic inflammatory diseases as well as for maintaining general good health. They can reduce inflammation and the risk of cardiovascular disease, reduce insulin resistance in cells, inhibit platelet aggregation (reducing the risk of thrombosis), and lower serum triglyceride levels. It can also help to suppress cell proliferation and induce apoptosis of cancerous cells.

Warnings: Not recommended where there is fatty congestion in the liver.

Usage: The best source of EPA/DHA fatty acids is to eat one pound a week of fatty, cold water fish like sardines, tuna, and wild salmon. These can be canned in water, fresh, or frozen. If you're not a fish fan, supplement with around 2,000 mg daily of combined EPA/DHA. Fish liver oil is an effective way to get EPA/DHA, while also getting the essential fat soluble nutrients vitamin A and D.

Used For: ADD/ADHD, addictions, addictions (drugs), addictions (sugar/carbohydrates), allergies (respiratory), **ALS**, Alzheimer's, amenorrhea, anxiety disorders, appetite (excessive), **arteriosclerosis**, **arthritis**, **arthritis (rheumatoid)**, **autism**, autoimmune disorders, Bell's palsy, **bipolar mood disorder**, **birth defect prevention**, **blood clot prevention**, BPH, breasts (swelling/tenderness), **burning feet/hands**, calcium deficiency, calcium deposits, cancer prevention, capillary weakness, **cardiovascular disease**, **cataracts**, cellulite, chemical exposure, **cholesterol (high)**, cholesterol (low), circulation (poor), cold hands/feet, cold sores, colitis, concentration (poor), confusion, **congestive heart failure**, constipation (children), convalescence, COPD, **cradle cap**, cramps (menstrual), croup, cystic breast disease, **dandruff**, debility, **dementia**, dental health, depression, **dermatitis**, diabetes, **diabetic retinopathy**, diverticulitis, dizziness, **down syndrome**, **eczema**, emotional sensitivity, **emphysema**, **endometriosis**, environmental pollution, **epilepsy**, **erectile dysfunction**, excess weight, exercise (recovery), failure to thrive, **fat cravings**, fibroids (uterine), fibromyalgia, food allergies/intolerances, gout, heart weakness, heavy metal poisoning, hot flashes, Huntington's disease, hypertension, **hypoglycemia**, hypotension, hypothyroidism, infertility, inflammation, inflammatory bowel disorders, interstitial cystitis, leaky gut, **lupus**, **macular degeneration**, **memory/brain function**, menopause, menstrual irregularity, **mental illness**, mercury poisoning, **metabolic syndrome**, mood swings, multiple sclerosis, **myasthenia gravis**, narcolepsy, nephritis, **nerve damage**, nervous exhaustion, nervousness, **neuralgia & neuritis**, neurodegenerative diseases, nightmares, OCD, osteoporosis, **pain**, paralysis, **Parkinson's disease**, peripheral neuropathy, **pet supplements**, **PMS**, PMS Type C, pneumonia, polycystic ovarian syndrome, **pregnancy**, **prostatitis**, psoriasis, **puberty**, **rosacea**, **schizophrenia**, seasonal affective disorder, seborrhea, sex drive (low), **skin (dry/flaky)**, **skin problems**, spider veins, strokes, surgery (recovery), testosterone (low), traumatic brain injury, **triglycerides (high)**, **triglycerides (low)**, **vaccine side effects**, vaginal dryness, and **wrinkles**

Properties: **Anti-inflammatory**, antiarthritic, **antithrombotic**, and immune modulator

Omega-3 EPA (Eicosapentaenoic Acid) *Fatty Acid*

EPA in combination with GLA, an omega-6 essential fatty acid (EFA), helps to make eicosonoids that mediate inflammation, improve immune response, and otherwise promote good health. Without EPA, omega-6 EFAs tend to be converted to eicosonoids that lower immune response, increase inflammation, raise blood pressure and have other undesirable effects. See omega-3 EFAs for more information.

Omega-6 CLA (Conjugated Linolenic Acid) *Fatty Acid*

CLA is conjugated linoleic acid and is a special form of linoleic acid, a part of the omega-6 group of fatty acids, that has been shown to have beneficial effects in human health. It occurs naturally in meat and dairy products when animals are grass fed. It is not present in significant amounts in animals fed on commercial feed or silage.

CLA enhances the cell membrane's defense mechanism against attack by free radicals. It also stimulates the production of key immune system cells and inhibits the release of an immunoglobulin associated with allergies. CLA influences the PPAR-gamma agonist, a class of internal cell receptors that are capable of suppressing the manifestations of inflammatory conditions. It also produces important immune-suppressing compounds such as leukotrienes and prostaglandins. In contrast, regular linoleic acid can increase the body's immune response.

Other possible benefits for CLA include the following: It increases metabolic rate and may help thyroid patients. It decreases abdominal fat, helping to balance adrenal hormones. It enhances muscle development and lowers cholesterol, and triglycerides. It reduces insulin resistance, enhances the immune system, and reduces food-induced allergic reactions.

Usage: Take 1 capsule (750 mg) with a meal three times daily.

Used For: Allergies (respiratory), depression, excess weight, exercise (performance), exercise (recovery), fat metabolism (poor), food allergies/intolerances, inflammation, metabolic syndrome, and triglycerides (high)

Properties: Anti-inflammatory, immune modulator, and nutritive

Omega-6 GLA (Gamma Linolenic Acid) *Fatty Acid*

GLA is formed from the basic omega-6 essential fatty acid, linolenic acid. Along with adequate levels of the omega-3 fatty acid EPA, it helps to reduce inflammation and modulate immune responses. The synthesis of GLA may be inhibited by nutritional deficiencies, alcohol or tobacco use, overconsumption of trans fatty acids or saturated fats, or by stress, illness, or aging. Supplementation with oils high in GLA may be helpful in a wide variety of disorders, but it is essential to obtain adequate amounts of EPA at the same time.

Usage: GLA is naturally found in evening primrose oil (8–10 percent), borage oil (20–24 percent) and black currant oil (15–18 percent).

Used For: Allergies (respiratory), arthritis, autoimmune disorders, bipolar mood disorder, **dermatitis**, diabetes, eczema, epilepsy, hypertension, menopause, multiple sclerosis, neuralgia & neuritis, Parkinson's disease, **PMS**, psoriasis, and skin (dry/flaky)

Properties: Nutritive

Omega-6 LA (Linoleic Acid) *Fatty Acid*

Linoleic acid is the basic plant-based omega-6 essential fatty acid. It is abundant in vegetable oils and needs to be balanced with omega-3 essential fatty acids.

Ophiopogon *Bitter & Sweet Herb*

Ophiopogon japonicus

A superior tonic herb in Chinese herbalism that affects the heart, lung, and kidney meridians. It moistens the lungs, eases thirst, and helps clear phlegm.

Look for *ophiopogon* in *Chinese Yin-Increasing* and *Dry Cough Syrup Formulas*

Energetics: Cooling and moistening

Used For: Constipation (adults), cough (dry), fever, and nervousness

Properties: Anti-inflammatory, antibacterial, antitussive, cardiac, diuretic, expectorant, and febrifuge

Oral Chelation Formula

See also *Cardiovascular Nutritional Program*

This formula contains high doses of vitamins, minerals, and other nutrients to improve cardiovascular function. It can help reduce arteriosclerosis and detoxify the body of heavy metals. It is used in the *Oral Chelation* strategy, which can have many benefits beyond aiding circulation as shown in the list of conditions.

Use this formula with butcher's broom or a *Vein Tonic Formula* for varicose veins. Use it with bilberry or an *Antioxidant Eye Protecting Formula* for eye problems. To aid the brain use with it with ginkgo or a *Brain and Memory Formula*. For calcium deposits use it with hydrangea.

See the strategy *Oral Chelation* for suggested uses.

Warnings: Starting with a full dose (six tablets twice daily) may cause dizziness, headache, skin rashes, kidney stress, and intestinal gas. It may temporarily elevate blood pressure and cholesterol levels when first starting use. These problems subside with continued use. Taking this formula may require supplements to support liver detoxification and kidney function, as these organs are used to flush the toxins released during oral chelation.

Used For: **Alzheimer's**, **arteriosclerosis**, arteriosclerosis, blood clot prevention, **burning feet/hands**, calcium deposits,

cardiovascular disease, cataracts, **circulation (brain)**, **circulation (poor)**, cloudy thinking, **cold hands/feet**, concentration (poor), **dementia**, **diabetic retinopathy**, erectile dysfunction, eye health, **gangrene**, glaucoma, **heavy metal poisoning**, hypertension, **lead poisoning**, **macular degeneration**, **memory/brain function**, Ménière's disease, mercury poisoning, **numbness**, Parkinson's disease, **Peyronie's disease**, spider veins, **strokes**, tinnitus, **ulcerations (external)**, and **varicose veins**

Affects: Arteries, capillaries, **circulatory atrophy**, circulatory stagnation, **heart**, sight, and **veins**

The full dose is 5-6 tablets two times per day, mornings and evenings. However, it is best to start slowly with 1 tablet morning and evening and gradually increase the dose. It is also wise to taper off slowly after having been on this formula. As a vitamin/mineral supplement for seniors take 1-2 tablets twice daily. When mixing with other products for specific problems (like those listed above) you also take 1-2 tablets twice daily.

Ingredients: Vitamin A, vitamin C, vitamin d3, vitamin E, vitamin B$_1$, vitamin B$_2$, niacin, vitamin B$_9$, vitamin B$_6$, vitamin B$_{12}$, biotin, pantothenic acid, calcium, iron, phosphorus, iodine, magnesium, zinc, selenium, copper, manganese, chromium, potassium, p-aminobenzoic acid (paba), inositol, Co-Q10, cysteine hci, and methionine

Orange (Bergamot)   *Aromatic Herb*

Citrus bergamia

This orange is the source of the essential oil called bergamot. It provides the flavor for Earl Grey tea. The herb itself is not widely used, but there is a patented extract of it that is used to reduce cholesterol levels and to keep cholesterol from oxidizing. It aids digestion and relaxes spasms.

Look for *orange (bergamot)* in *Cardiovascular Antioxidant* and *Cardiovascular Nutritional Formulas*

Energetics: Warming, drying, and relaxing

Used For: Cardiovascular disease, cholesterol (high), metabolic syndrome, and **triglycerides (high)**

Properties: Digestive tonic and relaxant

Orange, Bitter   *Aromatic & Bitter Herb*

Citrus aurantium

Bitter orange acts as a pleasant bitter digestive tonic and can be used to treat heartburn, flatulence, and ingestion, as well as boosting the appetite. It also contains traces of the alkaloid synephrine, which helps to dry up mucus secretions in respiratory allergies.

Look for *orange (bitter)* in *Anti-Snoring*, *Antihistamine*, *Chinese Qi-Regulating*, *Herbal Bitters*, *Metabolic Stimulant*, and *Seasonal Cold* and *Flu Formulas*

Energetics: Warming and drying

Used For: Acid indigestion, **allergies (respiratory)**, **appetite (deficient)**, congestion (sinus), gas & bloating, low stomach acid, prolapsed uterus, and protein digestion

Properties: Adrenergic, antiallergenic, **antihistamine**, carminative, digestive tonic, and stimulant (appetite)

Orange, Sweet EO

Fruity & Sweet Essential Oil

Citrus sinensis

A sweet citrus fragrance, orange EO is mildly sedative. It reduces anxiety and nervousness, being especially helpful to children with indigestion or insomnia due to nervousness.

The essential oil of sweet orange is both antifungal and antibacterial. It helps settle the stomach, easing cramps, constipation, gas, and irritable bowel. It stimulates the flow of lymph and is helpful for soothing dry, irritated skin. It is sedative and antidepressant and may be helpful for easing anxiety and insomnia. It is a good oil to settle the digestive system and promote sleep in children as they tend to love the fragrance. Emotionally, the fragrance helps promote happiness and laughter and is good for those who take themselves too seriously. It aids cheerfulness and optimism and eases fears and self-doubts.

See the strategy *Aromatherapy* for suggested uses.

Warnings: Do not use internally without the supervision of a professionally trained aromatherapy practitioner. Nontoxic and nonirritating for topical use.

Used For: Angina, anxiety (situational), constipation (adults), depression, diarrhea, digestion (poor), dyspepsia, fat metabolism (poor), gas & bloating, heart fibrillation/palpitations, insomnia, irritability, menopause, and stress

Properties: Anti-inflammatory, antibacterial, anticancer, antidepressant, antifungal, antiseptic, antispasmodic, aphrodisiac, carminative, cholagogue, digestive tonic, digestive tonic, disinfectant, diuretic, expectorant, lymphatic, sedative, stomachic, and tonic

Oregano   *Aromatic Herb*

Origanum vulgare

Oregano is antiseptic and useful for infections of the respiratory and digestive tracts. It is a good remedy for fungal infections and respiratory problems.

Look for *oregano* in *Anti-Fungal* and *Seasonal Cold* and *Flu Formulas*

Warnings: Oregano should be avoided in large quantities during pregnancy.

Energetics: Warming and drying

Used For: Abscesses, antibiotic side effects, asthma, **athlete's foot**, bronchitis, congestion (lungs), cough, dysbiosis, infection (bacterial), **infection (fungal)**, infection (viral), parasites, pertussis, and tonsillitis

Properties: Antiamebic, **antifungal**, antimicrobial, condiment, expectorant, and stimulant (metabolic)

Oregano EO *Herbaceous & Spicy Essential Oil*

Origanum vulgare

Oregano essential oil is a camphorous and herbaceous scent with a woody undertone. It is a strong antimicrobial remedy for parasites, fungus, viruses and bacteria. Inhaled, it can be helpful for respiratory problems as it things secretions and fights infection. Topically it is effective for lice or for easing arthritic pain and fighting skin infections.

Emotionally, oregano helps with hypochondria. It is mood elevating, overcomes mental fatigue and promotes clarity of thought. It helps calm people who are overly emotional, promoting calm, rational thought. It can help deflect the sense of dependency on others and shifts responsibility to oneself.

See the strategy *Aromatherapy* for suggested uses.

Warnings: Do not use internally without the supervision of a professionally trained aromatherapy practitioner. Even diluted it should not be taken for more than seven to ten days. Oregano oil is hepatotoxic, so internal use can damage the liver. Symptoms of liver damage do not develop gradually and will show up suddenly. May irritate skin and mucous membranes, so dilute for topical use.

Used For: Antibiotic resistance, arthritis, athlete's foot, bronchitis, gas & bloating, hypochondria, infection (bacterial), infection (fungal), infection (viral), infection prevention, lice, parasites, pertussis, tonsillitis, and tuberculosis

Properties: Analgesic, anti-inflammatory, antiallergenic, antibacterial, anticancer, antidepressant, antimicrobial, antioxidant, antiparasitic, antispasmodic, antiviral, diuretic, expectorant, parasympathomimetic, preservative, and sympatholytic

Oregon Grape *Bitter Herb*

Berberris aquifolium

Oregon grape has antimicrobial properties, due to the presence of berberine, and is a good lymphatic-cleansing herb. It also stimulates bile flow and has been used with other alteratives for liver conditions. It can be used both internally and externally to relieve skin conditions such as acne, boils, and eczema and may reduce itching.

Look for *Oregon grape* in *Christopher's Gallbladder Formula*

Warnings: Not for use with emaciation or weak digestion. Use with caution during pregnancy.

Energetics: Cooling and drying

Used For: Abscesses, antibiotic resistance, appetite (deficient), **chicken pox**, cholesterol (low), congestive heart failure, cystic breast disease, **dermatitis**, **digestion (poor)**, hepatitis, **infection (bacterial)**, itching, jaundice (adults), **measles**, **rashes & hives**, **rheumatic fever**, staph infections, swollen lymph glands, syphilis, vaccine side effects, and vaginitis

Properties: Alterative, antipruritic, antiseptic, cholagogue, detergent, hepatic, and **lymphatic**

Osha *Aromatic Herb*

Ligusticum porteri

Osha is a great remedy for viral infections. It stimulates the digestive and immune systems and expels mucus. It is also used for settling the stomach after vomiting. It can be used with eyebright to prevent and treat earaches in children.

Look for *osha* in *Damp Cough Syrup Formula*

Warnings: Do not use during pregnancy.

Energetics: Warming and drying

Used For: Allergies (respiratory), **bronchitis**, **colds**, **cough (damp)**, earache, fever, **flu**, food allergies/intolerances, infection (viral), **pneumonia**, rhinitis, **sinus infection**, and sore throat

Properties: Antiallergenic, antiviral, decongestant, and expectorant

Paavo Airola's Cold Formula

See also *Elderberry Cold* and *Flu Formula*, *Seasonal Cold* and *Flu Formula*, and *Steven Horne's Children's Composition Formula*

This is a general remedy for colds and respiratory congestion. Take at the first sign of a cold with plenty of liquids. It also helps to fast until symptoms begin to improve. It naturally stimulates the body and helps to fight infection, calm coughing, improve circulation, and soothe scratchy throats and watery eyes. It is also helpful in combating nausea, headaches, congestion, chills, and fever, as well as chronic ear infections.

Used For: Colds and nausea & vomiting

Affects: Acute disease stage, immune system, and sweat glands

Paavo Airola's Common Cold Relief

Capsule version of the formula. Take 2 capsules every hour with a large glass of water until symptoms are relieved.

Ingredients: Rose hips, chamomile flower, yarrow aerial parts, capsicum fruit, goldenseal root extract, myrrh gum, peppermint leaf, and lemongrass aerial parts

Liquid Cold Decongestant Formula

Liquid version of the formula. Great remedy for children. Use 1/4–1/2 teaspoon with water every hour with a large glass of water until symptoms are relieved.

Ingredients: Rose hips, chamomile flower, yarrow flower, yerba santa leaf, goldenseal rhizome, myrrh gum, astragalus root, and lemongrass aerial parts

Pancreatin   *Enzyme*

Pancreatin is derived from the pancreas of animals. It contains all the enzymes found in human pancreatic secretions. This includes amylases to digest starch, proteases to digest protein, and lipases to digest fats. It also helps alkalize the environment of the small intestine.

Used For: Convalescence, debility, digestion (poor), fat metabolism (poor), indigestion, and protein digestion

Properties: Digestant

Pantothenic Acid   **see** *vitamin B*$_5$

Papaya   *Sweet & Mildly Sour Herb*

Carica papaya

Papaya fruit contains a protein-digesting enzyme, papain. It can aid digestion of proteins and help expel intestinal worms. The seeds of papaya are an even better antiparasitic agent than the fruit.

Look for *papaya* in *Christopher's Carminative, Natural Antacid, Papaya Enzyme,* and *Skinny Formulas*

Energetics: Cooling and nourishing

Used For: Acid indigestion, constipation (children), cystic fibrosis, **digestion (poor)**, **dyspepsia**, gas & bloating, indigestion, parasites (nematodes, and worms)

Properties: Antiparasitic, condiment, digestant, and food

Papaya Enzyme Formula

See also *Plant Enzyme Formula*

These chewable tablets aid digestion and ease digestive upset. They are an especially helpful digestive aid for children. They are also useful as a breath freshener.

Used For: **Acid indigestion**, **belching**, cystic fibrosis, digestion (poor), dyspepsia, gas & bloating, and **indigestion**

Affects: **Digestive depression**, **digestive stagnation**, small intestines, and stomach

Chew 1-3 tablets with each meal to aid in digestion. Chew 1-2 tablets every half hour in acute indigestion.

Ingredients: Papaya fruit and peppermint leaf

Parasite Cleansing Program

See also *Antiparasitic Formula*

This is an outstanding program for removing yeast, worms, and other parasites from the intestinal tract. For best results, use this program for ten days, wait seven days, and then do a second ten-day round of the program. The theory is that the first cleanse removes the parasites and the break in-between allows any eggs to hatch so that the second cleanse removes any newly-hatched parasites. It is a good idea to follow up with probiotics after completing the program. One can enhance the program by taking protease enzymes in between meals.

Warnings: Not for continuous or long-term use. Not recommended for children under the age of twelve or pregnant women or nursing mothers.

Used For: Fingernail biting, food allergies/intolerances, **parasites**, **parasites (nematodes, worms)**, **parasites (tapeworm)**, and teeth (grinding)

Affects: **Intestinal depression**, intestinal stagnation, and large intestines (colon)

Take 1 packet fifteen minutes before breakfast and fifteen minutes before dinner daily for ten days. Drink one eight-ounce glass of water with each pack.

Ingredients: Black walnut, standardized acetogenin formula, and antiparasitic artemesia blend

Parsley

Salty, Mildly Aromatic, & Mildly Bitter Herb

Petroselinum crispum

Parsley is rich in sodium and potassium necessary to regulate fluids in the body. It has a volatile oil that stimulates kidney function and has a mild alkalizing effect on the system. It also helps to lower blood pressure and slow the pulse.

Look for *parsley* in *Circulatory, Diuretic, Kidney Stone, Liver Cleanse,* and *Prostate Formulas*

Warnings: Not recommended in cases involving fluid deficiency, wasting or dryness. It is used to dry up breast milk, so it should be avoided while breast feeding.

Energetics: Mildly warming, mildly drying, and nourishing

Used For: Bedwetting, body odor, breast milk (surplus), breasts (swelling/tenderness), **edema**, halitosis, **interstitial cystitis**, and kidney stones

Properties: Antigalactagogue, condiment, **diuretic**, food, mineralizer, and nutritive

Partridge Berry *Mildly Sweet Herb*

Mitchella repens

Partridge berry was traditionally taken as a tea by Native American women during pregnancy. They used the plant to ease the difficulties of pregnancy in the later stages and make childbirth fast and easy. The herb's ability to soothe sore nipples has long been known, and a salve applied after breast-feeding is very helpful. It was believed to increase fertility, and it was used to bring about menstruation in irregular cycles. It also used to tone the uterus, which helps in painful, heavy menstruation or periods of irregularity.

Look for *partridge berry* in *Prebirth Formula*

Energetics: Warming and drying

Used For: Dysmenorrhea, infertility, labor & delivery, and postpartum depression

Properties: Emmenagogue and uterine tonic

Passion Flower *Mildly Salty & Sweet Herb*

Passiflora incarnata

A relaxing nervine, often combined with other nervines for reducing stress and tension and aiding sleep. It helps to quiet mental chatter. Passionflower is also used for restless agitation and exhaustion with or without muscular twitching and spasms. It may also have a positive effect on heart rhythm.

Look for *passion flower* in *Antidepressant, Antispasmodic Ear, Attention-Focus, Brain Calming, Christopher's Nervine, Herbal Sleep Aid,* and *Jeannie Burgess' Stress Formulas*

Energetics: Cooling, relaxing, and balancing

Used For: Addictions (drugs), anxiety disorders, arrhythmia, colic (adults), Cushing's disease, depression, dysmenorrhea, epilepsy, headache (tension), heart fibrillation/palpitations, heart weakness, hypertension, hysteria, **insomnia**, neuralgia & neuritis, Parkinson's disease, PTSD, **restless dreams**, rheumatic fever, seizures, stress, teething, Tourette's, and trauma

Properties: Analgesic, antiepileptic, antispasmodic, anxiolytic, bronchial dilator, calmative, **gaba-enhancing**, **nervine**, **relaxant**, sedative, serotonergic, **soporific**, and sympatholytic

Patchouli EO

Balsamic, Musky, Spicy, & Woody Essential Oil

Pogostemon cablin

Patchouli EO has a deep, woody, balsamic odor and a rich, musk-like earthiness. Topically, it helps damaged tissues heal and helps prevent the formation of scar tissue. It can be used topically for insect bites and acts as an insecticide. It tones the skin and can be used to ease various skin disorders.

Patchouli's strongest area of use, however, is for emotional imbalances. It helps with an energetic imbalance in the spleen/pancreas in Chinese herbalism—meaning it helps with chronic anxiety, over-thinking, and worry. Where excessive mental activity and nervous strain have caused people to lose touch with their body and their sensuality, patchouli is a relaxing aphrodisiac that helps ground a person and open their physical senses. It eases depression and helps with impotence, frigidity, and sexual anxiety. It also expands creative expression and imagination.

See the strategy *Aromatherapy* for suggested uses.

Warnings: Do not use internally. Nontoxic and nonirritating for topical use.

Used For: Aging, anger (excessive), anxiety (situational), apathy, bites & stings, cellulite, confusion, depression, edema, gas & bloating, impetigo, infection (fungal), insect repellant, mood swings, nervous exhaustion, nervousness, scars/scar tissue, sex drive (low), and wrinkles

Properties: Anti-inflammatory, antibacterial, antidepressant, antiphlogistic, antiseptic, antiviral, **aphrodisiac**, cicatrizant, deodorant, diuretic, febrifuge, insecticide, perfume, relaxant, and sedative

Pau D'arco

Mildly Astringent, Mildly Bitter, & Sweet Herb

Tabebuia spp.

Commonly used as an anticancer remedy and an antifungal remedy. It may be helpful for fighting infections in the digestive tract, both bacterial and fungal. Its active constituents include lapachol and beta-lapachone, which have demonstrated potent antifungal properties in laboratory tests.

Look for *pau d'arco* in *Anti-Fungal, Blood Purifier, H. Pylori-Fighting,* and *Yeast Cleansing Formulas*

Warnings: Contraindicated for blood clotting disorders. Do not use during pregnancy. High doses may cause nausea, vomiting, intestinal discomfort and anticoagulant effects.

Energetics: Mildly cooling, drying, and mildly constricting

Used For: AIDS, ALS, antibiotic side effects, athlete's foot, blood poisoning, body odor, cancer, cancer treatment side effects, cradle cap, dandruff, **dermatitis**, diarrhea, **dysbiosis**, eczema, endometriosis, Epstein-Barr virus, fever, **infection (fungal)**, inflammation, **itching**, itchy ears, **jock itch**, **leucorrhea**, leukemia, parasites, polyps, preeclampsia, psoriasis, rashes & hives, scabies, SIBO, **skin (infections)**, snakebite, sprains, thrush, vaginitis, and wounds & sores

Properties: Alterative, anti-inflammatory, antibacterial, **anticancer**, anticoagulant, **antifungal**, antiseptic, antiviral, astringent, hepatic, and tonic

Pawpaw   *Bitter Herb*
Asimina triloba

The spring twigs, unripe fruit, and mature seeds of the American pawpaw tree contain compounds called acetogenins, which inhibit energy production in cells. Since cancer cells have a much faster metabolic rate than normal cells, this induces cancer cells to self-destruct. Scientific research demonstrates that pawpaw extract is more effective than many chemotherapy drugs at destroying cancer cells, and yet it is completely nontoxic. In a clinical trial involving over one hundred people with cancer, a standardized extract of pawpaw was shown to reduce tumor markers and tumor sizes, usually within one to four weeks, with virtually no side effects. The extract has also been used to kill intestinal parasites and fight fungal and viral infections. Although Native Americans made preparations from the twigs, unripe fruit, and seeds, one should rely on the standardized extract for modern applications.

Look for *pawpaw* in *Standardized Acetogenin Formula*

Warnings: Avoid during pregnancy. The pawpaw extract is not toxic to people or animals in normal doses, but it may cause nausea and vomiting when ingested. It is not recommended for healthy people as it will reduce energy levels, causing fatigue. It should only be used by persons with cancer, viral disorders, parasites, or other specific health problems. Pawpaw may also induce a healing crisis or cleansing reaction if cell die-off occurs too rapidly, which may require cleansing herbs to help the body detoxify.

Energetics: Cooling

Used For: Athlete's foot, **cancer**, **cancer treatment side effects**, cervical dysplasia, **endometriosis**, **fleas**, infection (fungal), lice, **parasites**, parasites (nematodes, worms), **parasites (tapeworm)**, **psoriasis**, scabies, **shingles**, and tick

Properties: **Anticancer**, antifungal, antimicrobial, **antiparasitic**, antiviral, **cytotoxic**, **escharotic**, **insecticide**, **nauseant**, vermifuge, and **virostatic**

Peony   *Bitter Herb*
Paeonia spp.

Peony is used as a tonic for women in Chinese herbalism. It is also used for abdominal pain, amenorrhea, and to move blood. It is commonly blended with rehmannia, dong quai and ligusticum as a female tonic. It builds the blood and can be helpful for hot flashes or night sweats. It can also relieve abdominal cramps and pain.

Look for *peony* in *Chinese Qi-Increasing*, *Chinese Wood-Decreasing*, and *Chinese Wood-Increasing Formulas*

Warnings: Western peony (P. officinalis) should only be used by professionals.

Energetics: Cooling and relaxing

Used For: Amenorrhea, cramps (menstrual), hot flashes, night sweating, and PMS

Properties: Alterative, analgesic, anti-inflammatory, antispasmodic, and female tonic

Peppermint   *Aromatic Herb*
Mentha piperita

Peppermint is a soothing aromatic with primary effects on the nervous system, stomach, and colon. It is a very safe remedy and is an excellent ingredient in formulas for acute ailments. It settles the stomach, expels gas, and has a mild effect on easing colds, fevers, and headaches. It's also a good herb to add to liquid formulas and teas to improve their flavor.

Look for *peppermint* in *Christopher's Carminative*, *Papaya Enzyme*, *Pregnancy Tea*, and *Steven Horne's Children's Composition Formulas*

Energetics: Cooling and drying

Used For: Anorexia, apathy, **belching**, cancer treatment side effects, cloudy thinking, colds, colic (children), concentration (poor), **confusion**, dizziness, dysmenorrhea, fever, **flu**, food poisoning, **gas & bloating**, **gastritis**, halitosis, hysteria, ileocecal valve, indigestion, **irritable bowel**, lactose intolerance, **morning sickness**, motion sickness, mumps, **nausea & vomiting**, and perspiration (deficient)

Properties: Analgesic, antacid, **antiemetic**, antinausa, antiseptic, aperitive, **carminative**, condiment, diaphoretic, **digestive tonic**, stimulant (metabolic), and **stomachic**

Peppermint EO   *Minty & Sharp Essential Oil*
Mentha piperita

The familiar grassy, minty and slightly sweet fragrance of peppermint EO is very helpful for balancing mind and body. It is slightly warming or stimulating, but feels cooling or calming at the same time. It is very good for helping people digest things, physically, mentally, or emotionally. When one has indigestion accompanied by brain fog, peppermint will clear the congestion in the stomach, at the same time clearing the cloudy thought processes in the head. Peppermint oil can be helpful for staying alert while driving, studying, or doing mental work, as it overcomes mental fatigue improving alertness and concentration.

Apply peppermint essential oil full strength externally as a mild stimulant or antiseptic for healing minor injuries, bites and stings. Put one or two drops in a cup of warm water and sip slowly to relieve gas, heartburn, and indigestion. A drop can also be placed on the bottom of the thumb and sucked on or placed on the back of the tongue with the finger. Inhaling the oil helps promote mental alertness for study, late night driving, etc. It also relieves muscle spasms. Inhale for sinus and respiratory conditions.

See the strategy *Aromatherapy* for suggested uses.

Warnings: One of the safest essential oils for internal use but should ideally be diluted for internal use. Don't take daily, however. Only use it when it is needed. Don't give the oil internally to young children; peppermint tea is better. The undiluted oil can cause skin irritation if used excessively.

Used For: Acid indigestion, apathy, asthma, belching, bronchitis, burns & scalds, **cloudy thinking**, cold sores, **colic (adults)**, colic (children), **concentration (poor)**, confusion, corns, cysts, dementia, diarrhea, **digestion (poor)**, dizziness, **dysbiosis**, dysmenorrhea, **dyspepsia**, fatigue, fever, flu, food poisoning, **gas & bloating**, gastritis, **halitosis**, headache (cluster), headache (migraine), herpes, hot flashes, hypochondria, hysteria, impetigo, **indigestion**, infection (fungal), memory/brain function, menopause, menstrual irregularity, morning sickness, **motion sickness**, mumps, **nausea & vomiting**, pet supplements, rheumatic fever, shock (medical), SIBO, skin (dry/flaky), sore throat, ulcers, and varicose veins

Properties: Analgesic, anesthetic, anti-inflammatory, antibacterial, **antiemetic**, antifungal, antinausa, antiphlogistic, antiseptic, antispasmodic, **carminative**, cephalic, cholagogue, decongestant, emmenagogue, expectorant, febrifuge, hepatic, nervine, sialogogue, stimulant (metabolic), stomachic, vasoconstrictor, and vermifuge

Pepsin Intestinal Formula

This formula can help to break down any undigested proteins that may be clogging the small and large intestines. It can help improve absorption of nutrients.

See the strategy *Detoxification* for suggested uses.

Used For: Allergies (respiratory), dyspepsia, food allergies/intolerances, gastritis, indigestion, inflammatory bowel disorders, irritable bowel, and leaky gut

Affects: Intestinal irritation, intestinal stagnation, mucous membranes, and **small intestines**

Take 2 capsules two to three times daily between meals with a glass of water.

Ingredients: Marshmallow root and pepsin

Perilla   *Aromatic & Mildly Pungent Herb*

Perillae frutescentis

This member of the mint family is used in Chinese herbalism as a remedy for the lung and spleen meridians.

Look for *perilla* in *Chinese Qi-Regulating Formula*

Energetics: Warming, drying, and mildly relaxing

Used For: Colds (decongestant) and gas & bloating

Properties: Antibacterial, carminative, diaphoretic, febrifuge, and soporific

Periwinkle

Mildly Astringent & Stimulant Bitter Herb

Vinca major or minor

Periwinkle increases blood flow and oxygen to the brain. Clinical studies suggest it may also be helpful in treating dementia, Alzheimer's disease, short-term memory loss caused by some medications, high blood pressure, age-related hearing loss, vertigo, and reducing calcium buildup from dialysis. Used as an astringent against internal bleeding, it can also be helpful for migraines due to vasoconstriction.

Look for *periwinkle* in *Headache Formula*

Warnings: Do not use during pregnancy. Avoid with low blood pressure and liver and kidney diseases. Periwinkle is best used under professional supervision.

Energetics: Drying and relaxing

Used For: Alzheimer's, bleeding (internal), dementia, dizziness, headache (migraine), headache (tension), hearing loss, and hypertension

Properties: Astringent, hypotensive, sedative, and styptic

Personal Boundaries FE Blend

This is for people who feel that anger is such a negative emotion that they have a hard time allowing themselves to feel it. As a result, they have a hard time standing up for themselves and often suffer a lot of abuse from others. They become people pleasers and enablers to the neglect of their own self-interest. It helps them recognize abuse for what it is and stand up to it by helping them to set healthy boundaries with other people. It also helps them find the courage to communicate openly and honestly in relationships.

These people often have problems with their detoxification systems (liver, intestines, kidneys, and bladder) and their immune system because these are the systems that defend the body against toxins and microbes. As a result, they may have frequent infections or suffer from autoimmune disorders or cancer. The blend helps activate their immune system by activating their will to fight for themselves.

See the strategy *Flower Essence* for suggested uses.

Used For: Anger (excessive), **apathy**, autoimmune disorders, bladder (irritable), cancer prevention, **depression**, hiatal hernia, **shame & guilt**, and trauma

Affects: Immune system

Ingredients: Mariposa lily FE, pine FE, scarlet monkeyflower FE, centaury FE, fuchsia FE, pink yarrow FE, and goldenrod FE

Pet Supplement Formula

This herbal formula is a rich source of various trace elements. It makes an excellent supplement for animals. Mix it with their food. It is a general tonic for children and adults.

Used For: Anemia, fingernails (weak/brittle), and **pet supplements**

Affects: Blood, bones, and teeth

Take 1-2 capsules three times daily. For pets, mix 1 capsule with their food.

Ingredients: Kelp leaf & stem, dandelion root, and alfalfa aerial parts

Phytoestrogen Breast Formula

Xenoestrogens are a major culprit in the development of breast cancer. (See the *Avoid Xenoestrogens* strategy for more information). The ingredients in this formula help block estrogen receptors against xenoestrogens and may also help balance female hormones. Women with a family history of breast cancer may wish to use this formula, along with avoiding xenoestrogens, to reduce cancer risk. The formula may also have a protective effect against prostate cancer in men.

Used For: BPH, **breast lumps**, **cancer prevention**, cystic breast disease, and estrogen (low)

Affects: Breasts and immune system

Take 2 to 3 capsules daily with a meal.

Ingredients: Flax, ellagic acid standardized extract, kudzu root extract, and maitake mushroom

Picrorhiza   *Bitter Herb*
Neopicrorhiza scrophulariiflora

A bitter herb used in Ayurvedic herbalism, picrorhiza is used to aid liver and digestive system issues. It has been found helpful for viral hepatitis and may be helpful for cirrhosis of the liver.

Energetics: Cooling and drying

Used For: Allergies (respiratory), anorexia, asthma, cirrhosis of the liver, dyspepsia, **hepatitis**, jaundice (adults), and parasites

Properties: Antioxidant, hepatoprotective, and immune modulator

Pine   *Aromatic & Mildly Astringent Herb*
Pinus strobus

Pine bark is primarily used as an expectorant for coughs. It helps discharge mucus and fight infection. It is particularly helpful for coaxing old, thick green mucus up and out of the lungs and sinuses and in cases of chronic bronchitis.

The pine gum is a good agent for drawing pus and slivers and a valuable ingredient in drawing salves. It helps wounds to heal. Pine also strengthens muscles and tendons and helps tissue regeneration and repair. The pollen contains testosterone and is used as a male glandular tonic.

Look for *pine* in *Drawing Salve*, *Ed Millet's Herbal Crisis*, *Herbal Composition*, and *Proanthocyanidins Formulas*

Energetics: Warming and drying

Used For: Bronchitis, cough, **cough (damp)**, croup, **slivers**, strep throat, and testosterone (low)

Properties: Antiseptic, **decongestant**, **drawing**, expectorant, and testosterone-enhancing

Pine EO (Scotch Pine)
Balsamic, Fresh, & Woody Essential Oil
Pinus sylvestris

The distinctive turpentine-like odor of pine EO is refreshing and slightly sweet. It is a stimulant, helping to overcome fatigue, lethargy, weakness, and heavy feelings in the chest.

Pine oil is an effective expectorant and can be inhaled to open up the lungs, loosen mucus, and fight infection. It is antiseptic and eases cough. Inhaling the oil can also help relieve mental and physical exhaustion by stimulating the adrenal glands. Cleansing and invigorating, this oil is often chosen to scent cleaning solutions for that sense of freshness.

Emotionally, it disperses melancholy and counteracts pessimism. It reawakens our instinctive connection to life. For those who blame themselves and feel responsible for all the mistakes and sufferings of others, pine can help to establish appropriate boundaries and let go of toxic shame, guilt, and fear. It renews hope, confidence, and self-acceptance.

See the strategy *Aromatherapy* for suggested uses.

Warnings: Do not use internally without the supervision of a professionally trained aromatherapy practitioner. It may be irritating to the skin; dilute for topical use. When using as an inhalant, it is contraindicated in dry conditions of the lungs.

Used For: Addictions (tobacco), appetite (deficient), asthma, bronchitis, circulation (poor), cloudy thinking, colds (antiviral), **colds (decongestant)**, concentration (poor), confusion, **congestion**, **congestion (lungs)**, **congestion (sinus)**, **cough**, **cough (damp)**, depression, **diphtheria**, fatigue, fleas, flu, foot odor, gout, grief & sadness, infection prevention, insect repellant, laryngitis, nervous exhaustion, nervousness, parasites, pertussis, **shame & guilt**, shock (medical), **sinus infection**, **trauma**, and uric acid retention

Properties: Anti-inflammatory, antimicrobial, antirheumatic, **antiseptic**, antiviral, bactericidal, balsamic, decongestant, deodorant, diuretic, expectorant, insecticide, pectoral, rubefacient, stimulant (metabolic), sympatholytic, and tonic

Pipsissewa

Mildly Astringent, Mildly Bitter, & Sweet Herb

Chimaphila umbellata

An antibacterial and astringent remedy, pipsissewa is used primarily for urinary problems involving inflammation such as cystitis, prostitis, and urethritis. It is a great remedy for an irritable bladder with frequent urge to urinate. It has the same urinary disinfectant compounds as uva ursi, but less tannin, which makes it easier on the kidneys.

Energetics: Cooling and drying

Used For: Bladder (irritable), **bladder infection**, **interstitial cystitis**, **kidney infection**, **urethritis**, **urinary tract infections**, **urination (burning/painful)**, **urination (frequent)**, and urine (scant)

Properties: Antiseptic and diuretic

Plant Enzyme Formula

See also *Digestive Support Formula* and *Papaya Enzyme Formula*

This formula contains enzymes for breaking down fats, proteins and carbohydrates. This formula can assist in breaking down the fibers in foods that contribute to gas and bloating. It's a good product for anyone to take with meals who eats primarily cooked and processed foods. For people over 50, consider *Digestive Support Formula*.

Warnings: Do not use in cases of ulceration.

Used For: Appetite (deficient), **autoimmune disorders**, **belching**, **digestion (poor)**, dyspepsia, **failure to thrive**, fibromyalgia, **food allergies/intolerances**, **gas & bloating**, **halitosis**, ileocecal valve, **indigestion**, inflammatory bowel disorders, **leaky gut**, overalkalinity, pancreatitis, sore/geographic tongue, **underweight**, and wasting

Affects: Digestive atrophy, digestive stagnation, **immune system**, small intestines, and **stomach**

Take 1-2 capsules with meals as an aid to digesting all types of food.

Ingredients: Protease 4.4, protease 5.0, protease 3.0, amylase, glucoamylase, lipase, cellulase, invertase, malt diastase, alpha-galactosidase, and peptidase

Plantain   *Mildly Astringent & Sour Herb*

Plantago major

This common lawn and garden weed is a valuable remedy for bruises, insect bites, and injuries when applied topically. It is a common ingredient in poultices. Plantain is used internally for ulcers, inflammatory bowel disorders, and coughs. It is helpful for drawing sticky phlegm out of the lungs, especially when combined with gumweed.

Look for *plantain* in *Herbal Calcium, Intestinal Soothing, Liquid Kidney, Lymph Cleansing, Lymphatic Infection,* and *Vulnerary Formulas*

Energetics: Cooling, moistening, and mildly constricting

Used For: **Abrasions/scratches**, abscesses, anal fistula/fissure, **bites & stings**, bronchitis, burns & scalds, celiac disease, **colitis**, congestion (lungs), cough (dry), **cysts**, emphysema, fibrosis, food allergies/intolerances, **inflammatory bowel disorders**, leaky gut, ligaments (torn/injuried), **oral surgery**, **poison ivy/oak**, **snakebite**, **sprains**, **surgery (recovery)**, and **tooth extraction**

Properties: Anticatarrhal, antiseptic, **antivenomous**, astringent, cicatrizant, decongestant, **drawing**, emollient, mucilant, and **vulnerary**

Pleurisy Root

Mildly Bitter, Mildly Salty, & Mildly Sweet Herb

Asclepias tuberosa

Native American's used pleurisy root for ailments relating to the heart, bronchi, and lungs. As its name implies it is one of the best remedies for pleurisy. It eases chest pain and is good for hot, dry conditions of the chest. It also relaxes the peripheral capillaries, increasing perspiration, making it an excellent diaphoretic. It is helpful for respiratory problems where there is dryness in the lungs.

Warnings: Excessive doses may cause vomiting. Avoid during pregnancy.

Energetics: Cooling and moistening

Used For: Bursitis, congestive heart failure, **cough (dry)**, eczema, fever, flu, measles, perspiration (deficient), pertussis, **pleurisy**, and pneumonia

Properties: Anti-inflammatory, diaphoretic, diuretic, and expectorant

Polygala (Seneca Snakeroot)

Bitter, Mildly Pungent, & Mildly Sweet Herb

Polygala sp.

The Chinese species (*P. tenuifolia*) is used to calm the mind and emotions (shen in Chinese herbalism terms) and to expel excess mucus. It is helpful for restlessness and absent-mindedness. It also helps rid the body of mucus that is difficult to expel. Polygala can be applied topically for swelling and abscesses. The Western species (*P. senega*) was used for snakebite and as an expectorant.

Warnings: Large doses can cause nausea and vomiting.

Energetics: Warming, relaxing, and drying

Used For: Abscesses, anxiety disorders, bites & stings, boils, breasts (swelling/tenderness), colds, cough (damp), edema, heart fibrillation/palpitations, insomnia, irritability, rashes & hives, and seizures

Properties: Calmative and expectorant

Pomegranate   *Sour & Sweet Herb*

Punica granatum

Pomegranate is rich in antioxidants known as punicalagins, which are more potent than those found in red wine or green tea. It also contains punicic acid, a conjugated linoleic acid that may help in weight management. It may help protect against hormonally related cancers—prostate cancer in men and breast cancer in women. It also contains dietary nitrates, which help produce nitric oxide to improve blood flow.

Look for *pomegranate* in *Blood Pressure Reducing* and *Phytoestrogen Breast Formulas*

Used For: BPH, cancer prevention, erectile dysfunction, inflammation, and memory/brain function

Properties: Anti-inflammatory, antibacterial, anticancer, antifungal, cephalic, food, and hypertensive

Potassium   *Mineral*

Potassium ions are necessary for the function of all living cells. Potassium ion diffusion is a key mechanism in nerve transmission, and deficiency can result in muscle twitching and

tension. It is also important for kidney function as it is lost in urination. It is an alkalizing mineral and helps maintain proper acid-alkaline balance. Potassium is widely available in plant foods, but many people eat too much sodium (salt) and don't eat enough high potassium foods. Ensuring adequate levels can be important in overcoming a wide variety of health problems.

Used For: Acne, afterbirth pain, allergies (respiratory), Alzheimer's, autoimmune disorders, cancer, cardiac arrest, cardiovascular disease, confusion, copper toxicity, **cramps (leg)**, cramps (menstrual), cramps & spasms, dehydration, diarrhea, edema, **emotional sensitivity**, Epstein-Barr virus, exercise (recovery), giardia, gout, headache, **heart fibrillation/palpitations**, hypertension, insomnia, irritability, kidney stones, Ménière's disease, muscular dystrophy, nerve damage, nervous exhaustion, overacidity, **PMS Type H**, stress, strokes, tachycardia, tics, tinnitus, **tremors**, and **twitching**

Properties: Diuretic, kidney tonic, and nutritive

Prebirth Formula

Use these formulas to help induce labor and make childbirth easier. They can promote uterine contractions, tone the uterus and help improve circulation.

Warnings: Some midwives caution that using black cohosh during the last five weeks of pregnancy may increase bleeding during labor in some women. If a tendency towards heavy bleeding exists, do not use formulas with black cohosh. These formulas should not be taken during early pregnancy (first and second trimesters) or when trying to get pregnant.

Used For: Labor & delivery

5-Week Childbirth-Support Formula

A general formula for aiding labor and delivery. Take 2 capsules three times per day only during the last five weeks of pregnancy with plenty of water.

Ingredients: Black cohosh root, partridge berry whole plant, dong quai root, and red raspberry leaf

Birth-Prep Formula

A traditional formula used by Utah lay midwives to prepare the body for childbirth. Use as directed on the label.

Ingredients: Partridge berry herb, black cohosh root, pennyroyal herb, false unicorn root, and lobelia herb

Labor Inducing Formula

This is a stronger labor-inducing formula, which is best used after the due date. Use as directed on the label.

Ingredients: Angelica, blue cohosh, partridge berry, and pennyroyal

Pregnancy Tea Formula

See also *Joan Patton's Herbal Minerals Formula*

This do-it-yourself tea has been helpful for many women during pregnancy. It helps to tone the uterus and provides trace minerals and iron to help both the mother and baby have a healthy pregnancy. It seems to also reduce complications during pregnancy, such as morning sickness. It has been used by Utah midwives for many years to aid pregnancy and delivery.

Used For: Anemia, birth defect prevention, **labor & delivery**, miscarriage prevention, **morning sickness**, and **pregnancy**

Affects: Blood and stomach

Mix dry herbs together and make a strong tea using 3-4 teaspoons of herbs in a quart of boiling water. Steep for 30 minutes and drink one quart daily throughout pregnancy.

2 parts Red raspberry leaf

2 parts Nettle

2 parts Alfalfa

1 part Peppermint

Prenatal Support Formula

See also *Joan Patton's Herbal Minerals Formula*

A vitamin and mineral formula to aid pregnant and lactating women. It contains 800 micrograms of folic acid and ginger to soothe the stomach.

Used For: Birth defect prevention and **pregnancy**

Take 1 tablet daily.

Ingredients: Vitamin A, vitamin C, vitamin D, vitamin E, vitamin B_1, vitamin B_2, vitamin B_3, vitamin B_6, folate, vitamin B_{12}, biotin, vitamin B_5, iron, iodine, magnesium, zinc, and copper

Prickly Ash
Aromatic & Mildly Stimulant bitter Herb

Zanthoxylum americanum

Prickly ash is used internally primarily to aid circulation. It increases peripheral circulation and is indicated for people with cold extremities, Raynaud's disease, sciatica, or peripheral neuropathy with damaged, numb, tingling or extremely painful nerves that cause a person to writhe in agony.

Look for *prickly ash* in *Liquid Lymph Formula*

Warnings: Avoid during pregnancy.

Energetics: Warming and drying

Used For: Arthritis, arthritis (rheumatoid), burning feet/hands, canker sores, **cardiovascular disease**, **circulation (poor)**, cold hands/feet, edema, **narcolepsy**, nerve dam-age, **numbness**, pain, paralysis, **peripheral neuropathy**, **Raynaud's disease**, and sciatica

Properties: Alterative, analgesic, carminative, diaphoretic, and **stimulant (circulatory)**

Proanthocyanidins Formula

See also *Antioxidant Formula*

Proanthocyanidins are powerful antioxidants, fifty times more potent than vitamin E. Antioxidants help prevent cell damage believed to be responsible for cancer, hardening of the arteries, and aging. They may also help with inflammatory diseases such as arthritis.

Used For: Aging, arthritis, cancer, cancer prevention, easily bruised, free radical damage, lupus, macular degeneration, meningitis, pain, Parkinson's disease, and surgery (recovery)

Affects: Immune system, liver, and structural irritation

Antioxidant Blend with Proanthocyanidins

Proanthocyanidin formula in a base of antioxidant herbs and nutrients. Take 1–2 tablets of three times a day.

Ingredients: Vitamin C, Grape seed extract, pine bark extract, Grape skin extract, turmeric root, and bioflavonoids

Proanthocyanidins

Higher potency product containing only proanthocyanidins. Take 2 tablets once or twice daily.

Ingredients: Grape seed extract and pine bark extract

Probiotic Blend

Acidophilus, bifidophilus and other species of *Lactobacillis* are friendly bacteria necessary for colon health. (See the *Friendly Flora* strategy for more information.) Probiotics should always be taken after a round of antibiotics. They can be taken orally or used in enemas or douches for yeast infection. They may be sprinkled in the diaper for thrush-related diaper rash. Probiotics are especially helpful when traveling abroad because they help to prevent traveler's diarrhea. When traveling, double or triple the amount normally consumed.

Although probiotics can be taken orally, they can also be given via rectal injection. Empty 3–5 capsules into a cup of room temperature water, dissolve, and inject rectally using a bulb syringe. This implants the bacteria right where they are needed.

Used For: Acne, ADD/ADHD, addictions (sugar/carbohydrates), Addison's disease, anorexia, **antibiotic side effects**, autoimmune disorders, bladder (irritable), cancer, cancer treatment side effects, **celiac disease**, chemical exposure, cold sores, colitis, **colon (atonic)**, constipation (adults), **constipation (adults)**, **constipation (children)**, COPD, cradle cap, **cystic fibrosis**, depression, dermatitis, **diaper rash**, **diarrhea**, digestion (poor), diverticulitis, down syndrome, **dysbiosis**, dyspepsia, eczema, enteritis, environmental pollution, Epstein-Barr virus, **fibromyalgia**, food allergies/intolerances, food poisoning, giardia, gonorrhea, herpes, **infection (bacterial)**, **infection (fungal)**, infection prevention, **inflammatory bowel disorders**, interstitial cystitis, **itchy ears**, **jock itch**, **lactose intolerance**, **leaky gut**, leucorrhea, **lupus**, malaria, mononucleosis, nursing, overalkalinity, pancreatitis, parasites, prostatitis, **SIBO**, sinus infection, **sore/geographic tongue**, staph infections, **surgery (recovery)**, syphilis, **thrush**, and **vaginitis**

Affects: Immune system, **large intestines (colon)**, and vagina

Probiotic Blend

Contains eleven strains of probiotics. The best choice for most people. Take 2–3 capsules daily with food.

Ingredients: Lactobacillus rhamnosus, bifidobacterium bifidum, lactobacillus acidophilus, lactobacillus brevis, lactobacillus bulgaricus, lactobacillus plantarum, streptococcus thermophilus, bifidobacterium infantis, lactobacillus casei, and lactobacillus salivarius

Bifidophilus Blend

A good probiotic for children. Take 1 to 2 capsules daily with food.

Ingredients: Lactobacillus rhamnosus, lactobacillus casei, lactobacillus acidophilus, and bifidobacterium longum

Acidophilus

A basic probiotic. Take 1 to 2 capsules daily with food.

Ingredients: Lactobacillus acidophilus

Propolis   *Supplement*

Resina propoli

Propolis is not an herb. It is a substance made by bees that has powerful antibiotic and immune-enhancing effects. Warming and stimulating, its antimicrobial activity is due largely to its richness in phenolic aglycones.

Warnings: Avoid propolis if you have bee allergies.

Energetics: Warming and drying

Used For: Abscesses, **canker sores**, **gingivitis**, **halitosis**, herpes, infection (bacterial), infection (viral), and **ulcerations (external)**

Properties: Antibacterial, antifungal, expectorant, and immune modulator

Prostate Formula

The prostate gland is located just underneath the bladder and may swell due to irritation (prostatitis) or enlarge in benign prostatic hyperplasia or BPH. This can result in difficult or painful urination. *Prostate Support Formulas* may be helpful for these and other symptoms of prostate problems.

Used For: Bladder (irritable), **BPH**, erectile dysfunction, **prostatitis**, **urination (burning/painful)**, urination (frequent), and urine (scant)

Affects: **Prostate**, urinary constriction, and urinary stagnation

Prostate Support Formula

Contains herbs and nutrients that are helpful for BPH and may also have a protective effect against prostate cancer. To ease prostate problems and improve urination take 2–3 capsules twice daily. For maintenance, take 1 capsule twice daily.

Ingredients: Zinc, saw palmetto fruit extract, pumpkin seed, pygeum bark extract, gotu kola aerial parts, lycopene, nettle, and stinging root extract

Stan Malstrom's Prostate Formula

An all-herbal formula that can aid prostatitis, BPH, or urinary tract infections. For difficult urination or prostate issues, take 1–2 capsules three times daily.

Ingredients: Pumpkin seed, saw palmetto fruit, black cohosh root, gotu kola aerial parts, and goldenseal root & rhizome

Christopher's Prostate Formula

This blend is a mild diuretic and also helps with blood sugar and urinary problems. For prostate swelling or blood sugar problems, use 2 capsules three times daily with meals.

Ingredients: Juniper berry, goldenseal root & rhizome, parsley leaf, uva ursi leaf, meadowsweet leaf, and marshmallow root

Protease   *Enzyme*

Protease enzymes are produced in the body and are responsible for a variety of functions, from aiding digestion to inducing programmed cell death (*apoptosis*). They can be taken between meals to enhance immunity and as part of a natural anticancer program.

Warnings: Do not use when ulcers are present. If stomach burning or pain occurs, reduce dose or discontinue use.

Used For: AIDS, autism, autoimmune disorders, belching, blood clot prevention, **cancer**, **cancer treatment side effects**, celiac disease, cholesterol (low), congestion, **cystic fibrosis**, cysts, digestion (poor), fibromyalgia, **fibrosis**, floaters, food allergies/intolerances, hair loss/thinning, infection (fungal), inflammatory bowel disorders, leukemia, lupus, overacidity, overalkalinity, **parasites**, **parasites (nematodes, worms)**, parasites (tapeworm), **protein digestion**, psoriasis, and underweight

Properties: Anticancer, antilipemic, digestant, and immune modulator

Psyllium   *Herb*

Plantago psyllium

A mucilaginous herb used as a bulk laxative or anti-diarrhea remedy or to soothe intestinal irritation. It also helps to lower cholesterol. It is a mild laxative suitable for use by children and the elderly, as well as during pregnancy.

Look for *psyllium* in *Chinese Balanced Cleansing, Fat-Absorbing Fiber, Fiber, Gut-Healing Fiber, Intestinal Detoxification,* and *Ivy Bridge's Cleansing Formulas*

Warnings: Avoid in cases of bowel obstruction or perforations. It can cause constipation when a person is dehydrated.

Usage: Take first thing in the morning or right before going to bed or take before meals to help regulate appetite and blood sugar. Always take psyllium with plenty of water or juice.

Energetics: Cooling and moistening

Used For: Appetite (excessive), cholesterol (high), cholesterol (high), colon (atonic), **constipation (adults)**, diarrhea, excess weight, food poisoning, heavy metal poisoning, hemorrhoids, multiple sclerosis, and psoriasis

Properties: **Absorbent**, anticholesteremic, antidiarrheal, emollient, hypolipidemic, **laxative (bulk)**, mucilant, and soothing

Pumpkin   *Oily Herb*

Cucurbita pepo

Pumpkin seeds are a traditional remedy for intestinal worms, such as tapeworm and ringworm. The crushed seeds appear to immobilize worms and help the body expel them. The seeds are a rich source of zinc and magnesium and have also been used to help prostate problems in men.

Look for *pumpkin* in *Antiparasitic, Male Performance, Prostate,* and *Testosterone Formulas*

Energetics: Neutral, moistening, and nourishing

Used For: BPH, **parasites (nematodes, worms)**, and prostatitis

Properties: Antiparasitic, food, and nutritive

Purslane   *Sour & Mucilant Herb*

Portulaca oleracea

This common garden weed is a succulent plant with juicy leaves that are actually quite tasty. In fact, the whole plant is edible both raw or cooked. It is rich in carbohydrates, proteins, omega-3 fatty acids, antioxidants, and vitamin E. It also contains oxalic acid, which gives it a cooling action, which means it also helps reduce inflammation. It can be applied topically for minor injuries and bites and stings. In Chinese herbalism, it is said to enter the heart and large intestine meridians. It removes toxic heat, eases diarrhea, and kills intestinal parasites.

Look for *purslane* in *Chinese Wind-Heat Evil Formula*

Energetics: Cooling and moistening

Used For: Bites & stings, carbuncles, edema, fever, inflammation, parasites, and wounds & sores

Properties: Anti-inflammatory, diuretic, food, mucilant, and nutritive

Pygeum   *Bitter Herb*

Pygeum africanum

Pygeum is a urinary remedy from Africa that has been found to be helpful for prostate swelling. It is most often used in combination with other herbs.

Look for *pygeum* in *Prostate Formula*

Energetics: Cooling

Used For: BPH and prostatitis

Properties: Anti-inflammatory and diuretic

Pyridoxine   **see** *vitamin B$_6$*

Quassia   *Fragrant Bitter Herb*

Quassia amara

Quassia is used in combination with other herbs for parasites. It may also help control infections.

Look for *quassia* in *Antiparasitic Formula*

Warnings: Excessive doses of the bark may cause irritation of the digestive tract and vomiting. Do not use during pregnancy.

Energetics: Cooling and drying

Used For: Parasites

Properties: Antibacterial, antispasmodic, and antiviral

Quercetin   *Nutrient*

Quercetin is the most abundant flavonoid found in the plant world. It is found in significant amounts in onions, apples, berries and cruciferous vegetables. Quercitin is a strong antioxidant, reducing inflammation throughout the body. Supplemental quercetin is poorly absorbed, with studies showing only about 2 percent passing through the gut into the bloodstream. There is a distinct possibility that many of the beneficial effects of quercetin are from a reduction of gut inflammation. quercetin is most beneficial for people with allergies and allergy-induced asthma. However, studies also found that people with chronic prostatitis and interstitial cystitis saw an improvement in symptoms.

Usage: 400–500 mg three times daily.

Used For: **Allergies (respiratory)**, asthma, bites & stings, interstitial cystitis, **prostatitis**, **rhinitis**, and **sleep apnea**

Properties: **Mast cell stabilizer**

Quince, Asian   *Sour Herb*

Chaenomeles lagenaria

Asian or Chinese quince is a sour fruit containing citric, malic, tartaric, and abscorbic (Vitamin C) acids. It has a cooling effect on the liver and a relaxing effect on the ligaments and sinews, so it helps to increase flexibility. It affects the liver and spleen meridians.

Look for *quince (Asian)* in *Chinese Water-Decreasing Formula*

Energetics: Mildly relaxing and mildly warming

Used For: Cough, cramps & spasms, and injuries

Properties: Antibacterial, antioxidant, and diuretic

Quince, Bengal

Astringent, Bitter, & Pungent Herb

Aegle marmelos

Native to India, the unripe fruits are used as an astringent for diarrhea. The ripe fruit is demulcent and a mild laxative. It helps protect the body against radiation and chemical exposure.

Used For: Diarrhea, digestion (poor), earache, environmental pollution, indigestion, pneumonia, tachycardia, and ulcers

Properties: Anti-inflammatory, antidiarrheal, antifungal, antimicrobial, antiparasitic, antiviral, aperient, astringent, and mucilant

Ravensara EO

Herbaceous, Spicy, & Woody Essential Oil

Ravensara aromatica

Ravensara EO has a spicy, herbaceous odor with woody undertones that can be used in a similar manner to eucalyptus and cajeput. It is an excellent antiviral and expectorant oil. It is also a nerve tonic and mental stimulant that can be revitalizing to people who feel tired and worn-out.

See the strategy *Aromatherapy* for suggested uses.

Warnings: Do not use internally. Dilute for topical use.

Used For: Anxiety (situational), bronchitis, congestion (sinus), cough, depression, fatigue, **flu**, gas & bloating, herpes, pertussis, rhinitis, sinus infection, stress, and wounds & sores

Properties: Abortifacient, analgesic, antiallergenic, antibacterial, antidepressant, antifungal, antimicrobial, antimicrobial, antiseptic, antiseptic, antispasmodic, antiviral, aphrodisiac, diuretic, expectorant, and immune modulator

Ravintsara EO   *Woody Essential Oil*

Cinnamomum camphora

This oil has also been called ho leaf or camphor. It is anti-inflammatory and used topically for muscle and joint pain. It helps calm anxiety and restores courage and self-confidence. It is also helpful for respiratory congestion and infection when inhaled.

See the strategy *Aromatherapy* for suggested uses.

Warnings: Do not use internally. Don't use around the mouth and nose of children. Dilute well for topical use.

Used For: Acne, anxiety (situational), arthritis, bronchitis, colds, congestion (sinus), cough, fever, and stress

Properties: Analgesic, anti-inflammatory, antiarthritic, antibacterial, antidepressant, antifungal, antirheumatic, antiseptic, antiseptic, expectorant, and stimulant (circulatory)

Red Clover   *Salty Herb*

Trifolium pratense

A pleasant-tasting blood purifier that is used in combination with other blood purifiers for skin conditions, cancer, swollen lymph glands, and liver detoxification. Red clover also contains phytoestrogens that block estrogen receptor sites for the stronger xenoestrogens, possibly inhibiting estrogen-dependent cancers.

Look for *red clover* in *Alterative-Immune, Blood Purifier, Drawing Salve, Dry Cough Syrup, Jeannie Burgess' Thymus, Liquid Lymph,* and *Lymph Cleansing Formulas*

Warnings: Due to its phytoestrogen content, some herbalists recommend avoiding red clover during pregnancy.

Energetics: Cooling and balancing

Used For: **Abscesses**, **acne**, **adenitis**, blood poisoning, boils, breasts (swelling/tenderness), cancer, cancer prevention, chemical exposure, **congestion**, **congestion (lymphatic)**, cough, **cysts**, dermatitis, **eczema**, edema, estrogen (low), fibrosis, gout, leukemia, lymphoma, mastitis, **menopause**, mercury poisoning, mononucleosis, muscle tone, **pertussis**, **PMS Type S**, poison ivy/oak, polyps, **preeclampsia**, **psoriasis**, **skin (infections)**, surgery (recovery), **swollen lymph glands**, and tuberculosis

Properties: Alkalinizer, **alterative**, **anticancer**, antiparasitic, antiseptic, antitussive, deobstruent, detergent, expectorant, lymphatic, mineralizer, phytoestrogen, and tonic

Red Mandarin EO

Fruity & Sweet Essential Oil

Citrus reticulata

The fragrance of mandarin EO is a very sweet citrus aroma. It is a playful fragrance, promoting the inner child and helping to uplift the spirits and promote joy. It is a good oil for children who are restless, distressed, hyperactive, or suffering from upset tummies. It promotes a sweet, loving, and kind disposition. If you want to create a playful, happy mood, this is a good oil to choose.

Mandarin can be used in a massage oil for nervousness and tension and lymphatic stimulation. Massaged over the digestive organs, it helps with the breakdown of fats in the gallbladder and in relieving colic, hiccups and intestinal gas. It can also be applied topically as a skin toner or acne treatment and to prevent stretch marks and scarring.

Emotionally, it relieves depression, having an uplifting and freeing energy. It is calming and cheering, easing stress, grief, and hysteria. It promotes self-awareness and an improved self-image.

See the strategy *Aromatherapy* for suggested uses.

Warnings: Do not use internally. Dilute for topical use. May cause photosensitivity, so avoid sun exposure after topical use. Always mix with a carrier and never apply directly on the skin.

Used For: Acne, adrenal fatigue, asthma, belching, colic (children), cramps (menstrual), depression, digestion (poor), dyspepsia, gas & bloating, hiccups, nausea & vomiting, scars/scar tissue, skin (oily), and stretch marks

Properties: Analgesic, anti-inflammatory, antioxidant, antiseptic, antispasmodic, antitussive, carminative, cholagogue, cicatrizant, digestive tonic, diuretic, sedative, stomachic, and tonic

Red Raspberry   *Mildly Astringent Herb*

Rubus ideaus

Red raspberry leaves are rich in manganese, an essential element for the oxygenation of the cells. It has been used as a tonic to strengthen the uterine muscles for childbirth. It also helps to relieve and prevent morning sickness. They act as a very mild astringent for both topical and internal use, toning and strengthening tissue.

The berries contain anthocyanin, a compound found to contribute to heart health, protect the eyes, guard against cancer, and help protect against diabetes.

Look for *red raspberry* in *Antioxidant, Female Tonic, Herbal Eyewash, Joan Patton's Herbal Minerals, Prebirth, Pregnancy Tea,* and *Women's Aphrodisiac Formulas*

Energetics: Cooling, mildly drying, and mildly constricting

Used For: Acid indigestion, afterbirth pain, bedwetting, **birth defect prevention**, cancer treatment side effects, **diarrhea**, gastritis, **hernias**, interstitial cystitis, **labor & delivery**, menstruation (scant), miscarriage prevention, **morning sickness**, myasthenia gravis, nausea & vomiting, **pregnancy**, prolapsed colon, **prolapsed uterus**, puberty, rosacea, and vaginitis

Properties: Antacid, **antiabortive**, antidiarrheal, antiemetic, astringent, **female tonic**, hemostatic, parturient, tonic, **uterine**, and **uterine tonic**

Red Root (New Jersey Tea)

Astringent & Sweet Herb

Ceanothus americanus

A powerful lymphatic cleanser, red root helps to shrink swollen lymph nodes and reduce an enlarged spleen. It also helps to raise platelet counts. Combined with echinacea, it works well for tonsillitis, cysts, and infections in the lymph glands. It is very good for AIDS patients with low platelet count, enlarged spleen, and swollen lymph nodes.

Look for *red root* in *Lymph Cleansing Formula*

Warnings: Not for use during acute inflammation of the spleen.

Energetics: Drying and constricting

Used For: **Adenitis**, **AIDS**, **congestion (lymphatic)**, cysts, leukemia, **lymphoma**, **mononucleosis**, **mumps**, **sore throat**, **swollen lymph glands**, and **tonsillitis**

Properties: Astringent and **lymphatic**

Red Yeast Rice   *Sweet Herb*

Monoascus purpureus

Red yeast rice helps to lower cholesterol production in the liver, which can help to lower blood cholesterol levels. Read *cholesterol (high)* before using.

Warnings: Red yeast rice blocks the production of cholesterol in the liver, which also blocks the production of Co-Q10. It should always be taken with Co-Q10.

Usage: Take 2 capsules with meals two or three times daily.

Used For: **Cholesterol (high)** and triglycerides (high)

Properties: **Anticholesteremic,** antithrombotic, and **hypolipidemic**

Refreshing and Cleansing EO Blend

This is a very refreshing blend with a very uplifting quality to it. It's also a great natural disinfectant, which can be used for household cleaning. It brightens the mood and helps clear the mind.

See the strategy *Aromatherapy* for suggested uses.

Used For: Confusion and fatigue

Affects: Central nervous system and immune system

Ingredients: Blue spruce leaf, lemon fruit, lime peel, lemongrass leaf, and citronella leaf

Rehmannia   *Mildly Bitter & Sweet Herb*

Rehmannia glutinosa

This Chinese herb is used to cool the blood, reduce fever, and rebuild the blood from blood loss. It is also a liver and kidney tonic.

Look for *rehmannia* in *Chinese Yin-Increasing* and *Vulnerary Formulas*

Warnings: Contraindicated with loss of appetite and diarrhea.

Energetics: Cooling and nourishing

Used For: Aging, broken bones, hepatitis, and menorrhagia

Properties: Antibacterial, blood building, and immune modulator

Reishi   *Sweet & Mildly Bitter Herb*

Ganoderma lucidum

This medicinal mushroom has been shown to have immune-enhancing effects as well as acting as a general health tonic. Research suggests that reishi relaxes muscles, improves sleep, eases chronic pain, aids heart function, reduces cholesterol, and has antioxidant effects.

Look for *reishi* in *Adaptogen, Adaptogen-Immune, Children's Elderberry Cold* and *Flu, Chinese Qi* and *Blood Tonic, Chinese Wood-Increasing, Immune-Boosting,* and *Mushroom Immune Formulas*

Warnings: May be contraindicated with fluid deficiency and dryness.

Energetics: Mildly warming, balancing, and nourishing

Used For: Addison's disease, adrenal fatigue, arteriosclerosis, arthritis, autoimmune disorders, bronchitis, **cancer,** cancer prevention, **cancer treatment side effects,** chemical exposure, cholesterol (high), COPD, **fear, hepatitis,** hypertension, infection (bacterial), infection prevention, insomnia, multiple sclerosis, nervous exhaustion, pernicious anemia, **radiation,** and triglycerides (high)

Properties: Adaptogen, alterative, antiallergenic, antibacterial, anticholesteremic, antiviral, immune modulator, and nutritive

Relaxing and Soothing EO Blend

This is a blend of oils that have anti-inflammatory and relaxing benefits. It may be helpful for calming the mind and it can also be applied topically to areas where there is pain associated with inflammation. It may also be helpful for skin problems.

See the strategy *Aromatherapy* for suggested uses.

Used For: Anxiety attacks, inflammation, skin problems, and stress

Ingredients: Frankincense EO, vanilla bean extract, copaiba resin oil, atlas cedarwood EO, and lavender EO

Renewing and Releasing EO Blend

The citrus notes in this blend are invigorating and uplifting, helping to overcome sluggishness and fatigue. It stimulates the mind while calming the nerves. A good blend for someone who feels exhausted or depleted or for calming people with ADHD (parasympathetic nervous system dominance).

See the strategy *Aromatherapy* for suggested uses.

Used For: ADD/ADHD, concentration (poor), confusion, croup, and fatigue

Affects: Brain and central nervous system

Ingredients: Lemon EO, pink grapefruit EO, cypress EO, and rosemary EO

Resveratrol   *Phytochemical*

Resveratrol is commonly extracted from an Asian plant called *Polygonum cuspidatum* or from red wine or red grape. It is an antioxidant and used to reduce inflammation. It also lowers LDL cholesterol and makes it more difficult for the clots, which lead to heart attacks and strokes, to form. It may protect nerve cells and prevent insulin resistance in diabetes.

Researchers believe that resveratrol activates the SIRT1 gene. That gene is believed to protect the body against the effects of obesity and the diseases of aging.

Warnings: Resveratrol may interact with blood thinners like warfarin (Coumadin) and NSAID medications like aspirin and ibuprofen to thin the blood and increase your chance of bleeding.

Usage: A therapeutic dose would be 500–2,000 milligrams per day.

Used For: Alzheimer's, cancer prevention, cardiovascular disease, diabetes, and Huntington's disease

Properties: Anticoagulant and antioxidant

Rhodiola   *Astringent & Mucilant Herb*

Rhodiola rosea

An adaptogenic tonic, rhodiola aids mental clarity, memory, energy, production, and stress reduction. It helps the body withstand harsh environmental influences such as cold and radiation.

Look for *rhodiola* in *Adaptogen*, *Adaptogen-Immune*, *Antidepressant*, *Ashwagandha Complex*, and *Metabolic Stimulant Formulas*

Energetics: Cooling, drying, and constricting

Used For: Addison's disease, altitude sickness, cancer treatment side effects, erectile dysfunction, exercise (performance), exercise (recovery), fatigue, memory/brain function, radiation, and **stress**

Properties: Adaptogen, antidepressant, astringent, and mucilant

Riboflavin   **see** *vitamin B₂*

Rose   *Sweet & Mildly Sour Herb*

Rosa spp.

Rose hips (fruits) are rich in bioflavonoids and vitamin C and strengthen capillaries. They are mildly astringent and can be helpful for acute illnesses like colds.

Rose petals are an uplifting addition to herbal teas. They reduce stress and help heal heartache.

Look for *rose* in *Paavo Airola's Cold Formula*

Energetics: Cooling, drying, and mildly constricting

Used For: Addictions, age spots, aneurysm, anger (excessive), **apathy**, arteriosclerosis, **capillary weakness**, **easily bruised**, fever, inflammation, nervous exhaustion, **nosebleeds**, scurvy, and spider veins

Properties: Anti-inflammatory, antibacterial, antidepressant, antiscorbutic, astringent, food, nutritive, refrigerant, tonic, and vascular tonic

Rose EO   *Spicy & Sweet Essential Oil*

Rosa laevigata

The wonderful floral aroma of the rose is sweet with a warm, slightly spicy quality. Rose EO has a great affinity for the heart. It opens the heart and helps a person release the feeling of sadness, grief, anger, or fear. It promotes calm, peaceful, and loving feelings in their place. Rose oil is very helpful for anyone who is experiencing anxiety or depression due to emotional wounds, loss or heartache. It helps a person who has been isolating themselves rediscover friendship and love. It also promotes empathy and compassion for others. Rose is also an aphrodisiac, promoting warm, loving intimacy.

Rose essential oil helps to regulate hormones and menstruation, overcome infertility, stop uterine bleeding, strengthen the uterus, and relieve menstrual cramps. Historically, it is used for cooling hot conditions. Possessing rehydrating and emollient properties, it is applied topically for inflamed or dehydrated skin. Rose has been confirmed with clinical studies to help with herpes zoster and herpes simplex when applied neat (undiluted) to the afflicted area. Emotionally, rose brings joy to the heart. Offering comfort to help heal emotional wounds, rose opens the cold heart, rebuilds trust, and restores one's capacity for self-love and self-nurturing. It is often used with abused children to help with the deep despair and feeling of unworthiness and violation.

See the strategy *Aromatherapy* for suggested uses.

Warnings: Do not use internally without the supervision of a professionally trained aromatherapy practitioner. Nontoxic and nonirritating for topical use.

Used For: Afterbirth pain, age spots, alcoholism, amenorrhea, anger (excessive), anxiety (situational), apathy, arrhythmia, asthma, bleeding (external), boils, bronchitis, bruises, burns & scalds, cardiovascular disease, circulation (poor), depression, **dermatitis**, digestion (poor), eczema, erectile dysfunction, fever, gingivitis, **grief & sadness**, headache, herpes, hot flashes, hypertension, indigestion, insomnia, **irritability**, menopause, menstruation (scant), nervous exhaustion, nervousness, **PMS Type D**, **rashes & hives**, scars/scar tissue, **sex drive (low)**, shame & guilt, **skin (oily)**, skin problems, sprains, thrush, tuberculosis, ulcers, wounds & sores, and wrinkles

Properties: Antidepressant, antiphlogistic, antiseptic, antispasmodic, antiviral, aphrodisiac, astringent, bactericidal, cicatrizant, emmenagogue, food, hemostatic, hepatic, laxative (bulk), moistening, nervine, perfume, sedative, soothing, stomachic, and tonic

Rosemary
Aromatic Herb

Rosmarinus officinalis

This herb is considered a tonic for elderly people and may help improve circulation to the brain. In Germany, rosemary is approved by the Commission E for use in treating indigestion, joint ailments, and stomach problems. Rosemary also has antioxidant properties that protect the brain and blood vessels.

Look for *rosemary* in *Watkin's Hair, Skin,* and *Nails Formula*

Warnings: Avoid during pregnancy.

Energetics: Warming, drying, and mildly constricting

Used For: Alzheimer's, apathy, **bipolar mood disorder, circulation (brain), cloudy thinking**, colds, **concentration (poor), confusion**, congestion, cough, cough (damp), cough (spastic), croup, dandruff, **dementia**, digestion (poor), fever, free radical damage, gas & bloating, **hair loss/thinning**, hysteria, indigestion, infection (bacterial), **memory/brain function, multiple sclerosis**, nervous exhaustion, pertussis, pertussis, **skin (oily), skin problems**, and traumatic brain injury

Properties: Antidepressant, antilipemic, **antioxidant**, antirheumatic, antiseptic, carminative, **cerebral tonic**, expectorant, **stimulant (metabolic)**, and sympathomimetic

Rosemary EO
Balsamic, Fresh, & Woody Essential Oil

Rosmarinus officinalis

Rosemary EO has a fresh, herbaceous odor with woody, balsamic undertones. It is a central nervous system stimulant, aiding memory and concentration; hence the saying, "Rosemary for remembrance." It helps keep the mind alert, aware, and active, aiding blood flow to the brain. This makes it particularly helpful for preventing memory loss and easing depression in the elderly. It's a good oil for anyone who wants to sharpen their mind and memory.

When inhaled, rosemary is a valuable essential oil for respiratory problems. Applied topically, it stimulates blood flow and eases pain. It can be helpful for tired, sore, or weak legs. Rosemary has traditionally been used in shampoos and hair treatments to stimulate blood circulation to the scalp to help promote hair growth.

Emotionally it renews enthusiasm and bolsters self-confidence. In the nervous system, it promotes mental clarity and awareness, stimulates the brain, and helps improve memory. For those who lack faith in their own potential and tend to doubt their every action, rosemary can help boost their confidence and help develop a sense of self-worth. It helps one find his or her purpose in life. It is thought to enhance the spiritual dedication of love, as in helping one be faithful to their partner.

See the strategy *Aromatherapy* for suggested uses.

Warnings: Do not use internally without the supervision of a professionally trained aromatherapy practitioner. Nontoxic and nonirritating for topical use. Not recommended for people with epilepsy or high blood pressure. Avoid during pregnancy or breast-feeding.

Used For: Alcoholism, apathy, arthritis, bronchitis, cancer, cardiovascular disease, cellulite, cholera, circulation (brain), circulation (poor), colds (decongestant), concentration (poor), confusion, congestion, cough, cough (spastic), croup, **dandruff**, dementia, **depression**, fatigue, fever, **fleas**, flu, gas & bloating, hair loss/thinning, headache (cluster), hepatitis, hypochondria, hypotension, hysteria, indigestion, **infection prevention, insect repellant**, lice, menstrual irregularity, pertussis, sinus infection, skin (infections), tachycardia, vaginitis, and varicose veins

Properties: Analgesic, antidepressant, antimicrobial, antiseptic, astringent, carminative, cephalic, cholagogue, cholinergic, decongestant, digestive tonic, diuretic, emmenagogue, hepatic, hypertensive, nervine, parasympathomimetic, pectoral, preservative, rubefacient, sympathomimetic, and tonic

Safflower
Mildly Aromatic Herb

Carthamus tinctorius

Safflowers aid digestion and neutralize waste acids in the body, particularly lactic acid. A tea of safflowers is a very dependable remedy for relieving muscle soreness from overexertion. It also reduces swelling in breasts, brings on delayed menses, helps move stagnant blood (as in bruises and blood clots), and heals injuries.

Look for *safflower* in *Hypoglycemic* and *Skinny Formulas*

Warnings: Do not use with excessive menstrual bleeding.

Energetics: Cooling

Used For: Acid indigestion, arthritis, body building, chicken pox, colic (children), cysts, digestion (poor), **exercise (recovery)**, gas & bloating, gout, hypoglycemia, indigestion, jaundice (adults), **jaundice (infants)**, pain, **tendonitis**, and **uric acid retention**

Properties: Alterative, **antacid**, anti-inflammatory, antiobesic, carminative, stimulant (appetite), stomachic, and vulnerary

Sage
Aromatic & Mildly Astringent Herb

Salvia officinalis

Sage can be helpful for colds and fever, especially involving intermittent chills and fever, hoarseness, or sweating at night. It is best taken as a cool tea for night sweats and as a hot tea for inducing perspiration. You can also use the tea for sore or horse throat and laryngitis and as a mouthwash or gargle for irritation of the throat or mouth. Sage's antiseptic properties make it helpful in treating wounds to prevent infection and inflammation. It acts as a nerve tonic, increasing your capacity to handle stress.

Look for *sage* in *Watkin's Hair, Skin,* and *Nails Formula*

Warnings: Avoid during pregnancy. Do not use while nursing; sage will dry up breast milk.

Energetics: Warming, drying, and mildly constricting

Used For: Anorexia, body odor, **breast milk (surplus)**, colds with fever, dementia, hair (graying), hair loss/thinning, headache, indigestion, **laryngitis**, memory/brain function, narcolepsy, nervous exhaustion, **night sweating**, parasites (nematodes, worms), **perspiration (excessive)**, sore throat, and wounds & sores

Properties: Antacid, antibacterial, antidiarrheal, **antigalactagogue**, antioxidant, antiseptic, **antisudorific**, astringent, carminative, cephalic, cholinergic, condiment, diaphoretic, emmenagogue, febrifuge, fumigant, insecticide, nervine, stimulant (metabolic), stomachic, **sympathomimetic**, vermifuge, and vulnerary

Saint John's Wort
Mildly Oily & Mildly Sweet Herb

Hypericum perforatum

St. John's wort became a popular herb when research suggested it could be helpful for mild to moderate depression. It is helpful for some cases of depression, especially those accompanied by anxiety, but the herb has many other valuable properties. It is a nervine herb that helps to regulate the solar plexus, the nerves which regulate digestion. It can be helpful for insomnia, fear, nerve pain, and nerve damage. It stimulates nerve regeneration and repair, especially when used homeopathically or applied topically in oil form to injured areas.

It has antiviral properties and has been used for viral infections such as shingles, herpes, mononucleosis, and flu. It also helps to heal wounds.

Look for *Saint John's wort* in *Antidepressant, Attention-Focus, Ear Drop, Healing Salve,* and *Topical Injury Formulas*

Warnings: The fresh plant is photo-toxic. It contains a chemical that changes to a toxin in the body after exposure to sunlight. This does not appear to be a problem when taking St. John's wort internally. Avoid when taking SSRI antidepressants.

Energetics: Cooling and mildly relaxing

Used For: Abrasions/scratches, addictions, addictions (drugs), **addictions (tobacco)**, AIDS, **alcoholism**, anorexia, autism, bedwetting, **Bell's palsy**, bunions, burning feet/hands, bursitis, **chicken pox**, cold sores, deafness, **depression**,

dermatitis, earache, fear, **frozen shoulder**, gastritis, hangover, headache (sinus), **hearing loss**, **herpes**, incontinence, **infection (viral)**, inflammation, inflammatory bowel disorders, insomnia, irritability, jaundice (adults), leaky gut, meningitis, menopause, mood swings, myasthenia gravis, narcolepsy, **nerve damage**, **neuralgia & neuritis**, **numbness**, pain, **paralysis**, peripheral neuropathy, PMS Type D, restless leg, **sciatica**, seasonal affective disorder, **shingles**, sprains, stress, **tinnitus**, **traumatic brain injury**, tuberculosis, ulcerations (external), and wounds & sores

Properties: **Antidepressant**, antiseptic, antismoking, antiviral, digestive tonic, expectorant, febrifuge, hypotensive, nervine, relaxant, sedative, serotonergic, styptic, tonic, vermifuge, and vulnerary

Salvia (Red Sage)   *Bitter Herb*
Salvia miltiorrhiza

The root of this Chinese species of sage is used to aid the circulation of blood, remove heat or irritation from the blood, and improve blood composition. It is used as a tonic for women for menstrual pain, lack of periods, or heavy periods. It is also a mild sedative.

Energetics: Cooling and mildly drying

Used For: Amenorrhea, angina, circulation (poor), dysmenorrhea, heart fibrillation/palpitations, insomnia, and irritability

Properties: Anti-inflammatory, antibacterial, calmative, hypotensive, and stimulant (circulatory)

SAM-e   *Nutrient*
S-adenosylmethionine (abbreviated as SAM-e or SAMe) is a natural substance the body makes to facilitate certain chemical reactions. It is synthesized from the amino acid methionine using adenosine triphosphate (ATP). First discovered in Europe and available there by prescription since 1975, SAM-e has a number of potential therapeutic benefits, primarily based on its ability to act as a methyl donor for people who are undermethylating.

It may be helpful for mood problems, some cases of mental illness, Gilbert's syndrome, and some types of pain. It helps the body produce more mood-enhancing neurotransmitters such as dopamine and serotonin. It works in conjunction with folic acid, B_{12}, and B_6 to produce these neurotransmitters, so it would be wise to use a B complex supplement when taking SAM-e. It can also aid energy production.

The dose required to manage depression is quite high. European studies typically use 1,200 mg daily. SAM-e can move a person from depression to mania and is therefore contraindicated with bipolar disorder.

SAM-e helps to increase the production of glutathione, a major antioxidant, which helps protect the liver (and other tissues) from free radical damage. It also helps in liver detoxification through a process called glutathione conjugation.

SAM-e shows particular promise in the treatment of osteoarthritis. In large, well-controlled studies, it has been shown to be as effective as nonsteroidal anti-inflammatories in relieving pain without the side effects. It may also prevent damage to cartilage and may help rebuild cartilage when taken for long periods (more than three months).

Several studies have been conducted using SAM-e with fibromyalgia. Patients taking SAM-e reported improvements in pain, fatigue, morning stiffness, and mood.

Warnings: Side effects are rare but may include heartburn, dry mouth, restlessness, diarrhea, headaches, and mania. SAM-e is contraindicated in bipolar disorders and is not recommended for use by children. Be cautious when using SAM-e with antidepressant medications or other drugs as negative interactions have been reported. SAM-e should be considered a medicinal supplement and is not recommended for healthy people, only for assisting people with specific health problems. If you are taking prescription antidepressants, consult your physician before or during the use of this product. Pregnant or lactating women should consult their healthcare provider prior to taking it. SAMe will make conditions caused by over-methylation worse. If SAM-e makes the problem worse, try a Methylated B9 and B12 Formula.

Usage: The longer SAM-e is taken, the better the effects. To prevent nausea start with 200 mg twice daily for the first day, increased to 400 mg twice daily on day three, then increase to 400 mg three times daily on day ten. Maintain this dose for depression. For all other conditions, after three weeks at 1,200 mg daily, reduce to 200 mg twice daily

Used For: Addison's disease, **alcoholism**, apathy, blood poisoning, chemical exposure, cholesterol (low), **cirrhosis of the liver**, **depression**, dysmenorrhea, fibromyalgia, gallbladder problems, headache (migraine), **hepatitis**, hypothyroidism, irritability, **jaundice (adults)**, mental illness, **methylation (under)**, mood swings, PMS Type D, and **seasonal affective disorder**

Properties: Dopamine-enhancing, hepatic, and lipotropic

Sandalwood EO
Balsamic & Woody Essential Oil

Santalum album

A soft, woody, but sweet fragrance, sandalwood EO has a lingering balsamic quality. It is relaxing to the nerves and calming to agitated emotions. Sandalwood's dominant action is on the mucous membranes. It eases dry cough and is especially effective in deep, painful coughs. It also helps with vaginal discharge. It is also very effective as a gargle for sore throats. Topically, sandalwood helps dry, irritated skin. It also helps dehydrated and oily skin.

Emotionally, sandalwood has a calming, harmonizing effect helping to reduce tension and confusion. A cooling oil, it is helpful for hot-headed people who tend to be angry, aggressive, and irritable. It promotes a serene, aware state of mind by calming down mental chatter, helping a person to have control of their emotions and their direction in life. It is considered one of the best oils for aiding prayer and meditation and developing a spiritual nature that is also grounded and practical. For those who feel a neurotic need for security and manipulation of outcomes, it helps to reestablish acceptance of reality. It is considered an aphrodisiac because it promotes openness, warmth, and understanding between partners.

See the strategy *Aromatherapy* for suggested uses.

Warnings: Do not use internally. Nontoxic and nonirritating for topical use.

Used For: Acne, aging, anxiety disorders, bronchitis, cancer, colic (adults), COPD, **cough (dry)**, **cough (spastic)**, diarrhea, **eczema**, erectile dysfunction, **fear**, gastritis, interstitial cystitis, nightmares, psoriasis, sex drive (excessive), **sex drive (low)**, skin problems, sore throat, and stress

Properties: Anti-inflammatory, antiphlogistic, antiseptic, antispasmodic, antiviral, aphrodisiac, astringent, carminative, diuretic, emollient, expectorant, expectorant, moistening, mucilant, nervine, perfume, sedative, and tonic

Saw Palmetto
Sweet, Oily, & Mildly Acrid Herb

Serenoa repens

Widely used for prostate enlargement and urinary problems in men, saw palmetto is a general tonic for elderly men and may be helpful with other problems associated with aging. It aids digestion and weight gain in wasting conditions and has a slight effect in stimulating breast tissue in women.

Look for *saw palmetto* in *Prostate Formula*

Warnings: Avoid during pregnancy. Avoid while nursing as this herb inhibits prolactin and may interfere with lactation.

Energetics: Moistening and nourishing

Used For: Anorexia, BPH, breasts (undersized), cysts, digestion (poor), Hashimoto's disease, hypothyroidism, muscular dystrophy, prostatitis, **underweight**, and wasting

Properties: Antigalactagogue, digestive tonic, expectorant, glandular, and **spleen chi tonic**

Schisandra
Astringent, Pungent, Sour, & Sweet Herb

Schisandra chinensis

Used as an adaptogen and general tonic, schizandra improves circulation, strengthens the heart, aids digestion, and increases bile secretion. In Chinese herbalism, it is thought to harmonize the body and help one retain energy. It helps to keep the nervous system balanced, increasing both excitatory and inhibitory action. It has hepatoprotective effects like milk thistle.

Look for *schisandra* in *Adaptogen, Adaptogen-Immune, Adrenal Glandular, Anti-Stress B-Complex, Ashwagandha Complex, Chinese Fire-Increasing, Colloidal Mineral,* and *Hypothyroid Formulas*

Warnings: Contraindicated with acute ailments like colds, flu and fevers.

Energetics: Cooling and moistening

Used For: **ADD/ADHD**, **addictions (coffee, caffeine)**, addictions (drugs), cancer treatment side effects, chemical exposure, cirrhosis of the liver, cough (dry), environmental pollution, exercise (performance), fear, hepatitis, mental illness, narcolepsy, nervous exhaustion, nervousness, **night sweating**, OCD, Parkinson's disease, **perspiration (excessive)**, **premature ejaculation**, PTSD, surgery (preparation), and **urination (frequent)**

Properties: **Adaptogen**, antisudorific, antitussive, **hepatic**, hepatoprotective, immune modulator, lung tonic, and moistening

Seasonal Cold and Flu Formula

See also *Elderberry Cold* and *Flu Formula* and *Paavo Airola's Cold Formula*

This formula helps decongest the sinuses, reduce sinus inflammation, combat allergic responses, and fight respiratory infections. It has a mild antihistamine effect.

Used For: Allergies (respiratory), colds, colds (decongestant), congestion (sinus), flu, rhinitis, and snoring

Affects: Immune system, lungs, respiratory irritation, and respiratory stagnation

Take 1 capsule with a meal three times daily.

Ingredients: Andrographis whole plant, thyme leaf, orange (bitter) fruit, eleuthero root, and oregano leaf

Selenium
Mineral

Selenium is an essential trace mineral that is toxic in large doses. Nevertheless, it is essential to good health because it functions as a cofactor in the reduction of antioxidant enzymes such as glutathione peroxidase. Research suggests that adequate levels help to protect the body against cancer. People with autoimmune thyroid conditions may be deficient. It also works well with vitamin E to mitigate the development of rheumatoid arthritis, elevated blood pressure, impaired thyroid function, loss of hair color, whitened fingernail beds, weakened immune system, increased risk of joint inflammation, and increased risk of atherosclerosis.

Usage: 5–55 mcg per day.

Used For: Aging, **AIDS**, allergies (respiratory), arsenic poisoning, arthritis, **cancer prevention**, cardiovascular disease, dandruff, exercise (performance), **Graves' disease**, hair (graying), **Hashimoto's disease**, hypertension, and **hypothyroidism**

Properties: Antioxidant, immune modulator, and nutritive

Self-Responsibility FE Blend

When people deny healthy fears, they can engage in self-destructive habits and form unhealthy addictions and compulsions. This is a flower essence blend I formulated to help people who are reckless and careless to be more careful and thoughtful about their actions. It is particularly helpful for making people aware of the fears and inner emotional issues that are driving their addictions, compulsions, and self-defeating behaviors. This enables them to recognize and heal these issues so they can break free from this cycle of self-destructive behavior.

This blend promotes inner integrity, self-awareness, and self-responsibility. It can help people who are trying to lose weight to avoid binges, aid people who are trying to quit smoking or break free from addictions to drugs and alcohol, and help people who have obsessive or compulsive behaviors to identify what drives this behavior so they can change.

See the strategy *Flower Essence* for suggested uses.

Used For: Addictions, addictions (coffee, caffeine), **addictions (drugs)**, addictions (sugar/carbohydrates), addictions (tobacco), alcoholism, anorexia, anxiety disorders, **OCD**, PTSD, sex drive (excessive), and trauma

Affects: Dopamine

Ingredients: Black cohosh FE, black-eyed susan FE, milkweed FE, california poppy FE, agrimony FE, joshua tree FE, and mullein FE

Senna   *Bitter Herb*

Senna alexandrina

A strong stimulant laxative; best used as part of a formula.

Look for *senna* in *Stimulant Laxative Formula*

Warnings: Can be gripping and habit-forming but is generally considered safe.

Energetics: Drying and cooling

Used For: Colon (atonic) and constipation (adults)

Properties: Laxative

Shepherd's Purse

Mildly Astringent & Pungent Herb

Capsella bursa-pastoris

One of the best herbs to use for hemorrhaging and heavy bleeding during menstruation. It is an important herb in midwifery because it helps deliver the placenta during childbirth and cuts down on postpartum bleeding. It is one of the few remedies that will increase blood pressure because it helps to constrict blood vessels. It can also be used to soothe the bladder and treat blood in the urine.

Look for *shepherd's purse* in *Internal Bleeding Formula*

Warnings: Not for use during pregnancy.

Energetics: Warming, drying, and constricting

Used For: Hypotension, interstitial cystitis, labor & delivery, menorrhagia, and nosebleeds

Properties: Astringent, **hypertensive**, styptic, and vasoconstrictor

Shitake   *Sweet Herb*

Lentinula edodes

This mushroom is finding increasing use as a medicinal treatment for cancer and other health problems. It can be helpful in lowering cholesterol and fighting various types of cancer. It stimulates the immune system to increase the body's ability to fight infections.

Look for *shitake* in *Colostrum-Immune Stimulator* and *Mushroom Immune Formulas*

Energetics: Balancing and nourishing

Used For: AIDS, cancer, cancer prevention, cancer treatment side effects, hepatitis, herpes, infection (viral), infection prevention, and triglycerides (high)

Properties: Adaptogen, alterative, antiallergenic, and restorative

Shock and Injury FE Blend

The only flower essence blend created by the originator of flower essences, Dr. Edward Bach, this blend has been successfully used to ease shock, both physically and emotionally. It is a general remedy for restoring presence and awareness during any kind of physical or emotional trauma. It helps a person stay calm in a crisis situation and helps people with healing and recovery. It can be used both internally and topically when a person has been physically injured to relieve shock and promote more rapid healing of tissues.

See the strategy *Flower Essence* for suggested uses.

Used For: Abrasions/scratches, **anxiety (situational), anxiety attacks**, bulimia, burns & scalds, **fainting**, fear, **injuries, jet lag, mental illness, nervous exhaustion, OCD, phobias, PTSD**, seizures, shame & guilt, **shock (medical)**, sprains, and **trauma**

Affects: Adrenal irritation, **adrenal medulla**, skin, and structural irritation

Steven Horne's Distress Flower Remedy

My modified version that adds two additional flower remedies. Works better on relieving unresolved trauma from the past.

Ingredients: Arnica FE, star of bethlehem FE, rock rose FE, impatiens FE, clematis FE, cherry plum FE, and red clover FE

Rescue Remedy

The original Bach formula. Helpful for any kind of acute shock or trauma.

Ingredients: Impatiens FE, rock rose FE, star of bethlehem FE, cherry plum FE, and clematis FE

Siler   *Acrid, Pungent, & Sweet Herb*

Saposhnikovia divaricata

Primarily used as an antispasmodic in Chinese herbalism to dispel "wind" conditions such as stiff neck, tension headache, tremors and convulsions.

Look for *siler* in *Chinese Water-Decreasing Formula*

Warnings: Do not use with blood deficiency (anemia) or if you are suffering from Parkinson's disease.

Energetics: Mildly warming and relaxing

Used For: Colds, cramps & spasms, epilepsy, headache, headache (migraine), stiff neck, and tremors

Properties: Analgesic, anti-inflammatory, antispasmodic, diaphoretic, and febrifuge

Silicon   *Mineral*

Silicon, the fourteenth element of the periodic table and the second most element on the planet, is surprisingly important for both computing and human health. It is important for healthy hair, skin, nails, joints, bones, and nerves. And while there is no US RDA for silicon, it's quite likely that many people aren't getting enough of this element. Some of the health issues that may involve silicon deficiency include brittle fingernails, getting split ends, dull lusterless skin, and brittle bones. Silicon deficiency may also be a factor in joint deterioration in osteoporosis and in the breakdown of nervous system tissue (especially the myelin sheath) in multiple sclerosis and neurodegenerative disorders.

Silicon is often found in the form of silicon dioxide (SiO_2), which also known as silica or quartz. Sand is primarily composed of silica. Plants rich in silica can help detoxify aluminum from the body. They may also aid the pineal gland.

Usage: Grains, legumes, fruits and vegetables with peelings and seeds, and raisins are good dietary sources of silicon. The average intake of silicon in adults is 14–21 mg per day. Horsetail and dulse are two herbs rich in silicon. Watkin's Hair, Skin, and Nails Formula is a good silicon source.

Used For: Aluminum toxicity, arthritis, broken bones, calcium deficiency, **fingernails (weak/brittle)**, **hair loss/ thinning**, nerve damage, **osteoporosis**, pancreatitis, and **skin problems**

Properties: Nutritive, tonic, and vulnerary

Sinus Formula

See also *Anti-Snoring Formula* and *Christopher's Sinus Formula*

This formula is particularly effective for sinus headaches, although it can be used as a general decongestant and expectorant for sinus problems.

Used For: Allergies (respiratory), colds (decongestant), congestion, **congestion (sinus)**, **headache (sinus)**, **sinus infection**, smell (loss of), and **snoring**

Affects: Mucous membranes, **respiratory stagnation**, **sinuses**, and smell

Take 2 capsules three times a day or 6 capsules every two to three hours for sinus congestion and sinus headaches.

Ingredients: Fenugreek seed and thyme leaf

Skeletal Support Formula

This formula combines calcium with other vitamins and minerals needed for healthy bones. It can be used to help prevent osteoporosis or as an aid to healing broken bones.

For women concerned about maintaining bone health after menopause, it works better than plain calcium supplements.

Used For: Arthritis, backache, **broken bones**, cramps (leg), **dental health**, menopause, **osteoporosis**, overacidity, scoliosis, **teeth (grinding)**, and twitching

Affects: Bones, parathyroid, **structural atrophy**, and structural relaxation

Use 1-2 tablets two times per day.

Ingredients: Vitamin C, vitamin d3, calcium, magnesium, zinc, copper, manganese, boron, horsetail stem & strobilus, and betaine hydrochloric acid (hcl)

Skinny Formula

This formula acts as a diuretic and mild laxative to aid the process of weight loss. It also contains herbs that aid digestive and glandular function. It can be taken with extra chickweed for better fat-burning results and as an aid to fatty liver disease or fat deposits.

Used For: Acne, appetite (excessive), arteriosclerosis, **cellulite**, cholesterol (high), excess weight, **fat metabolism (poor)**, **fatty liver disease**, **fatty tumors/deposits**, seborrhea, and triglycerides (low)

Affects: Liver

Take 2 capsules 1/2 hour prior to meals each day. Begin with smaller doses and work up. Add 1-2 chickweed per dose for fatty deposits or fatty liver disease.

Ingredients: Cascara sagrada bark, hawthorn berry, papaya fruit, licorice root, safflower flower, chickweed leaf, and dandelion root

Skullcap   *Bitter Herb*

Scutellaria lateriflora

A relaxing nervine, skullcap helps to calm brain function helpful for insomnia and chronic stress. It is also a good remedy for vasoconstrictive (or tension) headaches and migraines. It was used by 19th century herbalists for hysteria, epilepsy, convulsions, and schizophrenia. The person who needs skullcap often has an inability to pay attention or a dull headache in the front or base of the skull. Symptoms are worse with noise, odors, and light but improve with rest. Skullcap also seems to work well when people feel as if every sound, touch, and ray of light is personally attacking them. They are oversensitive to any stimulation, being twitchy even during sleep.

Look for *skullcap* in *Antispasmodic* and *Herbal Sleep Aid Formulas*

Energetics: Cooling and relaxing

Used For: **Addictions (tobacco)**, **adrenal fatigue**, anxiety disorders, arrhythmia, backache, **bipolar mood disorder**, cold hands/feet, concentration (poor), **cramps & spasms**, emotional sensitivity, **epilepsy**, **headache (cluster)**, **headache (tension)**, **hysteria**, **insomnia**, **mental illness**, **mood swings**, **myasthenia gravis**, nerve damage, **nervous exhaustion**, Parkinson's disease, peripheral neuropathy, **PTSD**, **restless leg**, **schizophrenia**, **seizures**, **stress**, **trauma**, and **tremors**

Properties: Analgesic, anticephalalgic, antispasmodic, **nervine**, **sedative**, and **soporific**

Skunk Cabbage   *Acrid Herb*

Symplocarpus foetidus

Skunk cabbage is a powerful antispasmodic, making it useful for cramps and muscle spasms of all kinds. It is a specific remedy for severe bronchial asthmatic spasms associated with emotional distress and coughing to the point of vomiting. It may also be helpful for fluid retention, headache, irritability, nervousness, tightness in the chest, and whooping cough.

Look for *skunk cabbage* in *Antispasmodic Formula*

Warnings: The fresh root can be irritating to mucous membranes. It should be used cautiously by people with a history of kidney stones.

Energetics: Mildly warming and relaxing

Used For: Asthma, bronchitis, cough (spastic), cramps & spasms, headache (tension), irritability, nervousness, pertussis, and **whiplash**

Properties: **Antispasmodic**, emetic, and expectorant

Sleep Support Formula

See also *Herbal Sleep Aid Formula*

These are formulas that combine relaxing herbs with various sleep supporting compounds like melatonin, l-threanine, CBD and GABA. They are generally more powerful than *Herbal Sleep Aid Formulas*.

Used For: **Insomnia**, **jet lag**, nervous exhaustion, nervousness, and nocturnal emission

Power Sleep Formula

A useful formula for helping a person fall asleep. Use 2 capsules prior to bedtime.

Ingredients: Valerian standardized extract, ashwagandha standardized extract, hops standardized extract, passion flower standardized extract, GABA, L-theanine, melatonin, and magnesium

Power Sleep Formula with CBD

A great sleep formula that includes CBD. Use 2 capsules prior to bedtime.

Ingredients: Hemp extract, ashwagandha standardized extract, GABA, L-theanine, melatonin, and magnesium

Power Sleep Formula with 5-HTP

A great sleep formula with 5-HTP and adaptagens for lack of sleep due to stress. Use 2 capsules prior to bedtime.

Ingredients: Lemon balm extract, magnesium, L-theanine, 5-HTP, melatonin, passion flower extract, rhodiola standardized extract, and ashwagandha root

Slippery Elm   *Mucilant & Mildly Sweet Herb*

Ulmus rubra

A soothing and nourishing mucilaginous herb that helps absorb acid and irritants in the stomach, slippery elm is used internally for irritation of the stomach and intestines and diarrhea (especially in children). It is also a mild, nourishing food for weak and debilitated persons.

Look for *slippery elm* in *Essiac Immune Tea*, *Intestinal Soothing*, *Irritable Bowel Fiber*, *Natural Antacid*, and *Vulnerary Formulas*

Warnings: Not recommended for external ulcers or purulent sores.

Usage: Works best in bulk form. Mix 1–2 teaspoons bulk powder with a cup of hot water or juice (mixes best using a blender). Sweeten to taste and drink (may be slightly thick depending on how much powder is used). Slippery elm can also be mixed with applesauce, cereal, or yogurt to feed to children. You can also take 2-4 capsules with plenty of water. Externally, slippery elm makes an excellent base for a poultice.

Energetics: Cooling, moistening, and nourishing

Used For: Acid indigestion, **cancer treatment side effects**, celiac disease, cholera, colitis, constipation (children), **convalescence**, cough (dry), debility, **diaper rash**, **diarrhea**, **diverticulitis**, **enteritis**, failure to thrive, food poisoning, gastritis, hemorrhoids, hiatal hernia, ileocecal valve, indigestion, **inflammatory bowel disorders**, interstitial cystitis, leprosy, mastitis, **sore throat**, **tickle in throat**, tonsillitis, ulcerations (external), **ulcers**, **wasting**, and wounds & sores

Properties: **Absorbent**, **antidiarrheal**, balsamic, drawing, emollient, expectorant, food, laxative (bulk), **mucilant**, nutritive, soothing, and **vulnerary**

Sodium Alginate   *Phytochemical*

Sodium alginate is the sodium salt of alginic acid, also referred to as algin. Sodium alginate is an anionic polysaccharide distributed widely in the cell walls of brown algae, where it, through binding water, forms a viscous gum. In extracted form it absorbs water quickly, capable of absorbing two hundred to three hundred times its own weight in water, which makes it useful as a thickening agent in foods.

As a dietary supplement, algin is used to lower serum cholesterol levels and to reduce the absorption of strontium, barium, tin, cadmium, manganese, zinc, and mercury. It may also help to lower cholesterol and slow the absorption of fats in the digestive tract.

Usage: 1–2 capsules two or three times daily.

Used For: Acid indigestion, cadmium toxicity, cholesterol (high), excess weight, **heavy metal poisoning**, lead poisoning, **mercury poisoning**, and **radiation**

Sodium Bicarbonate   *Nutrient*

Also known as baking soda, sodium bicarbonate can use used to settle an acid stomach and help to alkalize an over acidic system. It can be applied topically for insect bites and stings and is also helpful in baths for itching skin. People who have problems taking vitamin C because of its acidic nature can mix a little sodium bicarbonate with powdered vitamin C to buffer the acid.

Used For: **Acid indigestion**, **bites & stings**, itching, and **overacidity**

Properties: **Alkalinizer**, **antacid**, and soothing

Solomon's Seal   *Mildly Acrid & Sweet Herb*

Polygonatum multiflorum

A remedy for the musculoskeletal system. It helps tone up loose ligaments and tendons. It helps to heal broken bones and strengthen other bones. It is a kidney tonic and builds reproductive organs.

Energetics: Cooling, balancing, and moistening

Used For: **Arthritis**, **arthritis (rheumatoid)**, autoimmune disorders, **bunions**, **bursitis**, **carpal tunnel**, **cartilage damage**, **dislocation**, inflammation, **ligaments (torn/injuried)**, prolapsed colon, **spinal disks**, **sprains**, and **tendonitis**

Properties: Emollient and mucilant

Spearmint EO

Herbaceous & Minty Essential Oil

Mentha spicata

Spearmint EO has the same fresh, minty aroma as peppermint but is milder and sweeter. It's a great oil for children. Like peppermint it can be used to settle the stomach and increase mental alertness.

See the strategy *Aromatherapy* for suggested uses.

Warnings: Like peppermint, spearmint is very safe for internal use but should be diluted and taken in drop doses for only short periods. Don't use internally with young children. Nontoxic and nonirritating for topical use.

Used For: Anxiety (situational), belching, cloudy thinking, **colic (children)**, digestion (poor), fever, flu, **gas & bloating**, halitosis, headache, **indigestion**, motion sickness, nausea & vomiting, and stress

Properties: Analgesic, anesthetic, anti-inflammatory, antibacterial, antidepressant, antifungal, antiseptic, antispasmodic, carminative, decongestant, diuretic, emmenagogue, expectorant, insecticide, nervine, and restorative

Spilanthes   *Acrid & Pungent Herb*

Spilanthes acmella

An antibacterial and antifungal herb, spilanthes stimulates mucous membrane secretions and the immune system to fight respiratory infections. It acts as a local anesthetic to ease pain while reducing inflammation. One of its common names is toothache plant because it has been applied to the gums around an infected tooth to ease pain and help fight the infection.

Look for *spilanthes* in *Anti-Fungal Formula*

Energetics: Warming and constricting

Used For: Earache, flu, **gingivitis**, herpes, infection (bacterial), infection (fungal), interstitial cystitis, **toothache**, and urethritis

Properties: Analgesic, antibacterial, antifungal, and astringent

Spirulina   *Sweet Herb*

Spirulina sp.

Spirulina is an algae that is rich in essential amino acids, the building blocks of protein. It is considered a superfood and helps to stabilize energy and blood sugar levels. It has been used as an appetite suppressant to control food cravings. Its high amino acid content has also given it a reputation as a brain food, since amino acids are the building blocks of neurotransmitters.

Look for *spirulina* in *Algae, Brain Calming,* and *Whole Food Green Drink Formulas*

Energetics: Neutral and nourishing

Used For: ADD/ADHD, **addictions (sugar/carbohydrates)**, alcoholism, aluminum toxicity, **appetite (excessive)**, cartilage damage, convalescence, cystic fibrosis, **debility**, electromagnetic pollution, **fatigue**, glaucoma, hepatitis, **hypoglycemia**, jet lag, **mania**, mood swings, **radiation**, reversed polarity, triglycerides (high), underweight, and wasting

Properties: Antilipemic, appetite suppressant, corrects polarity, food, food, glandular, and nutritive

Spruce, Blue EO   *Woody Essential Oil*

Picea pungens

The Colorado or blue spruce tree is a native of the Western United States and has a woody, earthy, and evergreen aroma. Its sharp nettles suggest its ability to enhance a sense of security and its upright growth pattern a sense of self-dignity. It fosters self-acceptance and forgiveness. It is helpful as a topical disinfectant.

See the strategy *Aromatherapy* for suggested uses.

Warnings: Skin sensitization if oxidized. Old or oxidized oils should be avoided.

Used For: Arthritis, arthritis (rheumatoid), Graves' disease, and stress

Properties: Anti-inflammatory, antiseptic, antispasmodic, disinfectant, and expectorant

Spruce, Hemlock EO   *Woody Essential Oil*

Tsuga canadensis

The oil from this large evergreen tree, known as hemlock spruce. Spruce is applied topically for pain and inhaled for respiratory problems.

See the strategy *Aromatherapy* for suggested uses.

Warnings: Do not use internally.

Used For: Adrenal fatigue, arthritis (rheumatoid), asthma, bronchitis, cough, and pain

Properties: Antimicrobial, antiseptic, antitussive, expectorant, and rubefacient

Stabilized Allicin Formula

Garlic has many benefits, but when fighting infection, freshly crushed garlic works better than dry garlic powder in capsules. This is because the allicin in garlic rapidly degrades after the garlic is crushed. (See garlic for more information.) These tablets contain stabilized allicin, which makes this product more useful for fighting infections than garlic in capsules.

Warnings: See warnings under garlic.

Used For: AIDS, **antibiotic resistance**, **appendicitis**, **arsenic poisoning**, arteriosclerosis, **blood poisoning**, bronchitis, **cholera**, circulation (poor), colds with fever, **congestion (lungs)**, **cough**, cough (damp), **diphtheria**, fever, gangrene, hypertension, **infection (bacterial)**, infection (viral), insect repellant, itchy ears, lead poisoning, leucorrhea, mercury poisoning, **mumps**, **parasites**, parasites (nematodes, worms), **pertussis**, pet supplements, **pneumonia**, rheumatic fever, sore throat, **staph infections**, **strep throat**, tinnitus, tonsillitis, and **tuberculosis**

Affects: Arteries, digestive depression, **respiratory depression**, and tonsils

For acute infections take 1 tablet every two to four hours until relief is experienced. To help prevent infection or to improve cardiovascular health, take 1 tablet two or three times daily.

Ingredients: Garlic bulb and turmeric rhizome

Stan Malstrom's Herbal Aspirin Formula

See also *Analgesic Nerve Formula, General Analgesic Formula,* and *Headache Formula*

This is a mild pain reliever when compared to OTC pain relievers but is unlikely to cause side effects. It is best used to take the edge off pain.

Warnings: Not for emaciation or weak digestion (however, it does not irritate stomach, like synthetic aspirin). This formula does have mild blood-thinning properties and should be used with caution by those on blood-thinners or having a bleeding disorder.

Used For: Afterbirth pain, angina, **arthritis**, backache, Hashimoto's disease, **headache**, inflammation, lupus, pain, and tooth extraction

Affects: Nerve irritation (pain), prostaglandins, and structural irritation

Take 1-2 capsules every hour as needed for minor pain. Not recommended for severe pain.

Ingredients: White willow bark, valerian root, and capsicum fruit

Standardized Acetogenin Formula

See also *Alterative-Immune Formula* and *Essiac Immune Tea Formula*

Acetogenins, which are found in pawpaw and other related plants, inhibit the production of ATP in the mitochondria of cells. Since cancer cells have a much faster metabolic rate than normal cells, this induces cancer cells to self-destruct. Scientific research demonstrates that pawpaw extract is more effective than many chemotherapy drugs at destroying cancer cells and yet is completely nontoxic. In a clinical trial involving over one hundred people with cancer, pawpaw was shown to reduce tumor markers and tumor sizes, usually within one to four weeks, with virtually no side effects.

Acetogenins may also be helpful in fighting chronic viral conditions such as shingles and herpes because viruses require ATP to reproduce. These compounds also have antifungal and antibacterial activity. The acetogenins from pawpaw are also antiparasitic.

Some herbalists have found that alternating taking this formula for two to four weeks, followed by one to two weeks of building with antioxidants and other nutrients may increase the effectiveness of the program.

Acetogenins works better when taken with *Immune Boosting Formulas* and *Protease Enzymes*. It may also be combined with traditional anticancer herbs and formulas such as pau d'arco and Essiac tea.

Acetogenins be applied topically as a poultice to warts and for fungal, bacterial, or viral infections. Five to ten capsules can be mixed with a tablespoon of a salve. Acetogenins and tea tree oil can be added to shampoo to help kill head lice. This mixture can also be used as a flea and tick shampoo for dogs and cats.

Warnings: Only use paw paw with cancer, viral disorders, parasites, or other specific health problems. It is not for cancer prevention and may cause fatigue. Paw paw is not toxic to people or animals in normal doses, but it may cause nausea and vomiting when ingested. Excessive doses will cause nausea and vomiting. This formula may also induce a healing crisis or cleansing reaction if cancer cell die-off is too quick, which may require cleansing herbs to help the body detoxify. Pregnant women and nursing mothers should avoid using it without the advice of their health practitioner. Cancer is a serious illness. Seek professional assistance and advice.

Used For: Athlete's foot, **cancer**, **cancer treatment side effects**, **cervical dysplasia**, **endometriosis**, fleas, **herpes**, infection (fungal), infection (viral), lice, **parasites**, parasites (nematodes, worms), **parasites (tapeworm)**, **psoriasis**, **scabies**, **shingles**, and **warts**

Affects: Breasts and immune system

Take 1 capsule four times daily. Start with 1 capsule per day the first week, increasing 1 capsule for each week until reaching the full dose. Higher amounts can be taken if desired, but nausea and vomiting, dizziness, fatigue, or light headedness can occur.

Ingredients: Acetogenins and pawpaw twig extract

Steven Horne's Anti-Allergy Formula

See also *Antihistamine Formula*

This is formula helps to reduce symptoms of respiratory allergies. It works well for allergies to pollen, dust, and animal dander. It doesn't completely stop allergic reactions, but it does help to reduce them. It does not dry out the sinuses like antihistamines. Directions for this make-it-yourself formula can be found in the book *Modern Herbal Dispensatory*.

Used For: Allergies (respiratory), food allergies/intolerances, and rhinitis

Affects: Hyperactive immune activity, **respiratory irritation**, and respiratory stagnation

Take 1/2 to 1 teaspoon of the extracts two or three times daily with lots of water. The blend can also be made as a tea. Drink 1–3 cups daily.

4 parts Eyebright
4 parts Stinging nettle leaf
2 parts Goldenrod
2 parts Burdock root
1 part Blessed thistle
1 part Bitter orange peel

Steven Horne's Children's Composition Formula

See also *Herbal Composition Formula*

I developed this formula almost forty years ago when I had young children. It has worked very well for colds, flu, and other acute viral infections, especially when there is fever present. It's quite tasty, and kids don't usually object to taking it. Directions for this make-it-yourself formula can be found in the book *Modern Herbal Dispensatory*.

Used For: Chicken pox, **colds**, colds with fever, **fever**, **flu**, infection (viral), measles, mumps, **perspiration (deficient)**, sore throat, and **vaccine side effects**

Affects: Digestive stagnation, immune system, and **sweat glands**

Give small doses 1/8-1/2 teaspoon, depending on the age and weight of the child every one to two hours with lots of water until the child shows signs of improvement. This blend can also be used in an enema for fevers.

1 part Yarrow
1 part Elder flower
1 part Peppermint

Steven Horne's Horehound Cough Formula

See also *Damp Cough Syrup Formula*

This is adapted from one of herbalist Michael Moore's recipes. It's a great cough syrup for any kind of coughs where there is abundant mucus drainage. Horehound also has a tonic effect on the heart and stimulates digestion. Directions for this make-it-yourself formula can be found in the book *Modern Herbal Dispensatory*.

Used For: Appetite (deficient), congestion (bronchial), congestion (lungs), cough, cough (damp), and heart weakness

Affects: Respiratory constriction, respiratory depression, and respiratory stagnation

Take 1/2 to 1 teaspoon as needed for cough.

1 oz Horehound leaf

2 cups Honey or brown sugar

1 Tablespoon Lime juice

Steven Horne's Sinus Snuff Powder

This is a simple formula for clearing severe sinus congestion. It can cause brief discomfort as the powders are sniffed into the sinuses, but this is typically followed by rapid drainage and a clearing of the sinuses. This can shrink nasal polyps and help with severe chronic sinusitis. You can make this powder by mixing the powders from capsules together

Used For: Congestion (sinus), headache (sinus), nosebleeds, **polyps**, **sinus infection**, and smell (loss of)

Affects: Respiratory relaxation and **sinuses**

Sniff the mixture up the sinuses or make into a tea and wash the sinuses using a neti pot.

1 part Goldenseal root

1 part Bayberry root bark

Stevia   *Sweet Herb*

Stevia rebaudiana

Stevia is three hundred times sweeter than sugar and can be safely used to sweeten herbal teas for children or diabetics. It can also be used in baking, but you need to figure out the right conversions for recipes.

Energetics: Mildly cooling and mildly moistening

Used For: Diabetes, hypoglycemia, and metabolic syndrome

Properties: Antidiabetic, hypoglycemic, and sweetener

Stillingia (Queen's Root)

Sweet & Mildly Acrid Herb

Stillingia sylvatica

Stillingia, also known as queen's root, is an herb in some traditional anticancer formulas. It is used primarily to improve lymphatic drainage.

Look for *stillingia* in *Liquid Lymph Formula*

Energetics: Warming and balancing

Used For: Adenitis, **congestion (lymphatic)**, cough (dry), sore throat, and ulcers

Properties: Lymphatic and moistening

Stimulant Laxative Formula

See also *Senna Laxative Formula*

These are stimulant laxative formulas based on herbs that contain anthraquinone glycosides. Anthraquinones are yellow-brown dyes that intestinal bacteria metabolize into anthranols. These, in turn, inhibit the absorption of water, sodium, and chloride in the colon, which helps to hydrate the stool. They also cause a localized stimulation of prostaglandins, which increase the force and rate of peristalsis. So in small amounts, anthraquinone glycosides act as tonics to the colon. In larger doses they act as laxatives.

It takes about eight hours for these herbs to take effect, which means that an ideal time to take them is right before bed. This helps ensure a normal movement when you wake up the next morning. According to traditional Chinese medicine, the colon meridian is most active from 5:00 to 7:00 a.m., which is why many people have a bowel movement first thing in the morning. That's why bedtime is an ideal time to take these formulas.

An alternate time is to take them first thing in the morning before breakfast, along with your fiber and water. Depending on what time you wake up, this should result in a bowel movement in the late afternoon or early evening.

Ideally they should be used as part of a cleanse or for occasional relief from constipation. For long term relief try to use a *Fiber Blend* and/or the *Gentle Laxative Formula*. (See the condition *constipation* for more information.)

Warnings: The anthranols produced by the intestinal bacteria are absorbed into the bloodstream and can enter breast milk in nursing mothers. For that reason, they shouldn't be used when nursing. Many herbalists also recommend avoiding them during pregnancy but I've personally seen no harm from using them occasionally during pregnancy.

Also, anthraquinones are dyes, so they stain the colon if you use them regularly. While there is no evidence that this harms the colon, it does raise concerns with doctors giving colonoscopies.

Used For: Anal fistula/fissure, colon (atonic), **constipation (adults)**, hemorrhoids, parasites, parasites (nematodes, worms), parasites (tapeworm), prolapsed colon, and SIBO

Affects: Intestinal depression, **intestinal stagnation**, and **large intestines (colon)**

Lower Bowel Liquid Extract

A liquid stimulant laxative for children (over 2) and adults who can't swallow capsules.

Ingredients: Cascara sagrada bark, senna leaf, buckthorn bark, rhubarb root, and barberry bark

Stan Malstrom's Lower Bowel Formula

A popular stimulant laxative formula. Take 2–4 capsules before bedtime or 1–2 capsules twice daily, preferable first thing in the morning and before bedtime.

Ingredients: Cascara sagrada bark, buckthorn bark, Oregon grape root & rhizome, turkey rhubarb root, and red clover flower

Stimulant Laxative with Senna

A senna-based stimulant laxative. Take 2–4 capsules with water and a late evening snack for occasional relief from severe constipation.

Ingredients: Senna leaf, fennel seed, ginger rhizome, and catnip leaf

Christopher's Lower Bowel Formula

An alternative to Stan Malstrom's formula that's a little milder in action. Alternating formulas can help reduce dependency. Take 2–4 capsules before bedtime or 1–2 capsules twice daily, preferable first thing in the morning and before bedtime.

Ingredients: Cascara sagrada bark, turkey rhubarb root, goldenseal root & rhizome, Oregon grape root & rhizome, and lobelia aerial parts

Stimulating Energy Formula

See also *Chinese Qi-Increasing Formula* and *Vandergriff's Energy Booster Formula*

A healthier alternative to the popular energy drinks. It contains guarana, a natural source of caffeine. It may helpful for people with a parasympathetic-dominant nervous system. See the condition *ADHD*.

Warnings: Too much caffeine may cause nervousness, irritability, sleeplessness, and occasionally rapid heartbeat. Not recommended for use by young children or people with adrenal exhaustion or anxiety.

Used For: ADD/ADHD, addictions (coffee, caffeine), and fatigue

Affects: Epinephrine and **parasympathetic-dominant ANS**

Empty the contents of one packet into 14-16 ounces of cold water, mix and drink.

Ingredients: Vitamin B_1, vitamin B_2, vitamin B_3, vitamin B_6, vitamin B_{12}, pantothenic acid, potassium, guarana seed, and ginseng (Asian/Korean) root extract

Sugar Craving Reducer Formula

See also *Appetite Reducer Formula*

This formula helps to manage sugar cravings during weight loss, by balancing blood sugar levels. It contains L-arabinose, which helps block absorption of sugar. The amino acid L-theanine also helps to reduce feelings of stress, which may help reduce cravings for sweets that are emotionally based.

Used For: Addictions (sugar/carbohydrates), appetite (excessive), and excess weight

Take 3 capsules once daily, preferably before your largest meal (usually dinner).

Ingredients: Cinnamon bark extract, chromium, L-arbinose, and L-threonine

Suma   *Sweet Herb*

Pfaffia paniculata

This herb has a panacea-like reputation among natives of the Brazilian rain forest. It is believed to have adaptogenic and immune-stimulant effects similar to that of eleuthero root. It is helpful for menopause as it enhances estrogen levels. It aids sex drive in both men and women and enhances the immune system to fight viral disorders and cancer.

Look for *suma* in *Suma Adaptogen Formula*

Warnings: Contraindicated with acute disease, severe inflammation and high fever.

Energetics: Mildly cooling and balancing

Used For: Cancer, diabetes, erectile dysfunction, fatigue, menopause, sex drive (low), and stress

Properties: Adaptogen, antioxidant, aphrodisiac, cytotoxic, estrogenic, immune stimulant, and tonic

Suma Adaptogen Formula

See also *Adaptogen-Immune Formula*

This formula combines several adaptogenic herbs that help the body cope with stress and resist disease. They also help to stimulate the immune response.

Used For: ADD/ADHD, Addison's disease, adrenal fatigue, aging, AIDS, anxiety disorders, convalescence, Cushing's disease, endurance, Epstein-Barr virus, fatigue, Graves' disease, and sex drive (low)

Affects: Brain, central nervous system, and pineal

Use 2-4 capsules three times daily.

Ingredients: Echinacea aerial parts, suma bark, astragalus root, and eleuthero root

Sweet Annie
Fragrant Bitter Herb

Artemesia annua

A close relative of wormwood, sweet annie is used for malaria and intermittent fevers. It is also a good remedy for parasites.

Warnings: Do not use while pregnant or nursing. All artemesia species can be toxic in large doses.

Energetics: Cooling and drying

Used For: Cancer, fever, **lyme disease**, **malaria**, **parasites**, **parasites (nematodes, and worms)**

Properties: Anthelmintic, antibacterial, **antimalarial**, **antiparasitic**, and antiseptic

Tangerine (Mandarin)
Aromatic & Bitter Herb

Citrus reticulata

The peelings of citrus fruits like this one are used in Chinese herbalism to regulate qi and strengthen the spleen (digestive) meridian. It also aids respiratory congestion.

Energetics: Warming and drying

Used For: Cough (damp), diarrhea, and nausea & vomiting

Properties: Antibacterial, antiemetic, digestive tonic, expectorant, hypertensive, and stimulant (circulatory)

Tansy, Blue EO
Floral, Herbaceous, & Sweet Essential Oil

Tanacetum annuum

A sweet, floral fragrance of the oil of tansy is also camphorous with herbaceous undertones. It has a dark blue color due to it's chamazulene content, which also makes it very anti-inflammatory.

See the strategy *Aromatherapy* for suggested uses.

Warnings: Do not use internally.

Used For: Allergies (respiratory), anger (excessive), anxiety (situational), asthma, eczema, insect repellant, pain, skin problems, and stress

Properties: Analgesic, anti-inflammatory, antiallergenic, antibacterial, antidepressant, antifungal, antihistamine, antimicrobial, antioxidant, antiparasitic, antirheumatic, antispasmodic, antiviral, relaxant, and sedative

Target Mineral Thyroid Formula
See also *Hypothyroid Formula* and *Thyroid Glandular Formula*

This is a traditional thyroid formula that contains minerals chelated to amino acids. These direct the minerals to the pituitary, where they stimulate the production of thyroid releasing hormone (TRH). TRH then stimulates the thyroid gland. It can be used to boost metabolism to aid weight loss.

Used For: Excess weight, fatigue, and hypothyroidism

Affects: **Pituitary (anterior)**, thyroid depression, and thyroid-stimulating hormone

To stimulate the thyroid and as an aid in weight loss use 2 capsules before breakfast and 1 before lunch.

Ingredients: Zinc, manganese, Irish moss, kelp leaf & stem, L-glutamine, L-proline, and L-histadine

Tea
Mildly Astringent & Mildly Stimulant Bitter Herb

Camellia sinensis

Tea is the commonly consumed beverage in the world. It contains compounds that reduce cancer risk and protect the liver. Green tea contains powerful antioxidants and is generally considered healthier to drink. Black tea is made from fermented tea leaves. Tea contains caffeine, but is not as likely to cause jittery feelings because it also contains a relaxing amino acid, L-threonine.

Tea is also an astringent, so tea bags can be moistened with hot water and used topically as compresses for insect bites and stings or other skin irritations where astringents may be helpful. They can also be used as a compress for red, irritated eyes. Place the warm moistened tea bag over the closed eyelid.

Look for *tea* in *Antioxidant, Cardiovascular Antioxidant, Cortisol-Reducing, Green Tea Polyphenols, Headache,* and *Metabolic Stimulant Formulas*

Warnings: Excessive caffeine consumption can lead to anxiety and adrenal exhaustion.

Energetics: Warming, mildly drying, and mildly constricting

Used For: ADD/ADHD, aging, Alzheimer's, arteriosclerosis, autism, bedwetting, bites & stings, cancer, dental health, **excess weight**, eyes (red/itching), **eyes, bloodshot**, free radical damage, inflammation, psoriasis, and skin problems

Properties: Anticarious, antimutagenic, **antioxidant**, astringent, and stimulant (metabolic)

Tea Tree EO   *Spicy & Vaporous Essential Oil*

Melaleuca alternifolia

Best known for its antimicrobial activity, tea tree essential oil has a warm, spicy, vaporous odor. It is primarily used for its disinfectant and antifungal properties. Externally, apply full strength to aid healing and fight infection injuries to the skin. It usually does not sting.

It is also useful as a gargle; add 2–4 drops per pint of warm water. It can be used in an enema or douche; use 2–4 drops per pint of water. It can be used in baths; add 5–20 drops to the bath water. Use sparingly in baths as it can irritate the skin. As a skin cleanser and acne cream, combine with jojoba oil or other fixed oil. Mix with shampoo for lice, dandruff, and itching scalp.

Emotionally, tea tree dispels "cold," meaning it helps to awaken and invigorate a person. It uplifts the spirit and promotes confidence, making it helpful for people who are shy, timid, fearful, and struggling with feelings of victimhood and weakness. It can help these people a lack of vitality and help improve general health.

See the strategy *Aromatherapy* for suggested uses.

Warnings: Do not use internally without the supervision of a professionally trained aromatherapy practitioner. Generally safe and nonirritating for topical use, but may cause skin irritation in some people when used long term.

Used For: Abrasions/scratches, abscesses, acne, antibiotic resistance, asthma, athlete's foot, bites & stings, blisters, body odor, **boils**, bronchitis, burns & scalds, canker sores, carbuncles, chicken pox, cold sores, colds (decongestant), **corns**, cough, cuts, cysts, **dandruff**, denture sores, **earache**, eczema, fleas, flu, foot odor, gangrene, gingivitis, herpes, hypochondria, impetigo, **infection (bacterial)**, **infection (fungal)**, infection prevention, injuries, insect repellant, itching, itchy ears, jock itch, laryngitis, leucorrhea, **lice**, poison ivy/oak, rashes & hives, rosacea, **scabies**, scars/scar tissue, **seborrhea**, shingles, shock (medical), sinus infection, **skin (infections)**, skin (oily), skin problems, slivers, sore throat, staph infections, strep throat, sunburn, swollen lymph glands, **tetanus**, thrush, **tick**, tonsillitis, toothache, tuberculosis, **ulcerations (external)**, vaginal dryness, vaginitis, warts, and **wounds & sores**

Properties: Analgesic, anti-inflammatory, **antibacterial**, **antifungal**, **antimicrobial**, antioxidant, antiparasitic, **antiseptic**, antiviral, bactericidal, balsamic, **cicatrizant**, decongestant, deodorant, digestive tonic, disinfectant, expectorant, immune stimulant, insecticide, and vulnerary

Teasel   *Bitter Herb*

Dipsacus asper

Teasel root has been used for muscle and joint pain and as a tonic to aid repair of damaged tissues. It is also employed in the management of Lyme disease symptoms. It does not cure Lyme but is helpful in the relief of muscle pain and related symptoms. In Chinese herbalism, it enters the lung and kidney meridians and supports the tendons and muscles.

Look for *teasel* in *Chinese Water-Increasing Formula*

Energetics: Cooling and mildly moistening

Used For: Bursitis, inflammation, kidney weakness/failure, **lyme disease**, pain, and tendonitis

Properties: Anti-inflammatory, kidney tonic, and vulnerary

Testosterone Formula

See also *DHEA with Herbs Formula*

These are formulas to help enhance testosterone in men. See the condition *testosterone (low)*.

Used For: Depression, **erectile dysfunction**, infertility, **sex drive (low)**, **testosterone (low)**, and underweight

David Winston's Male Tonic

Take 40–60 drops one to three times daily

Ingredients: Ashwagandha root, maca root, red ginseng root, and epimedium

Testoserone-Libido Formula

Use 1 capsule four times daily

Ingredients: Ashwagandha standardized extract, maca root, epimedium standardized extract, muira puama bark extract, and ginseng (Asian/Korean) root extract

Testosterone Performance Formula

Aids blood flow for erectile dysfunction as well as enhancing testosterone. Take 2 soft-gels with food. Do not exceed four capsules a day.

Ingredients: Vitamin B_3, zinc, ashwagandha extract, pumpkin, tribulus extract, L-arginine, yohimbe extract, tongkat ali, cordyceps, and ginseng (Asian/Korean)

Thiamine   **see** *vitamin B_1*

Thlaspi   *Bitter & Pungent Herb*

Thlaspi arvense

Thiaspi is used in Chinese herbalism to dispell toxic heat, drain pus and expel phlegm. It clears toxic heat and fights infection.

Look for *thlaspi* in *Chinese Wind-Heat Evil Formula*

Energetics: Cooling and drying

Used For: Abscesses, appendicitis, and carbuncles

Properties: Alterative, anti-inflammatory, antibacterial, and decongestant

Thuja   *Fragrant Bitter Herb*
Thuja occidentalis

The leaves of thuja are a strong antifungal remedy, useful for candida, athlete's foot and jock itch. They also have antiparasitic effects against ringworm, amoebic dysentery, and giardia. They also have strong antiviral activity. Thuja homeopathic is good for side effects from vaccinations.

Warnings: In the 1930s, thuja was used as an abortifacient in Europe and North America. Do not use during pregnancy. Do not use long-term as it may irritate the kidneys.

Energetics: Warming and drying

Used For: Athlete's foot, blood poisoning, **gangrene**, giardia, **infection (bacterial)**, infection (fungal), infection (viral), jock itch, parasites (nematodes, worms), and vaccine side effects

Properties: Abortifacient, anthelmintic, antifungal, antiparasitic, emmenagogue, and expectorant

Thyme   *Aromatic Herb*
Thymus vulgaris

Thyme is a very powerful remedy for infections of all kinds, especially in the lungs and digestive tract. It is indicated for spasmodic conditions of the respiratory and urinary tract with infectious symptoms. It is a good antifungal remedy and can also be used to treat intestinal parasites in children. The combination of fenugreek and thyme is excellent for clearing sinus congestion. Applied topically, it helps with insect bites, stings and minor pain.

Look for *thyme* in *Herbal Tooth Powder, Seasonal Cold* and *Flu*, and *Sinus Formulas*

Warnings: Avoid large doses while pregnant. Culinary use and standard dosages found in formulas are safe.

Energetics: Warming and drying

Used For: Bronchitis, colds, confusion, congestion, congestion (lungs), **congestion (sinus)**, COPD, **cough**, cough (damp), cough (spastic), cramps (menstrual), croup, cystic fibrosis, dental health, dyspepsia, emphysema, fever, flu, **gas & bloating**, headache, **headache (sinus)**, hysteria, indigestion, infection (bacterial), infection (viral),

infection prevention, parasites (nematodes, worms), pertussis, **sinus infection**, smell (loss of), **snoring**, spinal disks, toothache, and wounds & sores

Properties: Antibacterial, antifungal, antilipemic, antiviral, carminative, decongestant, emmenagogue, and stimulant (circulatory)

Thyme EO
Herbaceous, Spicy, & Woody Essential Oil
Thymus vulgaris

Thyme EO has a turpentine-like aroma that is spicy, woody, and herbaceous. It is a nerve tonic and mental stimulant helping to increase circulation to the brain, promoting mental focus, clarity, and memory.

Thyme was used by the ancient Egyptians for embalming. It is a very good household disinfectant and home deodorizer. It can be applied topically to minor injuries as a natural disinfectant. It can be inhaled or diffused for respiratory problems such as spastic, dry coughs.

Emotionally, thyme helps mental focus, creating an alert, focused state of mind. It revives low spirits, combats exhaustion and stimulates the mind while calming mental chatter. Thyme can be used to help overcome confusion, fear and to regulate instinctive reactions. It dispels discouragement and despondency, aiding fortitude and vigor. It can be helpful for children who are disturbed because of family disharmony. It helps a person to be less dreamy and detached and more focused and logical.

See the strategy *Aromatherapy* for suggested uses.

Warnings: Do not use internally without the supervision of a professionally trained aromatherapy practitioner. May irritate skin and mucus membranes and cause a rash in sensitive individuals. Dilute for topical use.

Used For: Alcoholism, antibiotic resistance, asthma, athlete's foot, bites & stings, bronchitis, circulation (poor), colds (antiviral), colds (decongestant), colic (adults), colitis, confusion, **congestion**, congestion (lymphatic), cough (dry), **cough (spastic)**, dermatitis, digestion (poor), dyspepsia, earache, fatigue, flu, gastritis, hypochondria, **infection (bacterial)**, infection (fungal), infection (viral), **infection prevention**, insect repellant, interstitial cystitis, laryngitis, lice, pertussis, pleurisy, psoriasis, **scabies**, sciatica, shock (medical), sinus infection, skin (infections), sore throat, swollen lymph glands, tetanus, thrush, **tonsillitis**, tuberculosis, and warts

Properties: Antibacterial, anticarious, antifungal, antimicrobial, antioxidant, **antiseptic**, antiviral, astringent, carminative, counterirritant, diaphoretic, disinfectant, emmenagogue, expectorant, parasympatholytic, pectoral, preservative, stimulant (circulatory), sympathomimetic, and tonic

Thyroid Calming Formula

When the thyroid is irritated and/or hyperactive, this formula may be helpful. It has a calming effect on the thyroid gland and also helps reduce the nervousness, anxiety, and tachycardia that often accompany a hyperthyroid condition like Graves disease.

Used For: Anxiety (situational), **Graves' disease**, nervousness, and tachycardia

Affects: Thyroid irritation

Ingredients: Bugleweed herb, lemon balm flowering tops, and motherwort flowering tops

Thyroid Glandular Formula

See also *Hypothyroid Formula*

This product contains nutrients necessary to help the thyroid gland produce thyroxine, the major thyroid hormone. It contains a thyroid glandular which can help rebuild the thyroid gland.

Warnings: Not recommended for use with hyperthyroid (Graves disease). This formula will not work if the thyroid gland is missing or is destroyed. Not recommended for long-term use, especially in high doses. Use a Hypothyroid Formula for long-term thyroid support.

Used For: Amenorrhea, apathy, **cholesterol (low)**, **cold hands/feet**, **depression**, fat metabolism (poor), fibrosis, **goiter**, **hair loss/thinning**, **Hashimoto's disease**, **hypothyroidism**, menstrual irregularity, sex drive (low), skin (dry/flaky), and skin problems

Affects: Thyroid depression, **thyroxin**, and **tri-iodothyronine**

Take 1 capsule once or twice daily with food for low thyroid.

Ingredients: Vitamin B$_6$, zinc, copper, manganese, L-tyrosine, kelp leaf & stem, thyroid substance, nettle, and stinging leaf

Tienchi Ginseng   *Astringent Herb*

Panax notoginseng

Tienchi ginseng is used to control bleeding and hemorrhaging of all kinds. It is also a mild circulatory stimulant and may be helpful for angina.

Look for *tienchi ginseng* in *Myelin Sheath Formula*

Energetics: Warming and constricting

Used For: Bleeding (external), **bleeding (internal)**, blood in urine, and bruises

Properties: Hemostatic, stimulant (circulatory), and **styptic**

Topical Analgesic Formula

See also *Analgesic EO Blend* and *MSM Topical Analgesic Formula*

This is a blend of essential oils for easing pain. Both the lotion and essential oil can be massaged into the skin for relief of sore muscles or cramps. Massage into the throat for sore throats and into the chest for congestion. Massage into the neck and shoulders to relieve headaches.

Apply these essential oils to the temples for relief from headaches or to insect bites, beestings, bruises, and other minor injuries to aid healing. Inhale the oil for relief of sinus congestion. One drop of oil can be used on the back of the tongue to promote mental alertness while driving. Apply oil directly to canker sores to promote healing.

Warnings: This blend is not intended for internal use. If you do use it internally, do not use more than a drop and no more than once a day for only two or three days. Avoid contact with eyes and genitals. Do not apply after a hot shower as it will cause a severe burning sensation.

Used For: Allergies (respiratory), **arthritis**, backache, **bites & stings**, **bruises**, **bursitis**, **canker sores**, **carpal tunnel**, cold sores, **colds (decongestant)**, concentration (poor), congestion, **congestion (sinus)**, cough, cuts, dislocation, **exercise (recovery)**, **headache**, **headache (cluster)**, **headache (migraine)**, **headache (sinus)**, **headache (tension)**, **injuries**, laryngitis, ligaments (torn/injuried), motion sickness, **pain**, sciatica, sinus infection, sprains, **stiff neck**, **tendonitis**, and toothache

Affects: General depression, lungs, muscles, respiratory depression, sinuses, skin, spinal discs, structural depression, structural irritation, structural stagnation, and **substance P**

Topical Analgesic Essential Oils

My favorite topical analgesic. Use topically to ease aches and pains. Apply to temples for migraines. Inhale to ease respiratory congestion and promote mental alterness.

Ingredients: Menthol EO, eucalyptus EO, camphor EO, wintergreen EO, lavender EO, and clove EO

Topical Analgesic Lotion with Arnica

The same blend of analgesic oils in a cream base with other healing ingredients like arnica.

Ingredients: Camphor, menthol, methyl salicylate, eucalyptus EO, clove EO, and arnica flower extract

Topical Injury Blend

See also *Analgesic EO Blend* and *Topical Analgesic Formula*

This is usually made as an oil, but is also found as a homeopathic cream. It is applied topically to help injuries like bruises and sprains to heal more quickly. It may also aid the healing of damaged nerves.

See the strategy *Aromatherapy* for suggested uses.

Used For: Bruises, bursitis, frozen shoulder, injuries, ligaments (torn/injuried), nerve damage, **sprains**, and wounds & sores

Ingredients: Calendula flower, arnica flower, and Saint John's wort flowering tops

Trichosanthes   *Sour & Sweet Herb*

Trichosanthes kirilowii

The root of this herb is used in Chinese herbalism for the lungs and stomach. It clears heat, moistens dry tissues, discharges pus, and relieves thirst.

Warnings: Do not use while pregnant.

Energetics: Cooling

Used For: Diabetes, edema, jaundice (adults), mastitis, and sore throat

Properties: Abortifacient, anti-inflammatory, anticancer, and hypoglycemic

Triphala Formula

See also *Gentle Bowel Cleansing Formula*

Triphala is a blend of three fruits used in ayurvedic medicine as a gentle laxative, bowel tonic, and blood purifier. Besides normalizing colon function, triphala improves liver function, protects the liver against environmental toxins, and improves digestion. It is antioxidant and anti-inflammatory, so it slows aging and protects the body from degenerative disease. It enhances circulation, lowers blood pressure, and protects the heart. It helps expel mucus from the respiratory passages and fights infection. In ayurvedic medicine, triphala is used as a general health tonic for many ailments. I mix triphala with equal parts fresh ground flax seeds and psyllium hulls to make a lubricating bulk laxative and intestinal tonic.

Used For: Allergies (respiratory), **colon (atonic)**, **colon (spastic)**, **constipation (adults)**, constipation (children), **diverticulitis**, gas & bloating, **inflammatory bowel disorders**, **irritable bowel**, **leaky gut**, and sinus infection

Ingredients: Chebulic myrobalan fruit, amalaki, and belleric myrobalan fruit

Turkey Rhubarb   *Bitter Herb*

Rheum palmatum

A common ingredient in stimulant laxatives, this bitter is also used as a digestive tonic.

Look for *turkey rhubarb* in *Essiac Immune Tea* and *Stimulant Laxative Formulas*

Warnings: Some people react with abdominal pain. Ginger or nervine herbs can help to counteract this.

Energetics: Drying and cooling

Used For: Acid indigestion, **colon (atonic)**, and **constipation (adults)**

Properties: Antacid and laxative

Turkey Tail   *Sweet Herb*

Trametes versicolor

Turkey tail grows on dead hardwood trees and is one of the most abundant mushrooms found in deciduous forests. Enzymes secreted from its mycelium are some of the most potent toxin-destroyers found in nature, which means it could be very helpful for cleaning up environmental pollution.

There are some good studies showing it contains various compounds having immune-boosting activity. Studies suggest various compounds in it inhibit the growth of various types of cancer cells, initiate apoptosis, and stimulate immune responses such as natural killer cells.

An extract, known as PSK or krestin, is an approved anti-cancer drug in Asia. PSK enhances the effect of chemotherapy and radiation, prevents metastasis, and has broad neoplastic activity. It is immune-enhancing and prolongs the activity of antibiotics. It is also antiviral and inhibits the HIV virus involved in AIDS.

Look for *turkey tail* in *Mushroom Immune Formula*

Used For: AIDS, autoimmune disorders, cancer, and infection (viral)

Properties: Antibacterial, anticancer, antiviral, and immune stimulant

Turmeric   *Aromatic & Mildly Bitter Herb*

Curcuma longa

Turmeric stimulates digestion and aids assimilation. It is a very good liver and gallbladder remedy. It aids liver function and helps dissolve and prevent gallstones. Its potent ability to reduce inflammation and ease chronic pain makes it useful for treating arthritis. Also see *curcumin*.

Look for *turmeric* in *Anti-Inflammatory Pain, Antioxidant, Cardiovascular Antioxidant, CBD Anti-inflammatory, CBD*

Joint, General Analgesic, Hemp Oil with Terpenes, Herbal Arthritis, and *Stabilized Allicin Formulas*

Energetics: Cooling and mildly drying

Used For: Alzheimer's, **arthritis**, **arthritis (rheumatoid)**, autoimmune disorders, **bipolar mood disorder**, bursitis, **cancer**, **cancer prevention**, cartilage damage, cholesterol (high), denture sores, **depression**, digestion (poor), dislocation, eczema, environmental pollution, fat cravings, fever, **gallbladder problems**, **gallstones**, **inflammation**, metabolic syndrome, overacidity, **pain**, **psoriasis**, rashes & hives, **Raynaud's disease**, skin (dry/flaky), spinal disks, **traumatic brain injury**, triglycerides (high), and triglycerides (low)

Properties: **Anti-inflammatory**, **antiarthritic**, anticancer, antimutagenic, **antioxidant**, antithrombotic, cholagogue, condiment, and hepatoprotective

Typhonium   *Pungent & Sweet Herb*

Typhonium flagelliforme

A rarely used herb in Chinese herbalism, typhonium is used primarily to remove cold and dampness and to relax spasms. It primarily affects the stomach meridian.

Look for *typhonium* in *Chinese Metal-Decreasing, Chinese Qi-Regulating,* and *Chinese Wood-Decreasing Formulas*

Energetics: Warming, drying, and relaxing

Used For: Congestion and headache (tension)

Properties: Analgesic

Uña de Gato   **see** *cat's claw*

Urinary Immune Formula

See also *Diuretic Formula* and *UTI Prevention Formula*

Parthenium has some mild immunostimulant action similar to echinacea and has an affinity for the urinary tract. Combined in this formula with goldenseal, it is a useful product for urinary tract infections. It may also be helpful for other bacterial infections.

Warnings: See warnings for goldenseal.

Used For: Bladder infection, infection (bacterial), and **urinary tract infections**

Affects: Bladder, immune system, and **urinary stagnation**

Use 1/2 to 1 teaspoon two to four times per day.

Ingredients: Goldenseal root extract and parthenium root extract

Urinary Support Formula

See also *Chinese Water-Decreasing Formula* and *Diuretic Formula*

This formula is a soothing urinary tonic and diuretic and suitable for kidney infections where juniper is contraindicated. It strengthens the kidney's ability to flush toxins as well as increasing the flow of urine. It is a good choice for long-term use as a general kidney tonic.

Used For: Bedwetting, bladder (irritable), bladder infection, edema, incontinence, interstitial cystitis, kidney infection, kidney weakness/failure, nephritis, **urethritis**, urination (burning/painful), and urine (scant)

Affects: Bladder, **kidneys**, urinary atrophy, and urinary irritation

For kidney or bladder infections, or as a diuretic, take 2 capsules three times daily with plenty of water.

As a general aid to strengthen the kidneys, take 1 capsule three times a day with meals.

Ingredients: Magnesium, potassium, asparagus stem, dandelion leaf, corn silk, watermelon seed, hydrangea root, and uva ursi leaf

Usnea   *Bitter Herb*

Tillandsia usneoides

Actually a lichen, or a symbiotic combination of algae and fungi, usnea has been used for thousands of years in Chinese, Greek, and Egyptian herbalism to treat a variety of health conditions. It has antibiotic and antifungal properties that may be helpful for treating lung and upper respiratory infections such as the common cold, sore throat, and cough and as an antibacterial for the mouth to promote oral hygiene. It inhibits the growth of gram-positive bacteria.

Look for *usnea* in *Anti-Fungal Formula*

Energetics: Cooling and drying

Used For: Abscesses, athlete's foot, **bladder infection**, blood poisoning, colds, flu, **gangrene**, gingivitis, impetigo, **infection (bacterial)**, **infection (fungal)**, lyme disease, pneumonia, sore throat, **strep throat**, **tuberculosis**, urinary tract infections, and vaginitis

Properties: Antibacterial and antifungal

UTI Prevention Formula

See also *Diuretic Formula* and *Urinary Immune Formula*

This diuretic formula is specifically for preventing urinary tract infections. Cranberry makes the lining of the urinary tract inhospitable for bacteria.

Warnings: Buchu may be contraindicated with severe kidney inflammation.

Used For: Bladder infection, edema, **incontinence, interstitial cystitis, kidney infection**, prolapsed uterus, **urinary tract infections**, urination (burning/painful), and urine (scant)

Affects: Bladder, prostate, **urinary irritation**, and urinary stagnation

To help prevent UTIs, take 1-2 capsules three times daily. When there is an acute infection take 1 capsule of goldenseal, berberine or uva ursi with 2 capsules of this formula and drink extra water.

Ingredients: Cranberry fruit and buchu leaf extract

Uva Ursi   *Astringent Herb*

Arctostaphylos uva-ursi

A reliable diuretic with strong disinfectant and infection-fighting properties, uva ursi is useful for kidney and bladder infections, irritated female organs, and other urogenital problems.

Look for *uva ursi* in *Diuretic* and *Female Tonic Formulas*

Warnings: Not for use in cases involving fluid deficiency, wasting or dryness. Not recommended for long term use because of strong astringency. Prolonged use may irritate the stomach and cause constipation. Not recommended during pregnancy.

Energetics: Drying, constricting, and mildly warming

Used For: Bedwetting, bladder (irritable), **bladder infection**, blood in urine, cuts, diabetes, **edema**, gout, **incontinence**, interstitial cystitis, **kidney infection**, kidney stones, pancreatitis, **poison ivy/oak**, prolapsed colon, prolapsed uterus, prostatitis, urethritis, **urinary tract infections**, urination (burning/painful), urination (frequent), and urine (scant)

Properties: Antiseptic, **astringent**, and **diuretic**

Valerian   *Aromatic & Bitter Herb*

Valeriana officinalis

Valerian is a popular and potent nervine with strong tranquilizing effects on the central nervous system. It has been used to treat a wide variety of nervous system conditions, insomnia, and mild pain.

Look for *valerian* in *Analgesic Nerve, Christopher's Nervine, Herbal Sleep Aid, Sleep Support*, and *Stan Malstrom's Herbal Aspirin Formulas*

Warnings: Not recommended with hot disorders (i.e., high strung, nervous and excitable—skullcap or passion flower are better for such individuals). Not for long-term use in large doses. It does not generally cause drowsiness that

could affect driving. Some people have an opposite reaction to valerian and find it stimulating rather than sedating. Low thyroid and dosage appears to be a factor. Some people using valerian may experience a light feeling as if floating in air, and they may experience hallucinations at night.

Energetics: Mildly warming and relaxing

Used For: Addictions (drugs), addictions (tobacco), afterbirth pain, alcoholism, anxiety disorders, cramps (leg), cramps & spasms, headache (tension), heart fibrillation/palpitations, **insomnia**, myasthenia gravis, neuralgia & neuritis, pain, Parkinson's disease, seizures, stress, tooth extraction, and twitching

Properties: Analgesic, anticephalalgic, antispasmodic, CNS depressant, gaba-enhancing, hypotensive, **nervine**, parasympatholytic, **relaxant, sedative, soporific, sympatholytic**, and tranquilizer

Vanadium   *Mineral*

Vanadium, like chromium, is helpful in regulating blood sugar. It also lowers blood fats and inhibits cholesterol synthesis. It is needed for healthy bones and teeth.

Used For: Angina, **cholesterol (high)**, **dental health**, **diabetes**, excess weight, hypoglycemia, metabolic syndrome, and sore throat

Properties: Anticarious, anticholesteremic, and antidiabetic

Vandergriff's Energy Booster Formula

See also *Chinese Qi-Increasing Formula*

Use this formula as a general tonic for more energy. It addresses the various problems that cause feelings of fatigue. It contains adaptogens (eleuthero, gotu kola, schizandra), yellow dock to supply iron to combat anemia, kelp for the thyroid and licorice for the adrenals, high-energy foods (bee pollen and barley greens), herbs for immune system weakness (eleuthero, barley greens, rose hips), and capsicum to stimulate circulation. It is a useful remedy for some children with ADHD.

Used For: ADD/ADHD, addictions (coffee, caffeine), circulation (poor), **endurance, exercise (performance)**, and fatigue

Affects: Epinephrine and **parasympathetic-dominant ANS**

Take 2 capsules with breakfast and lunch, or whenever extra energy is needed.

Ingredients: Bee pollen, eleuthero root, gotu kola aerial parts, licorice root, schisandra fruit, and kelp leaf & stem

Vanilla
Sweet Herb

Vanilla planifolia

Derived from the bean pods of orchids native to Mexico, vanilla is best known as a flavoring agent. The Aztecs started using it in 1500s. It has some valuable medicinal properties. Pure vanilla extract is a great remedy for burns. It quickly eases pain and helps the burn to heal more quickly.

In old medicinal literature, vanilla is described as an aphrodisiac. It may also have positive effects on digestion and help to reduce fevers. Vanilla increases levels of catecholamines (including adrenaline).

Look for *vanilla* in *Relaxing* and *Soothing EO Formula*

Energetics: Mildly constricting, balancing, and cooling

Used For: Burns & scalds, fatigue, fever, indigestion, and sex drive (low)

Properties: Analgesic, antibacterial, aphrodisiac, carminative, febrifuge, and vulnerary

Vein Tonic Formula

These formulas contain herbs that help to tone up veins, reducing the tendency for varicose veins, bruising, phlebitis, and spider veins. They can reduce pain in the legs associated with standing for long periods or poor circulation in the legs. They can also be helpful for hemorrhoids. You can use the topical products and an internal formula together for better results.

Used For: Bruises, **capillary weakness**, circulation (poor), **easily bruised**, **hemorrhoids**, **phlebitis**, **spider veins**, strokes, thrombosis, and **varicose veins**

Affects: Capillaries, **circulatory relaxation**, **circulatory stagnation**, general relaxation, hepatic relaxation, rectum, and **veins**

Michael Tierra's Vein Cream

A more astringent vein cream. Apply topically.

Ingredients: Horse chestnut seed extract, butcher's broom leaf extract, witch hazel berry extract, white oak bark extract, myrrh gum extract, and rosemary EO

Michael Tierra's Vein Formula

An internal version of a vein tonic formula. Use 1 tablet twice daily between meals.

Ingredients: Horse chestnut skin extract, witch hazel bark, butcher's broom root, and ginkgo

Vein Tonic Formula

Internal formula for toning veins and improving circulation. Use 1–2 capsules two times daily with meals.

Ingredients: Vitamin C, horse chestnut standardized extract, fenugreek seed, rutin, and bioflavonoids

Vein Tonic Topical Cream

A topical cream for direct application to varicose veins or hemorrhoids. Apply topically to affected areas.

Ingredients: Menthol, melilot leaf extract, butcher's broom root extract, aloe vera leaf juice, and horse chestnut seed extract

Velvet Bean
Mildly Bitter & Sweet Herb

Mucuna pruriens

Velvet bean contains L-dopa which converts into dopamine, a neurotransmitter involved in motivation, sexuality, and co-ordination. Research suggests it can be helpful for Parkinson's disease. It is also helpful for male infertility and impotency.

Look for *velvet bean* in *Male Performance Formula*

Energetics: Neutral, balancing, and relaxing

Used For: Diabetes, dyspepsia, erectile dysfunction, infertility, and **Parkinson's disease**

Properties: Antioxidant, antivenomous, aphrodisiac, diuretic, and **dopamine-enhancing**

Venus Fly Trap
Sweet & Mildly Astringent Herb

Dionaea muscipula

Venus fly trap is used in malignant conditions such as tumors in advanced stages (mammary, bladder, prostate carcinomas and osteosarcoma) and solid tumors. It is also used for Hodgkin's and non-Hodgkin's lymphoma and other related conditions.

Warnings: Do not use during pregnancy.

Energetics: Cooling

Used For: Cancer and **lymphoma**

Properties: Analgesic, antimutagenic, antiviral, **cytotoxic**, and immune stimulant

Vervain, Blue
Mildly Acrid & Bitter Herb

Verbena hastata

Both vervain and blue vervain can be used internally to relax the nerves and combat anxiety. It is very helpful for nervous exhaustion from long-term stress or fanatical, hard-driving personalities and for people who suffer from neck and shoulder pain, feeling like they're tied up in knots. It's helpful for rage and women who suffer from anger and tension just before their period. It can alleviate some types of headaches, including migraines associated with PMS. Detail-oriented people who suffer from surface and peripheral nervous system problems and have neuralgias and skin problems may also benefit from blue vervain. It is beneficial for many spasmodic nervous disorders and acute viral diseases.

Look for *vervain (blue)* in *Antispasmodic Formula*

Warnings: Extremely large doses may cause nausea and vomiting. Large doses could potentially stimulate a miscarriage, although in normal doses blue vervain was used traditionally to protect against miscarriage.

Energetics: Mildly cooling, drying, and relaxing

Used For: Addictions (drugs), **adrenal fatigue**, anger (excessive), **anxiety attacks**, **anxiety disorders**, asthma, backache, **Bell's palsy**, bronchitis, chicken pox, cold hands/feet, colds, convalescence, cough (spastic), **croup**, Cushing's disease, **cystic fibrosis**, digestion (poor), diphtheria, epilepsy, **fever**, food poisoning, **headache (tension)**, hypertension, indigestion, insomnia, irritability, myasthenia gravis, nervous exhaustion, **neuralgia & neuritis**, parasites (nematodes, worms), Parkinson's disease, **perspiration (deficient)**, **pertussis**, phobias, **stiff neck**, **stress**, **teeth (grinding)**, **tics**, tonsillitis, Tourette's, tremors, and **whiplash**

Properties: Alterative, detoxifying, diaphoretic, diuretic, emetic, emmenagogue, expectorant, hypotensive, **nervine**, and relaxant

Vitamin A   *Vitamin*

Vitamin A is not a single compound but a family of fat-soluble compounds, including retinol, retinal, retinyl ester, and retinoic acid. We also use the term vitamin A to talk about certain plant compounds called carotenoids that are dietary precursors of retinol. Vitamin A has many actions. It helps control the gene expression that governs the growth of epithelial cells found in the skin and membranes. It is essential for maintaining membrane integrity and also aids the surface immune system by helping the production of IgA antibodies.

It is also essential for eye health, and many eye diseases may involve vitamin A deficiency. Vitamin A deficiencies are common in the developing world and even in America where less than 50 percent of Americans get the suggested RDA of vitamin A.

Dietary sources of vitamin A include butter, egg yolks, liver, seafood, and fish liver oils. It is commonly thought that beta carotene can be converted to vitamin A in sufficient quantities to supply your body's requirements. However, in several small studies, up to 45 percent of healthy people could not convert beta carotene to vitamin A. The conversion is also limited by several other factors, including a low-fat diet, low thyroid function, diabetes, zinc deficiency, inflammatory bowel disorders, and small bowel surgery. It is particularly impaired in infants and children. This is not to say beta-carotene is bad; carotenoids decrease your risk for many diseases. However, many people need to supplement with actual vitamin A, not just its plant precursors.

Warnings: The toxicity of vitamin A from foods and supplementation is exaggerated by most sources. In fact, in the thirty years that the National Poison Data System has been keeping records, not a single death has ever been reported from taking vitamins and supplements. There is an average of thirty to sixty cases of vitamin A overdose reported each year. Most of these cases are in alcoholics who are more prone to the damaging effects of vitamin A because of liver problems and other nutrient deficiencies. In all of the overdose cases, Vitamin A toxicity is completely reversible. The primary side effects associated with taking excess vitamin A are headaches, hair loss, red itchy skin, enlargement of the liver, and joint pain. If these symptoms occur discontinue taking vitamin A.

Usage: Use a dose of 1,000–10,000 IU daily depending on dietary consumption. The balance of vitamins A and D, along with EPA and DHA, make cod liver oil or fermented cod liver oil the preferred form for daily vitamin A supplementation (try the orange or lemon flavored products). For short term high dose supplementation, emulsified Vitamin A works well. Vitamin A, as with all fat-soluble vitamins, should be taken with a fatty meal. and To guarantee that your vitamin A is in the optimal range, especially during pregnancy, ask your doctor for a serum retinol test. This should be done early in pregnancy and several times throughout. You should aim for the medium high to high side of the blood reference range.

Used For: Acne, adenitis, **age spots**, allergies (respiratory), athlete's foot, autism, **bronchitis**, **cancer prevention**, cataracts, cervical dysplasia, **colds**, congestion (lungs), congestion (sinus), **conjunctivitis**, cystic breast disease, cysts, dermatitis, **eczema**, emphysema, endometriosis, **eye health**, **eyes (red/itching)**, **floaters**, **flu**, free radical damage, **glaucoma**, headache (sinus), **impetigo**, infection (bacterial), **infection (viral)**, **infection prevention**, leucorrhea, lyme disease, **lymphoma**, **macular degeneration**, malaria, **measles**, mental illness, metabolic syndrome, multiple sclerosis, **mumps**, **night blindness**, **pertussis**, poison ivy/oak, polyps, **psoriasis**, radiation, rashes & hives, **rosacea**, **seborrhea**, **shingles**, **sinus infection**, **skin (infections)**, skin problems, sore throat, spinal disks, **staph infections**, strep throat, **sty**, swollen lymph glands, tonsillitis, **tuberculosis**, **typhoid**, **ulcers**, **vaccine side effects**, and wrinkles

Vitamin B-Complex *Vitamin*

B-complex vitamins are essential for the formation of red blood cells, metabolism, nervous system function, promotes normal growth and metabolism of nutrients and proteins. They are needed for the synthesis of RNA and DNA, growth and division of cells, and fetal development, especially neural tube development. This group of vitamins also reduces blood levels of homocysteine, which is an amino acid that contributes to cardiovascular disease by damaging the endothelium (thin layer of cells that protect the artery walls).

Deficiencies of B vitamins in pregnant women may cause birth defects. Most of the B vitamins are excreted fairly quickly in the urine, so having a nutrient-dense diet or supplementing with B vitamins is essential for most people. Consider supplementation when dealing with high periods of stress, metabolic disease, or any nervous system disorder.

Usage: Take 1–3 capsules, three times a day, or as suggested on the label.

Used For: Acid indigestion, acne, addictions, **addictions (coffee, caffeine)**, **addictions (drugs)**, **addictions (sugar/carbohydrates)**, **addictions (tobacco)**, alcoholism, Alzheimer's, amenorrhea, anger (excessive), anorexia, anxiety (situational), anxiety disorders, apathy, asthma, **autism**, **Bell's palsy**, **birth control side effects**, body odor, **burning feet/hands**, burning feet/hands, cancer, **cancer treatment side effects**, canker sores, carpal tunnel, cholesterol (low), cirrhosis of the liver, cloudy thinking, cold sores, concentration (poor), copper toxicity, cramps (leg), **Cushing's disease**, cystic fibrosis, dandruff, **dementia**, dental health, **depression**, dizziness, down syndrome, dyspepsia, eczema, **epilepsy**, **fatigue**, fear, **fingernail biting**, Graves' disease, grief & sadness, hair (graying), hangover, **headache**, headache (tension), heart fibrillation/palpitations, **hypochondria**, hypotension, **hysteria**, inflammatory bowel disorders, insomnia, itching, lupus, **mania**, **memory/brain function**, **menopause**, **mental illness**, metabolic syndrome, **mitochondrial dysfunction**, mitral valve, morning sickness, **multiple sclerosis**, **muscular dystrophy**, myasthenia gravis, **narcolepsy**, nausea & vomiting, **nerve damage**, **nervous exhaustion**, **nervousness**, **neuralgia & neuritis**, numbness, OCD, pancreatitis, paralysis, Parkinson's disease, peripheral neuropathy, pernicious anemia, phobias, PMS Type C, PMS Type S, psoriasis, PTSD, Raynaud's disease, **restless leg**, **schizophrenia**, sore/geographic tongue, **stress**, surgery (preparation), surgery (recovery), tics, tinnitus, Tourette's, **trauma**, uric acid retention, and vitiligo

Properties: Adrenal tonic, nervine, and nutritive

Vitamin B1 (Thiamine) *Vitamin*

Thiamine is a water-soluble B vitamin that is required for the metabolism of fats, carbohydrates, and amino acids. Thiamine is used in every cell of the body to make ATP and aids in the production of acetylcholine and GABA. It is necessary to maintain and repair myelin sheaths and is essential to the nervous system. A deficiency of thiamine can manifest as Wernicke-Korsakoff psychosis or beriberi. Dry beriberi is characterized by weight loss, intestinal pain and constipation, nerve damage, sleep disturbance, and memory loss. Wet Beriberi causes cardiac failure, congestive heart disease, edema, and palpitations.

A thiamine deficiency was thought to only occur in severe malnutrition and alcoholism. However we now know that many drugs deplete thiamine and a diet high in simple carbohydrates and processed food, gastrointestinal surgery, dialysis, longer-term diuretic use, and cancer can all lead to a deficiency. Supplementing with thiamine can improve mood, peripheral neuropathy, memory, congestive heart failure, and multiple sclerosis.

Usage: 50–200 mg daily, normally as part of a B-complex.

Used For: Alcoholism, burning feet/hands, cataracts, **congestive heart failure**, heart weakness, insect repellant, memory/brain function, **mitochondrial dysfunction**, multiple sclerosis, myasthenia gravis, numbness, **peripheral neuropathy**, and tremors

Vitamin B12 *Vitamin*

B_{12} is essential for the normal formation of red blood cells, metabolism, and the nervous system. It acts as a cofactor or essential component in DNA synthesis. This makes B_{12} important for the production of all cells in the body, the development of red blood cells, normal myelination or covering of nerve cells and the production of neurotransmitters. The current accepted blood level range for B_{12} in the US is 200–900 ng/ml. Many experts think this is far too low, and standard ranges in most of Europe and Japan are 550–1800 ng/ml. When using these more appropriate healthy ranges, studies find that almost 40 percent of Americans, regardless of age or diet are deficient in B_{12}.

B_{12} is not found in plant foods, so vegetarians and vegans are more prone to B_{12} deficiency. Other factors like intestinal dysbiosis, gut inflammation, low stomach acid, excessive alcohol consumption, pernicious anemia, and acid-suppressing drugs can also cause a B_{12} deficiency. If you have memory loss, fatigue upon waking, tingling or numbness in the fingers or toes, cardiovascular disease, depression, migraines, infertility, cancer, or any autoimmune disease you should get your B_{12} levels checked.

Usage: The most common form of B12 on the market is cyanocobalamin. This is a cheap synthetic form of B12. Supplementation with methylcobalamin is preferable at a dose of 5,000 mcg sublingually a day. If your serum B12 level is below 350 or your MCV is over 96, shots of methylcobalamin are often necessary.

Used For: **Adrenal fatigue**, AIDS, **Alzheimer's**, **anemia**, anxiety disorders, body odor, **burning feet/hands**, canker sores, **celiac disease**, cervical dysplasia, cholesterol (low), cystic fibrosis, dehydration, **depression**, dermatitis, diabetes, dizziness, down syndrome, **epilepsy**, **fatigue**, hair loss/thinning, hangover, headache (cluster), heart fibrillation/palpitations, **hemochromatosis**, **memory/brain function**, methylation (under), **multiple sclerosis**, nervousness, **neuralgia & neuritis**, **numbness**, **paralysis**, **peripheral neuropathy**, **pernicious anemia**, **Raynaud's disease**, restless leg, **schizophrenia**, **sore/geographic tongue**, tics, tinnitus, Tourette's, tremors, and **vitiligo**

Properties: Nutritive

Vitamin B2 (Riboflavin)   *Vitamin*

Riboflavin is a B vitamin used in many pathways of the body and helps the breakdown of fats, carbohydrates, and amino acids. Overt deficiency is not common in the US because riboflavin is found in a variety of foods and is added to many foods. However around 10 percent of the population shows signs of a subclinical deficiency, most likely due to malabsorption issues. It takes three to eight months of inadequate dietary intake for clinical signs and symptoms to appear. Symptoms of a riboflavin deficiency include cracked lips and sides of the mouth, painful inflammation of the tongue and mouth, sore throat, dry skin, and iron deficient anemia. Those with anemia, elevated homocysteine levels, migraines, cataracts, and carpal tunnel syndrome should consider supplementing with B_2.

Usage: 30–50 mg daily, normally as part of a B-complex; 400 mg daily to help prevent migraines.

Used For: Anemia, carpal tunnel, cataracts, **headache (migraine)**, and myasthenia gravis

Vitamin B3 (Niacin)   *Vitamin*

Vitamin B_3 or niacin is an important nutrient for a variety of functions in the body. A severe niacin deficiency manifest as a disease called pellagra. Pellagra is characterized by the four Ds: diarrhea, dermatitis, dementia and death. While pellagra is less common now than one hundred years ago thanks to the fortification of foods, it still exists, and its early symptoms are often overlooked. In addition to reversing pellagra, niacin helps improve circulation, as evidenced by the red flushing of the skin from capillaries dilating when a big dose of niacin is taken. It also helps lower cholesterol and is used as a prescription drug for its cholesterol-lowering effects.

Niacinamide, the form of B_3 that doesn't cause skin flushing, doesn't seem to help with circulation, but it does help prevent pancreas cell damage from type 1 diabetes, while improving joint function in people with arthritis. Niacinamide also has a long history of use in treating schizophrenia. Psychiatric journals from the 1940's showed many people with schizophrenia being cured when food began being fortified with niacin. Since then studies have shown conflicting results using niacinamine for schizophrenia. It appears that when given in high doses in the initial stages of schizophrenia, niacinamide can prove an effective cure, but people who have had schizophrenia for a long time don't see any improvement with supplementation. Niacinamide also helps with skin disorders, the metabolism of nutrients, and the production of hydrochloric acid.

Warnings: A flushing (reddening) can occur when taking niacin, but this is harmless and passes. Avoid high amounts if you have gout, peptic ulcer, glaucoma, liver disease, or diabetes, or if you are pregnant. Taking too much niacinamide can cause nausea, heartburn, vomiting, flatulence, and diarrhea.

Usage: For circulatory issues or high cholesterol, start with 50 mg of niacin (nicotinic acid) three times a day. Once a week increase your dose by 50 mg three times daily until you reach 200 mg three times daily. Niacin (in the form of nicotinic acid) should not be taken if you drink alcohol or have liver disease, stomach ulcers or gout. Niacin can cause an elevation of liver enzymes and liver damage in high doses. For type 1 diabetes, schizophrenia, and arthritis, niacinamide (a flush-free form of niacin) is used in doses ranging from 1.75 grams to 3.5 milligrams daily. The dosage for children with diabetes is 150–300 mg per year of age, up to 3 grams daily.

Used For: Addictions (drugs), alcoholism, Alzheimer's, **arteriosclerosis**, arthritis (rheumatoid), backache, cataracts, cholesterol (high), **cholesterol (high)**, circulation (poor), cold hands/feet, depression, diabetes, fatigue, halitosis, headache (migraine), hypertension, mental illness, osteoporosis, postpartum depression, **schizophrenia**, sore/geographic tongue, stress, and teeth (grinding)

Vitamin B5 (Pantothenic Acid) *Vitamin*

Vitamin B_5 is essential for the production of coenzyme A, an enzyme responsible for cellular energy production and liver detoxification. It also aids in the formation of some fats, participates in energy metabolism, plays a role in the formation of antibodies, and is important for the production of adrenal hormones. Dietary pantothenic acid is found in a wide variety of foods including meats, vegetables, and fruits, making a deficiency rare. However supplemental pantothenic acid has been shown to help with stress, adrenal health, acne, arthritis, chronic fatigue, and Parkinson's.

Usage: Therapeutic dose is 50–100 mg.

Used For: Acne, ADD/ADHD, Addison's disease, **adrenal fatigue**, aging, anger (excessive), antibiotic side effects, anxiety disorders, arrhythmia, asthma, bedwetting, congestion (bronchial), cramps & spasms, Cushing's disease, dermatitis, eczema, fatigue, Graves' disease, hair (graying), hiccups, **hot flashes**, irritability, itching, menopause, nervous exhaustion, neuralgia & neuritis, **Parkinson's disease**, PTSD, seasonal affective disorder, stress, surgery (recovery), tachycardia, and teeth (grinding)

Properties: Adrenal tonic and nutritive

Vitamin B6 (Pyridoxine)   *Vitamin*

B_6 is the primary cofactor for over one hundred enzymes that control amino acid metabolism. It is responsible for producing many of the amine-based neurotransmitters and hormones, including serotonin, that the body uses to control mood and energy production. B_6 is also involved in the formation of antibodies, hemoglobin production, and sodium/phosphorus balance in the body. B_6 is found in a variety of foods, so severe deficiency is uncommon. However your body doesn't store B_6, so you need a constant supply from your diet.

Supplemental B_6 may help improve certain types of anemia, carpal tunnel syndrome, morning sickness, elevated homocysteine levels, and PMS. Elderly and alcoholics along with people that have liver disease, rheumatoid arthritis, type 1 diabetes, and those infected with HIV are most prone to a B_6 deficiency. The metabolically active and most safe form of vitamin B_6 is pyridoxal-5-phosphate (P5P).

Warnings: High doses of pyridoxine hydrochloride can cause neuropathy. This is not been observed with P5P supplementation.

Usage: 50–100 mg three times daily. B6 is commonly taken as part of a B-complex.

Used For: Acne, anemia, anxiety disorders, autism, birth control side effects, breasts (swelling/tenderness), breasts (swelling/tenderness), burning feet/hands, **carpal tunnel**, cramps (leg), **cramps (menstrual)**, dental health, depression, diabetes, estrogen (low), fatigue, **hemochromatosis**, kidney stones, lyme disease, **mental illness**, **methylation (over)**, methylation (under), morning sickness, motion sickness, nausea & vomiting, **OCD**, peripheral neuropathy, **PMS**, **PMS Type A**, PMS Type C, **PMS Type D**, **PMS Type H**, **psoriasis**, puberty, and sore/geographic tongue

Properties: Adrenal tonic, nervine, and nutritive

Vitamin B9 (Folic Acid, Folate)   *Vitamin*

Folic acid or vitamin B_9 is a water soluble member of the B-vitamin family. Folic acid technically refers to the synthetic compound used in dietary supplements and food fortification. Folate is the correct term for the naturally occurring tetrahydrofolate derivatives found in food. Folic acid must undergo reduction and methylation in the liver utilizing the enzyme dihydrofolate reductase, unlike natural folates that are metabolized in the small intestines. The reduced activity of dihydrofolate reductase in the liver, combined with ingesting high levels of folic acid in fortified foods may result in high levels of synthetic folic acid in the body.

Epidemiological studies have linked elevated levels of synthetic folic acid in the body to an increase in all forms of cancer. If you supplement with folic acid, by itself or in a multi, it is best to take products that contain 5-MTHF or folate, not folic acid.

Folate prevents and treats folate deficient megaloblastic anemia, helps prevent neural tube defects, reduces miscarriages and reduces the risk of colorectal and cervical cancer. Folate also reduces homocysteine levels, decreasing cardiovascular risk, and improves age-related cognitive decline.

Warnings: Avoid high doses in hormone-related cancer or convulsive disorders.

Usage: B9 is readily available in green leafy vegetables and organ meats, particularly liver. Unless folate levels are low (easily checked with blood work), most people don't need to supplement. Women trying to become pregnant, and pregnant women should supplement with 800–1,000 mcg of 5-MTHF daily. Dosage to reduce homocysteine levels range from 2–5 mg daily. Women with cervical dysplasia should supplement with 10 mg of 5-MTHF daily. Supplementing with folate might mask an underlying B12 deficiency. It is advisable to supplement with B12 and folate together, as in the Methy.

Used For: Anemia, angina, anxiety disorders, arteriosclerosis, autism, **birth defect prevention**, **burning feet/hands**, cancer, canker sores, cardiovascular disease, cataracts, **cervical dysplasia**, cholesterol (low), depression, dizziness, **down syndrome**, gingivitis, hearing loss, **hemochromatosis**, insomnia, macular degeneration, memory/brain function, **mental illness**, methylation (under), **numbness**, **peripheral neuropathy**, pernicious anemia, polyps, **pregnancy**, **restless leg**, **schizophrenia**, **sore/geographic tongue**, and **vitiligo**

Vitamin C   *Vitamin*

Vitamin C is extremely important for tissue integrity (healthy gums, wound healing, etc.), adrenal function (stress, fatigue), the immune system, and much more. Vitamin C acts as an antioxidant, protecting the body from the oxidative damage linked to heart disease, diabetes, and many chronic inflammatory conditions. Consuming vitamin C from foods or supplements increases iron absorption and the healing rate of wounds and burns. Vitamin C also stabilizes mast cells and improves immune function, reducing allergic reactions, and when taken daily shortens the duration of common viral infections like colds. Vitamin C in very high doses might play a positive role in cancer treatment.

Unlike most mammals, humans don't synthesize their own vitamin C and must obtain it from their diet. Aspirin, most pain medications, alcohol, some antidepressants, steroids, and oral contraceptives may reduce vitamin C levels in the body.

Usage: 250–10,000 mg daily. Vitamin C may be taken to bowel tolerance, meaning you can increase the dose until it starts causing diarrhea. If diarrhea occurs with large doses of vitamin C reduce the dose until the diarrhea stops.

Used For: Abrasions/scratches, abscesses, addictions (coffee, caffeine), addictions (drugs), addictions (tobacco), Addison's disease, adenitis, **adrenal fatigue**, age spots, alcoholism, **allergies (respiratory)**, ALS, anemia, anger (excessive), apathy, appendicitis, appetite (deficient), arteriosclerosis, athlete's foot, autism, backache, bites & stings, bladder infection, bleeding (external), bleeding (internal), blood in urine, blood poisoning, broken bones, **burns & scalds**, cadmium toxicity, **cancer prevention**, cancer treatment side effects, **capillary weakness**, **cardiovascular disease**, cartilage damage, cataracts, cervical dysplasia, colds, colon (atonic), congestion, copper toxicity, cough, cough (damp), cough (spastic), COVID-19, cystic breast disease, dermatitis, **diabetic retinopathy**, **easily bruised**, electromagnetic pollution, **eye health**, eyes (red/itching), eyes, bloodshot, fatigue, fear, **floaters**, **free radical damage**, **gangrene**, **gingivitis**, **glaucoma**, grief & sadness, hemochromatosis, **hemorrhoids**, hepatitis, hypertension, infection (bacterial), **infection (viral)**, **infection prevention**, injuries, **insomnia**, irritability, jaundice (adults), labor & delivery, leaky gut, leukemia, ligaments (torn/injuried), lupus, lyme disease, **lymphoma**, **macular degeneration**, **meningitis**, mental illness, mercury poisoning, metabolic syndrome, **mitochondrial dysfunction**, myasthenia gravis, **nosebleeds**, osteoporosis, **overalkalinity**, Parkinson's disease, peripheral neuropathy, pernicious anemia, pertussis, phobias, pleurisy, PMS Type S, pneumonia, poison ivy/oak, poisoning, polyps, postpartum weakness, **preeclampsia**, prolapsed colon, prolapsed uterus, psoriasis, **rhinitis**, **schizophrenia**, **scurvy**, **sinus infection**, skin (infections), skin problems, **sleep apnea**, snakebite, sore throat, **spider veins**, sprains, **staph infections**, strep throat, **stress**, **stretch marks**, strokes, sun-

burn, **surgery (preparation)**, **surgery (recovery)**, **teeth (loose)**, tick, tonsillitis, tooth extraction, **tuberculosis**, **typhoid**, **ulcerations (external)**, **ulcers**, **vaccine side effects**, **varicose veins**, vitiligo, warts, **wounds & sores**, and wrinkles

Properties: Adrenal tonic, adrenergic, antiabortive, **antiallergenic**, antibacterial, antihistamine, **antioxidant**, **antiscorbutic**, antiseptic, antitoxic, antivenomous, hepatoprotective, mast cell stabilizer, nutritive, vascular tonic, and vulnerary

Vitamin D   *Vitamin*

Vitamin D is a fat-soluble vitamin that the body naturally synthesizes during exposure to sunlight. Vitamin D is primarily known for its role in promoting calcium absorption from the intestinal tract. It helps to maintain adequate levels of calcium and phosphorus in the blood to enable the mineralization of bone. Without sufficient vitamin D, bones become thin, brittle, or misshapen. A severe deficiency produces the disease known as rickets in children and osteomalacia in adults. Vitamin D is needed to prevent osteoporosis in the elderly as well.

However, the benefits of vitamin D do not end with the role it plays in maintaining proper calcium and phosphorous levels for bone health. Vitamin D also affects the immune system. It promotes phagocytosis (anti-tumor activity) and helps modulate the immune system. Some evidence suggests it may play a role in protecting the body against cancer. Insufficient levels of vitamin D may also be linked to an increased susceptibility to other chronic diseases. Since wintertime levels

Supplemental vitamin D is found in two forms, vitamin D_2 and vitamin D_3. Vitamin D_2 is not naturally present in the human body and has actions within the body different than those of vitamin D_3. Vitamin D_3 is formed in Vitamin D_3 is the form of vitamin D that the body naturally produces and is most effective at treating vitamin D deficiency. Adequate vitamin D_3 blood levels have been shown to help prevent osteoporosis and bone loss, diabetes, cancer, low thyroid, and autoimmune disorders. Expert opinions vary on what an adequate blood level of vitamin D_3 is. A review of the published literature shows that a blood level of 35-45 ng/ml is the ideal range for most people.

Warnings: Blood levels of vitamin D over 70 ng/ml show no concrete benefits and increase your risk of kidney stones.

Usage: The dose of supplemental vitamin D3 varies. Some people, with normal sun exposure, only need 2000 IU a day of D3. However some people require up yo 10,000 IU daily to achieve adequate blood levels. It's best to supplement with 5,000 IU daily of vitamin D3 and after one month check your blood level. If your blood level of vitamin D is too low, increase your dose. If your blood level is too high, decrease your dose. Vitamin D3 and all other fat soluble vitamins absorb better when taken with the largest meal of the day.

Used For: Abscesses, **acne**, addictions, adenitis, **adrenal fatigue**, age spots, **ALS**, arteriosclerosis, arthritis, **arthritis (rheumatoid)**, athlete's foot, autism, autoimmune disorders, **broken bones**, bronchitis, **calcium deficiency**, **cancer prevention**, **cancer treatment side effects**, colds, congestion (sinus), conjunctivitis, cough (damp), **COVID-19**, croup, cystic breast disease, cysts, **dental health**, depression, dermatitis, **diabetes**, down syndrome, eczema, emphysema, **endometriosis**, floaters, **flu**, **free radical damage**, gingivitis, glaucoma, **Hashimoto's disease**, **headache (sinus)**, hypertension, impetigo, infection (bacterial), infection (viral), **infection prevention**, insomnia, leucorrhea, leukemia, **lupus**, **lyme disease**, **lymphoma**, **macular degeneration**, **menopause**, mental illness, mitochondrial dysfunction, **multiple sclerosis**, **mumps**, nervousness, **osteoporosis**, **peripheral neuropathy**, **pertussis**, poison ivy/oak, polyps, **psoriasis**, radiation, rashes & hives, **rosacea**, **schizophrenia**, **seasonal affective disorder**, seborrhea, skin (infections), skin problems, sore throat, spinal disks, **staph infections**, **sty**, swollen lymph glands, Tourette's, **tuberculosis**, **typhoid**, **vaccine side effects**, vitiligo, and wrinkles

Properties: Anticancer and nutritive

Vitamin E   *Vitamin*

Vitamin E refers to a family of fat-soluble vitamins called tocopherols. Alpha-tocopherol is considered the most active form of Vitamin E, but plants also contain beta-, gamma- and delta-tocopherol, all of which have beneficial actions. Vitamin E's primary action is to prevent oxidative damage to cell membranes, but vitamin E also prevents the oxidation of polyunsaturated fatty acids, helps control gene expression, and inhibits platelets from sticking together.

While studies have found that people who consume more vitamin E from foods have less heart disease, studies have also shown that supplementing with d-alpha-tocopherol doesn't seem to increase longevity or decrease heart disease. Small studies indicate that supplementing with mixed tocopherols, instead of just d-alpha-tocopherol, might reduce heart disease in addition to improving blood flow in intermittent claudication. Vitamin E taken with selenium may reduce the risk of blood clotting. Vitamin E is protective against prostate, bladder, and colon cancer.

Warnings: Use caution when taking Vitamin E with prescription blood thinners.

Usage: 400–800 IU daily of mixed tocopherols.

Used For: Abrasions/scratches, age spots, aging, ALS, angina, arteriosclerosis, **blood clot prevention**, breast lumps, breasts (swelling/tenderness), burns & scalds, cancer treatment side effects, cardiac arrest, **cardiovascular disease**, cataracts, chicken pox, circulation (poor), copper toxicity, **corns**, **cradle cap**, cramps (menstrual), croup, cuts, **cystic breast disease**, dandruff, denture sores, dermatitis, eczema, endometriosis, erectile dysfunction, eye health, fibroids (uterine), **fibrosis**, **free radical damage**, glaucoma, Hashimoto's disease, heart fibrillation/palpitations, hemorrhoids, **Huntington's disease**, hypertension, infertility, itching, menopause, miscarriage prevention, mitochondrial dysfunction, multiple sclerosis, muscle tone, muscular dystrophy, myasthenia gravis, narcolepsy, neurodegenerative diseases, nursing, Parkinson's disease, **peripheral neuropathy**, Peyronie's disease, **phlebitis**, PMS, PMS Type H, **psoriasis**, restless leg, rosacea, **scars/scar tissue**, sex drive (low), skin problems, stretch marks, strokes, **surgery (recovery)**, **thrombosis**, and vaginal dryness

Properties: Anticoagulant, **antioxidant**, **antithrombotic**, cicatrizant, and nutritive

Vitamin K   *Vitamin*

Vitamin K refers to a family of fat-soluble vitamins that include K_1 and K_2. Vitamin K_1 is found in a variety of green vegetables and is essential for normal blood clotting. Healthy gut bacteria can transform K_1 into K_2, and new research suggest that K_1 to K_2 conversion can occur in the testes, pancreas, and arterial walls as well. K_2 helps with blood clotting as well as playing an important role in bone and immune health.

There are several subtypes of K_2, the most researched being MK4 and MK7. MK4 is the most common type of K_2 that the body creates from K_1. MK4 strengthens the bones and prevents fractures and bone loss from normal aging as well as bone loss associated with steroid medications, anorexia, post-menopausal bone loss, and cirrhosis of the liver. MK7, the form of K_2 derived from fermented soy (natto), seems to have some of the beneficial actions on bone health as MK4. Both MK4 and MK7 in sufficient doses seem to prevent and even reverse the deposition of calcium in the arteries associated with heart disease.

Vitamin K_2 (MK4) has a strong action on the immune system. In several studies K_2 (MK4) was found both in test tubes and in humans to reduce the growth of several types of cancer. Broad-spectrum antibiotics, aspirin, and the fat substitute Olestra reduce the synthesis of Vitamin K in the gut.

Usage: The standard dose for the treatment of osteoporosis in studies is 45 mg of K2 daily. However doses as small as

1.5 mg of K2 a day help prevent osteoporosis in healthy people. The normal dose in studies for cancer ranges from 25–140 mg daily of K2, but the most common dose is 45 mg a day of K2. Vitamin K1 and K2, even at very high doses, have no known toxicity. There is a possibility that a high intake of vitamin A and/or vitamin E could interfere with vitamin K utilization, but more studies are needed to confirm this. Vitamin K1 and to a lesser extent, K2 interfere and should not be taken with blood thinning medications that are vitamin K antagonist (such as warfarin). Vitamin K1 and K2 do not interfere with heparin, antiplatelet agents (aspirin, Plavix etc.) and direct thrombin inhibitors (hirudin, argatoban).

Used For: **Broken bones**, **calcium deficiency**, calcium deposits, **dental health**, down syndrome, gingivitis, Hashimoto's disease, **osteoporosis**, and swollen lymph glands

Properties: Coagulant

Vulnerary Formula

These formulas are best used topically as a poultice (see *Poultice* strategy). Apply the poultice to swellings, minor injuries, and minor injuries to promote healing. Poultices should be changed at least twice a day. Taken internally, they can also aid tissue healing, having cooling soothing effects.

See the strategy *Poultice* for suggested uses.

Used For: **Abrasions/scratches**, arthritis, bites & stings, broken bones, cartilage damage, colitis, cuts, dislocation, diverticulitis, **hernias**, **injuries**, **ligaments (torn/injuried)**, menorrhagia, **spinal disks**, sprains, surgery (preparation), **surgery (recovery)**, tendonitis, ulcers, and **wounds & sores**

Affects: Bones, **general atrophy**, intestinal atrophy, lungs, mucous membranes, **muscles**, respiratory atrophy, **skin**, and spinal discs

Bone and Skin Formula

May be helpful for healing injuries such as broken bones and sprains. Use as a poultice or take 2–3 capsules two or three times daily.

Ingredients: Plantain leaf, rehmannia root, mullein leaf, and yarrow aerial parts

Stan Malstrom's Poultice Blend

Primarily for healing the mucus membranes of the GI tract and respiratory system. The best choice for making a poultice for topical application. Helpful for respiratory and digestive irritation. Use as a poultice or take 2–3 capsules two or three times daily.

Ingredients: Slippery elm bark, marshmallow root, goldenseal root & rhizome, and fenugreek seed

Watkin's Hair, Skin, and Nails Formula

See also *Joan Patton's Herbal Minerals Formula*

This formula contains two of the richest sources of organic silicon in the plant kingdom, horsetail and dulse. (See *silicon* for more information.) It is helpful for strengthening structural tissues like skin, hair, bones, and joints. It is also helpful for the nervous system. The other two ingredients, sage and rosemary, are antioxidants for the brain and nerves. They also enhance acetylcholine, the neurotransmitter responsible for memory. This is a great supplement for people to take as they grow older to keep both their brain and their structural system healthy. It may also help with parathyroid and pineal gland problems.

Used For: **Aluminum toxicity**, **arthritis**, bleeding (internal), **blood in urine**, **broken bones**, **calcium deficiency**, **calcium deposits**, capillary weakness, cramps (leg), dandruff, **dental health**, **dislocation**, eczema, **fingernail biting**, **fingernails (weak/brittle)**, **hair loss/thinning**, hemochromatosis, injuries, memory/brain function, menopause, **multiple sclerosis**, **nerve damage**, **osteoporosis**, Parkinson's disease, pregnancy, scoliosis, **skin problems**, **surgery (preparation)**, surgery (recovery), **teeth (grinding)**, vitiligo, and wrinkles

Affects: Acetylcholine, **bones**, brain, brain atrophy, **central nervous system**, **general relaxation**, **hair**, joints, **nails**, **parathyroid**, **pineal**, **skin**, structural relaxation, and urinary relaxation

Take 1–2 capsules two to three times per day.

Ingredients: Horsetail stem & strobilus, dulse fronds, rosemary leaf, and sage leaf

Weight Loss Cleansing Program

This cleanse was designed for the beginning of a weight loss program. It not only cleanses the colon, liver, and lymphatics, it also contains ingredients to balance metabolism.

Warnings: Do not use if diarrhea, loose stools, or abdominal pain are present or develop. Not intended for prolonged use.

Used For: **Excess weight** and leaky gut

Affects: Large intestines (colon)

As a cleanse to begin a weight loss program, take the contents of one (1) AM packet with breakfast, one (1) PM packet with evening meal with 8 oz. of pure water daily for seven days.

Ingredients: Intestinal detoxification formula, general glandular formula, environmental detoxifying formula, paavo airola's liver cleanse, stan malstrom's lower bowel formula, chromium blend, and skinny formula

White Oak   *Astringent Herb*

Quercus alba

A powerful astringent, white oak bark is used internally for hemorrhoids and varicose veins. A decoction can be used as a rectal injection for hemorrhoids or as a douche to stop bleeding. The decoction can also be used as a fomentation for swelling, varicose veins, and other injuries and as a gargle for sore throat or a mouthwash for bleeding gums. Use white oak bark powder with black walnut powder as a tooth powder for bleeding gums and loose teeth. The powder may be sprinkled into cuts to stop bleeding.

Look for *white oak* in *Drawing Salve*, *Herbal Tooth Powder*, and *Vein Tonic Formulas*

Warnings: Can be constipating when taken internally. Can interfere with digestion (take between meals). Contains large amounts of tannin, which may be associated with mouth and stomach cancer with consistent, long-term use. Use only for short periods internally. No warnings for external use.

Energetics: Drying and constricting

Used For: Anal fistula/fissure, bedwetting, **bites & stings**, bleeding (external), blood in stool, **blood in urine**, colon (atonic), cuts, **dental health**, diarrhea, **gingivitis, hemorrhoids**, injuries, menorrhagia, nervous exhaustion, oral surgery, phlebitis, poison ivy/oak, prolapsed colon, prolapsed uterus, **sprains, teeth (loose)**, tonsillitis, **tooth extraction, varicose veins**, and wounds & sores

Properties: Anticarious, antidiarrheal, antiemetic, antiseptic, antivenomous, **astringent**, dentifrice, hemostatic, styptic, and vermifuge

White Pond Lily   *Astringent Herb*

Nymphaea odorata

A cooling and constricting remedy, white pond lily and white water lily (*N. alba*) have been used to reduce restlessness, inflammation, and irritation in tissues. They also have a calming effect on libido (sex drive).

Energetics: Cooling and constricting

Used For: Prolapsed uterus, sex drive (excessive), and vaginal dryness

Properties: Anaphrodisiac, anti-inflammatory, astringent, and **uterine tonic**

White Sage

Aromatic & Mildly Astringent Herb

Salvia apiana

White sage is most commonly used for smudging and produces a delightful uplifting smoke. It can be applied locally to reduce pain and fight infection. Internally, it is used to aid BPH and prostatitis, as well as to dry up breast milk.

Energetics: Warming, drying, and mildly constricting

Used For: BPH, breast milk (surplus), laryngitis, **prostatitis**, and strep throat

Properties: Antiseptic and carminative

Whole Food Green Drink Formula

This bulk powder of whole foods and herbs is a convenient way to improve general nutrition or take as a meal replacement for a weight loss program. It is good for balancing the immune system and is a great nutritional supplement for pregnancy.

Used For: Aging, AIDS, anemia, appetite (excessive), **autoimmune disorders**, birth defect prevention, **body building**, body odor, **cancer, convalescence, debility**, failure to thrive, **infertility**, muscle tone, **overacidity, postpartum weakness, pregnancy**, psoriasis, puberty, triglycerides (high), and wasting

Affects: Hyperactive immune activity, immune system, muscles, **nails**, pancreatic irritation, and pituitary (anterior)

Mix 2 scoops in 8 to 12 ounces of water or juice once daily. (You may want to start with 1/2 scoop and work up to 2 scoops, as this product can be very detoxifying.)

Ingredients: Rice, flax seed, spirulina, quinoa, chia seed, chlorella, millet seed, alfalfa leaf, broccoli flower, kale leaf, asparagus stem, beet root, chicory root, and acerola fruit

Whole Food Protein Formula

Protein supplements containing herbs and whole foods can be useful for weight loss, body building, or general nutrition. A smoothie made with one of these whole food protein supplements is a good way to start the day for people who are too busy to eat breakfast. It helps set the metabolism for the day.

Used For: Appetite (excessive), **body building**, diabetes, **excess weight**, exercise (performance), hypoglycemia, **muscle tone, pregnancy, puberty**, and underweight

Affects: Brain, **muscles**, nails, and **pancreatic irritation**

Pea and Rice Protein Powder

Pea and rice protein powder with fiber, vitamins, minerals, and antioxidants. Dairy-free, lactose-free and gluten-free and vegan certified. Mix 2 level scoops (45 grams) with approximately 12–16 ounces of cold water or juice or use as part of a smoothie.

Ingredients: Pea protein, rice protein, adzuki bean powder, black bean powder, garbonzo bean flakes, flax seed, rice bran, and multi vitamins and minerals

Green Food Protein Powder

Pea and bean proteins with rice, blended with powdered fruits, vegetables and seeds. It provides essential fatty acids, fiber and 75% of the daily value (DV) for eighteen essential vitamins and minerals. Vegan, dairy-free, and lactose-free. Mix 2 level scoops (45 grams) with approximately 12–16 ounces of cold water or juice or use as part of a smoothie.

Ingredients: Pea protein, adzuki bean, black bean, garbonzo bean, rice protein, amaranth, brown rice grain, spirulina, quinoa, flax seed hull lignans, chia seed, chlorella, millet, rice, flax seed, and mulit vitamins and minerals

Wild Lettuce   *Bitter Herb*

Lactuca serriola

The milky sap of the wild lettuce contains a compound with a mild opiate-like activity that can help relieve pain. The dried herb has very little pain relieving activity, but does have some sedative activity. You need to tincture the fresh white sap to get a stronger pain-relieving effect. I've also blended the fresh leaves with alcohol to preserve the juice for a stronger analgesic action. The dried herb can aid sleep and reduce anxiety when combined with other herbs.

Energetics: Cooling and drying

Used For: Headache (tension), insomnia, and pain

Properties: Analgesic and anaphrodisiac

Wild Yam   *Sweet Herb*

Dioscorea villosa

Wild yam is a valuable antispasmodic and anti-inflammatory remedy. It has been used to ease menstrual cramps and ovarian pain, and is also helpful for irritable bowel and intestinal cramps (gripping). It has also been used in conditions like arthritis and neuralgia. Contrary to popular myth, wild yam is not a source of progesterone and is not a reliable herb for birth control. However, it does seem to tip the hormonal balance in women in favor of progesterone, especially when used in combination with herbs like chaste tree or false unicorn.

Look for *wild yam* in *Antispasmodic, DHEA with Herbs, Female Cycle,* and *Intestinal Soothing Formulas*

Warnings: Overdose may cause nausea, vomiting, and diarrhea.

Energetics: Cooling, mildly moistening, and relaxing

Used For: Appendicitis, **colic (adults)**, colon (spastic), **cramps (menstrual)**, cramps & spasms, dermatitis, diverticulitis, **dysmenorrhea**, estrogen dominance, **gallbladder problems**, **gallstones**, inflammation, inflammatory bowel disorders, irritable bowel, jaundice (adults), leaky gut, lupus, miscarriage prevention, neuralgia & neuritis, nocturnal emission, ovarian pain, and progesterone (low)

Properties: Analgesic, **anti-inflammatory**, antiemetic, antirheumatic, **antispasmodic**, cholagogue, contraceptive, diaphoretic, and diuretic

Willow   *Mildly Astringent & Sour Herb*

Salix spp.

Willow bark has long been used for pain, fevers, and inflammation. Its active compound, salicin, is the original source of the synthetic derivative aspirin. The action of white willow is much weaker than that of the synthetic drug, but is less likely to cause stomach problems. Willow generally works best at easing pain when combined with other analgesic herbs.

Look for *willow* in *Analgesic Nerve, Anti-Inflammatory Pain, General Analgesic,* and *Stan Malstrom's Herbal Aspirin Formulas*

Warnings: Avoid with ulcers or a weak digestive system. Avoid during pregnancy.

Energetics: Cooling and mildly drying

Used For: **Arthritis**, bursitis, fever, **headache**, **pain**, spinal disks, sprains, and tendonitis

Properties: Analgesic, anti-inflammatory, anticephalalgic, antiseptic, and **febrifuge**

Wintergreen EO

Minty, Sharp, Sweet, & Woody Essential Oil

Gaultheria procumbens

Wintergreen essential oil contains salicylic acid (a natural aspirin), which can help to reduce inflammation and pain. The plant itself has been taken internally as a tea to ease pain, but it is seldom used internally today. The oil of wintergreen, however, is frequently used as a topical analgesic and is a common ingredient in topical analgesic formulas.

See the strategy *Aromatherapy* for suggested uses.

Warnings: Do not use internally. May trigger contact dermatitis in some people, so dilute for topical use. People who are sensitive to aspirin should avoid wintergreen.

Energetics: Cooling

Used For: **Arthritis**, backache, congestion (sinus), cough, cramps & spasms, dislocation, exercise (recovery), gas & bloating, **headache**, hypertension, inflammation, **pain**, shock (medical), and tendonitis

Properties: Analgesic, **anesthetic**, anti-inflammatory, antirheumatic, antiseptic, antispasmodic, deodorant, diuretic, febrifuge, and relaxant

Women's Aphrodisiac Formula

This formula is used to support the female reproductive organs and to increase sexual desire in women. It will also have some general hormone balancing actions.

Warnings: Avoid during pregnancy.

Used For: Amenorrhea, infertility, and **sex drive (low)**

Take 2 capsules with a meal three times daily.

Ingredients: L-arginine, maca root extract, eleuthero root, oat straw, red raspberry leaf, and damiana leaf

Wood Betony *Aromatic & Sweet Herb*

Betonica officinalis or Stachys officinalis

Wood betony is an analgesic nervine that relaxes tension in the muscles. It is frequently used in formulas for headaches and is used to relieve middle back pain and tension, facial pain, and muscle tension. It is helpful for people whose minds are overactive and stressed and helps ease tension in one's thoughts and emotions.

Look for *wood betony* in *Analgesic Nerve Formula*

Warnings: Avoid during pregnancy.

Energetics: Cooling and relaxing

Used For: ADD/ADHD, backache, **Bell's palsy**, cramps & spasms, headache (migraine), headache (sinus), headache (tension), indigestion, nerve damage, neuralgia & neuritis, nosebleeds, Parkinson's disease, peripheral neuropathy, **stiff neck**, tics, tinnitus, **tremors**, twitching, and whiplash

Properties: Analgesic, anticephalalgic, antispasmodic, **nervine**, parasympathomimetic, and sedative

Wormwood *Fragrant Bitter Herb*

Artemisia absinthium

As the name implies, wormwood is a powerful antiparasitic herb used for expelling tapeworms and other intestinal worms and parasites. It is also used to stimulate digestion and appetite.

Look for *wormwood* in *Antiparasitic Formula*

Warnings: A very strong and potentially toxic herb, wormwood should not be used by pregnant women, nursing mothers, or weak, emaciated persons. It should only be used for short periods of time and preferably as part of a formula.

Energetics: Cooling and drying

Used For: Belching, **parasites**, **parasites (nematodes, worms)**, parasites (tapeworm), and pet supplements

Properties: Abortifacient, **anthelmintic**, **antiparasitic**, stomachic, and **vermifuge**

Xylitol *Food*

Xylitol is a useful sweetener that does not spike blood sugar levels. It is usually made from the fibers of corn husks or birch tree bark but can also be found in beets and other foods. Xylitol has been used in Europe and China for over twenty years and has an excellent track record for safety.

It has about the same sweetness as table sugar (sucrose) so it can substituted for equal amounts of sugar in most cases. It does have caloric value, but it has 40 percent fewer calories than sugar. It has a glycemic index of 7, which means it does not trigger insulin production. This means that xylitol can be used safely by both hypoglycemics and diabetics.

The bacteria which cause cavities and gum disease can't live on xylitol. This means that using xylitol regularly will actually reduce cavities and prevent gum disease. It helps the body bind calcium, which actually aids remineralization of the teeth and bones.

Xylitol also inhibits the bacteria that cause middle ear infections and sinus problems. It also helps reduce unfriendly bacteria in the intestines.

Warnings: Some people experience gas or diarrhea using xylitol because of the changes it makes in gut flora.

Used For: **Addictions (sugar/carbohydrates)**, **dental health**, dental health, diabetes, infection (fungal), and sinus infection

Properties: Antibacterial, antidiabetic, food, hypoglycemic, low glycemic, and sweetener

Yam, Chinese *Sweet Herb*

Dioscorea oppositifolia

Chinese yam is used in Chinese herbalism to support digestion and strengthen the lungs and kidneys. It acts as a tonic for general weakness and poor appetite.

Look for *yam (Chinese)* in *Chinese Earth-Increasing Formula*

Energetics: Mildly warming, nourishing, and balancing

Used For: Cough (dry), diabetes, diarrhea, and nocturnal emission

Properties: Nutritive and tonic

Yarrow

Aromatic, Astringent, & Mildly Fragrant Bitter Herb

Achillea millefolium

Yarrow's hemostatic properties (ability to stem bleeding) made it the medication of choice for treating war injuries in ancient times. The leaves may be applied topically to bleeding wounds, and the herb can be taken internally to stop internal bleeding.

Yarrow flowers are also a strong diaphoretic and are used to cool high fevers and help the body fight infection. A warm tea of yarrow is one of the best remedies for inducing a sweat and breaking a fever. Add a little peppermint to improve the flavor.

Look for *yarrow* in *Internal Bleeding, Lymphatic Infection, Paavo Airola's Cold, Steven Horne's Children's Composition,* and *Vulnerary Formulas*

Energetics: Cooling, drying, and constricting

Used For: Abrasions/scratches, abscesses, **aneurysm**, bites & stings, **bleeding (external)**, **bleeding (internal)**, blisters, **blood in stool**, blood in urine, **bruises**, capillary weakness, celiac disease, chicken pox, colds, colds (antiviral), **colds with fever**, COVID-19, **cuts**, diarrhea, **dysmenorrhea**, easily bruised, **fever**, **fibroids (uterine)**, **flu**, infection (fungal), infection (viral), inflammation, **injuries**, kidney infection, **measles**, meningitis, **menorrhagia**, mumps, **nosebleeds**, **perspiration (deficient)**, pleurisy, pneumonia, scars/scar tissue, **shingles**, skin (infections), swollen lymph glands, traumatic brain injury, vaccine side effects, varicose veins, and **wounds & sores**

Properties: Alterative, anti-inflammatory, antibacterial, antifungal, **antiphlogistic**, antiseptic, **antiviral**, **astringent**, cicatrizant, **coagulant**, **diaphoretic**, diuretic, emmenagogue, **febrifuge**, **hemostatic**, hypotensive, lymphatic, nervine, **parasympatholytic**, stimulant (metabolic), stomachic, **styptic**, tonic, uterine, and **vulnerary**

Yeast Cleansing Program

See also *Anti-Fungal Formula*

This is an effective cleanse for yeast and fungal overgrowth. This pack contains three antifungal products that reduce yeast overgrowth and enzymes that help break down dead yeast cells. Combined with some dietary changes, it can improve the balance of friendly flora in the digestive tract and improve overall health. Avoid sugar, white flour, and other refined carbohydrates when doing this cleanse. Eat more fresh fruits and vegetables.

Used For: Addictions (sugar/carbohydrates), antibiotic side effects, **athlete's foot**, **dysbiosis**, **infection (fungal)**, **itchy ears**, jock itch, **leucorrhea**, and **vaginitis**

Affects: **Chronic disease stage**, digestive stagnation, immune system, intestinal stagnation, and large intestines (colon)

There are two packets in this program. One contains Pau d'Arco and two Anti-Fungal Formulas. The other contains enzymes. Take the pack with the pau d'arco three times daily with meals and enzyme packet twice times daily between meals on an empty stomach.

Ingredients: Zinc, selenium, caprylic acid, pau d'arco bark, anti-fungal blend with caprylic acid, and anti-fungal formula

Yellow Dock   *Bitter & Mildly Sour Herb*

Rumex crispus

Yellow dock is high in organic iron compounds and liberates iron stored in the liver. This makes it useful for anemia, especially when combined with alfalfa, beets, and other iron-rich herbs. It is also used as a blood purifier for skin disorders (acne, boils, etc.) and general liver problems. It stimulates the flow of bile and acts as a mild laxative while reducing heat and irritation in the digestive tract. It is especially indicated where a person has a geographic tongue (a tongue with heavily coated patches and bare bright red areas) and intestinal inflammation with constipation.

Look for *yellow dock* in *Christopher's Herbal Iron, Gentle Bowel Cleansing, Herbal Bitters,* and *Liver Cleanse Formulas*

Warnings: Large doses can cause nausea and diarrhea.

Energetics: Cooling and mildly drying

Used For: **Acid indigestion**, acne, **anemia**, cancer, **chicken pox**, cholesterol (high), cirrhosis of the liver, constipation (adults), constipation (children), cysts, depression, diarrhea, gallbladder problems, hemochromatosis, hemorrhoids, hepatitis, inflammatory bowel disorders, **itching**, jaundice (adults), leprosy, myasthenia gravis, poison ivy/oak, pregnancy, **prolapsed colon**, **prolapsed uterus**, **rashes & hives**, **sore/geographic tongue**, and wounds & sores

Properties: Alterative, **antipruritic**, **aperient**, astringent, blood building, **cholagogue**, hepatic, laxative (gentle), and mineralizer

Yerba Maté

Mildly Astringent & Stimulant Bitter Herb

Ilex paraguariensis

An astringent and bitter herb containing caffeine. It is used primarily as a beverage to stimulate energy.

Look for *yerba maté* in *Blood Sugar Control* and *Metabolic Stimulant Formulas*

Warnings: Excessive consumption of caffeine can lead to anxiety, insomnia, and adrenal exhaustion.

Energetics: Warming, drying, and mildly constricting
Used For: Fatigue
Properties: Stimulant (metabolic) and sympathomimetic

Yerba Santa   *Pungent Herb*

Eriodictyon californicum

A warming and stimulating expectorant, yerba santa clears phlegm from the chest and opens air passages. It is a reliable herb for most respiratory problems but is especially helpful for asthma, profuse expectoration and respiratory complaints with obscure symptoms. It is also an effective diuretic and urinary antiseptic.

Look for *yerba santa* in *Damp Cough Syrup* and *Paavo Airola's Cold Formulas*

Energetics: Warming and drying

Used For: Allergies (respiratory), **asthma**, **bronchitis**, bruises, **congestion**, congestion (bronchial), congestion (lungs), **cough**, **cough (damp)**, cuts, laryngitis, poison ivy/oak, sinus infection, and urinary tract infections

Properties: Decongestant, **expectorant**, and pulmonary

Ylang Ylang EO   *Floral & Sweet Essential Oil*

Cananga odorata

This sweet, floral oil has a calming effect on the mind and body. It reduces the rapid breathing and heart rate associated with irritability and stress, producing a more calm, relaxed state. It is helpful for people who are too harsh on themselves. It opens up sensual feelings and is considered an aphrodisiac ylang ylang is a wonderfully exotic and enticing floral essential oil. The name ylang ylang means "flower of flowers." In Indonesia they spread the delicate and sweet-smelling flower petals on the bed of a newly married couple. Ylang ylang is a sweet flora scent that helps to balance the nervous system, inhibiting excess adrenal activity and symptoms of anxiety like rapid breathing and heart rate. It can be used in a massage oil for muscle cramps and spasms, high blood pressure, intestinal gas and diarrhea, PMS, and stress. It can be used in a shampoo to stimulate hair growth. It also stimulates breast growth.

Emotionally, ylang ylang arouses the senses and draws out sensuality and passion. It eases fear and anxiety and inspires confidence and joy. It replaces jealousy, doubt, frustration and guilt with a feeling of caring and contentment.

See the strategy *Aromatherapy* for suggested uses.

Warnings: Do not use internally. Nontoxic and nonirritating for topical use. Excessive use may lead to headaches and nausea.

Used For: Aging, anger (excessive), anxiety (situational), anxiety disorders, appetite (excessive), asthma, bites & stings, breasts (undersized), cardiovascular disease, colic (adults), cramps (leg), **cramps & spasms**, depression, diabetes, fatigue, **fear**, gas & bloating, hair loss/thinning, headache (migraine), heart fibrillation/palpitations, hypertension, indigestion, insomnia, menopause, mood swings, nervous exhaustion, nervousness, Peyronie's disease, PMS Type C, PTSD, sex drive (excessive), **sex drive (low)**, shame & guilt, skin (oily), skin problems, stress, and tachycardia

Properties: Anti-inflammatory, antibacterial, antidepressant, antiseptic, antispasmodic, **aphrodisiac**, cardiac, hypotensive, nervine, **sedative**, and sympatholytic

Yohimbe   *Stimulant Bitter Herb*

Pausinystalia yohimbe

Yohimbe causes dilation of blood vessels, including those in the genitalia, thus helping men to maintain an erection. This effect also lowers blood pressure.

Look for *yohimbe* in *Testosterone Formula*

Warnings: Avoid long term use, as it can irritate the urinary tract. Contraindicated in cases of emaciation or inflammation.

Energetics: Warming

Used For: Erectile dysfunction and sex drive (low)

Properties: Stimulant (circulatory) and vasodilator

Yucca   *Bitter Herb*

Yucca spp.

Yucca is a blood purifier with anti-inflammatory, antioxidant, antifungal and detergent properties. It is helpful as an analgesic and anti-inflammatory in arthritis, neuralgia, and other inflammatory conditions.

Warnings: Excessive consumption may cause diarrhea, nausea, upset stomach and vomiting. Use only under professional supervision during pregnancy.

Energetics: Cooling and moistening

Used For: Arthritis, arthritis (rheumatoid), **dermatitis**, eczema, fibromyalgia, **inflammation**, **lupus**, myasthenia gravis, **neuralgia & neuritis**, overacidity, and uric acid retention

Properties: Alterative, analgesic, **anti-inflammatory**, antirheumatic, antiseptic, and detergent

Zeaxanthin   *Phytochemical*

Zeaxanthin is one of the most common carotenoids found in nature. It is the pigment that gives paprika, corn, saffron, wolfberries, and many other plants their characteristic color.

Zeaxanthin is one of the two primary carotenoids contained within the retina of the eye. Within the central macula, zeaxanthin is the dominant component, whereas in the peripheral retina, lutein predominates. Several research studies have connected high dietary intake of foods providing zeaxanthin with a lower incidence of age-related macular degeneration (AMD).

Usage: The best way to obtain zeaxanthin is from dietary foods such as vegetables, fruits and berries.

Used For: Cataracts, eye health, free radical damage, glaucoma, and **macular degeneration**

Properties: Antioxidant

Zhu-Ling (Polyporus) *Sweet Herb*

Polyporus sclerotium

A parasitic herb that grows on oak and liquidambar trees that is used in Chinese herbalism as a tonic to the kidneys and bladder.

Energetics: Drying and cooling

Used For: Edema and leucorrhea

Properties: Anti-inflammatory, antibacterial, and diuretic

Zinc *Mineral*

Zinc is important for immune system function, male reproductive function and tissue healing. Zinc is essential for the production of superoxide dismutase, a potent antioxidant, and helps protect vitamin E stores and prevents LDL and VLDL oxidation. Severe deficiencies of zinc are rare but mild to moderate deficiency occurs regularly in children, the elderly, and those with eating disorders, diabetes, renal disease, and gastrointestinal disease. Zinc has been shown to help slow the progression of Alzheimer's, improve sperm count, reduce prostate swelling in BPH, and increase the speed of healing from both gastric ulcers and lower limb ulcers. Zinc also helps the body fight viral infections and helps in the production of calming neurotransmitters. Along with vitamin C it is essential for wound healing.

Warnings: Daily doses over 100 mg. can depress the immune system. Copper and zinc levels should be balanced.

Usage: 10–100 mg. If you supplement above 50 mg take 2 mg of copper to prevent a copper deficiency. Zinc supplementation can reduce the absorption of some antibiotics. Birth control medications and tetracycline can reduce zinc levels in the body. Take zinc supplements separate from acid-reducing medications.

Used For: Abrasions/scratches, acid indigestion, **acne**, ADD/ADHD, adenitis, aging, allergies (respiratory), anemia, anxiety disorders, appetite (deficient), arteriosclerosis, athlete's foot, body odor, **BPH**, burns & scalds, **cad-**mium toxicity, calcium deficiency, **cancer prevention**, cataracts, cervical dysplasia, cold sores, colds, **copper toxicity**, **COVID-19**, cramps & spasms, croup, cystic breast disease, dandruff, dermatitis, diabetes, diarrhea, **down syndrome**, eczema, **erectile dysfunction**, floaters, **flu**, free radical damage, gingivitis, Graves' disease, **hair (graying)**, hair loss/thinning, Hashimoto's disease, **hemochromatosis**, herpes, **hypothyroidism**, **infection (viral)**, **infection prevention**, inflammation, injuries, interstitial cystitis, laryngitis, **lead poisoning**, lupus, lyme disease, **macular degeneration**, **mental illness**, metabolic syndrome, **methylation (over)**, **methylation (under)**, mitochondrial dysfunction, **OCD**, osteoporosis, PMS Type C, pneumonia, premature ejaculation, prostatitis, psoriasis, **rosacea**, **schizophrenia**, sickle cell anemia, **smell (loss of)**, strep throat, **stretch marks**, **surgery (recovery)**, testosterone (low), tinnitus, **ulcerations (external)**, **ulcers**, **vaccine side effects**, vitiligo, and **wounds & sores**

Properties: Anxiolytic and virostatic

Aromatic Properties Appendix

This appendix contains the definition of the various properties used to describe the aroma and effects of essential oils.

Aromas

Balsamic: A sweet, but earthy aroma, like balsamic vinegar. The opposite of *minty*.

Camphorous: A camphor-like smell, the opposite of *earthy*.

Floral: A light, flowery smell. The opposite of *sharp*.

Fresh: A refreshing aroma, like the earth after a rain or the predawn morning. The opposite of *resinous*.

Fruity: A sweet, fruit-like aroma, such as found in oranges and pink grapefruit. The opposite of *spicy*.

Herbaceous: A grassy, hay-like, or green smell found in meadows and freshly mown lawns. The opposite of *woody*.

Minty: A smell like peppermint or spearmint, typically characteristic of members of the mint family. It is mildly stimulating and helps to wake up the mind and body. The opposite of *balsamic*.

Musky: A mossy or moldy smell. The opposite of *vaporous*.

Musky: A rich, deep dirt-like aroma. The opposite of *camphorous*.

Resinous: The earthy odor of resinous substances excreted by trees like pines and myrrh. The opposite of *fresh*.

Sharp: The sour citrus smell of lemons and limes. The opposite of *floral*.

Spicy: The odor of hot spices and pungent herbs. The opposite of *fruity*.

Sulfuric: The odor associated with garlic, onions and mustard due to the presence of sulfur compounds. The opposite of *sweet*.

Sweet: A pleasant, sugary aroma. The opposite of *sulfuric*.

Vaporous: A penetrating fragrance that has an opening, clearing effect. The opposite of *musky*.

Woody: The odor of cut trees and forests. The opposite of *herbacious*.

Aromatic Effects

Calming: Peaceful, flexible, relaxed, patient, tolerant, open hearted, yielding. Counters: Irritability, anger, impatience, feeling stressed, workaholic, intolerance, fanaticism, restlessness.

Ethereal: Qualities: Fluid, expansive, creative, imaginative, light, uplifted, open heart and mind. Counters: Rigidity, dogmatism, materialism, addiction, obsession, feeling stuck, uninspired.

Grounding: Solid, practical, realistic, solid, stable, firm, physically connected. Counters: Impractical, unrealistic, spacey, unaware, blinded, head in the clouds, ungrounded.

Invigorating: Enthusiastic, determined, outgoing, active, busy, driven, focused. Counters: lack of direction, being wishy-washy, overly pleasing or yielding to others, discouraged, low energy and motivation.

Refreshing: Qualities: Renewed, revived, replenished, awake, unburdened, open, emotional free, generous, giving. Counters: Self-pity, toxic shame, victim-hood, emotional paralysis, feeling burdened and weighed down, stifled, stingy.

Soothing: Relaxed, calm, restful, quiet, still, peaceful, happy, playful, yielding, open. Counters: Feeling overwhelmed, feeling over-stimulated, excessively busy, restless, nervous, agitated, stressed, burned-out.

Stimulating: Excited, stimulated, inspired, motivated, moving, outgoing, active. Counters: Coldness, fatigue, feeling stuck, discouraged, unmotivated, procrastination, laziness.

Sultry: Sensual, seductive, passionate, embodied, stable, strong, solid, rooted. Counters: Tense, flighty, changeable, airy, air headed, disconnected, ungrounded, overly idealistic, unembodied.

Properties Appendix

This appendix contains the definition of the various properties used to describe the therapeutic actions of natural remedies. Indications and contraindications are included with many properties.

Abortifacient: May cause abortion or miscarriage. Trying to abort a baby with herbs is not recommended.

Absorbent: A substance used to absorb irritating toxins both internally and externally. May be applied topically as a poultice for bites, stings, or other irritations. Can also be taken internally to absorb toxins. Must be used with large amounts of water to be effective.

Adaptogen: Adaptogens help the body adapt to stressful situations and maintain normal function under mental or physical stress. Strengthen and support adrenal function by adjusting the hypothalamus/pituitary/ adrenal axis to reduce the output of stress hormones. Helps to build the immune system because stress hormones reduce the immune response.

Adrenal tonic: A substance that builds up and strengthens the function of the adrenal glands.

Adrenergic: Stimulates the production of or mimics the action of epinephrine. Useful for ADD where parasympathetic dominance is involved. Not recommended in anxiety and stress-related disorders. See also *sympathomimetic*.

Adsorbent: An adsorbent causes other substances to stick to it. It is different from an *absorbent*, in that substances adhere to the surface of it, instead of being drawn into it. Used topically and internally to eliminate poisons and irritants. May be helpful to counteract chemical poisoning from caustic agents. Contact your poison control center for advice. Should not be taken with other nutritional supplements as they tend to inhibit nutrient absorption.

Alkalinizer: An agent that neutralizes acid or causes alkalization; a substance used to raise the pH level of the body, especially urine and/or saliva.

Alterative: Cleanses (or alters) the internal environment of the body without producing noticeable laxative or diuretic effects. Helps remove toxins from the blood, probably by strengthening liver and/or lymphatic function. Purifies the blood, helping to combat impurity in the blood and organs. Used to treat torpid or stagnant conditions in the body. Traditionally used to clear up morbid conditions in the body, especially skin diseases, skin eruptions, cancer, and wounds with pus.

Analgesic: Helps to relieve pain without causing loss of sensation. An *anodyne* is a mild analgesic. Useful for minor pains. Don't expect herbal analgesics to have the strength of prescription pain-killing drugs. Often they simply take the "edge" off the pain so it is bearable.

Anaphrodisiac: Decreases sex drive.

Androgenic: An agent that produces or enhances masculine characteristics.

Anesthetic: A drug or agent that is used to abolish the sensation of pain by numbing nerve endings.

Anodyne: See *Analgesic*.

Antacid: Neutralizes excess stomach acid and/or relaxes the stomach and prevents or treats acid indigestion.

Anthelmintic: A vermifuge, destroying or expelling intestinal worms; an agent that is destructive to parasitic worms. See *vermifuge*.

Anti-inflammatory: Reduces inflammation (heat, swelling, redness, and pain). Used to reduce inflammatory conditions in the body. Anti-inflammatories vary widely in their mode of action, and hence in their specific applications. Almost any herb that heals tissue damage will also act as an anti-inflammatory agent.

Antiabortive: Helps stop miscarriage or spontaneous abortion. Opposite of abortifacient. Used when bleeding or cramping starts in the early stages of pregnancy to help avoid a miscarriage.

Antiadrenergic: Of or pertaining to a substance that opposes the physiological effects of epinephrine; an agent that reduces production or uptake of epinephrine (adrenaline) and other related compounds secreted by the adrenal glands. See *sympatholytic*.

Antiaging: Helps to counter the effects of aging

Antiallergenic: Reduces allergic reactions. Includes herbs listed under antihistamine and mast cell stabilizers. These remedies are used to reduce the allergic responses in mucous membranes of the digestive and respiratory tract. They are useful for hay fever, allergy-induced asthma and earaches.

Antiamebic: An agent that destroys or suppresses the growth of amebas.

Antiarrhythmic: Combating an irregular heartbeat; an agent that prevents or alleviates cardiac arrhythmia.

Antiarthritic: An agent that combats joint pain or arthritis (rheumatism).

Antibacterial: Destroys or inhibits bacteria. Used to fight infection both internally and externally. Many of these remedies do not directly kill bacteria but act in indirect ways to inhibit their growth or enhance the body's own ability to destroy them.

Anticancer: Remedies that help to fight cancer and shrink tumors.

Anticarious: Preventing or suppressing the development of dental caries (cavities).

Anticatarrhal: Help the body remove excess catarrh, whether in the sinus area or other parts of the body.

Anticephalalgic: Curing or preventing headache.

Anticholesteremic: Agent that helps to reduce cholesterol.

Anticholinergic: Cholinergic receptors in the nervous system respond to acetylcholine. Anticholinergic remedies block the action of acetylcholine. This may be helpful in relaxing muscle spasms.

Anticoagulant: Inhibits coagulation of blood and blood clotting. Opposite of blood tonic. Used where there is a risk of thrombosis (blood clots forming in the circulatory system). These remedies also help blood stagnation (thick, heavy blood) which in natural medicine is believed to contribute to a wide variety of conditions, including varicose veins, uterine fibroids, and liver congestion. These remedies may be contraindicated in anemia or when the person is already using blood thinners.

Antidepressant: Relieves depression. Helps alleviate depression. Used to help lift the spirits and relieve depression. Caution: do not take people "cold turkey" off antidepressant drugs.

Antidiabetic: An agent that prevents or alleviates diabetes.

Antidiarrheal: Arrests diarrhea.

Antidote: A remedy for counteracting a poison.

Antiemetic: Suppresses vomit reflex, relieves nausea. Used for flu, morning sickness, motion sickness, nausea, etc.

Antiepileptic: Opposed to epilepsy; relieving fits.

Antifungal: Kills or inhibits the growth of fungus and yeast. Used for candida and other yeast infections both topically and internally. Similar to *fungicide.*

Antigalactagogue: Inhibits lactation (flow of breast milk). Opposite of galactagogue. Used for nursing mothers to help dry up breast milk when it is time to stop nursing.

Antigonadotropic: Inhibiting the secretion or actions of the gonadotropins (lutenizing and follicle stimulating hormones).

Antihemorrhagic: See *hemostatic.*

Antiherpetic: An agent that inhibits or counteracts the herpes virus.

Antihistamine: Helps dry up sinus congestion by counteracting histamine. Similar to *antiallergenic,* but more specific. Histamine produces swelling in mucous membranes, leading to itchy, watery eyes, runny nose, swollen eustachian tubes, intestinal inflammation, and other allergic reactions.

Antihypertensive: An agent that reduces high blood pressure. See also *hypotensive.*

Antilipemic: An agent that counteracts high levels of lipids in the blood.

Antilithic: An agent that prevents the formation of stone or calculus; preventing the formation of calculi in the urinary organs.

Antimalarial: An agent that is therapeutically effective against malaria.

Antimicrobial: An agent that kills microorganisms or suppresses their multiplication or growth.

Antimutagenic: Helps prevent the formation of cancer cells.

Antinausa: Helps to relieve nausea. See also *antiemetic.*

Antiobesic: A remedy used in the treatment of weight reduction for persons suffering from obesity.

Antioxidant: Helps prevent free radical damage by scavenging oxygen radicals, which may help prevent aging and decay.

Antiparasitic: Remedies that destroy parasites.

Antiphlogistic: An agent that counteracts inflammation and fever.

Antipruritic: An agent, usually applied topically, that relieves or prevents itching.

Antirheumatic: An agent that relieves or prevents rheumatism; any substance applied topically or taken internally that reduces pain and inflammation of the joints or other connective tissue.

Antiscorbutic: Effective in the prevention or relief of scurvy, a disease caused by vitamin C deficiency.

Antiseptic: Destroys or inhibits microorganisms (germs). This term is usually used in reference to herbs that are used on wounds or injuries rather than for internal infections.

Antismoking: An agent that helps a person quit smoking.

Antispasmodic: Relaxes or prevents muscle cramping or spasms. Used for muscle spasms in a variety of applications including: cramps and charley horses, intestinal cramps (spastic bowel), bronchial spasms in asthma, menstrual cramps, pain during childbirth, pain due to muscle tension, and tension headaches.

Antisudorific: Decreases perspiration and elimination through the skin. Used to stop night sweats and/or excessive perspiration. Closes skin pores.

Antithrombotic: An agent that prevents or interferes with the formation of blood clots within vascular walls.

Antithyrotropic: Inhibiting the secretion or actions of thyrotropin.

Antitoxic: Effective against a poison.

Antitussive: Suppresses the cough reflex, reducing coughing. Used to arrest coughing when excessive coughing causes chest pain or loss of sleep.

Antiurolithic: An agent that prevents the formation of urinary calculi (kidney stones).

Antivenomous: Counteracts venom from bites and stings by absorbing it or neutralizing it. Used primarily topically for spider bites, bee stings, snake bites, etc. For topical use, moisten powders and apply as a poultice directly to the affected area. It may be necessary to change the poultice several times to obtain the full effect. (Caution: this is a first aid measure and should not replace appropriate medical assistance, especially in the case of allergies to bee stings or the bite of poisonous snakes and spiders.)

Antiviral: Destroys, inhibits or helps the body to destroy viruses.

Anxiolytic: An agent that reduces anxiety.

Aperient: A very mild laxative. Used to create a gentle laxative action, especially in children or elderly persons.

Aperitive: Stimulating the appetite. This term is frequently applied to a premeal cocktail or drink.

Aphrodisiac: Increases sex drive. Used for low sex drive, impotency, or frigidity. Not recommended for teenagers.

Appetite suppressant: Suppresses hunger and the desire to eat. Opposite action of appetite stimulant. Remedies may supply nutrients that give satisfaction and allay appetite. They may also be bulking agents that swell in the stomach and provide a feeling of fullness. A few may affect neurotransmitters that control appetite.

Astringent: Herbs that are astringent contain tannins (and sometimes other compounds) that contract and tone muscle fiber and other tissue. They are used to stop bleeding, arrest discharges (diarrhea, excess mucus, pus, etc.), tone up soft or spongy tissue (varicose veins, hemorrhoids), reduce swelling, and/or counteract venom (see *antivenomous*). They are contraindicated in tension and dryness.

Bactericidal: Destructive to bacteria. See also *antibacterial*.

Balsamic: Healing or soothing to inflamed parts.

Blood building: A concept from Chinese and traditional medicine. Refers to herbs that help overcome anemia and build up the blood. Traditionally used for weak, thin pulse, pale complexion, general weakness.

Blood purifier: See *alterative*.

Blood thinner: See *anticoagulant*.

Bronchial dilator: Remedies that relax and dilate the bronchi. Used for asthma that is induced by muscular constriction of the air passages due to nervous reactions. These remedies are also good for deep cough, especially whooping cough, where there is constriction of the airways.

Calmative: A mild sedative.

Cardiac: A remedy that tones and strengthens the heart muscle. Used to prevent heart disease or to strengthen the heart when heart disease is already present.

Carminative: Expels gas from the bowel or relieves bloating. Used for people who suffer from severe gas and poor digestive function. These remedies act by stimulating blood flow to the digestive organs, increasing digestive secretions, and increasing motility (movement) in the digestive tract.

Catalyst: A catalyst is a substance that causes or speeds a chemical reaction without being affected itself. A synergist is a plant medicine that increases blood flow, digestive activity, and absorption of other herbs or nutrients. These are often used in small amounts in herbal formulas to enhance their effectiveness.

Cathartic: A substance that stimulates the movement of the bowels, a powerful laxative. See also *laxative*.

Cell proliferant: An agent that speeds tissue growth to enhance the repair of wounds and injuries. Used to speed healing in injuries.

Cephalalgic: An agent that can cause a headache but may also be used as a remedy to treat headache.

Cephalic: Relating to diseases of the head; an agent to treat disorders that affect the head.

Cerebral tonic: Improves memory and brain function. Used for loss of memory or concentration due to aging or senility. Also useful for increasing mental alertness and concentration in students or others who need better memory or focus. May be helpful in some cases of ADD.

Cholagogue: Increases the flow of bile; helps prevent or dissolve gallstones. Indicated for clay-colored stools, some cases of constipation, and in gall bladder problems where the gallbladder is congested or has stones. Contraindicated in duodenal ulcers and intestinal inflammation. May also be contraindicated with inflammatory liver diseases.

Cholinergic: Pertaining to the parasympathetic portion of the autonomic nervous system and the release of acetylcholine as a transmitter substance. See *parasympathomimetic*.

Cicatrizant: A remedy that helps tissues heal without scarring.

CNS depressant: A remedy that can suppress the activity of the central nervous system; generally used to promote sleep or reduce pain.

Coagulant: An agent that promotes or accelerates the coagulation of blood. See also *styptic*.

Condiment: Herbs or nutrients used as seasonings to improve the flavor of food. Condiment herbs are generally safe for long-term use in low doses.

Contraceptive: Helps prevent conception. Should be avoided when trying to get pregnant. Caution: Herbs are not a very reliable method of birth control.

Corrects polarity: An agent that acts upon the thymus gland to correct energy flow when the polarity is reversed so that a person can be accurately muscle-tested. Also helps a person who is attracted to negative influences to be attracted to more positive influences.

Counterirritant: A remedy that causes irritation (redness) and thus draws blood away from one area of the body to another. Used topically for temporary relief of pain associated with arthritis, gout, rheumatism, strained muscles, etc. Helps to relieve pain by depleting or blocking substance P neurotransmitters. Pain relief is usually temporary, although increased blood flow may help to stimulate healing. Contraindicated with redness and swelling on the surface of the skin or when the surface of the skin is broken. Not recommended for application after a hot shower or bath. Avoid contact with sensitive areas of the body (eyes, genitals).

Cytotoxic: Kills cancer cells

Decongestant: Relieves (breaks up or loosens) respiratory congestion. Used primarily where mucus has become thick and stuck, causing difficult breathing, sinus pressure, or thick drainage. These remedies tend to thin mucus, making it easier to expel.

Demulcent: See *mucilant*.

Dentifrice: A preparation, usually a paste, gel, or powder, used with a toothbrush for cleaning the accessible surfaces of the teeth.

Deobstruent: Removes obstructions from the body.

Deodorant: Preparations used to eliminate, prevent, or mask unpleasant odor.

Detergent: A remedy that is cleansing to wounds, boils, or ulcers. This is different from commercial detergents used for laundry and household cleaning.

Detoxifying: Cleanses the body of toxins by promoting elimination. Related to deobstruent or lymphatic and alterative or blood purifier, but may also involve mild diuretic and/or laxative actions. Also used for remedies that aid liver pathways of detoxification.

Diaphoretic: Increases perspiration and elimination through the skin. Used to bring down fevers. In Chinese medicine, these are called "surface-relieving" herbs and are used to relieve "superficial" conditions, such as colds, flu, coughs, asthma, and edema. Warming sudorifics are used for "wind chill" (mild fever with chills, lack of sweating, white phlegm), and cooling sudorifics are used for "wind-heat" (high fever with chills and sweating, thirst, yellow phlegm).

Digestant: Aids digestion of food, generally applied to remedies that contain enzymes or other elements that directly aid in the breakdown of food. Used to supplement digestive secretions and aid in the digestion of food where people are having difficulty manufacturing sufficient hydrochloric acid, enzymes, and/or bile salts to break down their food. These remedies are especially helpful for older people with poor digestion or people in a wasting condition (where they are losing weight).

Digestive tonic: Herbs, generally bitter or aromatic, that promote the flow of digestive secretions to aid digestion. They are generally taken about twenty to thirty minutes prior to meals in a liquid form.

Disinfectant: An agent that disinfects; applied particularly to agents used on inanimate objects; a substance that destroys noxious properties of decaying organic matter. See *antiseptic*.

Diuretic: Increases flow of urine to expel excess fluids from the body. Diuretics are used for water retention and various types of kidney problems. They vary widely in their mode of action.

Dopamine-enhancing: Remedies that enhance the action of the neurotransmitter dopamine. Dopamine helps to lift mood and aids in muscle movement and muscle coordination. Loss of dopamine receptors in the brain causes Parkinson's disease.

Drawing: Refers to agents that pull morbid material out of the body.

Emetic: Induces vomiting. Used for food or chemical poisoning. Call poison control center for advice before inducing vomiting in cases of chemical poisoning. With caustic agents like lye, vomiting should not be induced. Emetics are also used to expel excess phlegm from the system to halt asthma attacks and relieve severe respiratory congestion.

Emmenagogue: Increases (stimulates) and regulates menstrual flow. These herbs have also been called female correctives because they help to regulate the menstrual cycle. They are generally contraindicated during pregnancy.

Emollient: A preparation that soothes and softens external tissue.

Emulsifier: An agent that helps break down fats to make them water-soluble.

Escharotic: An agent that is applied topically to destroy morbid tissue. Harsh escharotics should be used with caution and are best used by experienced professional herbalists as they can cause redness, swelling, pain, drainage, and scarring. The milder drawing agents will not do this (see *drawing*).

Estrogenic: Mimics estrogen in the body. Used to help women during menopause or during the menstrual cycle when PMS symptoms are related to excess progesterone and deficient estrogen. May also have a protective effect against estrogen-dependent cancers.

Euphoretic: An agent that produces an exaggerated feeling of physical and mental well-being, especially when not justified by external reality.

Expectorant: Expels phlegm or mucus from the lungs and sinuses. Increases coughing and sneezing and stimulates drainage.

Febrifuge: Reduces fever and inflammation.

Female tonic: A rather-vague action referring to remedies that regulate the female hormonal cycle. See *emenogogue*. These remedies help menstrual irregularities of various kinds such as heavy menstruation, scant menstruation, delayed menstruation or irregularities of the cycle. They act in different ways and an understanding of the specific types of menstrual irregularities and the specific actions of remedies is necessary for dependable results. These remedies are generally contraindicated in pregnancy, especially in the early stages. Some herbalists called them female correctives.

Food: These herbs have been eaten food or have parts that are used as food.

Fungicide: Prevents and combats fungal infection; an agent that destroys fungi. See also *antifungal*.

Gaba-enhancing: Remedies that increase the calming neurotransmitter GABA, helping to calm the mind, reduce anxiety, and aid sleep.

Galactagogue: Enriches and/or increases the flow of breast milk. Opposite of antigalactagogue. Used for nursing mothers to enrich and promote the flow of breast milk. These remedies may also ease colic in nursing babies when taken by the mother to "sweeten" the milk.

Germicide: Destroys germs or microorganisms such as bacteria, etc. See also *antimicrobial*.

Glandular: Influences the glands to produce more of certain hormones. May also mimic hormones. This is a very vague and general term, since specific herbs act on specific glands.

Hemostatic: Stops internal bleeding or hemorrhage. Similar to styptic but generally used internally. **Caution:** Seek medical assistance for serious bleeding.

Hepatic: Strengthens liver function. Useful for people who have been exposed to chemicals or whose livers are inherently weak or damaged. Very helpful as preventatives for people who work around chemicals (i.e., painters, lab workers, farmers) to protect the liver against damage.

Hepatoprotective: Protects the liver from toxic chemicals.

Hydrating: See *moistening*.

Hypertensive: Help to increase blood pressure when it is low.

Hypnotic: See *soporific*.

Hypoglycemic: An agent that acts to lower the level of glucose in the blood.

Hypolipidemic: Promoting the reduction of lipid concentrations in the serum (blood).

Hypotensive: Decreases blood pressure.

Immune modulator: Remedies that help to normalize the function of the immune system whether it is underactive (immune weakness) or overactive (autoimmune disorders). These remedies are particularly useful for autoimmune disorders. They appear to enhance communication in the immune system so that it works better without a general stimulating effect that would aggravate autoimmune conditions.

Immune stimulant: Stimulates the function of the immune system. Used for frequent colds and infection, lowered resistance. Many are helpful for cancer. May be contraindicated in autoimmune disorders.

Insecticide: A substance that destroys insects.

Kidney tonic: Strengthens kidney function and tone. In Chinese medicine, the kidneys are thought to be connected to the health of the structural system, so these remedies are helpful for structural weakness too. They stabilize the structure of the body by acting to balance mineral electrolytes through the kidneys.

Laxative: A remedy that stimulates bowel movements to relieve constipation. These herbs contain anthraquinone glycosides, which increase peristalsis in the colon and inhibit absorption of water and electrolytes. Long-term use of stimulant laxatives can be habit-forming.

Laxative (bulk): Stimulates elimination through the lower bowel by adding fiber to the intestinal tract; best laxatives for long-term use. Indicated in high cholesterol, sluggish elimination, elimination problems during pregnancy, and general detoxification.

Laxative (gentle): A medicine that acts gently on the bowels, without gripping; stimulates bowel movement; an agent that acts to promote the evacuation of the bowel.

Lipotropic: Promoting the flow of lipids to and from the liver; acting on fat metabolism by hastening the removal of it or by decreasing its deposits in the liver.

Lithotriptic: Helps dissolve kidney stones. Used to help people pass kidney stones and/or to prevent their formulation. Will probably help with calcifications elsewhere in the body, such as bone spurs.

Low glycemic: A low-glycemic carbohydrate is one that does not spike blood sugar levels and therefore does not trigger a strong insulin response in the blood. Low-glycemic carbohydrates can reduce sugar cravings, stabilize blood sugar in hypoglycemia and diabetes, aid in weight loss, and help reduce chronic inflammation.

Lung tonic: Strengthens lung tissue and function. Used where the lungs are weak and prone to frequent infection, also for conditions where the lungs are dry and leathery and have sustained a loss of elasticity.

Lymphatic: Remedies that act on the lymphatic system. They cleanse, tone, or improve the function of the lymph glands and vessels. Indicated with lymphatic swellings, sore throats, mumps, tonsillitis, some cases of breast swelling or tenderness, and other problems where there is lymphatic congestion or stagnation.

Mast cell stabilizer: Stabilize mast cells to reduce allergic reactions. Used in hay fever, allergenic asthma, and other respiratory allergies to reduce allergic reactions.

Mineralizer: Mineralizer is a term I termed to describe nutritive herbs that supply trace minerals to aid in tissue healing. They are used to build up structural tissues in the body by supplying nutrients to aid tissue regeneration and repair. These herbs are generally rich in calcium and silica.

Moistening: Helps body tissues retain moisture. Used when tissues are dry and don't rehydrate by just drinking water.

Mucilaginous: See *mucilant*.

Mucilant: Demulcents contain complex polysaccharides, which are indigestible but hold water and absorb irritants. *Mucilant* is a term coined by myself and Steve Smith in the 1980s to describe this action. It is not found in traditional texts. Applied topically herbs with this property act as a drawing poultice to absorb irritants, reduce inflammation and swelling, and keep tissues moist and pliable. Taken internally, they absorb irritants in the digestive tract, help to reduce cholesterol, act as bulk laxatives, and moisten dry

tissues. They also tend to act as mild nourishing foods to counteract weight loss (wasting). They are indicated in hard, dry, irritated tissue states, including inflammation of the digestive tract, dry and irritating coughs, burning or painful urination, and redness and swelling of the skin. Also indicated in conditions where a person needs mild nourishing foods when recovering from debilitating illnesses.

They are contraindicated with bowel obstruction and should not be applied topically to deep wounds.

Mucolytic: Dissolving or breaking down mucus.

Narcotic: A painkiller that numbs or depresses the central nerves to reduce pain sensations. Do not confuse with *hallucinogenic*. Narcotics are used for more serious pain than analgesics or anodynes.

Nauseant: Causing an inclination to vomit.

Nervine: A remedy that strengthens the nervous system. Generally used to refer to remedies that inhibit sympathetic nerves and stimulate parasympathetic nerves to have a calming or relaxing effect. Technically speaking, an agent that does the opposite (stimulates sympathetic nerves and inhibits parasympathetic nerves) could also be called a nervine, but the term is not generally used in this manner. These remedies are used to relax muscles, reduce anxiety and tension, ease stress, and aid sleep and relaxation

Neuroprotective: Protects neurons from damage due to chemicals and inflammation. May also help damaged nerve cells to heal faster.

Nutritive: An herb, food, or supplement that supplies essential nutrition.

Opthalmicum: A remedy for diseases of the eye.

Oxytocic: Refers to remedies that have an oxytocin-mimicking effect. Oxytocin is the hormone responsible for uterine contractions during labor.

Panacea: A remedy that has been recommended for so many different problems it appears to cure "everything."

Parasiticide: Destroys parasites. See also *antiparasitic*.

Parasympatholytic: An agent that blocks or inhibits the parasympathetic nerves. These herbs are indicated in conditions where there is excess parasympathetic nervous system activity. Small pupils are a good indication of excess parasympathetic activity.

Parasympathomimetic: Stimulates the parasympathetic nervous system. Relaxes the nervous system. Fairly synonymous with nervine.

Parturient: Stimulates uterine contractions to start or assist labor and delivery. If an herb has this property, it should also be considered a potential *abortifacient*. These remedies are used during the last five weeks of pregnancy or during labor to assist uterine contractions and the delivery of the baby. See also *oxytocic*.

Perfume: Used for its fragrance.

Phytoestrogen: A plant substance that mimics estrogens is called a phytoestrogen. Plants that contain phytoestrogens may or may not enhance estrogenic effects in the body. Some phyoestrogens are very weak, but by binding to estrogen receptor sites, they can reduce the risk of estrogen-dependent cancers or aid in estrogen-dominant PMS.

Pulmonary: An agent specific to the treatment of the lungs.

Purgative: Purgatives and cathartics are strong laxatives. See also *laxative*.

Refrigerant: Lowers body temperature and relieves thirst. For fever and "hot" conditions, where a person feels hot, thirsty, dry, or flushed, but fluids don't seem to hydrate or cool the body.

Relaxant: An agent that reduces tension and helps muscles to relax. Used for muscle tension and stress.

Rubefacient: Produces redness of the skin; generates a localized increase in blood flow when applied to the skin, helping healing, cleansing and nourishment. These are often used to ease pain and swelling of arthritic joints.

Sedative: Sedates the nervous system. Has a calming effect on the body.

Serotonergic: Enhances the action of serotonin, a neurotransmitter involved in appetite, depression, pain regulation, and sleep. These remedies can reduce anxiety, lift depression, and reduce cravings for carbohydrates.

Soothing: A remedy that reduces tissue irritation. Used when tissues are inflamed and irritated.

Soporific: Producing or inducing sleep; an agent that acts to induce sleep.

Spleen chi tonic: Chinese term for aiding the entire digestive process of turning food into flesh. Refers to herbs that improve appetite and digestive function and promote weight gain. *Stomachic* is a Western term for herbs that improve digestive function in the stomach and is probably closely related; however, these remedies do more than promote digestion. They promote anabolic function. Indicated when a person is pale and thin and unable to gain muscle mass. They may lose weight during or following a debilitating illness like cancer or AIDS. This may also happen to elderly people with poor digestive function.

Stimulant (appetite): Stimulates hunger and the desire to eat. Opposite action of appetite suppressant. Used for people who are anorexic or bulimic and for children with poor appetites. They may also be helpful in wasting conditions and poor digestive function as they tend to stimulate digestive secretions. Bitters and aromatics taken in a liquid form or chewed (so they can be tasted and smelled) will generally help stimulate both appetite and digestive secretions.

Stimulant (circulatory): An agent that stimulates circulation. Used for cold hands and feet or other symptoms of poor circulation to the extremities. Also used to aid blood flow to various areas of the body to promote tissue healing.

Stimulant (metabolic): An agent that stimulates metabolism, increasing heat and energy.

Stomachic: A digestive aid and tonic, which improves stomach function and appetite.

Styptic: A powerful astringent action that closes wounds and stops bleeding. Used to stop internal and external bleeding. Caution: With serious external bleeding one should use these remedies by putting them into a wound and then applying the standard first aid practice of applying pressure directly to the injury.

Sweetener: An agent used to sweeten foods or beverages.

Sympatholytic: Inhibits the sympathetic nervous system. Has a calming effect in cases of stress and tension.

Sympathomimetic: Stimulates activity of sympathetic nervous system. Could also be called a sympathetic nervine. Used to promote alertness, relieve fatigue, and aid in mental concentration. Generally contraindicated with heart palpitations, anxiety, high blood pressure, and high levels of stress.

Synergist: See *catalyst*.

Taenicide: An agent that destroys tapeworms. See also *antiparasitic*.

Testosterone-enhancing: Helps increase testosterone levels.

Thrombolytic: An agent that dissolves or splits up blood clots. See also *anticoagulant*.

Thyrotropic: Having an influence on the thyroid gland.

Tonic: Refers to remedies with a general anabolic effect; they build up and strengthen organs and tissues, often causing greater structural density or greater functional strength. Used for weakened conditions of the body or specific organs.

Toxic: An herb that can be poisonous if used incorrectly.

Tranquilizer: Agents that have calming, mildly sedating, and/or a muscle-relaxing effect.

Uterine: Agents that have an affinity for uterine tissue or maladies thereof.

Uterine tonic: Strengthens and tones the uterine muscle in preparation for childbirth.

Vascular tonic: Tone up varicose veins. Used for varicose veins, hemorrhoids, pain and swelling in the legs, and other conditions where venous circulation is impaired.

Vasoconstrictor: Constricts blood vessels to reduce circulation. Opposite of *vasodilator*. Used to raise low blood pressure or help reduce bleeding. Some of these remedies may also aid vasodilative headaches. Contraindicated in high blood pressure.

Vasodilator: Opens and relaxes blood vessels to increase circulation. Opposite of vasoconstrictor. Used for high blood pressure. Contraindicated with low blood pressure and vasodilative headaches.

Vermifuge: Destroys intestinal worms. See also *antiparasitics*.

Virostatic: An agent that inhibits the replication of viruses.

Vulnerary: Helps injured tissues to heal, usually without scarring

Help Us Share the Message

Millions of people are stuck just managing disease symptoms without getting better. They need help to learn how they can heal and experience life without disease by removing the root cause of their health problems. You can help them! If you:

Enjoy helping people
Believe in the power of nature's remedies
And, want to make a difference in the world

Go to stevenhorne.com/signup to become a part of Steven's member program and start making a difference.

As a member you'll have access to hundreds of webinars on important health topics with new webinars every month, a searchable database of health conditions and natural remedies, and information you can share in emails and social media to spread the message about natural health.

Want to Learn More?

Subscribe to Steven's free newsletter at stevenhorne.com to receive regular articles about herbs and natural healing

You can also follow Steven at

facebook.com/stevenhhorne
youtube.com/herbaleducation
twitter.com/abcherb
instagram.com/abcherb
vimeo.com/abcherb

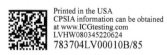

Printed in the USA
CPSIA information can be obtained
at www.ICGtesting.com
LVHW080345220624
783704LV00010B/85

9 781637 102534